CHILD ABUSE

Medical Diagnosis & Management

3rd Edition

Editors

Robert M. Reece, MD, FAAP
Clinical Professor
Department of Pediatrics
Tufts University School of Medicine
Director, Child Protection Program
Department of Pediatrics
The Floating Hospital for Children at Tufts Medical Center
Boston, MA
Editor, *The Quarterly Update*
North Falmouth, MA

Cindy W. Christian, MD, FAAP
Associate Professor
Department of Pediatrics
The University of Pennsylvania School of Medicine
Chair, Child Abuse and Neglect Prevention
Co-director, Safe Place: The Center for Child Protection and Health
The Children's Hospital of Philadelphia
Philadelphia, PA

American Academy of Pediatrics
DEDICATED TO THE HEALTH OF ALL CHILDREN™

Editor: Diane Beausoleil
Marketing Manager: Linda Smessaert
Copy Editor: Kate Larson
Production Manager: Theresa Wiener
Designer: Linda J. Diamond

Library of Congress Control Number: 2005936502
ISBN-13: 978-1-58110-208-6
MA0341

The recommendations in this publication do not indicate an exclusive course of treatment or serve as a standard of care. Variations, taking into account individual circumstances, may be appropriate.

Brand names are furnished for identification purposes only. No endorsement of the manufacturers or products mentioned is implied.

Printed in China

9-156/0808

Last digit is the print number: 10 9 8 7 6 5 4 3 2 1

To my wife Betsy Kyle Reece, my children, and my grandchildren.
RMR

To my family, for their unconditional love.
To my professional mentors:
Steve Ludwig, MD, for the opportunities and support;
Tina Duhaime, MD, for her objectivity and critical thinking; and
Catherine Manno, MD, for her guidance and friendship.
CWC

Table of Contents

Contributing Authors

Tom Andrew, MD
Assistant Professor, Dartmouth Medical College
Chief Medical Examiner, State of New Hampshire
Concord, NH

Abby Berenson, MD
Professor, Departments of Obstetrics/Gynecology and Pediatrics
Director, University of Texas Medical Branch Center for Interdisciplinary Research
in Women's Health
The University of Texas Medical Branch
Galveston, TX

Elizabeth Benzinger, PhD
DNA Quality Assurance Administrator
Ohio Bureau of Criminal Identification and Investigation
Office of the Attorney General
London, OH

Carol D. Berkowitz, MD, FAAP
Professor of Clinical Pediatrics
Executive Vice Chair Department of Pediatrics
Harbor-UCLA Medical Center David Geffen School of Medicine at UCLA
Torrance, CA

Maureen Black, PhD
John A. Scholl Professor, Department of Pediatrics
Director, Growth and Nutrition Clinic
University of Maryland School of Medicine
Baltimore, MD

Stephen Boos, MD, FAAP
Medical Director, Pediatric Forensic Assessment Consultation Team, Inova Fairfax
Hospital for Children
Falls Church, VA

Roger W. Byard, MD
Marks Chair of Pathology
Department of Pathology
University of Adelaide
Australia

Cindy W. Christian, MD, FAAP
Associate Professor, Department of Pediatrics, University of Pennsylvania
    School of Medicine
Chair, Child Abuse and Neglect Prevention
Co-director, Safe Place: The Center for Child Protection and Health
The Children's Hospital of Philadelphia
Philadelphia, PA

Arthur Cooper, MD
Professor of Surgery, Columbia University College of Physicians & Surgeons
Director, Trauma & Pediatric Surgical Services
Harlem Hospital Center
New York, NY

Daniel R. Cooperman, MD
Professor of Orthodpedic Surgery, Case Western Reserve University School
    of Medicine
Chief of Pediatric Orthopedics at the MetroHealth Medical Center
Rainbow Babies and Childrens Hospital and the MetroHealth Medical Center
Cleveland, OH

Allan R. DeJong, MD
Clinical Professor of Pediatrics, Jefferson Medical College, Philadelphia
Director, Children at Risk Evaluation Program
Nemours–Alfred I. duPont Hospital for Children
Wilmington, DE

Melissa Desai, MD, MPH
Pediatrics Resident, Children's Hospital of Philadelphia
Philadelphia, PA

Marcella M. Donaruma-Kwoh, MD
Assistant Professor of Pediatrics
Section of Emergency Medicine
Baylor College of Medicine
Houston, TX

Dennis Drotar, MD
Department of Pediatrics
Case Western Reserve University
Cleveland, OH

Howard Dubowitz, MD, FAAP
Professor of Pediatrics, University of Maryland School of Medicine
Chief, Division of Child Protection,
University of Maryland Hospital
Baltimore, MD

Christine-Ann Duhaime, MD
Professor of Surgery (Neurosurgery) and Pediatrics
Director, Pediatric Neurosurgery and Neuroscience
Children's Hospital at Dartmouth, Dartmouth Hitchcock Medical Center
Lebanon, NH

Kenneth W. Feldman, MD
Clinical Professor of Pediatrics, University of Washington School of Medicine
Medical Director, Children's Protection Program & Team
Children's Hospital and Regional Medical Center
Seattle, WA

Kathleen Coulborn Faller, PhD, ACSW, DCSW
Marion Elizabeth Blue Professor of Children and Families
Director, Family Assessment Clinic
University of Michigan School of Social Work
Ann Arbor, MI

James A. Feinstein, MD
Pediatric Resident, Children's Hospital of Philadelphia
Philadelphia, PA

Martin A. Finkel, DO, FACOP, FAAP
Professor of Pediatrics
Medical Director CARES (Child Abuse Research Education & Service) Institute
University of Medicine and Dentistry of New Jersey
School of Osteopathic Medicine
Stratford, NJ

Deborah A. Frank, MD
Professor of Pediatrics, Boston University School of Medicine
Director, Grow Clinic for Children
Boston Medical Center
Boston, MA

Lori Frasier, MD, FAAP
Medical Director, Child Protection Team
Center for Safe and Healthy Families
Primary Children's Medical Center
Salt Lake City, UT

Jordan Greenbaum, MD
Medical Director, Child Protection Center
Children's Healthcare of Atlanta
Atlanta, GA

Frederick M. Henretig, MD, FAAP
Director, Section of Clinical Toxicology
The Children's Hospital of Philadelphia
Medical Director, The Poison Control Center
Philadelphia, PA

Kent P. Hymel, MD, FAAP
Visiting Associate Professor of Pediatrics and Instructor in Pediatrics
Medical Director, Child Advocacy and Protection Program
Dartmouth-Hitchcock Medical Center
Lebanon, NH

Carole Jenny, MD, FAAP
Professor of Pediatrics, Brown University School of Medicine
Director, Child Protection Program, Hasbro Children's Hospital
Providence, RI

Heather T. Keenan, MDCM, PhD
Associate Professor of Pediatrics, University of Utah Pediatric Critical Care
University of Utah Health Sciences Center
Salt Lake City, UT

Nancy Kellogg, MD
Professor of Pediatrics, University of Texas Health Science Center at San Antonio, TX
Chief, Division of Child Abuse

Henry F. Krous, MD
Director, Department of Pathology, Children's Hospital-San Diego
Adjunct Professor, Departments of Pathology and Pediatrics
University of California at San Diego
La Jolla, CA

Alex V. Levin, MD, FAAP, FAAO, FRCSC
Professor, Departments of Paediatrics, Genetics, and
Ophthalmology & Vision Science
Staff Ophthalmologist, Staff Child Abuse
Pediatrician
The Hospital for Sick Children, University of Toronto
Toronto, Ontario Canada

John Leventhal, MD, FAAP
Professor of Pediatrics, Yale University School of Medicine
Medical Director of the Child Abuse Programs and the Child Abuse
Prevention Programs
Yale-New Haven Children's Hospital
New Haven, CT

Heather Littleton, PhD
Assistant Professor of Psychology, Sam Houston State University
Huntsville, TX

Kathi L. Makoroff, MD
Assistant Professor of Pediatrics, University of Cincinnati School of Medicine
Child Abuse Pediatrics Fellowship Director
Mayerson Center for Safe and Healthy Children
Cincinnati Children's Hospital Medical Center
Cincinnati, OH

David F. Merten, MD
Emeritus Professor of Radiology and Pediatrics
Chief, Section of Pediatric Radiology (retired)
School of Medicine, University of North Carolina
Chapel Hill, NC

Yair Morad, MD
Department of Ophthalmology
Assaf Harofeh Medical Center
Tel Aviv University
Tel Aviv, Israel

Lynn Douglas Mouden, DDS, MPH, FICD, FACD
Associate Clinical Professor, University of Missouri Kansas City School of Dentistry
Assistant Professor, University of Tennessee College of Dentistry
Director, Office of Oral Health, Arkansas Department of Health
Little Rock, AK

John E. B. Myers, JD
Distinguished Professor and Scholar, University of the Pacific, McGeorge School
    of Law
Sacramento, CA

Michael L. Nance, MD
Associate Professor of Surgery, University of Pennsylvania School of Medicine
Director, Pediatric Trauma Program
Children's Hospital of Philadelphia
Philadelphia, PA

Robert T. Paschall, MD
Medical Director, Child Protection Program
Washington University in St Louis School of Medicine
St Louis, MO

Robert M. Reece, MD, FAAP
Clinical Professor of Pediatrics, Tufts University School of Medicine
Director, Child Protection Program,
The Floating Hospital for Children at Tufts Medical Center
Boston, Massachusetts
Editor, The Quarterly Update
North Falmouth, MA

Lawrence R. Ricci, MD, FAAP
Associate Clinical Professor of Pediatrics, University of Vermont College of Medicine
Co-director Spurwink Child Abuse Program
Portland, ME

Lucy B. Rorke-Adams, MA, MD
Clinical Professor of Pathology, Neurology and Pediatrics, University of Pennsylvania
    School of Medicine
Senior Neuropathologist, The Children's Hospital of Philadelphia
Former Forensic Neuropathologist, Office of the Medical Examiner
City of Philadelphia
Philadelphia, PA

Donna Andrea Rosenberg, MD
Associate Clinical Professor of Pediatrics,
University of Colorado Health Sciences Center
Denver, CO

David Rubin, MD, MPH
Assistant Professor of Pediatrics, University of Pennsylvania School of Medicine
Co-director, Safe Place: The Center for Child Protection and Health
Children's Hospital of Philadelphia
Philadelphia, PA

Desmond K. Runyan, MD, DrPH
Director, Robert Wood Johnson Clinical Scholars Program, The University
    of North Carolina School of Medicine
Professor of Social Medicine and Pediatrics
University of North Carolina School of Medicine at Chapel Hill
Attending Physician, Department of Pediatrics
North Carolina Children's Hospital
Chapel Hill, NC

Robert Shapiro, MD
Professor of Pediatrics, University of Cincinnati School of Medicine
Medical Director , Mayerson Center for Safe and Healthy Children
Cincinnati Children's Hospital Medical Center
Cincinnati, OH

Wilbur L. Smith, MD
Professor and Chairman
Department of Radiology
Wayne State University
Detroit, MI

Rebecca R. Socolar, MD, MPH
Professor of Pediatrics and Social Medicine
Director, Child Medical Evaluation Program
University of North Carolina-Chapel Hill
Chapel Hill, NC

John Stirling, MD, FAAP
Clinical Professor (Affiliated), Stanford University
Director, Center for Child Protection
Santa Clara Valley Medical Center
San Jose, CA

Preface

Since the publication of the first 2 editions of this book, there have been hundreds of peer-reviewed articles appearing in the world's English-language medical literature about child maltreatment or related conditions. Some of these articles have been significant enough to alter our concepts about the medical aspects of child maltreatment. Some have added persuasive information to bolster past concepts. Others have described new manifestations or presented clinical cases to clarify our thinking. These contributions have been found in a broad range of publications encompassing the field of pediatrics and the pediatric subspecialties in radiology, neurosurgery, orthopedics, infectious disease, genetics, surgery, gynecology, dermatology, and psychiatry. Other critical contributions have been made from the fields of mental health, general medicine, pathology, forensic pathology, and the law. Moreover, a new subspecialty in pediatrics—child abuse pediatrics—is now recognized by both the American Board of Pediatrics and the American Medical Association.

All professionals working in the evaluation and treatment of abused or neglected children need resources that incorporate this new information. The contents of this book emphasize the pediatric approach to diagnosis and management of child maltreatment, but the book is "user-friendly" to all who seek to help the maltreated child. The first 2 editions of this book have been used extensively by social workers, law enforcement, lawyers, judges, physicians, dentists, nurses, and mental health professionals. The book is designed to provide a guide through the medical, surgical, radiographic, and laboratory terrain of child abuse and neglect as well as clarifying the complex psychological dynamics that invariably happen in the context of abuse. For the medical practitioner, the book advises about the best diagnostic and therapeutic approaches to diagnose and treat victims of child abuse. For nonmedical professionals, it provides authoritative information about the state of the art and science of the field of child abuse pediatrics. For those who must present their findings and opinions in court, it offers the collective knowledge and experience of the contributing authors, all experts in the field of child maltreatment.

In this third edition, new chapters are presented on the epidemiology of maltreatment, abusive head trauma, interviewing of child victims, adolescent sexual assault, the role of forensic analysis, unusual manifestations of abuse, the pathology seen in fatal child abuse, the neurobiology of abuse, and the long-term consequences of abuse and neglect. New images are used to illustrate cases. We have striven to make this textbook current and relevant and hope it will be as useful as the past 2 editions have been.

Robert M. Reece, MD, and Cindy W. Christian, MD

Acknowledgments

The editors are profoundly grateful for the unselfish and painstaking work of the authors whose expertise shines in these pages. Thanks in particular go to Diane Beausoleil, an editor whose patience in the face of delays in manuscripts was biblical in proportion. Thanks also to Mark Grimes, the director of the Division of Product Development at the American Academy of Pediatrics, for recognizing the importance and value of this book to the community of professionals who care for children. Thank you all.

Introduction

The Evolution of Child Abuse Research

Heather T. Keenan

Department of Pediatrics, University of Utah

John M. Leventhal

Yale University School of Medicine
Child Abuse Programs, Yale-New Haven Children's Hospital

Introduction

Epidemiological studies of child maltreatment and its consequences have become increasingly larger in scope and sophisticated in design since Kempe et al's[1] landmark article on the battered child in 1962. The increased volume of quality research is due partially to a greater societal understanding of child maltreatment as both a medical and social problem. This introduction will review briefly the historical and legal framework that has led to the development of several large federal data sources for the study of child maltreatment. It also will review the epidemiological features of different types of child maltreatment and highlight several studies that illustrate either study design or relevant aspects of child maltreatment.

Historical Overview

The rights of children in the United States are based in English Common Law, which obligated fathers to provide for their children's education, religious upbringing, maintenance, and support. The law had a social intent: keeping poor children off of the streets. Colonial American law expanded on the English tradition. In early 17th century Massachusetts, fathers had a duty to train their children to be literate, religious, and economically productive citizens. In return for the maintenance and education of his child, the father was entitled to the custody of the child's person and to the value of his labor and service.[2] If the father failed in his duty toward the child, the state was allowed to intervene and place a child to work elsewhere. Thus the legal relationship of father to child was not one of property, but more one of master and servant. These laws were not intended to protect children, but to maintain social order and provide useful labor to the states.[3]

In the late 19th century the physical well-being of children was brought to social attention by the celebrated case of Mary Ellen Connolly in New York City.[4] Connolly had been severely abused and her legal case was brought before the New York Society for the Protection of Cruelty to Animals because no organization existed to protect children. This case, widely publicized, reportedly galvanized the first social response to child abuse and was instrumental in the creation of the New York Society for Prevention of Cruelty to Children. By 1900 there were 161 such societies in the United States. However, it was not until the 1940s that that the Supreme Court confirmed the state's authority to intervene in family relationships to protect children.[5]

Child maltreatment changed from a purely social problem into both a social and medical issue in 1962 with the publication of C. Henry Kempe's "The Battered Child Syndrome" in the *Journal of the American Medical Association*.[1] This article is credited with raising both public and professional awareness of child abuse and leading to the Children's Bureau recommendation for a model child abuse reporting law. By 1967, 44 states had mandatory child abuse reporting laws. In 1974 Congress passed the federal Child Abuse Prevention and Treatment Act (CAPTA), which provided states with federal funding for the investigation and prevention of child maltreatment under the condition that states adopt mandatory reporting laws.[6] It also required guaranteed immunity for reporters, confidentiality, and the appointment of a guardian ad litem to represent children. All states now have mandated reporting laws that require physicians and other state-named mandatory reporters to report reasonable suspicion of child maltreatment. The act also created the National Center on Child Abuse and Neglect, which serves as an information clearinghouse. A 1988 amendment to CAPTA directed the US Department of Health and Human Services (DHHS) to establish a national data collection and analysis program: the National Child Abuse and Neglect Data Systems (NCANDS).[7]

Current US law regarding child maltreatment rests on the basic premise that the family is best suited to provide for the interests of children. This premise, however, relies on 2 basic assumptions: that parents act in the best interests of their children and that parents have the judgment to make decisions for their children, which the children themselves lack. Thus case law has been shaped to allow children more decision-making capacity as they mature and gain judgment, and to examine whether parents are acting in the best interests of their children. Intervention into family life by the state remains uneasily balanced between what is perceived to be the best interest of the child based on the assessment of medical and social agencies and a parent's right to make decisions for their child.

Study Design

There are many types of data now available about child maltreatment in the United States, including data collected at national, state, and institutional levels. Each data set has it own strengths and weaknesses arising from the way in which the data are collected, including how the study population is chosen, whether the data are retrospective or prospective, study definitions, why the data are collected (eg, research, clinical, or legal proceedings), and how research questions are phrased.

Most data sets contain some systematic error in collecting data (bias). Child abuse research is particularly vulnerable to both selection and misclassification bias. Selection bias may result from the way in which individuals are ascertained and selected for study. This may include differential surveillance, diagnosis, or referral into the study group.[8] It may start with whether a child is seen for care and continue on through the final legal disposition of a case.[9]

Systematic misclassification of exposure (eg, exposed to maltreatment or not) is considered misclassification bias. There may be systematic differences in what is considered abuse, in whether abuse is considered in the differential diagnosis of a child seen for care (with minority children more frequently reported)[10] in reporting to child protective services (CPS) agencies, and in how CPS agencies classify substantiated cases. These systematic errors may lead to erroneous conclusions from the data. Misclassification bias may be mitigated by the type of study design chosen.

Studies that are population-based minimize bias by identifying an entire community (eg, a county, state, or province) for study. Population-based research gives the investigator the ability to calculate either the incidence (the number of new cases per population per unit time) or the prevalence (the number of existing cases within a population) of a problem using the population chosen as the denominator. Both of these types of data (incidence and prevalence) are useful for different purposes. Incidence data may help to determine whether a problem is increasing or decreasing. They may be used to tell whether a prevention effort is successful (ie, has the number of new cases decreased over time since an intervention was put into place). Prevalence data are useful when trying to estimate the need for services for children or to determine the number of adults who may have experienced a certain type of maltreatment. For example, if one wished to set up counseling services for victims of sexual abuse, it would be necessary to know the number of cases existing in the population to determine the resources necessary to care for them.

There are multiple study designs used in research of child maltreatment (Table 1). Each has its own strengths and weaknesses, thus the use of different study designs to address the same problem may be useful. Often, less expensive study designs identify a hypothesis that can then go on to be addressed with a larger, more comprehensive study.

Randomized, controlled trials are considered one of the strongest epidemiological designs because the

TABLE 1
Study Designs With Advantages and Disadvantages

Study Design	Advantages	Disadvantages
Randomized controlled trials	• Investigator assigns exposure/intervention • Unsuspected confounders equally distributed • Establish causality	• Very expensive • Ethical considerations • Selection of study population difficult
Cohort studies	• Selected on exposure history • Ability to follow children over many years • Collection of multiple outcomes • Establish temporal relationships • Measure incidence of disease • May be prospective or retrospective	• Very expensive • Loss of follow-up hurts validity • Inefficient for rare diseases • Difficult to choose comparison group
Case-control studies	• Good for rare diseases • Less expensive and quick • Examine multiple etiologic factors • Selected on outcome	• Problems with selection and recall bias • Temporality hard to establish
Cross-sectional surveys	• Establish prevalence at a point in time • Hypothesis generating • Early reporting of new problem	• Descriptive only • Exposure and outcome ascertained together • Cannot make statistical associations

research subject is randomly assigned to a study or control arm of the trial. Random assignment of the subject minimizes bias by helping to ensure that non-measured characteristics of the subjects are similar across study groups. This type of study, in which the investigator controls the exposure, is not practical for measuring the outcome of child maltreatment, but could be used to establish the best therapy for a specific type of maltreatment, or to determine whether a prevention program is effective.

Cohort studies, which select children based on presence or absence of an exposure, are another strong study design. Cohort studies follow children over time and can collect detailed outcome information. One advantage of a cohort design is the ability to establish a cause and effect relationship. Good surveillance mechanisms are required to follow a population-based cohort because these types of studies are susceptible to bias from children dropping out of the study. These studies were difficult to perform before the advent of federally funded programs because they tend to be expensive. An example of this type of study is the Longitudinal Study of Child Abuse and Neglect (LONG-SCAN), which is following 5 groups of children at multiple time points with very detailed questionnaires and psychometric testing.[11] Another example of a cohort that has followed maltreated and comparison children from childhood to adulthood has been described by Widom.[12]

Case-control studies are generally good for studying rare outcomes. These studies choose a subject based on the outcome (eg, physical abuse) and controls who come from a similar population and are at risk of the outcome. The investigators then compare cases and controls for the experience of the exposure (eg, prematurity or teen pregnancy).[13] Choosing appropriate controls is one of the biggest challenges for case-control studies and needs to be carefully considered when judging the results of an analysis.

Large cross-sectional studies that ask about children's or adults' current or past experiences also are useful.[14] Data from surveys can give descriptive information or, if the survey participants are selected to be representative of the state or nation, the data can be statistically manipulated to give population estimates.[15] Children or their parents may be asked about what happened to them in the past year or in the past month. Cross-sectional studies are limited in that they cannot show causality because the exposure and outcome are determined at the same point in time.

Data collected from a single institution, such as case series, may reflect that institution's population and referral pattern, thus the data may lack the generalizability of broader-based studies. Single institution studies, however, may provide detailed case-level data that give

valuable insights into a problem and are often hypothesis-generating studies.

Ethical Issues in Child Abuse Research

The conduct of child maltreatment research is bounded by ethical obligations toward children and families, including the obligations of informed consent and mandated reporting. These obligations make some types of research, such as surveys in which children and parents are directly asked about maltreatment, quite difficult because such research may place the child at risk of being removed from the home or the parent at risk of legal proceedings if there is a clear statement of ongoing maltreatment that has not been recognized previously. The potential for reporting maltreatment also may make some families reluctant to participate in research, potentially skewing the study sample. Some investigators have used innovative techniques to gather contemporaneous data in an ethical manner without putting children or parents at risk. LONGSCAN, a multiyear study of child maltreatment, directly asked 12-year-olds about their experiences via computer questionnaire.[16] The computer allows the children either to encrypt their replies or to flag their replies depending on whether the child wants help. Encrypted replies are divorced from identifying data and thus not subject to report.[17] This methodology allows the children to report honestly without forcing them to bring social services agencies into their homes. Other investigators have used questionnaires in young adult populations to ask about their past experiences of maltreatment.[18] Finkelhor and colleagues[19] directly surveyed children as young as 10 years about victimization. They built follow-up mechanisms into their design that ensure any history of ongoing abusive behavior is followed until reported to the proper authorities.

National Sources of Child Abuse Data

The US Congress requires the DHHS to track national trends in child abuse and neglect. Two such data collection systems exist currently: the National Incidence Study of Child Abuse and Neglect (NIS) and NCANDS. Each system employs a different methodology and different definitions of child maltreatment, which has resulted in disparate survey results. Definitions of child maltreatment can depend on whether the data gathered are intended for research or for legal reasons. For example, Runyan et al[20] compared the CPS definition of maltreatment to that used in NIS-2 at 4 separate study sites. They found that definitions were consistent for the same type of maltreatment 81% of the time, with the least consistency in definitions of emotional maltreatment.

NIS

The NIS collects population-based data on the incidence, severity, and demographic distribution of child maltreatment in the United States.[21] Data are collected in specified counties over 1 of 2 three-month periods (to lessen the effect of seasonality). The DHHS has now funded 3 waves of the NIS: the first in 1979 and 1980, the second in 1986 and 1987, and the third between 1993 and 1995 and published in 1997. The NIS is currently in its fourth cycle of data collection (2005–2006), with reporting likely in 2008.[22]

The NIS offers a number of advantages. Data are gathered from multiple counties chosen to be representative of the US population. It is an active, prospective surveillance system that uses standard research definitions for all of its reporters and has a high level of quality control. The NIS is an inclusive system that collects data from multiple sources including local CPS agencies and agencies and individuals who have contact with children younger than 18 years. Other agencies may include schools, hospitals, child care centers, police departments, community mental health clinics, and shelters for abused women. Reporters from these agencies are asked to serve as "sentinels" by providing descriptive information about children with whom they come into contact during the study period and whom they believe are maltreated. This approach is used to attempt to include children who are identified as maltreated in the community but may not have been reported to CPS. After data collection, all reports are unduplicated using probabilistic matching techniques, and trained coders review and code the type and severity of the maltreatment from descriptions on the form according to the NIS guidelines (available at www.NIS4.org). The sample is weighted using common statistical techniques to arrive at national incidence estimates.

Therefore, NIS contains data on cases accepted for referral by a CPS agency and suspected cases of child maltreatment from sentinels using definitions that do not necessarily correspond to each state's legal definition of child maltreatment. The methods used to define a case for NIS result in incidence estimates that are higher than estimates of maltreatment from cases that require substantiation of maltreatment. Because the NIS uses the same standardized definitions during each period of data collection and follows the same study procedures, it is useful to characterize whether there is an increase or decrease in the number of new cases of child maltreatment in the population.

The NIS also reports the severity of maltreatment according to a harm standard and an endangerment standard.[23] To reach the level of the harm standard, children must have already experienced harm from maltreatment. The endangerment standard includes children who experienced abuse or neglect that put them at risk of harm.

NCANDS

The DHHS also collects annual information on child maltreatment from all of the states and the District of Columbia. Beginning in 1976 data were collected from many state CPS agencies by the American Humane Association. The 1988 amendment to CAPTA provided for the first report from NCANDS, which was based on data from 1990.[7] Data are submitted to NCANDS voluntarily by state CPS agencies about children who received either an assessment or investigation by the agency regarding alleged abuse where the disposition was substantiated. Only substantiated cases are counted as victims of maltreatment. States may report aggregate or case-level data. Case-level data (44 states) include characteristics of the referral, the alleged abuse or neglect, the disposition of the case, and characteristics of the children and the caregivers, as well as characteristics of the perpetrators.

NCANDS counts a child each time he or she is a victim of maltreatment, so that the same child could be counted more than one time in 1 year. Therefore it reports the incidence of episodes of maltreatment per population per year. Referrals to and acceptance and substantiation of cases by CPS may be open to many influences. In a system that is at times overwhelmed, only the most egregious referrals may be accepted for investigation. Additionally, states may code different types of abuse in a way that will meet legal scrutiny per each state's regulations. Because NCANDS receives data from the state's CPS agencies, it does not give standardized definitions of maltreatment to the states and is a voluntary system. Like NIS, NCANDS probably provides reasonable trends as long as the rules for reporting, accepting and substantiating referrals, and defining types of maltreatment in the states remain relatively constant.

Overview of Incident Maltreatment From NIS and NCANDS

The NIS data report an increase in the national incidence of children harmed by maltreatment in each cycle since the inception of data collection (Figure 1).[23] When considering children harmed,

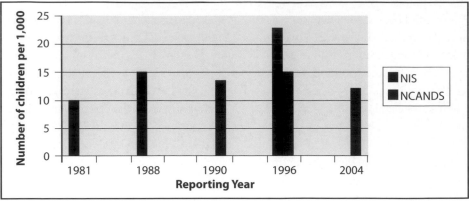

FIGURE 1

Comparison of incidence of child abuse between the National Incidence Study of Child Abuse and Neglect (NIS) and the National Child Abuse and Neglect Data Systems (NCANDS).

the incidence of maltreatment from abuse or neglect was elevated 1.5 times in NIS-3 compared with NIS-2. Between 1988 and 1996, the incidence of physical abuse almost doubled; sexual abuse was more than twice as frequent; and emotional abuse, emotional neglect, and physical neglect were more than 2.5 times as frequent.

NCANDS reported that 872,000 children were determined to be victims of abuse or neglect in their most recent year of reporting (2004), or an incidence of 11.9 per 1,000 children (www.acf.hhs. gov/programs/cb/pubs/cm04/index. htm). This reflected a decrease in the incidence since the first NCANDS report of 13.4 per 1,000 children in 1990. The incidence did not steadily decrease, but peaked in the early 1990s and then declined (Figure 1).

To compare the incidence from NCANDS with NIS-3, the rate of reported maltreatment from 1996 was used from both data sources. The incidence rate of 15 per 1,000 children in 1996 from NCANDS was approximately

one-third lower than that estimated by NIS-3 (23.1 per 1,000 children).[24] This comparison would suggest that the use of sentinel reporters by NIS captures a broader range of maltreatment or that approximately a third of the cases of child maltreatment are either not reported to or not substantiated by CPS agencies.

Data from NIS-1 through NIS-3 report a rise in incident cases of maltreatment, while NCANDS reports a decrease (Figure 1). It is not known why this discrepancy is so large. The rate of children receiving an investigation or assessment by CPS agencies increased from 36.1 per 1,000 children to 42.6 per 1,000 children between 1990 and 2004, while the rates of substantiation fell.[25] Possible explanations include overreporting or the saturation of the CPS system so that less serious maltreatment is not substantiated and considered victimization. NIS-3 reports that only 28% of children who met the harm standard were investigated by CPS, down from 44% in NIS-2.[26] The reasons for this decline are unknown, but need to be taken into account when comparing incident child abuse across studies.

Risk Factors for Child Maltreatment

Risk factors for child maltreatment vary by the population under study, but commonalities in risk factors across studies do exist. Risk factors may be put into a multilayered ecological framework that encompasses interactions among the child, the parents, the family, the social setting, and the social context.[27]

Child factors that may make children more likely to be victims of abuse include premature birth and disability.[28,29] In general, boys are more likely to be physically abused and girls sexually abused.

Parental risk factors include both specific parental behaviors and abnormalities within the parent-child relationship. Bavolek[30] noted 4 abnormalities that can lead to child abuse or neglect: inappropriate parental expectations of the child, lack of empathy to the child's needs, the parents' belief in physical punishment, and parental role reversal. Specific parental problems that have been identified include mental health problems and substance abuse.[31,32] Children born to young mothers (≤18 years) have been shown to be at higher risk of experiencing maltreatment both in an index-comparison study of inner-city women and in a statewide cohort focused on inflicted traumatic brain injury.[33,34]

Domestic violence is an example of a family-level risk for children.[35] Examples of social risk factors associated with child maltreatment are poverty and high levels of drug use and alcohol availability in neighborhoods.[36–38] In all 3 waves of NIS, child race, which could be considered a societal-level risk, has not been associated with child maltreatment.[26] Child maltreatment also needs to be considered within its cultural context. Societies and communities may differ on what is considered child maltreatment.[39]

Many of the risk factors for child maltreatment are associated with each other, such as poverty, drug abuse, mental health problems, and young maternal age, which makes it difficult to determine which risk factors are the most important or whether the danger to children lies in the cumulative effect of multiple risk factors. To know whether a specific risk factor is associated independently with child maltreatment, the study should use an appropriate comparison group (in case-control or cohort studies), and results should be adjusted for other known risk factors using common statistical techniques.

Types of Maltreatment

Neglect

Child neglect is generally defined in terms of caretaker omissions that result in harm or potential harm to a child. This may include the failure of parents to provide adequate physical care (including food, clothing, and shelter), ensure appropriate medical and dental care or education, provide adequate supervision, or provide emotional support. Exposure to familial violence is also considered a form of psychological neglect. It is difficult to separate the terms *psychological maltreatment* and *emotional abuse* from definitions of neglect. The American Academy of Pediatrics includes in its definition of psychological maltreatment neglecting mental health, medical, and educational needs as well as making a child feel unsafe, humiliating a child in public, and a child witnessing domestic violence.[40] How neglect is defined may depend on whether the data are intended for research, reporting, or treatment.

Some authors feel that the definition of child neglect should be broad and considered in the context of a child's development.[41] English et al[42] found that factors not usually considered neglectful, such as the quality of child-adult communication, stability of living situation, and cleanliness of the house, are markers of neglectful behavior that are associated with child functioning. This broader concept of neglect is appealing because it incorporates factors that seem to affect the child's welfare and may arise from either parental or societal omissions or commissions. This approach also adopts a nonpunitive attitude toward parents who may have social circumstances that make appropriate child care impossible; such broad definitions, however, are difficult for CPS agencies that focus on the more extreme deficiencies of caretaking.

The NCANDS data (2004) report that of the 872,000 children found to be victims of child maltreatment, 64.5% were victims of neglect. An additional 7.0% were emotionally or psychologically maltreated, and 2.1% experienced medical neglect.[25] The incidence of neglect has been relatively stable over the past 5 reporting cycles of NCANDS between 7.1 and 7.5 per 1,000 children. Data for medical neglect (0.3 per 1,000 children) and psychological maltreatment (0.9 per 1,000 children) are reported separately.

Physical Abuse

Physical abuse is defined as a physical injury inflicted on a child. It may include hitting, shaking, burning, beating, or other forms of direct physical contact. It may also include harsh physical punishment that is inappropriate for the child's age. The difference between what is considered physical abuse and what is considered appropriate physical punishment has changed over time and is perceived differently across cultures.[43]

The Parent-Child Conflict Tactics Scale has become a useful research tool for quantifying physical abuse as well as other types of child maltreatment.[44] It asks parents specific questions about actions that they may or may not have taken in the past year, including nonviolent discipline and varying degrees of physical discipline/assault, some of which are considered socially acceptable (spanked on the bottom with bare hand) and some of which are not (hit with fist). It differs from other methods of measuring physical maltreatment because it measures parental actions as opposed to a child's injury. Because children's injuries are probably underreported, this approach of asking parents may give a more clear representation of child maltreatment. Of course, parents may underreport what they perceive as socially unacceptable behaviors. The Parent-Child Conflict Tactics Scale also has subscales for sexual maltreatment and neglect.

There are multiple data sources for child physical abuse including national and statewide studies. The NIS-3 reported an increase in child physical abuse in each reporting cycle. NCANDS data reported rates of physical abuse at approximately 2.1 per 1,000 children in 2004. The incidence of child physical abuse has not changed substantively in the NCANDS data over the 5-year period of 2000 to 2004.

A prevalence study of child physical and sexual abuse was conducted in Ontario, Canada from 1990 to 1991. The study used a random subsample of respondents to the Ontario Health Survey who were aged 15 years or older.[45] Respondents were asked questions about physical abuse by an adult when they were "growing up." Questions used were based on the Parent-Child Conflict Tactics Scales.[46] The prevalence of having been a victim of child physical abuse was higher for males (31.2%, 95% confidence interval [CI], 28.8–33.7) than females (21.1%, 95% CI, 19.3–22.9); however, estimates for severe physical abuse were similar in males and females, respectively (10.7%, 95% CI, 9.1–12.3 vs 9.2%, 95% CI, 7.9–10.5).

Specific types of physical abuse have been studied in more depth. Inflicted traumatic brain injury has received attention secondary to its serious potential for harm and in the hopes of being able to measure the outcomes of prevention programs. The first population-based study collected data from all pediatric departments, neurosurgical departments, and pediatric intensive care units in Scotland for an 18-month period in 1998 and 1999. It reported an incidence of 24.6 per 100,000 children younger than 1 year annually (95% CI, 14.9–38.5).[47] A statewide study performed in North Carolina over a 2-year period, which required intensive care admission or death for entrance to the study, reported an incidence of 29.7 per 100,000 (95% CI, 22.9–36.7) for children younger than 1 year and 3.8 per 100,000 (95% CI, 1.3–6.4) for children between ages 1 and 2 years. Boys were injured more frequently than girls.[34]

Ellington and colleagues[48] found rates similar to those found in North Carolina using an administrative database compiled by the Healthcare Cost and Utilization Project (the Kid Inpatient Database) of children hospitalized in the United States during 3 discrete 1-year periods (1997, 2000, 2003).[48] Traumatic brain injury was identified from the database with *International Classification of Diseases, Ninth Revision, Clinical Modification (ICD-9-CM)* codes, and mechanism of injury was specified with external cause of injury codes (E-codes). The incidence of inflicted traumatic brain injury varied from 21.0 to 23.6 per 100,000 in children younger than 1 year. These rates are comparable to the results in North Carolina for children younger than 1 year, excluding children who died prior to hospitalization (23.5/100,000). This comparison of a prospective population-based study and a study using a hospital-based data set show that such national databases may be useful for following the incidence of inflicted traumatic brain injury resulting in hospitalization.

As with many types of child maltreatment, the shaking of infants as a problem is probably broader than these data suggest. For example, Theodore et al,[49] in a study of harsh child physical discipline in North and South Carolina, directly asked parents in a telephone survey about shaking children younger than 2 years as a form of discipline. The authors estimated that for every child sustaining a life-threatening or fatal inflicted traumatic brain injury, 152 children may be shaken by their caregivers and sustain subclinical brain trauma. These data are consistent with the finding that many children are found to have both old and new injuries when they are brought to medical attention.[50,51]

Abdominal injury due to abuse has also been studied in some detail. While the incidence of this type of abuse is relatively rare (2.3 cases per million children <5 years per year, 95% CI, 1.4–3.8), it is difficult to detect and has a high case fatality rate. Small bowel injury is frequent among children who have sustained abusive abdominal trauma.[52]

Sexual Abuse

Sexual abuse is the involvement of adults, older children, or adolescents in sexual activities with children who cannot give appropriate consent and who do not understand the significance of what is happening to them, or that violate the social taboos of society.[53] To be considered abuse by CPS, the acts have to be committed by a person who is responsible for the child's care. If the acts are committed by a stranger, it is considered sexual assault. The CPS definition presents a problem when sexual abuse is committed by a 15-year-old cousin. It is unclear how CPS agencies code such episodes of sexual abuse by a non-caretaker.

Contrasting data are available about the changes in the reported incidence of sexual abuse over the last 2 years. In each cycle of the NIS, the incidence of child sexual abuse has risen. In contrast, in the NCANDS data, there was a sharp decline from 1992 to 1999, with a plateau (1.2 per 1,000 children per year) in the years 2000 through 2004. In 2004 NCANDS reported that 9.7% of children who were victims of abuse were victims of sexual abuse.

Estimates of the incidence of child sexual abuse in North and South Carolina were obtained from direct telephone interviews of mothers. Mothers were chosen at random and asked to respond to a questionnaire on child rearing and discipline. The incidence of child sexual abuse reported by mothers (10.5 cases per 1,000 children) was approximately 10 times higher than that reported by NCANDS for the year 2002.[49] Data reported to NCANDS from North and South Carolina showed a rate of 0.6 per 1,000 children. While it seems likely that the NCANDS data underreport the actual incidence of child sexual abuse, it is unclear whether the decrease in the national incidence from 1992 to 1999 represents an actual drop, a decrease in reporting of sexual abuse, or a change in the way that CPS handles cases.[54,55]

Prevalence data on sexual abuse have been obtained via retrospective studies of adults about their experiences in childhood in many developed countries. In general, these studies show a substantial minority of men and women report having a history of child sexual abuse. For example, a study in the United Kingdom employing random probability sampling of young adults found that 11% of men and 21% of women reported experiences that the investigators classified as consistent with sexual abuse, or 16% overall.[56] Only 6% of the sample considered themselves to be abused. The difference between how individuals and researchers perceive abuse highlights the importance of including questions about specific behaviors in surveys of sexual abuse.

In the United States, a 1990 population-based telephone survey of the prevalence of child sexual abuse in which adults older than 18 years were interviewed about their experiences in childhood revealed a prevalence of 16% for men and 27% for women.[57] This is slightly higher than the prevalence found in the UK study.

The results of the Ontario Health Supplement reported a population prevalence of child sexual abuse of 4.3% in men and 12.8% in women.[45] These figures are lower than both the UK and US studies. Discrepancies in the prevalence of sexual abuse among studies may be due to actual differences of prevalence rates or differences in the study methodology: The UK study surveyed young adults aged 18 to 24 years while the Ontario study and the US study surveyed adults of all ages.[58] The Ontario and US studies showed a decrease in reported prevalence for sexual abuse in the group 65 years or older. This differential in reporting by age may reflect generational differences in the willingness to report sexual abuse, differences in recall, or changes in the prevalence of sexual abuse over time. Another factor that could lead to differences in response among studies is the specificity of the survey instrument: The US study used very imprecise and broad screening questions, which might lead to a high prevalence of reported abuse. Unlike the US study, the Ontario study chose to use 4 precise questions to establish sexual abuse. The UK study used precise definitions but had a broader scope of activities that were considered abusive behavior than the Ontario study. Thus the differences in both populations studied and survey instruments make the direct comparisons of prevalence rates among countries difficult.

The previous studies collected data about the prevalence of sexual abuse by asking adults about their childhood experiences. In a different approach to understanding the problem, investigators asked parents about their child's experiences. In the United States, the Gallup Organization conducted a survey of a representative sample of parents that asked questions about their child-rearing and discipline practices.[59] The 1995 survey found that by parent report,

1.9% of children had been victims of child sexual abuse in the past year, and 5.7% of children had been victims of sexual abuse during their lifetime. Children aged 9 to 12 years had a higher rate of abuse (6.6% per year) than children younger than 9 years (5% per year). The rate of sexual abuse for boys and girls was approximately the same. Risk factors for child sexual abuse included living in a family with a lower income (≤$50,000), a single head of household, and parental education not exceeding high school graduation.[59] The prevalence of child sexual abuse in this study (ever abused) is lower than that reported by studies that ask adults about lifetime experience as children. This difference may be explained by the study design. Children in the Gallup Poll survey had fewer years at risk to experience abuse than the studies that interviewed adults, and parents may not know about or choose to report on their child's experience with sexual abuse.

Fatalities

Fatalities from child maltreatment are widely recognized to be underreported. In 2004 NCANDS reported that 1,490 children died from abuse or neglect (approximately 2 children per 100,000 per year). Fatality statistics were collected from child welfare agencies, health departments, and child fatality review boards. Most fatalities were in children younger than 4 years (81.0%). Deaths in the 0- to 4-year age group occurred disproportionately in children younger than 1 year (45.0%). Children aged 4 to 7 years accounted for 11.5% of deaths, and children aged 8 to 11 years

and 12 to 17 years comprised 4.1% and 3.4% of deaths, respectively. Neglect is reported as the most frequent type of maltreatment leading to death (35.5% of fatalities).[25]

The Centers for Disease Control and Prevention (CDC) National Center for Injury Prevention and Control tracks injury-related morbidity and mortality. Its Web-based Injury Statistics Query and Reporting System (WISQARS) reports violence-related injury deaths identified by *ICD-10* (www.cdc.gov/ncipc/wisqars/). For the same year (2003) as NCANDS, WISQARS reported fewer (1,180 vs 717, respectively) violence-related deaths in children younger than 4 years, with most (48%) of those deaths in children younger than 1 year. The WISQARS fatality data do not include deaths secondary to neglect because it is not violence-related. Data for older children are more difficult to compare because violence-related death is not specific to child abuse.

Several studies show that both NCANDS and the CDC underreport fatalities secondary to maltreatment. Reasons for underreporting include deficiencies in hospital discharge reporting and lack of information on the death certificate.[60,61] When *ICD-9-CM*[62] coding of deaths for children aged 10 years and younger were compared with the records of the Office of the Chief Medical Examiner in North Carolina, almost 60% of the homicides found to be due to abuse were not coded as abuse in the North Carolina vital records.[63] This finding is consistent with the report by Crume et al,[61] who found that only one-half of children in Colorado who died from maltreatment had maltreatment listed as a cause on the death certificate.[61] This report also found that vio-lent deaths were more likely to be reported as maltreatment than deaths from neglect, and that black race and female gender were associated with reporting death from maltreatment. Therefore, data systems that rely on death certificates or *ICD-9-CM* coding are both likely to underreport and to present skewed sociodemographic profiles of children who die from maltreatment.

Poly-victimization

Studies of child maltreatment often concentrate on only one aspect of abusive behavior: bullying, traumatic brain injury, sexual abuse, etc. Unfortunately, many children who suffer from one type of maltreatment often suffer from repeated episodes of maltreatment or differing types of maltreatment.[15,45] In a recent nationally representative survey, Finkelhor and colleagues[57] asked children or their parents about episodes of victimization that they had experienced over the past year. The results of this study showed that children who experience one type of victimization often experience repeated victimization or multiple types of victimization.[15] Children who experienced poly-victimization, defined as at least 4 different kinds of victimization in the past year, were those most likely to suffer from traumatic symptomatology.[19]

Conclusion

There is a need for accurate data on the scope of child maltreatment. Such data are needed to explore the root causes of the problem that may be amenable to change, guide prevention programs, and leverage resources for prevention and treatment. What is clear from the data is that child maltreatment is more prevalent than what is identified in the current surveillance systems, it has adverse effects on children, and those adverse effects extend through adulthood.

References

1. Kempe CH, Silverman FN, Steele BF, Droegemueller W, Silver HK. The battered-child syndrome. *JAMA*. 1962;181:17–24
2. Brenner R. *Children and Youth in America: A Documentary History.* Cambridge, MA: Harvard University Press; 1970–1974
3. Mason M. *From Father's Property to Children's Rights: The History of Child Custody in the United States.* New York, NY: Columbia University Press; 1994
4. Ashby L. *Endangered Children: Dependency, Neglect, and Abuse in American History.* New York, NY: Twayne Publishers; 1997
5. *Prince v Commonwealth of Massachusetts,* 313 Mass 223, 46 NE2d 755 (1944)
6. Child Abuse Prevention and Treatment Act. Pub L No. 93-273
7. Child Abuse Prevention and Treatment Act; Pub L No. 100-294
8. Hennekens C, Buring J. *Epidemiology in Medicine.* Boston, MA: Little, Brown and Company; 1987
9. Zellman GL. The impact of case characteristics on child abuse reporting decisions. *Child Abuse Negl.* 1992;16:57–74

10. Lane WG, Rubin DM, Monteith R, Christian CW. Racial differences in the evaluation of pediatric fractures for physical abuse. *JAMA*. 2002;288:1603–1609

11. Consortium for Longitudinal Studies of Child Abuse and Neglect. Longitudinal Studies of Child Abuse and Neglect. http://www.iprc.unc.edu/longscan/. Accessed February 28, 2006

12. Widom CS. Posttraumatic stress disorder in abused and neglected children grown up. *Am J Psychiatr*. 1999;156:1223–1229

13. Leventhal JM. Risk factors for child abuse: methodologic standards in case-control studies. *Pediatrics*. 1981;68:684–690

14. Felitti VJ, Anda RF, Nordenberg D, et al. Relationship of childhood abuse and household dysfunction to many of the leading causes of death in adults. The Adverse Childhood Experiences (ACE) Study. *Am J Prev Med*. 1998;14:245–258

15. Finkelhor D, Ormrod R, Turner H, Hamby SL. The victimization of children and youth: a comprehensive, national survey. *Child Maltreat*. 2005;10:5–25

16. Runyan DK. Prevalence, risk, sensitivity, and specificity: a commentary on the epidemiology of child sexual abuse and the development of a research agenda. *Child Abuse Negl*. 1998;22:493–498; discussion 499–502

17. Runyan D. Maltreatment in families: a research dilemma. In: King N, Henderson G, Stein J, eds. *Beyond Regulations: Ethics in Human Subjects Research*. Chapel Hill, NC: University of North Carolina Press; 1999:163–170

18. Fergusson DM, Lynskey MT. Physical punishment/maltreatment during childhood and adjustment in young adulthood. *Child Abuse Negl*. 1997;21:617–630

19. Finkelhor D, Ormrod RK, Turner HA, Hamby SL. Measuring poly-victimization using the Juvenile Victimization Questionnaire. *Child Abuse Negl*. 2005;29:1297–1312

20. Runyan DK, Cox CE, Dubowitz H, et al. Describing maltreatment: do child protective service reports and research definitions agree? *Child Abuse Negl*. 2005;29:461–477

21. Child Welfare Information Gateway Web site. http://www.childwelfare.gov/. Accessed October 18, 2006

22. Administration for Children and Families, US Department of Health and Human Services. 4th National Incidence Study of Child Abuse and Neglect: Project Summary. http://www.nis4.org/DOCS/ProjectSummary.pdf. Accessed February 21, 2006

23. Administration for Children and Families, US Department of Health and Human Services. 4th National Incidence Study of Child Abuse and Neglect: Sentinel Guide. https://www.nis4.org/DOCS/SentinelGuide.pdf. Accessed June 6, 2006

24. Administration for Children and Families, US Department of Health and Human Services. Highlights of Findings. http://www.acf.hhs.gov/programs/cb/pubs/ncands96/highligh.htm. Accessed February 24, 2006

25. US Department of Health and Human Services Abuse of Children, Youths, and Families. *Child Maltreatment 2004*. Washington, DC: US Government Printing Office; 2006

26. Sedlack A, Broadhurst D. *Executive Summary of the Third National Incidence Study of Child Abuse and Neglect*. Washington, DC: US Department of Health and Human Services; 1996

27. Belsky J. The determinants of parenting: a process model. *Child Dev*. 1984;55:83–96

28. Murphy JF, Jenkins J, Newcombe RG, Sibert JR. Objective birth data and the prediction of child abuse. *Arch Dis Child*. 1981;56:295–297

29. Spencer N, Devereux E, Wallace A, et al. Disabling conditions and registration for child abuse and neglect: a population-based study. *Pediatrics*. 2005;116:609–613

30. Bavolek S. *The Nurturing Parenting Programs.* Washington, DC: Office of Juvenile Justice and Delinquency Prevention, US Department of Justice; 2000

31. Leventhal JM, Forsyth BW, Qi K, Johnson L, Schroeder D, Votto N. Maltreatment of children born to women who used cocaine during pregnancy: a population-based study. *Pediatrics.* 1997;100:e7

32. Walsh C, MacMillan HL, Jamieson E. The relationship between parental substance abuse and child maltreatment: findings from the Ontario Health Supplement. *Child Abuse Negl.* 2003;27:1409–1425

33. Stier DM, Leventhal JM, Berg AT, Johnson L, Mezger J. Are children born to young mothers at increased risk of maltreatment? *Pediatrics.* 1993;91:642–648

34. Keenan HT, Runyan DK, Marshall SW, Nocera MA, Merten DF, Sinal SH. A population-based study of inflicted traumatic brain injury in young children. *JAMA.* 2003;290:621–626

35. Lee LC, Kotch JB, Cox CE. Child maltreatment in families experiencing domestic violence. *Violence Vict.* 2004;19:573–591

36. Sidebotham P, Heron J, Golding J, ALSPAC Study Team. Child maltreatment in the "Children of the Nineties": deprivation, class, and social networks in a UK sample. *Child Abuse Negl.* 2002;26:1243–1259

37. Sedlak A. *Third National Incidence Study of Child Abuse and Neglect (NIS-3).* Washington, DC: US Department of Health and Human Services; 1996

38. Freisthler B, Needell B, Gruenewald PJ. Is the physical availability of alcohol and illicit drugs related to neighborhood rates of child maltreatment? *Child Abuse Negl.* 2005;29:1049–1060

39. Ferrari AM. The impact of culture upon child rearing practices and definitions of maltreatment. *Child Abuse Negl.* 2002;26:793–813

40. Kairys SW, Johnson CF. The psychological maltreatment of children—technical report. *Pediatrics.* 2002;109:e68

41. Dubowitz H. *Neglected Children: Research, Practice, and Policy.* Thousand Oaks, CA: Sage; 1999

42. English DJ, Thompson R, Graham JC, Briggs EC. Toward a definition of neglect in young children. *Child Maltreat.* 2005;10:190–206

43. Maker AH, Shah PV, Agha Z. Child physical abuse: prevalence, characteristics, predictors, and beliefs about parent-child violence in South Asian, Middle Eastern, East Asian, and Latina women in the United States. *J Interpers Violence.* 2005;20:1406–1428

44. Straus MA, Hamby SL, Finkelhor D, Moore DW, Runyan D. Identification of child maltreatment with the Parent-Child Conflict Tactics Scales: development and psychometric data for a national sample of American parents. *Child Abuse Negl.* 1998;22:249–270

45. MacMillan HL, Fleming JE, Trocme N, et al. Prevalence of child physical and sexual abuse in the community. Results from the Ontario Health Supplement. *JAMA.* 1997;278:131–135

46. Straus M. The Conflict Tactics Scales and its critics: an evaluation and new data on validity and reliability. In: Strauss M, Gelles R, eds. *Physical Violence in American Families: Risk Factors and Adaptations to Violence in 8,145 Families.* New Brunswick, NJ: Transaction Publishers; 1990:49–73

47. Barlow KM, Minns RA. Annual incidence of shaken impact syndrome in young children. *Lancet.* 2000;356:1571–1572

48. Ellington KD, Leventhal JM, Weiss HB. Using hospital discharge databases to track the incidence of inflicted traumatic brain injury in infants. Presented at: Pediatric Academic Societies Annual Meeting; May 2, 2006; San Francisco, CA

49. Theodore AD, Chang JJ, Runyan DK, Hunter WM, Bangdiwala SI, Agans R. Epidemiologic features of the physical and sexual maltreatment of children in the Carolinas. *Pediatrics*. 2005;115:e331–e337

50. Jenny C, Hymel KP, Ritzen A, Reinert SE, Hay TC. Analysis of missed cases of abusive head trauma. *JAMA*. 1999;281:621–626

51. Keenan HT, Runyan DK, Marshall SW, Nocera MA, Merten DF. A population-based comparison of clinical and outcome characteristics of young children with serious inflicted and noninflicted traumatic brain injury. *Pediatrics*. 2004;114:633–639

52. Barnes PM, Norton CM, Dunstan FD, Kemp AM, Yates DW, Sibert JR. Abdominal injury due to child abuse. *Lancet*. 2005;366:234–235

53. Kempe CH. Sexual abuse, another hidden pediatric problem: the 1977 C. Anderson Aldrich lecture. *Pediatrics*. 1978;62:382–389

54. Jones LM, Finkelhor D, Kopiec K. Why is sexual abuse declining? A survey of state child protection administrators. *Child Abuse Negl*. 2001;25:1139–1158

55. Leventhal JM. A decline in substantiated cases of child sexual abuse in the United States: good news or false hope? *Child Abuse Negl*. 2001;25:1137–1138

56. May-Chahal C, Cawson P. Measuring child maltreatment in the United Kingdom: a study of the prevalence of child abuse and neglect. *Child Abuse Negl*. 2005;29:969–984

57. Finkelhor D, Hotaling G, Lewis IA, Smith C. Sexual abuse in a national survey of adult men and women: prevalence, characteristics, and risk factors. *Child Abuse Negl*. 1990;14:19–28

58. Widom CS, Raphael KG, DuMont KA. The case for prospective longitudinal studies in child maltreatment research: commentary on Dube, Williamson, Thompson, Felitti, and Anda (2004). *Child Abuse Negl*. 2004;28:715–722

59. Gallup Organization. *Disciplining Children in America: A Gallup Poll Report*. Princeton, NJ: Gallup Organization; 1995

60. Olsen SJ, Durkin MS. Validity of hospital discharge data regarding intentionality of fatal pediatric injuries. *Epidemiology*. 1996;7:644–647

61. Crume TL, DiGuiseppi C, Byers T, Sirotnak AP, Garrett CJ. Underascertainment of child maltreatment fatalities by death certificates, 1990–1998. *Pediatrics*. 2002;110(2 Pt 1):e18

62. *International Classification of Diseases, 9th Revision, Clinical Modification*. 5th ed. Los Angeles, CA: Practice Management Information Corporation; 1998

63. Herman-Giddens ME, Brown G, Verbiest S, et al. Underascertainment of child abuse mortality in the United States. *JAMA*. 1999;282:463–467

Cutaneous Manifestations of Child Abuse

Carole Jenny

Child Protection Program, Hasbro Children's Hospital
Department of Pediatrics, Brown University School of Medicine

Robert M. Reece

Child Protection Program, The Floating Hospital for Children at Tufts
Medical Center
Tufts University School of Medicine

Incidence of Abusive Cutaneous Injuries

Cutaneous injuries include bruises, petechiae, burns, bite marks, lacerations, and abrasions. In 2004 data from the National Child Abuse and Neglect Data System of the US Department of Health and Human Services indicated that physical abuse constituted 17.5% of the total substantiated reports for child maltreatment.[1] Data from the first Canadian incidence study of child maltreatment showed that 49% of 7,672 child protection investigations in 1998 were substantiated. More than 13% of these involved moderate injuries, defined as cases in which physical harm was observed. Two thirds of these injuries were due to bruises, cuts, or scrapes.[2] In other studies, 50% to 60% of all physical abuse cases had skin injuries, either in isolation or in combination with other abusive injuries.[3,4] Cutaneous injuries are the single most common presentation of physical child abuse.

Skin: An Overview

Human skin is an extraordinary organ, accounting for 16% of the weight of the human body.[5] It serves many important functions, including control of thermoregulation, regulation of blood pressure, protection from microorganisms and toxins, and maintenance of hydration. Normal skin is supple, allowing facial expressions and joint mobility. The skin interfaces with the environment, providing many of our sensory experiences as well as the unique visage with which we interact with our environment.[6]

Skin varies in thickness, depending on the location of the body. On the eyelid, it is 0.5 mm thick. On the soles of the feet, it can be up to 4 mm thick and can tolerate constant abrasion.[5] Skin consists of 2 basic layers, the epidermis and dermis.

Epidermis

The epidermis is the outer protective layer. It is made up of 5 cellular layers, all of which gradually migrate to the surface from the most basilar layer impinging on the basement membrane. In addition to epithelial cells and their main product, keratin, the epidermis contains melanocytes, providing melanin to protect and color the skin. Keratin constitutes 85% of the mass of the epidermis. The epidermis is replaced every 2 to 4 weeks.[7]

Dermis

The underlying dermis provides the skin's elasticity and strength. The dermis itself is composed of 2 layers containing the proteins collagen, elastin, and reticulin and permeated by a mucopolysaccharide ground substance. Blood vessels, lymph vessels, and nerve fibers traverse the dermis. Fibroblasts, macrophages, and mast cells reside in the dermis. Hair follicles, sweat glands, and sebaceous glands protrude from the dermis to the epidermis and skin surface, providing regenerative potential after loss of the epidermis through illness or injury. Below the dermis, a subcutaneous layer attaches to fascia. This layer contains immune cells, blood and lymph vessels, nerves, and fatty tissue, and also protects the body.

Properties of Skin

Skin has biomechanical properties that affect its function and healing. It has a distinctly nonlinear deformation response to loading. Small loads produce great deformation, but as the load increases, skin becomes progressively stiffer. Within limits it also is elastic, and ideally reverts to its original state when loads are removed. Skin is viscoelastic and capable of both deformation and flow with load. If held in a stretched position, the tension on the skin decreases with time. Thus it exhibits a time-dependent response to load. Temperature, humidity, and pH affect the biomechanical properties of skin. Skin is thinner but more dense on the extremities. It increases in stiffness from the head to the foot.[8]

Human skin is constantly under tension in most areas of the body. If a portion of skin is removed from the body, the wound edges retract, and the excised skin shrinks. The lines of tension on the human body were first described by Langer in 1861. Langer noticed that if round pieces of skin were removed from cadavers, the wound contracted into a slit-shaped opening along the long axis of the elastic tension on the skin. Langer lines are often used to guide the choice of sites and directions for surgical incisions to minimize scarring and stretch on the wound. If healed by secondary intention, a circular or elliptical excision will form a linear scar. If a square of skin is removed, the resulting scar will take on the shape of a 4-pointed star.[9]

Dermal fibers in children are tortuous, unbranched, and loosely arranged. The lack of connection among fibers gives young skin greater mobility and elastic properties. When skin is strained, dermal fibers reorient to the direction of the load, becoming straightened and compact to minimize strain. With excess stress, the fibers fail and rupture, causing tissue failure. Young skin is less protected against large strains than is older skin. It is more viscous and less elastic.[10]

The upper layers of the bloodless epidermis are relatively colorless. Skin coloration comes from the melanin (brown pigment) in the basilar layers of the epithelium, as well as from chemicals in the dermal tissues, including oxygenated hemoglobin (red), deoxygenated hemoglobin (blue), and bilirubin (yellow).[11] Normal skin can appear erythematous because of either increased blood flow through capillaries or increased number of capillaries.

Injuries of the Skin

When sufficient force is delivered to skin, deformation and injury result. The injury experienced depends on the nature of the insult, the amount of force or energy applied, and the extent of surface area experiencing the force.[12] Injuries are categorized into 4 types by the nature of disruption to the tissues.

1. Abrasions: Abrasions result from friction removing superficial layers of skin. They are also called scrapes. Skinned knees are a typical example of abrasions.[13]
2. Contusions: Contusions cause discoloration of the skin because of hemorrhage into the skin after blunt trauma. Contusions can be diffuse (bruise) or focal (hematoma).
3. Lacerations: Lacerations are tears into the skin caused by shearing or crushing forces. Sharp or blunt objects can lacerate the skin, depending on the amount of force applied.
4. Burns: A burn is destruction of tissue by a physical agent applied to skin.

Burns can result from the application of heat, chemical agents, or electromagnetic radiation. Although burn injuries caused by different types of agents can appear similar, their basic pathophysiology at the cellular level is quite different. This is described in more detail in a later section.

Healing of Injured Skin

Once skin is injured, the complex process of wound healing begins. This is a dynamic process involving soluble mediators, blood cells, extracellular material, and parenchymal cells.[14] A procession of overlapping steps occurs in healing, including formation of a blood clot; infiltration of the site with neutrophils, macrophages, and monocytes; progressive migration of epithelial cells over the healing area; wound contraction; fibrinolysis of the original clot; formation of granulation tissue; and neovascularization of the healing wound.

Clot formation and inflammation begin almost immediately to preserve the integrity of the body after the skin is injured. Within hours, epidermal cells from the skin appendages begin to remove clotted blood and damaged tissues. Epithelial cells at the wound edges dissolve their bonds to each other, and by 1 to 2 days after injury, begin proliferating. Granulation tissue begins to invade the wound space approximately 4 days after injury. The fibroblast-rich granulation tissue establishes the matrix to support the migration of epithelial cells across the scar.[14] Angiogenesis begins within 2 to 3 days. During the second week of healing, fibroblasts are transformed into myofibroblasts, which aid in wound contraction.

The healing area gains 20% of its strength in the first 3 weeks. As time goes on, the tensile strength of a wound increases slowly as collagen accumulates and remodels. A fully healed wound, however, is only 70% as strong as uninjured skin.[9]

Many factors can slow the rate of healing, including hypoxia, ischemia, chronic shear forces, hyperthermia, infection, foreign bodies in the wound, use of anti-inflammatory medications, use of tobacco, poor nutrition (including deficiencies of vitamins A, B, C, and E; zinc; copper; calcium; methionine; proteins; and essential fatty acids), and metabolic diseases (such as diabetes) and other systemic disease.[15] Wound desiccation and eschar formation also are detrimental to healing.

The central nervous system and the cutaneous sensory nerves play a role in healing. Pain within the healing region provides protection for the healing wound. In addition, cutaneous sensory neurons secrete neuropeptides that actually modulate the healing process. Denervated tissue heals more slowly than enervated tissue.[16] Better blood supply facilitates more rapid healing. The mouth, anus, and genitals heal most quickly, followed by the head and trunk. Healing of the extremities is slowest.[17] Rewounding an injury causes acceleration of the healing process.[18]

Healing of skin injuries is faster in children than in adults. Human fetal tissue in the first 6 months of pregnancy heals perfectly, without scar formation.[19] Larger wounds require longer healing

time than smaller, less deep wounds, and crush injuries cause more devitalization of tissue than do shear injuries, thus delaying healing.[20] The compressive force of crush injuries delivers more energy to larger amounts of tissue, causing more tissue disruption and greater risk of infection.[21] A scar (cicatrix) results from the deposition of fibrous tissue in the healed wound. A hypertrophic scar is limited to the original wound margin. A keloid, conversely, results from collagen deposited beyond the margins of the original wound. Keloids form when fibroblasts are less responsive to tissue-modulating agents, resulting in excess collagen formation during the remodeling phase.[18] Keloids are more likely to form on darkly pigmented children and on certain areas of the body, including the earlobes, sternum, back, shoulder, and upper arm.[22]

Healing of Bruises

Bruises differ from other wounds because the skin itself remains intact. Bruises are the result of the rupture of blood vessels and seepage of blood into interstitial spaces. In addition, local inflammation and capillary dilation may add to the bright red color of a fresh bruise. As the blood cells and hemoglobin break down, the bruise exhibits a succession of colors, including red, violet, black, blue, yellow, green, and/or brown. However, there does not seem to be a predictable order or chronology of color progression.[23] One study of visible bruises concluded that a bruise with any yellow coloration must be older than 18 hours; the colors red, blue, purple, or black may appear in the bruise at any time from 1 hour of injury to resolution of the bruise; red can appear in the bruise at any time and does not predict age; and bruises of identical age and cause on the same person may not appear the same and may change colors at different rates.[24] In a recent review of peer-reviewed articles on the subject of bruise color and its relation to the age of the bruise, Maguire and colleagues[25] found only 3 articles out of 167 that fit their criteria for summarizing acceptable scientific evidence for bruise age determination. Timing of yellow bruising remained unclear in their review. They found that the accuracy of physician determination of the age of a bruise within 24 hours is less than 40%. In addition, interobserver and intra-observer reliability was poor. They concluded that the use of color to determine how old a bruise is should be avoided.

Many factors affect the rate of bruise resolution, including the amount of blood extravasated after the injury, the distance of the leakage of the blood from the skin surface, the amount of force applied and the amount of tissue damage incurred, the vascularity of the underlying tissue, the age of the person injured, and the underlying color of the injured person's skin.[26] Bruises are often less obviously noted on the skin of more darkly pigmented children.[27] The location of the bruise also can be a factor. Loosely attached skin, such as the skin around the eyes or genitals, will bruise more readily than skin that is under more tension. Drugs (eg, corticosteroids) can alter the rate of bruise dispersion. Aspirin or other anti-inflammatory drugs can increase susceptibility to bruising by platelet inhibition, and the bruised person's underlying clotting mechanisms can increase or decrease the size of the initial bruise that must be cleared.[26] Given the many variables involved, the aging of bruises is an inexact process requiring redundant caution and healthy skepticism.

Bruises in Abused and Non-Abused Children

There are 2 common characteristics separating abusive from non-abusive bruises: location and pattern. Bruises, lacerations, abrasions, and soft tissue swelling are commonly found in both abused and non-abused children. Table 1.1 summarizes several studies of skin injuries in non-abused children. The studies show that bruises are extremely uncommon in children younger than 6 months and increase in frequency as children become older and more adventurous. Bruising in normal children also relates to developmental stage (Table 1.2). Infants who do not pull to standing are highly unlikely to suffer bruises. Studies have shown that infants who do not yet "cruise" holding onto furniture are unlikely to be bruised.[27,30–32] The amount of bruising in toddlers increases as their motor skills increase.

The distribution of bruises on the body also differs by age and developmental stage, and abusive bruises have been found to be located on parts of the body where bruises are not found due to normal daily activities. Roberton et al[28] found injuries on the lower legs to be uncommon in children younger than 18 months. Head and face injuries were more common in 10- to 18-month-olds

TABLE 1.1
Studies of Skin Trauma in Normal Children by Age

Location	Study	Population	Lesions Studied	Age	% With Lesions
Health clinics (UK)	Roberton et al[28] (1982)	Normal children (N = 400)	Bruises and abrasions	2 wk–2 mo 3–9 mo 18 mo–11 y	3.3 0.1 50–65
Health clinics (UK)	Mortimer and Friedrich[29] (1983) N = 620	Normal children	Bruises	<1 y	0.9
Physician offices (USA)	Sugar et al[27] (1999) N = 930	Well-child visits	Bruises	0–2 mo 3–5 mo 6–8 mo 9–11 mo 12–14 mo 15–17 mo 18–23 mo 24–35 mo	0.04 0.7 5.6 19.3 22.6 42.8 49.4 60.9

TABLE 1.2
Studies of Skin Trauma in Normal Children by Developmental Stage

Location	Study	Population	Lesions Studied	Motor Development	% With Lesions
Hospital (UK)	Wedgwood[30] (1990) N = 24	Hospitalized children, not suspected of being abused	Bruises	Pre-cruisers Walk up stairs	0 100
Physician offices (USA)	Sugar et al[27] (1999) N = 930	Well-child visits	Bruises	Pre-cruisers Cruisers Walkers	2.2 17.8 51.9

and uncommon in children older than 4 years. Whereas fewer than 1% of children younger than 3 years had lumbar bruises, the lumbar areas of 14% of school-aged children were bruised (Table 1.3). Sugar et al[27] also found lower leg bruising to be common in children who could pull to standing or walk (Table 1.3). They found bruising to be rare on the hands, buttocks, cheek, nose, forearms, or chest of non-abused children. In their review of 167 published articles on this subject, Maguire et al[31] concluded that bruising in babies is uncommon; most bruises in walking children are small and occur over bony prominences, and on the front of the body. Abusive bruises tend to be away from bony prominences and involve the head, neck, and face, followed by the buttocks, trunk, and arms. Abusive bruises tend to be larger and multiple and occur in clusters, some carrying the imprint of an implement.

While facial injury has been shown to be uncommon in non-abused children, it is a frequent finding in abused children[33] (Box 1.1).

TABLE 1.3

Studies of Location of Skin Trauma in Normal Children by Developmental Stage or Age

Location	Study	Population	Location of Injury	Age or Stage of Motor Development	% With Lesions
Health clinics (UK)	Roberton et al[28] (1982)	Normal children N = 400	Lower leg	18 mo–3 y 3–11 y	>40.0 34.3
			Thigh and buttocks	<18 mo >18 mo	2.4 17.0
			Arms	<18 mo >18 mo	2.4 15.4
			Face and head	18 mo–3 y >3 y	16.6 <5.0
Health clinics (UK)	Mortimer and Friedrich[29] (1983) N = 620	Normal children	Face	<1 y	0.6
Physician offices (USA)	Sugar et al[27] (1999) N = 930	Well-child visits	Lower leg	Pre-cruiser Cruiser Walker	0.6 11.9 44.7
			Forehead	Pre-cruiser Cruiser Walker	0.6 3.0 5.7
			Scalp	Pre-cruiser Cruiser Walker	0.6 5.0 0.6
			Upper leg	Pre-cruiser Cruiser Walker	0.2 1.0 4.4

BOX 1.1

Comparison of Accidental and Inflicted Bruises by Location

Accidental	Inflicted
Shins	Upper arms
Lower arms	Upper anterior thighs
Under chin	Trunk
Forehead	Genitalia
Hips	Buttocks
Elbows	Face
Ankles	Ears
	Neck

Accidental bruises are very unlikely to occur in children who are not yet standing or walking. As children learn to walk and climb, they are more susceptible to injuries of all kinds, especially bruising. The distribution of bruises, however, tends to be different than that in abused children, with bruises to "exploratory surfaces" such as the lower legs being common, and bruises to the trunk less common.[34]

Variations of Bruises in Abused Children

Although many non-abused children will manifest injuries, certain patterns of injury have been recognized to be frequently caused by the abuse of children.

Pattern Marks

Injury inflicted with an object will often leave marks that reflect the outline of that object. The hand itself can leave a negative imprint, particularly on the face, when capillaries break between the fingers as blood is pushed away from the point of impact (Figure 1.1).[35] Cords, ropes, shoes, kitchen implements, and belt buckles can leave notable outlines on the skin (Figure 1.2).[36,37] Loop marks are generally worse at their extreme ends because the far end of the flexible cord travels at a faster rate of speed around the hand of the batterer.

Subgaleal Hematomas

Violently pulling on a child's hair can cause subgaleal hematomas (hemorrhage under the scalp).[38] The scalp is lifted off the calvarium at the aponeurotic junction. In addition to scalp swelling, traumatic alopecia (traumatic hair loss) can occur.[39] The hair loss is usually seen on the top of the head and is patchy. The underlying scalp can appear normal, or petechial bruising can be seen (Figure 1.3).

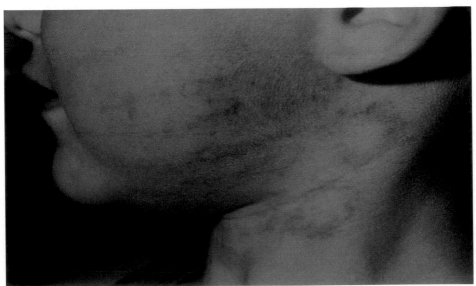

FIGURE 1.1
Inflicted handprint on the face of a child, leaving an outline of the fingers.

Petechiae on the Face and Neck Resulting From Strangulation

Conjunctival hemorrhages and facial and neck petechiae (masque ecchymotique) can result from compression of the chest and neck, causing increased venous pressure (Figure 1.4). In one case, the petechial eruption resulted from folding the child in half at the waist by applying pressure to the neck and buttocks.[40] Strangulation or suffocation by occlusion of the airway can cause similar lesions.

Bite Marks

Human bite marks are sometimes an abusive injury. They appear most frequently on the upper extremities.[41] The incisal edges of the mandibular teeth will be more clearly delineated than those of the maxillary teeth because as the upper and lower incisors meet through the tissues, the

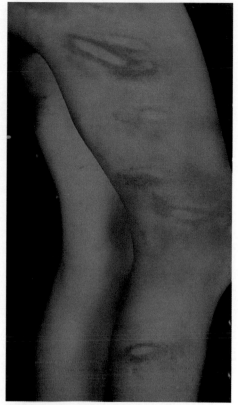

FIGURE 1.2
Inflicted pattern mark on a child's body.

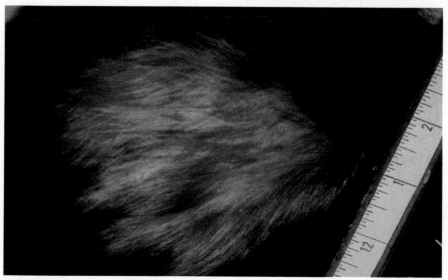

FIGURE 1.3
Traumatic alopecia.

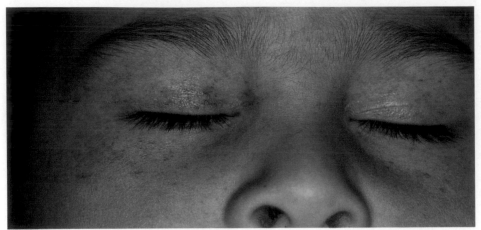

FIGURE 1.4
Facial petechiae caused by strangulation.

skin is often impacted by the lower incisor edges against the lingular surface of the upper teeth.[42] Bite marks should be carefully photographed with and without a size standard and swabbed with sterile water or saline to recover genetic markers left behind from saliva.

Purpura of the External Ear

Blows to the side of the head can cause purpuric or petechial hemorrhages to occur on the external ear, often in the interior folds of the ears.[43] Pulling or pinching the top of the ear leaves bruises on the helix or behind the pinna. If a blow sharply folds and crimps the pinna at the apex of the helix, petechiae can result.[44]

Vertical Bruises of the Gluteal Cleft

Blows to the buttocks can leave vertical marks at the junction where the buttocks curve into the gluteal cleft.[44]

Subungual Hematomas

Abusive biting of a child's fingers can cause chronic subungual hematomas. Leukonychia and swelling of the hands and feet also can be seen.[45] Hitting a child's fingers with an object might leave subungual hemorrhages as well.

Tattooing

Purposely disfiguring a child's skin by tattooing the skin with an ink-filled needle has been reported.[46]

Factitious Dermatitis (Dermatitis Artefactia)

Many different types of skin injuries can be purposefully inflicted on children by their caretakers to gain medical attention.[47,48] This factitious disorder by proxy often presents with chronic dermatitis or skin ulcers that heal poorly. They are more likely found on the face, chest, anterior surfaces of the legs, and dorsal surfaces of the arms. The condition resolves when the child is removed from the abuser.

Children who have been victims of abuse (especially sexual abuse) are more likely to inflict injuries on themselves, cutting or burning themselves to distract themselves from emotional pain.[49]

Air Rifles or Pellet Guns

These weapons are unregulated and readily available. They propel pellets at adequate velocities to penetrate human skin. A pellet-gun pellet has been reported to traverse the skin and lodge in the sagittal sinus in a purposefully inflicted injury to an infant.[50]

Skin Conditions That May Mimic Abuse

Many different pathologic conditions have been described as lesions confused with inflicted injury. Table 1.4 lists these lesions by type of wound. The more common conditions are described.

Dermal Melanosis (Mongolian Spots, Slate Gray Nevi)

These slate-blue or blue-green patches with indistinct borders are commonly seen in newborns. From 80% to 90% of African American infants, 75% of Asian infants, and 10% of white infants have dermal melanosis. They are most often found on the lumbosacral region, but can occur anywhere on the body. Most fade by age 5 years.[51] These lesions are uniformly the same blue-gray color from one side of the lesion to the other, and the absence of swelling and erythema helps differentiate dermal melanocytosis from bruising (Figure 1.5). Whereas bruises fade over a few weeks, mongolian spots remain unchanged during that time. Moreover, when asking parents when they first noticed these lesions they will usually say that they were there at birth, and some will know the name mongolian spots. Newborn records can help corroborate their presence at birth.

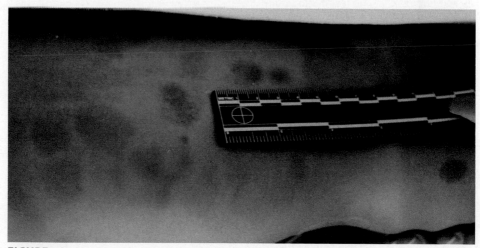

FIGURE 1.5
Child with extensive, dark mongolian spots (dermal melanosis) and many red, inflamed, inflicted bruises on her back.

TABLE 1.4

Skin Lesions Confused With Inflicted Injuries

Injury	Other Lesions Confused With Type of Injury	Reference
Bruises, ecchymoses, and petechiae	Dermal melanosis (mongolian spots)	51
	Chilblain (pernio)	52
	Bleeding disorders (leukemia, von Willebrand disease, idiopathic thrombocytopenic purpura, hemophilia)	53,54,55
	Henoch-Schönlein purpura	56,57
	Phytophotodermatitis	58,59
	Hemangiomas	60
	Maculae ceruleae (secondary to pediculosis)	61
	Cao gio (coin rolling)	62,63
	Cupping	62,63
	Quat sha (spooning)	63
	Erythema nodosum	64,
	Ink, paint, or dye to the body	65
	Hypersensitivity vasculitis	66
	Cystic lymphangiomas	
	Osteoma cutis (Albright hereditary osteodystrophy)	67
	Urticaria pigmentosa	68
	Popsicle panniculitis	69
	EMLA cream application	70
	Epidermal nevi	71
	Prominent facial veins	65
	Subconjunctival hemorrhages from pertussis	65
	Facial bruising from dental treatment	65
	Disseminated intravascular coagulation	66
	Meningococcemia	66
	Congenital indifference to pain	72
Contusions, hematomas, and ulcerated lesions	Erythema multiforme	73
	Erythema nodosum	64
	Angioedema	74
	Loxosceles reclusa (brown recluse spider) bite	75
	Calcium chloride necrosis	76
	Eczema	65
	Hemangiomas	60
	Hypersensitivity vasculitis	66
	Phytophotodermatitis	58,59
	Streptococcal toxic shock syndrome	77
	Chilblain (pernio)	52
	Postmortem insect bites	78
	Congenital indifference to pain	72
	Osteoma cutis (Albright hereditary osteodystrophy)	67
	Urticaria pigmentosa	68
Abusive scarring and lacerations	Striae	79
	Ehlers-Danlos syndrome	80
	Self-injurious behavior	49
	Epidermolysis bullosa	81
Traumatic alopecia	Loose anagen syndrome	39
	Trichotillomania	82
	Alopecia areata	65

TABLE 1.4
Skin Lesions Confused With Inflicted Injuries, *continued*

Injury	Other Lesions Confused With Type of Injury	Reference
Bite marks	Defibrillator injuries	83
Abusive tattoos	Religious tattoos associated with Afro-Caribbean religions such as Santeria and Palo Mayombe; cultural body ornamentation (Maori culture)	46 84
Intentional banding	Accidental banding of digits Ainhum (dactylosis spontanea)	85
Sexual abuse	Perianal streptococcal cellulitis and vaginal streptococcal infections	86
	Lichen sclerosus	87
	Hemangiomas	60
	Lymphangioma circumscriptum	88
	Chronic bullous disease of childhood	89
	Perianal Langerhans cell histiocytosis	90
	Crohn disease	90
	Lichen planus	90
	Hemolytic uremic syndrome	90
	Bullous pemphigoid	91

Chilblain (Pernio)

Chilblain occurs when tissues are exposed to wet, cold weather.[52] Bluish discoloration, erythema, and swelling occur, especially on the hands, feet, and face. Blistering or ulceration also can develop. Vasospasm induced by the cold leads to hypoxemia and localized inflammation of the tissues. "Popsicle pernio" occurs in some children secondary to holding popsicles in the corner of the mouth.

Bleeding Disorders

One study found that 16% of children evaluated for child abuse because of excessive bruising had a bleeding disorder.[55] The most common inherited bleeding disorder is von Willebrand disease, affecting about 1% of the population.[53] It is caused by a deficiency of the protein von Willebrand factor and a variable deficiency of factor VIII:C. In some cases, impaired platelet adhesiveness occurs. The severity of symptoms in patients with von Willebrand disease varies. Some patients are completely asymptomatic, whereas others experience epistaxis, gingival bleeding, severe postoperative bleeding, menorrhagia, and easy bruisability. Idiopathic thrombocytopenia purpura and the hemophilias also have been confused with child abuse.[54]

When extensive unexplained bruising occurs, particularly in the absence of associated injuries, bleeding disorders should be considered. A complete blood count with platelet count, an activated partial thromboplastin time, a prothrombin time, a bleeding time (in children >1 year), and levels of von Willebrand factor antigen and ristocetin cofactor are useful in screening for unrecognized bleeding disorders. In some cases, a fibrinogen level, thrombin time, clotting factor levels, and platelet kinetic studies may be helpful. Of note, patients with bleeding disorders should exhibit ongoing problems with bruising, rather than an isolated episode, although the severity of von Willebrand disease is known to wax and wane over time.

Henoch-Schönlein Purpura

Henoch-Schönlein purpura causes a non-thrombocytopenic purpuric rash that can be complicated by abdominal pain and bleeding, nephritis, and/or arthritis that can be confused with abusive injury.[56] The symmetrical rash tends to be more common over the buttocks and lower extremities, but can be found in other places as well, including the face or ears. The lesions can look like multiple bruises, especially early in the course of the disease. Patients often have a thrombocytosis and an elevated erythrocyte sedimentation rate. Lesions occur in crops over time.[57]

Phytophotodermatitis

Phytophotodermatitis is an acute phototoxic skin eruption occurring after contact with certain fruits or plants followed by sun exposure. The lesions often have bizarre configurations, making them appear to be inflicted burns or contusions (Figure 1.6).[58] As the lesions heal, they often become hyperpigmented and can mimic bruises. Citrus fruits and fruit juices, bergamot oil, figs, angelica, cow parsley, scurf pea, celery, wild parsnips, and rue are among the plants that can photosensitize the skin. Furocoumarins (psoralens) are the agents in the plants that cause the reaction.[59]

Hemangiomas

Hemangiomas can look like bruises and also can ulcerate. They are not always obvious at birth and can become obvious later in infancy. On the genitals, they can mimic sexual abuse–related trauma.[60]

Maculae Ceruleae

Flat, purpuric macules can be associated with pediculosis. They occur distant from the actual site of the lice infestation. The exact cause of the lesions is unknown. Although maculae ceruleae are more commonly seen on the body as a complication of pubic crab lice, they have been associated with head lice as well.[61]

Folk Remedies

Cao gio (coin rolling) is a Southeast Asian remedy for fever, chills, and headache. The back or chest is massaged with

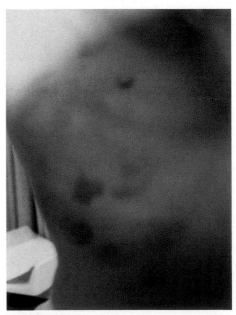

FIGURE 1.6
Phytophotodermatitis caused by exposure to lemon juice, mimicking inflicted injury.

mentholated oil and then vigorously rubbed with the edge of a coin until petechiae or purpura appear.[62] *Cupping* (glass leaching) is used by Mexican and Eastern European immigrants to treat a variety of ailments. Alcohol is ignited in a cup. The cup is then placed on the skin. As it cools, a round vacuum forms in the cup, causing an ecchymotic lesion to develop at the site. *Quat sha* (spooning) is a Chinese remedy used to relieve pain and headaches. Skin is scratched with a porcelain spoon until ecchymotic lesions appear.[63]

Erythema Multiforme

Erythema multiforme often presents with red skin blotches that then darken. The lesions resemble traumatic contusions and bruises. The lesions evolve into the classic target lesions with central clearing associated with the disease.[73]

Erythema Nodosum

Erythema nodosum presents as tender erythematous nodules that can evolve to bruise-like marks. It occurs most commonly on the lower limbs, and lesions can mimic trauma.[64]

Angioedema

Thakur and Kaplan[74] described in an infant a case of recurrent angioedema limited to the scalp and face. The diagnosis of trauma to the head and face was initially considered.

Loxosceles (Brown Recluse Spider) Bites

Loxosceles reclusa (brown recluse spiders) are widespread in the United States.[75] They commonly live in homes, barns, and garages, where they come in contact with humans. The bite itself is often painless, and the biting spider is rarely captured or identified. The bite becomes extremely painful and pruritic over 6 to 12 hours. The lesion enlarges and can develop into a significant necrotic ulcer. By day 6 or 7 an eschar develops over the lesion. Because the lesion is so dramatic and usually unexplained, it could be confused with an inflicted injury.

Calcium Chloride Necrosis

Exposure to calcium chloride can cause progressive, necrotic skin ulcers. A case was reported of a child who came into contact with calcium chloride used to melt ice on sidewalks, causing an initially unexplained necrotic ulcer.[76]

Striae

Physiological striae (stretch marks) are common and are sometimes found in adolescents who are growing rapidly. Striae in the lumbar area can occur horizontally across the back and hips, appearing to be linear inflicted pattern marks.[79] Over time they fade and take on a sclerotic appearance.

Ehlers-Danlos Syndrome

Ehlers-Danlos syndrome is an inherited disease caused by the production of defective collagen. Various types of the disease have been described, ranging from dramatic to subtle skin findings.[80] The defective collagen causes skin to be soft, friable, and easily traumatized. Injured skin heals with wide scars, appearing to have healed by secondary intention. Scars are thin and shiny (cigarette paper scars). Other findings include hyperextensible joints, history of premature rupture of membranes at birth, and ocular fragility. Late complications include heart valve defects, ruptured bowel, or aortic aneurysms. Ehlers-Danlos syndrome also has been reported to cause subdural bleeding.[92]

Loose Anagen Syndrome

Loose anagen syndrome is a genetic disease frequently causing abrupt, patchy hair loss.[39] There is a lack of cohesion between the hair root sheaths and the cuticle during the growth phase of the hair-growth cycle (anagen). Anagen hairs can be pulled out easily and painlessly. The affected hair has a characteristic microscopic appearance, with dystrophic roots, longitudinal groove, lack of root sheaths, and a ruffled cuticle. It is more commonly seen in young, fair-haired children.[82]

Ainhum (Dactylosis Spontanea)

This disease of tropical countries causes fibrous bands of tissue to encircle the toes and fingers, leading to autoamputation of the digit. It can be confused with intentional banding.[85]

Skin Conditions Confused With Sexual Abuse (See also Chapter 7)

Streptococcus pyogenes infections can cause erythema of the anus and vagina, as well as vaginal and anal discharge, anal fissuring, pain on defecation, and blood-streaked stools, simulating sexual abuse injuries.[86] Lichen sclerosus, a skin disease, causes subepidermal bleeding around the genitals and anus that can be confused with genital and anal bruising.[87] Perianal lymphangioma circumscriptum (dilated lymph channels formed from maldeveloped, sequestered lymphatic sacs) are difficult to distinguish from perianal condylomata.[88] Other conditions confused with child abuse–related skin diseases are listed in Table 1.5.

Burns

The term *burn* is used to describe a variety of physical and chemical insults to tissue, including thermal, electrical, chemical, and radiation. Although the injuries caused by these insults can appear quite similar, their molecular basis and biological consequences are quite different. They all can lead to tissue inflammation.

Thermal burns cause damage by coagulating tissue proteins. As temperature rises, the number of molecular collisions and the transferred molecular momentum increase in tissues. The transmitted energy deforms proteins and other macromolecules, causing denaturation and structural breakdown. The cell membrane is the most vulnerable component of the cell to heat damage.[93]

Damage from electrical burns is not actually mediated by the heat generated by supraphysiological electrical currents alone. Whereas the passage of electrical current produces damage by the generation of Joule heating effects, additional damage results from the direct action of electrical forces on electrically charged or polarized molecules in tissues. Both mechanisms lead to alteration of molecular conformation and disruption of macromolecular structures. Although thermal forces are random in direction, electric forces produce vectorial electrical coupling in tissues. These vectorial forces can cause changes in protein conformation.[94]

Electrical burns cause damage to tissues above the macromolecular level. The bilayer cell membrane acts as an insulating shell for the intracellular contents. As electrical field strengths outside the cell increase, the cell membrane can no longer maintain its integrity, and electroporation occurs. Structural defects, or pores, are formed in the membrane, which makes it permeable to ions and molecules, leading to cellular breakdown. In thermal injury, all components of cells are damaged, whereas in electrical injuries, only the cell membrane is damaged.[94]

Radiation injuries also are called burns, but heating has no role in the tissue damage caused by ionizing radiation.[94] Ionizing particle beams and electromagnetic irradiation alter atomic structures, which mediate damaging chemical reactions in tissues. The most common radiation burn is caused by excessive ultraviolet (UV) light exposure (sunburn). Ionizing UV light penetrates only the most superficial layers of the epidermis. High-frequency ionizing radiation (x-rays or gamma rays) can penetrate the entire body. High-energy irradiation causes damage to proteins, polysaccharides, nucleic acids, and lipids.

Chemicals (acids and alkalis) can cause direct tissue damage by chemically altering the extracellular matrix, cellular membranes, and intracellular structures and molecules. In addition, chemical reactions are exothermic or endothermic and can result in damaging changes in tissue temperature.

All of these mechanisms (thermal burns, electrical burns, radiation injury, and chemical burns) have in common the disruption of cell membranes and the loss of their barrier functions. In addition, cold injury and barotrauma disrupt cell membrane integrity.[93] Whereas the biochemical denaturation caused by heat and chemical burns is usually obvious to the observer, the physicochemical effects of ionizing radiation and electricity may not be observable, even though tissue damage has occurred.[94]

Evaluating Thermal Burns

The severity of a thermal burn depends on many factors, including the thickness of the skin, temperature of the burning agent, length of time the agent contacted the skin, and heat-dissipating capacity of the burned tissue (the tissue blood flow). Skin thickness varies with the age and gender of the individual, as well as by the location of the tissue on the body. A scald burn in an infant will be more severe than the identical burn inflicted on an adult.[95] Infant skin in many parts of the body is less than half as thick as adult skin.[96] Skin thickness reaches adult levels by age 5 years. The dermis is thickest on the palms and soles, whereas that of the eyelids and genitals is the thinnest.

Heat is most effectively removed from tissues by vascular perfusion. If the burn wound is poorly perfused, the heat affects the tissues for a longer period. In addition, if shock and hypotension occur after a burn, potentially viable tissue may die. Infection is more likely to become established, and the burn depth increases. In abusive burns, a delay in seeking care can turn a more superficial burn into a deeper, more serious burn by delaying fluid resuscitation and pain and infection control. Tissue burns are dynamic, and a burn that appears shallow initially can worsen with time, and later appear to be a deep burn.

Early experimental work determined burn tolerances in adult tissues.[97] At 44°C (111.2°F), 6 hours is required to cause a superficial epidermal burn. For each degree centigrade above 44°C, and up to 51°C (123.8°F), the time required to produce a burn of given depth decreases by approximately one half. Infants and young children can sustain partial- and full-thickness burns after 10 seconds of exposure at 54.4°C (130°F), 4 seconds at 57°C (135°F), 1 second at 60°C (140°F), and 0.5 seconds at 64.9°C (149°F).[98] Thus very transient exposures to high temperatures can cause serious burns.

Superficial epidermal burns cause redness of tissues without blister formation. They heal quickly and spontaneously. Superficial dermal burns include only the upper layers of the papillary dermis. They often form blisters at the interface of the dermis and epidermis. The wound is pink and hypersensitive once blisters are removed. These burns heal completely within a few weeks. Charred, full-thickness burns are leathery, firm, and insensitive to touch. They often appear white and dry. Non-charred full-thickness burns are more difficult to evaluate. They may be mottled and dry, and sometimes clotted vessels are visible. Full-thickness scald burns may be red in appearance and can be confused with partial-thickness burns, although capillary refill is not demonstrated.[96]

When deaths occur from flame burns, several mechanisms may be at work. Often the death itself is caused by the inhalation of soot or poisonous gases or from heat exposure, and actual tissue burns occur after death. Physical injuries can occur when buildings collapse on the victims before or after death. Burns occurring after death will not show vital reaction. Skin and soft tissues can contract and split, causing lesions that resemble incised wounds. Muscle proteins contract and coagulate, causing rigid flexion of the extremities (a pugilistic attitude) resembling attempts at self-protection. Spontaneous bony fractures can occur in desiccated bones, including skull fractures. Extradural hemorrhage can occur as brain tissue contracts from the heat, causing hemorrhage that resembles traumatic injury.[99]

Epidemiology of Inflicted Burns in Children

Reported proportions of inflicted burns in all children with burns vary greatly, depending on the study sample and diagnostic criteria used for abuse. Table 1.5 reviews several studies determining the proportion of abusive or neglectful burns in children. Abusive burns have been found to be more common in younger children[100–105] and in children from single-parent families.[55,100,102,103,105] Abuse-related burns are generally more serious and more likely to require excision and grafting, be full-thickness burns,[103,104,106] and have longer hospital stays than accidental burns.[102] Parents of abused burned children are more likely to be poor and unemployed than are parents of non-abused children with burns.[100,102] Two studies found that children who were small for their ages using standardized growth charts were at increased risk of abusive burns.[107,108] Ninety-five percent of tap-water scalds occur in the home.[109] In the United States, burns from tap water are the most common form of abusive burns,[103,104] and the most common form of all burns,[110] whereas in Africa, flame burns and burns with hot objects are the most common forms of abusive burns.[111]

Healing of Burns

Burns that heal within 3 weeks generally leave no scars or functional impairment. More serious burns require early excision and grafting.[96] Many of the physiological, immunologic, and biochemical processes involved in healing burns are the same as those found in other skin injuries, with some essential differences. First, a full-thickness burn actually forms an eschar of coagulated tissue rather than a scab or crust of clotted blood. Surrounding this zone of necrosis is a zone of stasis, where impaired blood supply is caused by leukocytes sticking to damaged capillary endothelium. Around this zone is a zone of increased blood flow (hyperemia). Important in burn healing, if deep skin structures are preserved (glands and hair follicles), epithelial migration can occur from these structures as well as from the wound edges.[116]

TABLE 1.5
Proportion of Burns Caused by Abuse or Neglect

Location	Population	Burns Caused by Abuse and/or Neglect	Reference
Detroit, MI	431 emergency department patients	19.5% abuse or neglect	105
San Francisco, CA	60 inpatients	25% abuse or neglect	103
Cincinnati, OH	1,203 inpatients	4.3% abuse	102
Chicago, IL	321 inpatients	24.6% abuse or neglect	100
Dallas, TX	678 inpatients	10.5% abuse	104
Plymouth, UK	269 inpatients	<1% abuse	112
Seattle, WA	56 inpatients admitted for tap-water scalds	28.6% abuse	106
Columbus, OH	872 inpatients	16% abuse	101
Columbus, OH	139 inpatients and outpatients	10% abuse	113
Sydney, Australia	507 inpatients	8% abuse or neglect	114
Miami, FL	47 inpatients	12% abuse	115

Systemic responses to serious burns include diffuse tissue edema (probably caused by cytokines and growth factors spilling over into the circulatory system) and a generalized, hypermetabolic inflammatory response causing fever and hyperdynamic circulation. If large areas of skin are burned, severe fluid and electrolyte disturbances can occur from dehydration and protein loss. After extensive burns, the body's immune system also is impaired, increasing the risk of serious infection.[117] Not only is the body's skin barrier to microbial invaders broken down, but actual immune suppression occurs, decreasing the body's ability to fight infection.[118]

Children who sustain abusive burns are at risk for long-term emotional problems.[119,120] Some researchers have hypothesized that families with severe emotional problems are more likely to have a child sustain a serious burn than are other families.[121,122] The preexisting and complicating emotional problems of abusively burned children complicate their management in the burn unit and in long-term rehabilitation.[123,124] Abusive burns and genital and buttocks burns in children are more likely to be complicated by depression than are other types of burns.[125]

Certain characteristics are considered to be more likely to indicate an abusive burn rather than an accidental burn. Table 1.6 reviews the common patterns thought to be associated with abusive burns. In some of these studies, abusive burns were diagnosed based on the presence of these factors.

Variations of Burn Injuries in Abused Children

Similar to lacerations and abrasions, some patterns of burns are highly correlated with abuse. This section reviews burns more commonly seen as abusive rather than accidental.

Scald Burns

Accidental Scald Burns

Children who accidentally pull hot liquids down onto themselves will usually scald the anterior face and head, neck, palmar surfaces of the hand, arms, and anterior shoulder and chest. The burns generally become less intense as the liquid runs down the body and dissipates heat.[98,104] Oily or viscous substances can cause full-thickness burns because they stick to the body and hold heat for longer periods.

The fragile skin of infants and young children can be accidentally burned by bathing the child in hot water. Mirowski et al[127] reported a case of a newborn bathed in a hospital nursery where the hot water temperature from the nursery faucet was between 56°C (132.8°F) and 59°C (138.2°F). The newborn sustained superficial partial-thickness burns. As part of the case report, they asked nursery nurses to estimate appropriate water temperature for bathing babies using an ungloved hand or brief immersion of the elbow. On days when the water temperature in the nursery was higher, the nurses' estimates of correct temperature for bathing babies was also higher. The authors speculated that because of repeated hand washing, the nurses became accustomed to higher

TABLE 1.6
Case Characteristics Attributed to Burns Caused by Abuse

Characteristic	References
Historic Factors	
Discrepant history	114,126,115,101,105
Burn incompatible with developmental age of child	114,126,115,101,112,105
Vague, inconsistent history	114,126,115,101,112,105
Unwitnessed burn	101,105
Denial that lesion is a burn	105
Speculative account of what occurred	112,105
Burn attributed to sibling or babysitter not present at time of presentation	114,126,115,101,112,105
Child contradicts history	114,105
Burn Patterns	
Cigarette burn	105
Iron or radiator grill	105
Stocking- or glove-pattern burn	114,105
Mirror-image burns of the extremities	126,115,101,105
Symmetric burns on buttocks	105
Sparing of flexor creases	105
Burns of posterior head, chest, neck, or extremities	105
Burns localized to perineum, genitalia, or buttocks	114,115,101,112,103,104,105
Absence of splash marks in immersion burn	114,105
Crisp margins of burned surface	114,105
Central sparing on buttocks and perineum (doughnut appearance)	114,104,105
Deep scald with running water appearance	105
Multiple burn sites	105
Other Factors	
Unexplained delay in seeking care	114,106,115,101,112,103,105
Associated or previous injuries	114,126,115,101,112,105
Previous burns or evidence of previous abuse or neglect	105
Inappropriate level of concern by (affect of) caretakers	114,126,115,101,105
Child excessively withdrawn, submissive, or fearful	114,115,101,112,105
Malnourished child	114,105
Child left with inappropriately young caretaker	105
Unkempt, dirty child	114,105
Inappropriate behavior of caretaker (drunk, impaired, euphoric, depressed)	112,105
Parents do not accompany child to hospital	114,106,115,101,112
Patient is male	106
Adult in the room when victim is scalded	106

temperatures. Higher estimates also were associated with nurses who held their hand or elbow in the bath for less than 10 seconds. The authors recommended that a thermometer be used to measure water temperature before babies are bathed. The correct temperature for infant bathwater is between 36°C (96.8°F) and 39°C (102.2°F).

Burns sustained in the kitchen are more likely to be accidental. Drago[128] found 704 case reports of kitchen scalds that had been filed with the US Consumer Product Safety Commission (CPSC) from emergency departments (EDs) from January 1, 1997, to December 31, 2002. Two thirds of these cases were scalds and one third were thermal. Approximately half of the cases involved a child pulling a pot onto himself. In another one quarter of the cases, the pot contents splashed onto the child. In 8%, the child collided with the person carrying the pot of hot liquid. Hot water was the burning agent in 49%, grease in 20%, soups in 13%, food in 12%, and hot drinks in 4%. Titus et al[129] reported on three 18-month-old children with bilateral lower extremity burns where the history was that the toddlers had climbed into the bathroom sink and turned on the hot water. The burns were symmetrical, with irregular depth and margins, not a stocking appearance. Scene examinations showed that there were climbing aids to the sinks and that these children were developmentally able to climb into the sinks. Measurement of the water temperature showed a very high temperature that was consistent with burns within one half to 1 second. A child protection team was consulted and concluded that the burns were accidental.[129] Accidental scald burns are rarely full-thickness burns,[101] and the burn margins are more likely to be irregular and asymmetrical.[130]

To determine the developmental capabilities of young children to get into and out of a bathtub, Allasio and Fischer[131] placed a 15-inch high bathtub in an outpatient clinic. One hundred seventy-six children, ranging in age from 10 to 18 months, were placed standing holding onto the tub. Thirty-five percent of these children got into the tub, and as expected the older ones did better in getting in than the younger ones. The biggest jump in ability came between 13 and 14 months. Seventy-three percent got in leg first and 27% headfirst.

Abusive Scald Burns

Immersion scald burns are the most common inflicted burns and are usually the easiest to diagnose. These burns usually involve the lower trunk, buttocks, perineum, arms, and legs. They can appear as stocking or glove burns involving the feet and hands. Abusive burns are more likely to have a clear demarcation between burned and normal skin and to have an absence of splash marks[108,98] (Figure 1.7). Sometimes sparing of the buttocks and soles of the feet is seen if the child's body is pushed down against the cooler surface of the tub or sink. The flexor creases also may be spared, reflecting the body's flexed position in the hot water.[132] In accidental scald burns, the child is less likely to have a clear tide mark at the top of the burn.

Daria and colleagues[133] reviewed the records of 195 cases of scald burns in children younger than 5 years in a multicenter study. Five percent of these (9/195) were inflicted burns. Six children ranging in age from 5 weeks to 5 years had been plunged headfirst into hot water, resulting in scald burns to the head. Three of the children died. In a study of perineal burns, Angel et al[134] reported on 78 children who were between the ages of 3 months and 17 years with second-degree or worse burns of perineum or genitals, usually in context of a more extensive burn. Isolated genital and perineal burns were seen only in 3.8% of accidental burns. In these cases, 64% were hot liquid scalds, 30% caused by flames, 4% contact, and 2.6% electrical. Forty-eight percent of the girls and 46% of the boys younger than 2 years had scald burns to the perineum or genitalia that were due to child abuse, as determined by a child protection team. The team concurred with the recommendation that there should be a child abuse investigation when any child younger than 2 years has isolated burns to the perineum or genitals. As a cautionary note, however, there have been at least 2 reports linking laxative use, especially laxatives with senna content, to severe diaper dermatitis secondary to acidic diarrhea and breakdown of skin of the diaper area.[135,136]

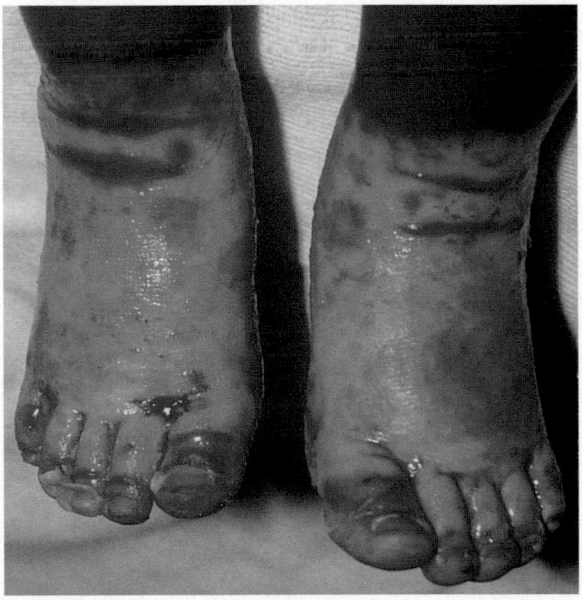

Cigarette Burns

Inflicted cigarette burns are circular, uniform-sized, deep burns ranging from 0.75 to 1.0 cm in diameter. They are often grouped, and often found on the hands and feet.[137] Accidental contact with cigarettes usually causes brushed lesions, which appear ovoid, and causes superficial burns instead of deep burns.

Hair Dryer and Other Appliance Burns

Hair dryers can reach very high temperatures in a short time. In one study, the metal grids of hair dyers remained at temperatures above 68°C for up to 2 minutes after the dryers were turned off.[138] In normal use, a hair dryer is in constant motion to avoid hot spots. When a hair dryer or other appliance is held on the skin, deep pattern burns can result in just a few seconds (Figure 1.8)

During a 5-year period between 1992 and 1996, reports to the CPSC from EDs allowed Qazi et el[139] to project an incidence of 82,151 curling iron injuries during the 5 study years. The median age at injury was 8 years. In the group of children younger than 4 years, 56% of the incidents occurred when the child grabbed the hot iron, 14% pulled on the cord, and 30% had unintentional contact with the

FIGURE 1.7
Immersion burn of the extremities.

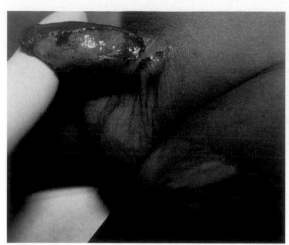

FIGURE 1.8
Burn inflicted with a curling iron.

curling iron. Fifty-eight percent of the younger children had hand and finger burns, while the older children had more ocular burns. No abuse was described in the article.

Domestic irons are another source of burns in children. Gaffney[140] described burns in 62 children secondary to irons over a 36-month period in an ED. Sixty had contact burns, 2 were due to scalds. Boys were twice as likely to be victims, as were children younger than 2 years. Fifty-five percent of the children were younger than 2 years; 63% had burns on the hands. Burns were linear or triangular in pattern. Irons had been left on the floor or on low surfaces or iron electrical cords were left dangling. Nine of these cases were considered abusive, with multiple injuries, burns to the face or dorsal hand injuries, delays in seeking care, and discrepant history being the determinants.[140]

Stun Gun Injuries

Stun guns administer an electric shock with a high-voltage, low-amperage impulse, causing the victim to experience muscular tetany, numbness, confusion, and loss of balance. With a longer administration of current, the victim can be paralyzed for up to 15 minutes.[141] The characteristic lesion resulting from a stun gun injury is a pair of superficial, symmetrical, circular burns about 0.5 cm in diameter, located about 5 cm apart. Two additional marks may be seen between the round lesions if the recessed spark-gap pins contact the skin.[137]

Microwave Oven Burns

Inflicted microwave oven burns to young infants have been reported.[142] Microwave radiation spans the electromagnetic spectrum between radiofrequencies and infrared light. Microwaves cause tissue destruction by dielectric heating of tissues. Water molecules act as dipoles and oscillate rapidly in a microwave field, causing heat by molecular agitation.[94] Tissues with high water content will be more affected by microwave heating than will those with low water content. Microwave burns typically show damage to skin and muscle layers, sparing the fatty tissue layers.

Burns Secondary to Supervisory Neglect

House Fires

Many house-fire burns are associated with a lack of adequate smoke detectors. Children and the elderly are particularly vulnerable in house fires. Children can die in house fires resulting from their own unsupervised play, being left home alone, in fires deliberately set by adults, and in fires caused by negligence because of drug or alcohol use by an adult.[143] Smoking-related fires are often linked to alcohol use by the smoker.

Walker-Related Burns

Infants in walkers are upright and have increased access to surfaces. Burns have been reported from infants pulling down hot liquids or objects onto themselves when they are in walkers. These burns often resemble hot liquid splash burns.[144]

Electrical Burns and Electrocution

Electrical burns and electrocution injuries have not been described in the literature as a mechanism of child abuse. However, when unexplained death or loss of consciousness occurs, electrocution should be considered as a possible cause of injury. Signs of electrocution and electrical burns may be quite subtle. Skin lesions can be inconspicuous or completely absent. The hands are the most common sites of lesions. A thermal blister can be present if the hand actually touched the current source. With intermittent contact or if an arc forms between the hand and current source, a spark burn will occur, with a central core of coagulated keratin surrounded by a blanched halo. With high-voltage burns, multiple spark lesions can be seen, causing crocodile skin.[145] Exit wounds can be seen on the foot. Death occurs secondary to thermal injury to organs, electrical shock to the heart or brain, or paralysis of the respiratory muscles, depending on the nature of the current and location of contact.[94]

Skin Conditions Confused With Abusive Burns

Many different pathologic conditions have been described as lesions confused with inflicted burns. Table 1.7 lists these lesions by type of burn. The more common conditions are described.

Accidental Contact Burns

Accidental contact with hot objects can leave burns on children. These burns usually have indistinct margins and do not occur in multiples. They are unlikely to occur on parts of the body that are normally clothed.

Accidental home radiator burns also have been found to be more frequent in houses served by steam radiators versus hot-water radiators.[156] Steam radiators operate at 82°C (179.6°F) to 109°C (228.2°F), whereas hot-water radiators operate at about 49°C (120.2°F). The difference in temperature means that very brief contact with steam radiators can cause serious burns.

Innocent Pressure Injuries

Pressure injuries to infant skin can be confused with dry contact burns. Feldman[151] described 4 cases in which patterned lesions in parallel lines with

TABLE 1.7
Skin Lesions Confused With Inflicted Burns

Type of Burn	Other Lesions Confused With Type of Burn	Reference
Circular or patterned burns	Enuresis blanket burn	146
	Moxibustion	62,63
	Maquas	63
	Garlic burns	147
	Therapeutic burns for convulsions by African healers	111,148
	Accidental contact burns	137
	Dermatitis herpetiformis	81
	Impetigo and bullous impetigo	149,84,65
	Phytophotodermatitis	59
	Fixed drug eruption	65
	Varicella	137
	Guttate psoriasis	137
	Pityriasis lichenoides	137
Other burns	Congenital indifference to pain	72
	Epidermolysis bullosa	81
	Staphylococcal scalded skin syndrome	149
	Allergic contact lesions	150
	Innocent pressure injuries	151
	Car safety seat burns	152
	Chemical burns from home remedies	153
	Dishwasher effluent burns	154
	Accidental scald burns	106
	Chilblain	52,65
	Sunburn	155

sharply demarcated edges were caused by ischemia from pressure of objects on the skin. These lesions resembled burns.

Staphylococcal Toxin Syndromes

Infections with *Staphylococcus aureus* can release toxins that affect the desmosomes holding epidermal cells together, causing bullous lesions or areas of red, denuded skin (staphylococcal scalded skin syndrome and bullous impetigo). These lesions can be confused with burns (Figure 1.9).[149,84]

Car Seat Burns

Car seats left in hot cars can reach high temperatures on warm days. When infants' and toddlers' skin contacts the

hot upholstery or buckles, pattern marks can result (Figure 1.10).[153]

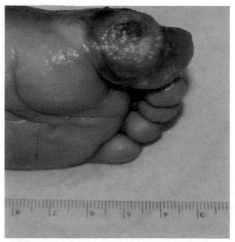

FIGURE 1.9
Bullous impetigo resembling a burn.

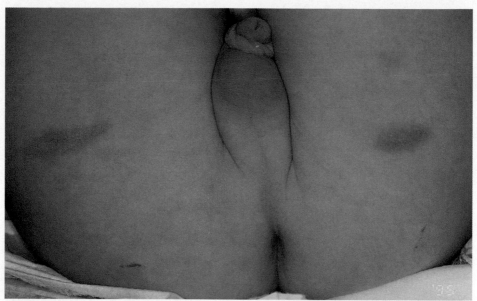

FIGURE 1.10
Accidental car safety seat burn.

Enuresis Blanket Marks

Circular scars from enuresis blankets have been reported. The marks are linear and 0.4 to 0.6 cm in diameter. They occur on the same side of the body.[146]

Folk Remedies

Moxibustion is a variant of acupuncture. The moxa herb (*Artemisia vulgaris)* is burned on the skin with a piece of yarn, incense, or even with a cigarette to draw out illness.[62] The burns appear as circular full- or partial-thickness burns. Bedouins, Arabs, Druses, Russians, and Oriental Jews use the folk remedy *Maquas,* deep burns caused by hot metal spits, to cure illness.[63] The belief is that when pus oozes from the burn, the disease drains out. Garlic is sometimes used as a remedy for infections. Garty[147] reported an infant with partial-thickness chemical burns of the wrist caused by the caustic effect of garlic taped to the wrist to treat fever. Other home remedies can cause chemical burns, such as topical methyl salicylate for sprains.[153] In some African countries, burning of the skin is an accepted treatment for convulsions.[111,148]

Postmortem Insect Bites

Insect bites can be confused with burns or abrasions. Cockroaches (*Dictyoptera blattaria)* are notorious for scavenging bodies, particularly after death. They bite hands, toes, eyelashes, and areas of the skin with thin epidermis such as the face and ears. The bites are small and well circumscribed, but irregular. They can sometimes be inflicted in a row. Smaller bites can coalesce into larger lesions.[78]

Conclusion

The cutaneous manifestations of abuse are varied and often nonspecific. Careful consideration by the practitioner, including the medical history, physical examination, and psychosocial context, is necessary to diagnose child abuse accurately.

References

1. US Department of Health and Human Services, Administration on Children, Youth and Families. *Child Maltreatment 2004.* Washington, DC: US Government Printing Office; 2006. http://www.ACF.DHHS.GOV/PROGRAMS/CB/PUBS/CM04. Accessed April 30, 2007
2. Trocme N, MacMillan H, Fallon B, De Marco R. Nature and severity of physical harm caused by child abuse and neglect: results from the Canadian Incidence Study. *Can Med Assoc J.* 2003;169:911–915
3. Johnson CF, Showers J. Injury variables in child abuse. *Child Abuse Negl.* 1985;9:207–215
4. Johnson CF. Inflicted injury versus accidental injury. *Pediatr Clin North Am.* 1990;37:791–814
5. Wilkes GL, Brown IA, Wildnauer RH. The biomechanical properties of skin. *CRC Crit Rev Bioeng.* 1973;1:453–495
6. Smith KL, Dean SJ. Tissue repair of the epidermis and dermis. *J Hand Ther.* 1998;11:95–104
7. Fuchs E. Keratins and the skin. *Annu Rev Cell Dev Biol.* 1995;11:123–153
8. Ryan TJ. Mechanical resilience of skin: a function of blood supply and lymphatic drainage. *Clin Dermatol.* 1995;13:429–432
9. Bernstein G. Healing by secondary intention. *Dermatol Clin.* 1989;7:645–660
10. Edward C, Marks R. Evaluation of biomechanical properties of human skin. *Clin Dermatol.* 1995;13:375–380
11. Kollias N. The physical basis of skin color and its evaluation. *Clin Dermatol.* 1995;13:361–367
12. DiMaio DJ, DiMaio VJ. *Forensic Pathology.* New York, NY: Elsevier; 1989:87–88
13. Evans RC, Jones NL. The management of abrasions and bruises. *J Wound Care.* 1996;5:465–468
14. Singer AJ, Clark RAF. Mechanism of disease: cutaneous wound healing. *N Engl J Med.* 1999;341:738–746
15. Stadelmann WK, Digenis AG, Tobin GR. Impediments to would healing. *Am J Surg.* 1998;176(2A suppl):39S–47S
16. Ansel JC, Kaynard AH, Armstrong CA, et al. Skin-nervous system interactions. *J Invest Dermatol.* 1996;106:198–204
17. Rowell LB. Reflex control of the cutaneous vasculature. *J Invest Dermatol.* 1977;69:154–166
18. Cohen BH, Lewis LA, Resnik SS. Wound healing: a brief review. *Int J Dermatol.* 1975;14:722–726
19. Martin P. Wound healing—aiming for perfect skin regeneration. *Science.* 1997;276:75–81
20. Hollander JE, Singer AJ. Laceration management. *Ann Emerg Med.* 1999;34:356–367
21. Cardany CR, Rodeheaver G, Taacker J, et al. The crush injury: a high risk wound. *J Am Coll Emerg Physicians.* 1976;5:965–970
22. Laude TA. Approach to dermatologic disorders in black children. *Semin Dermatol.* 1995;14:15–20
23. Schwartz AJ, Ricci LR. How accurately can bruises be aged in abused children? Literature review and synthesis. *Pediatrics.* 1996;97:254–257
24. Langlois NEI, Bresham GA. The aging of bruises: a review and study of the color changes with time. *Forensic Sci Int.* 1991;50:227–238
25. Maguire S, Mann MK, Sibert J, Kemp A. Can you age bruises accurately in children? A systematic review. *Arch Dis Child.* 2005;90:187–189
26. Stephenson T. Aging of bruising in children. *J R Soc Med.* 1997;90:312–314
27. Sugar NF, Taylor JA, Feldman KW. Bruises in infants and toddlers. *Arch Pediatr Adolesc Med.* 1999;153:399–403

28. Roberton DM, Barbor P, Hull D. Unusual injury? Recent injury in normal children and children with suspected non-accidental injury. *Br Med J.* 1982;285:1399–1401

29. Mortimer PE, Friedrich M. Are facial bruises in babies ever accidental? *Arch Dis Child.* 1983;58:75–76

30. Wedgwood J. Childhood bruising. *Practitioner.* 1990;8:598–601

31. Maguire S, Mann MK, Sibert J, Kemp A. Are there patterns of bruising in childhood which are diagnostic or suggestive of abuse? A systematic review. *Arch Dis Child.* 2005;90:182–186

32. Labbe J, Caouette G. Recent skin injuries in normal children. *Pediatrics.* 2001;108:271–276

33. McMahon P, Grossman W, Gaffney M, et al. Soft-tissue injury as an indication of child abuse. *J Bone Joint Surg Am.* 1995;77:1179–1183

34. Ellerstein NS. The cutaneous manifestations of child abuse and neglect. *Am J Dis Child.* 1979;133:906–909

35. Raimer BG, Raimer SS, Hebeler JR. Cutaneous signs of child abuse. *J Am Acad Dermatol.* 1981;5:203–214

36. Showers J, Bandman RL. Scarring for life: abuse with electric cords. *Child Abuse Negl.* 1986;10:25–31

37. Solomon BA, Laude TA. A peculiar annular eruption in a child with AIDS. *J Am Acad Dermatol.* 1995;33:513–514

38. Hamlin H. Subgaleal hematoma caused by hair-pull. *JAMA.* 1968;204:129

39. Whiting DA. Traumatic alopecia. *Int J Dermatol.* 1999;38(suppl 1):34–44

40. Perrot J. Masque ecchymotique: specific or nonspecific indicator for abuse. *Am J Forensic Med Pathol.* 1989;10:95–97

41. Vale GL, Noguchi TT. Anatomical distribution of human bite marks in a series of 67 cases. *J Forensic Sci.* 1983;28:61–69

42. Sperber ND. Bite marks, oral and facial injuries: harbingers of severe child abuse? *Pediatrician.* 1989;16:207–211

43. Hanigan WC, Peterson RA, Njus G. Tin ear syndrome: rotational acceleration in pediatric head injuries. *Pediatrics.* 1987;80:618–622

44. Feldman KW. Patterned abusive bruises of the buttocks and pinnae. *Pediatrics.* 1992;90:633–636

45. Gavin LA, Lanz MJ, Leung DY, et al. Chronic subungual hematomas: a presumed immunologic puzzle resolved with a diagnosis of child abuse. *Arch Pediatr Adolesc Med.* 1997;151:103–105

46. Johnson CF. Symbolic scarring and tattooing. *Clin Pediatr.* 1994;33:46–49

47. Jones DP. Dermatitis artefactia in mother and baby as child abuse. *Br J Psychiatry.* 1983;143:199–200

48. Stankler L. Factitious skin lesions in a mother and two sons. *Br J Dermatol.* 1977;97:217–219

49. Gupta MA, Gupta AK. Dermatitis artefacta and sexual abuse. *Int J Dermatol.* 1993;32:825–826

50. Campbell-Hewson GL, D'Amore A, Busuttil A. Non-accidental injury inflicted on a child with an air weapon. *Med Sci Law.* 1998;38:173–176

51. Cordova A. The mongolian spot. *Clin Pediatr.* 1981;20:714–722

52. Giusti R, Tunnessen WW. Picture of the month. *Arch Pediatr Adolesc Med.* 1997;151:1055–1056

53. Falaki NN. Case 3 presentation of facial bruises. *Pediatr Rev.* 1998;19:247–248

54. Johnson CF. Bruising or hemophilia: accident or abuse? *Child Abuse Negl.* 1988;12:409–415

55. O'Hare AE, Eden OB. Bleeding disorders and non-accidental injury. *Arch Dis Child.* 1984;50:860–864

56. Brown J, Melinkovich P. Schönlein-Henoch purpura misdiagnosed as suspected child abuse. *JAMA.* 1986;256:617–618

57. Lanzkowsky S, Lanzkowsky L, Lanzkowsky P. Henoch-Schöenlein purpura. *Pediatr Rev.* 1992;13:130–137

58. Goskowicz MO, Friendlander SF, Eichenfield LF. Endemic "lime" disease: phytophotodermatitis in San Diego County. *Pediatrics.* 1994;93:828–830

59. Hill PF, Pickford M, Parkhouse N. Phytophotodermatitis mimicking child abuse. *J R Soc Med.* 1997;90:560–561

60. Levin AV, Selbst SM. Vulvar hemangioma simulating child abuse. *Clin Pediatr.* 1988;27:213–215

61. Ragosta K. Pediculosis masquerades as child abuse. *Pediatr Emerg Care.* 1989;5:253–254

62. Feldman KW. Pseudoabusive burns in Asian refugees. *Am J Dis Child.* 1984;138:768–769

63. Stewart GM, Rosenberg NM. Conditions mistaken for child abuse: part II. *Pediatr Emerg Care.* 1996;12:217–221

64. Labbe L, Perel Y, Maleville J, et al. Erythema nodosum in children: a study of 27 patients. *Pediatr Dermatol.* 1996;13:447–450

65. Wheeler DM, Hobbs CJ. Mistakes in diagnosing non-accidental injury: 10 years' experience. *Br Med J Clin Res Ed.* 1988;296:1233–1236

66. Waskerwitz S, Christoffel KK, Hauger S. Hypersensitivity vasculitis presenting as suspected child abuse: case report and literature review. *Pediatrics.* 1981;67: 283–284

67. Kappy M, Kummer M, Tyson RW, et al. Pathological case of the month. *Arch Pediatr Adolesc Med.* 1999;153:427–428

68. Gordon EM, Bernat JR Jr, Ramos-Caro FA. Urticaria pigmentosa mistaken for child abuse [letter]. *Pediatr Dermatol.* 1998;15:484–485

69. Day S, Klein BL. Popsicle panniculitis. *Pediatr Emerg Care.* 1992;8:91–93

70. Calobrisi SD, Drolet BA, Esterly NB. Petechial eruption after the application of EMLA cream. *Pediatrics.* 1998;101:471–473

71. Sekula SA, Tschen JA, Duffy JO. Epidermal nevus misinterpreted as child abuse. *Cutis.* 1986;37:276–278

72. Spencer JA, Grieve DK. Congenital indifference to pain mistaken for non-accidental injury. *Br J Radiol.* 1990;63:308–310

73. Adler R, Kane-Nussen B. Erythema multiforme: confusion with child battering syndrome. *Pediatrics.* 1983;72:718–720

74. Thakur BK, Kaplan AP. Recurrent "unexplained" scalp swelling in an eighteen-month-old child: an atypical presentation of angioedema causing confusion with child abuse. *J Pediatr.* 1996;129:163–165

75. Newcomer VD, Young EM Jr. Unique wounds and wound emergencies. *Dermatol Clin.* 1993;11:715–727

76. Zurbuchen P, LeCoultre C, Calza AM, et al. Calcium necrosis after contact with calcium chloride: a mistaken diagnosis of child abuse. *Pediatrics.* 1996;97:257–258

77. Nields H, Kessler SC, Boisot S, et al. Streptococcal toxic shock syndrome presenting as suspected child abuse. *Am J Forensic Med Pathol.* 1998;19:93–97

78. Denic N, Huyer DW, Sinal SH, et al. Cockroach: the omnivorous scavenger. Potential misinterpretation of postmortem injuries. *Am J Forensic Med Pathol.* 1997;18:177–180

79. Cohen HA, Matalon A, Mezger A, et al. Striae in adolescents mistaken for physical abuse. *J Fam Pract.* 1997;45:84–85

80. Owens SM, Durst RD. Ehlers-Danlos syndrome simulating child abuse. *Arch Dermatol.* 1984;120:97–101

81. Winship IM, Winship WS. Epidermolysis bullosa misdiagnosed as child abuse: a report of 3 cases. *S Afr Med J.* 1988;73:369–370

82. Baden HP, Kvedar JC, Magro CM. Loose anagen hair as a cause of hereditary hair loss in children. *Arch Dermatol.* 1992;128:1349–1353

83. Grey TC. Defibrillator injury suggesting bite mark. *Am J Forensic Med Pathol.* 1989;10:144–145

84. Oates RK. Overturning the diagnosis of child abuse. *Arch Dis Child.* 1984;59:665–666

85. Johnson CF. Constricting bands. Manifestations of possible child abuse. Case reports and a review. *Clin Pediatr.* 1988;27:439–444

86. Duhra P, Ilchyshyn A. Perianal streptococcal cellulitis with penile involvement. *Br J Dermatol.* 1990;123:793–796

87. Jenny C, Kirby P, Fuquay D. Genital lichen sclerosis mistaken for child sexual abuse. *Pediatrics.* 1989;83:597–599

88. Darmstadt GL. Perianal lymphangioma circumscriptum mistaken for genital warts. *Pediatrics.* 1996;98:461–463

89. Coleman H, Shrubb VA. Chronic bullous disease of childhood: another cause for potential misdiagnosis of sexual abuse? *Br J Gen Pract.* 1997;47:507–508

90. Papa CA, Pride HB, Tyler WB, et al. Langerhans cell histiocytosis mimicking child abuse. *J Am Acad Dermatol.* 1997;37:1002–1004

91. Levine V, Sanchez M, Nestor M. Localized vulvar pemphigoid in a child misdiagnosed as sexual abuse. *Arch Dermatol.* 1992;128:804–846

92. Beighton P, Horan F. Orthopaedic aspects of the Ehlers-Danlos syndrome. *J Bone Joint Surg.* 1969;51:444–453

93. Lee RC, Astumian RD. The physico-chemical basis for thermal and non-thermal burn injuries. *Burns.* 1996;22:509–519

94. Lee RC. Injury by electrical forces: pathophysiology, manifestations, and therapy. *Curr Probl Surg.* 1997;34:677–764

95. Spillert CR, Vernese NA, Suval WD, et al. The effect of age on severity of murine burns. *Am Surg.* 1984;50:660–662

96. Heimbach D, Engrav L, Grube B, et al. Burn depth: a review. *World J Surg.* 1992;16:10–15

97. Moritz AR, Henriques FC. Studies of thermal injury: the relative importance of time and surface temperature in the causation of cutaneous burns. *Am J Pathol.* 1947;23:695–720

98. Renz BM, Sherman R. Child abuse by scalding. *J Med Assoc Ga.* 1992;81:574–578

99. Lawler W. Bodies associated with fires. *J Clin Pathol.* 1993;46:886–889

100. Bennett B, Gamelli R. Profile of an abused burned child. *J Burn Care Rehabil.* 1998;19:88–94

101. Hight DW, Bakalar HR, Lloyd JR. Inflicted burns in children: recognition and treatment. *JAMA.* 1979;242:517–520

102. Hummel RP III, Greenhalgh DG, Barthel PP, et al. Outcome and socioeconomic aspects of suspected child abuse scald burns. *J Burn Care Rehabil.* 1993;14:121–126

103. Montrey JS, Barcia PJ. Nonaccidental burns in child abuse. *South Med J.* 1985;78:1324–1326

104. Purdue GF, Hunt JL, Prescott PR. Child abuse by burning: an index of suspicion. *J Trauma Injury Infect Crit Care.* 1988;28:221–224

105. Rosenberg NM, Marino D. Frequency of suspected abuse/neglect in burn patients. *Pediatr Emerg Care.* 1989;5:219–221

106. Feldman KW, Schaller RT, Feldman JA, et al. Tap water scald burns in children. *Pediatrics.* 1978;62:1–7

107. Barillo DJ, Burge TS, Harrington DT. Body habitus as a predictor of burn risk in children: do fat boys still get burned? *Burns.* 1998;24:725–727

108. Renz BM, Sherman R. Abusive scald burns in infants and children: a prospective study. *Am Surg.* 1993;59:329–334

109. Baptiste MS, Feck G. Preventing tap water burns. *Am J Public Health.* 1980;70:727–729

110. Smith EI. The epidemiology of burns: the cause and control of burns in children. *Pediatrics.* 1969;44:S821–S827

111. Forjuoh SN. Pattern of intentional burns to children in Ghana. *Child Abuse Negl.* 1995;19:837–841

112. Hobson MI, Evans J, Stewart IP. An audit of non-accidental injury in burned children. *Burns.* 1994;20:442–445

113. Showers J, Garrison KM. Burn abuse: a four-year study. *J Trauma Injury Infect Crit Care.* 1988;28:1581–1583

114. Andronicus M, Oates RK, Peat J, et al. Non-accidental burns in children. *Burns.* 1998;24:552–558

115. Hammond J, Perez-Stable A, Ward CG. Predictive value of historical and physical characteristics for the diagnosis of child abuse. *South Med J.* 1991;84:166–168

116. Greenhalgh DG. The healing of burn wounds. *Dermatol Nurs.* 1996;8:13–23

117. Griswold JA. White blood cell response to burn injury. *Semin Nephrol.* 1993;13:409–415

118. Heideman M, Bengtsson A. The immunologic response to thermal injury. *World J Surg.* 1992;16:53–56

119. Woodward JM. Emotional disturbances of burned children. *Br Med J.* 1959;1:1009–1013

120. Woodward JM, Jackson DM. Emotional reactions in burned children and their mothers. *Br J Plast Surg.* 1961;13:316–324

121. Long RT, Cope O. Emotional problems of burned children. *N Engl J Med.* 1961;264:1121–1127

122. Vigliano A, Hart LW, Singer F. Psychiatric sequelae of old burns in children and their parents. *Am J Orthopsychiatry.* 1964;34:753–761

123. Galdston R. The burning and the healing of children. *Psychiatry.* 1972;35:57–66

124. Holter JC, Friedman SB. Etiology and management of severely burned children: psychosocial considerations. *Am J Dis Child.* 1969;118:680–686

125. Campbell JL, LaClave LJ, Brack G. Clinical depression in burn cases. *Burns.* 1987;13:213–217

126. Clark KD, Tepper D, Jenny C. Effect of a screening profile on the diagnosis of non-accidental burns in children. *Pediatr Emerg Care.* 1997;13:259–261

127. Mirowski GW, Frieden IJ, Miller C. Iatrogenic scald burn: a consequence of institutional infection control measures. *Pediatrics.* 1996;98:963–965

128. Drago DA. Kitchen scalds and thermal burns in children five years and younger. *Pediatrics.* 2005;115:10–16

129. Titus MO, Baxter AL, Starling SP. Accidental scald burns in sinks. *Pediatrics.* 2003;111:e191–e194

130. Yeoh C, Nixon JW, Dickson W, et al. Patterns of scald injuries. *Arch Dis Child.* 1994;71:156–158

131. Allasio D, Fischer H. Immersion scald burns and the ability of young children to climb into a bathtub. *Pediatrics.* 2005;115:1419–1421

132. Lenoski EF, Hunter KA. Specific patterns of inflicted burn injuries. *J Trauma.* 1977;17:842–846

133. Daria S, Sugar NF, Feldman KW, Boos SC, Benton SA, Ornstein A. Into hot water head first. Distribution of intentional and unintentional immersion burns. *Pediatr Emerg Care.* 2004;20:302–319

134. Angel C, Shu T, French D, et al. Genital and perineal burns in children: 10 years of experience at a major burn center. *J Pediatr Surg.* 2002;37:99–103

135. Spiller HA, Winter ML, Weber JA, et al. Skin breakdown and blisters from senna-containing laxatives in young children. *Ann Pharmacotherapy.* 2003;37:636–639

136. Leventhal JM, Griffin D, Duncan KO, Starling SP, Christian CW, Kutz T. Laxative-induced dermatitis of the buttocks incorrectly suspected to be abusive burns. *Pediatrics.* 2001;107:178–180

137. Frechette A, Rimsza ME. Stun gun injury: a new presentation of the battered child syndrome. *Pediatrics.* 1992;89:898–901

138. Prescott PR. Hair dryer burns in children. *Pediatrics.* 1990;86:692–697

139. Qazi K, Gerson LW, Christopher NC, Kessler E, Ida N. Curling iron-related injuries presenting to US emergency departments. *Acad Emerg Med.* 2001;8:395–397

140. Gaffney P. The domestic iron: a danger to young children. *J Accid Emerg Med.* 2000;17:199–200

141. Burdette-Smith P. Stun gun injury. *J Accid Emerg Med.* 1997;14:402–404

142. Alexander RC, Surrell JA, Cohle SD. Microwave oven burns to children: an unusual manifestation of child abuse. *Pediatrics.* 1987;79:255–260

143. Squires T, Busuttil A. Child fatalities in Scottish house fires 1980–1990: a case of child neglect? *Child Abuse Negl.* 1995;19:865–873

144. Johnson CF, Ericson AK, Caniano D. Walker-related burns in infants and toddlers. *Pediatr Emerg Care.* 1990;6:58–61

145. Knight B. Forensic problems in practice: XI. Injury from physical agents. *Practitioner.* 1976;217:813–818

146. Diez F, Berger TG. Scarring due to an enuresis blanket. *Pediatr Dermatol.* 1988;5:58–60

147. Garty BZ. Garlic burns. *Pediatrics.* 1993;91:658–659

148. Oluwasanmi JO. Burns in Western Nigeria. *Br J Plast Surg.* 1969;22:216–223

149. Ginsburg CM. Staphylococcal toxin syndrome. *Pediatr Infect Dis J.* 1991;10:319–321

150. Inman JK. Cetrimide allergy presenting as suspected child abuse. *Br Med J.* 1982;284:385

151. Feldman KW. Confusion of innocent pressure injuries with inflicted dry contact burns. *Clin Pediatr.* 1995;34:114–115

152. Schmitt BD, Gray JD, Britton HL. Car seat burns in infants: avoiding confusion with inflicted burns. *Pediatrics.* 1978;62:607–608

153. Nunez AE, Taft ML. A chemical burn simulating child abuse. *Am J Forensic Med Pathol.* 1985;6:181–183

154. Sheridan RL, Sheridan M, Tompkins RG. Dishwasher effluent burns in infants. *Pediatrics.* 1993;91:142–144

155. Wardinsky T, Vizcarrondo F. The mistaken diagnosis of child abuse: a three-year USAF Medical Center analysis and literature review. *Milit Med.* 1995;160:15–20

156. Quinlan KP. Injury control in practice: home radiator burns in inner-city children. *Arch Pediatr Adolesc Med.* 1996;150:954–957

Chapter 2

Head Trauma

Lucy Rorke-Adams
University of Pennsylvania School of Medicine
The Children's Hospital of Philadelphia

Christine-Ann Duhaime
Children's Hospital at Dartmouth
Dartmouth Hitchcock Medical Center

Carole Jenny
Brown University School of Medicine
Child Protection Program, Hasbro Children's Hospital

Wilbur L. Smith
Department of Radiology
Wayne State University

Traumatic brain injury is the most common cause of fatal inflicted injury in childhood. The past decade has led to increasing recognition of this entity around the world, both as a cause of death and of lasting disability in survivors. This chapter will review the epidemiology, clinical presentation, evaluation and management, pathophysiology, differential diagnosis, biomechanics, radiology, and neuropathology of inflicted head injury in infants and young children.

Terminology and Definitions

There have been a number of physical abuse syndromes with clusters of common findings that have included injury to the head and brain. A number of terms have been used to describe these, the earliest of which implied mechanistic etiologies, including *battered child syndrome*[1] and *whiplash shaken infant syndrome.*[2] The most enduring term has been *shaken baby syndrome,* or its later iteration, *shaken impact syndrome.*[3-6] Because of the recognition that a specific mechanism is rarely known with certainty and that a variety of forces and mechanisms may be at play in a specific patient or among different patients, nonmechanistic terms including *non-accidental head injury, abusive head trauma (AHT),* or *inflicted injury* are probably more accurate and inclusive. In this chapter, these non-mechanistic terms will be used interchangeably. Typical injuries most often include subdural and/or subarachnoid hemorrhage, with or without discernible impact phenomenon, such as scalp hematomas, skull fractures, facial trauma, and focal brain contusions, and with or without evidence of focal or diffuse brain swelling.

Epidemiology

Unlike research on other, more objectively defined disease entities, inflicted injury studies differ widely on basic criteria, including how the entity is defined, thereby making comparisons among studies difficult. While early, classic studies focused on describing constellations of findings in non-accidental injuries, including head injuries, in more recent years investigators have tried to ascertain the extent of the problem with population-based data. Table 2.1 provides an overview of a number of studies of the incidence of inflicted head injuries in infants and young children. Variation in methods and inclusion criteria likely contribute to the range of values noted, but it seems clear that children younger than 1 year are at highest risk for inflicted head injuries, ranging from approximately 14 in 100,000 to 30 in 100,000 in various series.[6–11] The risk is lower in children

between 1 and 2 years of age and decreases thereafter.

Mortality is significantly higher for children with inflicted injury compared with those with accidental injury (16.8% compared with 10.7%, $P<0.001$), and more children with inflicted injury die in the hospital than in the prehospital setting compared with those with accidental trauma.[10] Most population-based studies show a slight male predominance or equal gender distribution,[6–8,10] and some have noted an increased incidence in urban regions and during the autumn and winter months.[6] Risk factors include young parents, lower socioeconomic status, urban location, unstable family situations, single parents, presence of extended family or an unrelated adult in the home, having a parent in the military, disability or prematurity of the child, history of abuse toward the caretaker, and psychiatric and substance abuse histories.[8,12–16] Starling et al[17] found that perpetrators are most likely to be fathers, followed by boyfriends, female babysitters, and mothers, in descending order.

Clinical Presentation

History

The 2 most common histories given for infants with inflicted head injuries in multiple series include (1) a low-height fall and (2) no specific history of trauma, that is, the child is brought to attention because of specific symptoms or findings. These symptoms may include lethargy, irritability, vomiting, seizures, apnea or other breathing difficulties, and unresponsiveness.[3,18–21]

TABLE 2.1
Incidence Studies of Inflicted Head Injuries in Infants and Young Children

Reference	Inclusion Criteria	N (Non-Accidental Injuries)	Incidence	Critique
Jayawant et al, 1998[7]	Retrospective study of hospitalized children age < 2 with subdural hemorrhage in South Wales and southwest England from 1995–1998	27	12.8 non-accidental subdurals per 100,00 children age <2; 21/100,000 age <1 (1/4,761)	Does not include children with other types of head injuries; specific criteria for deciding that injury was non-accidental are not described.
Barlow and Minns, 2000[6]	Prospective survey of inpatient pediatric units and death records in Scotland for all cases of non-accidental head injury from 1998–1999	19	24.6 non-accidental head injuries per 100,000 children age <1 year (1/4,065)	Criteria for deciding that injury was non-accidental are not described.
Keenan et al, 2003[8]	Prospective review of inpatient pediatric intensive care and medical examiner records for children age <2 in North Carolina in 2000–2001	80	17 non-accidental head injuries per 100,000 person-years in children age <2, 30 per 100,000 age <1	Less seriously injured children might be missed; determination of inflicted injury based on records or case review.
Hobbs et al, 2005[9]	Monthly retrospective reporting survey of physicians and pathologists in UK and Ireland of all children with subdural hematomas or effusions in 1998–1999	106	7.1 non-accidental subdurals per 100,000 age <2; 14.2 per 100,000 age <1	Etiology of injury determined by individual physicians' contributing cases.
Sills et al, 2005[10]	Retrospective case review from traumatic brain injury surveillance system in children 0–36 months old in Colorado	340	16.1 intentional traumatic brain injuries per 100,000 children 0–36 months old	Intentional injury determined by *ICD-9* or *ICD-10* codes.
Sun et al, 2006[11]	Retrospective single-center review of children with subdural hemorrhage age <5 in Hong Kong	11	1.5 non-accidental subdurals per 100,000 children age <5	Authors note not all possible cases underwent investigation.

Seizures are common, being reported in 40% to 71% of patients in various series, and hypoventilation or apnea in more than half.[3,22] Children also may come to attention because of other injuries, with head injury being diagnosed by screening, or because of physical findings such as macrocephaly in the setting of chronic subdural collections.[23,24]

Because the initial history is often the most reliable and helpful, it is important that the clinician who first has contact with the caretaker is thorough in the interview. After obtaining the presenting history, specific questions will clarify the circumstances under which the child's symptoms became apparent. The clinician should ask exactly what happened, at what time, who was present, what the child looked like and sounded like immediately and over time, who did what in response, what happened next, and so on. If a history of a fall is given, a detailed description of the exact event is needed, including how the child fell, how far the trajectory was, on what and in what position the child landed, exactly what happened next, and so on until the present time. A detailed medical and family history is also necessary, including antecedent symptoms, birth and delivery history, prior injuries or illnesses, bleeding tendencies in the child or family (including at delivery), developmental history, and questions to begin to screen for possible genetic or metabolic disease. This information helps to clarify the possible mechanism and severity of the injury and helps guide the initial management.

Because most low-height falls in children are well tolerated and cause only minor injuries, the finding of a more severe clinical picture with this history is a common reason for which suspicion for non-accidental injury is raised (see Differential Diagnosis).[25-33] Skull fractures can occur from low-height falls, but usually are not associated with major intracranial injuries, with the exception of epidural hematoma.[34-36] The concept of "history insufficient to explain the injury" is one on which the ascertainment of non-accidental injury often is initiated. However, because of remaining uncertainty as to what mechanism is necessary to cause what specific injury in what age child, the diagnosis often depends on a constellation of supportive findings, including associated acute injuries and/or evidence of prior trauma. The institution's child protection team should be notified as soon as any suspicion of non-accidental injury is encountered. Early involvement by these specialists is both crucial for appropriate evaluation and invaluable to the treating physician in helping to interact with and support the child's family.

Physical Examination

The initial approach to the child with head injury of any etiology is to follow the basic scheme of airway, breathing, and circulation. Infants who present with apnea must be considered for intubation because hypoventilation may exacerbate the primary brain injury. As in all trauma, the spine should be immobilized until it can be assessed for injury on clinical and/or radiologic grounds. Intravenous access is essential both for laboratory studies and for administration of medications, including anticonvulsants in many cases.

Blood gases may be needed in children with more severe injuries, and an arterial catheter should be considered. In most cases of severe injuries requiring intubation, short-acting pharmacologic agents can be used for this procedure so that the neurologic examination is not eliminated for more than a very brief period.

Once the child has been assessed and resuscitated as needed, a more thorough examination can ensue. The neurologic examination can be performed even in an intubated child if sedation is minimized. The Glasgow Coma Scale (GCS) has significant drawbacks as an assessment tool for preverbal children and may underestimate the severity of injury. Other scales designed for infants may be more reliable and objective.[37] It may be useful to note that an infant who does not grimace or cry when exposed to noxious stimulation is likely to have significant cortical impairment reflective of serious damage, even in the face of extremity movement and eye opening.[37] Limb movements may reflect seizure activity rather than normal motion, and this possibility should be kept in mind. Seizures in infants with brain injury may be subtle or even subclinical. Finally, it should be noted that even in the face of major hemispheric injury, young infants may not exhibit lateralized neurologic findings on examination.

Retinal hemorrhages are highly associated with inflicted injuries, being reported in 65% to 95% of cases in various series. They may be unilateral or bilateral and are most reliably detected with the use of mydriatics.[38,39] While accidental trauma can cause retinal hemorrhages, when these are seen in association with witnessed low-height falls, they are usually sparse and/or unilateral.[40,41] In contrast, severe bilateral hemorrhages, as well as retinal folds or detachments, are seen in association with major forces and have not been reported with simple low-height falls.[4,42,43,44]

The other major part of the constellation of inflicted head injury is associated extracranial injuries. Visceral and other injuries can also occur, and therefore all children with inflicted injuries should have a trauma consult to screen for additional injuries. These include long-bone (especially metaphyseal) fractures, rib fractures, and soft-tissue injuries, especially those in patterns characteristic of abuse. The latter include hand marks from slapping or forceful grabbing, bite marks, patterns suggestive of striking with an object, and burns. Both skeletal and soft-tissue injuries may be acute or in various stages of healing, denoting repeated episodes of trauma. However, extracranial injuries are not identified in all cases of AHT. A thorough physical examination of all skin surfaces for trauma, all extremities to assess for swelling, the scalp for contusions or local swelling, and the frenulum for tears should be performed. A radiographic skeletal survey is indicated for any child who may be a victim of inflicted head injury.

Laboratory Studies

Routine laboratory studies for all patients with significant head injury include complete blood count with differential, electrolytes, blood gases in ventilated patients or those with questions of respiratory distress, and coagulation studies. Coagulation studies may be difficult to interpret in the setting of acute, severe injury because the injury alone may elevate the coagulation values.[45] A formal hematology consult may be helpful to advise on the specific studies to be sent and the time at which they should be obtained (such as von Willebrand panel, various clotting factors, and newer methods of detecting possible platelet dysfunction and/or vitamin K deficiency). Timing of specialized studies may depend on the child's age, transfusion history, and time since injury. Finally, certain screening studies for metabolic diseases, such as glutaric aciduria, are appropriate in some patients depending on the presentation and radiologic findings.

Management

Once the initial resuscitation, evaluation, and stabilization have occurred and the initial radiologic studies have been performed, including computed tomography (CT) and/or magnetic resonance imaging (MRI) of the brain as well as spine imaging in the unconscious or unexaminable infant (often most efficiently accomplished by MRI), management of the head injury ensues depending on the clinical and radiologic findings. Children with significant mass lesions are taken for surgical evacuation of the clot. The use of hemicraniectomy for severe brain swelling has been reported, but outcomes using this approach have not been tested prospectively.[46] The role of intracranial pressure (ICP) monitoring in the setting of severe traumatic brain injury in

infancy remains unclear.[47,48] However, at present, routine management of elevated ICP is generally applied to infants by most clinicians. The exception may be for those infants in whom severe, diffuse, bilateral brain injury is identified (the so-called bilateral black brain).[49] In this group, no therapy has been shown to make a difference in mortality or long-term outcome in survivors, which is dismal.[50,51]

While there are few prospective data, most authors advocate consideration of prophylactic treatment of seizures because these occur so commonly in traumatized infants and may be subclinical. Which agent should be used remains uncertain and probably varies with age.[52]

During this phase of management, it is helpful for the clinician to call on social services support for the family because the stress and suddenness of a severe injury can be overwhelming. The fact that the suspicion of inflicted injury has been raised typically adds to the stress of all parties. Decisions may need to be made regarding level of aggressiveness of care, and understanding the prognostic variables for the individual child and the range of possible outcomes is essential. As a general rule, the degree of parenchymal hypodensity correlates inversely with outcome.[50,53–55]

Children with less severe injuries, who do not require treatment for increased ICP, typically undergo a complete clinical and radiologic evaluation (the latter outlined as follows), and are treated symptomatically for seizures or other neurologic signs. Rehabilitation or early intervention services may be helpful, and children should be followed for resolution of extra-axial collections. Late complications include chronic subdural hematomas; hydrocephalus; seizures; visual impairment; and a variety of cognitive, neuromotor, and behavioral problems.[56-58] Follow-up with neurodevelopmental specialists can facilitate obtaining appropriate services and rehabilitative interventions.

Pathophysiology of Brain Damage

Subdural hematomas are significantly more common in non-accidental than in accidental injuries in infants, but both mechanisms can lead to a unique, age-dependent pattern of brain injury. There is evidence to suggest that the combination of subdural hemorrhage and some additional insults, such as increased ICP, hypoxia or hypercarbia, seizures, or hypotension, may lead to a peculiar mismatch between metabolic demand and substrate delivery, which affects the infant brain in a unique manner. This may be in part related to microvascular spasm or compression over the cerebral hemisphere in the face of increased metabolism due to excitotoxicity related to ischemia or seizure activity. The brain regions that are affected look hypodense on CT scan and have the gross appearance of an infarction on CT, MRI, and neuropathologic examination.[53,54,58-60] This phenomenon does not seem to be due to large-vessel occlusion and crosses vascular distributions, but may respect the midline as well as the tentorium cerebelli. It is the cause of the so-called reversal sign when bilateral.[61] When it is unilateral, it occurs on the side of the larger subdural hemorrhage.[39] The exact pathophysiology of this injury remains unclear at present, and although the phenomenon by itself does not connote that an injury was inflicted, it occurs more frequently in victims of inflicted injury.[49,62]

Mechanisms of Injury in Abusive Head Trauma

To understand how head injuries occur, it is helpful to know some basic terminology regarding injury types and mechanisms. In some instances terminology is straightforward, but in other settings similar words can be used to encompass different concepts and meanings, leading to confusion. This can be particularly troublesome in the legal arena, when terms are used by different specialists with varying implications.

First, it is helpful to understand that there are various classifications of head injuries. These include classification by injury severity, injury type, and injury mechanism. Even within these realms of classification, assumptions can be made both about the terms themselves and about their correlation and relationships, which lead to misunderstanding if not clarified, as will be discussed in more detail below.

Injury Severity

The most common classification of head injury severity is the subclassification of various injuries as *mild, moderate,* and *severe.* In many hospitals, these terms are assigned using the GCS, which is designed to assign a severity of injury in the acute post-injury period, after trauma resuscitation. This scale ranges from 3 to 15 points, depending on the patient's degree of eye opening, motor, and verbal responses. Patients with a score of 13 to 15 are considered to have mild injuries, those with scores of 9 to 12 are considered to have moderate injuries, and those with scores of 3 to 8 are considered to have severe injuries.

While this classification is of use in comparing severity of injury of patient populations between centers, it has a number of drawbacks in assigning injury severity to the population of patients who are the subject of this chapter. The GCS was not designed for nor is it clearly validated in infants. Many patients have received pharmacologic interventions that make assigning the score difficult. Many infants with non-accidental trauma present with seizures, which may confound the initial assessment. In others, the cortex may be significantly damaged but because of preservation of brain stem reflexes, the severity of injury may be underestimated in this age group. For this reason, some workers have modified the GCS to try to more accurately assess infants.[37,63–65]

In addition to the difficulties in assigning severity of injury based on bedside clinical assessment tools in infants, there is difficulty in translating this definition of severity to that used in common conversation. For instance, while most clinicians understand that a skull fracture is, in itself, not an injury with long-term consequences nor necessarily associated with significant primary brain injury, to a layperson a fractured skull is a serious or even severe injury. Similarly, an epidural hematoma, while often not associated with a severe primary brain injury, can cause severe brain damage if unrecognized or untreated. That such an injury can happen by what one might consider routine or mild mechanisms, including low-height falls, can cause great confusion among nonmedical learners who struggle to understand these unfamiliar concepts. This may lead to the incorrect certainty that such an injury "had to" occur from a dramatic or forceful or inflicted causation.

Injury Type

The most common terminology used for classification of injury type is based on the anatomy of the lesion or lesions as seen on radiologic studies or at autopsy. Most lesions are described with "where and what" terminology. Thus a skull fracture is a broken bone in the calvarium, a subdural hematoma is a clot in the subdural space, and so on. It should be kept in mind that most patients with head injuries have more than one injury type, that most injury types can occur in a gradation of severities, and that most injury types can occur by more than a single mechanism. Failure to understand these distinctions can lead to erroneous assumptions about the possible causes of a given injury. This variability will be discussed in more detail below.

Injury Mechanisms

The study of what mechanisms cause what injuries has a long and evolving history. When one adds in the variable of age-dependent response to injury forces, the picture becomes even more complex. A full discussion of the entirety of this field is beyond the constraints of this chapter and has been the subject of a number of reviews.[58,66-68] However, some generalizations can be made that may be of use to the clinician called to assess and care for children presenting with head injuries of various possible etiologies.

Forces Acting on the Head and Brain

The anatomical components of the head, including the brain, can be injured by direct contact to the head, as well as by motion of the structures within the intracranial compartment. *Contact* (also called *impact)* forces occur when the head is struck by or impacts an object or surface. Contact events cause damage at the site at which the contact occurs. Examples include scalp hematomas or lacerations, skull fractures, epidural hematomas, and brain surface contusions under the site at which the head was impacted or contacted.

In contrast, *inertial* forces occur due to the structures inside the skull being set in motion, or stopping when the head is already in motion. Motion of intracranial structures results in acceleration and/or deceleration of the tissues, which causes them to deform. The occurrence of deformation over time, or *strain,* can result in tissue injury when it exceeds the tolerance of that particular tissue to being stretched or deformed at a particular rate. Concussion, rupture of parasagittal bridging veins leading to subdural hematoma, and traumatic axonal injury result from inertial forces.

Inertial events can occur with or without actual contact of the head. Examples of noncontact inertial events include those instances of automotive whiplash in which the head moves but does not strike any surface, or shaking in which there is no impact of the head. Likewise, contact events can occur with or without the head also moving. Thus a "pure" contact event might occur when an immobilized head is struck by a moving object, for instance, if a person lying on the ground were struck by falling debris. However, while the distinction between contact and inertial forces is useful in understanding how injuries occur and in modeling specific injury types in the laboratory, it should be stressed that in most clinically occurring injury events, *both contact and inertial forces occur.* A seated person who is struck in the head by a rock sustains mostly contact forces, but the head also will be set in motion, and some inertial strains will result. Likewise, most patients with serious head injuries from motor vehicle crashes have sustained both head impact events and high-magnitude inertial force from the head striking a surface and rapidly decelerating. An infant falling from a height who strikes the head may show contact injuries, such as scalp bruising, skull fracture, and contusion, along with inertial events, such as concussion or shear (axonal) injury, due to head deceleration. Whether these various types of forces result in a specific injury depends on the magnitude and direction of the force and the tolerance of the tissue, as will be discussed in more detail on the following page.

The absence of signs of visible contact injury often causes confusion in interpreting injury events. This is because while contact-type physical signs clearly indicate that contact has occurred, absence of contact signs does not mean that contact has not occurred. The reason is that when contact force is applied over a wide, deformable surface, like the infant head, the contact forces may be distributed such that no visible injury to the surface structures themselves may be seen, even though considerable deceleration to the cranial contents may have occurred. For this reason, the absence of visible surface injury should not be interpreted as indicating that no contact event could have occurred. In infant injuries, many authors conclude that shaking had to have been the mechanism of injury simply because no contact injuries were seen on the child, an assumption which, for the reasons above, may not be correct.

In inertial events, tissue can be injured equivalently whether it is subject to acceleration or deceleration, so these terms often are used interchangeably. Subtypes of inertial injuries include translational deceleration, in which structures move in a straight line, and rotational or angular deceleration, in which brain structures rotate around a center of rotation. The distinction between rotational and angular deceleration depends on whether the structure, in this case the brain, rotates around its center of gravity (rotational) or rotates around a fulcrum outside the brain (angular). In most clinical injuries, the fulcrum of rotation is in the cervical spine, although exceptions occur (eg, a punch to the jaw may cause horizontal rotation around the center of gravity of the brain itself). In most clinical injuries in which inertial events occur, a combination of translational and angular deceleration forces occur simultaneously.

Magnitude of Force

Besides the specific *type* of force (impact, inertial, translational, or rotational deceleration), the injury resulting from a specific event is highly dependent on the *magnitude* of the force acting on specific structures. Impact forces can be small or large, depending on such factors as the velocity of the impacting object that strikes the head or the height of a fall. In inertial injuries, the greater the velocity of the head and the more rapidly it stops, the greater the magnitude of deceleration. This is why trauma involving high speeds, such as motor vehicle crashes, tends to cause more severe injuries. It also explains why a head stopping rapidly when it impacts a surface experiences significantly greater deceleration force than one without an impact event, which stops more slowly. Injury researchers often try to measure the exact forces that may occur under various injury mechanism scenarios, but other factors also influence whether an injury will occur, as noted below.

Effect of Type and Direction of Inertial Force

In general, translational (straight-line) decelerations are associated with more focal injuries, while rotational decelerations are associated with more diffuse injuries. This is because straight-line motion generally is dampened by the contact of the brain surface moving through the cerebrospinal fluid (CSF) in the subarachnoid space and contacting the dura and skull, typically leading to relatively focal surface injury. This is the mechanism, for instance, of so-called contrecoup contusions. In contrast, the rounded shape of the brain and the surrounding fluid-filled subarachnoid space allow the brain to rotate and stretch significantly under conditions of rotational deceleration, resulting in potentially injurious strains to surface vessels and more diffusely distributed brain tissue, especially the white matter. This typically leads to the spectrum of concussion, subdural hematoma, and traumatic axonal injury, depending on the magnitude and durations of the forces involved. Primate experiments have shown that the direction of rotational (or angular) deceleration is also important in determining the resulting injury type because different structures are deformed. High-magnitude angular deceleration in the sagittal plane in primates results in rupture of the parasagittal bridging veins, leading to acute subdural hemorrhage. Rotation in the coronal plane results in the classic distribution of diffuse axonal injury in the subcortical white matter, corpus callosum, and midbrain, with deeper structures being involved at successively greater magnitudes of deceleration. Torsional rotation (such as from a lateral punch to the jaw) leads to a somewhat different pattern of axonal injury, including various brain stem structures. It should be kept in mind that most clinical injury scenarios will include a combination of these various vectors and that injuries rarely cause rotation only in a single plain of rotation.

Tissue Tolerance

The final factor influencing what injuries result from a specific mechanism is the tolerance of the specific tissues subjected to the forces involved. Thus patients with temporal arachnoid cysts may sustain subdural hemorrhages from relatively minor impacts, presumably due to bridging veins that are stretched over a long distance and more prone to tearing. Some children with shunted hydrocephalus and enlarged subarachnoid spaces seem to have a lower threshold for sustaining subdural hemorrhage,[69] as do some elderly individuals with brain atrophy.

Infants and small children have specific biomechanical features that influence injury susceptibility. One of the most important is skull deformability. Infants sustaining impact events can have significant deformation of the underlying brain and vessels, leading to different types of injuries. Tearing of surface or deep vessels can occur from skull deformation, such as in subdural hemorrhages related to vaginal delivery.[70] There is evidence to support both increased susceptibility to inertial events and decreased susceptibility to focal brain surface deformation in infant gyrencephalic animals compared with more mature animals.[71,72] Mechanically, immature tissue has a higher water content, which causes it to be more resistant to deformation.[73]

Mechanisms of Specific Injuries

Data from clinical series, accident reconstructions, and experimental models have furthered the understanding of what mechanisms generally cause what injury types.[25–33,40,66,74] However, what specific mechanism causes what injury in what age child remains at present incompletely understood. In general, the greater the magnitude of the force, the more extensive the injury is, and the more deeply it extends into the cranium. Table 2.2 outlines the typical mechanisms and magnitude of the various injury types seen in children.

Scalp and skull injuries and brain surface contusions are caused by contact forces, although some brain surface contusions can be caused by inertial events (eg, contrecoup contusions caused by the brain moving within the skull). Subdural hematomas in adults and primate experiments are caused by inertial events. This requires large angular deceleration of a magnitude, which in adults usually requires impact to occur (ie, rapid stopping of the rotating head against a surface). In infants, models have shown that the inertial forces generated when the head is stopped suddenly against a surface are many times greater than those that seem to be generated by shaking alone, and that shaking does not generate force sufficient to reach the threshold of brain injury.[18,74] However, due to limitations in physical models and the unknown effect of repeated injuries, many authors believe that shaking alone, without impact, also can lead to brain injury.[75] The role of injury to the brain stem and cervical spine also remains as possible contributors to the pathophysiology of injury in shaking or forceful inflicted impact, although this does not explain the presence of cortical subdural hemorrhage.[76]

In addition, in the clinical world, especially in infants and young children, contact events that lead to significant deformation of the skull and underlying cortical surface also can lead to rupture of surface vessels, resulting in subdural hemorrhage. Similarly, subdural hemorrhage can result from static, or slow, application of skull deformation, with tearing of venous sinuses or other venous structures, such as occurs in birth injuries.

It is also worth noting that some lesions interpreted as subdural hematomas on CT scan actually represent epidural collections, especially when associated with overlying skull fracture (venous epidurals). Focal subarachnoid hemorrhages can also mimic subdural hemorrhage.[76]

Finally, traumatic axonal injury results from high-magnitude inertial (angular acceleration-deceleration) events.

Summary of Mechanism of Injury

In determining whether a specific injury or constellation of injuries may have occurred from a specific mechanism, it is helpful to know that the clinical data cited previously have shown consistently that apart from epidural hematoma, life-threatening primary brain injuries do not occur in otherwise healthy children from low-height falls. *Low height* in most studies is defined as a distance less than 3 ft from the head to the contact surface, which encompasses most household falls. In children with normal bones, skull fractures require a contact event. Subdural hematomas generally require large forces to occur, with the caveats noted

TABLE 2.2
Injury Types and Mechanisms

Injury Type	Mechanism	Magnitude of Force
Scalp laceration	Contact	Variable (low to high)
Scalp hematoma	Contact	Variable (low to high)
Skull fracture	Contact or crush (static loading)	Variable (low to high)
Epidural hematoma	Contact	Variable (low to high)
Cortical contusion	Contact or inertial (contrecoup)	Usually moderate to high
Cortical laceration	Contact	High
Focal subarachnoid hemorrhage	Contact (usually) or inertial	Moderate to high
Subdural hematoma	Inertial (usually, especially in older children/adults); contact (cortical vessel or venous tear); static loading (eg, birth injuries)	Moderate to high
Diffuse axonal injury	Inertial	High

above regarding different causes and mimics of subdural hematoma.

In general, the level of suspicion for inflicted injury rests on the relationship between the injury type, the best history describing how the injury occurred (or lack thereof), and associated physical and radiologic findings. Children who are otherwise healthy and who have no history of trauma or a history of a low-height fall who present with subdural hemorrhage and unexplained skeletal injuries, soft tissue–patterned inflicted injuries, or severe bilateral retinal hemorrhages generally are presumed by most physicians to have a non-accidental mechanism of injury. Other patterns of history, injury type, and associated findings are analyzed on a case by case basis to determine whether an injury seems consistent with an accidental, indeter-

minate, or non-accidental mechanism. Such determinations require experience in the field and familiarity with the literature, and are optimally undertaken by individuals or teams with specific expertise to render the best care to the affected child and family.

Differential Diagnosis of AHT

Distinguishing between AHT and numerous other causes of brain injury can be challenging. The signs of AHT are often subtle, and sometimes a victim of head injury will have injuries that have occurred at different times, complicating the diagnostic decision about etiology.[78,79] One study, for example, found that 31.2% of children found to have AHT had evidence of previous head injury episodes, where the children had been seen by a physician and the diagnosis of AHT missed.[80] Another study found that 45% of children diagnosed with AHT had evidence of previous injury on imaging studies.[56] A careful history, a thorough physical examination, and thoughtful laboratory and imaging evaluations are needed to arrive at the correct diagnosis. It is particularly difficult to make the diagnosis in younger infants who have a limited range of normal behavior and fewer neurologic signs to assess. Thus an infant who is evaluated for irritability and vomiting could have any number of diagnoses, such as gastroenteritis, milk protein allergy, or a viral infection.[3] Often physicians do not consider the possibility of head injury, particularly if the caretaker of the child gives no history of injury.

The clinical presentation of AHT varies, and the diagnostic considerations will vary depending on the child's clinical presentation.[81]

1. Children whose presentation triggers a high suspicion of AHT because they are encephalopathic or have signs of obvious trauma in the absence of an adequate history of trauma. For children with clear evidence of trauma, the primary distinction to be made is between accidental and abusive injury. For children who present with acute encephalopathy, the differential diagnosis includes both traumatic and medical causes.
2. Children with nonspecific presentations, such as abnormal head growth, suspected meningitis, or other symptoms that lead to imaging studies, revealing subdural hemorrhages or other signs of head injury. Diagnostic

considerations for children with this type of presentation include accidental trauma and medical explanations including hematologic, anatomical, or metabolic diseases.
3. Children who have unexplained illness with no signs of neurologic problems and a negative or nonspecific neurologic examination. The children in this third category are the most difficult to diagnose, and the differential diagnoses are considerable.

While any child with suspected AHT should be carefully evaluated for other types of physical injury, the lack of associated injury does not rule out AHT. For example, one study found that 29% of 24 fatal AHT cases had no acute bruises and 21% had no bruises anywhere on the body.[82]

Jaspan and colleagues[81] describe 3 phases of injury resulting from AHT. In each phase the presentation will be different, depending on how the injury has evolved. The first phase, the acute phase, occurs immediately after the injury has occurred. Children present with anatomical disruptions of the brain and cranium, including extra- or intra-axial hemorrhage, and anatomical disruptions such as contusions or shearing tears, often involving cardiorespiratory depression secondary to brain stem dysfunction. The second phase, the early subacute phase, occurs when the primary injury has set off a cascade of events resulting in a disruption of cerebral autoregulation and perfusion and chemically mediated tissue damage. This stage evolves over time. Subdural hematomas may enlarge and brain swelling and infarction can occur. The third phase, the late subacute or chronic phase, presents with hydrocephalus due to impaired CSF resorption, chronic subdural hematomas, cerebral scarring and atrophy, leptomeningeal cysts, and/or impaired head growth. In the first 2 phases children usually appear acutely ill. In the later phase, they might be more likely to present developmentally delayed or with poor or excessive head growth. Again, the diagnostic considerations will vary depending on the presentation of the child to care.

The evaluation of the child with AHT requires a careful and objective investigation into alternative diagnoses that can mimic the presentation of child abuse. In some cases, an extensive evaluation for metabolic, genetic, or hematologic diseases is required, but for others, the constellation of injuries identified at the time of hospitalization negates the need for an exhaustive search for alternative explanations. The medical team caring for child abuse victims needs to have an understanding of mechanisms of injury and of conditions known to mimic AHT. For many patients, the primary consideration is distinguishing accidental from inflicted injury.

Distinguishing Between Abusive and Accidental Head Trauma

As has been stated earlier in this chapter, the preponderance of the literature on childhood falls indicates that short falls rarely result in serious or life-threatening head injuries, despite their frequency. Falls are the most common cause of injury bringing children to emergency departments (EDs) and requiring hospital admission.[83,84] In one population-based study, falls accounted for one-third of pediatric hospital admissions due to trauma but were an infrequent cause of death.[83] However, differences are substantial between traumatic injuries suffered in falls and other accidents and those inflicted abusively.[56] Each credible study supports the conclusion that severe head injuries purported to be accidental, unless related to a moving vehicle accident or a fall from a significant height, are very likely to be the result of abuse, particularly if injuries are ascribed to falls from short heights that occur at home, unwitnessed by objective observers. Difficulty remains in sorting out accidental from abusive injury when the head injuries are less severe. But studies of head injuries in children due to falls are difficult to compare. Some studies are based on all children ages 0 through 18 years in whom a greater proportion of outdoor accidents are represented. Others address a public health threat by focusing on young children who fall down stairways in walkers or from open windows in high-rise buildings.

Despite these limitations, there are studies that collectively describe injuries of more than 4,600 children. For comparison these can best be divided into short falls (n = 1,732), stairway falls (n = 1,037), and falls greater than one story (n = 1,902).[25,26,28,31,83–90] In the short fall category, Helfer and colleagues[25] studied the injuries of 246 children younger than 6 years who had fallen from their beds or sofas. One hundred seventy-six of these falls took place in the children's homes and 85 occurred in the hospital. The children generally fell from beds or sofas that were elevated 3 ft or less, although several were from heights up to 5 ft. Two of the children sustained linear skull fractures from these falls, but none of the children had central nervous system (CNS) damage. Drawing on these findings, Helfer and co-workers asserted that serious injuries attributed to an accidental fall from a bed or low height should be considered unlikely and, in most instances, are due to child abuse. Nimityongskul and Anderson[26] replicated the findings of Helfer and colleagues, describing 76 children who were injured as the result of a fall while in the hospital. These children experienced minor injuries and only one patient had a skull fracture. This study also scrutinized the surface onto which the child fell, comparing their data with existing literature on playground safety.[91] The authors hypothesized that a carpeted floor or thick rug could cushion falls from high places sufficiently that injury was unlikely, but that a child falling onto a tiled or concrete surface would be more likely to sustain injury. Other investigators reached similar conclusions after studying the outcomes of accidental head trauma in situations where the histories were reliable. Focusing only on falls in children younger than 3 years that were witnessed by a person other than the child's caretaker, Williams[92] described 44 children who fell less than 10 ft and 62 who fell 10 ft or more. Those who fell less than 10 ft sustained serious but not life-threatening injuries, including small, depressed skull fractures from falling against sharp edges. In contrast,

2 children died from falls from reportedly less than 5 ft among the 53 uncorroborated falls. The only other death was in a child who fell 70 ft. Relying on the accurate history from incident reports in hospital-related falls, Lyons and Oates[90] found no serious, multiple, visceral, or life-threatening injuries in children younger than 6 years, 124 of whom fell from cribs and 83 from beds. Falls from beds ranged from 25 to 41 in. (over the side rails) and up to 54 in. over the top of the crib railing. One 21-month-old child who climbed over the top of the crib rail sustained a fractured clavicle and one 10-month-old who fell from his crib had a simple linear skull fracture. Studying the safety of bunk beds, Selbst et al[93] found only 6 of 68 children who fell from a top bunk required admission to the hospital. Of these, 4 had concussions, 1 had a skull fracture with a subdural hematoma, and 1 had a laceration near the eye.

Chadwick and Salerno[86] studied serious head injuries occurring at child care centers. Reviewing 338 records, they found only one child, age 2½ years, who sustained a somewhat serious head injury at child care, falling a distance of 5 ft from a tree onto a concrete walk. The child was temporarily unconscious, a CT of the head was negative, and he recovered completely within a few hours. Tarantino et al[31] limited their study to infants younger than 10 months presenting to the ED after falling from distances of up to 4 ft. Twelve of the 167 infants had skull fractures and 7 had long-bone fractures. No intracranial hemorrhages were attributed to the short vertical fall;

however, 2 infants with intracranial hemorrhages initially presented with a false history of falling only a short distance. Mayr and colleagues[94] found no intracranial injuries or neurologic sequelae due to falls from high chairs in 103 young children whose ages ranged from 7 to 30 months. Almost all of the children were unrestrained, half were trying to stand up when they fell, and 14% tipped the high chair over as they fell. Joffe and Ludwig[87] studied 363 stairway falls presenting to their ED in children younger than 11 years. Although injuries to the head and neck were the most common, most of the injuries were superficial and none of the children required intensive care. The authors found that the injuries in the children who fell more than 4 steps were of no greater severity or number than those who fell fewer than 4 steps. Four of 10 infants who fell with their caretakers while being carried on the stairway sustained skull fractures. Infant walkers were involved in 24 of the 40 injuries of children 6 to 12 months of age. Excluding falls downstairs in walkers, and likely abusive trauma, Chiavello et al[30] found that the most serious injuries from falls occurred in infants who were being carried by their caretakers who then fell on the child against the stairs. Of 3 infants who fell under these circumstances, 2 sustained skull fractures. One of these 2 infants also had a subdural hematoma and cerebral contusion as well as a fracture of the second cervical vertebra. Overall the authors concluded that stairway-related injuries were much less severe than free falls from the same vertical height. Chiavello et al[95] studied stairway falls in walkers

and found that most of these falls result in only minor injuries. However, of 46 stairway walker falls in this study, there was one fatally injured child who suffered a cervical spine fracture, skull fracture, and subdural hematoma and 4 other infants with intracranial hemorrhages. Smith et al[96] noted that intracranial injuries were rare among 260 minor injuries of infants sustained when they fell downstairs in walkers. They also found that the number of stairs the child fell was significantly associated with the seriousness of the injury. Only 10 patients were admitted to the hospital, all 10 of whom had skull fractures. Three of the skull fractures were depressed and 3 had accompanying intracranial hemorrhages. In contrast, Mayr et al,[97] in a study from Austria, found 19 infants had skull fractures but no intracranial injuries among 143 infants falling downstairs in walkers.

In comparison, Plunkett[32] conducted a retrospective review of the US Consumer Product Safety Commission (CPSC) National Injury Clearinghouse data. There were 18 deaths secondary to short playground falls from more than 75,000 cases reviewed. There were no infants reported in this study; there were 5 children between 12 and 24 months; 5 between 25 and 60 months; and 8 between 6 and 13 years of age. Distances were all "felt" to be between 2 and 10 ft. Autopsies showed one extra-dural hematoma, 2 cerebral infarctions, 10 subdural hematomas, and 12 with cerebral edema. The author concluded that short falls can cause death. The incidence of fatality due to short falls in this study—18 out of

75,000 cases—suggests the extreme rarity of a fatal outcome from a short fall. Several major methodological problems exist in this study: absence of infants, the age group of most importance in inflicted head injury; data sets relying on histories of the injuries accepted at face value by hospital personnel; a variety of mechanisms of falling, depending on the playground equipment being used at the time of fall; and variable reporting practices over a 10-year period by those submitting the data to the clearinghouse.[98]

Falls from extreme heights are expected to cause serious head injury, but mortality in this group is surprisingly low. Combining the data of studies involving 1,902 children younger than 18 years, there were 23 deaths.[28,83,85,89,91,99,100] Nineteen deaths involved falls of greater than 3 stories. Most long-fall studies do not describe in detail the morbidity associated with the falls, so correlations between the heights of the falls and the incidence of severe intracranial injuries are not available. One study from Saudi Arabia of 104 children younger than 13 years reported no brain injuries in those children who fell fewer than 7 m (23 ft).[85] Fatalities and neurologic morbidity were related to falls from second- and third-floor balconies. Three of 44 children died, 2 falling from the second floor and one from the third floor. Five other children sustained multiple skull fractures and hemorrhagic cerebral contusions resulting in moderate neurologic sequelae, such as monoparesis, ataxia, or seizures from falls of 7 to 12 m.

In comparison to the data on falls, convincing evidence supports AHT as a leading cause of serious head injury in infants.[101] Billmire and Myers[102] reported that 95% of fatal or life-threatening head injuries in infants admitted to an intensive care unit were the result of abuse. Duhaime et al[40] reported 100 children younger than 2 years who were hospitalized with head injury. An initial history of household falls was provided in 73 cases. Twenty-four were found to be due to AHT and another 32 had injuries suggestive of abuse. Epidural hematomas occurred in 3 children who fell fewer than 4 ft. Falls greater than 4 ft resulted in focal parenchymal contusions in 4 children and focal subarachnoid hemorrhages in 2 others, all of whom had good outcomes. In contrast, abusive injuries had a disproportionately high incidence of intracranial hemorrhage (13 of 24 children), with 3 deaths.

Despite the differences in severity and outcomes for infants with accidental head trauma and AHT, both mechanisms can cause intracranial injury, complicating diagnostic decision-making. Young infants can sustain intracranial injury after accidental trauma and can be asymptomatic at presentation. Greenes and Schutzman[103] reviewed the medical records of children younger than 2 years hospitalized over a 6½-year period with intracranial hemorrhage, cerebral contusion, or cerebral edema. They found that 19 of 101 infants had asymptomatic intracranial injuries, and 14 of these 19 infants sustained their injuries in short falls or downstairs. Only one of these infants was thought to be a victim of abuse. None of the 19 infants were seriously injured, and all were neurologically normal at the time of hospital discharge.

The studies cited here, taken in totality, support the conclusion that not only are accidental falls from heights of less than several stories unlikely to result in death, but also that severe intracranial injuries ascribed to short falls likely indicate abusive injury. Accidental household falls from furniture or downstairs most commonly result in minor trauma, but these falls, particularly when from the arms of a caretaker, may cause skull fractures, some of which may be complex or depressed, epidural hematomas, focal subdural and/or subarachnoid hemorrhage, or small parenchymal contusions. Falls downstairs in walkers infrequently cause clinically severe intracranial injury and rarely can cause fatal injury. High-velocity impact injuries, falls from significant heights, or falls onto extremely hard surfaces provide the opportunity for more severe injury. Rarely do these catastrophic events occur without a corroborated history. If these factors are not present to account for severe head injury, the examining physician must strongly consider the possibility of AHT.

Other household accidents occur rarely in young children, but can have severe neurologic consequences and can be fatal. One such injury is when a television set topples from an unstable table, crushing a child. Bernard et al[104] reported that the CPSC received 73 reports of falling televisions resulting in 28 deaths over a 7-year period. Head injuries accounted for 72% of the injuries. A crushing injury of the head was found in 13 of 14 deaths further investigated by the commission. Duhaime et al[105] described crush injuries to the head in 7 children, 4 of whom were run over by a motor vehicle in a driveway or parking lot. In the other 3, children pulled heavy objects onto their heads. All children had basilar skull fractures, and calvarial fractures were often multiple, complex, and associated with subarachnoid and intraparenchymal hemorrhage. All surviving children made good cognitive recoveries despite their alarming histories and initial clinical condition.

The most frequent explanation offered by adults when children present with AHT is accidental injury, which requires careful consideration of injury biomechanics, epidemiology of childhood injury, a thorough search for occult injury, and a careful investigation into the cause of injury for each child.

When comparing factors that assist in distinguishing accidental from abusive injury, those that are found more often for AHT victims include young age (<1 year), lack of history of a significant traumatic event, a changing history from the caretaker, the presence of head injury symptoms and seizures at the time of presentation, poor outcome, and the belief by the caretaker that home resuscitation caused the injury.[21,106–108] Retinal hemorrhages are more commonly found after AHT compared with accidents.[109] Several studies have shown that extensive multilayered retinal hemorrhages extending from the ora serrata to the posterior pole of the eye are almost always found only in AHT.[40,106,108,110] Retinoschisis and bleeding into the orbital contents (fat, muscle) and optic nerve sheath are also more common in abused children.[110-112] Certain MRI and CT findings are also correlated with abuse. These include subdural hematomas (especially in the region of intrahemispheric falx) and mixed-density subdural collections.[113]

Other Conditions in the Differential Diagnosis of AHT

While many disorders can cause subdural hematomas and encephalopathy, most can be discerned with a careful physical examination, past medical and family history, and imaging and screening laboratory studies.[114] The medical diseases commonly listed in the differential diagnosis of inflicted neurotrauma include congenital or acquired coagulopathies; metabolic diseases; intracranial structural anomalies, such as arterio-venous malformations (AVMs); unintentional asphyxiation; and birth trauma.

Strangulation, Suffocation, and Asphyxia

Anoxic damage must be considered in the differential diagnosis in inflicted neurotrauma. Rauschschwalbe and Mann[115] retrospectively analyzed CPSC data on window-cord strangulations in the United States between 1981 and 1995. They found a total of 183 fatal strangulations, with 93% of the victims 3 years of age or younger. In 1997 Drago and colleagues[116] reported 47 children injured by clothing drawstrings, 8 of whom died. In 1999 they cited 2,178 cases of suffocation in infants that occurred in 1995 in the United States, a prevalence rate of 29 in 100,000.[117] The patterns of suffocation were wedging (879), oronasal obstruction (512), overlaying (180), entrapment by suspension (145), and hanging (142). Both hypoxia and circulatory compromise can result from either strangulation or shaking; however, subdural hemorrhage does not result from suffocation or asphyxial injury in children.

Prenatal and Perinatal Trauma

Akman and Cracco,[118] in a review of the literature on intrauterine subdural hematomas, found 7 cases of spontaneous intrauterine subdural hematomas and 24 cases of intrauterine subdural hematomas with associated risk factors. Trauma was the most suspected cause of intrauterine subdural hematomas, but other etiologies, such as thrombocytopenia, other coagulation disorders, and liver disease, need to be considered. Towner and colleagues[119] studied the records of 583,340 singleton births to nulliparous women. Ten percent of these were vacuum-assisted births, 2.7% were forceps-assisted births, and 0.5% had both forceps and vacuum assistance. Between 0.02% and 0.26% of operative deliveries resulted in recognized and reported subdural or intracerebral hemorrhage. Whitby et al[120] screened 111 asymptomatic full-term babies for subdural hematomas. Eight percent were found to have subdural hematomas, all of which resolved within 4 weeks. None of the infants were symptomatic. Complicated deliveries (eg, vacuum extractions, forceps deliveries) can lead to retinal and subdural hemorrhages.[121-123] These hemorrhages clear within a few weeks of delivery.

Glutaric Aciduria Type I (GAI)

This rare autosomal-recessive inborn error of metabolism is due to a deficiency of glutaryl-CoA dehydrogenase, an enzyme required for the metabolism of lysine, hydroxylysine, and tryptophan. The clinical course is characterized by an unremarkable early history and development, followed by an acute dystonic-dyskinetic syndrome in infancy or early childhood. Macrocephaly may be present at birth or it may develop within the first few weeks of life.[124,125] The diagnosis depends on the demonstration of large amounts of glutaric acid and its metabolites in the urine and/or a deficiency of glutaric acid dehydrogenase in leukocytes or fibroblasts. Computed tomography and MRI show widening of the insular cisterns and frontotemporal atrophy, diffuse cortical atrophy, changes in the basal ganglia, white matter hypodensities, internal and external hydrocephalus and, in some cases, subdural effusions.[126] Subdural hemorrhage may be the initial sign of GAI disorder. In some cases, retinal hemorrhages have been described.[127] Because of this, some cases of GAI disorder have initially been considered to be due to inflicted injury. Morris et al[127] stress that when subdural hematomas are found in children with GAI, they occur in conjunction with significant frontotemporal cerebral atrophy and there are no associated injuries, such as fractures.[127]

Cerebral Sinovenous Thrombosis

This is a rare but serious disorder in children. A collaborative study from 16 tertiary pediatric care centers in Canada showed that the prevalence in all children younger than 18 years was 0.67 cases per 100,000 children per year.[128] Acute systemic illness was present in 84% of the neonates, most of these being perinatal complications (51%) and dehydration (30%). In a recent series of 42 children between the ages of 3 weeks and 13 years with cerebral sinovenous thrombosis, all children had underlying clinical risk factors, including preexisting medical diseases, infection, and/or dehydration.[129] Diagnosis is best made by MRI with venography, and evaluation for thrombotic disorders, anemia, or infection is indicated based on the clinical situation.

Congenital Malformations

Congenital malformations such as intracranial arteriovenous malformations and aneurysms can cause intracranial bleeding, although the pattern of bleeding is usually recognizably different than that seen in AHT.[130-132]

Disorders of Coagulation

Few of the common pediatric coagulopathies have been reported to cause intracranial hemorrhage in infants. Moderate or severe hemophilia (Factor VIII or IX deficiency) is a well-known cause of spontaneous intracranial hemorrhage, including isolated subdural hemorrhage.[133-135] Conversely, mild hemophilia is not associated with spontaneous intracranial bleeding. Although hemophilia has been misdiagnosed as child abuse, cutaneous injuries, not intracranial hemorrhage, have been the focus of medical reports.[136,137]

Unlike hemophilia, child abuse has been misdiagnosed in infants with intracranial hemorrhage due to vitamin K deficiency, with recent reports in the medical literature.[138-140] Vitamin K deficiency due to lack of vitamin K administration at birth can lead to severe intracranial and intraretinal bleeding.[141,142] With the routine use of prophylactic vitamin K at delivery, clinicians are often unaware of the presentation of late hemorrhagic disease of the newborn, which can include subdural hemorrhage. Both hemophilia and vitamin K deficiency are identifiable by routine screening tests. Intracranial hemorrhage associated with hemophilia is associated with a markedly prolonged partial thromboplastin time (PTT), and vitamin K deficiency causes a prolonged prothrombin time (PT) and PTT. A more sensitive measure of vitamin K deficiency can be obtained by measuring levels of abnormally carboxylated prothrombin (protein induced by vitamin K absence [PIVKA II]) and can be helpful in identifying vitamin K deficiency in infants who present with intracranial hemorrhage and abnormal PT/PTT.[143] Although PIVKA II is detectable in plasma before changes occur in conventional coagulation tests, the clinical significance of an isolated PIVKA II level without abnormal PT/PTT is uncertain. Additionally, the location of hemorrhage in coagulopathic infants is often (but not always) different than that seen in child abuse, with intraparenchymal and intraven-

tricular hemorrhage more common with coagulopathy.[144,145]

Symptomatic intracranial bleeds are uncommon in children with known clotting disorders such as von Willebrand disease and factor deficiencies.[146] For example, a review of cases of more than 300 children with idiopathic thrombocytopenic purpura showed only 2 had intracranial hemorrhage and both recovered without sequelae.[147]

Additional hematologic causes of spontaneous intracranial hemorrhage in infants include neonatal alloimmune thrombocytopenia, disseminated intravascular coagulation, and Factor XIII deficiency. Factor XIII (fibrin-stabilizing factor) is responsible for clot stabilization and cross-linking of fibrin polymers. Deficiency of Factor XIII is associated with severe, characteristic bleeding, including umbilical stump bleeding in more than 80% of affected newborns and spontaneous intracranial hemorrhage in approximately 25% of infants.[148-150] Laboratory evaluations, including PT, PTT, bleeding time, and thrombin time are all normal in affected infants, and a fibrin clot solubility test should be considered in infants with a history suggestive of excessive neonatal bleeding. Factor XIII deficiency has been mistaken for child abuse.[151]

Accidental and inflicted head trauma can cause a secondary coagulopathy, and the degree of hemostatic abnormality generally correlates with the severity of brain injury.[152] Abnormalities in coagulation occur frequently in children after head trauma, even those with mild injury.[152] However, major hemostatic abnormalities, such as disseminated intravascular coagulopathy (DIC), generally accompany severe injury and are associated with high mortality rates in the setting of trauma.[91] Disseminated intravascular coagulopathy secondary to disseminated herpes simplex virus infection has been mistaken for inflicted trauma.[138] Hymel et al[45] have shown that PT prolongation and activated coagulation are strongly related to the presence of parenchymal brain injury in abused infants.

The hematologic evaluation for children with intracranial hemorrhage serves 2 purposes: to identify a treatable coagulopathy that results from trauma and to identify the child whose intracranial hemorrhage is the result of a primary bleeding diathesis. In the setting of suspected abuse, guidelines for appropriate laboratory screening do not exist, and recommendations for screening tests vary considerably. Universal recommendations include a complete blood count, platelet count, PT, and PTT. For ill-appearing infants, additional DIC evaluation, including a fibrinogen, D-dimer, blood type, and crossmatch, is warranted. Factor XIII assay may also be indicated. Additional testing should reflect the results of the initial screening tests and a search for diseases that are known to mimic the intracranial findings seen in AHT.

Infectious Diseases

Hemorrhagic subdural effusions can result from *Haemophilus influenzae* meningitis and other bacterial meningitis. The onset of disease and unique laboratory findings in these infectious conditions easily differentiate infection from trauma.[153]

Malignancies

Leukemia and solid tumors can cause intracranial bleeding. The diagnosis is made on imaging studies and blood tests.[154,155]

As in all of clinical medicine, every possibility must be considered when making a diagnosis and instituting treatment. In the case of AHT, treatment has social and legal implications as well as medical ones. The responsibility of the physician is to identify victims of abuse to ensure their protection while recognizing the medical conditions that can mimic AHT.

Neuroimaging

Neuroimaging has been an essential feature of the diagnosis of AHT since John Caffey's seminal description of "shaken baby" in 1974.[2] In the early days of recognition of AHT, neuroimaging was primitive by current standards, consisting of invasive techniques of pneumoencephalography, subdural aspiration, and arteriography. The diagnosis and understanding of AHT dramatically improved in the 1970s with the widespread adoption of CT and was further revolutionized by the application of MRI in the late 1980s.[156] Advances in both of these technologies have refined and improved the detection and understanding of AHT and enhanced clinical prediction of the clinical consequences of AHT. New pulse sequences for MRI, volume-rendered CT, CT and MRI non-invasive angiography, hydrogen

MRI spectroscopy, and a myriad of other noninvasive neuroimaging techniques will undoubtedly further our understanding, assessment of outcomes, and even treatment options for AHT. This section discusses imaging applications as they exist now and suggests protocols for the evaluation of abused infants and children with head injury. It is certain that these protocols will evolve perhaps radically before the next edition of this book.

Radiographs

A number of approaches exist for imaging skull fractures, including plain radiographs and volumetric data acquisition with spiral CT (Figures 2.1 and 2.2). Cervical spine radiographs are used to evaluate for neck injury in selected cases; however, the enhanced specificity of MRI versus plain radiographs of the cervical spine makes it unlikely that cervical spine films will endure. This comment is not intended to denigrate radiographs for extremity or rib fractures; the skeletal survey should be obtained in all cases of AHT because about half of these infants will exhibit skeletal injuries.

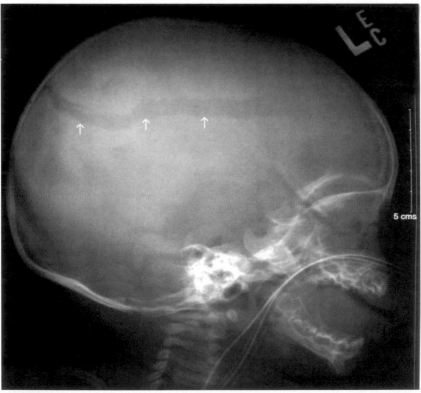

FIGURE 2.1
Lateral view of the skull demonstrates linear diastatic parietal fracture.

CT Scan

Computed tomography is a technique that measures the absorption of x-ray photons by tissues. The absorption is measured in the X and Y axis by detectors circumferentially arrayed about an x-ray source to give digital cross-sectional pictures of the body part, in the case of this discussion the brain. The tissue differences are displayed over a range of x-ray photon absorption measured in reproducible values (Hounsfield units), each assigned a shade of gray ranging from white to black. By convention, high photon absorbers such as bone and localized blood collections were whiter, and lower absorbers such as CSF were blacker. These static, high spatial resolution images of the brain became the gold standard of the 1970s, 1980s, and even into the 1990s for the diagnosis of AHT; however, the conventional CT technique had limited tissue contrast and spatial resolutions. These limitations were recognized in the mid-1980s[157,158]

and a gradual shift in emphasis has occurred toward MRI for evaluation of AHT.

A major advance in CT technology and reassertion of its importance in AHT occurred with the advent of spiral multi-detector techniques. These developments allowed very short scan times and enhanced temporal and spatial resolution because of volumetric acquisition of data. Put simply, one can now use standard CT scan techniques noninvasively to observe changes over large volumes of tissue in a short period, allowing physiological measurements of cerebral perfusion (cerebral regional blood volume, cerebral blood flow, flow velocity) as predictors of brain tissue viability. The same scan can produce dynamic high-resolution CT angiograms of the arteries and veins of the brain and high-detail 3-dimensional reconstructions of the brain and its surrounding structures all from a less than 5-second scan (Figures 2.3 and 2.4). Computed tomography scanning

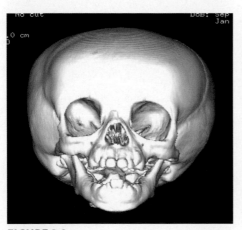
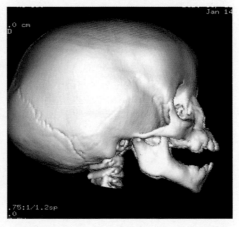

FIGURE 2.2
Three-dimensional volume-rendered reformat of the skull showing normal anatomy obtained by reformatting volumetric computed tomography scanning.

has gone from a diagnostic screening tool to a highly specific technique with major implications for predicting severity and extent of brain injury and even predicting the success of treatment decisions.

MRI

An imaging technique that does not involve ionizing radiation and that provides superb tissue contrast, MRI has become the neuroimaging method of choice for the comprehensive evaluation of AHT. In the past, access problems related to the availability of MRI devices and the difficulties of providing adequate physiological monitoring and life support for critically ill children in high magnetic field work areas limited MRI use in the acutely ill AHT victim; however, the documented enhancements in sensitivity and specificity of MRI neurodiagnosis have driven life support improvements such that early MRI for children with AHT may soon become the standard of care in the United States.

Magnetic resonance imaging is based on shifts in energy levels of unbalanced protons, principally hydrogen, when placed in a high magnetic field then

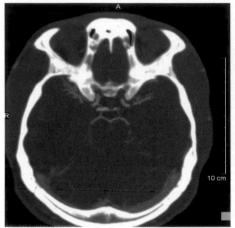
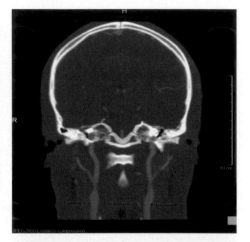
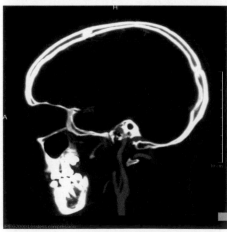

FIGURE 2.3
Axial-coronal-sagittal computed tomography arteriogram of the head and neck demonstrates normal arterial supply of the brain after intravenous contrast injection.

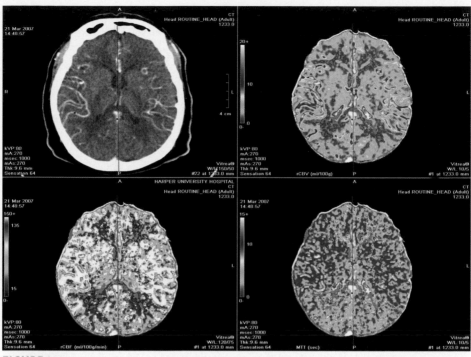

FIGURE 2.4
Computed tomography perfusion image after single intravenous injection of contrast with volumetric scanner shows cerebral blood volume, cerebral blood flow (mL/100 g/min), and mean transit time.

excited by radiofrequency energy. The excitement causes an energy field shift of the protons that in turn emit a signal that can be "read" according to certain temporal and spatial parameters. Varying the radiofrequency signal duration, repetition interval (TR) and the time at which one measures the signals from changed energy states (TE[time to echo]) gives a number of parameters (T1-weighted [T1W], T2-weighted [T2W], proton density) by which the tissues of the brain, spinal cord, and surrounding structures can be visualized. Although this is a gross oversimplification of MRI technology, it provides a framework to approach the enhancements in MRI described in this section.

Water, or more specifically the unbalanced hydrogen proton contained in water, predominates in the current clinical MRI neuroimaging. Two general types of tissue edema ("free water") are seen in AHT of the tissues of the brain, vasogenic (best seen on T2W) edema, and cytotoxic edema (best seen on diffusion-weighted imaging [DWI]). In general the former is reversible, while the latter implies cell death and is not reversible. Magnetic resonance imaging techniques for the diagnosis of brain tissue injury generally employ T2W sequences in a number of variations to show the edema associated with cell injury. T2-weighted imaging shows free water as white (by convention)

(Figure 2.5). A problematic limitation when imaging the brains of children younger than 6 months with T2W sequences is that babies have "wet brains" owing to physiologically incomplete myelin production. Neuronal myelination, virtually completed by age 3, is "hydrophobic" in that it decreases water content about the axons and facilitates visualization of edema. Special supplementary sequences such as DWI are needed to document injury in very young infants where the conventional "adult" sequences may be misleading. We now use DWI for all infants suspected of suffering brain injury (Box 2.1).

Blood contains hemoglobin and iron in various states of oxygenation and constitutes the other major component of AHT demonstrated by MRI. The sensitive detection of blood involves

techniques called *susceptibility imaging,* which takes advantage of gradient echo recall techniques emphasizing the magnetic susceptibility of protons and optimally visualizing tissue inhomogeneity[159] (Figure 2.6). These sequences are the most sensitive for detection of hemorrhage but are less specific for timing of hemorrhage. Magnetic resonance imaging dating of extra-axial bleeding depends on the degeneration of the hemoglobin-oxygen bond and the cellular integrity of the clot. There are a number of complexities that impact MRI dating including pulse sequences, magnet strength, and imaging plane. The original dating of hemorrhage work was done on an in-vitro model (Table 2.3); the results are still valid as a general rule, but there are sufficient exceptions that MRI dating of blood is still an area

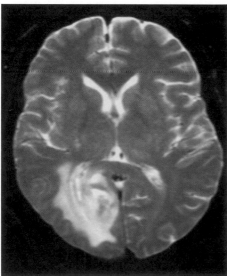

FIGURE 2.5
Axial T2-weighted image shows extensive vasogenic edema (white) within the occipital lobe on the right.

BOX 2.1
Age and Preference of Magnetic Resonance Imaging Techniques

Age <6 months
T1-weighted (inversion recovery) sagittal and axial
T2-weighted coronal
Diffusion-weighted imaging
Susceptibility-weighted imaging
Age >6 months
T1-weighted sagittal
T2-weighted axial and coronal
Fluid-attenuated inversion-recovery imaging
Susceptibility-weighted imaging
Diffusion-weighted imaging

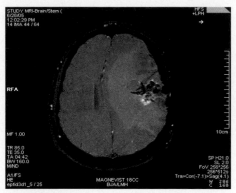

FIGURE 2.6
Susceptibility-weighted image shows
evidence of blood.

requiring expert consultation. Even in
expert hands, there are inherent limitations in the dating of hemorrhage by
MRI, in part due to mixing of blood
and CSF, layering, and loculation of
blood products.

Magnetic resonance imaging spectroscopy takes advantage of the chemical
properties of unpaired protons, particularly hydrogen, and presents a graphic
quantitative depiction of various chemical components of brain tissue (Figure
2.7). The limiting factor in the technique
is the ability to separate the chemical
components of the voxel of tissue in-

terrogated. This is a function of field
strength (the higher the better), the gradient sequencing, and the detector components of the scanner. The complexity
of the process has limited the usefulness of the data but the potential is
tremendous. Current work emphasizes
the area of the lactate peak as a predictor of poor outcome. Higher field magnets and better techniques will allow
splitting of tissue peaks, the one of
most immediate interest being for
AHT GLX (glutamine, glutamate, and
glutaric acid), compounds prominent
in hypoxic-ischemic brain injury as
measures of tissue damage.

Imaging Appearance of AHT Lesions

Subdural Hematoma

Subdural fluid collections occur
between the dura and the pia/arachnoid
membrane in a potential extra-axial
space. In AHT, the most common fluid
is blood, often in various stages of resolution. Subdural hematoma is the most
common single lesion identified in
AHT. While subdural hematoma can
occur after accidental trauma it is more
frequent with AHT.[15,67,160] Magnetic
resonance imaging is the most sensitive and specific test for the detection

TABLE 2.3
Magnetic Resonance Imaging Dating of Extra-Axial Bleeding

Time (d)	RBCs	Hemoglobin State	T1 Signal	T2 Signal
<1	Intact	Oxyhemoglobin	Iso/dark	Bright
0–2	Intact	Deoxyhemoglobin	Iso/dark	Dark
2–14	Intact	Methemoglobin (intracellular)	Bright	Dark
10–21	Lysed	Methemoglobin (extracellular)	Bright	Bright
>21	Lysed	Hemosiderin/ferritin	Iso/dark	Dark

Abbreviation: RBCs, red blood cells.

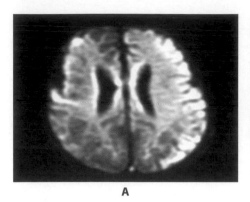 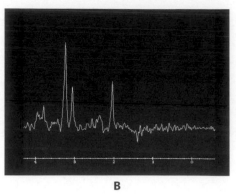

A   B

FIGURE 2.7
A. Diffusion-weighted image shows cytotoxic edema (white) within the left cerebral hemisphere. **B.** Magnetic resonance spectroscopy obtained from left cerebral hemisphere shows evidence of lactate (arrow) in a patient with non-accidental trauma; this indicates poor prognosis.

of subdural fluid collections, documenting 50% more than CT scan in the same patient population and detecting subdural hematomas in several instances where CT scans were even in retrospect normal.[157]

The imaging signs of subdural hematoma include a layer of fluid paralleling the dura-covered surfaces of the brain, usually with a convex configuration paralleling the course of the dura (Figure 2.8). Most subdural hematomas in AHT tend to be small and do not require neurosurgical drainage. The presence of the subdural hematoma is rather a "marker" of the trauma inflicted to the brain and its coverings.

Dating of subdural hemorrhage is complex. In general, on CT scans fresh subdural hemorrhage is high density for the first week after injury then becomes gradually more isodense with brain (gray) over the ensuing several weeks to 1 month and finally the blood

becomes low density, similar to CSF after 1 or 2 months (Figure 2.8A). Dating by MRI signal allows some refinement, particularly in the early stages after bleeding (Table 2.2); however, as noted in the technical discussion, there are a number of variables that can affect the appearance of the hemorrhage.[161]

Computed tomography scanning revolutionized the detection of subdural fluid collections. Since CT is not as specific as MRI in defining the subdural lesion, a number of confusing terms arose in the older literature. One such is the *benign subdural fluid of infancy*, a term that actually describes a large subarachnoid space, often associated with megalencephaly and not related to AHT. Although some controversy exists, there is evidence that a large subarachnoid space predisposes to subdural hematoma formation.[162]

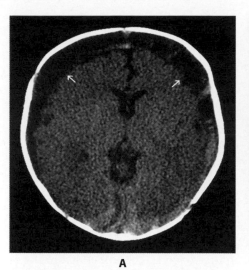
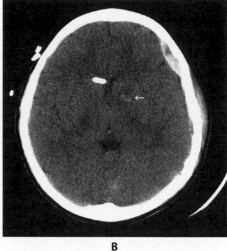

A   B

FIGURE 2.8
A. Axial computed tomography of the head shows acute and chronic bilateral subdural hematoma. **B.** Small left frontal acute subdural hematoma (black arrow) with hemorrhagic shearing injury to left internal capsule (white arrow).

Subdural bleeding is almost always venous in nature and therefore grows slowly. This allows the brain and fontanelles to accommodate, thereby allowing the subdural hemorrhage to become chronic and the head circumference to enlarge. Large chronic subdural hematomas are difficult to date precisely and may be relatively asymptomatic when discovered (Figure 2.9). There is some uncertainty regarding the extent to which a preexisting chronic subdural hematoma can predispose to re-hemorrhage with less trauma; the data in older adults (with atrophic brains) are suggestive and clinical experience suggests this sometimes occurs in children as well.

In the "hyperacute" subdural hematoma, seen very early after injury, the subdural hemorrhage appears mixed density (gray) on CT, and is sometimes

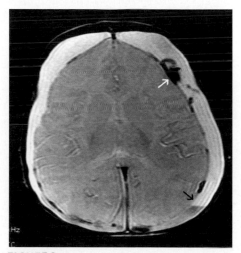

FIGURE 2.9
Gradient echo recall T2-weighted image shows large bilateral chronic subdural hematoma with new acute subdural hemorrhage on the left (black arrow) with blood sediment level.

a cause of confusion in timing.[163] The issue is easily resolved with either use of MRI or a close interval follow-up CT scan where the blood becomes more typical (white) in appearance.

Subarachnoid Hemorrhage

The pia-arachnoid are membranes that lie deep to the dura, although in the normal state the arachnoid parallels the dura creating a potential space while the pia covers the gyri of the brain. These membranes cannot be resolved by imaging and therefore are lumped into a single term: *subarachnoid space*. Subarachnoid bleeding (subarachnoid hemorrhage) is the second most common form of hemorrhage in AHT. Subarachnoid hemorrhage is diagnosed by either CT or susceptibility-weighted MRI as hemorrhage in the cisterns about the base of the brain or a hemorrhage conforming to the patterns of the gyri of the cerebral cortex (Figure 2.10). Unlike subdural hemorrhage, suba-rachnoid hemorrhage is rapidly re-sorbed, usually disappearing on CT scan within 2 to 3 days after the bleeding but detectable longer by susceptibility-weighted MRI.

Epidural Hematoma

The epidural hematoma is an infrequent AHT lesion and almost always implies direct contact impact, often but not always with associated skull fracture (Figure 2.11). Most epidural hematomas occur when a fracture traverses the course of an artery embedded in the inner surface of the skull causing bleeding into the potential space between the dura and the bone. The dura, being the periosteum of the skull, contains the hemorrhage, creating a convex hematoma that rapidly increases in size leading to mass effect on the brain. Epidural hematoma is the lesion classically described with a "lucid interval" where the victim originally suffers a concussion from the impact, briefly

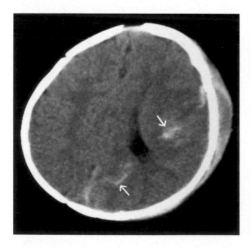

FIGURE 2.10
Multifocal contusions involving the left frontal and parietal lobe with evidence of subarachnoid hemorrhage (white arrow).

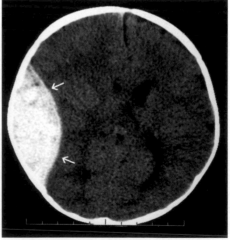

FIGURE 2.11
Axial computed tomography of the head demonstrates right frontal epidural hematoma with mass effect and midline shift to the left side.

recovers, then lapses again into coma owing to the mass effect of the growing hematoma. Surgical intervention is necessary in many but not all instances.

There is a variant of epidural hematoma that may be seen after relatively minor trauma, the venous epidural. In this instance the bleeding is slow and generally self-limited.

Parenchymal Brain Injuries

Contusions are direct impact injuries. If the contusion is associated with bleed-

ing, hemorrhagic contusion results and blood products are present on CT or MRI (Figures 2.12A and 2.12B). The symptoms of contusion depend on the severity, location, and associated injuries.

The tissues of the brain are of differing density and when associated with rapid deceleration tend to shear at the interfaces of zones of sharply differing tissue concentrations (Figure 2.12C). In animal models, high magnitude angular acceleration is the prototype mechanism

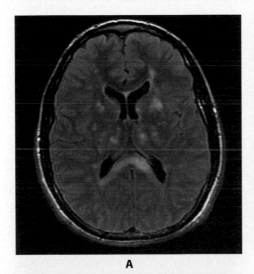

A

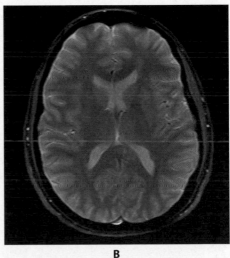

B

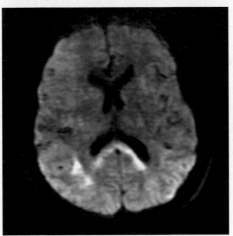

C

FIGURE 2.12
A. Axial flair T2-weighted image shows multiple foci of shearing injury. **B.** Axial gradient echo recall T2-weighted images obtained immediately after trauma demonstrates no obvious evidence of hemorrhage. **C.** Axial diffusion-weighted image of the brain shows diffusion restriction along the corpus callosum (black arrow) (shearing injury) and right posterior parietal subcortical white matter (white arrow) (contusion).

of injury for inflicting this shearing of tissue planes. Imaging shows these injuries as regions of edema or bleeding at the interface between the gray and white matter of the brain (Figure 2.13). Characteristic locations of shear injuries seen on imaging are at the peripheral edges of the centrum semiovale, corona radiata, pericallosal region, and the perithalamic region. Cerebellar and brain stem shearing are also possible. Historically, the hallmark of a shear injury was severe clinical symptoms of head injury that is out of proportion to the size of the apparent region of bleeding. With greater sensitivity of imaging, particularly with specific MRI sequences (susceptibility weighted imaging and FLAIR), these injuries can be detected in patients with milder clinical symptoms. Shearing injury evident by imaging is almost always rapidly symptomatic.

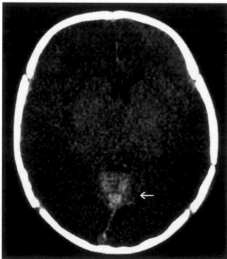

FIGURE 2.13
Diffuse low attenuation involving the bilateral frontal temporal parietal gray and white matter secondary to non-accidental trauma.

Hypoxic-ischemic injury is, unfortunately, the final pathway of many AHT injuries. The term *hypoxic-ischemic* stresses that these factors are generally interrelated; blood carries the tissue nutrient oxygen so that deprivation of either blood flow or deoxygenating of blood with normal flow can contribute to worsening of AHT. Although in some mechanisms of injury it is possible to identify predominantly ischemia or hypoxia, in most instances of AHT the mechanisms overlap and a combination of hypoxic and ischemic changes result. Increases in metabolic demand, as may occur with excitotoxic stress or seizures, may contribute to these findings even when substrate delivery would normally be sufficient. Diffuse hypoxic-ischemic injury is permanent and generally associated with a poor outcome. Computed tomography scanning shows diffuse cortical hypodensity, the "big black brain" (Figure 2.13), and diffusion sequences of MRI are most sensitive for defining the critically injured tissues[62] (Figures 2.14 and 2.15).

Magnetic resonance imaging spectroscopy demonstrating a large lactate peak predicts a poor outcome for the injured tissue. In a few days after the injury, CT scan may show enhanced gyral density in areas of injured cortex and T1W MRI will show high gyriform signal owing to cortical necrosis. These are irreversible processes with grave outcomes.

The imaging appearance of specific lesions must always be considered in conjunction with the clinical picture and history of injury to the child. In general, severe injuries present with

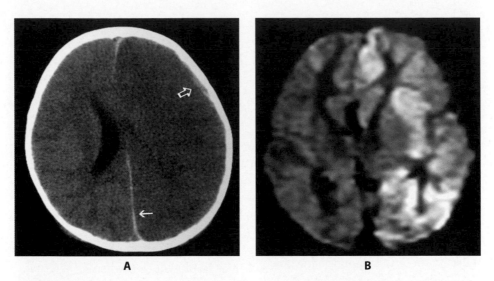

A   B

FIGURE 2.14
A. Axial computed tomography of head shows small left frontal and interhemispheric acute subdural hematoma with mass effect. **B.** Diffusion-weighted image demonstrates extensive diffusion restriction secondary to shearing injury of left frontal temporoparietal lobes.

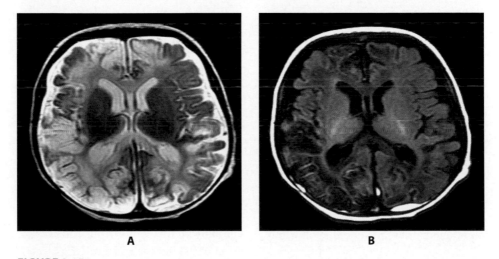

A   B

FIGURE 2.15
Shows extensive pseudo-laminar necrotic areas along the frontal temporoparietal lobes—this shows extensive areas of encephalomalacia and poor outcome. Magnetic resonance imaging is more sensitive and specific than computed tomography of the brain.

severe symptoms. It is unreasonable to believe that an infant with a fatal head injury was asymptomatic for a long time. In other instances only synthesis of the imaging, neurologic examination, and detailed history of trauma and child behavior will assist in timing the injury.[23,164]

Pathologic Features of Abusive CNS Trauma

The pathologist faced with postmortem evaluation of a victim of alleged abuse must approach this responsibility objectively. Before the examination is started, all investigative findings and available clinical records must be reviewed in detail, followed by a complete autopsy that includes a detailed and carefully documented external examination; radiologic studies (if they were not done previously); internal examination of body cavities and any soft tissue or bony injury; and a systematic study of the cranium and its contents, spine and cord, and eyes.

A decision relative to whether the allegation of abuse is valid can only be made after a series of questions is answered once these studies have been completed. These include the following:

1. Are the investigative findings consistent with the clinical and pathologic findings?
2. Is there clinical and/or pathologic evidence of a natural disease that could account for all findings?
3. If traumatic injury is present, could it have been accidental?

If the answer to these questions is negative, there is a high likelihood of abusive injury.

Examination of the CNS may be separated into 3 major divisions: external, internal, and microscopic. A detailed procedure for gross and microscopic examination of the CNS may be found in the article by Judkins et al[165] and, hence, will not be repeated here except to emphasize several issues.

Since bruises may not become apparent immediately, there may not be documentation of such injuries in the medical record. Further, it is important to note that injury to the deep tissues and skull may be present even when no external abnormality is identified. Finally, it cannot be too strongly emphasized that the technique for removal of the brain and spinal cord in continuity, as described in the article by Judkins et al,[165] should be followed in cases of alleged abuse. If this is not done, injury to the rostral cervical spinal cord and/or caudal medulla may be obscured.

Neuropathologic Features of Trauma

The CNS lesions to be described may occur consequent to both accidental and inflicted trauma. Hence the decision as to whether these injuries occurred because of an accident or were inflicted can only be made following consideration of the history and clinical aspects of the case. For example, if postmortem examination documents external head injuries, subdural hematoma, a swollen brain, and partial transection of the cervical spinal cord, and the pathologist is told that the 9-month-old decedent was thrown from a speeding automobile and struck a concrete abutment, a decision regarding the etiology of the injuries is not problematic. On the other hand, if the same combination of lesions is identified in a 5-month-old infant who was apparently well but who was said to have collapsed suddenly while at home, and died shortly thereafter in spite of vigorous treatment, there is a reasonable degree of medical certainty that these injuries are non-accidental or inflicted.

Whereas most fatally injured infants/children who have been victims of severe inflicted neurotrauma die shortly after their injury occurred, a small number survive for weeks, months, or even years. Hence lesions may be acute, subacute, or chronic.

External Injuries

External injuries of face, head, neck, and back may be absent altogether; subtle or striking; and include contusions, lacerations, and bruises (sometimes patterned), so-called black eye(s), lesions of 1 or both ears, or lesions behind the ears.[166] Injuries of the mouth may also include tears of the frenulum

or, if the victim has teeth and was smothered, bite marks of the mucosal surface of one or both cheeks may be present.[167]

Internal Soft Tissue Injury

As noted previously, internal soft tissue injury may be present, and in fact often is present even when there is no obvious external injury. Scalp hemorrhages may involve the deep layers of the scalp, galea, and periosteum (Figure 2.16). Uncommonly, the temporalis muscles may be injured. Hemorrhages into cervical musculature and soft tissue, or in the muscles of the back, are occasionally present in blunt trauma or severe whiplash injury. Periosteal hemorrhage is generally, but not necessarily, associated with a fracture.

Fractures

Uncomplicated, linear fractures may result from accidental falls, are not usually associated with significant cli-

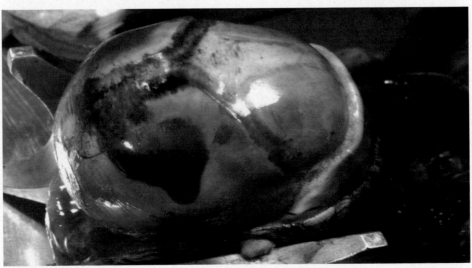

FIGURE 2.16
Skull of a 4-month-old infant showing striking diastasis of coronal and sagittal sutures and periosteal hematoma in midline/paramedian region.

nical problems, and do not require treatment.[168] In contrast, those occurring from serious accidental or inflicted trauma are often more severe. They develop when the victim's head is either struck forcefully by a hard object or is itself struck against the hard object. Frequency varies from 25% to 40% in victims of inflicted trauma.[59,169-171] Skull fractures are most commonly located in the parieto-occipital bones, but may be anywhere. The entire thickness of the skull is typically affected, but the fracture may be missed unless the dura is stripped. Massive brain swelling or, rarely, blunt trauma may lead to sutural diastasis, which should be distinguished from fractures (Figure 2.16). Fractures of the spine are rare, even in severe whiplash injury. If present, identification is facilitated by radiologic studies.

Intracranial Hemorrhage

Blood within the cranial cavity may be found in one or more "spaces," within brain parenchyma and/or the ventricles.

Epidural hemorrhage in the supratentorial epidural space is seen infrequently in inflicted CNS injury. Lateral blows to the head of infants/children that might be of sufficient strength to fracture the temporal bone are rare in abusive trauma, although fracture may not always be found in epidural hemorrhage in the young.[174] Epidural hemorrhage along the sagittal sinus is often seen and is usually associated with subdural hemorrhage. Epidural hemorrhages in the posterior fossa are typically associated with fracture of the occipital bone.[175] However, the most frequent sites of epidural hemorrhage in victims of inflicted CNS injury include rostral cervical levels and the region of the foramen magnum. Epidural hemorrhages may also be found if the victim has been subjected to blunt trauma at any level of the back (Figure 2.17). Care should be taken not to conclude that epidural hemorrhage at cervicothoracic levels is traumatic in origin if there is no other evidence of injury. Such hemorrhage may be found in young infants who have had severe cardiorespiratory dysfunction and results from back pressure and stasis of the venous system.

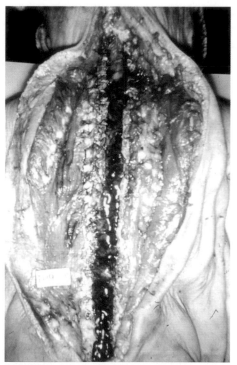

FIGURE 2.17
Extensive spinal epidural hemorrhage and cervical soft tissue hemorrhage in a traumatized infant.

Subdural Hematoma

The most characteristic postmortem finding in victims of inflicted neuro-trauma is subdural hemorrhage.[58,174,175] It is typically in a paramedian location at the vertex of the posterior frontal-parietal lobes, as well as in the inter-hemispheric region along the posterior falx cerebri. In most instances, the volume of blood is small and there is no necessity to treat this surgically (Figures 2.18 and 2.19). Blood may also pool on the floor of the skull. The blood in infants/children who die within a few days of the traumatic event is liquid or in the form of a dark, reddish-purple "currant jelly" clot. The color of this clot confirms its venous origin.

Although hemorrhage into the subdural space is almost always consequent to trauma, it may develop in infants who have a bleeding disorder, leukemia, met-abolic disorders, or rarely from a rup-tured vascular malformation.[176-184] In these situations, the hemorrhage is located in an atypical site (ie, it is not necessarily at the posterior paramedian cerebral vertex), a finding that should alert the prosector to consider the pos-sibility of a natural cause. Infants with bleeding disorders may not only have subdural hemorrhage, but there may be hemorrhage within cerebral paren-chyma, eyes, skin, soft issue, or other organs of the body. If such an infant is observed in the hospital to have new hemorrhages either in the intracranial/intraspinal regions or in other sites or organs, it is incumbent on the physi-cian to look vigorously for evidence of a non-traumatic etiology. In other words, infants whose injury occurred prior to hospitalization do not generally continue to bleed days later.

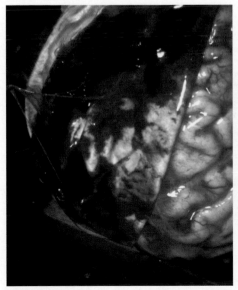

FIGURE 2.18
In situ brain with dura. The dura overlying the right hemisphere has been reflected to reveal presence of diffuse "currant jelly" clots.

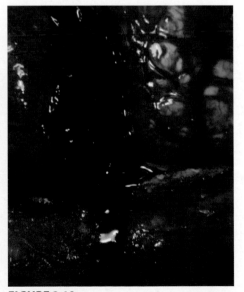

FIGURE 2.19
Brain in situ showing "currant jelly" clot in posterior interhemispheric fissure. Note severe venous congestion and cerebral swelling.

Most experts involved in diagnosis and treatment of victims of traumatic injury regard the hemorrhage into the subdural space to result from tearing of the bridging veins that normally enter the sinuses after leaving the brain parenchyma and subarachnoid space (Figure 2.20). Rarely, the source of blood may be a torn sinus. Hemorrhages may also be found within the leaves of the falx adjacent to the sinuses. The bridging veins are vulnerable to tearing because of a combination of anatomical and biomechanical factors called into play when trauma occurs.[172–174,180,184,185] These are outlined as follows: (1) the dura is firmly attached to the inner table of the skull and hence does not move, (2) the sinuses are located between the layers of the dura, (3) in order for the cerebral veins to drain into the sinuses they must leave the protection of the meninges and traverse the minimal "space" between the arachnoid and the sinus, (4) if there is no shift in the relationship of brain to sinus there is no problem. However, if a force is exerted on the head, the brain is free to move, whereas the sinuses are not: (5) movement of the brain places stress on the walls of the veins and subjects them to shearing forces causing tears. Whereas torn ends of veins are not easily identified during postmortem examination, neurosurgeons do observe them during surgical procedures.[186] Maxeiner[187] has outlined a technique that may be used to identify them postmortem as well.

It has been claimed by some that subdural hematomas result from hypoxia that initially produces bleeding within the dura that then leaks into the subdural space.[188] There is, however, no credible scientific evidence to support such an opinion. At the same time, however, intradural hemorrhage is frequently seen in infants with subdural hematoma.

If the victim survives the acute episode of bleeding, a membrane forms to encapsulate the hemorrhage. The mem-

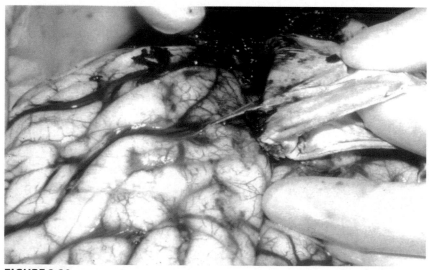

FIGURE 2.20
Brain of a 3-year-old girl with vertex dura and bridging vein showing cerebral contusions/lacerations. The child was beaten.

brane, by necessity, has 2 layers: an inner and outer membrane. The outer membrane adjacent to the dura is composed of fibrous granulation tissue, whereas the inner membrane adjacent to the arachnoid consists of denser fibrous tissue. The new vessels that form in the outer membrane are delicate structures, which, at times, may bleed without significant provocation. Such bleeds are rarely of clinical importance, although this mechanism is often cited to explain sudden collapse of an otherwise apparently well infant. In other words, it is claimed that an acutely neurologically decompensated infant with subdural hematoma actually sustained a primary injury days or weeks before the sudden collapse and that the current acute problem developed because of bleeding from a previously organized subdural hematoma.

Such arguments are untenable for several reasons. First, by its nature, a clinically silent subdural hemorrhage would not be large enough to produce a membrane with a luxuriant vascular growth that could subsequently lead to a subdural bleed of sufficient volume to manifest symptoms. Second, if the hemorrhage were of sufficient volume to become clinically apparent, the symptoms of increased ICP would develop over time and would be noticeable to the caretaker(s). If unattended to, the infant might then become unconscious, develop cardiorespiratory problems, and die. In that case, the postmortem examination would reveal the large, offending hematoma, evidence of mass effect causing compression of one cerebral hemisphere with uncal and para-hippocampal herniation, herniation of cerebellar tonsils, and brain stem swelling. Such findings, in fact, are exceedingly rare in infants in whom inflicted trauma is suspected. On the other hand, some children who sustain accidental trauma may die consequent to mass effect from a large, acute subdural hematoma.[32]

If the postmortem examination reveals presence of an organized subdural membrane without clinical evidence of an acute episode that might have produced a hematoma, there is no justification for assuming that the decedent, particularly if it is an infant, was victimized in the past. Small subdural and/or subarachnoid hemorrhages are not uncommon in association with vaginal deliveries, especially if forceps or vacuum extraction were used.

Subarachnoid Hemorrhage

Subarachnoid bleeding is almost universally found in fatal cases of inflicted neural trauma and in conjunction with subdural hematoma.[173] It may be located anywhere but is most common in the parasagittal region of the cerebral hemispheres or perivascularly (Figure 2.21). Subarachnoid hemorrhage may have various causes, such as a bleeding disorder, venous thrombosis, ruptured vascular malformation, or aneurysm (giant or mycotic). Distinguishing these conditions from trauma is not usually difficult except for the bleeding disorder, which may also be associated with subdural hematomas, as noted previously.

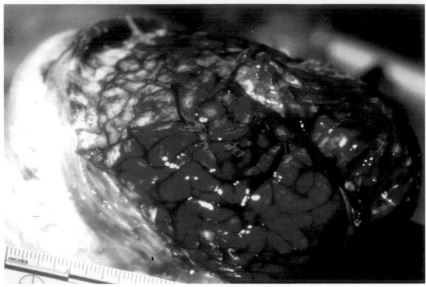

FIGURE 2.21
Extensive bilateral subarachnoid hemorrhage in a 3-month-old infant. Note bilateral, severe cerebral swelling.

Parenchymal/Intraventricular Hemorrhage

Isolated or large parenchymal or intra-ventricular hemorrhages, unassociated with other lesions suggestive of trauma, are generally caused by a bleeding disorder or rupture of a vascular malformation. If traumatic in origin, they are typically small, may be multiple, and occur in association with deep contusions or lacerations described as follows.

Vein of Galen Tears

Tears of the vein of Galen are rare but should be suspected when blood is pooled in the spaces around the pineal-brain stem tectal region. Some may pool around the lateral brain stem and dissect into the posterior (especially atrial) ventricular cavities. Documentation of such tears requires microscopic study of clots and structures in the area.

Contusions/Lacerations

Contusions/lacerations are by definition traumatic in origin and may be superficial and/or deep and single or multiple. Superficial contusions/lacerations caused by blunt trauma are generally located over the vertex and convexities of the cerebral hemispheres. They may be single or multiple and of varying ages as those shown in Figure 2.22.

Contusions/lacerations of the olfactory bulbs and tracts and underlying gyrus rectus are often seen in AHT. They are usually bilateral and associated with a small amount of free blood in the olfactory grooves.

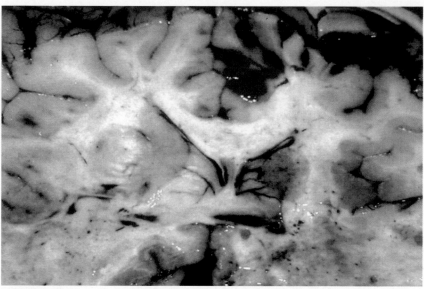

FIGURE 2.22
Coronal section through frontal lobes showing cerebral contusions and lacerations, subarachnoid hemorrhage plus hemorrhage into corpus callosum, deep white matter, and right caudate nucleus. Victim was 3 years old and severely beaten.

A typical coup contusion is often seen immediately beneath a fracture line. The mechanism for coup/contrecoup injuries in infants is similar to that in older children and adults. Specifically, superficial coup contusions are most obvious when a moving object strikes the stationary head, while a contrecoup injury in this circumstance is much less conspicuous or may be absent altogether; a fracture is not necessarily present. When the moving head strikes a blunt object (eg, if it is hit against a wall, table, or other hard object), the contrecoup contusion is larger or more prominent than the coup lesion.

The appearance is a function of the age of the lesion. Acute lesions are recognized by presence of hemorrhage into the tissue with or without swelling or pinkish discoloration. As the lesions age, the tissue begins to retract and the red hemoglobin is changed into hemosiderin, which changes the color to a golden hue. In the chronic stage it is typically a golden-brown color or may be bright yellow because of late transformation of the pigment into hematoidin (Figure 2.23).

The depth of a contusion cannot be discerned solely on external examination. Right-angled incisions are required to measure the depth accurately. The injury may involve deeper layers of the cortex or even extend into subcortical white matter (Figure 2.22).

Traumatic lesions that can only be identified when the brain is sectioned, or sometimes only on microscopic study, are consequent to shearing forces and tend to occur in particular sites, namely

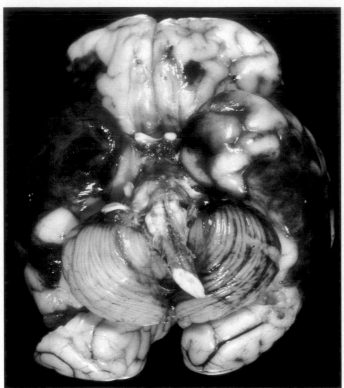

FIGURE 2.23
Basal view of a 2-month-old infant showing multiple contusions/lacerations of differing ages.

cerebral white matter, corpus callosum, internal capsule, brain stem and, less commonly, cerebellar white matter. Although rare, the ependyma may be torn, allowing ingress of fragmented brain tissue into the ventricular cavity where it may be seen on microscopic study, especially in the aqueduct, where it tends to get stuck. Otherwise, the deep traumatic injuries may be separated into 2 general groups: gliding contusions and axonal injury.

Gliding contusions/lacerations, well-described by Lindenberg and Freytag,[189] consist of dorsoventral slits in white matter, typically in the frontal lobes, although in severe cases they also occur more posteriorly. They are characteristically found in dorsal paramedian white matter and may have a hemorrhagic component, although if hemorrhage is present, it is not usually abundant (Figure 2.24). As noted, the acute lesions in infants generally consist of a dorsoventral slit in the white matter, with or without a small amount of hemorrhage. Microscopic features vary with the length of survival of the infant. If the lesion is less than 24 hours, only red blood cells and a few inflammatory cells are seen, but after a few days, the cellular reaction becomes more obvious and

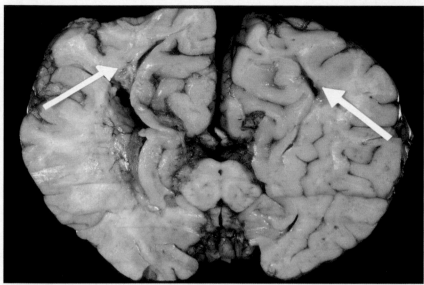

FIGURE 2.24
Coronal section of posterior parietal lobes of a 9-month-old who was repeatedly shaken by his mother. There are bilateral gliding contusions (white arrows), and the one on the left has torn the ependyma of the lateral ventricle.

consists of a mixture of mononuclear cells including lymphocytes and gitter cells with and without hemosiderin; astrocytes proliferate in the margins. The lesion in those who survive for months or years consists of a sharply defined cavity (Figure 2.25).

White matter lesions sometimes consist of acute swelling and necrosis of oligodendroglia, as manifested by pyknosis and karyorrhexis. Because edema is a frequent complication of craniocerebral trauma, it is unclear whether these findings are primarily traumatic or secondary.

Detection of callosal injury may be difficult if the victim has been maintained on a respirator for more than a day. Under the circumstances it is best to evaluate the callosum in situ by careful separation of the hemispheres and

examination of the structure to identify irregular tears with or without associated hemorrhage. Callosal tears are most frequently located in the posterior third of the body and splenium. If changes of respirator brain are advanced, it may not be possible to identify lesions, even if microscopic study is attempted. The term *respirator brain* is used to describe a postmortem state of the brain of individuals who have sustained global damage and have diminished or absent blood flow but who are maintained on a respirator for longer than 12 to 24 hours. Under these circumstances the tissue undergoes intravitam autolysis and becomes acidotic. Severity of the disintegration increases parallel with time on the respirator. If autolysis is advanced, microscopic evaluation, in particular, is compromised.

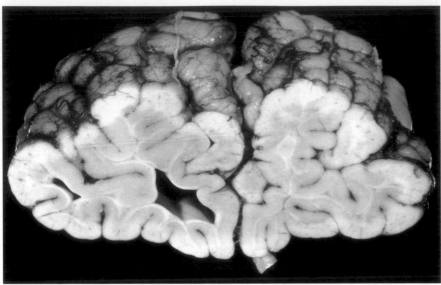

FIGURE 2.25
Coronal section through frontal lobes of a 4-year-old boy who was injured at 4 months of age. Note sharply demarcated cavity in white matter on the left.

Lesions of the callosum are best seen on coronal section of preserved specimens and vary from total transection to partial transection, the injury beginning dorsally and extending for a variable distance into the structure, to scattered hemorrhages, which may be oriented in a horizontal plane. The adjacent cingulate gyrus(i) is often contused as well (Figure 2.26). Microscopic study of the callosum is mandatory, especially of the midline and paramedian regions, even if nothing is seen on gross examination.

A contusional type of lesion that is easily missed unless carefully sought consists of incomplete subpial necrosis of the ventrolateral brain stem characterized by accumulation of lipid-laden macrophages and necrotic oligodendroglia with or without associated hemorrhage. Damage may extend for a variable distance into the parenchyma, in which case there is axonal injury

Shearing injury of axons may occur in one or more sites: the cerebral white matter and fiber tracts, including the corpus callosum, internal capsule and descending tracts in the brain stem, white matter of the spinal cord, and/or cranial and spinal nerve roots. Injury may or may not be visible grossly. It is most easily identified by the naked eye if there is a hemorrhagic component or by the presence of small tears.[59,60,190–192]

Primary traumatic lesions are typically localized to the upper, outer quadrant of the rostral pons at the level of the locus ceruleus and involve both axons and other tissue components. Axonal injury may be seen on routine hematoxylin-eosin (H & E)–stained sections by identification of small, eosinophilic,

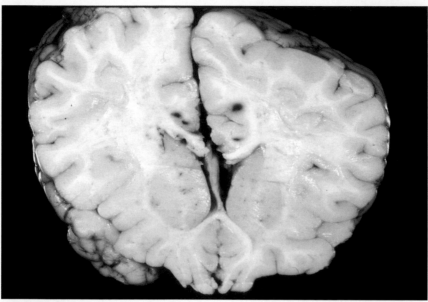

FIGURE 2.26
Coronal section through frontal lobes of a 1-year-old child who was struck repeatedly over the occiput. Note complete transection of corpus callosum and presence of small hemorrhages in that structure and dorsally placed cortex and white matter.

round structures called *retraction balls* (Figure 2.27). However, the extent of axonal damage is more accurately assessed if immunohistochemical tech niques for expression of ß-amyloid precursor protein (ß-APP) are used (Figure 2.28).

Axonal damage may result from causes other than trauma such as ischemia or even metabolic disturbances.[193] Distinction between traumatic versus non-traumatic axonal damage is sometimes difficult, especially if located in cerebral or cerebellar white matter, whereas it is less problematic in corpus callosum, fiber tracts, brain stem, spinal cord, and nerve roots, especially because these are unlikely sites of ischemic necrosis. It is important to note that axonal injury is not caused by tissue autolysis associated with the respirator brain phenomenon.

Spinal Injuries

In general, postmortem examination of the spinal cord is neglected unless there is a specific indication to examine it. When dealing with infants alleged to have been abused, such an omission is inexcusable, particularly because a component of the injury may be caused by spinal trauma. The role of injury to the brain stem and rostral cervical spinal structures in the clinical manifestations of AHT remain unclear, but may be significant. Lesions may include axonal tears of brain stem structures, contusions and lacerations of the spinal cord, avulsion of nerve roots, and tears of one or both vertebral arteries.

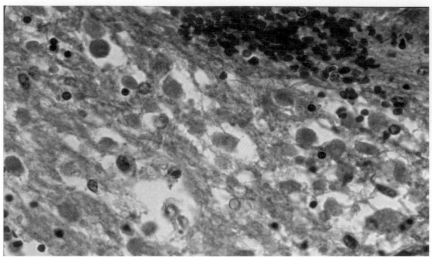

FIGURE 2.27
Photomicrograph of cerebral white matter of a severely battered 2-year-old girl
showing multiple retraction balls (hematoxylin-eosin stain x 250).

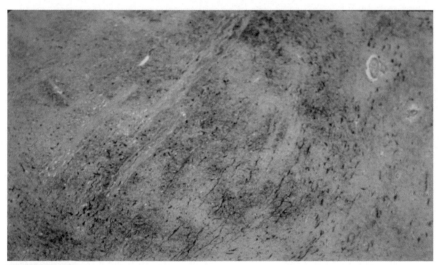

FIGURE 2.28
ß-amyloid precursor protein preparation of axonal injury in the midbrain of a
1-year-old infant (magnification x 250).

One hypothesized mechanism is that of a whiplash phenomenon.[59,169,173–175,192,194,195] It has long been known that the disproportionately heavy head of an infant must be supported until there has been sufficient growth and strengthening of spinal ligaments and cervical musculature to support it. The upper 2 cervical vertebrae are particularly mobile, and damage of the cervical spinal cord, for example, is a well-known sequela of hyperextension of the infant head in other situations, such as breech deliveries.[196]

It may be that forceful flexion in an impact scenario, distraction, or some other mechanism is at play in causing spinal injuries in AHT. Work in this area is ongoing.

In the setting of alleged abuse, a common report by the caretaker includes the statement that the infant had difficulty breathing and became limp. In some cases, the caretaker admits that this occurred after the infant was shaken, but more often there is no such admission. What is being described here may be the phenomenon of spinal shock, a phenomenon familiar to any biology student who has pithed a frog.[197]

The lesions that are seen in this region in association with AHT may be found in the pons, medulla, spinal cord, nerve roots (and ganglia), meningeal coverings, and/or one or both of the vertebral arteries (Figure 2.29). Fractures are rare, although subluxation probably occurs during the infliction of the injury. This, however, is not identifiable postmortem. There may be hemorrhage in cervical musculature and/or ligaments but this is an inconsistent finding.

Most frequent is meningeal hemorrhage, which may be epidural, intradural, subdural, and/or subarachnoid. Such hemorrhages typically accompany the damaged nerve roots that contain hemorrhage, and when studied for expression of beta APP, exhibit axonal damage (Figures 2.17 and 2.30). Hemorrhage is often also located in dorsal root ganglia.

The spinal cord injury varies from contusions/lacerations, often tissue fractures, to complete transection. Traumatic injury may involve several levels and must be distinguished from hypoxic-ischemic damage secondary to cardiorespiratory failure and shock (Figure 2.31).

It has been suggested that what appear to be traumatic spinal cord lesions are in reality secondary to compression of subarachnoid vasculature by fragments of necrotic and/or autolyzed cerebellum that may drift into both subarachnoid and subdural space when the victim has been maintained for some hours on a respirator. In this situation, the brain begins to autolyze and fragment. This assertion is untenable because the volume of displaced tissue is never great enough to fill the perispinal (cord) spaces and it is too soft to exert sufficient external pressure on the muscular arterial walls to compress them and thereby impede their flow. Moreover, these putative traumatic lesions are identified in sections containing no necrotic cerebellar tissue and, conversely, this type of spinal cord damage is not consistently found in cases containing an abundance of displaced cerebellar tissue.

Identification of the spinal injuries by gross and microscopic study is not challenging because the accompanying hemorrhages make them obvious. Occasionally retraction balls are identifiable with routine H & E stains, but confirmation of axonal injury in the cord and/or nerve roots rests on immunohistochemical techniques for identification of ß-APP antigen (Figure 2.32).

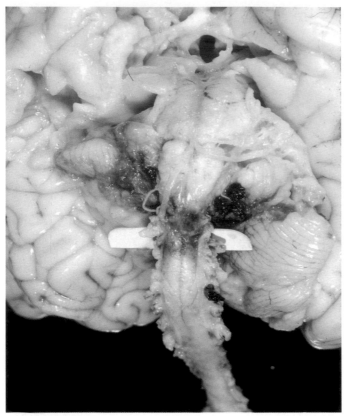

FIGURE 2.29
Acute hemorrhagic contusion/laceration of the cervico-medullary
region in a 3-month-old male.

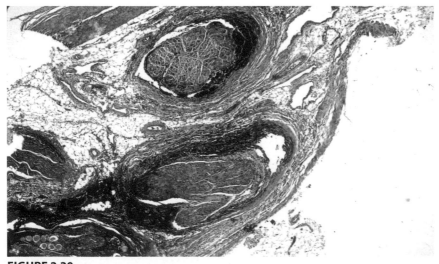

FIGURE 2.30
Photomicrograph of spinal nerve root injury in a 3-year-old girl. Note prominent
hemorrhage in the nerve and surrounding membranes (hematoxylin-eosin stain x 4).

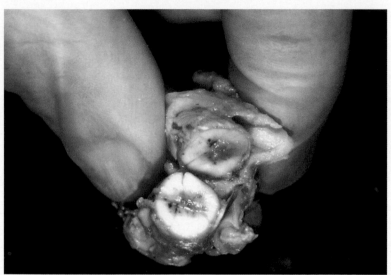

FIGURE 2.31
Transverse section of cervical spinal cord of a 2-year-old girl showing central contusion/laceration.

A unique spinal cord injury results when the primary force is applied to the top of the head, as when the victim is held by the feet or ankles and pounded against a hard surface, somewhat like a yo-yo. Damage of this type may also occur in older children or adults who dive into shallow water, striking the top of the head. The force generated on impact under these conditions moves from the vertex of the head directly into the spinal cord, producing a central cone-type contusion/laceration as it travels from cervical to lumbosacral levels. Other mechanisms of spinal injury include slamming the victim's back or coccyx against a tree, pole, or other hard object with sufficient force to fracture the spine and injure the spinal cord.

While autopsy series have found a high incidence of meningeal hemorrhage and root or cord injuries, MRIs in living children with AHT have rarely found evidence of spinal cord injury.[198] It is also uncommon to diagnose spinal cord injury on clinical grounds in children with AHT who survive, although milder injuries might be masked by the effects of intracerebral damage. Thus the role of these pathologic findings in understanding the mechanisms and pathophysiology of the AHT constellation remains an encouraging area for further investigation.

Brain Swelling

Unless the traumatized infant dies within 6 hours of injury, the likelihood of finding cerebral edema/swelling is high.[58,60] The cause is often multifactorial, and in the context of pediatric injury it has been called *malignant brain edema*.[199] The mechanisms involved are complex. Minns and Brown[183] provide a detailed, lucid discussion of this

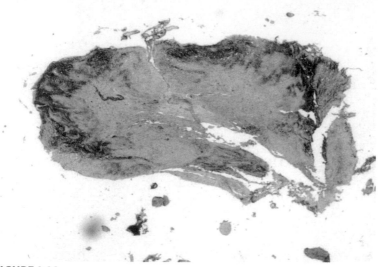

FIGURE 2.32
ß-amyloid precursor protein preparation of spinal cord of a 1-year-old infant. Note disruption of tissue and widespread peripheral expression of antigen (brown) (magnification x 1).

phenomenon, and reference to it is recommended.

Hypoxic-Ischemic Injury

Secondary hypoxic-ischemic lesions of the brain and/or spinal cord are common and have been found in at least three-quarters of abused infants/children.[60] At first glance, it might appear that identification and interpretation of these lesions is straightforward, whereas in reality, sorting out the range of abnormalities that fall under this general rubric is complex. These can be separated into several general categories, but by nature of the general pathophysiological features they overlap somewhat. For the purposes of this discussion they will be divided into 2 major groups: those that are primarily hypoxic and those that are primarily ischemic.

Hypoxic Lesions

Many children with AHT present with respiratory insufficiency, which causes a decrease in oxygen partial pressure (pO_2) in the blood and an increase in carbon dioxide partial pressure (pCO_2). This sets into motion a chain of events, one of the most important of which is the phenomenon of cerebral autoregulation.[200] The cerebral arteries dilate and capillaries open to allow for maximal flow to compensate for the lower oxygen concentration being delivered to the tissues. If this condition prevails for a time, the cardiac muscle is also deprived of oxygen and eventually begins to fail. This, in turn, leads to ischemia in both brain and heart (as well as other organs, of course), and tissue in-jury increases in severity. These events, resulting in cellular necrosis, precipitate swelling of damaged brain tissue, which can be diagnosed by neuroimaging studies.[22,202]

When abused infants come to post-mortem study, the brain (aside from whatever other abnormalities might be present) generally shows severe swelling, as manifested by gyral widening and flattening with associated effacement of sulci. It seems likely that respiratory insufficiency plays an important role in the pathogenesis of this brain swelling, although alternative mechanisms may also be responsible. Pressure cones are rarely seen in infants, presumably because the sutures are still open. There may, however, be obliteration of the cisterna magnum by swollen cerebellar tonsils, and the brain stem may be swollen, either because of primary injury or secondary to vascular compression. Durét hemorrhages do not occur in infants.

If the infant has been on a respirator, intravitam autolysis occurs and increases in severity commensurate with the length of time this is continued. In such instances, the pathologist is at a considerable disadvantage because the tissue becomes increasingly fragile and accurate microscopic study is seriously hindered. On the other hand, if tissue is sufficiently preserved, microscopic study assists in defining the damage, which varies in extent based on the severity of the hypoxia and subsequent ischemia and survival time.

In this connection, it may be pertinent to insert a discussion of primary hypoxic injury consequent to smothering as the mechanism of abuse. It is impossible to derive reliable statistics regarding the incidence of homicidal fatal smothering. Most such cases are placed in the category of sudden infant death syndrome (SIDS) because they typically exhibit no external evidence of trauma, and if the victim is edentulous, the possibility of mucosal trauma from teeth does not exist.[203] The general necropsy examination is typically negative, but careful examination of the brain may provide evidence of premortem asphyxia. Occasionally, however, a confession of smothering is obtained.[203]

Under the circumstances of homicidal smothering or severe asphyxia from any cause, the decreased pO_2 is associated with an increase in pCO_2 in the arterial blood. This calls into play autoregulatory mechanisms, which cause dilatation of the vascular bed. As long as the brain remains perfused, the gray matter then changes color from the usual light pink-gray color in the fresh state to one that varies in color from dark pink to purple, the intensity being a function of the severity of the asphyctic state. There may be some degree of associated brain swelling, but this is inconsistent. In addition, subarachnoid vasculature including the tiniest vessels and parenchymal vessels of both gray and white matter are prominent because of congestion (Figure 2.33).

Microscopic study may not be helpful if death occurs within a short time. On the other hand, acute neuronal necrosis may be identified in scattered sites, most typically in cerebellar Purkinje cells, neurons of the dentate nucleus, and/or pyramidal cells in the Sommer sector of the hippocampus. This combination of findings is not a feature of SIDS except possibly in the small number falling into the category of "near-miss SIDS" (ie, those who respond briefly to resuscitative efforts but who die a short time later).

Ischemic Lesions

Hypotensive brain stem necrosis falls into this category and is a condition that was described and named by Gilles[204] to reflect unique pathologic findings in individuals who experience profound shock and generally succumb in spite of a temporary response to resuscitation (Figure 2.34). In this circumstance, there is usually global necrosis, but the gross pathology of the brain stem is striking, being characterized by prominent duskiness of specific structures including inferior colliculi, pontine and medullary tegmentum, and olivary and dentate nuclei. It should not be confused with primary brain stem injury. Moreover, this pathologic picture is not unique to infants but may be seen at any age in consequence of the pathophysiological events noted above.

Extreme states of hypoxia-ischemia lead to frank infarction, pathologic features of which vary according to post-injury survival. The cellular reaction in the subacute stage may be confusing, particularly in infants, because such infarctive lesions often elicit a remarkable outpouring of fat-laden histiocytes (ie, gitter cells), which have occasionally suggested to the uninitiated the diagnosis of a histiocytosis.

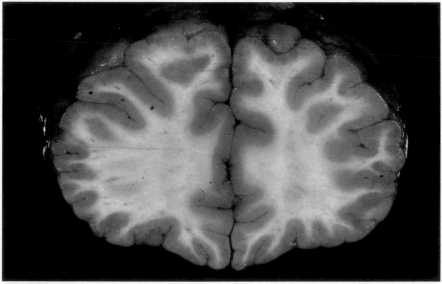

FIGURE 2.33
Coronal section through frontal lobes demonstrating bright dusky-pink color of gray matter, characteristic of acute asphyxia.

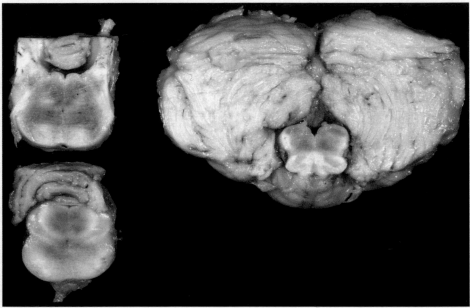

FIGURE 2.34
Three levels of brain stem demonstrating striking duskiness of tegmental tissues, characteristic of hypotensive brain stem necrosis.

Chronic Lesions

If the victim survives for months or years, the evidence of primary trauma is sometimes overshadowed by the secondary hypoxic-ischemic injury. However, subdural membranes or at least golden discoloration of the subdural surface, as well as pigmentary changes of leptomeninges, are often identifiable. If they are not grossly visible, iron deposition may be identified microscopically by use of a routine iron stain. At the same time, identification of iron in these tissues is not a sine qua non of inflicted trauma, particularly in a baby, because small hemorrhages are common in infants delivered by the normal vaginal route and in those delivered with the assistance of forceps or by vacuum extraction. Prematurely born infants are especially vulnerable to such small or even large hemorrhages, especially over the lateral temporal lobes.

It is difficult to identify retraction balls and damaged axons months or years after injury. Examples of chronic lesions are demonstrated in Figure 2.35.

Retinal and Optic Nerve Lesions

Although there is considerable debate regarding pathogenesis of retinal and optic nerve lesions, which are primarily hemorrhagic in nature, the fact remains that such lesions are common in infants who are considered to be victims of inflicted neurotrauma.[205-207] Discussion of various arguments relating to this issue

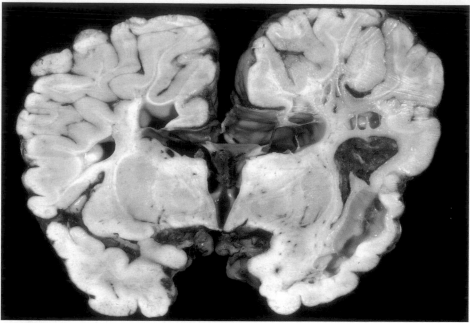

FIGURE 2.35
Coronal section through the mid-hemispheric level of brain. Note destruction of corpus callosum, reduction in volume of cerebral white matter with cysts, and patchy cortical sclerosis.

can be gleaned from the references and will not be discussed. Instead, focus is directed to the purely pathologic aspects of these lesions.

As noted in the article by Judkins et al,[165] the postmortem examination must include a thorough examination of the optic nerves and their coverings, soft tissue of the orbits, eye muscles, and external and internal features of the globe. Examination of these structures in situ most commonly reveals hemorrhage along the epidural and subdural regions of the nerve. This typically begins at the junction of the optic nerve and globe and extends for a variable distance posteriorly (ie, toward the brain). In some cases there is hemorrhage in soft tissue around the globe. In those who die shortly after the injury, the blood is red, but in those who survive for weeks or months, the characteristic rust color of hemosiderin or even the yellow of hematoidin is found (Figure 2.36).

Microscopic study of the nerve and its covering must include both cross-section and longitudinal section. Whereas hemorrhage is most commonly subdural and intradural, it may also be found clinging to the epidural surface and/or in the subarachnoid space (Figure 2.37). Rarely, there is injury to the nerve itself, with or without hemorrhage.

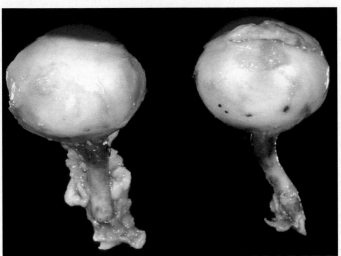

FIGURE 2.36
Eyes with optic nerves showing hemorrhage at junction of the
nerve with the globe and extension posteriorly (toward the brain).

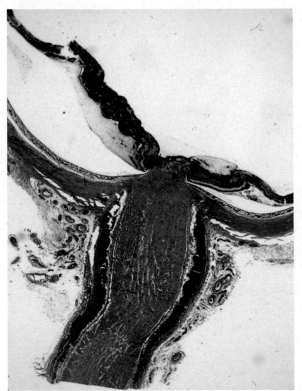

Gross examination of the
globe itself allows identification of vitreous and retinal
hemorrhages, or retinal tears.
These lesions are identified
without difficulty on microscopic study, which allows
more precise localization
in terms of the distribution
(ie, which retinal layers are
involved and the anterior
extent toward the ora serrata
from the optic disc).

If the victim survives for
weeks or months, these lesions
undergo organization of the
hemorrhage and scarring of
the retina.

FIGURE 2.37
Photomicrograph of optic nerve at its entrance into the
globe of a 5-month-old boy. Note subdural/intradural
hemorrhage adjacent to the nerve and prominent
retinal hemorrhage (hematoxylin-eosin stain x 4).

Closing Comments

There is a considerable body of forensic documentation of all of the lesions described herein in infants whose clinical history is discordant with the postmortem findings and who are therefore considered to be victims of inflicted trauma.[207] If careful investigation has excluded the presence of a bleeding disorder or other natural disease, it is reasonable to conclude that the findings are traumatic in origin. It was noted at the outset that one or more of the lesions may be a consequence of accidental trauma, in which case a straightforward history is typically available and the suspicion of inflicted trauma is a non-issue. In spite of these facts, there are those who suggest a variety of other causes for the characteristic constellation of clinical and pathologic findings, most of which enjoy no scientific credibility.

References

1. Kempe CH, Silverman FN, Steele BF, Droegmueller W, Silver HK. The battered-child syndrome. *JAMA.* 1962;181:105–112

2. Caffey J. The whiplash shaken infant syndrome: manual shaking by the extremities with whiplash-induced intracranial and intraocular bleedings, linked with residual permanent brain damage and mental retardation. *Pediatrics.* 1974;54:396–403

3. Ludwig S, Warman M. Shaken baby syndrome: a review of 20 cases. *Ann Emerg Med.* 1984;13:104–107

4. Gaynon MW, Koh K, Marmor MF, Frankel LR. Retinal folds in the shaken baby syndrome. *Am J Ophthalmol.* 1988;106:423–425

5. Bruce DA, Zimmerman RA. Shaken impact syndrome. *Pediatr Ann.* 1989;18:482–489

6. Barlow KM, Minns RA. Annual incidence of shaken impact syndrome in young children. *Lancet.* 2000;356:1571–1572

7. Jayawant S, Rawlinson A, Gibbon F, et al. Subdural haemorrhages in infants: population based study. *BMJ.* 1998;317:1558–1561

8. Keenan HT, Runyan DK, Marshall SW, Nocera MA, Merten DF, Sinal SH. A population-based study of inflicted traumatic brain injury in young children. *JAMA.* 2003;290:621–626

9. Hobbs C, Childs AM, Wynne J, Livingston J, Seal A. Subdural haematoma and effusion in infancy: an epidemiological study. *Arch Dis Child.* 2005;90:952–955

10. Sills MR, Libby AM, Orton HD. Pre-hospital and in-hospital mortality. A comparison of intentional and unintentional traumatic brain injuries in Colorado children. *Arch Pediatr Adolesc Med.* 2005;159:665–670

11. Sun DTF, Zhu XL, Poon WS. Non-accidental subdural haemorrhage in Hong Kong: incidence, clinical features, management and outcome. *Childs Nerv Syst.* 2006;22:593–598

12. Klein M, Stern L. Low birth weight and the battered child syndrome. *Am J Dis Child.* 1971;122:15–18

13. Sills JA, Thomas LJ, Rosenbloom L. Non-accidental injury: a two-year study in Central Liverpool. *Dev Med Child Neurol.* 1977;19:26–33

14. Hunter RS, Kilstron N, Kraybill EN, Loda F. Antecedents of child abuse and neglect in permature infants: a prospective study in a newborn intensive care unit. *Pediatrics.* 1978;61:629–635

15. Dashti SR, Decker DD, Razzaq A, Cohen AR. Current pattern of inflicted head injury in children. *Pediatr Neurosurg.* 1999;31:302–306

16. Schnitzer PG, Ewigman BG. Child deaths resulting from inflicted injuries: household risk factors and perpetrator characteristics. *Pediatrics.* 2005;116:e87–e693

17. Starling SP, Holden JR, Jenny C. Abusive head trauma: the relationship of perpetrators to their victims. *Pediatrics.* 1995;95:259–262

18. Duhaime AC, Gennarelli TG, Thibault LE, Bruce DA, Margulies SS, Wiser R. The shaken baby syndrome. A clinical, pathological, and biomechanical study. *J Neurosurg.* 1987;66:409–415

19. Meservy CJ, Towbin R, McLaurin RL, Myers PA, Ball W. Radiographic characteristics of skull fractures resulting from child abuse. *Am J Radiol.* 1987;149:173–175

20. Alexander R, Sato Y, Smith W, Bennett T. Incidence of impact trauma with cranial injuries ascribed to shaking. *Am J Dis Child.* 1990;144:724–726

21. Hettler J, Greenes DS. Can the initial history predict whether a child with a head injury has been abused? *Pediatrics.* 2003;111:602–607

22. Johnson DL, Boal D, Baule R. Role of apnea in nonaccidental head injury. *Pediatr Neurosurg.* 1995;23:305–310

23. Rubin DM, Christian CW, Bilaniuk LT, Zazyczny KA, Durbin DR. Occult head injury in high-risk abused children. *Pediatrics.* 2003;111:1382–1386

24. Laskey AL, Holsti M, Runyan DK, Socolar RS. Occult head trauma in young suspected victims of physical abuse. *J Pediatr.* 2004;144:719–722

25. Helfer RE, Slovis TL, Black MB. Injuries resulting when small children fall out of bed. *Pediatrics.* 1977;60:533–535

26. Nimityongskul P, Anderson L. The likelihood of injuries when children fall out of bed. *J Pediatr Orthop.* 1987;7:184–186

27. Hall JR, Reyes HM, Worvat M, Meller JL, Stein R. The mortality of childhood falls. *J Trauma.* 1989;29:1273–1275

28. Musemeche CA, Barthel M, Cosentino C, Reynolds M. Pediatric falls from heights. *J Trauma.* 1991;31:1347–1349

29. Reiber GD. Fatal falls in childhood. How far must children fall to sustain fatal head injury? Report of cases and review of the literature. *Am J Forensic Med Pathol.* 1993;14:201–207

30. Chiaviello CT, Christoph RA, Bond GR. Stairway-related injuries in children. *Pediatrics.* 1994;94:679–681

31. Tarantino CA, Dowd MD, Murdock TC. Short vertical falls in infants. *Pediatr Emerg Care.* 1999;15:5–8

32. Plunkett J. Fatal pediatric head injuries caused by short-distance falls. *Am J Forensic Med Pathol.* 2001;22:1–12

33. Johnson K, Fischer T, Chapman S, Wilson B. Accidental head injuries in children under 5 years of age. *Clin Radiol.* 2005;60:464–468

34. Weber W. Experimental studies of skull fractures in infants [in German]. *Z Rechtsmed.* 1984;92:87–94

35. Greenes DS, Schutzman SA. Infants with isolated skull fracture: what are their clinical characteristics, and do they require hospitalization? *Ann Emerg Med.* 1997;30:253–259

36. Shugerman RP, Paez A, Grossman DC, Feldman KW, Grady MS. Epidural hemorrhage: is it abuse? *Pediatrics.* 1996;97:664–668

37. Durham S, Clancy RR, Leuthardt E, et al. CHOP Infant Coma Scale ("Infant Face Scale"): a novel coma scale for children less than two years of age. *J Neurotrauma.* 2000;17:729–737

38. Harcourt B, Hopkins D. Ophthalmic manifestations of the battered-baby syndrome. *Br Med J.* 1971;3:398–401

39. Gilles EE, McGregor ML, Levy-Clark G. Retinal hemorrhage asymmetry in inflicted head injury: a clue to pathogenesis? *J Pediatr.* 2003;143:494–499

40. Duhaime AC, Alario AJ, Lewander WJ, et al. Head injury in very young children: mechanism, injury types, and ophthalmologic findings in 100 hospitalized patients younger than 2 years of age. *Pediatrics.* 1992;90:179–185

41. Christian C, Taylor AA, Hertle R, Duhaime AC. Retinal hemorrhages due to accidental household trauma. *J Pediatr.* 1999;135:125–127

42. Greenwald MJ, Weiss A, Oesterle CS, Friendly DS. Traumatic retinoschisis in battered babies. *Ophthalmology.* 1986;93:618–625

43. Morad Y, Kim YM, Armstrong DC, Huyer D, Mian M, Levin AV. Correlation between retinal abnormalities and intracranial abnormalities in the shaken baby syndrome. *Am J Ophthalmol.* 2002;134:354–359

44. Lantz PF, Sinal SH, Stanton CA, Weaver RG. Perimacular folds from childhood head trauma. *Br Med J.* 2004;328:754–756

45. Hymel KP, Abshire TC, Luckey DW, Jenny C. Coagulopathy in pediatric abusive head trauma. *Pediatrics.* 1997;99:371–375

46. Cho D, Wang Y, Chi C. Decompressive craniotomy for acute shaken/impact baby syndrome. *Pediatr Neurosurg.* 1995;23:192–198

47. Keenan HT, Nocera M, Bratton SL. Frequency of intracranial pressure monitoring in infants and young toddlers. *Pediatr Crit Care Med.* 2005;6:537–541

48. Duhaime AC. Do we and should we monitor intracranial pressure in infants with closed head injury? *Pediatr Crit Care Med.* 2005;6:611–612

49. Duhaime AC, Durham S. Traumatic brain injury in infants: the phenomenon of subdural hemorrhage with hemispheric hypodensity ("big black brain"). *Prog Brain Res.* 2007;161:293–302

50. Duhaime AC, Christian C, Moss E, Seidl T. Long-term outcome in children with the shaking-impact syndrome. *Pediatr Neurosurg.* 1996;24:292–298

51. Graupman P, Winston KR. Nonaccidental head trauma as a cause of childhood death. *J Neurosurg.* 2006;104:245–250

52. Jensen FE. Developmental factors regulating susceptibility to perinatal brain injury and seizures. *Curr Opin Pediatr.* 2006;18:628–633

53. Gilles EE, Nelson MD Jr. Cerebral complications of nonaccidental head injury in childhood. *Pediatr Neurol.* 1998;19:119–128

54. Dias MS, Backstrom J, Falk M, Li V. Serial radiography in the infant shaken impact syndrome. *Pediatr Neurosurg.* 1998;29:77–85

55. Ewing-Cobbs L, Prasad M, Kraer L, Landry S. Inflicted traumatic brain injury: relationship of developmental outcome to severity of injury. *Pediatr Neurosurg.* 1999;31:251–258

56. Ewing-Cobbs L, Kramer L, Prasad M, et al. Neuroimaging, physical, and developmental findings after inflicted and noninflicted traumatic brain injury in young children. *Pediatrics.* 1998;102:300–307

57. Bonnier C, Nassagne MC, Evrard P. Outcome and prognosis of whiplash shaken infant syndrome: late consequences after a symptom-free interval. *Dev Med Child Neurol.* 1995;37:943–956

58. Duhaime AC, Christian CW, Rorke LB, Zimmerman RA. Nonaccidental head injury in infants—the "shaken baby syndrome". *N Engl J Med.* 1998;338:1822–1829

59. Geddes JF, Hackshaw AK, Vowles GH, Nickols CD, Whitwell HL. Neuropathology of inflicted head injury in children. I. Patterns of brain damage. *Brain.* 2001;124:1290–1298

60. Geddes JF, Hackshaw AK, Vowles GH, Nickols CD, Whitwell HL. Neuropathology of inflicted head injury in children. II. Microscopic brain injury in infants. *Brain.* 2001;124:1299–1306

61. Whyte KM, Pascoe M. Does "black" brain mean doom? Computed tomography in the prediction of outcome in children with severe head injuries: "benign" vs "malignant" brain swelling. *Australas Radiol.* 1989;33:344–347

62. Ichord R, Naim M, Pollock A, Nance ML, Margulies S, Christian CW. Hypoxic-ischemic injury complicates inflicted and accidental traumatic brain injury in young children: the role of diffusion weighted imaging. *J Neurotrauma.* 2007;24:106–118

63. Raimondi AJ, Hirschauer J. Head injury in the infant and toddler. Coma scoring and outcome scale. *Childs Brain.* 1984;11:12–35

64. Yager JY, Johnston B, Seshia SS. Coma scales in pediatric practice. *Am J Dis Child.* 1990;144:1088–1091

65. Simpson DA, Cockington RA, Hanieh A, Raftos J, Reilly PL. Head injuries in infants and young children: the value of the Paediatric Coma Scale. *Childs Nerv Syst.* 1991;7:183–190

66. Hymel KP, Bandak FA, Partington MP, Winston KR. Abusive head trauma? A biomechanics-based approach. *Child Maltreat.* 1998;3:116–128

67. Reece RM, Sege R. Childhood head injuries: accidental or inflicted? *Arch Pediatr Adolesc Med.* 2000;154:11–15

68. Pierce MC, Bertocci G, Berger RP, Vogeley E. Injury biomechanics for aiding in the diagnosis of abusive head trauma. *Neurosurg Clin North Am.* 2002;13:155–168

69. McNeely PD, Atkinson JD, Saigal G, et al. Subdural hematomas in infants with benign enlargement of the subarachnoid spaces are not pathognomonic for child abuse. *AJNR Am J Neuroradiol.* 2006;27:1725–1728

70. Menezes A, Smith D, Dell W. Posterior fossa hemorrhage in the term neonate. *Neurosurgery.* 1983;13:452–456

71. Raghupathi R, Mehr MF, Helfaer MA, Margulies SS. Traumatic axonal injury is exacerbated following repetitive closed head injury in the neonatal pig. *J Neurotrauma.* 2004;21:307–316

72. Duhaime AC, Margulies SS, Durham SR, et al. Maturation-dependent response of the piglet brain to scaled cortical impact. *J Neurosurg.* 2000;93:455–462

73. Prange MT, Margulies SS. Regional, directional, and age-dependent properties of the brain undergoing large deformation. *J Biomech Eng.* 2002;124:244–252

74. Prange MT, Coats B, Duhaime AC, Margulies SS. Anthropomorphic simulations of falls, shakes, and inflicted impacts in infants. *J Neurosurg.* 2003;99:143–150

75. Gilliland MGF, Folberg R. Shaken babies—some have no impact injuries. *J Forensic Sci.* 1996;41:114–116

76. Hadley MN, Sonntag VKH, Rekate HL, Murphy A. The infant whiplash-shake syndrome: a clinical and pathological study. *Neurosurgery.* 1989;24:536–540

77. Duhaime AC, Christian C, Armonda R, Hunter J, Hertle R. Disappearing subdural hematomas in children. *Pediatr Neurosurg.* 1996;25:116–122

78. Ricci L, Giantris A, Merriam P, Hodge S, Doyle T. Abusive head trauma in Maine infants: medical, child protective, and law enforcement analysis. *Child Abuse Negl.* 2003;27:271–283

79. Alexander R, Crabbe L, Sato Y, Smith W, Bennett T. Serial abuse in children who are shaken. *Am J Dis Child.* 1990;144:58–60

80. Jenny C, Hymel KP, Ritzen A, Reinert SE, Hay TC. Analysis of missed cases of abusive head trauma. *JAMA.* 1999;281:621–626

81. Jaspan T, Griffiths PD, McConachie NS, Punt JA. Neuroimaging for non-accidental head injury in childhood: a proposed protocol. *Clin Radiol.* 2003;58:44–53

82. Atwal GS, Rutty GN, Carter N, Green MA. Bruising in non-accidental head injured children; a retrospective study of the prevalence, distribution and pathological associations in 24 cases. *Forensic Sci Int.* 1998;96:215–230

83. Rivara FP, Alexander B, Johnston B, and Soderberg R. Population-based study of fall injuries in children and adolescents resulting in hospitalization or death. *Pediatrics.* 1993;92:61–63

84. Tarantino CA, Dowd MD, Murdock TC. Short vertical falls in infants. *Pediatr Emerg Care.* 1999;15:5–8

85. Annobil SH, Binitie B, Ranganayakulu Y, Ogunbiyi O, Al-Malki T, Bassuni W. A hospital-based study of falls from heights in children in southwestern Saudi Arabia. *Saudi Med J.* 1995;16:133–138

86. Chadwick DL, Salerno C. Falls in day care [letter]. *J Trauma.* 1993;35:968

87. Joffe M, Ludwig S. Stairway injuries in children. *Pediatrics.* 1988;82:457–461

88. Kravitz H, Criessen C, Gomberg R, Korach A. Accidental falls from elevated surfaces in infants from birth to one year of age. *Pediatrics.* 1969;44:869–876

89. Lehman D, Schonfeld N. Falls from heights: a problem not just in the northeast. *Pediatrics.* 1993;92:121–124

90. Lyons T, Oates RK. Falling out of bed: a relatively benign occurrence. *Pediatrics.* 1993;92:125–127

91. Haviland J, Russell RIR. Outcome after severe non-accidental head injury. *Arch Dis Child.* 1997;77:504–507

92. Williams RA. Injuries in infants and small children resulting from witnessed and corroborated free falls. *J Trauma.* 1991;31:1350–1352

93. Selbst SM, Baker MD, Shames M. Bunk bed injuries. *Am J Dis Child.* 1990;144:721–723

94. Mayr J, Gaisl M, Purtscher K, et al. Baby walkers—an underestimated hazard for our children? *Eur J Pediatr.* 1994;153:531–534

95. Chiavello CT, Christoph RA, Bond GR. Infant walker-related injuries: a prospective study of severity and incidence. *Pediatrics.* 1994;93:974–976

96. Smith GA, Bowman MJ, Luria JW, Shields BJ. Babywalker-related injuries continue despite warning labels and public education. *Pediatrics.* 1997;100:e1

97. Mayr J, Gaisl M, Purtscher K, et al. Baby walkers—an underestimated hazard for our children? *Eur J Pediatr.* 1994;153:531–534

98. Reece RM. Differential diagnosis of inflicted childhood neurotrauma. In: Reece RM and Nicholson CE, eds. *Inflicted Childhood Neurotrauma.* Elk Grove Village, IL: American Academy of Pediatrics; 2003:17–31

99. Barlow B, Niemirska M, Gandhi RP, Leblanc W. Ten years of experience with falls from a height in children. *J Pediatr Surg.* 1991;31:1353–1355

100. Smith MD, Burrington JD, Woolf AD. Injuries in children sustained in free falls: an analysis of 66 cases. *J Trauma.* 1975;15:987–991

101. DiScala C, Sege R, Li G, Reece RM. Child abuse and unintentional injuries: a 10-year retrospective. *Arch Pediatr Adolesc Med.* 2000;154:16–22

102. Billmire M, Myers PA. Serious head injury in infants: accident or abuse? *Pediatrics.* 1985;75:340–342

103. Greenes DS, Schutzman SA. Occult intracranial injury in infants. *Ann Emerg Med.* 1988;32:680–686

104. Bernard PA, Johnston C, Curtis SE, et al. Toppled television sets cause significant pediatric morbidity and mortality. *Pediatrics.* 1998;102:e32

105. Duhaime AC, Eppley M, Margulies S, et al. Crush injuries to the head in children. *Neurosurgery.* 1995;37:401–407

106. Bechtel K, Stoessel K, Leventhal JM, et al. Characteristics that distinguish accidental from abusive injury in hospitalized young children with head trauma. *Pediatrics.* 2004;114:165–168

107. Ettaro L, Berger RP, Songer T. Abusive head trauma in young children: characteristics and medical charges in a hospitalized population. *Child Abuse Negl.* 2004;28:1099–1111

108. Vinchon M, Defoort-Dhellemmes S, Desurmont M, Dhellemmes P. Accidental and non-accidental head injuries in infants: a prospective study. *J Neurosurg.* 2005;31:302–306

109. Levin AV. Retinal haemorrhage and child abuse. In: David TJ, ed. *Recent Advances in Paediatrics.* Edinburgh, UK: Churchill Livingstone; 2000:151–220

110. Johnson DL, Braun D, Friendly D. Accidental head trauma and retinal hemorrhage. *Neurosurgery.* 1993;33:231–234; discussion 234–235

111. Wygnanski-Jaffe T, Levin AV, Shafiq A, Smith C, Enzenauer RW, Elder JE, et al. Postmortem orbital findings in shaken baby syndrome. *Am J Ophthalmol.* 2006;142:233–240

112. Budenz DL, Farber MG, Mirchandani HG, Park H, Rorke LB. Ocular and optic nerve hemorrhages in abused infants with intracranial injuries. *Ophthalmology.* 1994;101:559–565

113. Tung GA, Kumar M, Richardson RC, Jenny C, Brown WD. Comparison of accidental and nonaccidental traumatic head injury in children on noncontrast computed tomography. *Pediatrics.* 2006;118:626–633

114. Hymel KP, Jenny C, Block RW. Intracranial hemorrhage and rebleeding in suspected victims of abusive head trauma: addressing the forensic controversies. *Child Maltreat.* 2002;7:329–348

115. Rauschschwalbe R, Mann NC. Pediatric window-cord strangulations in the United States, 1981–1995. *JAMA.* 1997;277:1696–1698

116. Drago DA, Winston FK, Baker SP. Clothing drawstring entrapment in playground slides and school buses. *Arch Pediatr Adolesc Med.* 1997;151:72–77

117. Drago DA, Dannenberg AL. Infant mechanical suffocation deaths in the United States, 1980–1997. *Pediatrics.* 1999;103:e59

118. Akman CI, Cracco J. Intrauterine subdural hemorrhage. *Dev Med Child Neurol.* 2000;42:843–846

119. Towner C, Castro M, Eby-Wilkins E, Gilbert W. Effect of the mode of delivery in nulliparous women on neonatal intracranial injury. *N Engl J Med.* 1999;341:1709–1714

120. Whitby EH, Griffiths PD, Rutter S, et al. Frequency and natural history of subdural haemorrhages in babies and relation to obstetric factors. *Lancet.* 2004;363:846–851

121. Egge K, Lyng G, Maltau JM. Effect of instrumental delivery on the frequency and severity of retinal hemorrhages in the newborn. *Acta Obstet Gynecol Scand.* 1981;60:153–155

122. Egge K, Lyng G, Maltau JM. Retinal haemorrhages in the newborn. *Acta Ophthalmol (Copenh).* 1980;58:231–236

123. Berkus MD, Ramamurthy RS, O'Connor PS, Brown KJ, Hayashi RH. Cohort study of Silastic obstetric vacuum cup deliveries: II. Unsuccessful vacuum extraction. *Obstet Gynecol.* 1986;68:662–666

124. Forstner R, Hoffman GF, Gassner I, et al. Glutaric aciduria type 1: ultrasonic demonstration of early signs. *Pediatr Radiol.* 1999;29:138–143

125. Amir N, El-Peleg O, Shalev R, Christiansen E. Glutaric aciduria type 1: clinical heterogeneity and neuroradiologic features. *Neurology.* 1987;37:1654–1657

126. Woelfle J, Kreft B, Emons D, Haverkamp F. Subdural hemorrhage as an initial sign of glutaric aciduria type a: a diagnostic pitfall. *Pediatr Radiol.* 1996;26:779–781

127. Morris AA, Hoffmann GF, Naughten ER, et al. Glutaric aciduria and suspected child abuse. *Arch Dis Child.* 1999;80:404–405

128. de Veber G, Andrew M, Adams C, et al. Cerebral sinovenous thrombosis in children. *N Engl J Med.* 2001;345:417–423

129. Sebire G, Tabarki B, Saunders DE, et al. Cerebral venous sinus thrombosis in children: risk factors, presentation, diagnosis and outcome. *Brain.* 2005;128:477–489

130. Oikawa A, Aoki N, Sakai T. Arteriovenous malformation presenting as acute subdural haematoma. *Neurol Res.* 1993;15:353–355

131. O'Leary PM, Sweeny PJ. Ruptured intracerebral aneurysm resulting in a subdural hematoma. *Ann Emerg Med.* 1986;15:944–946

132. Weissgold DJ, Budenz DL, Hood I, Rorke LB. Ruptured vascular malformation masquerading as shaken baby syndrome. *Surv Ophthalmol.* 1995;39:509–512

133. Yoffe G, Buchanan GR. Intracranial hemorrhage in newborn and young infants with hemophilia. *J Pediatr.* 1988;113:333–336

134. Eyster M, Gill F, Blatt P, Hilgartner M, Ballard J, Kinney T. Central nervous system bleeding in hemophiliacs. *Blood.* 1978;51:1179–1189

135. Bray GL, Luban NLC. Hemophilia presenting with intracranial hemorrhage: an approach to the infant with intracranial bleeding and coagulopathy. *Am J Dis Child.* 1987;141:1215–1217

136. Harley JM. Disorders of coagulation misdiagnosed as nonaccidental bruising. *Pediatr Emerg Care.* 1997;13:347–349

137. O'Hare AE, Eden OB. Bleeding disorders and non-accidental injury. *Arch Dis Child.* 1984;59:860–864

138. Fenton LZ, Sirotnak AP, Handler MH. Parietal pseudofracture and spontaneous intracranial hemorrhage suggesting nonaccidental trauma: report of 2 cases. *Pediatr Neurosurg.* 2000;33:318–322

139. Wetzel RC, Slater AJ, Dover GJ. Fatal intramuscular bleeding misdiagnosed as suspected nonaccidental injury. *Pediatrics.* 1995;95:771–773

140. Lane PA, Hathaway WE, Githens JH, Krugman RD, Rosenberg DA. Fatal intracranial hemorrhage in a normal infant secondary to vitamin K deficiency. *Pediatrics.* 1983;72:563–564

141. Shapiro AD, Jacobson LJ, Armon ME, et al. Vitamin K deficiency in the newborn infant: prevalence and perinatal risk factors. *J Pediatr.* 1986;109:675–680

142. Lane PA, Hathaway WE. Vitamin K in infancy. *J Pediatr.* 1985;106:351–359

143. Von Kreis R, Greer FR, Suttie JW. Assessment of vitamin K status of the newborn infant. *J Pediatr Gastroenterol Nutr.* 1993;16:231–238

144. Chaou WT, Chou ML, Eitzman DV. Intracranial hemorrhage and vitamin K deficiency in early infancy. *J Pediatr.* 1984;105:880–884

145. Shih SL, Lin JCT, Liang DC, Huang JK. Computed tomography of spontaneous intracranial haemorrhage due to haemostatic disorders in children. *Neuroradiology.* 1993;35:619–621

146. Dietrich AM, James CD, King DR, Ginn-Pease ME, Cecalupo AJ. Head trauma in children with congenital coagulation disorders. *J Pediatr Surg.* 1994;29:28–32

147. Medeiros D, Buschanan GR. Major hemorrhage in children with idiopathic thrombocytopenic purpura: immediate response to therapy and long term outcome. *J Pediatr.* 1998;133:334–339

148. Francis J, Todd P. Congenital factor XIII deficiency in a neonate. *Br Med J.* 1978;2:1532

149. Abbondanzo S, Gootenberg J, Lofts RS, McPherson RA. Intracranial hemorrhage in congenital deficiency of factor XIII. *Am J Pediatr Hematol Oncol.* 1988;10:65–68

150. Duckert F. The fibrin stabilizing factor, factor XIII. *Blut.* 1973;26:177–179

151. Newman RS, Jalili M, Kolls BJ, Dietrich R. FXIII deficiency mistaken for battered child syndrome: case of "correct" test ordering negated by a commonly accepted qualitative test with limited negative predictive value. *Am J Hematol.* 2002;71:328–330

152. Miner ME, Kaufman HH, Graham SH, Haar FH, Gildenberg PL. Disseminated intravascular coagulation fibrinolytic syndrome following head injury in children: frequency and prognostic implications. *J Pediatr.* 1982;100:687–691

153. Ogilvy CS, Chapman PH, McGrail K. Subdural empyema complicating bacterial meningitis in a child: enhancement of membranes with gadolinium on magnetic resonance imaging in a patient without enhancement on computed tomography. *Surg Neurol.* 1992;37:138–141

154. Mashiyama S, Fukawa O, Mitani S, et al. Chronic subdural hematoma associated with malignancy: report of three cases [in Japanese]. *No Shinkei Geka.* 2000;28:173–178

155. Ozhan S, Tali ET, Isik S, Saygili MR, Baykaner K. Haematoma-like primary intracranial malignant fibrous histiocytoma in a 5-year-old girl. *Neuroradiology.* 1999;41:523–525

156. Alexander RC, Schor DP, Smith WL. Magnetic resonance imaging of intracranial injuries from child abuse. *J Pediatr.* 1986;109:975–979

157 Sato Y, Kao SC, Smith WL. Radiographic manifestations of anomalies of the brain. *Radiol Clin North Am.* 1991;29:179–194

158. Sato Y, Smith WL. Head injury in child abuse. *Neuroimaging Clin N Am.* 1991:1475–1492

159. Bital R, Perng R, Moody AR, et al. MR pulse sequences: what every radiologist wants to know but is afraid to ask. *Radiographics.* 2006;26:513–537

160. Tung GA, Kumar M, Richardson RC, Jenny C, Brown WD. Comparison of accidental and non-accidental traumatic head injury in children on noncontrast computed tomography. *Pediatrics.* 2006;118:626–633

161. Vinchon M, Moule N, Tchofo PJ, Soto-Ares G, Fourier C, Dhellemmes P. Imaging of head injuries in infants: temporal correlates and forensic implications for the diagnosis of child abuse. *J Neurosurg.* 2004;101:44–52

162. McNeely PD, Atkinson JD, Saigal G, O'Gorman AM, Farmer JP. Subdural hematomas in infants with benign enlargement of the subarachnoid spaces are not pathognomonic for child abuse. *AJNR Am J Neuroradiol.* 2006;27:1725–1728

163. Sargent S, Kennedy JG, Kaplan JA. "Hyperacute" subdural hematoma: CT mimic of recurrent episodes of bleeding in the setting of child abuse. *J Forensic Sci.* 1996;41:314–316

164. Arbogast KB, Margulies SS, Christian CW. Initial neurologic presentation in young children sustaining inflicted and unintentional fatal head injuries. *Pediatrics.* 2005;116:180–184

165. Judkins AR, Hood IG, Mirchandani HG, Rorke LB. Technical communication. Rationale and technique for examination of nervous system in suspected infant victims of abuse. *Am J Med Pathol.* 204;25:29–32

166. Kornberg AE. Skin and soft tissue injuries. In: Ludwig S, Kornberg AE, eds. *Child Abuse. A Medical Reference.* 2nd ed. New York, NY: Churchill Livingstone; 1992:91–104

167. Hobbs CJ, Hanks HGI, Wynne JM. *Child Abuse and Neglect. A Clinicians Handbook.* London, UK: Churchill Livingstone; 2000:73–75

168. Raffel C, Litofsky NS. Skull fractures. In: Cheek WR, Margin AE, McLone DG, Reigel DH eds. *Pediatric Neurosurgery.* Philadelphia, PA: WB Saunders Co; 1994: 258

169. Case ME, Graham MA, Handy TC, Jentzen JM, Monteleone JA. Position paper on fatal abusive head injuries in infants and young children. *Am J Forensic Med Pathol.* 2001;22:112–123

170. Rorke LB. Neuropathology. In: Kornberg AE, ed. *Child Abuse. A Medical Reference.* New York, NY: Churchill Livingstone; 1992:403–422

171. DiRocco C, Velardi F. Epidemiology and etiology of cranio-cerebral trauma in the first two years of life. In: Raimondi AJ, Choux M, DiRocco C, eds. *Head Injuries in the Newborn and Infants.* New York, NY: Springer Verlag; 1986:125–139

172. Lindenberg R. Trauma of meninges and brain. In: Minckler J, ed. *Pathology of the Nervous System.* Vol 2. New York, NY: McGraw-Hill Book Co; 1972:1705–1763

173. Rorke LB. Neuropathology of inflicted childhood neurotrauma. In: Reece RM, Nicholson CE, eds. *Inflicted Childhood Neurotrauma.* Elk Grove Village, IL: American Academy of Pediatrics; 2003:165–179

174. Case ME. Central nervous system trauma. In: Nelson JS, Mena H, Parisi JE, Schochet SS, eds. *Principles and Practice of Neuropathology.* New York, NY: Oxford University Press; 2003:167–175

175. Tzioumi D, Oates RK. Subdural hematomas in children under 2 years. Accident or inflicted? A 10-year experience. *Child Abuse Negl.* 1998;22:1105–1112

176. Sutor AH, von Kries R, Cornelissen EAM, McNinch AW, Andrew M. Vitamin K deficiency bleeding (VKDB) in infancy. *Thromb Haemost.* 1999;81:456–461

177. Suzuki K, Fukushima T, Meguro K, et al. Intracranial hemorrhage in an infant owing to vitamin K deficiency despite prophylaxis. *Childs Nerv Syst.* 1999;15:292–294

178. O'Hare AE, Eden OB. Bleeding disorders and non-accidental injury. *Arch Dis Child.* 1984;59:860–864

179. Weissgold DJ, Budenz DL, Hood I, Rorke LB. Ruptured vascular malformation masquerading as shaken baby syndrome. *Surv Ophthalmol.* 1995;39:509–512

180. Minns RA. Subdural haemorrhages, haematomas, and effusions in infancy. *Arch Dis Child.* 2005;90:883–884

181. Woelfle J, Kreft B, Emons D, Haverkamp F. Subdural hemorrhages as an initial sign of glutaric aciduria type 1: a diagnostic pitfall. *Pediatr Radiol.* 1996;26:779–781

182. Payne NR, Hasegawa DK. Vitamin K deficiency in newborns: a case report in α-1-antitrypsin deficiency and a review of factors predisposing to hemorrhage. *Pediatrics.* 1984;73:712–716

183. Minns RA, Brown JK. Neurological perspectives of non-accidental head injury and whiplash/shaken baby syndrome: an overview. In: Minns RA, Brown JK, eds. *Shaking and Other Non-accidental Head Injuries in Children.* London, UK: MacKeith Press; 2005:1–105

184. Jellinger K. The neuropathology of pediatric head injuries. In: Shapiro K, ed. *Pediatric Head Trauma.* Mount Kisco, NY: Futura Publishing Co; 1983:143–194

185. Rowbotham GF. *Acute Injuries of the Head.* Edinburgh, UK: E&S Livingstone Ltd; 1964:120

186. Peet MM. Extradural hematoma, subdural hematoma and subdural hygroma. In: Brock S, ed. *Injuries of the Skull, Brain and Spinal Cord.* Baltimore, MD: Williams & Wilkins; 1943:130

187. Maxeiner H. Demonstration and interpretation of bridging vein ruptures in cases of infantile subdural bleedings. *J Forensic Sci.* 2001;46:83–93

188. Geddes JF, Tasker RC, Hackshaw AK, et al. Dural haemorrhage in non-traumatic infant deaths: does it explain the bleeding in 'shaken baby syndrome'? *Neuropathol Appl Neurobiol.* 2003;29:14–22

189. Lindenberg R, Freytag E. Morphology of brain lesions from blunt trauma in early infancy. *Arch Pathol.* 1969;87:298–305

190. Geddes JF, Whitwell HL, Graham DI. Traumatic axonal injury: practical issues for diagnosis in medico-legal cases. *Neuropathol Appl Neurobiol.* 2000;26:105–116

191. Gleckman AM, Bell MD, Evans RJ, Smith TW. Diffuse axonal injury in infants with non-accidental craniocerebral trauma: enhanced detection by beta-amyloid precursor protein immunohistochemical staining. *Arch Pathol Lab Med.* 1999;123:146–151

192. Shannon P, Smith CR, Deck J, Ang LC, Ho M, Becker L. Axonal injury and the neuropathology of shaken baby syndrome. *Acta Neuropathol.* 1999;95:625–631

193. Dolinak D, Smith C, Graham DI. Hypoglycemia is a cause of axonal injury. *Neuropathol Appl Neurobiol.* 2000;26:448–453

194. Lena G, Ballini G. Spinal injuries in children. In: Choux M, DiRocco C, Hockley AD, Walker ML, eds. London, UK: Churchill Livingstone; 1999:381–391

195. Sneed RC, Stover SL. Undiagnosed spinal cord injuries in brain-injured children. *Am J Dis Child.* 1988;142:965–967

196. Gilles FH, Bina M, Sotrel A. Infantile atlanto-occipital instability. *Am J Dis Child.* 1979;133:30–37

197. Nacimiento W, Noth J. What, if anything, is spinal shock? *Arch Neurol.* 1999;56:1033–1035

198. Feldman KW, Weinberger E, Milstein JM, Fligner CL. Cervical spine MRI in abused infants. *Child Abuse Negl.* 1997;21:199–205

199. Bruce DA, Alavi A, Bilaniuk L, Dolinskas C, Obrist W, Uzzell B. Diffuse cerebral swelling following head injuries in children: the syndrome of "malignant brain edema." *J Neurosurg.* 1981;54:170–178

200. Chillon J-M, Baumbach GL. Autoregulation of cerebral blood flow. In: Welch KMA, Caplan LR, Reis DJ, Siesjö, Weir B, eds. *Primer on Cerebrovascular Diseases.* New York, NY: Academic Press; 1997:51–54

201. Jaspan T. Ultrasound and computed tomography in the diagnosis of non-accidental head injury. In: Minns RA, Brown JK, eds. *Shaking and Other Non-accidental Head Injuries in Children.* London, UK: MacKeith Press; 2005:208–261

202. Chen CY, Zimmerman RA, Rorke LB. Neuroimaging in child abuse: a mechanism-based approach. *Paediatr Neuroradiol.* 1999;41:711–722

203. Firstman R, Talan J. *The Death of Innocents.* New York, NY: Bantam Books; 1997

204. Gilles FH. Hypotensive brain stem necrosis. Segmental symmetrical necrosis of tegmental neuronal aggregates following cardiac arrest. *Arch Pathol.* 1969;88:32–42

205. May K, Parson MA, Doran R. Haemorrhagic retinopathy of shaking injury: clinical and pathological aspects. In: Minns RA, Brown JK, eds. *Shaking and Other Non-accidental Head Injuries in Children.* London, UK: MacKeith Press; 2005:185–207

206. Budenz D, Farber M, Mirchindani H, Park H, Rorke LB. Ocular and optic nerve hemorrhages in abused infants with intracranial injuries. *Ophthalmology.* 1994;101:559–565

207. Minns RA. Shaken baby syndrome: theoretical and evidential controversies. *J Royal Coll Phys Edinburgh.* 2005;35:5–15

Chapter 3

Skeletal Manifestations of Child Abuse

Daniel R. Cooperman

Case Western Reserve University School of Medicine
Department of Orthopaedic Surgery, MetroHealth Medical Center and
Rainbow Babies and Childrens Hospital

David F. Merten

University of North Carolina School of Medicine

General Considerations

Historical Perspective

The first report of skeletal injury as a manifestation of maltreatment of children was published in Paris in 1860 by Ambroise Tardieu,[1] a specialist in pathology, public health, and forensic medicine, who described multiple fractures and other injuries in children that were inflicted by parents or others with authority over the victims. His report seems to be the first inclusive concept of the medical, demographic, social, and psychiatric features of child physical abuse that would be defined more than a century later as battered child syndrome.[2] The nidus for current concepts of a syndrome of child physical abuse was Caffey's[3] description in 1946 of clinically unsuspected fractures of the long bones associated with subdural hematomas in infants with no history of trauma. His suggestion that the injuries

were possibly inflicted by the child's caretaker was confirmed in 1953, when Silverman[4] determined that observed skeletal injuries were the result of repetitive trauma that was unrecognized through unawareness or deliberate denial on the part of the perpetrators. This and later reports led to the formal description and definition of battered child syndrome by Kempe et al[5] in 1962.

Incidence and Pathologic Characteristics of Inflicted Skeletal Injuries

The reported frequency of fractures associated with child abuse varies from 11% to 55%.[6-9] Inflicted skeletal trauma may involve virtually any part of the axial and appendicular skeleton. Many injuries (43%) are clinically unsuspected, and multiple fractures are found in more than one-half of physically abused children.[6,10] The true incidence of inflicted skeletal injury is, however, probably greater than these reports would indicate because radiologic examination is performed inconsistently in suspected cases of abuse and, when performed, it is frequently incomplete or of non-diagnostic quality. Post-mortem comparison of high-detail radiographic skeletal surveys, specimen radiography, and histopathologic analysis indicate that the yield of skeletal surveys can be increased from 5% to 92% by specimen radiography.[11]

Factors Increasing the Risk of Child Physical Abuse and Skeletal Injury

Age is the single most important risk factor in the incidence of abuse-related skeletal injuries,[12] with 55% to 70% of all inflicted skeletal trauma found in infants younger than 1 year.[6,10,13] Put another way, 80% of abuse fractures are found in infants younger than 18 months, whereas only 2% of accidental fractures are found in this age group.[14] Similarly, occult and multifocal skeletal trauma are in large part limited to the first 2 years of life.

Socioeconomic factors also influence the incidence and severity of physical abuse and skeletal injury. The classic picture of the battered child has been that of an infant with multiple skeletal as well as soft tissue and other injuries inflicted over the course of time by a depressed mother. This spectrum of serious physical abuse, resulting in death or requiring hospitalization, seems to be changing, with an increase in the severity of inflicted trauma (ie, intracranial injuries) and an increasingly prominent role of nonfamily male

friends who are babysitters as perpetrators.[15] Although overt physical child abuse is more often identified in lower socioeconomic levels, maltreatment of children crosses all social and economic boundaries. Reported statistics should be thought of as delineating the recognition of, rather than the true existence of, child abuse because better educated and more affluent members of society can more readily disguise physical injury and other forms of abuse.[16]

Developmental handicaps and prematurity also increase the risk for child abuse.[17-19] Infants and children with cerebral palsy and a variety of developmental disabilities are at increased risk for physical abuse, with the incidence of maltreatment in handicapped children reported in up to 70% of cases.[20] Preterm infants are also at increased risk for abuse because of early bonding failures. Low birth weight infants, although accounting for only 10% of the newborn population, constitute approximately 20% to 25% of the physically abused population.[19]

Associated Injury

The association of skeletal injuries with head and visceral trauma in the abused child has long been recognized,[3] and concurrent intracranial injuries and fractures are identified in up to 70% of infants presenting with abuse-related head injury.[6] Caffey's[3] original admonition that "the presence of unexplained fractures in the long bone warrants investigation for subdural hematoma" should not go unheeded. A screening radiologic skeletal examination should be carried out in all suspected victims of abuse with significant head injuries; conversely, cranial computed tomography (CT) should be performed in any infant with extensive inflicted skeletal injuries, even those without significant neurologic findings.

Diagnostic Considerations

Diagnostic Imaging

Diagnostic imaging plays a fundamental role in the evaluation of suspected child abuse, and judicious application of modern imaging techniques facilitates early and accurate diagnosis in such cases. Diagnostic imaging serves (a) to identify the presence and extent of trauma, and (b) to document, if possible, that observed injuries are the result of abuse.[21] In fulfilling this role, the radiologist must determine the location, nature, and extent of skeletal trauma, as well as attempt to determine when and how these injuries occurred. Fractures must be assessed in relation to the morphological response of the skeleton to specific mechanical forces and to established pathologic and radiologic features of accidental versus non-accidental skel-

etal injuries. Clinical findings and suspicions should be correlated with the findings of the radiologic evaluation, and the radiologist must be fully informed of the suspicion of abuse before the radiologic examination begins. It is as an integral part of the overall evaluation of suspected child abuse that radiologic imaging has its maximal diagnostic impact.

A complete radiographic skeletal survey (child abuse, trauma-X, SCAN series) remains the primary imaging study for suspected child abuse[22,23] and is mandatory in all cases of suspected child abuse in children younger than 2 years. The routine screening skeletal survey includes 19 separate radiographic exposures tightly collimated to each anatomical region, with axial images viewed in 2 projections (frontal and lateral) and specific anatomical regions of the extremities viewed in the single projection (frontal) (Box 3.1).[7,22] Additional views, including oblique projections, may be taken when abnormalities are identified or suspected on the screening survey and/or the clinical findings.

BOX 3.1
Radiographic Skeletal Survey for Suspected Child Abuse[a]

Skull: Frontal and lateral (lateral to include the cervical spine)

Spine: Frontal and lateral thoracolumbar spine

Chest: Frontal and lateral (lateral for sternum)

Extremities
    Upper: Humeri (frontal)
    Forearms (frontal)
    Hands (frontal, oblique as needed)

Lower: Pelvis (frontal, to include the mid and lower lumbar spine)
    Femora (frontal)
    Tibias (frontal)
    Feet (frontal, oblique as needed)

---

[a]At least 2 views of each fracture should be obtained.

A single radiograph of the entire infant ("babygram") is diagnostically inadequate and must not be substituted for a true skeletal survey. When child abuse is strongly suspected clinically and/or radiographically after the initial skeletal survey, a follow-up skeletal survey 2 weeks after the initial examination may facilitate a more accurate assessment of the presence and extent of skeletal injury.[22,24] All studies should be closely monitored by a radiologist for technical and diagnostic adequacy, and because fractures associated with child abuse are often subtle and easily overlooked, it is essential that skeletal surveys are carried out with a high level of technical excellence.

The diagnostic capacity of the skeletal survey depends on the spatial and contrast resolution of the radiographic imaging system. With conventional film-screen combination, the radiographic imaging system should have a limiting resolution of at least 10 line pairs per millimeter and a maximal film speed of 200. Although mammographic film-screen systems can provide optimal skeletal detail, newer high-detail double-screen/double-emulsion film systems seem to produce radiographs of comparable detail with lower radiation doses.[7,25] Digital (filmless) radiography has, in recent years, been replacing conventional film/screen radiography, with many radiology departments now using digitally acquired images for skeletal surveys. Although there was initial concern that digitized radiographic skeletal images may not be technically adequate for recognition of classic metaphyseal lesions of abuse because of lower image quality,[25,26] more recent experience indicates that digital radiography affords performance comparable to high-detail/film-screen imaging in the identification of abuse-related skeletal injuries.[27]

Postmortem radiographic skeletal examination also plays an important complementary role to autopsy in identifying fractures in fatal cases of child abuse,[28-30] and the forensic medical investigator should seek the advice and expertise of a radiologist familiar with the findings of child abuse when this diagnosis is suspected.[31] It is recommended that radiologic studies be obtained in all unexplained deaths that are suspicious for abuse in children younger than 2 years. The skeletal examination should consist of well-collimated views of the long bones, with additional views as necessary (postmortem). Where possible, studies should be performed by trained radiology technicians or personnel. It is essential that the radiographic images are reviewed promptly by a pediatric radiologist so that additional views can be obtained as needed.

Skeletal radionuclide scintigraphy (bone scan) in the evaluation of suspected child abuse is a complementary imaging modality to conventional radiographic examination in the diagnosis and management of child abuse.[32-37] As a general rule the bone scan is appropriate as a supplement to the initial skeletal survey when clinical suspicion of abuse is high in the absence of radiographic evidence of skeletal injury. Scintigraphy is sensitive in defining the extent of skeletal injury and identifying non-displaced or subtle healing fractures, especially acute rib fractures and periosteal injury inapparent radiographically.[22,33,38,39] At the same time there are a number of diagnostic limitations to the use of scintigraphy in the investigation of suspected child abuse. These include difficulty in identifying classic metaphyseal lesions of abuse, symmetrical fractures, subtle spinal injuries, and the inability to determine the age and type of fracture.[22] The diagnostic quality of scintigraphic imaging depends on proper immobilization of the child, correct positioning, magnification techniques in infants, and optimized imaging equipment.[33,40] When scintigraphy is performed as the initial imaging study, all areas of abnormal tracer uptake must be evaluated radiographically, and because scintigraphy is not sensitive for detecting skull fractures, at least 2 views of the skull must supplement the bone scan.[22]

Occasionally other imaging methods are needed to evaluate possible inflicted skeletal and soft tissue injury. Ultrasonography may be used to identify non-displaced fractures before the onset of callus formation and acute subperiosteal hemorrhage in the absence of overt fracture.[41,42] In patients with extensive muscle and soft tissue trauma, CT and magnetic resonance imaging (MRI) may further define the type and extent of injury.[23,43] On occasion, when plain radiographs may be insufficient to evaluate vertebral compression and spinous process fracture, thin-section CT with multiplanar reformatting may be required to define the extent of injury.[22] The efficacy of skeletal imaging in the evaluation of child abuse can be increased by clinical criteria based on the age of the child and the type of abuse.[6,22,44] Routine complete skeletal screening for occult fractures is indicated in all infants younger than 2 years with clinical evidence of physical abuse, and in infants younger than 1 year with evidence of significant neglect and deprivation. In older children (age 2–5 years), the frequency of occult skeletal injuries decreases, and a selective approach to a complete screening skeleton examination is indicated on the basis of clinical presentation and the results of radiographic examination for clinically evident skeletal injuries. Beyond age 5 years, complete skeletal screening has little value.[6] Victims of isolated sexual abuse and siblings of abused children (with the exception of twins) without clinical evidence of physical abuse do not require routine skeletal surveys.[22]

Fractures of the Appendicular Skeleton

Fractures of the extremities are the most common skeletal injuries occurring in abused children and have long been recognized as important indicators of child abuse.[2,3,10,12,45] Fractures may be isolated, involving a single bone, or they may be multifocal. In one study of skeletal trauma in abused children, 1 to 15 fractures per child were identified, with an average of 3.6 fractures.[17] Long-bone fractures may involve the diaphysis (shaft), as well as the metaphyseal-epiphyseal complex. Although diaphyseal fractures have been reported to be the most common extremity injury in abused children,[6,46,47] postmortem studies using a combination of high-detail skeletal surveys, specimen radiography, and histopathologic analysis show that metaphyseal fractures are identified more frequently than diaphyseal fractures, at least in the fatal cases included in this study.[11]

The mechanism of extremity fractures in abused children may be difficult to define in any single case because the trauma is often unobserved, is inflicted on more than one occasion by a variety of methods, is perpetrated by individuals who are reluctant to confess or discuss the mechanism of injury, and is sustained by children who lack the ability to describe what happened to them. An understanding of basic mechanics and the anatomical and developmental features of pediatric bone that determine the response to mechanical loading patterns are the basis for any practical approach to evaluating various fractures in suspected victims of abuse.[48] Such an approach substitutes science for speculation. A combination of mechanical forces is probably at play in most cases of abuse-related skeletal injury, reflecting repeated episodes of abuse over time that produce more than one fracture in multiple locations and a variety of fracture types in various stages of healing. The broad spectrum of biomechanical forces producing extremity injury results in a variable pattern of fractures: spiral fractures reflect torsional forces, buckle or cortical fractures result from axial loading (compressive forces transmitted down the long axis of the bone), transverse fractures are due to bending or direct blows to the extremity; oblique fractures are due to combined loading (compression and rotation, bending, or more complex loads), and the classic metaphyseal lesions (CML) and epiphyseal-complex injuries reflect shearing forces due to shaking or violent traction/twisting of the extremity.[48]

Metaphyseal fractures were described as part of the initial definition of battered child syndrome.[5] It was noted that the "classical radiologic features of the battered child syndrome are usually found in the appendicular skeleton" and include "irregularities of mineralization in the metaphysis of the bones of the major tubular bones with slight misalignment of the adjacent epiphyseal ossification centers." Meticulous pathologic-radiographic investigation has demonstrated that the classic metaphyseal lesion is not an avulsion at the site of periosteal attachment as was originally thought,[49] but rather a planar fracture through the region of the metaphysis abutting the physis.[50] Histologic examination reveals a series of subphyseal microfractures through the delicate primary spongiosa and calcified cartilaginous cores traversing this most immature portion of the metaphysis (Figure 3.1). The result is 2 contiguous mineralized regions: calcified cartilage in the adjacent subphyseal zone of the metaphysis separated from the calcified cartilage in the physeal-epiphyseal fragment. As the fracture plane extends peripherally to the cortex it veers away from the growth plate, undercutting a fragment of bone, the subperiosteal collar, producing a disk-like fragment that is thin centrally but has a thicker, mineralized peripheral rim.

Non-displaced metaphyseal injuries appear radiographically as planar lucencies traversing the subphyseal metaphysis for variable distances (Figure 3.2A).

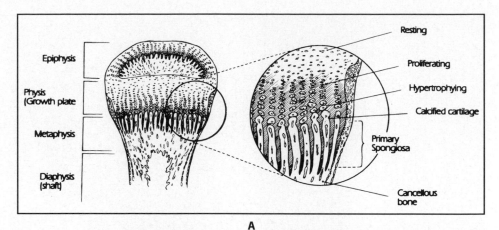

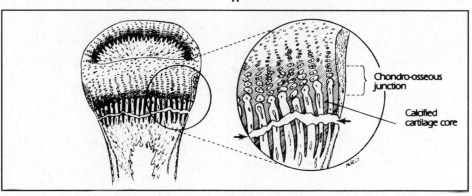

FIGURE 3.1

Skeletal manifestations of child abuse. **A.** Normal tubular bone consists of the diaphysis (shaft), metaphysis, physis (growth plate), and epiphysis. Longitudinal growth results from proliferation and calcification of cartilage cells at the chondro-osseous junction. The physis is a disk of cartilage extending from the zone of resting cartilage to the zone of calcified cartilage in the metaphysis. In the metaphysis, calcified cartilage is transformed in the bone in the primary spongiosa. **B.** Metaphyseal fracture in the primary spongiosa. The planar fracture separates a disk-like fragment of calcified subphyseal cartilage from the adjacent calcified submetaphysis.

With a complete fracture, inclusion of the subperiosteal bone collar within the periphery metaphyseal fracture fragment explains the radiographic picture of the corner fracture (Figure 3.2B) or bucket-handle pattern (Figure 3.2C), depending on the degree of displacement and the radiographic projection.[51] If no further injury occurs, the fracture will disappear in several weeks. If, however, trauma is continued, with additional trabecular disruption, a wider lucency and metaphyseal irregularity will be seen. The amount of periosteal disruption and subsequent new bone formation depends on the extent of metaphyseal injury and degree of displacement. Because the periosteum is

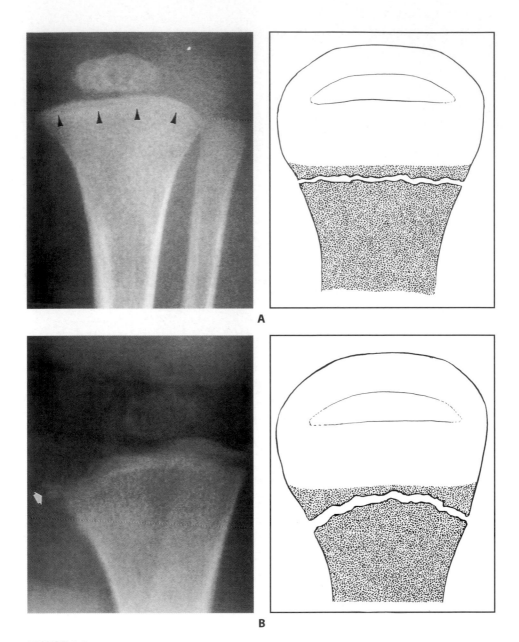

FIGURE 3.2

Radiographic appearance of metaphyseal fracture. **A.** Non-displaced fracture. The fracture line is seen as a subtle linear lucency (arrows). **B.** Corner fracture. As the fracture is viewed tangentially, the dense peripheral margin of the disk-like metaphyseal fragment may be seen as a discrete bony fragment (arrow).

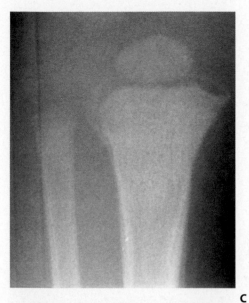

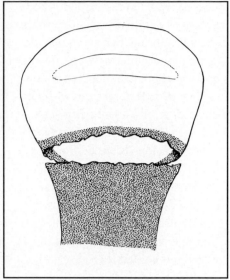

C

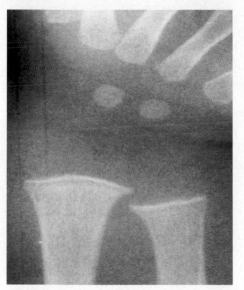

D

FIGURE 3.2, *continued*
Radiographic appearance of metaphyseal
fracture. **C.** Bucket-handle fracture. With
additional separation/displacement, the
dense margin of the disk-like fragment is
projected as a continuous arc-like density.
Although the disk contains calcified cartilage
throughout, only the dense peripheral margin
is seen radiographically. **D.** Lucent lines
reflecting disturbance in bone growth are
generalized and symmetrical, and traverse
the entire metaphysis.

loosely attached to the diaphysis and metaphysis but is very adherent to the perichondral ring that surrounds the growth plate, subperiosteal hemorrhage stops at that point, and it is common to see no periosteal reaction with non-displaced or only slightly displaced CML.[52] The transmetaphyseal planar lucency of a non-displaced fracture (Figure 3.2A) must be differentiated from metaphyseal lucent lines reflecting disturbance in normal bone growth (growth disturbance lines, Figure 3.2D). Fracture lines are usually asymmetrical and often incomplete, whereas the growth disturbance lines are generalized and symmetrical and traverse the entire metaphysis.

Metaphyseal fractures require biomechanical forces that are not produced by the usual accidental trauma of infancy. Rather, rotational forces are generated as the shaken infant is held by the trunk or when the extremities are used as convenient handles for violent shaking.[16,53] Rapid acceleration and deceleration delivers planar shearing forces to the metaphysis, resulting in fracture. Cartilaginous epiphyseal fracture with separation occurs when the limb is subjected to massive traction, compression, or

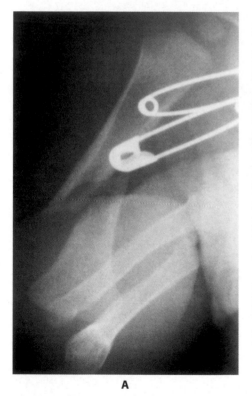

A

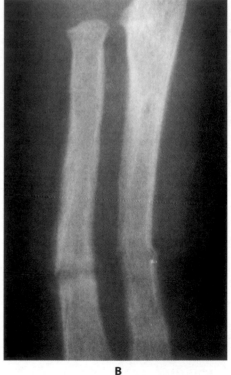

B

FIGURE 3.3
Diaphyseal fracture. Chest radiograph obtained in a patient with pneumonia identified an unsuspected acute oblique fracture of the right humeral diaphysis. **A, B.** A complete skeletal survey revealed older transverse diaphyseal fractures of the left radius and ulna, with evidence of healing.

rotation. Because of the specificity of metaphyseal fracture in infancy, it has been suggested that resection of high-risk metaphysis (proximal humeri, knees, distal tibia) followed by high-detail radiography and histologic examination be performed to verify the fracture in infants for whom cause of death is not determined and in fatal cases with central nervous system injuries or ocular signs of abuse.[54,55]

Diaphyseal (shaft) fractures may be transverse or oblique/spiral fractures. Although fractures of the humerus, femur, and tibia are found frequently in abused children, most authors agree that there are no specific types or locations of diaphyseal fractures in abused children.[8,15,46,56] In contrast to metaphyseal fractures, diaphyseal fractures may result from accidental injury.[57] A careful history and physical examination for other evidence of unexplained injury are necessary, and in cases in which abuse is suspected, a complete skeletal survey must be obtained to search for additional occult injuries (Figure 3.3). In this context, because extremity injuries are common initial presentations often involving an orthopedic surgeon, it is essential that this physician be familiar with the signs of abuse and make referral to the appropriate child protection agency.[51,58–60] Recognition of non-accidental fractures in children, and especially in young infants, is of paramount importance because these infants are at increased risk for further abuse.[61]

Periosteal injury may occur without radiographically evident diaphyseal fracture. The periosteum is most strongly attached to the metaphysis in infants and is loosely attached to the underlying diaphyseal cortex. As a result, twisting or torsion of the limb may result in stripping of the periosteum from the cortex with associated subperiosteal hemorrhage. These bone bruises can be detected radiographically only when periosteal new bone has begun to form 5 to 10 days after injury. Ultrasonographic examination can be used to demonstrate acute periosteal elevation and hemorrhage and, in some cases, the presence of acute non-displaced incomplete diaphyseal fractures.[31] On radionuclide scintigrams, tracer activity is increased in the area of acute periosteal stripping and hemorrhage well before periosteal new bone formation (Figure 3.4).[33]

Upper Extremities

Clavicular fractures have been reported in 3% to 10% of abused children.[17,46,62,63] Because the most common location for both accidental and inflicted clavicular fractures is the middle one third of the shaft, fractures in this location are by themselves of limited diagnostic significance. Clavicular fractures are the most common birth-related skeletal injury, and a healing fracture in the first 7 to 10 days of life must be regarded as accidental; however, any acute clavicular fracture identified after age 10 days without evidence of healing is suggestive of abuse. In older infants, recognition and treatment of both accidental and inflicted fractures of the midshaft may be delayed until abundant callus produces a palpable lump, and these fractures must be evaluated within the context of the history and other evidence of physical injury and/or abuse. By contrast,

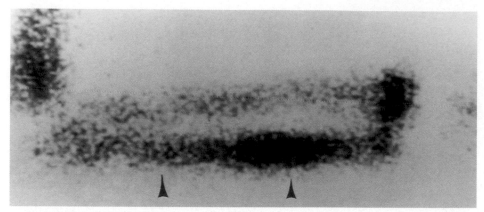

A

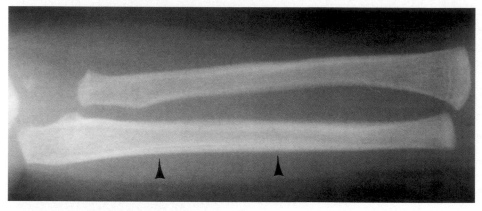

B

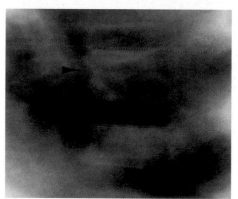

C

FIGURE 3.4
A. A radionuclide bone scan reveals increased tracer activity in the right forearm (arrowheads). **B.** Radiographic examination of the right forearm shows periosteal new bone along the shaft of the ulna (arrowheads). **C.** A lateral view of the thoracic spine shows anterior compression of the T8 and T9 vertebral bodies (arrows).

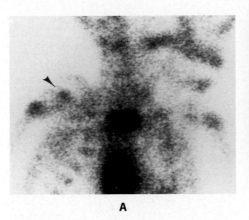
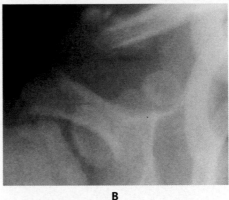

A   **B**

FIGURE 3.5
A. A radionuclide bone scan in a 10-month-old infant with a subdural hematoma reveals an area of tracer uptake in the distal right clavicle (arrowhead). **B.** A radiograph of the right shoulder reveals a healing distal clavicular fracture.

accidental fractures in the medial or lateral end of the clavicle are uncommon in children aged 3 years or younger.[47] These fractures are adjacent to the sternoclavicular and acromioclavicular articulations and are likely the result of shaking (Figure 3.5).

Scapular fractures are unusual in abused children.[17,46,47,62–64] Fracture or fragmentation of the acromion at the acromioclavicular articulation occurs most commonly and probably results from indirect shearing biomechanical forces generated by shaking or as traction is applied to the upper extremity (Figure 3.6D). Rare fractures of the body of the scapula are presumably the result of direct impact. Coracoid fractures are similarly uncommon.

Fractures of the humerus are reported in 12% to 57% of abused infants and children.[17,20,65–68] The frequency of these fractures in abused children is readily

explained: The arms offer a convenient handle to the assailant as the infant is pulled, swung, or shaken. Abuse-related transverse or oblique/spiral diaphyseal fractures are found most frequently in the middle or lower one third of the diaphysis. Supracondylar fracture, although a common accidental distal humeral injury in older children, should prompt consideration of possible child abuse when encountered in a child younger than 3 years.[42,68] Although less common than diaphyseal fractures of the humerus in abused children, proximal humeral metaphyseal fractures have been demonstrated by postmortem radiologic-histopathologic examination, stressing the need for careful examination of this area in the initial radiographic survey in cases of suspected abuse.[69] Inflicted epiphyseal fracture-separation of the proximal and distal epiphyses also may occur, and acute injuries may be difficult to identify

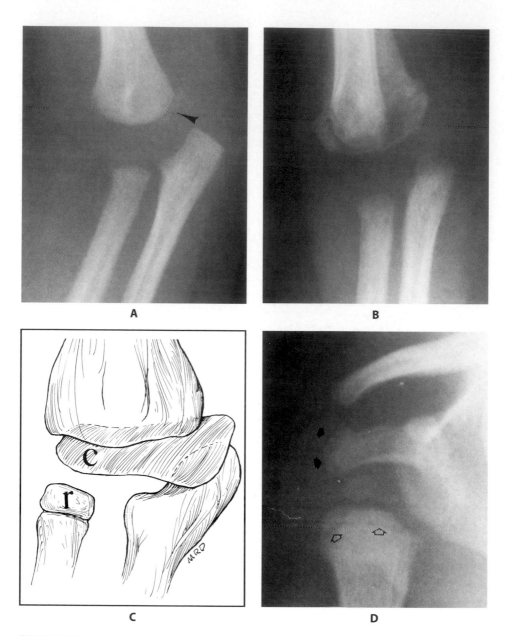

FIGURE 3.6

A. Extensive soft-tissue swelling is evident about the right elbow with a subtle curvilinear fragment of bone adjacent to the humeral metaphysis (arrowhead). **B.** Five weeks later, abundant callus formation is medially displaced about the distal humeral epiphysis. **C.** The diagram shows separation and displacement of the capitellum (c). The radial head (r) remains with the capitellum. **D.** A fracture of the right acromion process is shown (solid arrows), as well as the adjacent proximal humeral metaphysis (open arrows).

radiographically before periosteal new bone and callus formation (Figure 3.6).[70] Ultrasonography and MRI may be useful in establishing the diagnosis of these fractures before epiphyseal ossification and may obviate the need for arthrography.[43] Once the capitellum is ossified, the radiographic diagnosis of distal humeral fracture separation should be little trouble because the radius will remain aligned with the displaced capitellum.[71]

Fractures of the radius and ulna are common extremity injuries in abused children.[17] As with humeral fractures, their frequency reflects the use of the forearms as handles for shaking. Diaphyseal subperiosteal hemorrhage may be the only sequelae of abuse. Forearm fractures are most frequently paired fractures of the radius and ulna, are found in the distal one third of the shaft, and tend to be transverse (Figure 3.3) Accidental torus or buckle fractures of the distal radius and ulna are also relatively common in toddlers and small children, and are typically transverse. As in all nonspecific long-bone fractures, the history and age of the child must be used to determine the risk of child abuse in such injuries.[65]

Hand fractures have been reported only sporadically in abused children[6]; however, these fractures may be subtle, and a study of abused infants revealed both metacarpal and phalangeal fractures that are presumably the result of forced extension.[72] Abuse-related hand fractures also may result when older children attempt to shield themselves from a blow (Figure 3.7). Well-collimated initial radiographs with oblique views followed by reexamination in 2 weeks may aid in detection of these injuries. Fractures of the hands are often associated with more widespread musculoskeletal and soft tissue injury.

Lower Extremities

Fractures of the pelvis are seldom reported in abused children,[6,17,46,62] although the rarity of these fractures may well reflect underdiagnosis.[73] Fractures of the pubic bones and ischium are reported most frequently and require close radiographic scrutiny for identification.[12,23,74] Radionuclide scintigraphy also may aid in the identification of these fractures.[39] Considering the direct force required to produce such injuries, pelvic fractures without a history of vehicular or other severe trauma should be considered nonaccidental injuries.

Femoral fractures are reported in 12% to 29% of physically abused children.[17,46,75,76] In at least one study, these fractures were the most common long-bone injury identified in abused children.[63] Femoral shaft and distal metaphyseal fractures occur most commonly and may result from rotational force applied to the leg during twisting or shaking, torsion when the leg is used as a handle for shaking, or from a direct blow. Torus/buckle injuries at the end of the diaphysis probably occur at the end of a shaking episode as the infant is forcibly brought down against a hard surface.[77] Distal metaphyseal fractures initially involve the posteromedial aspect of the femur, with anterior and lateral extension in more extensive

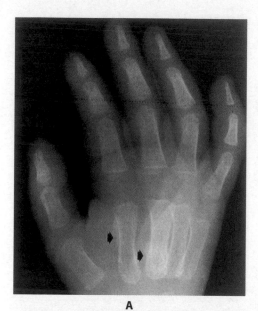

A

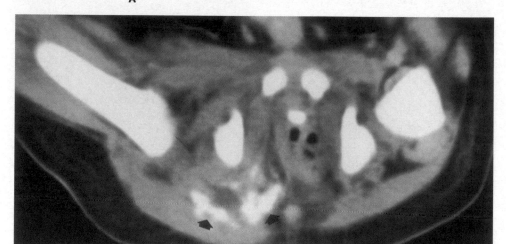

B

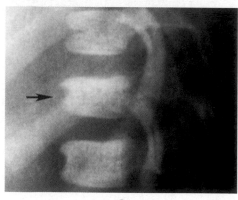

C

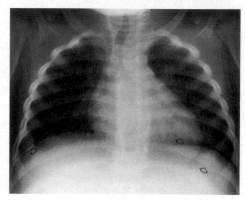

D

FIGURE 3.7
A 14-month-old child had multiple bruises
and a buttocks mass. **A.** Radiography reveals
healing fractures of the second and third
metacarpals (arrows). **B.** Computed tomography of the buttocks mass reveals a calcified right gluteal hematoma (arrows).
C. An anterior compression fracture of
the twelfth thoracic vertebral body.
D. Multiple healing rib fractures also
were identified.

lesions.[76] Fractures of the proximal femur occur less frequently than distal fractures.[8,78] Proximal femoral epiphyseal-metaphyseal fractures result from sudden compression or traction of the leg, producing shearing forces that are concentrated on the proximal femoral physis.[79] The radiographic diagnosis of the proximal metaphyseal-epiphyseal fractures before ossification of the femoral head is made on a basis of displacement of the femoral shaft relative to the femoral head and acetabulum (Figure 3.8). Ultrasonography, MRI, and/or arthrography may be necessary to define the fracture further.

With the exception of metaphyseal injuries, femoral fracture patterns cannot be used to rule in or rule out abuse.[78] Age is an important consideration in differentiating accidental from non-accidental femoral fractures.[8] In one study, 60% of fractures of the femur occurring in infants aged 1 year or younger were the result of abuse, whereas only 20% of fractures in children aged between 2 and 3 years were determined to be the result of abuse.[68] Significant blood loss or shock does not accompany isolated unilateral femoral fractures, and their presence should suggest the possibility of additional visceral injuries.[8]

Tibial fractures are the third most common extremity injury in abused children.[17,62] By contrast, fractures of the fibula are relatively uncommon as isolated injuries, and most occur in conjunction with a tibial fracture. Most inflicted tibial fractures occur in the distal metaphysis, less frequently in the proximal metaphysis, and only occasionally in the diaphysis.[49] Distal tibial metaphyseal fractures are initially seen along the medial aspect of the metaphysis and extend to the lateral metaphysis with more extensive injuries.[80] Proximal metaphyseal fractures show a similar pattern of medial involvement and lateral extension.[81] Distal fractures show the typical radiographic changes of metaphyseal lucency as well as corner and bucket-handle configurations (Figure 3.9). Inflicted diaphyseal fractures usually have less obliquity than do accidental spiral tibial fractures, which are relatively common in infants and young children between 9 months to 3 years (toddler fracture).[82,83] Toddler fractures are non-displaced spiral fractures. They are classically due to trivial or innocuous injuries in ambulatory infants and young children that are frequently unobserved. These fractures were initially described in the tibia; however, accidental fractures of the femur and bones of the feet in this age group are now included in the concept of the toddler fracture.[84,85] Soft tissue swelling and ecchymoses are unusual, with localized tenderness often being the only physical finding. These children are usually seen because of failure to bear weight, a limp, or the appearance of pain when forced to stand on the involved extremity.[86] Radiographic evidence of a toddler fracture is subtle and requires at least 2 (anteroposterior and lateral) and possibly 3 (oblique-internal/external rotation) views for diagnosis. Skeletal scintigraphy (bone scan) may be helpful in identifying these subtle fractures when radiographic findings are negative.[87,88] If fracture is suspected but not visualized, immobilization is indicated. Repeated radiographs obtained 7 to 10 days later usually show subperiosteal new bone formation.[83,89]

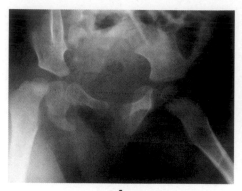

A

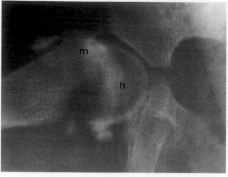

C

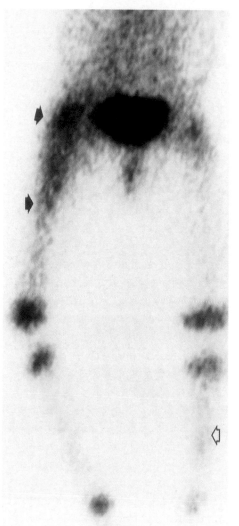

B

FIGURE 3.8

A 10-month-old boy refused to move his right leg. **A.** The right femoral head is mal-aligned relative to the adjacent metaphysis when compared with the normal left hip. **B.** A radionuclide bone scan reveals increased tracer uptake about the right hip, extending to the middle of the femur (solid arrows). An area of increased activity in the middle of the left tibial shaft (open arrow) was identified later as a healing diaphyseal fracture. **C.** An arthrogram of the right hip shows complete fracture-separation of the femoral head (h) from the metaphysis (m).

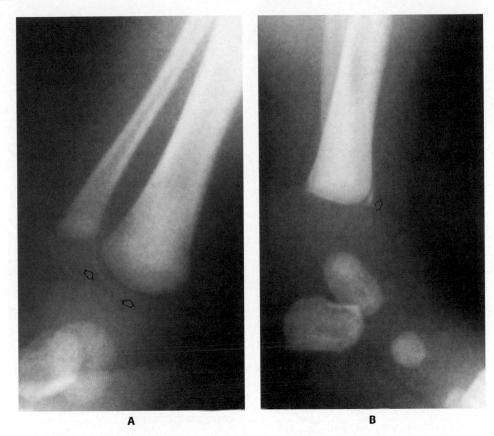

A   **B**

FIGURE 3.9
A 1-month-old infant had a swollen left leg. **A.** Radiography shows a bucket-handle fracture (arrows) of the distal tibial metaphysis. **B.** Viewed in a lateral projection it appears as a corner fracture (arrow).

Fractures of the feet are unusual injuries in abused children.[17,46,62] The mechanism is thought to be forced hyperextension with a tendency to involve the first metatarsals and phalanges with few clinical signs of injury.[72] Radiographic diagnosis requires careful, focused examination of the feet in at least 2 projections including oblique views.

Long-Term Sequelae of Long-Bone Fractures

In general, the outcome of a fracture is related to the position of the bone ends after the bone has healed. Three factors correlate with prognosis: (1) maintenance of length, (2) proper rotational alignment, and (3) angulation. If fractures are not displaced or are minimally displaced, the bone will usually be normal after healing, provided the physis (growth plate) has not been damaged. If the fracture alignment is nonanatomical at presentation, the goal of treatment is to align the bones appropriately with respect to length, angulation, and rotation. If children present with nonanatomical alignment but the bones are healed, remodeling can occur to a certain extent, depending on the location and plane of angular deformity. As a general rule, a child can remodel 3 to 4 degrees of flexion deformity at the distal femur with each year of remaining growth. Therefore, if a 3-year-old child's femur heals in 30 degrees of flexion just above the knee, this angulation will be completely remodeled, and the bone will be straight by the time the child has finished growth.

Length also is a plastic property in children. Increased nutrition delivered to the area of injury to aid in healing also stimulates the physes both proximally and distally, resulting in an increased rate of growth in the fractured bone. For example, overgrowth in a femur can range from a few millimeters to 4 cm in children aged 10 years and younger. Consequently, even fractures that heal with considerable shortening may normalize in length. Unfortunately, there is no good prognostic indicator in any individual case to predict the amount of overgrowth the patient will experience. Most overgrowth occurs within the first 2 years after injury. If a child has a functionally short limb 2 years after injury, further significant spontaneous correction should not be expected. If limb length inequalities cause problems, further treatment is required.

Rotational misalignment has less potential for remodeling. No good data exist on what can be reasonably expected in terms of rotational correction after fracture in children. Two mechanisms account for remodeling of bone: epiphyseal, relating to the longitudinal growth of the bone at the growth plate, and diaphyseal, related to the forces acting on the shaft of the bone. In child abuse, the diaphyseal mechanism is rarely disrupted. By contrast, the epiphyseal mechanism may be disrupted, with severe metaphyseal-epiphyseal fractures that damage the physis.[90] As a consequence, growth may cease altogether or may become asymmetrical, producing an angular deformity. Damage to the physis resulting from child abuse has been described with shortening and deformity of the injured limb, flaring of the metaphysis, and blurring of the growth plate.[91] All children with fractures in the epiphyseal region must be followed up carefully for 6 to 12 months to determine if the physis will grow normally.

A rarely encountered but devastating sequela to inflicted proximal femoral fracture is avascular necrosis of the proximal femoral epiphysis (head). If the epiphysis is displaced with respect to the femoral neck or the femoral neck is displaced with respect to the shaft of the femur, the blood vessels nourishing the femoral head can be damaged. If avascular necrosis occurs, the entire proximal femoral epiphysis may collapse, leading to flattening of the proximal femur and loss of longitudinal growth in the proximal femoral growth plate.[79]

Management of Long-Bone Fractures

The management of abuse-related skeletal injury differs little from treatment of accidental fractures. Simple immobilization in a cast is usually sufficient because the children are young, and most inflicted fractures are not displaced or are minimally displaced. Closed reduction and cast immobilization are required for displaced fractures to restore length as well as rotational and angular alignment. Operative management, either open reduction with internal fixation or closed reduction with percutaneous internal fixation, is rarely necessary, except in supracondylar elbow fractures and epiphyseal fracture-separation.

Fractures of the Axial Skeleton

Thoracic Cage

Rib fractures constitute between 5% and 27% of all skeletal injuries occurring in abused children,[42] with almost 90% seen in infants younger than 2 years.[6] Most fractures (80%) are located posteriorly near the costovertebral articulation (Figure 3.10).[6,92] In contrast to extremity fractures, most rib fractures in abused children are clinically unsuspected. Rib fractures are rarely if ever the result of minor accidental trauma in otherwise healthy infants and children because the compliance and mobility of the thoracic cage in childhood normally prevent rib fracture in situations other than massive vehicular or other major accidental trauma.[34,49,93] The positive predictive value for abuse of rib fractures is 100% in infants younger than 2 years without a history of massive accidental trauma.[94]

Rib fractures have not been found after cardiopulmonary resuscitation (CPR) in children, and only rarely from over-enthusiastic physiotherapy.[77,95,96] Even in children with increased bone fragility (osteogenesis imperfecta or other skeletal dysplasias) rib fractures are rarely if ever the result of CPR.[97]

Most rib fractures are thought to result from violent shaking[53] rather than from direct impact[38] or lateral compression of the chest.[49] As the infant is grasped, the assailant's palms are usually situated laterally, with the thumbs positioned anteriorly and the fingers placed posteriorly (Figure 3.11). Compression of the chest is from front to back, with levering of the proximal rib over the fulcrum of the

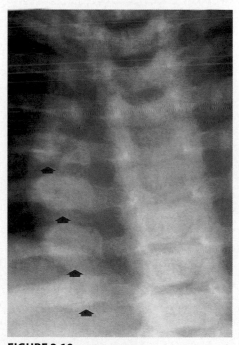

FIGURE 3.10
Multiple healing fractures of the right fourth through seventh ribs (arrows) at the costovertebral junction, adjacent to the tip of the transverse processes.

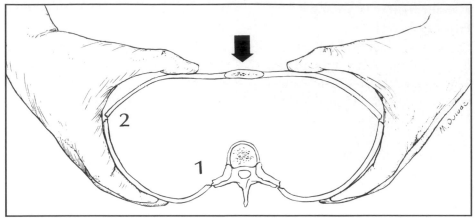

FIGURE 3.11
With anteroposterior compression of the chest, rib fractures occur initially in the proximal rib over the transverse process of the adjacent vertebrae (1) and more laterally along the posterior arc of the rib to the midaxillary line (2).

transverse process. Animal studies confirm that these fractures require excessive levering associated with massive forces that entail violent anteroposterior compression, as with child abuse or deceleration associated with motor vehicle crashes.[98] Posterior fractures are seen initially at the costovertebral junction and subsequently tend to occur laterally along the posterior arc of the rib as compressive force increases. Because these compressive forces are distributed more or less equally over the thoracic cage during shaking, rib fractures often are multiple and bilateral. Although anterior and costochondral junction fractures are identified less frequently,[6] these injuries are likely more common than reported because they are often difficult to detect.[99] Lateral and anterior arc fractures tend to occur along the inner cortex of the rib. Costochondral junction fractures are usually bilateral and symmetrical and tend to involve the sixth through ninth ribs.[100]

Costochondral junction fractures impact along the inner aspect of the osteochondral interface with an osseous fragment analogous to metaphyseal corner and bucket-handle fractures.[101] These fractures are almost always associated with major intra-abdominal injuries. Fracture of the first rib is less commonly seen in abused infants and may be due to impact force or acute axial load (slamming), producing an indirect fracture.[102]

Whereas rib fractures are readily detected radiographically with healing and callus formation, acute non-displaced rib fractures are difficult to identify.[101] Costovertebral fractures may be subtle, appearing only as slight expansion of the head and neck of the rib.[99] Asymmetry in the appearance of the ribs at the costovertebral junction may be the only radiographic evidence of fracture. In addition to the routine frontal and lateral thoracic views in the skeletal survey, right and left posterior oblique views should be obtained to define further rib fractures identified on initial examination.[94] Skeletal scintigraphy may contribute to the detection of acute and healing rib fractures in abused children.[33,36,38]

Fractures of the sternum are infrequently reported in abused infants and children.[45,47,103] These injuries result from direct blows or violent compression of the thorax with sternal displacement at the sternomanubrial articulation or along the cartilaginous margins of the sternal ossification centers. Although isolated, unexplained sternal fractures are not specific to abuse in children, and these fractures in infants or toddlers younger than 18 months without adequate explanation are highly suspicious if not diagnostic of abuse.[42,103] Detection requires careful inspection of the chest in the lateral projection.

Spine

Vertebral fractures are reportedly uncommon skeletal injuries with child abuse.[6,12,62] Personal experience and postmortem study of abused infants, however, suggest that these fractures are more common than reported previously.[104] In most cases, vertebral fractures are asymptomatic and may go unrecognized without complete radiographic screening and careful radiologic inspection of the spine in lateral projection.[105] Radionuclide scintigraphy can demonstrate fractures of the transverse and spinous processes, but it is relatively insensitive for vertebral body fractures.[22]

Most inflicted spinal injuries occur in the lower thoracic and upper lumbar vertebrae at the apex of an acute kyphotic angle resulting from hyperflexion.[47,105-109] Occasionally there may be a fracture/dislocation of the thoracolumbar spine with cord compression.[110] Reports of fracture and/or ligamentous injury to the cervical vertebrae are rare, although spinal injuries in abused infants are presumably a result of violent shaking.[111] Evidence exists, however, that cervical cord injuries may occur more frequently in shaken infants than previously recognized.[111-114] The paucity of cervical spine injuries in child abuse may reflect a lack of inquiry: subtle fractures may be occurring but are difficult to detect radiographically.[115] Abusive cervical spine injuries have been reported in up to 3% of pediatric cervical spine injuries, and all cases were found in infants younger than 1 year.[112] Pre-vertebral soft tissue swelling may be the only radiographic evidence of significant spinal injury. The craniocervical junction and upper cervical spine should be thoroughly evaluated in any shaken infant with an intracranial injury; however, cervical spine MRI is not indicated in children with abusive head injury without clinically evident spinal cord injury.[116]

Variable anterior compression deformity of the vertebral body is usually present (Figure 3.12A). The 3 histologic-radiographic patterns of vertebral body fracture are (a) pure compression of the anterior half of the vertebral body without disruption of the end plate, (b) compression fractures with extension into the end plate, and (c) combined lesions.[104] The vertebral end

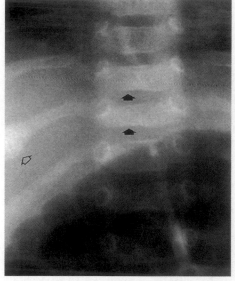

A

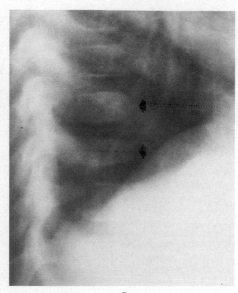

B

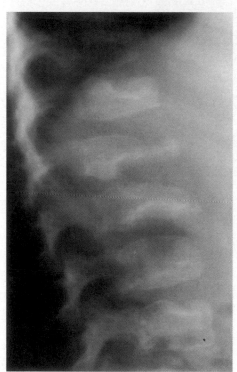

C

FIGURE 3.12
A, B. Frontal and lateral views of the thoracolumbar spine show anterior compression
of the 10th and 11th thoracic vertebrae (solid
arrows). Also evident is a healing fracture of
the right seventh rib at the costovertebral
junction (open arrow). **C.** Lateral view of
a 5-year-old child with history of abuse in
infancy shows anterior deformity of the
vertebral bodies at multiple levels, reflecting
old vertebral fracture.

plates are analogous to the metaphyseal-epiphyseal complex of the long bone, and end-plate injury often results in significant growth disturbance and persistent vertebral deformity (Figure 3.12B).[117] More violent hyperflexion may be associated with disk rupture and herniation along the anterior margin or the anterior-inferior margin of the vertebral end plates, resulting in a notched appearance. Uniform vertebral body compression is unusual in abused infants and should suggest weakened bone associated with intrinsic skeletal disease.

Injuries to the posterior vertebral elements most frequently involve the spinous process. These fractures are again related to severe hyperflexion and occur most frequently at or around the thoracolumbar junction.[108] These fractures may be solitary or multiple and seem to result from avulsion of cartilage and/or bone at the attachments of the interspinous ligaments.

Skull

Cranial fractures are the second most common skeletal injury in abused children.[6,118] The presence of a skull fracture indicates direct impact either from a blow to the head or the rapidly moving head of a shaken baby brought up against a static object. Skull fractures are classified radiographically as simple, non-displaced linear fractures involving a single calvarial bone or complex multiple fracture lines (eggshell fractures), which may be displaced, comminuted, or widened (diastatic) (Figure 3.13). Depressed skull fractures are uncommon in abused infants and young

children, perhaps reflecting the inherent plasticity of the infant skull.[98,111] The pattern of skull fractures as well as inconsistencies between the observed fracture and the alleged mechanisms of injury may be instrumental in confirming child abuse.[119] Occasionally bilateral non-diastatic linear skull fractures may be associated with a single midline impact due to short falls onto a hard surface.[9] Some investigators have suggested that complex fractures are more common in abused children,[120] although this possibility has not been borne out in other reports.[98] Skull fractures rarely result from accidental falls from up to 3 ft,[121-123] and when they do occur are linear and uncomplicated.

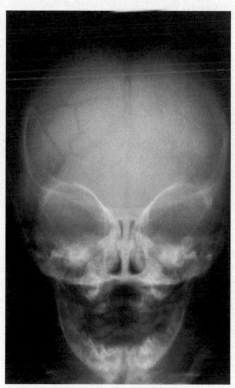

FIGURE 3.13
Complex right posterior parietal eggshell fracture.

Radionuclide scintigraphy (bone scan) is insensitive in identifying abuse-related skull fractures. Any patient undergoing CT scanning for head trauma should have images obtained at bone window settings to examine for unsuspected fractures. Fractures occurring in the same plane or at a shallow obliquity to the CT cut, however, may be undetectable.

Facial fractures constitute only 2% of all intentional injuries,[124] despite the frequency of injury to the soft tissues of the face in abused children. Most such reported injuries involve the mandible or, less commonly, the maxilla, and are found in older children.

Dating Fractures

The capacity to determine the age of skeletal injuries is important in documenting child abuse. Discrepancy between the age of fractures and the clinical history of injury is often the first indication of inflicted injury in abused children, and the presence of multiple fractures of different ages is evidence of repetitive inflicted injury. Although precise dating of fractures is impossible, it is usually possible to define a relatively narrow time frame in which the injury is likely to have occurred. In general, the longer from the time of injury, the more imprecise the dating process.[77] A prospective, well-controlled study to validate the current criteria used in the radiologic dating of fractures in children younger than 5 years is unlikely to be undertaken given the practical constraints of cost and radiation exposure that would be necessary to fully document the stages of fracture healing.

Without such a scientific study, those responsible for the investigation and prosecution of child abuse must continue to base clinical and radiologic judgments on personal and published experience, recognizing that fracture repair is a continuum with considerable overlap. Although not an exact science, radiologic dating of skeletal injuries may be approximated with relative accuracy using currently published criteria.[125,126]

Dating fractures is based on the radiographic appearance of the soft tissues, periosteum, fracture line, and callus formation.[126] Although there are well-established criteria for dating fractures, important differences exist between the pathophysiology of abuse-related fractures relative to usual accidental fractures in children. These differences are (a) abuse-related fractures occur predominantly in the infant younger than 2 years, (b) the fractures often reflect multiple episodes of trauma rather than a single incident, and (c) frequent delay in recognition and treatment of fractures results in additional repetitive injury to the original fracture site. The timetable and radiographic appearance for repair of fractures varies with the age of the child as well as the site and severity of injury. In general, the younger the infant is, the more rapid the healing process. Understanding the stages of healing and histopathologic responses associated with skeletal injury is important in accurate dating of fractures.

The first phase of healing (induction stage) extends from the moment of injury to the appearance of new bone in the area of the fracture. The initial inflammatory response is usually associated with pain and swelling; with non-displaced fractures, the inflammatory reaction may last only a few days. These infants may show no discomfort as early as 1 to 2 days after injury. Radiographically, initial findings are soft tissue swelling with displacement and obliteration of normal fat and fascial planes, which gradually recedes over the next 3 to 7 days (Figure 3.6). The initially sharp acute fracture line gradually becomes less well defined as healing progresses.

The second phase of healing (soft callus stage) begins with subperiosteal new bone formation approximately 7 to 10 days after injury in infants and slightly later (10–14 days) in older children. Recurrent injury at the same site within hours after initial trauma will produce more hemorrhage, but healing will then proceed normally. However, with repetitive injury more than 7 days later, additional bleeding and disruption of subperiosteal new bone leads to florid and exuberant callus formation.[127] Similarly, fracture instability is associated with exuberant subperiosteal new bone and callus formation around the fracture site.

The third phase of healing (hard callus stage) occurs when subperiosteal and endosteal bone begins to convert to lamellar bone. In children, particularly infants, the hard callus stage begins at 14 to 21 days at the earliest and peaks at 21 to 42 days. Radiographically, progressive solid union is noted at the fracture site.

The final phase (remodeling stage) begins with gradual restoration of bony configuration and correction of deformity. Remodeling begins at 3 months, with a peak at ages 1 to 2 years.

The classic metaphyseal fractures of child abuse pose a special diagnostic problem in radiologic dating of fracture. Unlike diaphyseal fractures with subperiosteal hemorrhage and new bone formation, metaphyseal fractures most frequently do not disrupt the tightly adherent periosteum, and subperiosteal new bone formation will be absent or produce only a haziness of the adjacent cortex.[52,127] More pronounced periosteal reaction is usually associated with periosteal shearing and/or more extensive injury to the metaphysis and displacement of the metaphyseal fragment.[128] Radiologic-histopathologic studies have shown that healing of usual metaphyseal fractures is characterized histologically by significant thickening of the zone of hypertrophic cartilage in the physis, with extension of chondrocytes into the calcified primary spongiosa that may be detected radiographically as a radiolucent extension into the adjacent metaphysis.[128] Because the relative rates of physeal growth of individual long bones are known, it may be possible to estimate more accurately the minimal age of a metaphyseal fracture based on radiologic appearance.[129] Healing of metaphyseal fractures may also present radiographically with a sclerotic band as endosteal callus obscures the fracture line.[127]

Differential Diagnosis

Before the diagnosis of non-accidental injury as a result of child abuse can be established, consideration must be given to possible preexisting medical conditions that may predispose structurally weak bones to injury with normal handling or minor trauma, and to disorders that may produce skeletal abnormalities that mimic the radiographic manifestations of inflicted trauma (Box 3.2).[45,130-132] Although these conditions are the exception rather than the rule, they must be excluded before establishing the diagnosis of child abuse. Careful clinical and radiologic evaluation usually permits accurate differentiation of skeletal abnormalities associated with these conditions from the skeletal injuries of child abuse. A variety of tests have been proposed to evaluate for osteopenia and fracture risk. Quantitative ultrasound of long bones may in time prove useful in evaluating bone strength, but experience in assessing risk for fracture is lacking.[133] Similarly, the evaluation of osteopenia by dual energy x-ray absorptiometry (DEXA) may be limited by potential diagnostic errors; however, with additional experience, DEXA may prove useful in assessing fracture risk in children.[134]

Obstetric Trauma

Breech and other traumatic deliveries are a well-recognized cause of certain skeletal injuries in otherwise healthy neonates.[135-137] Clavicular and humeral fractures occur most commonly with birth trauma. Both diaphyseal and metaphyseal fractures occur with the latter and are usually associated with breech positioning and difficult extraction.[138] Congenital neuromuscular disorders, such as arthrogryposis, that are associated with contractures also may

BOX 3.2

Child Abuse: The Differential Diagnosis of Skeletal Injury

Obstetric trauma

Prematurity

Nutritional/metabolic disorders
  Scurvy
  Rickets
  Renal osteodystrophy/secondary
    hyperparathyroidism
  Menkes syndrome

Drug-induced toxicity
  Methotrexate
  Prostaglandin E
  Hypervitaminosis A

Infection
  Osteomyelitis
  Congenital syphilis

Neuromuscular defect
  Spinal dysraphism (myelodysplasia)
  Cerebral palsy
  Congenital insensitivity to pain

Neoplasm
  Leukemia
  Metastatic (neuroblastoma)
  Langerhans cell histiocytosis
    (histiocytosis X)

Accidental trauma
  Toddler fracture

Normal variant
  Physiological periosteal new bone
    (infancy)
  Ossification center (acromial process)

Skeletal dysplasia
  Osteogenesis imperfecta
  Schmid/Schmid-like metaphyseal
    chondrodysplasia
  Metaphyseal dysostosis (Jansen type)
  Spondylometaphyseal chondrodysplasia
    (corner fracture type)

Miscellaneous
  Infantile cortical hyperostosis
    (Caffey disease)

result in fractures in an otherwise un-complicated delivery; fractures in such infants most frequently involve the lower extremities. Rib fractures are extraordinarily rare due to birth trauma. They were reported in one case where there was thoracic compression during mid-forceps or vacuum extraction delivery of a large neonate.[139,140] Obstetric fractures heal rapidly with early callus formation. It should be noted that birth-related fractures are often clinically overlooked in the delivery room.[141]

Prematurity

The delicate osteopenic bones of premature infants are at increased risk for fractures during normal handling. In addition, acquired nutritional deficiencies and infections also contribute to bone fragility. Long-bone fractures and rib fractures are most frequently observed. Skeletal injuries in the premature infant are usually not clinically evident. During passive exercises, the parent or caretaker may also inflict fractures.[142]

Nutritional and Metabolic Disorders

Certain acquired nutritional deficiencies as well as inborn metabolic errors may have skeletal manifestations suggestive of abuse-related injuries.

Scurvy is a rare disorder in our modern world, although sporadic cases continue to be reported.[143] Children with scurvy present with painful swollen limbs associated with radiographic evidence of extensive periosteal new bone formation as well as metaphyseal irregularity (Figure 3.14). Fracture-separation of the distal femoral epiphysis may occur,

reflecting the fibrous deficiency. The presence of a dense ring around an otherwise hyperlucent epiphysis (Wimberger ring) is a typical finding in children with scurvy.

Rickets is associated with metaphyseal irregularity and splaying, widening of the physis, and occasional pseudofractures (Milkman fracture).[144] Periosteal reaction and new bone formation are common and occasionally are extensive (Figure 3.15). The generalized distribution and symmetrical pattern of skeletal involvement are distinguishing features of rickets.

Menkes syndrome is a rare congenital defect of copper metabolism associated

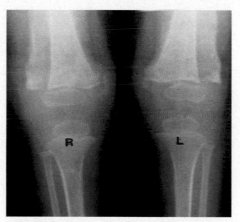

FIGURE 3.14
A 14-month-old child with painful swelling of both legs has symmetrical lateral dislocation of both femoral epiphyses with extensive periosteal new bone cloaking the distal femurs. The bones are generally demineralized with thin cortices. The growth plates are not widened, and the metaphyses are generally smooth. Dense zones of provisional calcification are evident. The femoral and tibial epiphyses are normally developed but have a relatively dense peripheral ossific rim (Wimberger sign). (Courtesy of J.C. Hoeffel, Hôpital Jeanne D'Arc, Dommartin les Toul, France.)

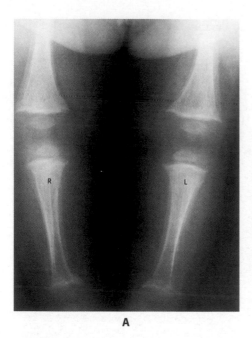

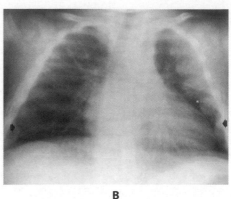

A   B

FIGURE 3.15
A 6-month-old infant had failure to thrive because of intestinal malabsorption. **A.** The long bones show generalized coarse demineralization with symmetrical flaring and irregularity of the femoral and tibial metaphyses and periosteal new bone along the shafts of the long bones. **B.** The chest also shows generalized skeletal demineralization with periosteal reaction and anterior enlargement of the ribs at the costochondral junction (rachitic rosary) (arrows).

with metaphyseal fractures and periosteal reaction, indistinguishable from abuse-related fractures. The presence of sparse, microscopically kinky hair, calvarial wormian bones, anterior rib flaring, along with failure to thrive and developmental retardation, are distinguishing features of this condition.

Other congenital metabolic disorders, such as mucolipidosis II (I-cell disease), may have radiographic features suggestive of abuse-related fractures. Again, the clinical and radiographic features suggest the correct diagnosis. Biliary atresia with diffuse skeletal demineralization may lead to fractures that mimic abuse.[145]

Drug-Induced Toxicity

A variety of therapeutic agents induce toxic osteopathics that resemble abuse-related lesions. The correct diagnosis is based on history of drug therapy.

Methotrexate therapy may be associated with an osteopathic condition characterized by periosteal reaction and impaction fractures of the metaphyses. Generalized and severe osteopenia is a prominent distinguishing feature of methotrexate toxicity.

Prostaglandin E therapy and hypervitaminosis A are associated with diaphyseal periostitis that may mimic skeletal trauma (Figure 3.16). In addition, acute vitamin A toxicity results

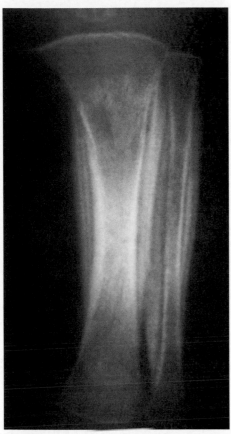

FIGURE 3.16
A 3-month-old infant with congenital heart disease receiving prostaglandin E therapy has symmetrical, uniform tibial and fibular diaphyseal periostitis. The metaphyses appear normal with smooth chondro-osseous junctions.

in increased intracranial pressure and sutural diastasis. A history of unusual vitamin intake or dietary habits and elevated serum vitamin A levels is diagnostic.

Infection

Osteomyelitis can result in metaphyseal irregularities and periosteal new bone growth that mimics metaphyseal and other fractures in infancy. Involvement of the physis in meningococcal infection may result in the shortening of affected limbs that is identical to long-term abuse-related traumatic sequelae.

Congenital syphilis usually manifests between ages 1 and 6 months with diffuse osteomyelitis that is characterized by symmetrical metaphyseal irregularities and diaphyseal fractures associated with extensive diaphyseal periostitis resembling traumatic lesions.[146] The diagnosis is suggested by the presence of focal erosion on the medial aspect of the proximal tibia (Wimberger sign) and is confirmed by serologic testing.

Neuromuscular Defects

Infants and children with a variety of congenital and acquired neuromuscular defects are at increased risk for accidental skeletal trauma. Spinal dysraphism and cerebral palsy are frequently associated with diffuse osteoporosis and contractures of the lower extremities. Distal femoral osteopenia is profound in such non-ambulatory children, and fractures are common.[147] In such cases, fractures of the metaphysis and diaphysis may occur with routine handling or during physical therapy.[142,148–150] Fracture risk is greatly exacerbated by cast immobilization. In infants being treated for equinovarus deformity, fractures secondary to forced eversion and dorsiflexion of the foot following casting of the clubfoot are similar to mechanical forces associated with abusive metaphyseal fractures.[149] Patients undergoing surgery for hip subluxation are at increased risk for fracture. This surgery is often followed by body cast (spica cast) immobilization. This provides a stable environment for healing of the hip sub-luxation but leads to joint stiffness and increased osteoporosis. Experience suggests 1 in 5 of these patients will evidence a lower extremity fracture within 3 months of cast removal.[151] Neurogenic sensory deficit with decreased or absent pain perception may result in non-displaced fractures that go undetected for prolonged periods.[152] As a result, these fractures lead to abundant callus formation. Given that these children are also at increased risk for child abuse because of their handicaps,[20] it is essential to consider the possibility of maltreatment in any handicapped infant or child with unexplained fractures. Careful medical and social evaluation as well as strong family support is required in such situations.

Congenital insensitivity to pain is a neurologic syndrome associated with bizarre skeletal lesions.[153] Radiographically, multiple fractures in different stages of repair in the absence of the history of trauma may at times be difficult to distinguish from child abuse.[154] Careful clinical history and neurologic sensory examination will establish the correct diagnosis.

Skeletal Dysplasia

Osteogenesis imperfecta (OI) is an inherited disorder of connective tissue with deficiency of type I collagen, leading to abnormal bone formation and increased bone fragility. As a result, trivial injuries may cause fractures in these patients. Of all the various conditions invoked by parents and their legal representatives to explain inflicted fractures, OI is cited most frequently. It is there-fore essential to be familiar with the classification of OI and the features that distinguish it from child abuse.[155]

The simple classification of OI into congenita and tarda types fails to consider the complex and heterogeneous nature of this disorder. The current classification identifies OI as 4 major types, depending on age of onset of fractures, extraskeletal manifestations, and mode of inheritance.[156] Infants with type I and II disease usually present no diagnostic problem and account for 80% of all cases of OI. Types I and II OI should not be confused with child abuse because all children with these types have blue sclerae and, with the exception of rare cases of type II OI with autosomal-recessive or dominant new mutation inheritance, are autosomal-dominant. Type II OI is lethal in the perinatal or neonatal period. Fractures associated with type I OI initially occur in the preschool period in most cases, although fractures may be seen in the neonate or at any time in childhood. Fractures heal at a normal rate, and their frequency declines after puberty. The bones are generally osteopenic with thin cortices. Rib fractures occur frequently. Bowing of the long bones of the lower extremities is characteristic, and wormian bones in the skull are present (Figure 3.17). Stature is normal or near normal. Dentinogenesis imperfecta is variable, and children commonly have hearing loss or a family history of hearing impairment. By contrast, mild cases of type III and IV OI may be confused with child abuse. In both instances, sclerae may be normal and with autosomal-dominant new mutations, the

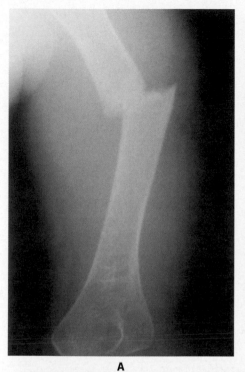

A

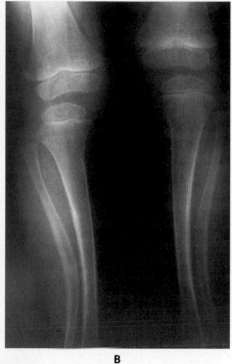

B

FIGURE 3.17
An 18-month-old child with clinically short stature (osteogenesis imperfecta) has a transverse fracture of the left humerus **(A)** with symmetric tibial and fibular bowing **(B).** The bones are generally demineralized with thin cortices. The skull shows multiple sutural (wormian) bones **(C).**

C

family history of OI is negative. In type III OI, however, patients should have wormian bones and osteoporosis, which, along with other features of OI, should help identify the child with OI. Cases of type IV OI pose greater diagnostic problems because skeletal involvement tends to be less severe than in type III disease. In these patients, however, a family history of wormian bones, osteoporosis, and characteristic clinical findings is often present. In rare cases of type IV OI, the potential for misdiagnosis exists. Given the rarity of this type of OI (1.1 in 3 million births), however, relative to the frequency of child abuse, the probability of error is minimal. It has been estimated that in a child younger than 1 year, with no family history and normal skull and teeth, the chance the fractures observed are related to type IV OI is less than 3 in a million.[157] Although metaphyseal fractures may occur in OI, the onset is typically late in such children.[158]

A variant form of OI has been described as temporary brittle bone disease (TBBD) and has been proposed as a cause for multiple fractures including classic metaphyseal and rib fractures.[159–162] Temporary brittle bone disease is claimed to be a condition of young infancy where a problem makes the bones susceptible to fracture for a short period, with spontaneous resolution leaving no identifiable pathology.[163] This hypothetical condition has frequently been cited by defense attorneys supported by purported expert witnesses to explain skeletal injury in cases of suspected child abuse. An international committee of pediatric radiologists; experts in pediatric forensics and pathology, and epidemiology; and legal professionals experienced with the diagnosis and prosecution of child abuse has evaluated the 2 different hypotheses that have been proposed to explain the pathogenesis of TBBD (copper deficiency and decreased fetal movement). The results of this evaluation clearly establish that the diagnosis of TBBD does not meet basic evidentiary standards due to lack of appropriate scientific methods and procedures, and that testimonial conjecture by "expert" witnesses based on speculation and subjective beliefs held by a miniscule number of health care professionals cannot help a judge or jury in understanding and evaluating medical evidence. In short, the concept of TBBD as a medical entity has been discredited as lacking any scientific data to support it.[164]

In addition to classic OI, there are other types of dysplastic bone disease that may be associated with osteopenia and fractures that have been recognized.[165]

In most cases, accurate differentiation is possible based on correlation of data from the clinical history, physical examination, family history, and radiographic examination. In atypical cases, the availability of biochemical analysis of synthesis and structure may be helpful in confirming the diagnosis of OI. Such studies should be obtained, however, only when diagnostic uncertainty persists after clinical and radiologic examinations have been carried out and there has been consultation with an expert in pediatric genetics. Biochemical testing is rarely necessary, and routine dermal biopsy for children suspected to have been abused is unwarranted.[166,167]

Unfortunately, children with OI also may be abused. In such cases, the diagnosis of child abuse may be made on the basis of typical inflicted injury fracture patterns that are inconsistent with the history and physical examination.[168]

Schmid and Schmid-like metaphyseal chondrodysplasia are characterized by mild to moderate metaphyseal flaring, irregularity, and sclerosis, as well as by enlarged capital femoral epiphyses, coxa vara, and cupping of the anterior ribs.[169] Spondylometaphyseal dysplasia, corner fracture type, may also occur with metaphyseal fragmentation as part of the larger spectrum of dysplastic skeletal fractures.[170] Similarly, Jansen-type metaphyseal dysostosis may manifest with metaphyseal irregularity and periosteal new bone resembling callus formation.[45] Despite the striking similarity of the metaphyseal fragmentation in these patients to the abuse-related corner fracture pattern of metaphyseal injury, a misdiagnosis can be avoided if a careful family history is taken and a complete radiographic skeletal survey is obtained.

Neoplasm

Patients with leukemia and metastatic neuroblastoma can present with localized osteolytic lesions, periosteal new bone and, occasionally, pathologic fractures. In addition, the metaphyseal lucency that can be the initial skeletal manifestation of leukemia may be indistinguishable from incomplete or non-displaced metaphyseal fractures. Non-traumatic leukemic lucencies are symmetrical and generalized, however, and are noted without additional skeletal evidence of abuse.[130] Careful clinical

and hematologic evaluation will establish the diagnosis of neoplasm.

Langerhans cell histiocytosis (histiocytosis X) is a proliferative rather than a true neoplasm that occasionally is associated with long-bone or rib lesions complicated by an unsuspected pathologic fracture and periosteal new bone suggestive of child abuse. The diagnosis of histiocytosis is established by a complete radiographic skeletal survey with identification of appendicular and axial skeletal lesions that are typically lytic, without reactive sclerosis or periosteal reaction.

Accidental Trauma

Almost invariably, caretakers attribute the injuries identified as suspected child abuse to accidental trauma. Frequent explanations include falls from bed or other pieces of furniture, dropping the infant, rough "play" by a parent or sibling, or being struck by a falling object.[78,122,123,171,172] It would be useful in such cases to be able to state that, based on scientific data, the fractures identified required a specific amount of biomechanical force to produce the observed injuries. With the exception of skull fractures, however, there is a paucity of experimental data relating to skeletal injuries in infants and children. With regard to skull fracture, the occurrence of fractures as a result of falls depends on the contact surface, drop height, and resultant gravitational force (g).[173] Some data indicate an increasing risk of skull fracture and concomitant intracranial injury with an impact force of greater than 50g. A head-on fall to a concrete surface of 1 ft or more can generate an impact force of 160g; at the same time, a 3-ft fall height is required to produce the same force with a packed dirt surface. Carpeted floors soften the impact even more. In general, the incidence of fractures from accidental falls increases with the height of the fall.[174]

Unfortunately, no such experimental data exist for appendicular and other axial skeletal injuries. Attempts to develop computer simulation of falls as a reliable forensic tool in cases of childhood injury will depend on an empirically developed data set that defines children's "injurability" (knowing what physical force might have affected a child's body part in a fall).[175] Such data are useless unless damage to the tissue occurring as a result of the fall is known. Additional scientific data on what kind of forces cause what specific tissue damage is needed before a given history of injury is plausible.[176] Several reports, however, may prove helpful in determining the likelihood of extremity fracture occurring with accidental trauma.[121,122,137,173] A study of 38 infants younger than 2 years with accidental falls from cribs (38 in.), beds (23–34 in.), and wagons (12 in.) showed that there were no appendicular or axial fractures other than a single simple skull fracture.[173] Because most such falls are headfirst, variable soft tissue injury was limited to the head, and most children had no bruises or other cutaneous evidence of trauma. Another study of 81 children aged 5 years or younger with a fall height of 90 cm yielded similar results, with only one simple skull fracture and no appendicular fractures.[121] It is evident from the results of these admittedly uncontrolled studies that skeletal injuries in the pre-toddler age (9–10 months) are rarely of accidental origin, and that any fracture in children in this age group must be given prompt and thorough evaluation for possible child abuse. It is equally evident that once the infant is ambulatory, the frequency of accidental trauma resulting in skeletal injuries increases.[68] Thus, in the older infant and child with fractures that are not pathognomonic of non-accidental injury, differentiation between accidental and non-accidental injury must be judged relative to the history of trauma and the patient's age, the presence or absence of other skeletal and nonskeletal injuries, and the child's general state of health. One suggested multidisciplinary approach to distinguishing accidental from non-accidental fractures is based on the use of established clinical and radiographic criteria for abuse-related injuries, an independent rating by the radiologist without clinical data, and a separate review by clinicians before forming a consensus opinion.[68] This retrospective analysis of clinical and radiographic data offers the potential for minimizing diagnostic errors resulting from busy outpatient clinics and emergency departments as well as physician inexperience.

Normal Variants and Other Mimics of Inflicted Skeletal Injuries

Physiological periosteal new bone is a reflection of normal skeletal growth that appears along the shafts of the long bones in infants between ages 2 and 3 months and normally resolves by age 8 months. Careful examination of these areas is, however, necessary to exclude a coincidental fracture in abused infants.[2,177] Metaphyseal spurring and cupping without fragmentation may also be seen in healthy infants and should not be confused with abuse-related fractures.[178] In both cases, the radiographic changes are bilaterally symmetrical and are not associated with evidence of soft tissue injury.

Variation in the ossification of the scapular acromial process may also resemble an avulsion fracture.[64] These variants are localized to the inferior portion of the acromial process with well-defined margins, in contrast to acromial fractures, which frequently are associated with avulsive changes in the adjacent clavicle and abundant callus formation.

In the skull, normal parietal fissures may present as pseudofractures.[177]

Infantile cortical hyperostosis (Caffey disease) is an unusual condition of unknown etiology that is seen only rarely today. These infants, from ages 3 to 6 months, present with swollen, painful extremities, the appearance of chronic illness, and exuberant diaphyseal periostitis suggestive of child abuse. Absence of metaphyseal involvement and the presence of periosteal reaction involving the mandible establish the correct diagnosis.

Intraosseous vascular access defects of the tibia may also mimic fractures in the skeletal survey for suspected child abuse.[179]

Skeletal Injuries as Evidence of Child Abuse

If expert medical testimony is to be credible in court proceedings, physicians and other health care professionals must be able and willing to use radiographic and other findings of skeletal as well as non-skeletal trauma as evidence of inflicted injury. Some medical witnesses in civil or criminal legal proceedings in child abuse cases are reticent when presenting radiographic evidence under oath. Although it is not possible to differentiate accidental from inflicted injuries in every case of suspected child abuse, there are patterns of injury and certain fracture types that are either pathognomonic or strongly suggestive of non-accidental injury (Box 3.3). Under these circumstances, the expert witness must unequivocally describe the presence and diagnostic characteristics of skeletal injuries as evidence of child abuse.[180]

Specific skeletal injuries that permit a definitive diagnosis of non-accidental injury include metaphyseal-epiphyseal complex, thoracic, shoulder girdle, and vertebral fractures. The mechanical forces required to produce these fractures are not generated by simple accidental falls and normal handling in an otherwise healthy infant and child. Other fracture patterns are highly suggestive of abuse and increase in specificity when there is a lack of adequate clinical history of trauma relative to the observed injuries. Included in this category are occult skeletal injuries; fractures inconsistent with accidental trauma given the age of the infant or history provided by caretakers; multifocal fractures of different ages,

BOX 3.3
Specificity of Skeletal Injuries as Evidence of Child Abuse[a]

Specific fractures
    Metaphyseal-epiphyseal (<2 years of age)
    Thoracic cage
        Rib
        Sternum
    Shoulder
        Scapula
    Clavicle
        Medial (sternoclavicular)
        Lateral (acromioclavicular)
    Spine
        Vertebral body (anterior compression)
        Spinous process
Highly suggestive fractures/patterns
    Multiple: bilateral, symmetrical
    Repetitive/different age
    Hands and feet
    Skull, complex fracture line
    Associated nonskeletal injury;
        intracranial, visceral
Nonspecific fractures
    Diaphyseal (shaft of long bone)
    Clavicular, midshaft
    Skull, linear

[a]In otherwise healthy infant/child without major trauma (ie, vehicular).

indicating repetitive episodes of trauma; or a pattern of concurrent skeletal and nonskeletal injuries.

Finally, some nonspecific fractures occur as the result of accidental trauma and are not by themselves specific evidence of abuse. Nonspecific fractures include single diaphyseal fractures of long bones, linear skull fractures, and midclavicular shaft fractures. To distinguish between accidental and inflicted injuries, these fractures must be considered within the context of patient age, history of trauma (or lack thereof), radiographic evidence of additional fractures, and other clinical findings suggestive of abuse.[77]

References

1. Tardieu A. Etude medio-legale sur les services et mauvais traitments exerces surdes enfants. *Ann Hyg Publ Med Leg.* 1860;13:361–368

2. Silverman FN. Unrecognized trauma in infants, the battered child syndrome, and the syndrome of Ambroise Tardieu. *Radiology.* 1972;104:337–353

3. Caffey J. Multiple fractures in the long bones of infants suffering from chronic subdural hematoma. *AJR Am J Roentgenol.* 1946;56:163–173

4. Silverman FN. The roentgen manifestations of unrecognized skeletal trauma in infants. *Am J Roentgenol Radium Ther Nucl Med.* 1953;69:413–427

5. Kempe CH, Silverman FN, Steele BF, et al. The battered child syndrome. *JAMA.* 1962;181:17–24

6. Merten DF, Radkowski MA, Leonidas JC. The abused child: a radiological reappraisal. *Radiology.* 1983;146:377–381

7. American College of Radiology. *ACR Standards, Standards for Skeletal Surveys in Children.* Reston, VA: American College of Radiology; 1997:47–50

8. Anderson WA. The significance of femoral fractures in children. *Ann Emerg Med.* 1982;11:174–177

9. Arnholz D, Hymel KP, Hay TC, Jenny C. Bilateral pediatric skull fractures. *J Trauma.* 1998;45:172–174

10. Krishnan J, Barbour PJ, Foster BK. Patterns of osseous injuries and psychosocial factors affecting victims of child abuse. *Aust N Z J Surg.* 1990;60:447–450

11. Kleinman PK, Marks SC Jr, Richmond JM, Blackbourne BD. Inflicted skeletal injury: a postmortem radiologic-histopathologic study in 31 infants. *AJR Am J Roentgenol.* 1995;165:647–650

12. Leonidas JC. Skeletal trauma in the child abuse syndrome. *Pediatr Ann.* 1983;12:875–882

13. Gross RH, Stranger M. Causative factors responsible for femoral fractures in infants and young children. *J Pediatr Orthop.* 1983;3:341–343

14. Worlock T, Stower M, Barbor P. Patterns of fractures in accidental and non-accidental injury in children: a comparative study. *Br Med J.* 1986;293:100–102

15. Bergman AB, Larsen RM, Mueller BA. Changing spectrum of serious child abuse. *Pediatrics.* 1986;3:113–116

16. Caffey J. The parent-infant traumatic stress (Caffey-Kempe, syndrome battered babe) syndrome. *Am J Roentgenol Radium Ther Nucl Med.* 1972;114:218–229

17. Akbarnia B, Torg JS, Kirkpatrick J, et al. Manifestations of the battered-child syndrome. *J Bone Joint Surg Am.* 1974;56:1159–1166

18. Jaudes PK, Diamond LJ. The handicapped child and child abuse. *Child Abuse Negl.* 1985;9:341–347

19. Stern L. The high risk infant and battering. In: Child Abuse in Developmental Disabilities. Washington, DC: US Department of Health, Education and Welfare; 1980:20–24. Publication OH-DS 79-30226

20. Gelles RJ. Child abuse and developmental disabilities. In: *Child Abuse in Developmental Disabilities.* Washington, DC: US Department of Health, Education and Welfare; 1980:25–31. Publication OH-DS 79-30226

21. Merten DF. The battered child syndrome: the role of radiological imaging. *Pediatr Ann.* 1983;12:867–868

22. American Academy of Pediatrics Section on Radiology. Diagnostic imaging of child abuse. *Pediatrics.* 2000;105:1345–1348

23. Merten DF, Carpenter BLM. Radiologic imaging of inflicted injury in the child abuse syndrome. *Pediatr Clin North Am.* 1990;37:815–837

24. Kleinman PK, Nimkin K, Spevak MR, et al. Follow-up skeletal surveys in suspected child abuse. *AJR Am J Roentgenol.* 1996;167:893–896

25. Kleinman PK. Diagnostic performance of modern radiographic imaging systems in the detection of inflicted skeletal injury in infancy. *AJR Am J Roentgenol.* 1997;168(suppl):127

26. Youmans DC, Don S, Hildebolt C, Shackelford GD, Luker GD, McAlister WH. Skeletal surveys for child abuse: comparison of interpretation using digitized images and screen-film radiographs. *AJR Am J Roentgenol.* 1998;171:1415–1419

27. Kleinman PK, O'Connor B, Nimkin K, et al. Detection of rib fractures in an abused infant using digital radiography: a laboratory study. *Pediatr Radiol.* 2002;32:896–901

28. McGraw EP, Pless JE, Pennington DJ, White SJ. Postmortem radiography after unexpected death in neonate, infants and children: should imaging be routine? *AJR Am J Roentgenol.* 2002;178:1517–1521

29. Society for Pediatric Radiology, National Association of Medical Examiners Postmortem radiography in the evaluation of unexpected death in children less than 2 years of age whose death is suspicious for fatal abuse. *Pediatr Radiol.* 2004;34:675–677

30. Walker PL, Cook DC, Lambert PM. Skeletal evidence for child abuse: a physical anthropological perspective. *J Forensic Sci.* 1997;42:196–207

31. Kahana T, Hiss J. Forensic radiology. *Br J Radiol.* 1999;72:129–133

32. Berdon WE. Battered children: how valuable are bone scans in diagnosis [editorial]. *Appl Radiol.* 1981:981

33. Conway JJ, Collins M, Tanz RR, et al. The role of bone scintigraphy in detecting child abuse. *Semin Nucl Med.* 1993;23:321–333

34. Ellerstein NS, Norris KJ. The value of radiologic skeletal survey in assessment of abused children. *Pediatrics.* 1984;74:1075–1078

35. Howard JL, Barron DJ, Smith GG. Bone scintigraphy in the evaluation of extraskeletal injuries from child abuse. *Radiographics.* 1990;10:67–81

36. Jaudes PK. Comparison of radiography and radionuclide bone scanning in the detection of child abuse. *Pediatrics.* 1984;73:166–168

37. Mandelstam SA, Cook D, Fitzgerald M, Ditchfield MR. Complementary use of radiological skeletal survey and bone scintigraphy in detection of bony injuries in suspected child abuse. *Arch Dis Child.* 2003;88:387–390

38. Smith FW, Gilday DL, Ash JM, et al. Unsuspected costo-vertebral fractures demonstrated by bone scanning in the child abuse syndrome. *Pediatr Radiol.* 1980;10:103–106

39. Tan TX, Gelfand MJ. Battered child syndrome. Uncommon pelvic fractures detected by bone scintigraphy. *Clin Nucl Med.* 1997;22:321–322

40. Rossmuller B, Hahn K, Fischer S. Bone scintigraphy in non-neoplastic diseases in children. *Q J Nucl Med.* 1998;42:133–147

41. Graif M, Sonntag VK, Rekate HL, et al. Sonographic detection of occult bone fractures. *Pediatr Radiol.* 1988;18:383–385

42. Kleinman PK. *Diagnostic Imaging of Child Abuse.* St Louis, MO: Mosby; 1998:5–28

43. Nimkin K, Kleinman PK, Teeger S, Spevak MR. Distal humeral physeal injuries in child abuse: MR imaging and ultrasonography findings. *Pediatr Radiol.* 1995;25:562–565

44. Belfer RA, Klein BL, Orr L. Use of the skeletal survey in the evaluation of child maltreatment. *Am J Emerg Med.* 2001;19:122–124

45. Haller JO, Kassner EG. The "battered child" syndrome and its imitators: a critical evaluation of specific radiological signs. *Appl Radiol.* 1977;6:88–111

46. King J, Diefendorf D, Apthorp J, Negrete VF, Carlson M. Analysis of 429 fractures in 189 battered children. *J Pediatr Orthop.* 1988;8:585–589

47. Kogutt MS, Swischuk LE, Fagen CJ. Patterns of injury and significance of uncommon fractures in the battered child syndrome. *Am J Roentgenol Radium Ther Nucl Med.* 1974;121:143–149

48. Pierce MC, Bertocci GE, Vogeley E, Moreland MS. Evaluating long bone fractures in children: a biomechanical approach with illustrative cases. *Child Abuse Negl.* 2004;28:505–524

49. Cameron JM, Rae LJ. *Atlas of the Battered Child Syndrome.* Edinburgh, UK: Churchill Livingstone; 1975:20–77

50. Kleinman PK, Marks SC, Blackbourne B. The metaphyseal lesion in abused infants: a radiologic-histopathologic study. *AJR Am J Roentgenol.* 1986;146:895–905

51. Kleinman PK, Marks SC Jr. Relationship of the subperiosteal bone collar to metaphyseal lesions in abused infants. *J Bone Joint Surg Am.* 1995;77:1471–1476

52. Jacobsen FS. Periosteum: its relation to pediatric fractures. *J Pediatr Orthop.* 1997;6:84–90

53. Kleinman PK. Diagnostic imaging in infant abuse. *AJR Am J Roentgenol.* 1990;155:703–712

54. Kleinman PK, Blackbourne BD, Marks SC, et al. Radiologic contributions to the investigation and prosecution of cases of fatal infant abuse. *N Engl J Med.* 1989;320:507

55. Thomsen TK, Elle B, Thomsen JL. Post-mortem radiological examination in infants: evidence of child abuse? *Forensic Sci Int.* 1997;90:223–230

56. O'Neill JA Jr, Meacham WF, Griffin JP, Sawyers JL. Patterns of injury in the battered child syndrome. *J Trauma.* 1973;13:332–339

57. Hymel KP, Jenny C. Abusive spiral fractures of the humerus: a videotaped exception. *Arch Pediatr Adolesc Med.* 1996;150:226–227

58. Banaszkiewicz PA, Scotland TR, Myerscough EJ. Fractures in children younger than age 1 year: importance of collaboration with child protection services. *J Pediatr Orthop.* 2002;22:740–744

59. Oral R, Blum K, Johnson C. Fractures in young children: are physicians in the emergency department and orthopedic clinics adequately screening for possible abuse? *Pediatr Emerg Care.* 2003;19:148–153

60. Sinal SH, Stewart CD. Physical abuse in children: a review for orthopedic surgeons. *J South Orthop Assoc.* 1998;7:264–276

61. Shellern C, Wood D, Murphy A, Crawford M. Non-accidental fractures in infants: risk of further abuse. *J Pediatr Child Health.* 2000;36:590–592

62. Galleno H, Oppenheim WL. The battered child syndrome revisited. *Clin Orthop.* 1982;162:11–19

63. Herndon WA. Child abuse in a military population. *J Pediatr Orthop.* 1983;3:73–76

64. Kleinman PK, Spevak MR. Variations in acromial ossification simulating infant abuse in victims of sudden infant death syndrome. *Radiology.* 1991;180:85–86

65. Leventhal JM, Thomas SA, Rosenfield NS, et al. Fractures in young children: distinguishing child abuse from unintentional injuries. *Am J Dis Child.* 1993;147:87–92

66. Shaw BA, Murphy KM, Shaw A, et al. Humerus shaft fractures in young children: accident or abuse? *J Pediatr Orthop.* 1997;17:293–297

67. Strait RT, Siegal RM, Shapiro RA. Humeral fractures without obvious etiologies in children less than 3 years of age: when is it abuse? *Pediatrics.* 1995;96:667–671

68. Thomas SA, Rosenfield NS, Leventhal JM, et al. Long bone fracture in young children: distinguishing accidental injuries from child abuse. *Pediatrics.* 1991;88:471–476

69. Kleinman PK, Marks SC Jr. A regional approach to the classic metaphyseal lesion in abused infants: the proximal humerus. *AJR Am J Roentgenol.* 1996;167:1399–1403

70. Merten DF, Kirks DR, Ruderman RJ. Occult humeral epiphyseal fracture in battered infants. *Pediatr Radiol.* 1981;10:151–153

71. DeLee JC, Wilkins KE, Rogers LF, Rockwood CA. Fracture-separation of the distal humeral epiphysis. *J Bone Joint Surg Am.* 1980;62:46–51

72. Nimkin K, Spevak MR, Kleinman PK. Fractures of the hands and feet in child abuse: imaging and pathologic features. Radiology. 1997;203:233–236

73. Starling SP, Heller RM, Jenny C. Pelvic fractures in infants as a sign of physical abuse. *Child Abuse Negl.* 2002;26:475–480

74. Pendergast NC, deRoux SJ, Adsay NV. Non-accidental pediatric pelvic fracture: a case report. *Pediatr Radiol.* 1998;28:344–346

75. Hedlund R, Lindgren U. The incidence of femoral shaft fractures in children and adolescents. *J Pediatr Orthop.* 1986;6:47–50

76. Kleinman PK, Marks SC Jr. A regional approach to the classic metaphyseal lesion in abused infants: the distal femur. *AJR Am J Roentgenol.* 1998;170:43–47

77. Carty HM. Fractures caused by child abuse. *J Bone Joint Surg Br.* 1993;75:849–857

78. Beals RK, Tufts E. Fractured femur in infancy: the role of child abuse. *J Pediatr Orthop.* 1983;3:583–586

79. Jones JCW, Feldman KW, Bruckner JD. Child abuse in infants with proximal physeal injuries of the femur. *Pediatr Emerg Care.* 2004;20:157–161

80. Kleinman PK, Marks SC Jr. A regional approach to classic metaphyseal lesions in abused infants: the distal tibia. *AJR Am J Roentgenol.* 1996;166:1207–1212

81. Kleinman PK, Marks SC Jr. A regional approach to the classic metaphyseal lesion in abused infants: the proximal tibia. *AJR Am J Roentgenol.* 1996;166:421–426

82. Mellick LB, Reesor K. Spiral tibial fractures of children: a commonly accidental spiral long bone fracture. *Am J Emerg Med.* 1990;8:234–237

83. Tenebien M, Reed MH, Black GB. The toddler's fracture revisited. *Am J Emerg Med.* 1990;8:208–211

84. Halsey MF, Finzel KC, Carrion WV. Toddler's fracture: presumptive diagnosis and treatment. *J Pediatr Orthop.* 2001;21:475–481

85. John SD, Moorthy CS, Swischuk LE. Expanding the concept of the toddler's fracture. Radiographics. 1997;17:367–376

86. Oudjhane K. Occult fractures in preschool children. *J Trauma.* 1988;28:858–860

87. Schwend RM, Werth C, Johnston A. Femoral shaft fractures in toddlers: rarely from abuse. *J Pediatr Orthop.* 2000;20:475–481

88. Singer J, Towbin R. Occult fractures in the production of gait disturbance in childhood. *Pediatrics.* 1979;64:192–196

89. Shavrat BP, Harrop SN, Kane TP. Toddler's fracture. *J Accid Emerg Med.* 1996;13:59–61

90. Ogden JA. Injury to the growth mechanisms of the immature skeleton. *Skeletal Radiol.* 1981;6:237–253

91. Caffey J. Traumatic cupping of the metaphysis of growing bones. *AJR Am J Roentgenol.* 1970;108:451–460

92. Bullock B, Schubert CJ, Brophy PD, Johnson N, Reed MH, Shapiro RA. Cause and clinical characteristics of rib fractures in infants. *Pediatrics.* 2000;105:e48

93. Cadzow SP, Armstrong KL. Rib fractures in infants: red alert! The clinical features, investigations and child protection outcomes. *J Pediatr Child Health.* 2000;36:322–326

94. Barsness KA, Bernsard DD, Calkins CM, Patrick DA, Karrar FM, Strain JD. The positive predictive value of rib fractures as an indicator of non-accidental trauma in children. *J Trauma.* 2003;54:1107–1110

95. Feldman KW, Brewer DK. Child abuse, cardiopulmonary resuscitation and rib fractures. *Pediatrics.* 1984;73:339–342

96. Ryan MP, Young SJ, Wells DL. Do resuscitation attempts in children who die cause injury? *J Emerg Med.* 2003;20:10–12

97. Sewell RD, Steinberg MA. Chest compressions in an infant with osteogenesis imperfecta type II: no new rib fractures. *Pediatrics.* 2000;106:e71

98. Kleinman PK, Schlesinger AE. Mechanical factors associated with posterior rib fractures: laboratory and case studies. *Pediatr Radiol.* 1997;27:87–91

99. Kleinman PK, Marks SC, Adams VI, Blackbourne BD. Factors affecting visualization of posterior rib fractures in abused infants. *AJR Am J Roentgenol.* 1988;150:635–638

100. Ng CS, Hall CM. Costochondral junction fracture and intraabdominal trauma in non-accidental injury (child abuse). *Pediatr Radiol.* 1998;28:671–676

101. Kleinman PK, Marks SC Jr, Nimkin K, et al. Rib fractures in 31 abused infants: postmortem radiologic-histopathologic study. *Radiology.* 1996;200:807–810

102. Strouse PJ, Owings CL. Fractures of the first rib in child abuse. *Radiology.* 1995;197:763–765

103. Hechter S, Huyer D, Manson D. Sternal fractures as a manifestation of abusive injury in children. *Pediatr Radiol.* 2002;32:902–906

104. Kleinman PK, Marks SC. Vertebral body fractures in child abuse: radiologic-histologic correlates. *Invest Radiol.* 1992;27:715–722

105. Levin TL, Berdon WE, Cassell I, Blitman NM. Thoracolumbar fracture with listhesis—an uncommon manifestation of child abuse. *Pediatr Radiol.* 2003;33:305–310

106. Cullen JC. Spinal lesions in battered babies. *J Bone Joint Surg Br.* 1975;17:364–366

107. Gabos PG, Tuten HR, Leet A, et al. Fracture-dislocation of the lumbar spine in an abused child. *Pediatrics.* 1998;101:473–477

108. Kleinman PK, Zito JL. Avulsion of the spinal processes caused by infant abuse. *Radiology.* 1984;151:389–391

109. Swischuk LE. Spine and spinal cord trauma in the battered child syndrome. *Radiology.* 1969;92:733–738

110. Diamond P, Hansen CM, Christoferson MR. Child abuse presenting as a thoracolumbar spinal fracture dislocation: a case report. *Pediatr Emerg Care.* 1994;10:83–86

111. Kleinman PK, Shelton YA. Hangman's fracture in an abused infant: imaging features. *Pediatr Radiol.* 1997;27:776–777

112. Brown RL, Brunn MA, Garcia VF. Cervical spine injuries in children: a review of 103 patients treated consecutively at a level 1 pediatric trauma center. *J Pediatr Surg.* 2001;36:1107–1114

113. Hadley MN, Sonntag VK, Rekate HL, et al. The infant whiplash-shake syndrome: a clinical and pathological study. *Neurosurgery.* 1989;24:536–540

114. Rooks VJ, Sisler C, Burton B. Cervical spine injury in child abuse: report of two cases. *Pediatr Radiol.* 1998;28:193–195

115. Givens TG, Polley KA, Smith GF, Hardin WD Jr. Pediatric cervical spine injury: a three year experience. *J Trauma.* 1996;41:310–314

116. Feldman K, Weinberger E, Milstein J, Figner C. Cervical spine MRI in abused infants. *Child Abuse Negl.* 1997;21:199–205

117. Wenger DR, Rokicki RR. Spinal deformity secondary to scar formation in a battered child: case report. *J Bone Joint Surg Am.* 1978;60:847

118. Merten DF, Osborne DR, Radkowski MA, et al. Craniocerebral trauma in the child abuse syndrome: radiological observations. *Pediatr Radiol.* 1984;14:272–277

119. Saulsbury FT, Alford BA. Intracranial bleeding from child abuse: the value of skull radiographs. *Pediatr Radiol.* 1982;12:175–178

120. Hobbs CJ. Skull fracture and the diagnosis of abuse. *Arch Dis Child.* 1984;59:246–252

121. Helfer RE, Slovis TL, Black M. Injuries resulting when small children fall out of bed. *Pediatrics.* 1977;60:533–535

122. Kravitz H, Dreissen G, Gomberg R, et al. Accidental falls from elevated surfaces in infants from birth to one year. *Pediatrics.* 1969;44(suppl):867–876

123. Tarantino CA, Dowd MD, Murdock TC. Short vertical falls in infants. *Pediatr Emerg Care.* 1999;15:5–8

124. Tate RJ. Facial injuries associated with the battered child syndrome. *Br J Oral Maxillofac Surg.* 1971;9:41–45

125. O'Connor JF, Cohen J. Dating fractures. In: Kleinman PK, ed. *Diagnostic Imaging of Child Abuse.* 2nd ed. St Louis, MO: Mosby; 1998:168–177

126. Prosser I, Maguire S, Harrison SK, Mann M, Sibert JR, Kemp AM. How old is this fracture? Radiologic dating of fractures in children: a systematic review. *AJR Am J Roentgenol.* 2005;184:1282–1286

127. Chapman S. The radiological dating of injuries. *Arch Dis Child.* 1992;67:1063–1065

128. Kleinman PK, Marks SC Jr, Spevak MR, Belanger PL, Richmond JM. Extension of growth-plate cartilage into the metaphysis: a sign of healing fracture in abused infants. *AJR Am J Roentgenol.* 1991;156:775–779

129. Osier LK, Marks SC Jr, Kleinman PK. Metaphyseal extensions of hypertrophied chondrocytes in abused infants indicate healing fractures. *J Pediatr Orthop.* 1998;13:249–254

130. Brill PW, Winchester P, Kleinman PK. Differential diagnosis I: diseases simulating abuse. In: Kleinman PK, ed. *Diagnostic Imaging of Child Abuse.* 2nd ed. St Louis, MO: Mosby; 1998:178–196

131. Radkowski MA. The battered child syndrome: pitfalls in radiological diagnosis. *Pediatr Ann.* 1983;12:894–903

132. Radkowski MA, Merten DF, Leonidas JC. The abused child: criteria for the radiologic diagnosis. *Radiographics.* 1983;3:262–297

133. Falk B, Bronshtein Z, Zigel L, Constantini NW, Eliakim A. Quantitative ultrasound of the tibia and radius in prepubertal and early pubertal female athletes. *Arch Pediatr Adolesc Med.* 2003;157:139–143

134. Gafni RI, Barton J. Overdiagnosis of osteoporosis in children due to misinterpretation of dual-energy x-ray absorptiometry (DEXA). *J Pediatr.* 2004;144:253–257

135. Cumming WA. Neonatal skeletal fractures: birth trauma or child abuse. *Can Assoc Radiol J.* 1979;30:30–33

136. McBride MT, Hennrikus WL, Mologne T. Newborn clavicle fractures. *Orthopedics.* 1998;17:317–320

137. McClelland CQ, Heiple KG. Fractures in the first year of life: a diagnostic dilemma? *Am J Dis Child.* 1982;136:26–29

138. Lysack JT, Soboleski D. Classic metaphyseal lesion following external cephalic version and cesarian section. *Pediatr Radiol.* 2003;33:422–424

139. Hartman RW Jr. Rib fractures produced by birth trauma: radiological case of the month. *Arch Pediatr Adolesc Med.* 1997;151:947–948

140. Rizzolo PJ, Coleman PR. Neonatal rib fracture: birth trauma or child abuse. *J Fam Pract.* 1989;29:561–563

141. Morris S, Cassidy N, Stephens M, McCormack D, McManus F. Birth associated femoral fractures: incidence and outcome. *J Pediatr Orthop.* 2002;22:27–30

142. Helfer RE, Scheurer SL, Alexander R, et al. Trauma to the bones of small infants from passive exercise: a factor in the etiology of child abuse. *J Pediatr.* 1984;104:47–50

143. Hoeffel JCl. Fracture separation of the epiphysis and scurvy. Presented at: Congress of European Society of Pediatric Radiology; 1992; Budapest, Hungary

144. Paterson CR. Vitamin D deficiency rickets simulating child abuse. *J Pediatr Ortho.* 1981;1:423–425

145. DeRusso PA, Spevak MR, Schwarz KB. Fractures in biliary atresia misinterpreted as child abuse. *Pediatrics.* 2003;112:185–188

146. Lim HK, Smith WL, Sato Y, et al. Congenital syphilis mimicking child abuse. *Pediatr Radiol.* 1995;25:560–561

147. Henderson RC, Lark RK, Gurka MJ, et al. Bone density and metabolism in children and adolescents with moderate to severe cerebral palsy. *Pediatrics.* 2002;110:e5

148. Brunner R, Doderlein L. Pathological fractures in patients with cerebral palsy. *J Pediatric Orthop Br.* 1996;5:232–238

149. Grayev AM, Boal DK, Wallach DM, Segal LS. Metaphyseal fractures mimicking abuse during treatment of clubfoot. *Pediatr Radiol.* 2001;31:559–563

150. Torwalt CR, Balachandra AT, Youngson C, deNanassy J. Spontaneous fractures in the differential diagnosis of fractures in children. *J Forensic Sci.* 2002;47:1340–1344

151. Sturm PF, Almon BA, Christie BL. Femur fractures in institutionalized patients after hip spica immobilization. *J Pediatr Orthop.* 1993;13:246–248

152. Gyepes MT, Newbern DH, Neuhauser EB. Metaphyseal and physeal injuries in children with spina bifida and meningomyeloceles. *Am J Roentgenol Radium Ther Nucl Med.* 1965;95:168–177

153. Silverman FN, Gilder JJ. Congenital insensitivity to pain: a neurologic syndrome with bizarre skeletal lesions. *Radiology.* 1959;72:176–190

154. Spencer JA, Grieve DK. Congenital indifference to pain mistaken for nonaccidental injury. *Br J Radiol.* 1990;63:308–310

155. Ablin DS. Osteogenesis imperfecta: a review. *Can Assoc Radiol J.* 1998;49:110–123

156. Ablin DS, Greenspan A, Reinhart M, Grix A. Differentiation of child abuse from osteogenesis imperfecta. *AJR Am J Roentgenol.* 1990;154:1035–1046

157. Taitz LS. Child abuse and metabolic bone disease: are they often confused? *Br Med J.* 1991;302:1244

158. Astley R. Metaphyseal fractures in osteogenesis imperfecta. *Br J Radiol.* 1979;52:441–442

159. Ablin DS, Sane SM. Non-accidental injury: confusion with temporary brittle bone disease and mild osteogenesis imperfecta. *Pediatr Radiol.* 1997;27:111–113

160. Chapman S, Hall CM. Non-accidental injury or brittle bones. *Pediatr Radiol.* 1997;27:106–110

161. Dent JA, Patterson CR. Fractures in early childhood: osteogenesis imperfecta or child abuse? *J Pediatr Orthop.* 1991;11:1984–1991

162. Patterson CR, Burns J, McAllion SJ. Osteogenesis imperfecta: the distinction from child abuse and recognition of a variant form. *Am J Med Genet.* 1993;45:187–192

163. Mendelson KL. Critical review of "temporary brittle bone disease." *Pediatr Radiol.* 2005;35:1036–1040

164. Block RW. Child abuse—controversies and imposters. *Curr Probl Pediatr.* 1999;29:249–272

165. Widhe TL. A probable new type of osteopenic bone disease. *Pediatr Radiol.* 2002;32:447–451

166. Kleinman PK. Differentiation of child abuse and osteogenesis imperfecta: medical and legal implications. *AJR Am J Roentgenol.* 1990;154:1047–1048

167. Steiner RD, Pepin M, Byers PH. Studies of collagen synthesis and structure in the differentiation of child abuse from osteogenesis imperfecta. *J Pediatr.* 1996;128:542–547

168. Knight DJ, Bennett GC. Non-accidental injury and osteogenesis imperfecta: a case report. *J Pediatr Orthop.* 1990;10:542–544

169. Kleinman PK. Schmid-like metaphyseal chondrodysplasia simulating child abuse. *AJR Am J Roentgenol.* 1991;156:576–578

170. Langer LO Jr, Brill PW, Ozonoff MB, et al. Spondylometaphyseal dysplasia, corner fracture type: a heritable condition associated with coxa-vara. *Radiology.* 1990;175:761–766

171. Grant P, Mata MB, Tidwell M. Femur fracture in infants: a possible accidental etiology. *Pediatrics.* 2001;108:1009–1012

172. Warrington SA, Wright CM, ALSPAC Study Team. Accidents and resulting injuries in premobile infants: data from the ALSPAC study. *Arch Dis Child.* 2001;85:104–107

173. Nimituyongskul T, Anderson LD. The likelihood of injuries when children fall out of bed. *J Pediatr Orthop.* 1987;7:184–186

174. Sawyer JR, Flynn JM, Dormans JP, Catalano J, Drummond DS. Fracture patterns in children and young adults who fall from significant heights. *J Pediatr Orthop.* 2000;20:197–202

175. Sloan GD, Talbot JA. Forensic application of computer simulation of falls. *J Forensic Sci.* 1996;41:782–785

176. Pergolizzi R Jr, Oestreich AE. Child abuse fracture through physiologic periosteal reaction. *Pediatr Radiol.* 1995;25:566–567

177. Fenton LZ, Sirotnak AP, Handler MH. Parietal pseudofracture and spontaneous intracranial hemorrhage suggesting non-accidental trauma. *Pediatr Neurosurg.* 2000;33:318–322

178. Kleinman PK, Belanger PL, Karaellas A, Spevak MR. Normal metaphyseal radiologic variants not to be confused with findings of infant abuse. *AJR Am J Roentgenol.* 1991;156:781–783

179. Harty MP, Kao SC. Intraosseous vascular access defect: fracture mimic in the skeletal survey in child abuse. *Pediatr Radiol.* 2002;32:188–190

180. Norman MG, Smialek JE, Newman DE, Horembala EJ. The post-mortem examination of the abused child. Pathological, radiographic, and legal aspects. *Perspect Pediatr Pathol.* 1984;8:313–343

Chapter 4

Visceral Manifestations of Child Physical Abuse

Michael L. Nance

University of Pennsylvania
Pediatric Trauma Program, The Children's Hospital of Philadelphia

Arthur Cooper

Columbia University College of Physicians & Surgeons
Trauma & Pediatric Surgical Services, Harlem Hospital Center

Treatment of the abused child represents one of the most challenging aspects of pediatric medicine and trauma care. In addition to the complex medical issues, there are frequently daunting social and ethical problems that compound the care. The United States has one of the highest reported rates of child maltreatment death in the industrialized world, accounting for 17% of all injury deaths in the pediatric population.[1]

In 2004 an estimated 3.5 million investigations were launched into suspected child abuse and neglect. Of these, nearly 872,000 cases were substantiated, an average of one case every 10 seconds. Of the reported cases, there were 1,490 fatalities due to child abuse and neglect.[2] Despite these significant numbers, the recognition of death due to inflicted injury is often underappreciated. The under-ascertainment of child abuse homicides may be as high as 50% to 61% using traditional *International Classification of Diseases, Ninth Revision, Clinical Modification* coding strategies, making child abuse deaths a much greater problem than is generally understood.[3,4] Estimating the true incidence of child physical abuse in the non–fatally injured child may be harder still. It has been suggested that child abuse may be responsible for as many as 10% of all pediatric visits to the emergency department.[5] In a review of the National Pediatric Trauma Registry, more than 10% of children younger than 5 years entered into the dataset had inflicted injuries.[6] In large urban pediatric trauma centers, 1.4% of all admissions (all ages) were due to child abuse.[5] Because of the unacceptably high incidence of child physical abuse, health care professionals must be ever observant and questioning.

Informed estimates of the incidence of intrathoracic or intra-abdominal injuries resulting from inflicted injuries are limited. Major blunt trauma to the abdomen is an infrequent injury in abused children, accounting for less than 1% of all reported cases of abuse.[7] Despite this, abdominal trauma is among the leading causes of death from physical abuse. This high mortality rate reflects the young age of the victims, the severity of injuries sustained, delay in seeking appropriate medical care, and a characteristic delay in making a correct diagnosis that occurs with the typical misleading histories. Blunt abdominal trauma (both acute and chronic) has been demonstrated in 14% of fatally abused children in an autopsy series.[8]

In reported series of pediatric abdominal trauma, child abuse accounts for between 5% and 20% of abdominal injuries[9] (Table 4.1). Most children who sustain significant abdominal trauma are typically young (between 6 months and 3 years of age), younger than those with accidental abdominal injury.[7,10,11] For example, Ledbetter et al[11] reported that 11% of pediatric abdominal trauma cases were attributed to child abuse. However, in children younger than 4 years, abuse accounted for 44% of the abdominal injuries. The pattern of organ injury differs in children who are abused compared with those accidentally injured. Whereas single, solid organ injuries are most common in accidental trauma, injuries in abused children are often multiple owing to the small size of the toddler abdomen.[11–13] Additionally, injuries to hollow viscera are common in abused children. Injury to both solid organs and hollow viscera are highly specific for inflicted injury and are rarely seen with accidental trauma.[13] Compared with children who die of inflicted neurotrauma, those with fatal abdominal trauma tend to be slightly older, generally toddler-aged, suggesting a shift in

TABLE 4.1
Frequency of Visceral Injuries From Child Abuse in Selected Reports of Pediatric Thoracoabdominal Trauma

Author	Year of Publication	N	Injury Type	% Due to Abuse
Cooper et al	1988	22	Abdominal	0.5
Miller et al	1998	36	Liver	11.0
Sivit et al	1989	69	Abdominal/thoracic	20.0
Ng et al	1997	12	Visceral	4.0
Arkovitz et al	1997	26	Pancreas	19.0
Jobst et al	1999	56	Pancreas	17.9
Mehall et al	2001	89	Liver/spleen	4.5
Margenthaler et al	2002	55	Renal	7.0
Nance et al	2002	134	Liver/spleen	2.2
Nance et al	2004	101	Renal	5.3
Landau et al	2006	311	Hepatic	4.8

injury mechanism from the head to the abdomen with increasing age.

Unlike injuries in other anatomical locations, inflicted abdominal injuries frequently lack external evidence of trauma, making the recognition more challenging. Even with severe trauma, abdominal wall bruising is often absent.[11,14] It is likely that abdominal injury is more common than recognized. More subtle abdominal trauma often is undetected, and occult abdominal injury is identified in abused children.[15] Recognizing the need to uncover potentially subtle abdominal injuries in physically abused children, the American Academy of Pediatrics recommends screening tests for intra-abdominal injuries in all physically abused children (although the utility of this approach has yet to be confirmed).[16] Because rates of both intra-abdominal and intrathoracic injury have been shown to be significantly higher in abused children than in their unintentionally injured peers, there is a need for vigilance.[6]

Clinical Presentation

Most inflicted abdominal injuries caused by abuse are due to blunt trauma. Although penetrating injuries do occur (such as stabs or gunshot wounds), they are comparatively rare. One of 3 basic mechanisms of trauma account for the typical injuries identified. These include crushing of solid organs against the vertebral bodies or bony thorax, compression of the hollow viscera against the vertebral column, or shearing of the posterior attachments or vascular supply of the abdominal viscera. The symptoms and presentation of the child reflect the type and severity of the injuries sustained, the amount of time that has elapsed prior to seeking medical care, and the rate of bleeding (if present).

In the setting of abuse, the history provided by the parent or caregiver is almost always incomplete and misleading. Often, the child is brought to medical attention by a non-offending parent who may be unaware of the trauma and, therefore, unable to explain the etiology of the child's symptoms. The typical history provided by perpetrators may include minor trauma, such as falls down stairs, off a bed, or off a couch. In some cases, the chief complaint is apnea (as a consequence of hypovolemic or septic shock) or seizures, and medical attention focuses on possible central nervous system rather than abdominal causes. Other children sustain both abdominal and head trauma, which makes the clinical examination of the abdomen more difficult, leading to further delay in diagnosis.

Children often present to medical care with nonspecific abdominal complaints, such as vomiting, fever, or abdominal pain. Symptoms generally reflect the type of injury sustained, but infants and toddlers do not always show classic signs of injury. For example, intestinal perforation presents with signs of peritonitis, including fever, pain, abdominal distention, diminished bowel sounds, and leukocytosis, but these classic peritoneal signs are not always present in infants and young children. In one series, absent bowel sounds and non-localized tenderness were the only consistent physical findings in children with intestinal perforations.[10] Children with mesenteric tears or massive liver or spleen injuries typically present with signs of hypovolemic shock.

Mortality from inflicted abdominal trauma is greater than from accidental injury and is usually due to severe blood loss and/or a delay in seeking treatment.[11] These children present with either profound hemorrhagic shock or are dead on arrival to the hospital. Children who exsanguinate and die before reaching the hospital are often found to have more than 50% estimated blood volume loss at autopsy.[7] Peritonitis and sepsis account for most other deaths. The severity of the peritonitis and the rapidity with which signs and symptoms develop depend on the location and severity of the initial injury, the type of bacterial contamination of the peritoneal cavity, and the child's preexisting health. In general, signs of peritonitis develop within hours of the injury, although death may be delayed by a few days in untreated cases. It is worth noting, however, that while delay in presentation or recognition of an abdominal injury is concerning for child abuse, it can be seen in cases of accidental trauma, particularly in preverbal children.[13]

Initial Evaluation

Evaluation of the injured child, whether or not physical abuse is suspected, should proceed in accordance with the well-established guidelines developed by the American College of Surgeons Committee on Trauma and taught through the Advanced Trauma Life Support (ATLS)

course.[17] Such care should be rendered under the supervision of qualified emergency medical and surgical personnel in a center with appropriate equipment and support staff for managing pediatric trauma. The ATLS guidelines mandate a systematic assessment of the patient from head to toe with the goals of detecting life-threatening injuries early and, at the same time, minimizing the risk of missed injuries. In the initial phase, a primary assessment is performed focusing on airway, breathing, and circulatory issues (the ABCs). Once completed, a quick neurologic assessment is performed. It is during this primary assessment that the airway is controlled, intravenous (IV) access established, and fluid resuscitation initiated. The primary assessment is designed to identify life-threatening injuries necessitating immediate intervention. During the secondary survey, a complete physical examination is performed, carefully documenting all abnormalities. Appropriate laboratory and imaging studies are obtained based on the findings noted during the primary and secondary surveys.

For many victims of child abuse, the presenting history is not that of trauma but rather of the related symptoms (eg, irritability, gait disturbance) that might be attributable to an injury. It is with a high index of suspicion, often developed after a thorough history, that one recognizes the potential for inflicted trauma and proceeds with a more formal evaluation for detection of clinically occult injuries. This heightened index of suspicion cannot be understated, particularly when one realizes that more than 75% of child abuse victims are younger than 4 years, making accurate history taking a challenge.

Laboratory Studies

A complete blood count (CBC) including indices should be obtained in a child undergoing an evaluation for suspected visceral injury. The CBC may reveal anemia from ongoing blood loss due to injury or anemia due to chronic disease. The platelet count is valuable in the setting of unexplained chest or abdominal wall bruising to help exclude an underlying bleeding disorder. In addition, a coagulation profile (prothrombin time, partial thromboplastin time) should be obtained in any child with suspicious bruising to exclude the possibility of an underlying coagulopathy. A urinalysis should be performed to look for hematuria (a marker of genitourinary trauma). The finding of hematuria should be further investigated with computed tomography (CT) scan of the abdomen to exclude occult renal trauma or a congenital genitourinary anomaly. The utility of additional routine screening laboratory studies in the setting of blunt abdominal trauma is controversial. Several studies have demonstrated some benefit to the use of such studies in the setting of possible or suspected child abuse. Liver function tests have been found to be elevated in 8% of child abuse victims with a normal abdominal examination.[15] Elevated liver function studies (aspartate transaminase [AST] >400 IU/L, alanine transaminase [ALT] >250 IU/L) were found to be predictive of liver injury and, thus, the need for CT scan in children with inflicted abdominal trauma.[18] Liver function studies as a screening tool may be useful in identifying the need to perform a CT scan in the setting of suspected physical abuse. Support for the routine use of amylase and lipase as markers of abdominal trauma are lacking. Amylase and lipase have been shown to be poorly correlated with risk for abdominal injury.[19] In a review of 1,800 children evaluated for trauma, amylase and lipase did not improve the rate of detection of pancreatic injury above suspicion based on clinical examination.[20]

Imaging Modalities

Radiographic imaging is frequently used to assess the child with suspected inflicted injuries. Plain films of body regions with clinical evidence of injury are necessary to confirm or exclude fractures. In addition, in infants and younger children, a skeletal survey is useful to detect clinically occult or healing fractures. The skeletal survey includes 2 views of each extremity, anteroposterior (AP) and lateral skull, AP and lateral spine, chest, abdomen, pelvis, hands, and feet. It can be difficult to detect fractures in the ribs and, in cases of suspected abuse, oblique views or skeletal radionuclide scintigraphy (bone scan) has been recommended to optimize the rate of detection.[21,22] Assessment of the abdominal organs is best done with a contrast enhanced CT scan. This provides information about the solid organs, retroperitoneum, and osseus structures. It is not unusual to detect previously unrecognized rib fractures on an abdominal CT. If significant thoracic trauma is suspected, a CT scan of the chest is recommended to evaluate the lung fields, the major vasculature, and mediastinal structures.

An ultrasound may be useful in selected settings to detect fluid in the abdomen suggesting bowel injury or hemorrhage, but is less specific in identifying injuries and is not the first-line study in the pediatric patient.

Injuries to Specific Body Regions

Understanding the true incidence of abuse-related injuries and defining characteristic patterns of injury from abuse are difficult. This lack of understanding is in part due to the uncertainty of injury mechanisms that surround many of the cases of suspected abuse as well as the fact that many cases of abuse go unrecognized. The incidence of abdominal or thoracic injuries in children evaluated for child abuse may be as high as 20%, emphasizing the need to evaluate each child thoroughly (Table 4.1).[23] Further, the severity of inflicted injuries is often magnified by the fact that there is a delay in seeking medical treatment for often life-threatening conditions. Ongoing studies of cases of documented abuse will help identify injuries suggestive of abuse and better define thoracoabdominal injury patterns characteristic of abuse.

Soft Tissues

Injuries to the soft tissues of the chest wall and abdomen may include burns, contusions, and ecchymoses. Such injuries are rarely life-threatening. Rather, their importance lies in the fact that they may be indicative of more serious associated injury. The significance of a bruise must be interpreted within the context of the medical history and developmental level of the child. Bruising in any location in a non-ambulatory patient is concerning for abuse. In addition, bruising of the back or abdomen (ie, the torso) in infants and toddlers is extremely uncommon and rarer still in non-ambulatory children.[24,25] Such findings should stimulate further investigation for medical or traumatic causes. Bruising of the torso may be associated with internal injuries, which should be investigated in the appropriate clinical setting. Patterned bruises or marks may indicate beating with an object such as a rope or belt. Burns are a common mechanism of child abuse. Patterned or multiple burns may indicate inflicted injuries. Typically, soft tissue injuries represent little threat to life but are a marker of abuse and mandate further evaluation. Most soft tissue injuries are self-limited, requiring only comfort or topical care.

Thoracic Injuries

Injuries to the thoracic cavity are noted in 12.5% of abused children, compared with 4.5% of the general pediatric trauma population.[6] Due to the increased compliance of the pediatric chest wall, blunt forces are more readily transmitted to the underlying structures (eg, lung) and one must be cautious of serious intrathoracic injury without associated bony injury.

Rib Fractures

Due to the compliant nature of the pediatric skeletal system, the forces required to cause a fracture can be quite substantial. Thus the presence of a rib fracture (or other skeletal injury) without adequate explanation is highly suspicious for child abuse. In the infant, it has been demonstrated that 82% of rib fractures are due to child abuse, compared with 7.7% from accidental injury, 7.7% from bone fragility, and 2.6% from birth trauma.[26] Rib fractures have a 95% positive predictive value of non-accidental trauma in children younger than 3 years and are the only skeletal manifestation of inflicted injury in 29% of cases.[27] Anterior rib fractures are quite uncommon, and those along the costochondral junction have the added concern for associated intra-abdominal injury.[28] Rib fractures from abuse are frequently multiple (Figure 4.1). Posterior and lateral locations for the fracture are common features based on the suspected mechanism of AP compression of the thorax (Figure 4.2). Fractures of the first rib are exceedingly rare and are indicative of significant force. They should be considered highly suggestive of child abuse in the young child.[29] Flail chest as a result of inflicted injuries has been reported in an infant, but is quite unusual.[30] Some controversy exits about rib fractures detected in the child who has undergone cardiopulmonary resuscitation (CPR) for cardiac arrest. In this setting, rib fractures have been attributed to the chest compressions. However, rib fractures from CPR are very unusual (3 in 923 patients).[31] In those cases of fractures associated with CPR, all were noted to be anterior. Thus CPR is not an adequate explanation as a source for most rib fractures and in particular the classic posterolateral rib fractures often seen with child abuse.

While rib fractures are often markers for child abuse, they are not always visualized by standard imaging techniques such as skeletal surveys. In fact, only 36% of all rib fractures identified in a series of fatally abused children were

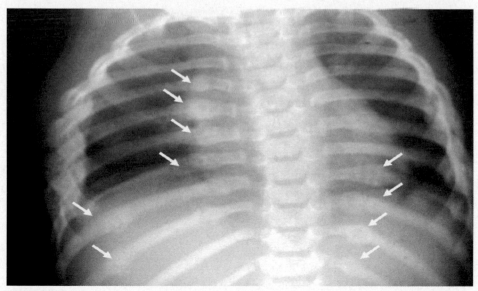

FIGURE 4.1
Chest radiograph demonstrating the characteristic rib fractures (white arrows) associated with child abuse. This child had a total of 23 fractures identified.

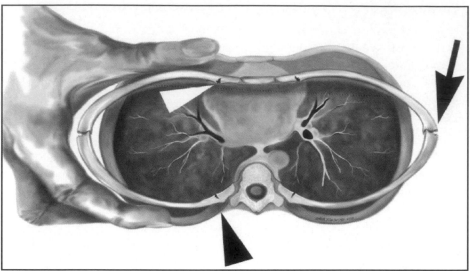

FIGURE 4.2
Characterization of rib fracture mechanism in inflicted injury. (From Lonergan GF, Baker AM, Morey MK, et al. Child abuse: radiologic-pathologic correlation. *Radiographics*. 2003;23:811.)

visible on standard imaging.[32] Skeletal radionuclide scintigraphy has been demonstrated to increase the detection of rib fractures in cases of suspected abuse and should be considered a complementary study (Figure 4.3).[22] More recent studies have recommended the routine addition of oblique views of the ribs to optimize the detection of rib fractures in cases of suspected child abuse.[21] The management of rib fractures is based on symptomatology. Nonsteroidal analgesics or narcotics will control the pain in most patients. On occasion, particularly with multiple fractures, IV or epidural pain management is necessary.

Hypopharynx/Esophagus

Subcutaneous emphysema and pneumomediastinum have been reported in child abuse secondary to perforation of the hypopharynx and esophagus.[33,34]

Ng and colleagues[28] reported cases of pharyngeal perforation with associated focal abscess and mediastinitis. In addition, mediastinitis with an associated

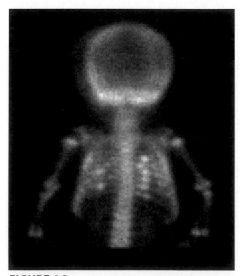

FIGURE 4.3
Bone scan of child with multiple rib fractures from physical abuse (white spots correlate with fractures).

mediastinal abscess has been documented as a result of inflicted injury.[35] Such injuries are typically the result of insertion of a foreign body forcefully into the esophagus; however, an acceleration/deceleration mechanism has also been reported.[36] Unexplained mediastinal findings should be thoughtfully investigated and abuse excluded. Management of hypopharyngeal or esophageal injuries depends on the location and extent of injury as well as the degree of contamination. Management may be expectant, with broad-spectrum antibiotics. In more severe cases, formal drainage procedures may be necessary.

Internal Chest Injuries

Inflicted blunt trauma to the heart and lungs is less common than abdominal injury. This may be due partly to the protection afforded by the pliable, cartilaginous ribs of the young child. It is likely, however, that internal chest injuries are underreported in the child abuse literature. On occasion, contusions and lacerations of the lower lungs are identified by abdominal CT.[23] As with significant abdominal trauma, external signs of trauma may be absent despite serious intrathoracic injury.[37]

Hemothorax/Pneumothorax

Hemothorax and pneumothorax are unusual injuries in the setting of child abuse. They may result from an injury to underlying, adjacent lung in the setting of rib fractures or from an inflicted penetrating mechanism. The diagnosis of hemothorax and/or pneumothorax can be made by chest radiograph. Management of hemothorax or pneumothorax in most cases requires only tube thoracostomy. In more severe cases, thoracotomy to control ongoing bleeding or a persistent air leak may be required.

Pulmonary Contusion

Pulmonary contusion, typically from compressive forces, has been reported in the abuse population. McEniery et al[38] reported a 6-week-old infant with pulmonary contusion, pulmonary edema, and a pneumomediastinum resulting from severe AP chest compression by the infant's father. Symptomatic pulmonary injury is unusual and presents with tachypnea and hypoxia. The contusions should be evident by chest x-ray within hours of the injury. Rib fractures may also be found in association with pulmonary contusion and are indicative of increased force. Most contusions will be of limited clinical significance. Large contusions, however, can result in respiratory failure. Because most contusions are self-limited, management is supportive. In cases of severe contusion, particularly when associated rib fractures impair respiration, mechanical ventilatory support may be necessary.

Cardiac Trauma

Cardiac injuries in pediatric trauma are quite rare.[39] Cardiac injuries as the result of abuse have been reported.[40–42] Several cases of commotio cordis—fatal dysrhythmia due to forces applied to the precordial chest—have been reported as causes of fatal child abuse.[43,44] External evidence of trauma was present in only one case (chest wall ecchymosis), and resuscitation efforts were unsuccessful. The diagnosis was made only after confessions by the perpetrators. Because physical evidence may be lacking, it may be a more common phenomenon than generally appreciated. Cardiac rupture has been reported in several cases of fatal child abuse.[45] The injury in 5 cases was to the right ventricle, and to the left ventricle in a sixth case. The mechanism was thought to be compression of the heart between the sternum and spine. In the 3 cases with a reported confession, the injury was a result of a blow with a fist, a kick, and a stomp.[45] The diagnosis of physical abuse should be strongly pursued in cases of cardiac rupture in young children without an obvious injury mechanism. Cumberland et al[42] reported intimal tears of the right atrium found at autopsy of 6 children, 3 of whom were teenagers who died in motor vehicle crashes and 3 of whom were young victims of abuse. All 6 children had associated liver lacerations and other signs of abdominal trauma. The authors postulate that the cardiac injuries were the result of transmitted hydrostatic forces from the abdomen, through the inferior vena cava, and to the fixed right atrium.[42] Traumatic ventricular septal defect (VSD) as a result of child abuse has also been reported.[40,46] These injuries may present in an acute or subacute fashion as a result of heart failure. Rees et al[40] reported a traumatic VSD that resulted from a kick to the chest of a 5-year-old girl, causing the heart to be crushed against the vertebrae. The child presented in cardiac failure and was initially treated medically, with eventual surgical repair. Injuries to the heart can result in electrical conduction abnormalities and are evaluated with chest x-ray, electrocardiogram, and echocardiogram. Creatine phosphokinase MB fractions have not been described in the evaluation of abused children with cardiac injuries but could potentially help diagnose cardiac muscle damage that results from severe blunt thoracic injury. Treatment of cardiac injuries resulting in structural abnormalities (eg, valvular disruption) requires operative intervention. The management of injuries resulting in functional abnormalities is usually supportive.

Abdominal Injuries

The abdomen is the leading site of death due to occult injury in the general pediatric trauma population. Abdominal injuries are the second leading cause of death (behind head injuries) in children with fatal physical abuse and tend to occur in characteristic patterns with vital signs unique to each such presentation[7,47] (Table 4.2). Major abdominal injuries were identified in 0.5% of all children hospitalized for evaluation of intentional injuries in one report, 45% of whom were fatally injured.[7] Abdominal injuries were identified in 11.4% of abused children (vs 6.8% of general pediatric trauma population) in a review of the National Pediatric Trauma registry that included more than 18,000 children younger than 5 years.[6] Abused children with abdominal injury are at a significantly greater risk of death due to injury than non-abused children with abdominal injury.[9] This fact may be due to the often extreme forces (eg, punch or

TABLE 4.2
Relationship of Vital Signs to Mortality Outcome in Major Blunt Abdominal Trauma.[7]

	T (°C)	P (bpm)	SBP (mm Hg)	Hct (%)	Mortality (n)
Pancreatic/duodenal hematoma	37.3	112	101	27	0/4
Duodenal/jejunal rupture	38.3	148	80	38	1/5
Minor solid visceral injuries	37.3	148	98	22	0/3
Major solid visceral injuries	35.2	133	62	22	9/10

Abbreviations: T, temperature; P, pulse; SBP, systolic blood pressure; Hct, hematocrit

kick) imparted on the small torso of an abuse victim. The young child is also at increased risk due to several anatomical factors. The intra-abdominal organs (eg, liver and spleen), which in the adult are protected by the thoracic cage, are larger proportionately in the child and extend beyond the costal margin. Because of increased compliance of the ribs, more energy is transmitted to the underlying structures. Also, the abdominal wall musculature is less well developed and affords relatively less protection to the internal organs. For these reasons, physical abuse directed at the torso can have devastating consequences. Cardiopulmonary resuscitation has on occasion been implicated as a cause of significant abdominal injuries detected in the setting of a traumatic arrest, although some reported cases predate widespread acknowledgment of child abuse.[48,49] More recent reviews indicate that the likelihood of CPR-related significant abdominal trauma in fatally injured children is extremely low.[50]

Stomach, Duodenum, Small Bowel

Hollow visceral injury associated with the battered child syndrome has long been reported.[12] In early reports, injuries were typically in the proximal small bowel (duodenum, jejunum), and patients presented with an abdominal crisis without adequate explanation. Eight of the 10 patients in the early McCort and Vaudagna[12] series had additional extra-abdominal injuries (as are common in the abused child). In general, injury to the duodenum is unusual (only 0.3% of all trauma admissions).[51] However, in one study, all cases of duodenal injury in children younger than 4 years were due to inflicted injury.[51] Similarly, the British Paediatric Surveillance Unit in the United Kingdom noted small bowel injuries to be significantly more common in abused children.[52] Thus a high index of suspicion for proximal intestinal injuries in the youngest age group is warranted. The duodenum is at risk of injury due to its central location in the abdomen and proximity to the spine (Figure 4.4). Forces applied anteriorly (eg, a punch) can crush the duodenum against the bony spine, resulting in injury. Inflicted injuries to the duodenum are frequently located at the junction between the third and fourth portion of the duodenum.[53] Such an injury may be the consequence of the fixation at the ligament of Treitz and usually results in perforation. In addition, compression

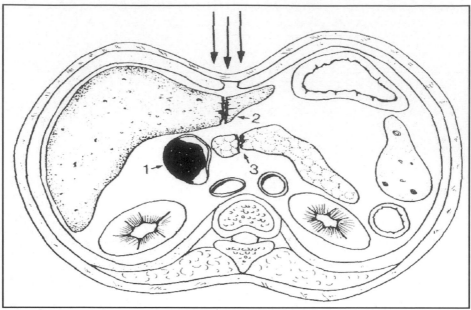

FIGURE 4.4
Common injury mechanism in child abuse. Blunt force (eg, from a fist) crushes organs against the rigid spine. Organs at risk include the duodenum (1), liver (2), and pancreas (3). (From Kleinman PK. *Diagnostic Imaging in Child Abuse*. Baltimore, MD: Williams & Wilkins; 1987.)

injury of the duodenum or jejunum against the spine can also result in an intramural hematoma. As the hematoma expands, the duodenal lumen narrows, leading to partial (or occasionally complete) obstruction (Figure 4.5). Children with duodenal hematomas may have delayed presentation because the signs of obstruction develop over time. Such injuries can be detected by upper gastrointestinal series revealing the characteristic "coiled spring" appearance of the bowel.[54] Other injuries noted in the gastrointestinal tract include mesenteric injuries resulting in a hematoma or free intraperitoneal blood. Mesenteric injuries can also lead to ischemia of the bowel with delayed perforation or stricture. Those injuries resulting in perfora-tion or suspected devitalized bowel require laparotomy and repair (Figure 4.6). A duodenal hematoma typically is managed with gastric decompression, IV nutrition, and time.

Gastric perforation is reported in the child abuse literature, although it is a rare injury.[12,55] Children are at higher risk for gastric perforation if the trauma occurs when the stomach is full. Gastric perforation results in rapid manifestations due to the pain associated with gastric spasms and the noxious effects of gastric acid in the peritoneum. Patients usually present with a distended, tense abdomen and pneumoperitoneum on plain radiograph. Gastric perforation has been reported as a complication of CPR, albeit rarely.[49]

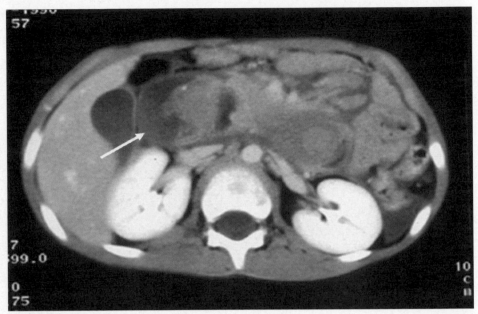

FIGURE 4.5
Computed tomography scan demonstrating a duodenal hematoma (white arrow) from a fist to the epigastrium.

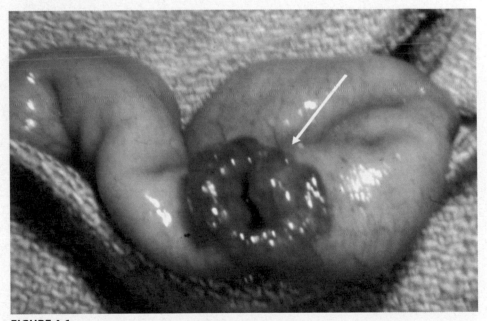

FIGURE 4.6
Intraoperative appearance of jejunal perforation (white arrow) following blunt trauma due to child abuse. This injury was inflicted with a baseball bat.

Colon, Rectal, and Anal Injuries

Anorectal injuries in young children are extremely uncommon and should raise suspicion for child abuse. There are occasional reports of colonic injury from blunt abdominal trauma.[56] More commonly, anorectal injury is the result of forced sexual intercourse or sodomy with a foreign object. Such abuse can lead to local lacerations or more serious perforations.[57,58] These injuries must be distinguished from injuries due to accidental impalement or straddle injuries. In inflicted anorectal injuries, typically only the rectum is involved (compared with evidence of other perineal trauma in the setting of accidental injury).[59] An examination under anesthesia is often beneficial to allow a more thorough assessment of the injuries. Severe perineal trauma or rectal perforation may require intestinal diversion to heal.

Solid Organ Injury

Injuries to the solid organs are relatively common in the general pediatric trauma population. The frequency of physical abuse as the mechanism of injury varies based on the organ injured (renal injuries, 5%–7%; liver/spleen injuries, 2%–11%).[60-64] Injuries to the solid organs can result from compression against the spine (Figure 4.4). Fractures to adjacent ribs may also penetrate the liver or spleen, resulting in injury. Because of the compliance of the ribs in the child, energy may be transmitted to the underlying organs, resulting in injury without associated rib fracture (Figure 4.7).

Hepatic Injuries

Although not specific for abuse, liver injuries are among the most common and potentially dangerous abdominal

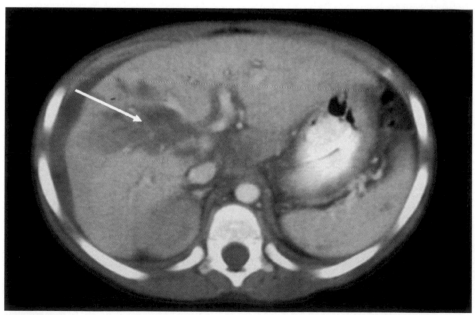

FIGURE 4.7
Computed tomography scan demonstrating grade 4 liver laceration (white arrow) in an 18-month-old child that presented in extremis with no reported trauma mechanism. The patient had elevated liver function tests stimulating the decision to scan the abdomen.

injuries identified in abused children. Liver injuries are most often due to blunt impact to the upper abdomen, although penetrating injuries occasionally result in liver laceration. Liver lacerations are a reported complication of CPR in adults, usually in association with rib fractures, and have been reported infrequently in association with CPR in young children.[49] Clinical manifestations of liver trauma depend on the extent and location of the laceration, as well as the presence or absence of free intraperitoneal blood.[65] Contusions may be contained by the liver capsule or may bleed freely into the peritoneal cavity.[66] Significant elevations of the hepatic enzymes ALT (>250 IU/L) and AST (>450 IU/L) have been shown to be a sensitive and reasonably specific marker of liver injury that can be detected by CT scan. An elevation of AST out of proportion to ALT may indicate significant muscle trauma. Hepatic enzyme values also rise after ischemic hepatic injury and are seen with some regularity in critically injured abused children, especially in those who have had a respiratory arrest. Computed tomography is the modality of choice for imaging the liver in cases of abdominal trauma and is obtained unless the child requires immediate surgical intervention (Figure 4.7). Most liver injuries are treated nonoperatively.

Splenic Injuries

Accidental trauma often results in splenic injury. It is infrequently reported as the result of abuse.[11,56] The reason for the lower rate of injury of this organ from inflicted trauma is likely the relative protection afforded by the ribs. Like liver injuries, the severity of splenic injuries ranges from minor to life-threatening. Evaluation of suspected splenic injuries is best done by contrast enhanced CT scan. Management depends on the extent of the injury, as well as other associated injuries, but operation is usually not necessary.

Pancreas

Because of its location in the center of the abdomen, draped across the spine, the pancreas is particularly vulnerable to inflicted injury to the torso (Figure 4.8). The true incidence of pancreatic injury in the setting of child abuse is unknown. However, child abuse may be the mechanism in as many as 18% of pancreatic injuries in the pediatric population.[67,68] The first report of a pancreatic pseudocyst resulting from physical child abuse was by Bongiovi and Logosso[69] in 1969. The initial presentation was not that of trauma but rather fever, anemia, and abdominal distention. Of concern in patients with pancreatic injury, particularly when due to child abuse, is the risk for associated hollow organ injury (eg, small bowel, duodenum). Injuries to the pancreas, whether in isolation or in combination with other solid organ injuries (eg, liver, spleen), are associated with a significantly increased risk of bowel injury.[61] Further, pancreatic injury due to child abuse is associated with a significantly higher risk of associated hollow organ injury than other injury mechanisms.[61] Management of pancreatic injuries is highly variable but generally is dictated by the integrity of the main duct. Disruption of the main pancreatic duct is

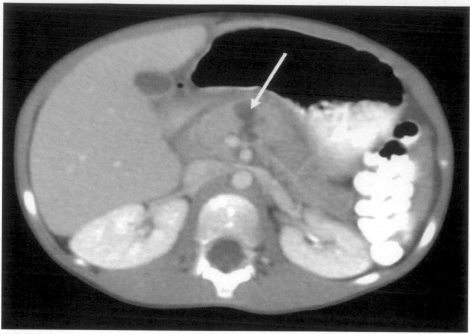

FIGURE 4.8
Typical findings in a transection of the pancreas due to blunt force. Note fracture line (white arrow) through the mid-body of the pancreas as it overlies the spine.

typically best managed operatively. Less severe pancreatic injury is managed by bowel rest, analgesics, and parenteral nutrition.

Vascular

Vascular injuries are quite rare in children. Inflicted vascular injuries have been reported in the literature, including an abdominal aortic transection from a suspected blow to the back.[70] Aortic pseudoaneurysms have also been observed in abused pediatric patients.[71,72] Such injuries are thought to be the result of direct trauma to the vessel. Injuries to other intra-abdominal vascular structures (including the renal artery) have been reported but are uncommon.[73] Vascular injuries to the torso represented just under 5% of all vascular injuries (16% of blunt injured) in a pediatric series.[74] Management of vascular injuries depends on the location and nature of the injury. Suspected injuries to the thoracoabdominal major vasculature may require interventional radiologic assessment for diagnostic purposes and, on occasion, endovascular treatment.[75,76] Other vascular injuries, for example pelvic fractures or solid organ injuries with associated hemorrhage, may also be amenable to interventional radiographic embolization.[77] Injuries in smaller children and injuries not correctable through interventional techniques generally require operative repair.

Urinary Tract Injuries

Physical abuse may result in injuries to the kidneys, ureters, and bladder. Severe blows to the flank may cause renal contusions or lacerations but are not common. Injuries that are severe enough to cause renal injury are often associated with injuries to other abdominal organs. Although children may present with flank pain and tenderness, these symptoms are not universally present. Hematuria (gross hematuria or >20 red blood cells per high-power field) generally indicates renal involvement in children with abdominal trauma. The severity of the renal injury is not reflected by the degree of hematuria, so that all children with hematuria require renal imaging by CT or other methods.[78] Both myoglobinuria (secondary to rhabdomyolysis and muscle injury) and hemoglobinuria may result from abuse and can be mistaken for hematuria.[79,80] Unlike hematuria, neither will show microscopic evidence of urinary red blood cells. Bladder injuries from abuse are unusual but have been reported.[81]

Injuries to the urinary bladder are typically limited to contusions resulting in self-limited hematuria. With significant forces (usually applied to a full bladder), however, rupture of the urinary bladder can occur. Such cases may present with abdominal pain and renal failure of unclear etiology.[82,83] The free extravasation of urine into the peritoneal cavity results in azotemia as the urine is reabsorbed. The management of bladder disruption is operative. Most renal injuries are managed conservatively and do not require surgery. Myoglobinuria and hemoglobinuria require aggressive medical treatment with hydration, alkalinization of the urine, and other supportive medications.

In addition to the previously enumerated thoracoabdominal injuries, other unusual injuries have been reported in the abused child, often in the absence of external evidence of trauma. Massive chylous ascites, presumably due to injury to the bowel mesentery, has been reported in children as an occult finding.[84,85] Similarly, a massive chylothorax, found in association with healing long bone fractures, presented with dyspnea but no outward manifestations of inflicted injury.[86] Portal venous gas was reported in a child undergoing CT scan of the abdomen for suspected child abuse.[87] Small bowel evisceration (from unclear mechanism) has been attributed to child abuse.[88] Adrenal injury has been reported (typically in association with other inflicted injuries) in confirmed child abuse.[89]

Conclusion

Visceral injury to the chest and abdomen are uncommon childhood injuries. Although uncommon in the abused child, they may be more prevalent than recognized. When obvious, they are often life-threatening. The manifestations of injury are varied and nonspecific, and may be attributed to more common pediatric diagnoses by unsuspecting physicians. By maintaining a high index of suspicion, the careful physician can use laboratory and radiologic techniques to make a diagnosis that may ultimately save a child's life. Children with significant visceral injury require hospitalization and coordinated care between the surgical and medical teams in order to ensure them proper treatment and protection.

References

1. UNICEF. *A League Table of Child Maltreatment Deaths in Rich Nations. Innocenti Report Card.* Florence, Italy: Innocenti Research Centre; 2003

2. Administration for Child and Families. Child abuse and neglect research. http://www.acf.hhs.gov/programs/cb/stats_research/index.htm#can. Accessed September 13, 2006

3. Crume TL, DiGuiseppi C, Byers T, et al. Underascertainment of child maltreatment fatalities by death certificates, 1990–1998. *Pediatrics.* 2002;110:e18

4. Herman-Giddens ME, Brown G, Verbiest S, et al. Underascertainment of child abuse mortality in the United States. *JAMA.* 1999;282:463–467

5. Chang DC, Knight V, Ziegfeld S, et al. The tip of the iceberg for child abuse: the critical roles of the pediatric trauma service and its registry. *J Trauma.* 2004;57:1189–1198

6. DiScala C, Sege R, Li G, et al. Child abuse and unintentional injuries: a 10-year retrospective. *Arch Pediatr Adolesc Med.* 2000;154:9–10

7. Cooper A, Floyd T, Barlow B, et al. Major blunt abdominal trauma due to child abuse. *J Trauma.* 1988;28:1483–1487

8. Pollanen MS, Smith CR, Chiasson DA, et al. Fatal child abuse-maltreatment syndrome: a retrospective study in Ontario, Canada, 1990–1995. *Forensic Sci Int.* 2002;126:101–104

9. Trokel M, DiScala C, Terrin NC, et al. Blunt abdominal injury in the young pediatric patient: child abuse and patient outcomes. *Child Maltreat.* 2004;9:111–117

10. Cobb LM, Vinocur CD, Wagner CW, Weintraub WH. Intestinal perforation due to blunt trauma in children in an era of increased nonoperative treatment. *J Trauma.* 1986;26:461–463

11. Ledbetter DJ, Hatch EI, Feldman KW, et al. Diagnostic and surgical implications of child abuse. *Arch Surg.* 1988;123:1101–1105

12. McCort J, Vaudagna J. Visceral injuries in battered children. *Radiology.* 1964;82:424–428

13. Wood J, Rubin DM, Nance ML, Christian CW. Distinguishing inflicted versus accidental abdominal injuries in young children. *J Trauma.* 2005;59:1203–1208

14. Hennes HM, Smith DS, Schneider K, et al. Elevated liver transaminase levels in children with blunt abdominal trauma: a predictor of liver injury. *Pediatrics.* 1990;86:87–90

15. Coant PN, Kornberg AE, Brody AS, et al. Markers for occult liver injury in cases of physical abuse in children. *Pediatrics.* 1992;89:274–278

16. Jenny C. Evaluating infants and young children with multiple fractures. *Pediatrics.* 2006;118:1299–1303

17. American College of Surgeons. *Advanced Trauma Life Support.* 7th ed. Chicago, IL: American College of Surgeons; 2004

18. Puranik SR, Hayes JS, Long J, et al. Liver enzymes as predictors of liver damage due to blunt abdominal trauma in children. *South Med J.* 2002;95:203–206

19. Capraro AJ, Mooney DP, Waltzman ML. The use of routine laboratory studies as screening tools in pediatric abdominal trauma. *Pediatr Emerg Care.* 2006;22:480–484

20. Adamson WT, Hebra A, Thomas PB, et al. Serum amylase and lipase alone are not cost-effective screening methods for pediatric pancreatic trauma. *J Pediatr Surg.* 2003;38:354–357

21. Kemp AM, Butler A, Morris S, et al. Which radiological investigations should be performed to identify fractures in suspected child abuse? *Clin Radiol.* 2006;61:723–736

22. Mandelstam SA, Cook D, Fitzgerald M, et al. Complementary use of radiological skeletal survey and bone scintigraphy in detection of injuries in suspected child abuse. *Arch Dis Child.* 2003;88:387–390

23. Sivit CJ, Taylor GA, Eichelberger MR. Visceral injury in battered children: a changing perspective. *Radiology.* 1989;173:659–661

24. Sugar NF, Taylor JA, Feldman KW. Bruises in infants and toddlers. *Arch Pediatr Adolesc Med.* 1999;153:349–403

25. Maguire S, Mann MK, Silbert J, et al. Are there patterns of bruising in childhood which are diagnostic or suggestive of abuse? A systematic review. *Arch Dis Child.* 2005;90:182–186

26. Bulloch B, Schubert JC, Brophy PD, et al. Cause and clinical characteristics of rib fractures in infants. *Pediatrics.* 2000;105:e48

27. Barsness KA, Cha E, Bensard DD, et al. The positive predictive value of rib fractures as an indicator of nonaccidental trauma in children. *J Trauma.* 2003;54:1107–1110

28. Ng CS, Hall CM, Shaw DG. The range of visceral manifestations of non-accidental injury. *Arch Dis Child.* 1997;77:167–174

29. Strouse PJ, Owning CL. Fractures of the first rib in child abuse. *Radiology.* 1995;197:763–765

30. Gipson CL, Tobias JD. Flail chest in a neonate resulting from nonaccidental trauma. *South Med J.* 2006;99:536–538

31. Maguire S, Mann M, John N, et al. Does cardiopulmonary resuscitation cause rib fractures in children? A systematic review. *Child Abuse Negl.* 2006;30:739–751

32. Kleinman PK, Marks SC Jr, Nimkin K, et al. Rib fractures in 31 abused infants: postmortem radiologic-histopathologic study. *Radiology.* 1996;200:807–810

33. Bansal BC, Abramo TJ. Subcutaneous emphysema as an uncommon presentation of child abuse. *Am J Emerg Med.* 1997;15:573–575

34. Ramnarayan P, Qayyum A, Tolley N, et al. Subcutaneous emphysema of the neck in infancy: under-recognized presentation of child abuse. *J Laryngol Otol.* 2004;118:468–470

35. Ablin DS, Reinhart MA. Esophageal perforation with mediastinal abscess in child abuse. *Pediatr Radiol.* 1990;20:524–525

36. Tavill MA, Trimmer WR, Austin MB. Pediatric cervical esophageal perforation secondary to abusive blunt thoracic trauma. *Int J Pediatr Otorhinolaryngol.* 1995;35:263–269

37. Lloyd-Thomas AR, Anderson I. ABC of major trauma. Paediatric trauma: secondary survey. *BMJ.* 1990;301:433–437

38. McEniery J, Hanson R, Grigor W, et al. Lung injury resulting from a nonaccidental crush injury to the chest. *Pediatr Emerg Care.* 1991;7:166–168

39. Dowd MD, Krug S. Pediatric blunt cardiac injury: epidemiology, clinical features, and diagnosis. *J Trauma.* 1996;40:61–67

40. Rees A, Symons J, Joseph M, et al. Ventricular septal defect in a battered child. *Br Med J.* 1975;5948:20–21

41. Marino TA, Langston C. Cardiac trauma and the conduction system: a case study of an 18-month-old child. *Arch Pathol Lab Med.* 1982;106:173–174

42. Cumberland GD, Riddick L, McConnell CF. Intimal tears of the right atrium of the heart due to blunt force injuries to the abdomen. *Am J Forensic Med Pathol.* 1991;12:102–104

43. Baker AM, Craig BR, Lonergan GJ. Homicidal commotio cordis: the final blow in a battered infant. *Child Abuse Negl.* 2003;27:125–130

44. Denton JS, Kalelkar MB. Homicidal commotio cordis in two children. *J Forensic Sci.* 2000;45:734–735

45. Cohle SD, Hawley DA, Berg KK, et al. Homicidal cardiac lacerations in children. *J Forensic Sci.* 1995;40:212–218

46. Karpas A, Yen K, Sell LL, et al. Severe blunt cardiac injury in an infant: a case of child abuse. *J Trauma.* 2002;52:759–764

47. O'Neill JA Jr, Meacham WF, Griffin JP, et al. Patterns of injury in the battered child syndrome. *J Trauma.* 1973;13:332–339

48. Thaler MM, Krause VW. Serious trauma in children after external cardiac massage. *N Engl J Med.* 1962;267:500–501

49. Krischer JP, Fine EG, Davis JH, Nagel EL. Complications of cardiac resuscitation. *Chest.* 1987;92:287–291

50. Price EA, Rush LR, Perper JA, et al. Cardiopulmonary resuscitation-related injuries and homicidal blunt abdominal trauma in children. *Am J Forensic Med Pathol.* 2000;21:307–310

51. Gaines BA, Shultz BS, Morrison K, et al. Duodenal injuries in children: beware of child abuse. *J Pediatr Surg.* 2004;39:600–602

52. Barnes PM, Norton CM, Dunstan FD, et al. Abdominal injury due to child abuse. *Lancet.* 2005;366:234–235

53. Bowkett B, Kolbe A. Traumatic duodenal perforations in children: child abuse a frequent cause. *Aust N Z J Surg.* 1998;68:380–382

54. Kleinman PK, Brill PW, Winchester P. Resolving duodenal-jejunal hematoma in abused children. *Radiology.* 1986;160:747–750

55. Schechner SA, Ehrlich FE. Gastric perforation and child abuse. *J Trauma.* 1974;14:723–725

56. Caniano DA, Beaver BL, Boles ET. Child abuse: an update on surgical management in 256 cases. *Ann Surg.* 1986;203:219–224

57. Shah PA, Pagare SK, Deshmukh VM, et al. Intra peritoneal rectal tear: delayed presentation in a battered baby. *Indian J Gastroenterol.* 1991;10:66

58. Gromb S, Lazarini HJ. An unusual case of sexual assault on an infant: an intra-peritoneal candle in a 20-month-old girl. *Forensic Sci Int.* 1998;94:15–18

59. Kadish HA, Schunk JE, Britton H. Pediatric male rectal and genital trauma: accidental and nonaccidental injuries. *Pediatr Emerg Care.* 1998;14:452–453

60. Miller K, Kou D, Sivit C, et al. Pediatric hepatic trauma: does clinical course support intensive care unit stay? *J Pediatr Surg.* 1998;33:1459–1462

61. Nance ML, Keller MS, Stafford PW. Predicting hollow visceral injury in the pediatric blunt trauma patient with solid visceral injury. *J Pediatr Surg.* 2000;35:1300–1303

62. Nance ML, Mahboubi S, Wickstrom M, et al. Pattern of abdominal free fluid following isolated blunt spleen or liver injury in the pediatric patient. *J Trauma.* 2002;52:85–87

63. Nance ML, Lutz N, Carr MC, et al. Blunt renal injuries in children can be managed nonoperatively: outcome in a consecutive series of patients. *J Trauma.* 2004;57:474–478

64. Margenthaler JA, Weber TR, Keller MS. Blunt renal trauma in children: experience with conservative management at a pediatric trauma center. *J Trauma.* 2002;52:928–932

65. Gornall P, Ahmen S, Jolleys A, et al. Intra-abdominal injuries in the battered baby syndrome. *Arch Dis Child.* 1972;42:211–214

66. Aoki Y, Nata M, Hashiyada M, Sagisaka K. Laceration of the liver with delayed massive intra-abdominal hemorrhage: a case report of child abuse. *Nihon Hoigaku Zasshi.* 1997;51:44–47

67. Jobst MA, Canty TG, Lynch FP. Management of pancreatic injury in pediatric blunt abdominal trauma. *J Pediatr Surg.* 1999;34:818–823

68. Arkovitz MS, Johnson N, Garcia VF. Pancreatic trauma in children: mechanisms of injury. *J Trauma.* 1997;42:49–53

69. Bongiovi JJ, Logosso RD. Pancreatic pseudocyst occurring in the battered child syndrome. *J Pediatr Surg.* 1969;4:220–226

70. Fox JT, Huang YC, Barcia PJ, et al. Blunt abdominal aortic transection in a child: case report. *J Trauma.* 1996;41:1051–1053

71. Pisters PW, Heslin MJ, Riles TS. Abdominal aortic pseudoaneurysm after blunt trauma. *J Vasc Surg.* 1993;18:307–309

72. Roche KJ, Genieser NB, Berger DK, et al. Traumatic abdominal pseudoaneurysm secondary to child abuse. *Pediatr Radiol.* 1995;25:S247–S248

73. Bolkier M, Moskovitz B, Levin DR. Renal artery injury in child abuse. *Child Nephrol Urol.* 1990;10:100

74. Klinkner DB, Arca MJ, Lewis BD, Oldham KT, Sato TT. Pediatric vascular injuries: patterns of injury, morbidity, and mortality. *J Pediatr Surg.* 2007;42:178–182

75. Szeto WY, Fairman RM, Acker MA, et al. Emergency endovascular deployment of stent graft in the ascending aorta for contained rupture of innominate artery pseudoaneurysm in a pediatric patient. *Ann Thorac Surg.* 2006;81:1872–1875

76. Milas Z, Milner R, Chaikoff M, Wulkan M, Ricketts R. Endograft stenting in the adolescent population for traumatic aortic injuries. *J Pediatr Surg.* 2006;41:e27–e30

77. Puapong D, Brown CV, Katz M, et al. Angiography and the pediatric trauma patient: a 10-year review. *J Pediatr Surg.* 2006;41:1859–1863

78. Levy JB, Baskin LS, Ewalt DH, et al. Nonoperative management of blunt pediatric major renal trauma. *Urology.* 1993;42:418–424

79. Mukerji SK, Siegel MJ. Rhabdomyolysis and renal failure in child abuse. *AJR Am J Roentgenol.* 1987;148:1203–1204

80. Rimer RL, Roy S. Child abuse and hemo-globinuria. *JAMA.* 1977;238:2034–2035

81. Halsted CC, Shapiro SR. Child abuse: acute renal failure from ruptured bladder. *Am J Dis Child.* 1979;133:861–862

82. Yang JW, Kuppermann N, Rosas A. Child abuse presenting as pseudorenal failure with a history of a bicycle fall. *Pediatr Emerg Care.* 2002;18:91–92

83. Sawyer RW, Hartenberg MA, Benator RM. Intraperitoneal bladder rupture in a battered child. *Int J Pediatr Nephrol.* 1987;8:227–230

84. Kleinman PK, Raptopoulos VD, Brill PW. Occult nonskeletal trauma in the battered-child syndrome. *Radiology.* 1981;141:393–396

85. Boysen BE. Chylous ascites: manifestation of the battered child syndrome. *Am J Dis Child.* 1975;129:1338–1339

86. Green HG. Child abuse presenting as chylothorax. *Pediatrics.* 1980;66:620–621

87. Wu JW, Chen MYM, Auringer ST. Portal venous gas: an unusual finding in child abuse. *J Emerg Med.* 2000;18:105–107

88. Press SP, Grant P, Thompson VT, et al. Small bowel evisceration: unusual manifestation of child abuse. *Pediatrics.* 1991;88:807–809

89. Nimkin K, Teeger S, Wallach MT, et al. Adrenal hemorrhage in abused children: imaging and postmortem findings. *AJR Am J Roentgenol.* 1994;162:661–663

Chapter 5

Maxillofacial, Neck, and Dental Manifestations of Child Abuse

Cindy W. Christian

Department of Pediatrics, The University of Pennsylvania School of Medicine
Child Abuse and Neglect Prevention and Codirector, Safe Place, The Center
*   for Child Protection and Health, The Children's Hospital of Philadelphia*

Lynn Douglas Mouden
University of Missouri Kansas City School of Dentistry
University of Tennessee College of Dentistry
Office of Oral Health, Arkansas Department of Health

Introduction

Physical injuries to the structures of the face, mouth, and neck are among the most common seen in abused children. Studies have shown that 65% to 75% of all physical abuse involves injuries to the head, neck, and face, with approximately half involving some form of orofacial injury.[1-3] For example, Willging et al[4] reviewed the medical records of 4,340 abused children seen at a large urban hospital over 5 years. Injuries to the head and neck were seen in 49% of physically abused children and, of those, the head or neck was the primary injury site in 82% of cases. In another retrospective analysis of hospitalized abused children, Leavitt et al[5] found the incidence of otolaryngologic findings to be 56%, more than half of which were directly related to physical abuse or neglect. Craniofacial injuries also are the most common injuries sustained by children who intervene in domestic violence.[6]

Abusive injuries to the face and mouth typically are due to blunt trauma by a hand or object, although penetrating trauma to facial cavities is well described. Most documented injuries are mild, with ecchymoses, abrasions, and lacerations most common.[4] Boys are more often victims than girls. Although many of the injuries are mild, requiring outpatient treatment only, early reports of battering often described extensive facial injuries.[7] Orofacial injuries are uncommonly isolated, and often are associated with more severe internal injuries. Certain injuries, such as those within the ear, nose, or throat, should arouse suspicion of abuse, especially in infants and young children. When recurrent, these injuries are almost always inflicted.[8] Cutaneous injuries are easily recognized, but injuries to the oral cavity may be overlooked by physicians who do not routinely examine the structures within the mouth.[2,9]

Injuries to the Face

Bruising and Burns

Contusions are the most common injury seen in abused children and are the most common injury sustained to the head and face.[1,2] The specificity of facial bruising for abuse is highest in young children. Facial bruising is notably uncommon during infancy and is even more atypical in non-ambulatory infants.[10-12] In contrast to accidental injuries, bruises to the head and face are common in abused infants.[13,14] These injuries should always elicit concern when identified. McMahon et al[15] reviewed soft tissue injuries in 341 hospitalized children reported for abuse and compared patterns of injury by age. Although infants averaged only one soft tissue injury, approximately 50% of those injuries were to the head and face. In contrast, children older than 2 years averaged 3 soft tissue injuries, of which 25% were to the head and face. Labbé and Caouctte[16] performed 2,040 physical examinations in a 1-year period on children 0 to 17 years old to identify patterns of recent skin injuries in non-abused children. While injuries in ambulatory children were common, less than 1% of all children examined had injuries to the chin, ears, or neck. Injuries in those locations, while not diagnostic of child abuse, should be scrutinized carefully. Non-ambulatory infants were least likely to have any

injury on the body, although in the 11% that did have an injury, most were self-inflicted fingernail scratches. Bruises were very uncommon in this age; only 1% of non-ambulatory infants had any bruise to the body at all. Facial bruising in infants may be the only external indication of trauma and is often associated with skeletal or other internal injuries.[11]

Inflicted facial burns may result from scalding or contact with hot objects and represent approximately 20% of inflicted burns identified. Immersion facial injuries are occasionally reported.[17] In a series of facial immersion burns, children's faces were submerged into sinks, bathtubs, or containers of hot liquids. Mortality from immersion in sinks or tubs was extremely high.

Fractures

Facial fractures are uncommon pediatric injuries. Approximately 5% of all facial fractures occur before the age of 12 years, and only 1% occur in the first 5 years of life.[18] During adolescence, the frequency of facial fractures increases, and the pattern of fractures begins to resemble that seen in adults. In preadolescent children, fractures to the mid-third of the facial skeleton are uncommon and are extremely rare in infants and preschool children.[12,19] Fractures of the zygoma or maxillary fracture of the LeFort type are rare pediatric injuries[20] and have not been reported in abused children. Mandibular fractures are more common. The pediatric mandible, however, is protected from fracture by the elasticity of the developing mandible; the relatively thick, soft tissue of the face; and the small size of the mandible compared with the cranium.[21] Because of the protection the frontal bone affords the smaller mandible, major head trauma is more likely to be transmitted to the frontal bone than the mandible.[12] When mandibular fractures occur, they are likely to be located in the premolar or subcondylar region, and more than one fracture site within the mandible is common throughout childhood (Figure 5.1).[14]

Mandibular fractures are uncommon but well described in abused children. Neonatal mandibular fracture inflicted by a mother suffering from postpartum psychosis has been reported.[22] Siegal et al[21] reviewed 73 mandibular fractures seen at an urban children's hospital over 10 years. Cases were divided by age and reflected the developing structure of the mandible and dentition. Mandibular fractures were most common in adolescents and least common in infants and preschoolers. Altercation, with direct blow to the jaw, was the most frequent cause of fracture. Child abuse accounted for 14% of the injuries, with an equal distribution throughout childhood. Surprisingly, although younger children had a higher incidence of extra-mandibular injuries than older children, none of the confirmed child abuse cases were associated with extra mandibular injuries. The authors concluded that child abuse should be strongly considered when infants present with isolated mandibular fractures.

Clinically, mandibular fractures in the premolar area are not severely painful. Those involving the subcondylar region are associated with trismus and pain and tenderness in the region of the temporomandibular joint. A contusion in the floor of the mouth may denote a fracture of the mandible. An irregularity in the mandibular arch may be noted, including alteration of the dental occlusion. Treatment varies by age and severity of the fracture.[15]

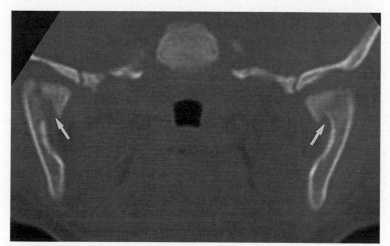

FIGURE 5.1
A 3-month-old baby with bilateral, displaced subcondylar fractures of the mandible (arrows). The baby had injury to the upper labial frenum, but no other injuries.

Injuries to the Ear

Injuries to the external and internal structures of the ear are well described in abused children and may result from either direct or penetrating trauma. Blows to the ear may cause bruising or hematomas of the pinna, abrasions, scarring or, less commonly, meatal wall lacerations, hemotympanum, or perforation of the tympanic membrane.[5] Bruises caused by pinching or pulling the ear may reveal a matching bruise on the posterior surface.[23] Other unusual injuries include a report of ossicular discontinuity (fractured stapes) from a blow to the ear and simulation of recurrent ear bleeding using beet juice.[8] Penetrating trauma with a pointed instrument may result in direct injury to the external meatus, tympanic membrane, or middle or inner ear. Repeated penetrating injuries are rarely accidental and are described in cases of Munchausen syndrome by proxy (MSBP).[24] Other aural manifestations of MSBP include trauma to the auditory canal resulting in bloody otorrhea or otitis externa and repeated placement of foreign bodies in the ear canal.[25–27] Like other orofacial injuries, aural injuries are unlikely to be isolated.

The tin ear syndrome is a pathognomonic triad of abuse consisting of unilateral ear bruising, radiographic evidence of ipsilateral cerebral edema with loss of the basilar cistern, and retinal hemorrhage.[28] The ear injuries described in the original report consisted of purpuric hemorrhages in the antitragus, helix, triangular fossa, and the interior folds of the ear. Internal ear injury was not present. All of the 3 children described died, and autopsy revealed the presence of an ipsilateral subdural hemorrhage. The mechanism postulated was blunt injury to the ear, resulting in rotational acceleration of the head and subsequent brain injury.

Injuries to the Nose

Abusive trauma to the nose, like other inflicted facial trauma, is often associated with extracranial injury. Blunt trauma to the nose can result in superficial abrasions, bruises, or nasal fractures.[4] The development of a hematoma and abscess of the nasal septum (HANS) after direct trauma is a rare complication of abuse. Canty and Berkowitz[29] noted 2 abused children in their case series of septal hematoma and abscess. Unlike the older children who developed HANS after minor, isolated nasal trauma, the abused children were young (<2 years); had severe facial, neck, and nasal injuries; and had a history of previous abuse. Nasal bone fractures are less common in children than soft tissue injuries because of the compliant nature of the pediatric bone.[30]

Collumella destruction and septal perforation, while uncommon, is documented in the abuse literature.[31,32] Fischer and Allasio[33] reported 6-month-old twins with traumatic destruction of the nose. One infant suffered loss of the nasal tip, columella, and distal nasal septum, with collapse of the nares. The other had loss of the alar rim and collapse of the nostril. Further investigation revealed nasal deformities in a 2-year-old sister. The nasal injuries to all 3 children were isolated and thought to be due to forceful, repeated nasal rubbing.

Injuries to the Pharynx, Larynx, and Esophagus

Iatrogenic pharyngeal and cervical esophageal perforation in infants is not uncommon and is usually related to instrumentation of the oropharynx. The anatomical weakness of the hypopharyngeal-esophageal junction predisposes this area to perforation.[34] Similar perforations due to child abuse are occasionally reported in the literature and are typically caused by penetrating trauma to the child's mouth.[35-37] Pharyngeal or esophageal lacerations introduce air, oral secretions, and bacteria into the soft tissues of the neck and mediastinum, with potentially life-threatening sequelae.[34] Such consequences of injury are well described. In 1971 Morris and Reay[38] described a battered baby with respiratory and feeding difficulties. Investigation revealed pharyngeal atresia, in which the soft palate was fused with the posterior pharyngeal wall. The authors suggest that the atresia was congenital, although they considered the (more probable) traumatic etiology. Inflicted tears to the palate, pharynx, tonsillar fossa, and high posterior cervical esophagus have resulted in the development of esophageal abscesses, pneumomediastinum, and a mediastinal pseudocyst.[39,40] Bansal and Abramo[41] reported a 2-month-old abused infant with severe subcutaneous emphysema of the scalp, neck, and anterior and posterior chest, with pneumomediastinum and subsequent *Moraxella catarrhalis* sepsis due to traumatic pharyngeal laceration.

Children with perforating injuries may present with fever, drooling, respiratory distress, (erythematous) cervical swelling, dysphagia, dysphonia, subcutaneous emphysema, or pneumomediastinum.[42] Infants with perforating pharyngeal injuries may have concomitant acute rib fractures, which may be missed on initial skeletal survey (Figure 5.2). Although not proven, these fractures are likely due to forceful chest squeezing during the oral trauma. Although most traumatic perforations associated with abuse occur in infants, exceptions exist.[43] Ablin and Reinhart[44] describe a 6-year-old abused child whose avulsed tooth was impacted in and/or through the esophageal wall, leading to a retropharyngeal and mediastinal abscess. The authors suggest the possibility of sexual assault as the cause of the initial injury.

Oral and esophageal foreign bodies in abused children are well described.[8] In a series of abusive ingestions and foreign bodies, Friedman[45] reported a 6-month-old child who was found to have a metallic foreign body in the esophagus and lower gastrointestinal tract and an 8-year-old boy who drank a glass of lye, causing extensive caustic burns and subsequent esophageal strictures. Foreign bodies being forced into the esophagus as a form of fatal child abuse is rare. Nolte[46] described repeated introduction of coins into the esophagus of a 5-month-old infant who ultimately died with multiple coins found in the esophagus.

Vocal cord paralysis can be a complication of strangulation or abusive head trauma.[47] The paralysis is due to either central or peripheral neuropathology. Children with unilateral paralysis may

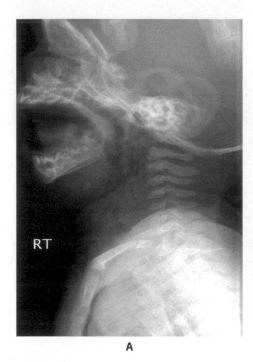
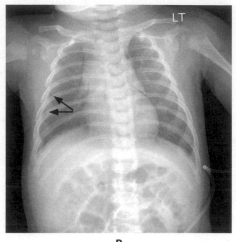

A   B

FIGURE 5.2
A. A 3-month-old infant who presented with hemoptysis, stridor, and respiratory distress. Lateral neck radiograph shows retropharyngeal swelling and air in the retropharyngeal space. In the operating room, the baby was found to have injury with eschar formation to the posterior pharynx. **B.** Chest x-ray of same 3-month-old infant shows pneumomediastinum and acute fractures of the right lateral 4th–6th ribs (arrows).

have few acute symptoms other than a weak voice or cry but are at risk for aspiration. Children with bilateral vocal cord paralysis usually have stridor or signs of upper airway obstruction. Bilateral cord paralysis can be an overlooked cause of extubation failure in patients with severe head injuries.

Injuries to the Neck

Neck injuries in abused children are less well studied than those of the head, although case reports of inflicted neck injuries are well documented. Cutaneous injuries, usually contusions or abrasions, are reported in a series of abused children.[48] More unusual injuries have also been documented. Ng et al[49] reported a 1-year-old who was found to have multiple needles imbedded in her neck. This was discovered after an autopsy of the child's 1-month-old sister revealed multiple needles in the brain and body. The authors speculate that the ethnic and cultural origins of the patients reported (Indian and African) may be relevant in this form of injury.[50] Although bruises are familiar injuries, Williams and colleagues[51] reported a child whose apparent cervical bruising was found to represent a cystic lymphangioma of the neck.

Strangulation is a well-described cause of child homicide.[52] The physical examination of a strangled child may reveal linear or circumferential ligature marks. Isolated venous obstruction from more mild neck compression may lead to petechiae over the skin of the face and postauricular region, the conjunctivae, or oral mucosa.[53] There also may be intense facial congestion, especially in fatal cases. The petechiae are due to increased vascular pressure, which ruptures small venules. Petechiae will not be seen if the strangulation causes simultaneous venous and arterial obstruction. Direct radiologic evidence of strangulation is rare. Carty[54] described the radiologic finding of calcification in the supraclavicular soft tissues of a 3-month-old battered infant. The calcification was thought to be due to fat necrosis from previous strangulation of the baby. Although strangulation or suffocation of a child may cause petechial hemorrhages of the face or neck, this is not a reliable finding. In a series of 14 patients who were intentionally suffocated during covert video surveillance, no child had facial markings that lasted more than 30 to 60 seconds after the attempted suffocation.[55] Meadow[56] reviewed the records of 81 children who were fatally smothered. Blood in the mouth or nose or on the face was reported in 39% of the children, and only 10 children had either bruises or petechiae on the face or neck. More than half of the victims had neither bruises, petechiae, nor a history or finding of bleeding. Accidental strangulation from a mother's long hair during co-sleeping also has been described in the literature.[57]

Injuries to the Cervical Spine

Cervical spine and spinal cord injury are uncommon findings in abused children.[58-60] In a review of 406 children with traumatic spinal injury, including isolated paravertebral soft tissue injuries, only one was noted to be a victim of child abuse.[61] In an early review of spinal and spinal cord injury in battered children, Swischuk[62] reported 7 children with spinal injury. While most injuries involved the lower spine, evaluation of a 2-year-old child with neck rigidity, flaccid extremities, and urinary incontinence revealed prevertebral edema and widening at the cervical spine consistent with trauma. Injuries to the cervical spine and cord may escape detection. Cervical spinal cord injury without radiographic abnormality is a well-known phenomenon in young children and is related to the mechanical tolerances of the young spine. Plain radiographs and computed tomography will fail to detect such cord injuries, although magnetic resonance imaging (MRI) may detect abnormalities.[61] Concomitant brain injury in some abused children may obscure signs of cervical cord injury.[60] Some injuries to the spine are asymptomatic and are identified at the time of a skeletal survey.

In recent years, an association of cervical cord injury and inflicted head injury has been noted, although to date this has not been extensively studied. In 1989 Hadley et al[63] reported subdural or epidural hematomas of the cervical spine with proximal spinal cord contusions in 5 of 6 autopsied infants with abusive shaking injuries. More recently, traumatic axonal injury to the cervical cord of fatally abused infants has been noted by both gross and microscopic autopsy studies.[64,65] The significance of these findings to the pathophysiology of brain injury or death in abused infants has yet to be completely delineated. To further investigate this relationship and determine the utility of screening the cervical spine with MRI, Feldman et al[66] prospectively imaged the cervical spine in abused infants with head injury. In cases of fatal injury, MRI findings were compared with autopsy data. None of the MRI scans in the 12 patients studied showed evidence of cervical cord injury or extra-axial cord blood. At autopsy, 1 of 5 infants who died had a thin subdural hemorrhage at the cervical cord and 3 had subarachnoid hemorrhage. No gross or microscopic changes were noted in the spinal cords of autopsied children, except for one cord with hypoxic neuronal changes. While this study confirms the finding of extra-axial hemorrhage in the cervical cord of infants dying of inflicted head injury, MRI was unable to detect these findings.

Fractures

Despite the frequency of abusive head trauma attributed to shaking, fractures to the cervical spine are rare. Cervical spine fractures associated with abuse are reported in infants and are postulated to be due to forced hyperflexion or hyperextension of the neck during shaking or a direct blow. The actual mechanism of these injuries remains speculative,

and concomitant intracranial injury is typically absent.[65] Cervical spine fractures may present with symptoms related to cord compression but are often asymptomatic, identified during skeletal survey.[67,68] In almost all case reports, additional skeletal injuries are present. Compression fractures, fracture dislocations, and anterior subluxations all may result from abuse. Hangman's fractures, which result from traumatic spondylolysis of C2, are a rare manifestation of abuse.[69-71] Like other cervical fractures, they are thought to be due to severe hyperflexion or hyperextension of the neck. Congenital spondylolysis can be confused with a Hangman's fracture, and serial radiographic studies may be needed to distinguish the two.[72,73]

Sexual Abuse

Oral injuries related to child sexual abuse are occasionally seen. Forced fellatio can cause palatal erythema, petechiae, and bruising; repeated fellatio can cause deep palatal ulcerations.[74] Similar injuries can also be seen on the floor of the mouth.[75] Sexually transmitted infections can have variable appearances in the oral cavity, making identification difficult for practitioners.[76] For example, oral gonorrhea may present with pharyngitis, exudative tonsillitis, or gingivitis but is most often asymptomatic in children.[77] Condyloma acuminatum may be found in the mucosa of the lip, cheek, palate, gingiva, or tongue but is infrequently considered in the differential diagnosis of oral lesions in children.[74,78]

The primary chancre of syphilis can be located on the lip, although this is rare in children. A careful examination of the oral cavity in sexually abused children is warranted and, on occasion, may reveal evidence to substantiate the diagnosis.

Dental Manifestations of Child Abuse

Many injuries to facial structures are within the scope of dentistry or easily observed by the dental professional in the course of routine dental treatment. Some types of injuries are pathognomonic for abuse and easily identified by the dentist. Injuries of this type include those that appear simultaneously on multiple body planes.[79] Injuries that exhibit patterned marks, implements, or an adult's hand, or bilateral injuries to the face, carry a high index of suspicion of abuse and can occur on easily observable areas of the child's body.[80] Various explanations for the mouth as a target of abuse are possible. Injuries to the mouth represent an assault on the communicative "self" of the child and can be a compelling reason behind abuse directed at the mouth. Another factor is the adult's easy access to the head of a child, which is often well within reach. Also, any physical injury or emotional trauma may elicit a cry from the child. Efforts to silence the crying often can result in injuries to the mouth.

While treatment of oral injuries is usually referred to the general dentist, pediatric dentist, or oral surgeon, proper evaluation of the abused child cannot be complete without a thorough visual examination by the primary care provider. Various types of oral injuries may be encountered in any clinical setting. The orofacial injuries that may be encountered in child abuse include trauma to the teeth, trauma to supporting structures, and trauma to surrounding tissues. The principal intraoral injuries of child abuse include missing and fractured teeth, oral contusions, oral lacerations, jaw fractures, and oral burns.

Oral Injuries to Infants

Inflicted injuries to oral structures of the infant should be considered separately from those of older children. Infants generally do not have teeth before 4 to 6 months of age. The pattern of eruption of primary teeth varies widely and is usually not important in deciding whether child abuse has occurred. Delayed eruption of primary teeth may, however, be seen in cases of child neglect resulting from poor nutrition, or may be as a result of poor prenatal nutrition during fetal development.

The difficulties and frustrations surrounding an infant's feeding may lead to abuse. Intraoral lacerations have long been recognized as possible indicators of forced feeding and abuse.[81] Injury can occur when excessive pressure is used while feeding with a nursing bottle or when a utensil is misdirected during feeding. If the adult feels that the child is uncooperative during bottle-feeding, the adult may use excessive force to introduce the nipple into the child's mouth or press too firmly against oral structures. This can cause mild to severe contusions of the lips and gingivae as well as lacerations of the labial frenum (Figure 5.3). Forced feeding with a utensil can lacerate the tongue, the floor of the mouth, or the lips (Figure 5.4).

Injuries to Teeth

All injuries to teeth and supporting structures should be referred to a dentist as soon as possible. The abuse-related injuries to teeth can include movement of the teeth within the socket, fracture, or loss. Any trauma to a tooth that does not result in loss of the tooth may, however, move the tooth sufficiently to result in loss of the tooth's vitality. Even relatively minor trauma may disrupt the neurovascular supply through the apex. Evidence of tooth injury may not be evident immediately after the trauma. However, after several weeks or months non-vital teeth are often characterized by slight to severe color changes of the tooth resulting from the necrotic pulp tissue within. The non-vital tooth appears discolored or markedly darker compared with the adjacent teeth. Dif-

ferential diagnosis of discolored teeth should also include a history of exposure to tetracycline or heavy metals during formation of the tooth enamel. Teeth affected in this manner, and not by trauma, will show similar discoloration for all teeth forming during the exposure.

Displaced or Avulsed Teeth

A tooth that has been moved within its socket often causes tears of the periodontal ligament and may bleed into the tooth's sulcus. Teeth traumatized in this way may also exhibit more mobility than normal. Normal, healthy teeth should move no more than 1 mm or less within the socket. Palpation to test tooth mobility must be conducted using 2 metal instruments or wooden tongue blades and the examiner should not rely on moving the tooth with fingers to judge the tooth's mobility. This is because the miniscule movement of teeth is virtually impossible to detect with the soft tissue of the fingers.

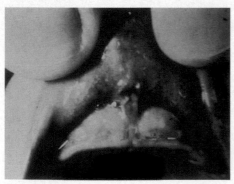

FIGURE 5.3
A 2-month-old baby with a laceration of the upper labial frenum from forced feeding.

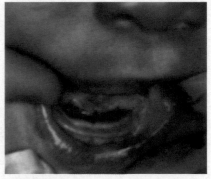

FIGURE 5.4
An unexplained lingular frenum injury in a 2-month-old infant. Lingular frenum injuries are occasionally misdiagnosed as hemangiomas by unsuspecting physicians.

A traumatized tooth can be displaced in any direction. Teeth can be bodily moved anteriorly or posteriorly, intruded into or avulsed from the socket, or moved mesially or distally if adjacent teeth are not in tight contact. This can happen with accidental injuries as well as with abuse. Contact directly on the tooth or from a blow to the face that transfers energy to the teeth can cause the displacement. Either the abuser's hand or an object can deliver sufficient force to displace one or several teeth.

In severe cases, the entire tooth can be forcefully expelled from the alveolar bone (Figure 5.5). The tendency for a tooth to be avulsed is related to the force and direction of the trauma as well as the anatomy of the tooth. Single-rooted teeth and teeth with conically shaped roots are more easily avulsed without being fractured. Therefore, anterior teeth, especially incisors, are most likely to be avulsed, but some premolars (bicuspids) also may have cone-shaped roots. Multi-rooted, posterior teeth are less likely to be avulsed, both because of their location in the mouth and because of the physics involved in forcing a

multi-rooted tooth bodily out of the alveolar bone. Because root anatomy of a primary tooth is likely to be less conical in form than its permanent counterpart, expulsion of teeth during physical violence is less common in children with primary dentition. Severe trauma can, of course, remove or shatter any tooth.

At least 2 cases have been reported of children who were abused by having permanent teeth extracted by the parents. In these cases, one adult held the child while another removed the intact teeth using pliers and without anesthesia.[82]

Traumatic tooth avulsion requires immediate dental consultation. The tooth must be kept moist in isotonic saline solution or milk. The chances for successful reimplantation are best if the procedure is accomplished within 30 minutes of the avulsion. No attempt should be made to clean or remove tissue tags from the tooth before the dentist reimplants it. Removing anything from the tooth may result in loss of tissue important for periodontal ligament regeneration. Reimplanted teeth must be stabilized for an absolute minimum of 7 to 10 days with intraoral fixation.

Tooth Fractures

Fractures of teeth can involve the crown, the root, or both. While tooth fractures are sometimes seen in abusive injuries, they can also be accidental. Fractures occur either when the tooth is struck with a hard object or when the face

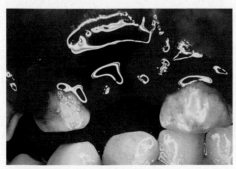

FIGURE 5.5
An 11-year-old child with a traumatic avulsion of a permanent central incisor from a beating.

comes into contact with a hard surface (Figure 5.6).

Fractures can involve only the enamel, extend into the dentin layer, or involve the tooth's pulp. Also, teeth may fracture, even bodily through the entire tooth, and still remain held in place by the surrounding bone, periodontal ligament, and gingival tissues. Timely referral to a dentist is mandatory for treatment of tooth fractures. Modern restorative materials and bonding procedures can save teeth with enamel or dentin fractures that only a decade ago would have required full crowns or extraction.

Injuries to Oral Soft Tissues

Gingiva

Trauma that affects teeth is also likely to affect the surrounding gingivae. In addition, trauma from an object striking the child can produce contusions or lacerations of the gingivae without apparent trauma to adjacent teeth. Radiographic examination is necessary in all cases of gingival trauma to properly diagnose

any damage to adjacent teeth or alveolar bone.

Lingual and Labial Frenula

Inflicted trauma can cause mild to extensive damage of the attachment tissues of the tongue and lips. Along with lacerations caused by forced feeding discussed previously, many forms of abusive trauma can tear these tissues. Blows to the face can displace the lip far enough to stretch the lip's attachment tissue beyond its elastic limit, causing laceration of the frenulum itself. Invasive trauma that introduces a hard or sharp object into the mouth can also lacerate these areas.

While accidental frenulum tears are common in the 8- to 18-month-old who is learning to walk, similar injuries in young infants (<6 months) and in older, more stable children should raise a suspicion of abuse. Lingular frenulum injuries in young infants may result in a hematoma under the tongue that can be misdiagnosed as a hemangioma or other non-traumatic finding. As they

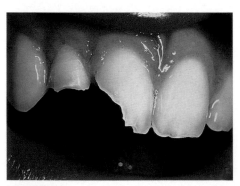

FIGURE 5.6
Fractured teeth sustained when a 16-year-old child hit his mouth against a piece of furniture during a beating.

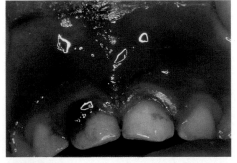

FIGURE 5.7
A 10-year-old with multiple oral injuries from an open-handed slap to the face, including laceration of the upper lip, contusions of the vestibule, laceration of the labial frenum, and subluxation of the right central incisor.

heal, they may form a sharply defined white eschar. In our experience, frenum injuries in very young infants are often associated with skeletal or other inflicted injuries and, when identified, require a thorough injury evaluation and involvement of child protective services (CPS) to ensure the future safety of the infant. Frenum tears will usually heal on their own, although they may require sutures if the wound is large, the alveolar bone is exposed, or the wound separates when the lip is pulled upward.[83]

Lips

Any trauma to the mouth can cause contusions and lacerations of the upper or lower lip. Inflicted injuries to the lips are evidenced by marks either from the offending object or the child's own teeth. When a blow is directed at the face or lips, the oral tissues can come into forceful contact with the child's teeth. The lips may show resulting "bite marks" from the child's own teeth. Bruising or laceration at the corners of the lips can also result from the use of a rope or other material to gag and silence the child. Scarring at the commissures of the lips may result from electrical burns from biting an electrical cord and is more likely to be caused accidentally. In addition, fixed and removable orthodontic appliances can damage lips during trauma. The clinician must exercise caution when examining the child's mouth if orthodontic appliances are in place because lips can become trapped in the wires or brackets.

Tongue

Laceration of the tongue can occur from abuse involving a sharp or hard object in the mouth. However, most abusive injuries to the tongue are a result of the child biting the tongue inadvertently. Any blow to the jaw can trap the tongue between upper and lower teeth. These injuries usually involve the lateral or anterior surfaces of the tongue and resemble jagged indentations seen with any bite mark in soft tissue. If the bite involves posterior areas of the tongue, the marks may appear more like crushed tissue and not show definite bite marks.

Bite marks to the tongue inflicted by the child's own teeth are likely to show a curvature consistent with the child's own arch. A bite mark on the tongue from an abuser may show a curve in the direction opposite to the curve of the child's dental arch.

Burns

Burns can affect any oral soft tissue. Abusive burns result from the introduction of a hot object into the mouth, forced feeding of a food or liquid that is too hot, or the use of caustic or acidic materials such as drain cleaner.

Bite Mark Analysis in Suspected Child Abuse

Bite marks can be important evidence in cases of suspected child abuse and should be evaluated by dentists with experience in forensic odontology. This evaluation can be expedited because most forensic odontologists work with medical examiners, coroners, and law enforcement agencies who are accustomed to working in cases involving non-accidental trauma and violence against persons of all ages.

Dental professionals are invaluable resources for identifying wound patterns that could be possible bite marks. When in doubt, health care professionals should seek the advice of a dentist to determine if an investigation should be made into the cause of the mark. The dental professional should be able to recognize the injury as a bite mark, determine and understand the significance, document basic information about the bite mark and, when necessary, contact the forensic odontologist for the definitive evidence collection and final determination.

Dentists and their staff members can often differentiate between bite marks and marks caused by different etiologies. If the injury is interpreted as a possible bite mark, the dentist should consider consulting with an experienced forensic dentist as soon as possible for analysis and collection of necessary evidence.

A "typical" bite mark can often be described as a "circular or oval (doughnut or ring-shaped) patterned injury consisting of 2 opposing symmetrical, U-shaped arches separated at their bases by open spaces. Following the periphery of the arches is a series of individual abrasions, contusions, and/or lacerations reflecting the size, shape, arrangement, and distribution of the class characteristics of the contacting surfaces of the human dentition."[84]

Bite marks can be inflicted by an adult, another child, an animal, or the patient.

Identifying the perpetrator is determined by size, dentition class characteristics seen in the wound, location of the wound, presence of puncture marks, arch form, and inter-cuspid distance. All of these characteristics may or may not be found in every bite mark.

Bite marks cannot only identify the attacker but may also be used to show evidence that the attacker was with the victim at or near the time of the injury, that a violent action was taken, or that the accused is not responsible for the injury.[85] Careful analysis may also show that bite marks are in various stages of healing. Repeated similar injuries can be a powerful indicator of continuing abuse. Therefore, any bite mark on a child should be immediately and clearly documented for court evidence and to aid CPS agencies in determining placement options for the child.

Those attempting to photographically record bite mark evidence should be well trained in forensic photography techniques. Multiple color photos, all including a known color and measurement index and taken perpendicular to each body plane, should be taken using various exposures to ensure adequate evidence collection. If a standard index, such as the American Board of Forensic Odontology No. 2 scale, is not available, any indexing item of known size and shape, such as a 25-cent piece, can be a suitable index for processing and analysis.

For proper investigation of suspected child abuse, or other forms of family violence, it is imperative that appropriate evidence collection be performed as soon as practical during the examination. Expedited, appropriate evidence collection will help the development of an accurate diagnosis as to the cause of the wound and assist in identifying the perpetrator. Health care professionals who are not forensic experts should seriously consider obtaining assistance and consultation from a forensic odontologist. Improper or inadequate collection and analysis of information can lead to faulty or misleading conclusions. Improper technique can also lead to exclusion of important evidence in a judicial proceeding. Practitioners are encouraged to contact the American Academy of Forensic Sciences for a list of forensic experts in North America *before* their services might be needed.

Bite mark evidence has provided critical information in child abuse cases. However, its usefulness is dependent on early examination, evidence collection, and proper analysis.[86] The dental team can provide critical assistance in this process to ensure accurate and complete documentation of the bite mark.

Dental Implications of Child Neglect

Typically dental neglect is but one manifestation of the general neglect of a child. It has been defined as lack of care that makes routine eating impossible, causes chronic pain, delays or retards a child's growth, or makes it difficult or impossible for a child to perform basic daily activities.[87] Untreated dental problems are as serious as an untreated wound to any other part of the body, in part because neglected oral health can lead to complications that affect the entire body.

The American Academy of Pediatric Dentistry (AAPD) has defined dental neglect as a willful failure on the part of the child's parent or caregiver to seek and follow through with treatment necessary to ensure a level of oral health essential for adequate function and freedom from pain and infection.[88] Previous definitions from the AAPD have included the caregiver's failure to seek treatment for a child's untreated rampant caries or untreated pain, infection, bleeding, or trauma. Rampant caries by definition involves gross carious lesions, including the mandibular anterior teeth. These teeth are the least likely to decay and are easily seen by even untrained observers.

Also included in the AAPD definition is the failure to follow through on treatment needs once the caregiver has been informed that treatment is needed. Many parents are unaware of conditions in their children's mouths. Often only following the dentist's diagnosis are they aware of even serious problems. However, if parents are informed of serious dental conditions and refuse to address these problems according to their personal resources, they have neglected their child. Therefore, parents' failure to follow through with necessary treatment is probably more important in determining reportable dental neglect than parents' lack of knowledge. Also, most practitioners would agree that no neglect may exist if parents are providing for their children's oral health needs in a manner consistent with their own financial situation or available economic existence. The argument has also been made that if parents have even taken the child to the dentist who diagnosed a dental problem, the parents are not neglecting the child. However, episodic pain relief is not appropriate dental care when adequate resources exist for more comprehensive care and definitive treatment.

The AAPD definitions of dental neglect serve neither as law nor as a standard of practice for reporting suspected cases of child neglect. They are merely a guideline for practitioners evaluating a patient's oral health in light of societal norms and fiscal realities. It is up to the health care professional to weigh the guidelines and legal definitions against such issues as money and access to care.

The most common form of dental neglect is failure to provide treatment for carious teeth. Multiple carious lesions can debilitate an otherwise healthy child, while untreated caries can lead to more serious problems of severe pain, fever, malaise, and lethargy. Pulpal infections can penetrate alveolar bone and exit through the gingiva, usually at or near the tooth's apex, resulting in a parulis or "gum boil." Severe untreated lesions can even lead to infection of fascial planes leading to serious, even fatal, consequences.

Baby bottle tooth decay (BBTD), a form of early childhood caries, is a severe form of rampant caries resulting from the habit of putting a child to bed with a nursing bottle or letting the child fall asleep at the breast. The remnants of milk in the child's mouth allow for bacterial growth, leading to carious lesions that can amputate teeth at the gingival crest. The clinical pattern of BBTD is typically different from other forms

of rampant caries because the most seriously affected teeth are the maxillary anterior teeth. While genetics does play a role in a person's susceptibility to caries, deleterious feeding habits can overcome even optimum genetic disposition. Practitioners should keep in mind that BBTD is totally preventable and recurrence could be considered a form of child neglect and reported as such.

Other conditions may constitute dental neglect if left untreated. These include severe malocclusions, abnormal tongue position, cleft lip or palate, missing teeth, or other manifestations that may lead to speech or eating difficulties.

Dentistry's Role in Preventing Abuse and Neglect

Dentists and other health care professionals in all 50 states and the District of Columbia are required by statute to report suspected cases of child abuse and neglect.[89] A 1995 national study of CPS agencies pointed out several facets of dentistry's involvement in the reporting process. Because only 8 states currently track the number of dentists making reports, the data on dentists' reporting of child maltreatment must be extrapolated from the small sample. In these states, from a total of 201,944 reports of child abuse and neglect, only 637 reports came from dentists. This figure represents a reporting rate of 0.32% of all reports.[90]

In an effort to change dentists' involvement with CPS agencies, the American Dental Association (ADA) added the required recognition and reporting of suspected child abuse to its Principles of Ethics and Code of Professional Conduct in 1993.[91] Official ADA policy states that dentists should become familiar with all physical signs of child abuse that are observable in the course of the normal dental visit. In 1999 the ADA further refined its policy to encourage dentists to become better educated about all forms of abuse and neglect and to learn about state-specific legal considerations for reporting suspected victims of abuse and neglect of all ages.[92]

In an effort to address prevention issues, the Prevent Abuse and Neglect through Dental Awareness (PANDA) Coalition was established in Missouri. The PANDA Coalition is a public-private partnership between the dental community, public health, social services agencies, and a dental insurance company.

The PANDA message is presented to diverse dental audiences, other health care providers, teachers, law enforcement staff, and child care workers. Another PANDA educational program targets 8th-grade students using a program that not only teaches about the problems of child abuse and neglect, but also discusses anger control, conflict resolution, and how to make decisions about proper discipline.

Increased reporting by dentists of suspected cases of child abuse and neglect since the coalition's educational program premiered in 1992 has proven the success of the initiative. Since the inception of the PANDA education and awareness programs, the reporting by dentists of suspected child abuse and

neglect has risen by 160%.[93] PANDA has further proven its success by having Missouri's program replicated in 46 other states; Ontario, Canada; Guam; the states of Timis and Mehedinti, Romania; Peru; Israel; and Finland. PANDA's founders are working with individuals in Mexico, South Africa, the Federated States of Micronesia, the Republic of Palau, Belgium, and Iceland to further replicate the program. Increased reporting of suspected cases of abuse and neglect encourages the PANDA volunteers around the world. However, true success of the initiative will be proven when the involvement of health care professionals in every discipline results in fewer cases to report and fewer children and adults who suffer from the ravages of family violence.

References

1. Becker D, Needleman HL, Kotelchuck M. Child abuse and dentistry: orofacial trauma and its recognition by dentists. *J Am Dent Assoc.* 1978;97:24–28
2. daFonesca MA, Feigal RJ, ten Bensel RW. Dental aspects of 1248 cases of child maltreatment on file at a major county hospital. *Pediatr Dent.* 1992;14:152–157
3. Cameron JM, Johnson HRM, Camps FE. The battered child syndrome. *Med Sci Law.* 1966;6:1–36
4. Willging JP, Bower CM, Cotton RT. Physical abuse of children. A retrospective review and otolaryngology perspective. *Arch Otolaryngol Head Neck Surg.* 1992;118:584–590
5. Leavitt EB, Pincus RL, Bukachevsky R. Otolaryngologic manifestations of child abuse. *Arch Otolaryngol Head Neck Surg.* 1992;118:629–631
6. Christian CW, Scribano P, Seidl T, Pinto-Martin JA. Pediatric injuries resulting from family violence. *Pediatrics.* 1997;99:8

7.   Tate FJ. Facial injuries associated with the battered child syndrome. *Br J Oral Surg*. 1971;9:41–45

8.   Grace A, Grace MA. Child abuse within the ear, nose and throat. *J Otolaryngol*. 1987;16:108–111

9.   Naidoo S. A profile of the oro-facial injuries in child physical abuse at a children's hospital. *Child Abuse Negl*. 2000;24:521–534

10. Sugar NF, Taylor JA, Feldman KW. Bruises in infants and toddlers: those who don't cruise rarely bruise. *Arch Pediatr Adolesc Med*. 1999;153:399–403

11. Carpenter RF. The prevalence and distribution of bruising in babies. *Arch Dis Child*. 1999;80:363–366

12. Mortimer PE. Are facial bruises in babies ever accidental? *Arch Dis Child*. 1983;58:75–80

13. Dunstan FD, Guildea ZE, Kontos K, Kemp AM, Sibert JR. A scoring system for bruise patterns: a tool for identifying abuse. *Arch Dis Child*. 2002;86:330–333

14. Maguire S, Mann MK, Sibert J, Kemp A. Are there patterns of bruising in childhood which are diagnostic or suggestive of abuse? A systematic review. *Arch Dis Child*. 2005;90:182–186

15. McMahon P, Grossman W, Gaffney M, Stanitski C. Soft-tissue injury as an indication of child abuse. *J Bone Joint Surg*. 1995;8:1179–1183

16. Labbé J, Caouette G. Recent skin injuries in normal children. *Pediatrics*. 2001;108:271–276

17. Daria S, Sugar MF, Feldman KW, Boos SC, Benton SA, Ornstein A. Into hot water head first: distribution of intentional and unintentional immersion burns. *Pediatr Emerg Care*. 2004;20:302–310

18. Rowe NL. Fractures of the facial skeleton in children. *J Oral Surg*. 1968;26:505–515

19. Kaban LB, Mulliken JB, Murray JE. Facial fractures in children. *Plast Reconstr Surg*. 1977;59:15–20

20. Waite DE. Pediatric fractures of jaw and facial bones. *Pediatrics*. 1973;51:551–559

21. Siegal MB, Wetmore RF, Potsic WP, Handler SD, Tom LWC. Mandibular fractures in the pediatric patient. *Arch Otolaryngol Head Neck Surg*. 1991;117:533–536

22. Chidzonga MM. Mandibular fracture in a neonate: report of a case. *Int J Oral Maxillofac Surg*. 2006;35:186–187

23. Welbury RR, Murphy JM. The dental practitioner's role in protecting children from abuse 2. The orofacial signs of abuse. *Br Dent J*. 1998;184:61–65

24. Grace A, Kalinkiewicz M, Drake-Lee AB. Covert manifestations of child abuse. *BMJ*. 1984;289:1041–1042

25. DiBiase P, Timmis H, Bonilla JA, Szeremeta W, Post JC. Munchausen syndrome by proxy complicating ear surgery. *Arch Otolaryngol Head Neck Surg*. 1996;122:1377–1380

26. Zohar Y, Avidan G, Shvili Y, Laurian N. Otolaryngologic cases of Munchausen's syndrome. *Larygngoscope*. 1987;97:201–203

27. Griffiths H, Cuddihy PJ, Marnane C. Bleeding ears: a case of Munchausen syndrome by proxy. *Int J Pediatr Otorhinolaryngol*. 2001;57:245–247

28. Hanigan WC, Peterson RA, Njus G. Tin ear syndrome: rotational acceleration in pediatric head injuries. *Pediatrics*. 1987;80:618–622

29. Canty PA, Berkowitz RG. Hematoma and abscess of the ansal septum in children. *Arch Otolaryngol Head Neck Surg*. 1996;122:1373–1376

30. Haug RH, Foss J. Maxillofacial injuries in the pediatric patient. *Oral Surg Oral Med Oral Pathol Oral Radiol Endod*. 2000;90:126–134

31. Orton CI. Loss of columella and septum from an unusual form of child abuse. Case report. *Plast Reconstr Surg*. 1975;56:345–346

32. Pincus RL, Bukachevsky RP. Medially based horizontal nasolabial flaps for reconstruction of columellar defects. *Otolaryngol Head Neck Surg*. 1990;116:973–974

33. Fischer H, Allasio D. Nasal destruction due to child abuse. *Clin Pediatr.* 1996;35:165–166

34. Tostevin PMJ, Hollis LJ, Bailey CM. Pharyngeal trauma in children— accidental and otherwise. *J Laryngol Otol.* 1995;109:1168–1175

35. McDowell HP, Fielding DW. Traumatic perforation of the hypopharynx—an unusual form of child abuse. *Arch Dis Child.* 1984;59:888–889

36. Golova N. An infant with fever and drooling: infection or trauma? *Pediatr Emerg Care.* 1997;13:331–333

37. Reece RM, Arnold J, Splain J. Pharyngeal perforation as a manifestation of child abuse. *Child Maltreat.* 1996;1:364–367

38. Morris TMO, Reay HAJ. A battered baby with pharyngeal atresia. *Laryngol Otol.* 1971;85:729–731

39. Ablin DS, Reinhart MA. Esophageal perforation with mediastinal abscess in child abuse. *Pediatr Radiol.* 1990;20:524–525

40. Kleinman PK, Spevak MR, Hansen M. Mediastinal pseudocyst caused by pharyngeal perforation during child abuse. *AJR Am J Roentgenol.* 1992;158:1111–1113

41. Bansal BC, Abramo TJ. Subcutaneous emphysema as an uncommon presentation of child abuse. *Am J Emerg Med.* 1997;15:573–575

42. Ramnarayan P, Qayyum A, Tolley N, Nadel S. Subcutaneous emphysema of the neck in infancy: under-recognized presentation of child abuse. *J Laryngol Otol.* 2004;118:468–470

43. Morzaria S, Walton JM, MacMillan A. Inflicted esophageal perforation. *J Pediatr Surg.* 1998;33:871–873

44. Ablin DS, Reinhart MA. Esophageal perforation by a tooth in child abuse. *Pediatr Radiol.* 1992;22:339–341

45. Friedman EM. Caustic ingestions and foreign body aspirations: an overlooked form of child abuse. *Ann Otol Rhinol Laryngol.* 1987;96:709–712

46. Nolte KB. Esophageal foreign bodies as child abuse. Potential fatal mechanisms. *Am J Forensic Med Pathol.* 1993;14:323–326

47. Myer CM III, Fitton CM. Vocal cord paralysis following child abuse. *Int J Pediatr Otorhinolaryngol.* 1988;15:217–220

48. Jessee SA. Physical manifestations of child abuse to the head, face and mouth: a hospital survey. *ASDC J Dent Child.* 1995;62:245–249

49. Ng CS, Hall CM, Shaw DG. The range of visceral manifestations of non-accidental injury. *Arch Dis Child.* 1997;77:167–174

50. Hadley GP, Bosenberg AT, Wiersma R, et al. Needle implantation ascribed to 'tikoloshe' (letter). *Lancet.* 1993;342:1304

51. Williams CM, Spector R, Braun M. Cervical bruises—a battered child? Cystic lymphangioma. *Arch Dermatol.* 1986;122:1066–1070

52. Fornes P, Druilhe L, Lecomte D. Childhood homicide in Paris, 1990–1993: a report of 81 cases. *J Forensic Sci.* 1995;40:201–204

53. Greenbaum J, Christian CW. Asphyxiation in children. In: David TJ, ed. *Recent Advances in Paediatrics.* London, United Kingdom: Royal Society of Medicine Press Ltd; 2006:93–112

54. Carty H. Case report: child abuse— necklace calcification—a sign of strangulation. *Br J Radiol.* 1993;66:1186–1188

55. Samuels MP, McClaughlin W, Jacobson RR, Poets CF, Southall DP. Fourteen cases of imposed upper airway obstruction. *Arch Dis Child.* 1992;67:162–170

56. Meadow R. Unnatural sudden infant death. *Arch Dis Child.* 1999;80:7–14

57. Milkovich SM, Owens J, Stool D, Chen X, Beran M. Accidental childhood strangulation by human hair. *Int J Pediatr Otorhinolaryngol.* 2005;69:1621–1628

58. Piatt JH, Steinberg M. Isolated spinal cord injury as a presentation of child abuse. *Pediatrics.* 1995;96:780–782

59. Towbin A. Sudden infant death (cot death) related to spinal injury (letter). *Lancet.* 1967;2:940

60. Sneed RC, Stover SL. Undiagnosed spinal cord injuries in brain-injured children. *Am J Dis Child.* 1988;142:965–967

61. Cirak B, Ziegfeld S, Knight VM, Chang D, Avellino AM, Paidas CN. Spinal injuries in children. *J Pediatr Surg.* 2004;39:607–612

62. Swischuk LE. Spine and spinal cord trauma in the battered child syndrome. *Radiology.* 1969;92:733–738

63. Hadley MN, Sonntag VKH, Retake HL, Murphy A. The infant whiplash-shake injury syndrome: a clinical and pathological study. *Neurosurgery.* 1989;24:536–540

64. Geddes J, Vowles G, Hackshaw A, Nickols C, Scott I, Whitwell H. Neuropathology of inflicted head injury in children. II. Microscopic brain injury in infants. *Brain.* 2001;124:1299–1306

65. Shannon P, Smith C, Deck J, Ang L, Ho M, Becker L. Axonal injury and the neuropathology of shaken baby syndrome. *Acta Neuropathologica.* 1998;95:625–631

66. Feldman KW, Weinberger E, Milstein JM, Fligner CL. Cervical spine MRI in abused infants. *Child Abuse Negl.* 1997;21:199–205

67. Rooks VJ, Sisler C, Burton B. Cervical spine injury in child abuse: report of two cases. *Pediatr Radiol.* 1998;28:193–195

68. Thomas NH, Robinson L, Evans A, Bullock P. The floppy infant: a new manifestation of nonaccidental injury. *Pediatr Neurosurg.* 1995;23:188–191

69. Kleinman P, Shelton Y. Hangman's fracture in an abused infant: imaging features. *Pediatr Radiol.* 1997;27:776–777

70. McGrory BE, Fenichel GM. Hangman's fracture subsequent to shaking in an infant. *Ann Neurol.* 1977;2:82

71. Ranjith RK, Mullett JH, Burke TE. Hangman's fracture caused by suspected child abuse. A case report. *J Pediatr Orthop B.* 2002;11:329–332

72. Parisi M, Lieberson R, Shatsky S. Hangman's fracture or primary spondylolysis: a patient and a brief review. *Pediatr Radiol.* 1991;21:367–368

73. Van Rijn RR, Kool DR, de Witt Hamer PC, Majoie CB. An abused five-month-old girl: hangman's fracture or congenital arch defect? *J Emerg Med.* 2005;29:61–65

74. Heitzler GD, Cranin AN, Gallo L. Sexual abuse of the oral cavity in children. *J Mich Dent Assoc.* 1994;76:28–30

75. Jessee SA. Orofacial manifestations of child abuse and neglect. *Am Fam Physician.* 1995;52:1829–1834

76. Casamassimo PS. Child sexual abuse and the pediatric dentist. *Child Abuse Negl.* 1986;8:1026

77. DeJong AR. Sexually transmitted diseases in sexually abused children. *Sex Transm Dis.* 1986;13:123–126

78. Kui LL, Xiu HZ, Ning LY. Condyloma acuminatum and human papilloma virus infection in the oral mucosa of children. *Pediatr Dent.* 2003;25:149–153

79. Schmitt BD, Kempe, CH. The pediatrician's role in child abuse and neglect. *Curr Probl Pediatr.* 1973;5:3–47

80. Mouden LD. The role of dental professionals in preventing child abuse and neglect. *J Calif Dent Assoc.* 1998;26:737–739, 741–743

81. Kempe CH. Uncommon manifestations of the battered child syndrome. *Am J Dis Child.* 1975;129:1265

82. Carrotte PV. An unusual case of child abuse. *Br Dent J.* 1990;168:444–445

83. Needleman HL. Orofacial trauma in child abuse: types, prevalence, management, and the dental profession's involvement. *Pediatr Dent.* 1986;8(1 Spec No):71–80

84. American Academy of Forensic Sciences. *American Board of Forensic Odontology Policies, Procedures and Guidelines.* Colorado Springs, CO: American Academy of Forensic Sciences; 1995

85. Kenney JP. Child abuse and neglect. In: Hardin JF, ed. *Clark's Clinical Dentistry.* Philadelphia, PA: Lippincott; 1993

86. Kenney JP, Spencer DE. Child abuse and neglect. In: Bowers CM, Bell G, eds. *Manual of Forensic Odontology.* 3rd ed. Colorado Springs, CO: American Society of Forensic Odontology; 1996

87. Malcecz RE. Child abuse, its relationship to pedodontics: a survey. *ASDC J Dent Child.* 1979;46:193–194

88. American Academy of Pediatric Dentistry. *1999–00 American Academy of Pediatric Dentistry Reference Manual.* Chicago, IL: American Academy of Pediatric Dentistry; 1999

89. Mouden LD, Bross DC. Legal issues affecting dentistry's role in preventing child abuse and neglect. *J Am Dent Assoc.* 1995;126:1173–1180

90. American Dental Association. Minutes of House of Delegates, November 6–10, 1993. In: *1993 Transactions.* Chicago, IL: 134th Annual Session; 1994

91. American Dental Association. Resolution 44-1999. Adopted by the 1999 ADA House of Delegates. October 1999, Honolulu, Hawaii

92. Mouden LD. Dentistry preventing family violence. *Mo Dent J.* 1996;76:21–22, 24, 27

Chapter 6

Ocular Manifestations of Child Abuse

Alex V. Levin

Department of Ophthalmology
The Hospital for Sick Children
University of Toronto

Yair Morad

Department of Ophthalmology
Assaf Harofeh Medical Center, Tel Aviv University

Ocular abnormalities may be found in all forms of child abuse. In one study, the eye was the presenting sign for physical child abuse in 4% to 6% of cases.[1] Ophthalmology consultations are an important tool in identifying child abuse or differentiating the child who is not abused. This is particularly important in physical abuse, although ocular abnormalities may be found as manifestations in nonorganic failure to thrive, child neglect, sexual abuse, Munchausen syndrome by proxy, and perhaps emotional abuse. The retinal hemorrhages of shaken baby syndrome (SBS) are the most common and familiar ocular sign of child abuse.

Shaken Baby Syndrome

Ocular involvement, in particular retinal hemorrhages, joins skeletal and brain injury as a cardinal manifestation of SBS. Retinal hemorrhages are seen in approximately 85% of shaken infants, with reports ranging from 30% to 100% depending on the population studied. For example, studies that included abusive head trauma not characterized by repetitive acceleration-deceleration are likely to have lower rates, whereas postmortem studies are likely to have higher rates.[2] The unique violent shaking that characterizes SBS results in abnormal shearing forces inside the eye and orbit. Elevation of intracranial pressure, intracranial hemorrhage, hypoxia, anemia, and increased intrathoracic pressure may also contribute to the intraocular abnormalities, although the unique mechanics of repetitive acceleration-deceleration forces seems to be the key factor, the other factors rarely resulting in significant hemorrhagic retinopathy. The reader is referred elsewhere for a more lengthy discussion of the pathogenesis of retinal hemorrhage.[2,3]

Perhaps the most important aspect of understanding the significance of retinal hemorrhage as a manifestation of SBS is a knowledge of the anatomical correlates used to describe them. The retina lines the inside of the eyeball up to and behind the posterior surface of the iris. It is a vascularized structure made up of multiple layers. It is separated from the sclera (white of the eye) by an interposed vascular layer called the *choroid*. That area straight back from the pupil and in the center of the visual axis has a specialized anatomy and is known as the *fovea* (Figure 6.1). The line of sight (visual axis) is along this pupil-fovea line. The optic nerve enters the globe just nasal to the fovea bringing with it the central retinal artery and vein. These vessels branch out over the superficial retinal layers, starting as 4 major branches (arcades): 2 temporal (superior and inferior) and 2 nasal (superior and inferior) (Figure 6.1). The area of retina that surrounds the fovea posteriorly, demarcated by the major vessels of the temporal half of the retina (the superior and inferior arcades), is known as the *macula* (Figure 6.1). The retina continues to extend along the inner surface of the globe almost up to the back of the iris. The retinal edge is known as the *ora serrata* and that area of retina leading up to the ora, not easily visible with the direct ophthalmoscope, is known as the *peripheral retina.*

Hemorrhage may be found lying on the retinal surface (preretinal hemorrhage), underneath the retina (subretinal hemorrhage), or within the retinal tissues proper (intraretinal hemorrhage) (Figure 6.2). Superficial intraretinal hemorrhage will lie within the nerve fiber layer of the retina, thus causing the blood to stream along the course of the neurons leading to "flame-shaped" or "splinter" hemorrhages (Figure 6.2). Deeper intraretinal hemorrhage tends to have a round or amorphous geographic appearance (Figure 6.2), which is arbitrarily referred to as a *dot* (smaller) or *blot* (larger) hemorrhage, although there is no specific size cutoff point for the use of either term. Retinal hemorrhages may have white centers. Although well recognized as a manifestation of endocarditis (Roth spots), this nonspecific sign may be observed in virtually any disorder associated with retinal hemorrhage including SBS.[4] Hemorrhage within the gel (vitreous) that fills the back part of the eye (in front of the retina but behind the iris and pupil) is called *vitreous hemorrhage* and may be

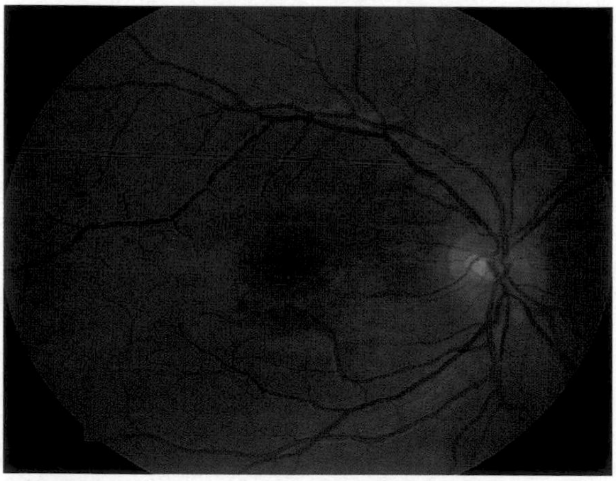

FIGURE 6.1
The posterior pole. This area of the retina encompasses the optic nerve and macula as well as the immediately surrounding retina.

mild, moderate, or severe and visually threatening.

The ophthalmologist can determine, through the use of indirect ophthalmoscopy, which types of hemorrhages are present. Likewise, the hemorrhages also may be described with regard to the number of hemorrhages observed (by counting or general description: few, moderate, many, or too numerous to count) and the distribution pattern. Hemorrhages may involve the entire retina or one or more specific regions such as the area immediately around the optic nerve (peripapillary), the area including the macula and peripapillary region (posterior pole), along major branches of the vascular tree (paravascular), the peripheral retina, or the area of retina posterior to the periphery but outside of the macula (midperipheral retina). The retinal hemorrhages of SBS may be unilateral or asymmetrical between the eyes.[3,5–11]

Describing the retinal hemorrhages in terms of type, number, and distribution is essential if one is to assess the specificity of any particular child's eye examination. A few intraretinal hemorrhages confined to the posterior pole may be very nonspecific and could result from numerous other causes (Figure 6.2). But massive retinal hemorrhage throughout the entire retina (subretinal, intraretinal, and preretinal) is rarely reported in any condition other than SBS, and those clinical scenarios are easily distinguished by the presence of other supportive signs (Figure 6.2). For example, a more severe hemorrhagic retinopathy can be seen in the first few days following normal birth or after severe motor vehicle crashes usually involving multiple impacts. In one report, a child who was allegedly killed when a television crushed his head had a severe hemorrhagic retinopathy,[12] but severe retinal

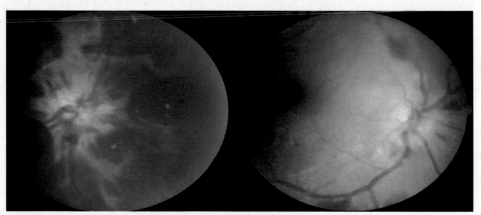

FIGURE 6.2
Retinal hemorrhages of various types in shaken baby syndrome. Note the asymmetry between the 2 eyes, as may sometimes occur, as well as the variety of hemorrhages. The image on the left demonstrates a severe hemorrhagic retinopathy that is virtually diagnostic of shaking injury. The image on the right is a more nonspecific retinopathy.

hemorrhages in head crush injury have not been found by other authors.[13]

Too often in the medical literature and other settings, comments are made about the specificity or implications of *retinal hemorrhages*. The use of this rather generic term is no more helpful in determining a diagnosis of non-inflicted versus inflicted injury than is the use of the term *fracture* without describing the involved bone and type of fracture. The non-ophthalmologist is at a distinct disadvantage in achieving an adequate description of intraocular hemorrhage because of infrequency of performing retinal examination, unfamiliarity with retinal anatomy, failure to dilate the pupil pharmacologically, and the optical limitations of the direct ophthalmoscope, particularly in the awake and noncooperative infant.

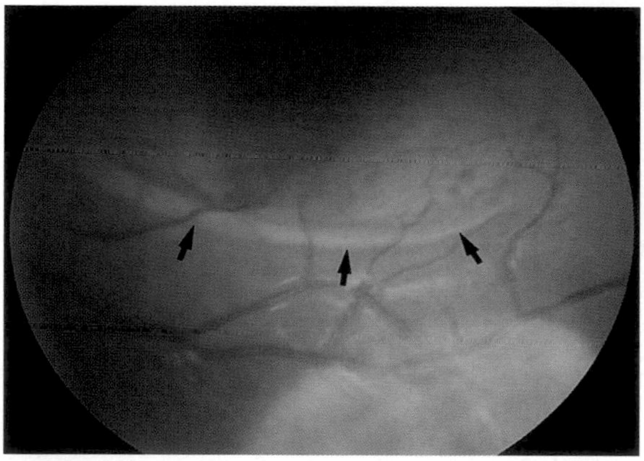

False-positive and false-negative examinations may occur that, if documented in the medical record, may lead to confusing evidence in a legal proceeding.[4,14]

It is essential that ophthalmology consultation be obtained in all cases in which SBS is suspected, and perhaps for all cases of unexplained sudden infant death. Except in those cases in which a child's pupils may be fixed and dilated because of imminent death, the pupils should always be pharmacologically dilated so that the entire retina may be viewed. If there are concerns about preserving pupillary reactivity for neurologic monitoring, options include the use of short-acting agents (phenylephrine, 2.5%; tropicamide, 1%), which will wear off within 4 to 6 hours; dilating one pupil at a time; or if no other options exist, using small pupil indirect ophthalmoscopy. Ideally, the examination should be conducted within 24 hours of presentation or recognition of the possibility of inflicted injury. The ophthalmologist should be encouraged to write a descriptive note and perform retinal photography by using either a standard handheld fundus camera, video indirect ophthalmoscopy, or the RetCam photographic unit. Such equipment is extremely costly and may not be available at many centers, but detailed drawings and scoring systems also can be useful.[2]

One specific retinal abnormality, traumatic retinoschisis (Figure 6.3), is essential to

FIGURE 6.3
Paramacular fold. Note the white line (arrows) over which blood vessels are elevated, caused by traction on the retina by the vitreous (vitreous not visible in photograph). This results in mechanical disruption of the pigment layer underlying the retina, resulting in the hypopigmentation. The paramacular fold is usually found at the edges of a traumatic retinoschisis cystic cavity.

recognize because it is highly specific for SBS and has never been described in any other condition of infants and young children in the usual shaken baby age range (<3 years old).[2,15] At these ages, the vitreous is quite firmly adherent to the macula and retinal blood vessels, much more so than in the adult.[16] As a result, the repetitive acceleration-deceleration forces applied indirectly to the vitreous exert shearing tractional forces on the retina, in particular the macula, causing it to split its layers, forming a cystic cavity that may be partially or completely filled with blood. It also is important to avoid the common error in identifying these blood collections as "preretinal" or "subhyaloid" (between the vitreous and retina).[17] Recognition of traumatic retinoschisis is aided by the identification of hemorrhagic or hypopigmented circumlinear ridges or lines at the edges of the lesion (Figure 6.3). These demarcations also have been called *paramacular folds.*

The folds may or may not be present and can also be observed in the absence of a schisis cavity or remain after a schisis cavity has settled. Folds were described in the controversial television head crush injury reported by Lantz and coworkers,[12] but not observed when larger samples of crush head injury patients were studied.[13] Schisis-like cavities also can form directly over blood vessels (Figure 6.4), although this is a less-specific finding that may be mimicked by virtually any disorder in which a major vessel can have a local bleed (eg, vasculitis, leukemia). The blood within a retinoschisis cavity may leak into the vitreous, making careful monitoring and follow-up essential.[18] In addition to schisis as evidence for the importance of vitreoretinal shearing and traction in the pathogenesis of retinal hemorrhage following repetitive acceleration-deceleration injury is the important presence of hemorrhage in the peripheral retina where the vitreous is also firmly attached.[2] In our ongoing computer-based finite element analysis of the eye in SBS, the importance of forces generated at the macula and in the peripheral retina has been observed.

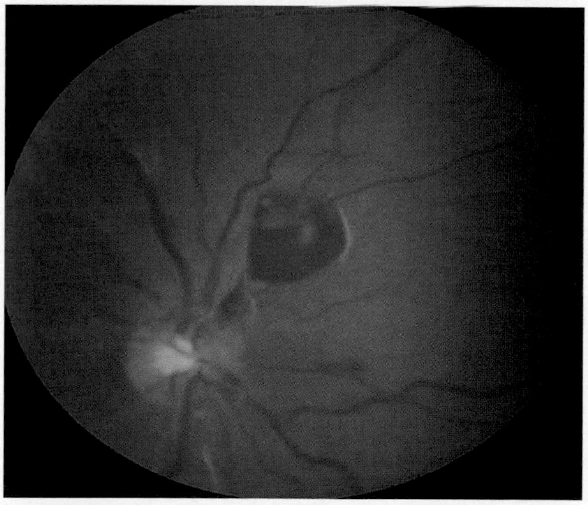

Peripapillary flame hemorrhages may be associated with papilledema, a very nonspecific finding, although certainly a marker for increased intracranial pressure (ICP) or orbital optic nerve compression. Yet many shaken babies do not have papilledema even when

FIGURE 6.4
A schisis-like blood collection in front of a blood vessel may be a sign of vessel shearing due to shaking but can also be due to other causes.

increased ICP is present.[3,4] Retinal hemorrhages are rarely associated with increased ICP from other causes in young children. When present, they tend to be few in number, intraretinal or pre-retinal, and confined to the posterior pole, in particular the peripapillary area. Likewise, intracranial hemorrhage alone, although not uncommonly associated with intraocular hemorrhage in adults (Terson syndrome), occurs in fewer than 8% of children with intracranial bleeding.[19] Retinopathy associated with increased intrathoracic pressure (Purtscher retinopathy) might be expected in view of the presence of rib fractures in many shaken babies. Yet Purtscher retinopathy is rarely reported in SBS.[3,20] Multiple studies show that retinal hemorrhage is extremely rare and, if at all possible, confined to a very limited number of retinal hemorrhages after cardiopulmonary resuscitation with chest compression.[2,21–24] The increased intrathoracic pressure produced by the Valsalva maneuver during cough or excessive vomiting can cause distinctive pre-retinal hemorrhage in the posterior pole of adults[25,26]; however, studies show that it is rare in children.[27,28] Shaking and other forms of severe repetitive acceleration-deceleration injury, such as a rollover multiple impact motor vehicle crash, induce unique shearing forces within the eye that cause intraocular hemorrhage to develop. This concept is additionally supported by the rare occurrence of retinal hemorrhage after other forms of non-inflicted head trauma. Retinal hemorrhages are observed in fewer than 3% of such children, and when they occur, the hemorrhages are almost always limited to the posterior pole, predominantly intraretinal and pre-retinal, and relatively few in number.[2,29] The mechanism for the accidental injury is usually so severe, life-threatening, and obvious (eg, motor vehicle crash) that child abuse would not even be considered. Only one paper has suggested that significant hemorrhagic retinopathy might develop following short falls,[22] but it suffers from many flaws including a lack of formal ophthalmology consultation.[2] Although the rate of retinal hemorrhage after severe trauma such as that from motor vehicle crashes is higher, the medical literature continues to confirm the rarity of hemorrhagic retinopathy due to other forms of non-inflicted trauma.[30,31] Yet it is perhaps the severe single acceleration-deceleration of extreme trauma that for a brief moment mimics the severe repetitive acceleration-deceleration of SBS, and leads to the comparatively mild retinopathy. Further evidence linking shaking to retinal hemorrhage comes from the studies at our center and others,[2] which reveal orbital injury at the optic nerve-scleral junction and the orbital apex: sites of fixation for the optic nerve, orbital vessels, and orbital nerves. The injuries observed to these structures may help to explain not only the retinal hemorrhage, but also the frequent observation of long-term optic atrophy, which is second only to cortical injury as the cause of permanent visual loss or blindness in survivors. Optic nerve sheath hemorrhage is not uncommon in shaken babies,[2,32] and although previously attributed to intracranial factors, may also reflect the direct effects of shaking. Optic nerve sheath hemorrhage and damage to vessels or nerves within the orbit all may play a role in generating intraocular bleeding. Postmortem examination of the entire orbital contents, preferably with sections taken after removal en bloc by a combined transconjunctival and intracranial route, may have specific utility in identifying pathophysiological mechanisms that identify the results of shaking.

There are many causes of retinal hemorrhages in children, and these are reviewed at length elsewhere.[2] Perhaps the most common cause is vaginal birth, which can result in an extensive hemorrhagic retinopathy in up to 45% of healthy babies at term examined in the first 24 hours of life. Studies in virtually every demographic setting have shown collectively that flame hemorrhages resolve within 7 days after birth, and intraretinal dot/blot hemorrhages usually resolve by 4 weeks. Rarely a large or deep intraretinal hemorrhage, particularly if it is in the fovea, may last to 6 weeks.[33] Preretinal and vitreous hemorrhage may also last longer. Although hemorrhagic retinopathy of normal birth may be difficult to distinguish from the shaken baby retina before 4 weeks of age, normal babies do not demonstrate traumatic retinoschisis, and other evidence of SBS is absent. In addition, subretinal hemorrhage is much more likely to occur after shaking as opposed to after vaginal birth. Retinal hemorrhage can occur after any type of delivery but is more common after spontaneous vaginal and vacuum-assisted parturition. After the time limitations for resolution of birth

hemorrhage have expired, inflicted neurotrauma is the most common cause of retinal hemorrhage in children younger than 4 years, with SBS itself being far more common than many of the disorders listed in the differential diagnosis of retinal hemorrhage in this age group. Nontraumatic causes of vitreous hemorrhage in infants and young children also are quite uncommon.[2,34]

Once the diagnosis of SBS has been made, there often is a request from criminal investigators to define a window of time within which the abuse may have occurred. Unfortunately, retinal hemorrhages cannot be used in this fashion with acceptable precision. Even though there are some data from adults[35,36] and clinical experience in abused children[7] that suggest perhaps a 2- to 3-day delay in the development of vitreous hemorrhage, particularly after traumatic retinoschisis, these data are "soft" and should not be used to rule out the possibility of vitreous hemorrhages occurring at the moment of shaking. This possibility of immediate vitreous hemorrhage must be true because retinal detachment can rarely be produced by the immediate effects of the shake. The timing of papilledema after increases in ICP also is not well understood.

Surprisingly, even the severe retinal hemorrhages and traumatic retinoschisis often resolve without long-term visual sequelae.[15] More often, long-term visual impairment results from optic atrophy or cortical damage, the latter being from autoinfarction of the occipital cortex, cortical contusion, occipital laceration, or intraparenchymal brain hemorrhage. It also is of note that in the awake and interactive child who is not experiencing central nervous system decompensation at the time of injury, no visual impairment may be noted by caretakers despite retinal hemorrhage. This is particularly true if only one eye has sustained the brunt of the ocular injury. Young children will seem to function normally unless both eyes have severe visual damage that is enough to interfere with the relatively few visual demands in their lives. Therefore, the history of normal visual function, as observed by caretakers in the home, does not rule out the possibility that hemorrhagic retinopathy has taken place. Our data and those from other centers[3,37,38] noted a positive correlation between the severity of retinopathy and the severity of intracranial injury.

Other ocular injuries are less common after shaking and include cataract, hyphema, ptosis, retinal edema, retinal detachment, or total disruption of the ocular contents.[2] Some of these injuries may reflect coincidental blunt trauma to the eye, either during or in addition to the shaking. Although some authors have suggested that blunt impact is necessary to generate enough acceleration-deceleration to cause severe, and in particular fatal, SBS injury,[39] numerous authors have concluded to the contrary that severe injury and death can result from shaking alone.[2,29] Not only does this hold true for retinal hemorrhage, but there also is strong empiric and reported evidence that "mild shaking" could result in a lesser hemorrhagic retinopathy that would go undetected because of the absence of a brain injury sufficient to bring the child to medical attention. Retinal hemorrhages due to shaking in the presence of normal neuroimaging have been reported,[40] and computed tomography scans showing edema without hemorrhage were also observed.[41] Shaken babies may make their first presentation to the medical system with relatively few or nonspecific symptoms and signs,[7] thus underscoring the importance of dilated retinal examination in situations in which a specific diagnosis is unclear, and "covert" shaking is a possibility.

Other Forms of Physical Abuse

Virtually any ocular injury could possibly result from an act of child abuse.[42] The face is involved in up to 45% of child abuse cases, with the eyes affected in up to 61%.[42] Like all forms of physical injury, a history and complete physical examination, with appropriate diagnostic testing, are essential to elucidate the cause. Yet certain eye injuries are virtually always indicators of trauma, whereas others must at least invoke the consideration of trauma. Table 6.1 offers some diagnostic guidelines for considering a possible traumatic nature of an observed ocular finding, although differentiating non-inflicted from abuse requires further investigation and evaluation beyond the eye examination. In the absence of intraocular surgery, avulsion of the vitreous base from its attachment to the peripheral retina is virtually diagnostic of trauma. Alternatively, trauma is a less likely cause of unilateral infantile cataract or ectopia lentis than non-traumatic etiologies.

There are many causes of optic atrophy in children, such as optic neuritis and Leber congenital neuropathy, but prior trauma must always be considered a possibility.

It is well beyond the scope of this chapter to discuss every possible physical injury to the eyeball. Many general references discuss ocular trauma,[43] but particular attention should be paid to the common error of attempting to date periocular hemorrhage in trying to establish a time of injury. The skin of the periorbita is loosely attached to the underlying tissues compared with other vulnerable body parts. As a result, large quantities of blood can accumulate, thus rendering dating systems,[42] which are already subject to inaccuracy and were designed with other body parts in mind, largely inaccurate. Periocular ecchymosis will often look darker for its age than subcutaneous accumulations of blood elsewhere on the body. This also will affect resolution time. In addition, the loose skin around the eye allows tracking of blood in the subcutaneous planes both to lower areas on the face and from areas on the forehead or scalp. A single blow to the forehead or anterior scalp can result in tracking of blood to the tissues around both eyes, thus giving the false impression of bilateral injury (Figure. 6.5).

A particularly troublesome situation arises when the eye is injured "accidentally" during physical discipline. I have seen 8 cases of hyphema (blood in the anterior chamber of the eye between the cornea and pupil) during a belt beating

TABLE 6.1
Specificity of Possibly Traumatic Ocular Abnormalities

Ocular Abnormality	Possible Trauma	Always Traumatic
Periocular ecchymosis	x	
Lid laceration	x	
Conjunctival abrasion/laceration		x
Corneal/scleral laceration	x	
Corneal scar	x[a]	
Iritis	x[a]	
Hyphema	x[a]	
Cataract	x[a]	
Ectopia lentis	x[a]	
Retinal detachment	x	
Commotio retinae (Berlin edema retinal bruise)		x
Avulsion of vitreous base	x	
Optic atrophy	x	

[a]Less likely to be traumatic when bilateral.

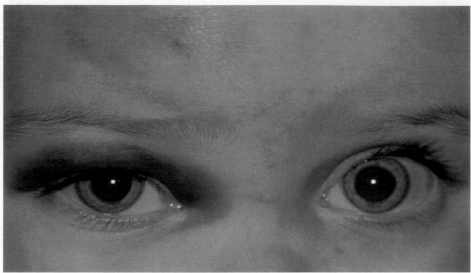

FIGURE 6.5
Bilateral periorbital ecchymosis from accidental blunt trauma to the central forehead.

in which the child had squirmed or the caretaker had lost positional control of the child and the belt or its buckle struck the eye. One child was rendered permanently blind in that eye, another lost the eye, and one did not experience sequelae until 30 years later when she presented with late-onset traumatic glaucoma (angle recession glaucoma). Although in each case the caretaker was remorseful, these situations do constitute reportable forms of child abuse.

One also may be confronted with a child who has sustained visual loss at some time significantly before the examination and now presents with sequelae that are otherwise of unknown etiology. Corneal scar or old retinal detachment or vitreous hemorrhage are examples. Further investigations, such as neuroimaging, may be useful. Old injuries may have particular morphology such as retinal pigmentary clumping, the fixed fold in a retinal detachment, or the whitened residual vitreous collection representing prior hemorrhage. A hypopigmented circumlinear line in the posterior pole may be a sign of prior retinoschisis due to SBS.

Munchausen Syndrome by Proxy

Ocular injury may be a primary or secondary manifestation of Munchausen syndrome by proxy (MSBP, also referred to as *factitious disorder by proxy*). This subject is reviewed elsewhere.[44] Direct ocular injury from MSBP has taken the form of covert instillation of a noxious substance onto the ocular surface, resulting in conjunctivitis or corneal scarring,[45] atropine sprayed onto the ocular surface resulting in factitious unilateral pupillary dilation,[46] and periorbital/orbital cellulitis due to the injection of noxious substances into the periorbita.[47]

In the first scenario, that of chronic idiopathic unilateral or bilateral conjunctivitis that is unresponsive to treatment, one might note a predominant involvement of the inferior half of the cornea and conjunctiva. This would result from the upgaze induced by forced opening of a resisting eye (Bell's phenomenon), thus exposing only the inferior corneal and conjunctival surfaces to the bulk of the noxious agent. Pharmacologic testing is available to help sort out the causes of anisocoria.[48] Careful inspection of the involved skin in an area of periorbital cellulitis may reveal needle-puncture marks.

Indirect manifestations may be more difficult to recognize. Subconjunctival hemorrhage or periocular petechiae may result from covert suffocation.[49] Although there are other possible causes, such as normal birth and pertussis (which often yields a more severe 360-degree hemorrhage), subconjunctival hemorrhage beyond the neonatal period is actually quite uncommon in the absence of direct blunt trauma to the eye. In any baby or child with sudden explained seizure, altered mental status, or unexplained signs of anoxia, a full eye examination should be requested to rule out not only the retinal hemorrhages of SBS but also the possibility of covert suffocation, as indicated by subconjunctival hemorrhage. This finding may otherwise go unobserved. The ophthalmologist must be alerted to inspect the conjunctiva before proceeding with retinal examination, which itself may induce subconjunctival hemorrhage if instrumentation is used.

Other indirect effects of MSBP would include those that result from covert poisoning that has an effect on the central nervous system. The pupils may become bilaterally constricted or enlarged.[50,51] Asymmetry of the pupils (anisocoria) may be the result from elevated ICP. Eye-movement disorders including strabismus[52] and nystagmus[53] can be seen. In addition, the covertly poisoned patient may be visually inattentive and seem to be "not focusing."

Neglect

Nonorganic failure to thrive has no specific ocular manifestations, although we have observed bilateral corneal erosions due to exposure in a severely wasted and neglected child who was left listless and unattended for a prolonged period before coming to medical attention. The lids were incompletely closed during this period and the blink rate reduced, thus leaving characteristic exposure desiccation injury involving the lower third of each cornea. We have also observed blindness due to bilateral corneal scarring in a child left to die in a latrine in a third-world country.

More commonly, the ophthalmologist is confronted with issues of less dramatic, chronic, medical neglect and noncompliance. For example, if the caretaker does not adhere to the prescribed regimen of patching to treat amblyopia, the child may be left with a permanently legally blind eye. Although noncompliance with patching regimens can be seen in normative families, complete failure to comply with patching is particularly troublesome when one considers that amblyopia is a treatable disorder. Failure to seek prompt medical attention for injury or other obvious ocular disorders also may result in blindness. The subject of child neglect is addressed elsewhere in this book (Chapter 14), but it is essential to note here the importance of consultations and collaboration between ophthalmologist and pediatricians/family physicians in managing such situations.

Sexual Abuse

Although there is one reported case of retinal hemorrhage presumably due to an extreme Valsalva effect in resisting a sexual assault, and we have observed children with severe retinal hemorrhages from fatal SBS in which sexual assault also occurred, ocular trauma is an uncommon manifestation of sexual abuse. Also uncommon is the occurrence of ocular involvement from sexually transmitted infection. Syphilis, "the great imitator," can result in a huge variety of ocular manifestations including keratitis, uveitis, retinal abnormalities, and optic nerve changes. It is always transmitted sexually, with the exception of transmission to the fetus or through the birth canal. Congenital syphilis has a different profile of ocular manifestations than does acquired infection and should be distinguishable by the ophthalmologist as well as other generalists and specialists. Although non-neonatal transmission of gonorrhea to the urethra, vagina, oropharynx, and rectum occurs exclusively through sexual contact, there is some evidence that the conjunctiva might represent a unique

"externalized" mucosal membrane that may make nonsexual transmission by fomites possible.[42,54] We are aware of one child who developed mild gonorrheal conjunctivitis after her mother, who had an active vaginal discharge later proven to be from gonorrhea, used a washcloth to clean her own genitals and then directly applied that same washcloth to her child's face during a joint shower. Full sexual abuse evaluation including examination and culture of other orifices and interview by a trained sexual abuse social worker and physician, as well as a child protective services investigation of the family and home, failed to uncover any evidence to support sexual abuse. However, the child was preverbal. Two other similar cases have been reported.[54]

If gonorrhea can possibly be transmitted to the conjunctiva in a nonsexual fashion, it raises the possibility that chlamydia conjunctivitis could be initiated in the same way. Human papillomavirus (HPV) can result in conjunctival lesions, and pubic lice can infest the eyelashes. Cases due to sexual abuse are known, but there are no studies evaluating the possibility of alternate routes of transmission. Human immunodeficiency virus (HIV) can have a wide range of primary and secondary ocular manifestations, but these are less common in infected children compared with infected adults. Of course, children may acquire HIV through routes other than sexual transmission. Herpes simplex and molluscum contagiosum, although occasionally transmitted by sexual contact, are so much more frequently transmitted by nonsexual routes that the consideration of sexual abuse is usually a low priority in the absence of other risk factors. In light of this information, it seems prudent that, in the absence of neonatal transmission or "consensual" sexual contact in an older adolescent, a full workup for sexual abuse be enacted for the ocular manifestations of syphilis, gonorrhea, chlamydia, HPV, pubic lice or, in the absence of other clear risk factors, HIV. At the very least, this intervention may have public health advantages in identifying infected adults in the child's home.

Emotional Abuse

Although perhaps not truly an ophthalmic manifestation of abuse, one must wonder about the psychosocial damage induced by harmful visual experiences in childhood. Children may be subjected to viewing sexual activity or drug-abuse behaviors by their caretakers or other adults. In a study of 1,000 Chicago high school students, 35% had witnessed a stabbing, 39% had witnessed a shooting, and 24% had witnessed a murder.[55] There is certain to be an adverse emotional impact of such experiences. Children also may present with functional visual loss and an otherwise normal eye examination as a result of unrevealed physical, emotional, or sexual abuse in the home.[56,57] Clearly such causes are far less common than the other stresses and strains of childhood, but it is important to include child abuse in the differential diagnosis.

References

1. Jensen A, Smith R, Olson M. Ocular clues to child abuse. *J Pediatr Ophthalmol.* 1971;8:270–272
2. Levin A. Retinal haemorrhage and child abuse. In: David T, ed. *Recent Advances in Paediatrics.* London, UK: Churchill Livingstone; 2000:151–219
3. Morad Y, Kim Y, Armstrong D, Huyer D, Mian M, Levin A. Are there correlations between retinal findings and intracranial findings in the shaken baby syndrome? *Am J Ophthalmol.* 2002;134:354–359
4. Kivlin J, Simons K, Lazoritz S, Ruttum M. Shaken baby syndrome. *Ophthalmology.* 2000;107:1246–1254
5. Ewing-Cobbs L, Kramer L, Prasad M, et al. Neuroimaging, physical, and developmental findings after inflicted and noninflicted traumatic brain injury in young children. *Pediatrics.* 1998;102:300–307
6. Harcourt B, Hopkins D. Ophthalmic manifestations of the battered-baby syndrome. *Br Med J.* 1971;3:398–401
7. Ludwig S, Warman M. Shaken baby syndrome: a review of 20 cases. *Ann Emerg Med.* 1984;13:51–54
8. Rao N, Smith R, Choi J, et al. Autopsy findings in the eyes of fourteen fatally abused children. *Forensic Sci Int.* 1988;39:293–299
9. Riffenburgh R, Sathyavagiswaran L. Ocular findings at autopsy of child abuse victims. *Ophthalmology.* 1991;98:1519–1524
10. Tyagi A, Willshaw H, Ainsworth J. Unilateral retinal hemorrhages in non-accidental injury. *Lancet.* 1997;349:1224
11. Weinberg H, Tunnessen W. Megacephaly: heeding the head. *Contemp Pediatr.* 1996;13:169, 172, 175
12. Lantz P, Sinal S, Stanton C, Weaver R. Perimacular retinal folds from childhood head trauma. *Br Med J.* 2004;328:754–756
13. Gnanaraj L, Gilliland MG, Yahya RR, et al. Ocular manifestations of crush head injury in children. *Eye.* 2007;21:5–10

14. Morad Y, Kim Y, Mian M, Huyer D, Capra M, Levin A. Non-ophthalmologist accuracy in diagnosing retinal hemorrhages in the shaken baby syndrome. *J Pediatr.* 2003;142:431–434

15. Greenwald M, Weiss A, Oesterle C, et al. Traumatic retinoschisis in battered babies. *Ophthalmology.* 1986;93:618–625

16. Sebag J. Age-related differences in the human vitreoretinal interface. *Arch Ophthalmol.* 1991;109:966–971

17. Weingeist T, Goldman E, Folk J, et al. Terson's syndrome: clinicopathologic correlations. *Ophthalmology.* 1986;93:1435–1442

18. Kuhn F, Morris R, Witherspoon D, et al. Terson syndrome: results of vitrectomy and the significance of vitreous hemorrhage in patients with subarachnoid hemorrhage. *Ophthalmology.* 1998;105:472–477

19. Schloff S, Mullaney P, Armstrong D, et al. Retinal findings in children with intracranial hemorrhage. *Ophthalmology.* 2002;109:1472–1276

20. Tomasi L, Rosman P. Purtscher retinopathy in the battered child syndrome. *Am J Dis Child.* 1986;93:1335–1337

21. Gilliland M, Luckenbach M. Are retinal hemorrhages found after resuscitation attempts? A study of the eyes of 169 children. *Am J Forensic Med Pathol.* 1993;14:187–192

22. Plunkett J. Fatal pediatric head injuries caused by short-distance falls. *Am J Forensic Med Pathol.* 2001;22:1–12

23. Goetting M, Sowa B. Retinal haemorrhage after cardiopulmonary resuscitation in children: an etiologic evaluation. *Pediatrics.* 1990;85:585–588

24. Kanter R. Retinal hemorrhage after cardiopulmonary resuscitation or child abuse. *J Pediatr.* 1986;180:430–432

25. Ladjimi A, Zaouali S, Messaoud R, et al. Valsalva retinopathy induced by labor. *Eur J Ophthalmol.* 2002;12:336–338

26. Chapman-Davies A, Lazarevic A. Valsalva maculopathy. *Clin Exp Optom.* 2002;85:42–45

27. Herr S, Pierce MC, Berger RP, Ford H, Pitetti R. Does Valsalva retinopathy occur in infants? An initial investigation in infants with vomiting caused by pyloric stenosis. *Pediatrics.* 2004;113:1658–1661

28. Goldman M, Dagan Z, Yair M, Elbaz U, Lahat E, Yair M. Severe cough and retinal hemorrhage in infants and young children. *J Pediatr.* 2006;148:835–836

29. Alexander R, Sato Y, Smith W, et al. Incidence of impact trauma with cranial injuries ascribed to shaking. *Am J Dis Child.* 1990;144:724–726

30. Bechtel K, Stoessel K, Leventhal JM, et al. Characteristics that distinguish accidental from abusive injury in hospitalized young children with head trauma. *Pediatrics.* 2004;114:165–168

31. Vinchon M, Defoort-Dhellemmes S, Desurmont M, Dhellemmes P. Accidental and nonaccidental head injuries in infants: a prospective study. *J Neurosurg.* 2005;102(4 suppl):380–384

32. Lambert S, Johnson T, Hoyt C. Optic nerve sheath hemorrhages associated with the shaken baby syndrome. *Arch Ophthalmol.* 1986;104:1509–1512

33. Sezen F. Retinal haemorrhage in newborn infants. *Br J Ophthalmol.* 1970;55:248–253

34. Dana M, Werner M, Viana M, et al. Spontaneous and traumatic vitreous hemorrhage. *Ophthalmology.* 1993;100:1377–1383

35. Muller P, Deck J. Intraocular and optic nerve sheath hemorrhage in cases of sudden intracranial hypertension. *J Neurosurg.* 1974;41:160–166

36. Vanderlinden R, Chisolm L. Vitreous hemorrhages and sudden increased intracranial pressure. *J Neurosurg.* 1974;41:167–176

37. Matthews G, Das A. Dense vitreous hemorrhages predict poor visual and neurological prognosis in infants with shaken baby syndrome. *J Pediatr Ophthalmol Strabismus.* 1996;33:260–265

38. Wilkinson W, Han D, Rappley M, et al. Retinal hemorrhage predicts neurologic injury in the shaken baby syndrome. *Arch Ophthalmol.* 1989;107:1472–1474

39. Duhaime A, Gennarelli T, Thibault L, et al. The shaken baby syndrome: a clinical, pathological, and biomechanical study. *J Neurosurg.* 1987;66:409–415

40. Morad Y, Avni I, Benton S, et al. Normal computerized tomography of brain in children with shaken baby syndrome. *J AAPOS.* 2004;8:445–450

41. Morad Y, Avni I, Capra L, et al. Shaken baby syndrome with no computerized tomography signs of intracranial bleeding on hospital admission. *J AAPOS.* 2004;8:521–527

42. Levin A. Ocular manifestations of child abuse. *Ophthalmol Clin North Am.* 1990;3:249–264

43. Levin A. Eye trauma. In: Fleisher G, Ludwig S, eds. *Textbook of Pediatric Emergency Medicine.* Philadelphia, PA: Williams & Wilkins; 2000:1561–1568

44. Levin A. Ophthalmic manifestations. In: Levin A, Sheridan M, eds. *Munchausen Syndrome by Proxy: Issues in Diagnosis and Treatment.* New York, NY: Lexington Books; 1995:207–212

45. Taylor D, Bentovim A. Recurrent nonaccidentally inflicted chemical eye injuries to siblings. *J Pediatr Ophthalmol.* 1976;13:238–242

46. Wood P, Fowlkes J, Holden P, et al. Fever of unknown origin for six years: Munchausen syndrome by proxy. *J Fam Pract.* 1989;28:391–395

47. Feenstra J, Merth I, Treffers P. A case of Munchausen syndrome by proxy. *Tijdschr Kindergeneeskd.* 1988;56:148–153

48. Levin A. Unequal pupils. In: Fleisher G, Ludwig S, eds. *Textbook of Pediatric Emergency Medicine.* Philadelphia, PA: Williams & Wilkins; 2000:237–244

49. Meadow R. Suffocation. *Br Med J.* 1989;298:1572–1573

50. Deonna T, Marcoz J, Meyer H, et al. Epilepsie factice: syndrome de münchausen par procuratio. Une autre facette de l'enfant maltraité: comas a répétition chez un enfant de 4 ans par intoxication non accidentelle. *Rev Med Suisse Romande.* 1985;105:995–1002

51. Rogers D, Tripp J, Bentovim A, et al. Non-accidental poisoning: an extended syndrome of child abuse. *Br Med J.* 1976;1:793–796

52. Kahn G, Goldman E. Munchausen syndrome by proxy: mother fabricates infant's hearing impairment. *J Speech Hear Res.* 1991;34:957–959

53. Rosenberg D. Web of deceit: a literature review of Munchausen syndrome by proxy. *Child Abuse Negl.* 1987;11:547–563

54. Lewis J, Glauser T, Joffe M. Gonococcal conjunctivitis in prepubertal children. *Am J Dis Child.* 1990;144:546–548

55. Bell C, Jenkins E. Community violence and children on Chicago's Southside. *Psychiatry.* 1993;56:46–54

56. Catalano R, Simon J, Krohel G, et al. Functional visual loss in children. *Ophthalmology.* 1986;93:385–390

57. Lim S, Siatkowski R, Farris B. Functional visual loss in adults and children patient characteristics, management, and outcomes. *Ophthalmology.* 2005;112:1821–1827

Chapter 7

Conditions Mistaken for Child Physical Abuse

Kent Hymel

Child Abuse Advocacy and Protection Program
Dartmouth Hitchcock Medical Center

Stephen Boos

Pediatric Forensic Assessment Consultation Team,
Inova Fairfax Hospital for Children

A child will grow best in a home that is safe, loving, and properly nurturing. This premise justifies intervention in homes and families that abuse and neglect their children. By the same reasoning, removing children from safe, loving, and nurturing homes on the basis of a misdiagnosis goes against the child's best interests. Therefore, identifying medical conditions that may mimic child abuse is as important as recognizing child abuse itself.

A complete list of conditions that have been, or may be, mistaken for child abuse is fairly long, and a thorough discussion of each potential pitfall is likely to be tedious. Such a catalog could potentially be misleading as well. Unusual conditions and unusual manifestations of more common conditions are likely to be overrepresented. Simple mistakes may go unreported in the literature as uninteresting, and thus be underrepresented. Searching the literature on medical misdiagnosis of abuse is difficult. Repeated searches using assorted synonyms for abuse and misdiagnosis fail to turn up known articles that are relevant to this topic. A recent search, excluding articles discussing inflicted versus non-inflicted trauma, abusive head trauma, and sexual abuse, identified 75 articles. Twenty-six dealt with the general issue of misdiagnosis. Of the rest, 10 dealt with coagulopathy, 7 with osteogenesis imperfecta (OI), and another 3 with temporary brittle bone disease. Another 7 reviewed folk medical practices, and 6 covered inflammatory conditions of the skin. Only one dealt with impetigo. Three articles detailed the authors' experiences with misdiagnosis of abuse.[1-3] Together they describe 81 children with 34 conditions (Table 7.1). Impetigo was the most common alternate diagnosis, followed by other inflammatory conditions of the skin, idiosyncratic non-inflicted trauma, mongolian spots, and vascular marks of the skin. All causes of coagulopathy combined were the fifth most common cause of difficulty. Twenty cases were diagnosed with conditions that appeared only once in the series, including the only case of OI.

Clearly, the volume of published literature does not accurately represent the spectrum of diagnostic confusion. Many misdiagnoses result from circumstances distinctive to the cases in which they arise. In addition to familiarity with conditions known or anticipated to cause diagnostic confusion, the provider evaluating possible child abuse would benefit from a systematic approach that will help recognize novel or idiosyncratic presentations that lead to the misperception of inflicted injury.

When considering conditions that may be mistaken for child abuse, it is instructive to consider how the diagnosis of child abuse itself is determined. The determination that physical abuse has occurred begins with the recognition of a traumatic injury. Once trauma is recognized, the health care professional must distinguish between inflicted trauma during child abuse and other forms of childhood trauma. In some cases, the identified injury will have an epidemiological association with child abuse. Awareness of this association will create a statistical expectation of child abuse. For the astute professional, objective findings will create expectations related to the history provided. For example, characteristics of the injury may form a pattern that indicates a particular causative mechanism that must be explained. Often an injury is felt to require trauma of a particular nature or severity, which should be known to the informant. The failure to report any trauma, or a trauma

that seems inadequately explained, will result in suspicion of inflicted injury. These 4 steps, recognizing trauma, reflecting on the collective experience with such trauma, looking for informative patterns, and drawing mechanistic inferences, present a good framework for both discussing known diagnostic pitfalls and thoughtfully constructing and resolving differential diagnoses in individual cases of suspected child abuse.

Finally, a discussion of conditions that may be confused with child abuse should proceed with caution. No underlying medical condition effectively protects a child from abuse. Children with disorders known to be confused with physical abuse in fact may also be abused.[4] Some of the children reported in the literature as examples of misdiagnosis may in fact have actually been abused. Each case must be evaluated on all of its merits, and the health care professional must consider abuse, conditions leading to misdiagnosis, and the possibility of abuse in a medically fragile child.

Recognizing Trauma

Non-Traumatic Skin Conditions That Mimic Trauma

The first step in diagnosing child abuse is identifying trauma. Whatever the means used to sort inflicted from non-inflicted trauma will be inadequate if the condition being evaluated is not, in fact, traumatic. Non-traumatic conditions that mimic trauma have been described as affecting both the skin and the bones. These include congenital conditions, developmental variants,

TABLE 7.1

Conditions Identified in 3 Consecutive Series of Children "Misdiagnosed" With Child Abuse

Diagnosis	No. of Cases
Impetigo	11
Inflammatory conditions of the skin	8
Non-abusive trauma	8
Mongolian spots	7
Vein of hemangioma	6
Non-traumatic intracranial fluid collection	4
Idiopathic thrombocytopenic purpura	3
Bone fragility with chronic disease	2
Chilblain	2
Folk medicine	2
Gonococcal infection (possibly) acquired from mother	2
Insect bites	2
Paint on face	2
Radiologic variant	2
Sunburn	2
Alopecia areata	1
Birth injury	1
Caffey disease	1
Chemical burn	1
Coagulopathy from cystic fibrosis	1
Congenital syphilis	1
Constricting band from tight clothing	1
Crohn disease	1
Ehlers-Danlos syndrome	1
Failure to thrive with chronic disease	1
Hemophilia	1
Hemorrhagic disease of the newborn	1
Intracranial hemorrhage from brain tumor	1
Medical treatment or misadventure	1
Osteogenesis imperfecta	1
Osteomyelitis	1
Rickets	1
Scoliosis	1
Subconjunctival hemorrhage with pertussis	1
Toddler's fracture	1

and pathologic conditions. We will discuss a number of these conditions. Beyond this list, however, professionals evaluating suspected abuse should make a practice of asking themselves: Is the patient's condition really traumatic? Often the answer to this question is made by following the child's clinical course. Bruises, burns, and fractures evolve and resolve over time. While bruise dating schemes have been shown to be inaccurate, the general expectations of color change and resolution over approximately 2 weeks is still valid. Most fractures will evolve through stages of subperiosteal new bone, soft callus, hard callus, and remodeling. Many conditions that mimic abuse will not follow these schemes. Failure to follow an expected pattern of resolution should prompt the health care professional to question whether a finding is traumatic in origin.

Naturally occurring markings of the skin may be mistaken for bruising, leading to concerns for child abuse. Mongolian spots, other pigmentary variants, and vascular markings have been mistaken as being caused by child abuse. Mongolian spots, also known as slate-gray or blue-black spots, are pigmentary marks of the skin that typically overlie the buttocks and low back (Figure 7.1). They occur in 75% to 90% of black and Asian, and 50% of Hispanic, but only 10% of white newborns.[5-7] While presacral and medial buttock location is most common, they may spread over the back, to the shoulders and arms, and across the buttocks onto the thighs. Involvement of as much as 15% of the body has been reported, with rare involvement of the face. A medical professional encountering mongolian spots for the first time, or an unusually extensive distribution, may mistake the condition for bruising.[2,3,8] The hue and evenness of color, and resolution over many years, rather than a few weeks, will distinguish these marks.

The brown or black color of nevi and the frequent occurrence of elevation or textural changes of the skin usually distinguish them from non-accidental trauma. We have seen a child reported for abuse on 2 separate occasions for a crescentic, flat, pigmented nevus lying under his eye. From a distance, or on casual inspection, the mark looked like a black eye (Figure 7.2). Epidermal nevi

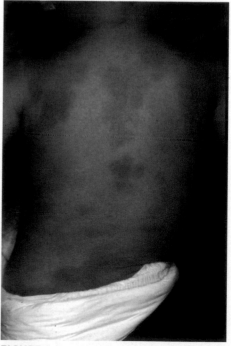

FIGURE 7.1
Mongolian spots, also known as slate-gray or blue-black spots, are pigmentary marks of the skin that typically overlie the buttocks and low back.

and hypopigmented macules may be mistaken for bruises, scars, or the hyperpigmented marks that sometimes follow trauma.[9] They may easily be distinguished from bruising by their persistence over time. The presence of normal dermal structures differentiates them from scarring. Differentiation from the hyperpigmentation that may follow trauma must be done by history and shape alone.

Vascular cutaneous markings have also been mistakenly attributed to abuse. Flame nevi and port wine stain create discrete areas of reddening and may become more visible when the child is crying. Because these marks occur on the face, where they are highly visible, mistaken reports of child abuse may occur (Figure 7.3).[10] A classic appearance, change in color with Valsalva maneuver, and the ability to blanch the lesion by stretching the skin will readily distinguish these conditions for the medical professional. Deeper, cavernous hemangiomas may pose more difficulty. Because of their deep location, a mixture of red and blue coloration occurs, and the edges are less discrete. The perception of a mass may suggest a deep hematoma. These lesions blanch less readily. Large lesions may ulcerate, creating concern for burning.[11] Capillary hemangiomas may be obvious initially, but as they resolve, their appearance changes and they may be mistaken for hemorrhage or scarring. Even single prominent facial veins have been mistaken as inflicted bruising.[1] The history of a long-standing lesion and persistence of the lesion beyond the lifespan of a bruise readily distinguishes each of these findings. The key to making the proper diagnosis is clinical follow-up.

The lesions discussed so far create the most diagnostic difficulty in very young children. At the opposite end of the pediatric age range, striae in adolescents have been suspected as a result of child abuse. Lesions may be raised or

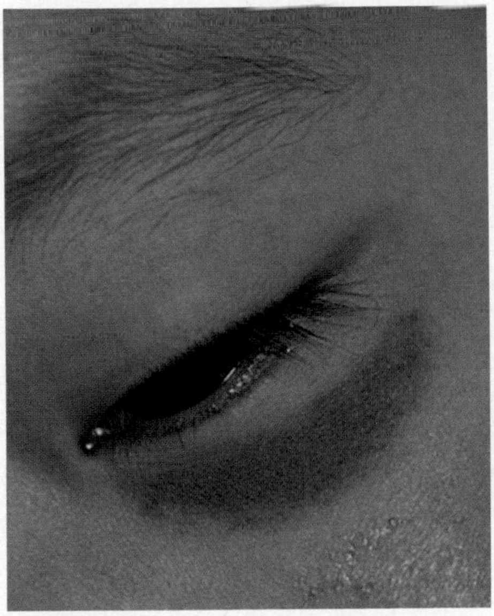

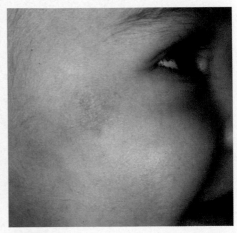

FIGURE 7.3
Facial hemangioma repeatedly mistaken for a bruise.

FIGURE 7.2
Intradermal nevus simulating a black eye.

depressed, flesh toned, pale, erythematous, or violaceous. They are usually multiple, often forming parallel ranks. They have been found in up to 35% of adolescents. Lesions of the low back and flanks have been mistaken for the effects of whippings or ritual abuse.[12-14] Obesity, steroid use and abuse, and body building are associated with striae, but they also may occur simply due to rapid growth. Their persistence over time will distinguish striae from acute welts of whipping, but not from scars. The characteristic appearance, orientation along Langer lines, and usual symmetrical distribution will help avoid misdiagnosis. Most adolescents are good historians, and a simple willingness to seriously consider their history should result in the health care professional dignosing this benign condition.

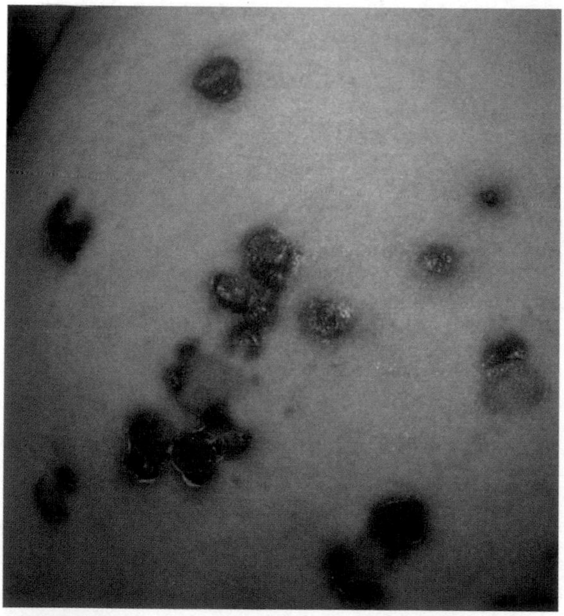

Inflammatory conditions of the skin may be more problematic. These conditions arise de novo and may resolve over a brief period, giving them a time course similar to trauma. The condition that most frequently simulates child abuse in case series is bullous impetigo (Figure 7.4).[1-3] The initial appearance of a few bullae may suggest cigarette burns. Impetigo lesions are very superficial and, once unroofed, exude a honey-colored crust. Culture will grow the typical mixture of *Streptococcus pyogenes* and *Staphylococcus aureus,* and if the lesions are not treated, they will grow and spread. Cigarette burns vary from circular bullae to a deep, punched-out crater with a raised edge. Most American cigarette brands produce a burn with an 8-mm diameter; impetigo lesions will vary in size from lesion to lesion and over time. At first glance, impetigo lesions and cigarette burns look similar, but distinguishing the two is not difficult if the examiner understands the difference in appearance of each. Another staphylococcal infectious syndrome, scalded skin syndrome, also simulates burns. Toxin-mediated desquamation may be extensive and the source infection may be covert, creating diagnostic difficulty. The Nikolsky sign, blistering of previously uninvolved skin during stroking, and progressive involvement of new skin differentiate the evolving process of scalded skin syndrome from a single event of burning. Fever and systemic signs point to an underlying infection.

FIGURE 7.4
Bullous impetigo. Note many lesions resemble cigarette burns, leading to the presumption of abuse.

Contact dermatitis and chemical burns may also simulate burning.[1] We have seen a child with a patterned, circular, bullous eruption that conformed to the circular pattern in which his mother applied a topical antifungal cream (Figure 7.5). The appearance suggested a patterned contact burn, but the history was clear and confirmed by the prescribing physician. Extensive dermatitis of the buttocks has been reported when children sustain prolonged contact with diarrheal stool following ingestion of senna-containing laxatives.[15] A desquamating lesion over both buttocks in a diaper distribution was noted, but the perianal area was spared, creating the appearance of an immersion burn. In both instances, a careful history and a willingness to consider a contact irritant allowed identification of the innocent cause.

An unusual form of contact dermatitis, phytophotodermatitis, is a reaction to ultraviolet light that is promoted by contact with certain fruit and vegetable juices. The result may be reddened, hyperpigmented, or bullous lesions of the skin. Because the lesions demonstrate the shape of the contact, they may be mistaken for an impact or contact burn.[16-19] Handprint patterns, in particular, have been reported. The history may reveal a day of partying in the sun and consumption of alcoholic drinks, further raising concerns for abuse. While the classic contacting agent is lime juice, other plants containing psoralens have been implicated, including lemons; certain oranges; figs; celery; parsley; carrots; several flowers, including ranunculus and euphorbia; and others. Some suspicion of child abuse will be allayed by careful consideration of the history and resulting findings. While handprints and contact burning are both child abuse concerns, a contact burn in the shape of a hand makes limited sense as a sign of abuse, and a bullous lesion in the shape of a hand should prompt broader thought. Once again, a careful history will steer the diagnosis in the direction of phytophotodermatitis.

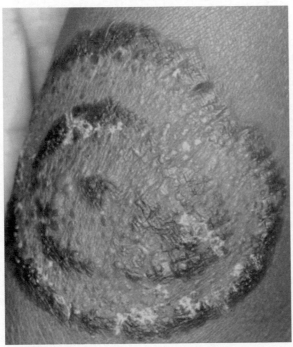

FIGURE 7.5
Patterned vesicular lesion from contact dermatitis due to sensitivity to antifungal cream.

Even the common inflammatory condition eczema has been reported as a condition mistaken as a result of child abuse.[1,20] In one patient, punctate lesions were confused with healing cigarette burns, and hyperpigmented marks from abrasions were suspected as inflicted injuries. Reviewing the case report; the social setting; and the unusual, non-inflicted injury set the stage for over-interpreting common findings that may have been exacerbated by eczema. This case stresses the need for the objective findings to be thoroughly evaluated on their own merits. Social risk factors have their place in an investigation, but should not hinder a thoughtful assessment of the objective medical evidence.

Henoch-Schönlein purpura is a small-vessel vasculitis characterized by abdominal pain, joint pain, and spontaneous purpura, particularly of the buttocks and lower extremities. The appearance of the many bruises, the tendency to develop lesions on the buttocks, and the absence of explanatory history might all be cited as reasons to consider abuse.[21,22] The accompanying joint and abdominal pain may also be attributed to injury during abuse, as may the presence of blood in the urine or stool. Young children may manifest swelling of the hands, feet, face, and scrotum. Rarely the skin lesions may ulcerate. Severe bowel involvement may cause shock or intussusception. Central nervous system involvement has produced seizure, coma, and subarachnoid hemorrhage. These unusual, severe cases may create further concern and confusion, but also present the opportunity for histologic diagnosis, which will reveal the presence of immunoglobulin A deposition and a leukocytoclastic vasculitis. The palpable purpura characteristic of this condition are usually denser, more discrete, and more indurated than typical traumatic bruises, and present a characteristic symmetrical appearance. Suspicion of abuse may be more likely when the social situation creates concern that distracts the examiner from the medical etiology.[22] Differentiation may be made by identifying the classic findings, by noting the presence of a viral illness in the preceding weeks, by observing the development of new crops of lesions in a supervised condition, or if the urinalysis shows evidence of nephritis.

Non-Traumatic Skeletal Conditions That Mimic Trauma

Radiographs may identify changes of bone that are non-traumatic in origin but that mimic traumatic changes. Perhaps the most classic of these findings is physiological, subperiosteal, new bone formation (Figure 7.6).[23,24] For incompletely understood reasons, infants often develop a visible layer of osseous density, under the periosteum but separated from the cortex, along the shaft of long bones. This may be seen in up to 35% of infants, involving the tibia, femur, humerus, ulna, and radius with decreasing frequency.[25] The finding is seldom seen in infants younger than 1 month and peaks at 2 to 3 months of age. Persistence to 8 months of age has been described, though most cases resolve by 4 months. Symmetrical involvement is most frequent, but a substantial minority of patients have asymmetrical involvement. Kwon et al[25] did meticulous study of 35 cases and found the maximal thickness of changes to be 1.8 mm of subperiosteal osseous density, separated from the cortex by a relatively radiolucent space of about a millimeter. While this finding has sometimes been described as physiological periostitis, there is no evidence that this represents an inflammatory process. Misdiagnosis has resulted when the finding is confused with changes typical of healing bone injury. The lack of an identifiable bone injury; the typical, often symmetrical, anatomical distribution; the appropriate thickness of changes; and the occurrence in a child of the appropriate age differentiates the physiological finding from trauma. A case of a child who suffered an inflicted fracture through physiological, subperiosteal new bone has been reported.[26] In this situation, the bone trauma was apparent, but the physiological changes were preexisting. Under these circumstances, it is important not to mistake the physiological finding for evidence of healing, which could create misunderstanding of the timing of the inflicted skeletal injury.

Other conditions produce subperiosteal new bone in the absence of bony trauma, including scurvy, rickets, Caffey disease, hypervitaminosis A, prostaglandin administration, congenital syphilis, leukemia, and osteomyelitis.[24,25] Several of these have been reported as conditions mistaken for child abuse.[1,2,27,28] Scurvy may also present with cutaneous and mucous membrane changes that simulate traumatic injury. Leukemia may result in thrombocytopenia, cutaneous bruising, or internal bleeding. Syphilis, osteomyelitis, and leukemia may actually destroy underlying bone, either in a pattern clearly distinct from fracture or resulting in pathologic fracture. Rickets results in genuine bone fragility and will be discussed later. At times these con-ditions produce patterns of new bone formation that do not resemble that seen following fracture. Caffey disease, scurvy, and prostaglandin administration sometimes produce extremely exuberant, subperiosteal new bone that balloons well away from the bony cortex. Caffey disease has a predilection for the mandible, a bone that is uncommonly fractured during abuse of infants. The absence of visualized skeletal injury as a cause of subperiosteal new bone should lead to consideration of non-traumatic causes. When other skeletal changes are seen, they will usually in-clude findings that are not typical of trauma. Systemic

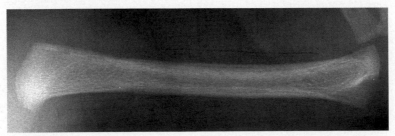

FIGURE 7.6
Physiological subperiosteal new bone formation in the humerus of an infant.

symptoms, such as fever, malaise, weight loss, and others, must be considered in the diagnostic paradigm. A thorough history and physical examination, and a search for   a diagnosis to explain all of the clinical findings, will lead to the correct, non-traumatic diagnosis.

Numerous normal variants of skeletal anatomy have been described, and some have led to the mistaken diagnosis of child abuse. Accessory skeletal sutures have been mistaken for skull fracture.[1,29] In the second reference, this error was made, in part, because another condition contributed to the confusion. Metaphyseal variants, such as metaphyseal step off, spurs, or beaking, could be mistaken for the classic metaphyseal lesion (CML).[30] Such an error is serious, as this finding is felt to be among the strongest radiologic associations with child abuse, but no case reports indicating such an error has occurred have ever been reported in the literature. Similarly, ossification defects and synostoses of the ribs may create confusion with fracture, though a report of this being confused with child abuse does not exist. Variations in the ossification pattern of the acromion process have been reported as mimics of inflicted trauma.[31,32] These variations have been well described, and may appear as an avulsion fragment at the tip of the acromion process. Once again, acromial and other scapular fractures in infants are strongly associated with inflicted trauma. Variation in ossification may occur in up to 13% of infants and can lead to misdiagnosis when high-quality skeletal x-ray surveys are taken during the evaluation of sudden infant death syndrome (SIDS). In living patients, there is no substitute for quality radiologic consultation. The use of qualified pediatric radiologists, either initially or to reinterpret important child abuse films, should reduce the misinterpretation of known pediatric radiologic variants. Single injuries unaccompanied by other traumatic findings should receive particular scrutiny. While an isolated skeletal finding may be the first sign of child abuse, subtle findings, such as CMLs or acromion fractures, are found more frequently in the battered child who has multiple injuries. In deceased patients, histologic evaluation of skeletal lesions identified during the skeletal x-ray survey should clarify the traumatic versus non-traumatic origin of the finding.

Several diseases may create changes in the metaphysis of long bones that might be confused with the CML. Copper deficiency from prematurity, total parenteral nutrition, or poor dietary intake; copper loss from peritoneal dialysis; and poor copper absorption associated with Menkes syndrome cause metaphyseal and other skeletal changes. The changes of rickets produce metaphyseal fraying and cupping that may create concern for fracture (Figure 7.7). A thorough clinical assessment and laboratory screening of mineral and vitamin status will uncover nutritional deficiencies; associated hematologic changes may prompt consideration of copper deficiency, and the characteristic hair and neurologic changes will raise the possibility of Menkes syndrome.

Misinterpretation of Epidemiology

Birth-Related and Accidental Fractures Mistaken for Abuse

When a specific injury is highly associated with abuse, it may come to be regarded by some practitioners as pathognomonic. Under such circumstances, exceptions to the abuse association can be overlooked. If the causal trauma was inapparent to the child's caretaker, resulting in the identification of injury without reported trauma, the likelihood of diagnostic error increases. Rib fracture during childbirth presents a good example of this problem. During infancy, rib fractures are the result of child abuse more than 80% of the time.[33,34] Most exceptions to this rule result from high-energy trauma. Rib fracture due to birth trauma has been repeatedly reported.[34–39] Most of these newborns were large with difficult vaginal births, though one weighed only 3,300 g. Clavicle fracture was commonly but not universally present. Signs of bruising, crepitus, and tachypnea were often present, but these findings may be biased by selection for publication. In the absence of associated clinical signs, rib fractures resulting from birth trauma can be missed. Subsequent identification of rib fracture outside the nursery could lead to a suspicion of abuse. Rib fractures heal rapidly in infants, though a reliable dating scheme has not been published. Difficulty distinguishing birth trauma from inflicted trauma is unlikely in children older than 3 months with healing fractures, or older than 1 week with acute rib fractures. Obvious

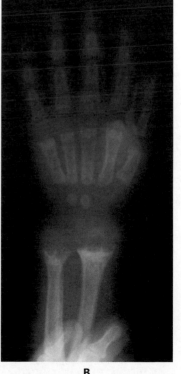

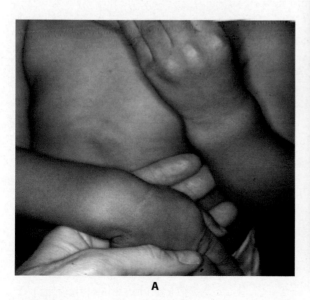

A   B

FIGURE 7.7
A. A 1-year-old with nutritional rickets. **B.** Metaphyseal fraying and cupping that result from rickets may create concern for fractures.

variation in the timing of multiple rib fractures excludes isolated occurrence during birth trauma.

Perinatal obstetrical manipulation can result in CMLs, also known as bucket-handle or corner chip fractures, of the infant metaphysis.[40,41] Two children demonstrated radiologic features typical of CMLs following cephalic version for breech presentation. Both developed fetal distress during the procedure, resulting in caesarean delivery, and both had symptoms of injury resulting in the radiologic evaluation of one knee. A CML-like appearance was identified in the distal femur of both infants and the proximal tibia of one. Follow-up x-ray demonstrated significant subperiosteal elevation and new bone formation in the femurs of both infants, a finding atypical of true CMLs. One infant's tibia, however, did heal consistent with the typical CML. Epiphyseal separation of both the proximal and distal femur have been reported as rare obstetrical injuries, and the CML-like appearance of the femur in these reported cases could represent a variation on that injury.[42,43]

Classic metaphyseal lesion has also been reported following serial casting for club foot. Grayev et al[44] reported 8 children with a CML appearance of the distal tibia during serial casting for club foot. Three of these children had additional issues of spina bifida or arthrogryposis, which may have complicated their situation. Consistent with our earlier contention that the identification of conditions that may be mistaken for child abuse does not rule out abuse in any one case, one child had 24 rib fractures and was thought to have been abused.

While the percentage varies with age and from study to study, there is general consensus that femur fractures in non-ambulatory children should be investigated for child abuse. In these children, the absence of a trauma history will predispose the clinician to the diagnosis of inflicted fracture. Considerations of unrecognized trauma, and/or accidental self-injury, are frequently dismissed in pre-ambulatory children. Grant and colleagues[45] reported 2 cases of children believed to be injured during use of an Exersaucer infant activity center.[45] Both children suffered fracture of the distal femur, in the same pattern, with a fracture line passing obliquely through the posterior metaphysis into the physeal lucency and subtle impaction of the bony fragments. Both children developed symptoms of tenderness and guarding, but there was no reported outcry at the time of injury, nor spontaneous pain when the leg was not stressed.

Humeral fractures have a somewhat weaker association with abuse, though this association has been defined in the literature out to 3 years of life.[46,47] Additionally, most non-inflicted humeral fractures are supracondylar in location, and humeral shaft fractures are more likely to be inflicted. Hymel and Jenny[48] reported a child who sustained a spiral fracture of the humeral shaft when she was rolled from prone to supine by a 2-year-old sister. The event was caught on videotape, which documented a loud snap followed immediately by a painful outcry. Torsional loading of the arm was apparent. One study of humeral fractures found that spiral and oblique morphology was associated with abuse.[44] The general belief that spiral fractures are somehow more suspicious than other fractures is widespread. Even in this source article, 42% of spiral fractures were non-inflicted. Spiral morphology in a humeral fracture has not always correlated with abuse, and is a common morphology for non-inflicted injury elsewhere, such as in the toddler's fracture of the tibia. Clearly this "folk epidemiology" is more biasing than informative.

Infanticide Misinterpreted as SIDS

Although decreasing in frequency over the past decade, sudden and unexpected death during infancy is still not rare. In many cases, these deaths are attributed to SIDS. Because there are no diagnostic findings that confirm SIDS, there is concern that some of these deaths are homicides by intentional suffocation, a form of infanticide that may leave no physical signs. This concern becomes greater when more than one SIDS death occurs in a family. The SIDS rate in Maryland was recently measured at 0.3 per 1,000 live births, or about one in 3,333 newborns.[49] If each SIDS death is an independent event, that would make the chance of 2 sudden infant deaths in a family about 1 in 11 million, and the chance of 3 SIDS deaths in a family about 1 in 37 billion. Such statistics have led to the aphorism "1 SIDS is a tragedy, 2 SIDS is suspicious, and 3 SIDS is homicide." But these statistics have been assailed. For instance, certain family and child care characteristics are associated with increased risk. If a family's risk is increased 10-fold, by a combination of unrelenting maternal tobacco abuse and prone infant sleep position, the risk for 2 sudden infant deaths in that family is about 1 in 111,000, and the risk of 3 is about 1 in 37 million. If only 1% of SIDS deaths are the result of an autosomal-recessive trait, the population risk rises to about 1 in 1 million for 2 sudden infant deaths in a family and to 1 in 5 million for 3 sudden infant deaths in a family. Additionally, the chance of a second sudden infant death in the family with the autosomal-recessive trait may be as high as 25% if they have a second child, 44% if they have 2 more children, and 58% if they have 3 more children. There is reason to believe that there are genetic syndromes that lead to death that can be confused with SIDS and genes that make some infants more vulnerable to the disorder we know as SIDS.[50,51]

Using epidemiological facts is an excellent way to describe population trends and generate suspicion of abuse in an individual patient. However, because epidemiological risk is defined over a population of children, it is not always easy to know whether a particular child is a classic example that epitomizes the described group, or is more consistent with the outliers that form exceptions to the group trend. Under these circumstances children with injuries that have demonstrated epidemiological risk for child abuse should be investigated to determine whether specific case factors support a diagnosis of abuse, conform to known exceptions, or represent unique variations that must be considered as a possible exception to the general epidemiological trend.

Creation of False Patterns

Skin Findings Misinterpreted as Abuse

Patterned injuries have played an important role in teaching about and recognizing inflicted injury. The presumption is that the pattern is a product of the weapon used against the child or its method of employment. At times, however, apparent patterns may be produced by the structure of the injured tissue, or by chance. It is unlikely that the given history will provide a credible explanation for such a pattern if it is assumed that the implement or its mode of employment must account for the pattern. This may lead to the mistaken assumption of a false history, and thus child abuse. We have not seen a report of false pattern leading to the mistaken diagnosis of child abuse in the literature, but have seen false and misleading patterns in our practices (see below).

While cutaneous trauma almost always results from forceful contact at the surface, injury can occur in deeper tissues while sparing superficial tissues. The deeper tissue hemorrhage that results does not become visible until it rises very close to the surface. This provides the opportunity for intervening tissue to influence the distribution of the blood, and the eventual appearance of the bruise. One classic example is impact to the scalp or forehead. Bleeding may often be subgaleal. While this can sometimes be felt as a bump or boggy area, blood in this location cannot be seen as a bruise. The galea may be impermeable to this blood. Blood collected below the galea can resolve in place without visible bruising, or move laterally and become

visible distant from the trauma site. Many providers have seen children who strike their foreheads and wake up the next day with a black eye or periorbital ecchymosis. The typical appearance is a swollen purple eye that appears as a bag of blood, without apparent superficial injury. Often the swelling and discoloration is worse in the lower lid, and there is no arc or accentuation at the orbital rim. Depending on the child's position during settling, the blood may settle into both eyes, creating 2 black eyes. We have also seen children who develop 2 black eyes and diffuse ecchymosis at the back of the neck. Once this phenomenon is recognized, diagnosis is easy. The history, absence of superficial trauma near the eye, and presence of an impact site on the head removes confusion.

Forceful impact injury to a large muscle mass may also result in deep bleeding, absent superficial injury. While a solid ovoid bruise may occur in some cases, tissue swelling and edema dilutes or displaces central blood, resulting in a circular bruise with central clearing.[52] We have witnessed similar patterns following impact by a spoon, and in older bites after individual teeth marks are lost. This creates the possibility for confusion. We have also seen the development of a striated pattern within extensive bruising of the buttocks. In each case, the buttocks were bruised during an abusive event in which the victims were beaten with a board or belt. Confusion resulted when investigators believed they should look for a specific weapon to explain the striation. We believe that tissue edema and connective tissue structures were responsible for the pattern, which should not be mistaken for an imprint of the injurious weapon. Another misleading pattern has been described on the buttocks. During abusive paddling, bruising often occurs at the margins of the paddle. This usually results in stripes crossing the buttock horizontally. Sometimes a vertical line of bruising will develop on both sides of and parallel to the intergluteal crease.[53] This has been explained as a line of bruising that occurs where the skin is abruptly folded during rapid compression in the coronal plane. Although several of these injury patterns resulted from inflicted force to the buttocks, these cases demonstrate the potential for overinterpretation of patterned injuries.

The occurrence of 2 to 5 oval bruises along a line or arc is sometimes recognized as a grip or grab mark—the imprint of fingertips when a child is forcefully grabbed by a hand. Similar bruising patterns can also occur if certain body regions, such as the ribs or spine, slide forcefully over a rigid edge. During such an event, while the skin is crushed between the rigid edge and the underlying bone, it is spared over the receding and yielding soft tissues. Because the skin is also pulled laterally, the bruises may not directly overlie the bony prominences. Movement and stretching of the skin will allow the examiner to align the bruises over the underlying bony prominences. Close inspection may reveal abrasion parallel to the line or arc of the bruises.

A similar occurrence may occur with loose soft tissues. We have personally examined a bruise that looked like a stack of coins, but originated from glancing contact against the back of a wooden chair. Very likely, the event resulted in a stuttering or intermittent contact—the chair dug in, crushing the tissue; released; then dug into a sequence of new catch points. The resulting bruise formed a distinct, though unrecognizable, pattern. We have heard anecdotes of a cat scratch that did the same thing. The claws caught and punctured, released, moved a distance, then caught and punctured again. This occurred repeatedly, creating rows of spaced puncture marks. Injury by a comb or brush was considered before the history of a cat scratch provided by the victim was accepted.

Patterns are read by clinicians to evaluate a history for consistency and to describe an injurious event when no history is provided. Many of these patterns are absolutely clear and can be specifically linked to the specific object that caused them. Some patterns are less distinct or do not conform to a known object. In these cases, the possibility exists that the bruising pattern was influenced by the structure of the underlying or intervening tissues, resulted from stuttering contact, or was due to some other chance event.

Mechanistic Assumptions and Fragility

Coagulopathies

Trauma is a daily life event. Toddlers sustain trauma each time they try to walk and fall. Many societies tolerate a certain level of inflicted trauma by spanking or slapping as discipline. Tissue damage is often used as a threshold in determining if trauma was too severe to be the result of typical incidents of daily life, or if discipline was too severe. When the body's ability to sustain trauma, injury-free, is altered, these determinations may be invalid. For this reason, medical conditions that convey vulnerability to traumatic injury are among the most discussed conditions that may be mistaken for child abuse. Sometimes the fragility is so exquisite that injury appears almost spontaneously. On other occasions, injurious trauma must be quite significant, just not quite as significant as in the well child. For this reason, abuse must still remain in the differential diagnosis, though the certainty of the diagnosis may be less.

The disruption of small blood vessels is a common occurrence, which is seldom recognized because normal hemostasis seals the rupture before hemorrhage can become significant, or even evident. Coagulopathies alter this. In the face of a coagulopathy, bruises appear where bleeding would otherwise have been imperceptible, and bleeding that would have been asymptomatic becomes problematic. Whenever the presence of blood serves as evidence of inflicted trauma, coagulopathy must be considered.

Vitamin K is a fat-soluble vitamin that is largely provided by symbiotic bacteria living in the human gut.[54,55] In the presence of vitamin K, precursors to clotting factors II, VII, IX, and X are γ-carboxylated, a necessary step in producing active factors. When vitamin K is deficient, proteins induced by vitamin K absence (PIVKAs) are produced and

appear in the circulation. Eventually the levels of active factors II, VII, IX, and X drop low enough that the extrinsic, intrinsic, and common coagulation pathways are affected, prolonging the prothrombin time (PT) and partial thromboplastin time (PTT). At some level of prolongation, abnormal hemorrhage will occur. Vitamin K levels are low in newborns, leaving them vulnerable to hemorrhage in the days following birth. Intramuscular or sometimes oral vitamin K is administered in obstetrical units to prevent this occurrence. Birth in the home or in a birthing center that does not administer vitamin K will increase the risk of hemorrhage. As the initial vitamin K dose wanes, the infant must acquire a new source of vitamin K. In formula-fed infants vitamin K is supplemented, but in breastfed infants vitamin K must come from the developing gut flora. Significant deficiency may develop in the transition period, posing serious risk of hemorrhage between 2 weeks and 6 months of age. The use of oral (rather than intramuscular) vitamin K, gastrointestinal (GI) conditions in the infant, and maternal use of certain medications (barbiturates, carbamazepine, isoniazid, phenytoin, rifampin, warfarin) increase this risk. This late-onset vitamin K– deficient bleeding may present as cutaneous, intracranial, GI, or other bleeding. Misdiagnosis of child abuse has principally occurred following presentation with unexplained intracranial bleeding.[1,54–56] Cutaneous and intramuscular bleeding have also caused misdiagnosis.[55,57] The birth, medical history, or family history may alert the provider to the child's risk of vitamin K deficiency. Recognition of clinically significant bleeding should trigger screening tests of coagulation function, which will demonstrate a coagulopathy. PIVKAs can identify vitamin K deficiency as a contributing factor to bleeding, possibly even post-mortem.[58]

The hemophilias are genetic disorders that compromise the production of clotting factors VIII or IX, leading to a bleeding diathesis. Factors VIII and IX are both coded on the X chromosome, and so classic (hemophilia A) and Christmas disease (hemophilia B) are both X-linked recessive traits, most commonly occurring in males. Both factors participate in the extrinsic pathway, and so deficiency greatly prolongs the PTT but not the PT. The classic presentation is with hemarthrosis, but cutaneous bruising, excess bleeding following cuts and lacerations, deep muscle hemorrhage, and internal bleeding all occur. Knowledge of a family history of hemophilia is helpful, but not always present because a significant minority of hemophilia A cases represent new mutations. Confusion with child abuse has been reported, but is easily avoided if routine screening for coagulopathy occurs, and abnormal screening tests are further investigated.[1,59-61] Johnson and Coury[4] reported 2 children reported for abuse, one with previously unknown hemophilia and one with known hemophilia. Both had complicated social situations and fluctuations in the frequency of bleeding based on changes in placement. These children were felt to suffer from the effects of abuse, neglect, and hemophilia. The simplicity of making this diagnosis with screening tests that should be routinely performed belies the complexity of this entire issue. Fragility does not provide protection from abuse, though it does contribute to diagnostic uncertainty. In these circumstances, a thoughtful collaboration with child protective services, or even with law enforcement, may be necessary to determine whether child protection is a necessary component of the child's medical management.

Von Willebrand disease is the most common of the inherited clotting disorders, affecting as much as 1% to 2% of the population. Although it is an autosomal-dominant trait, it is most commonly identified in adult women, because menorrhagia is the most common presenting complaint. The von Willebrand protein circulates bound to factor VIII, but is a separate protein coded by a separate gene. It is principally responsible for platelet adhesion and aggregation. Oozing from cuts, surgical incisions, and dental extraction sites may be the only bleeding issues for patients with von Willebrand disease, but epistaxis, bleeding gums, and easy or excessive bruising all occur. Serious internal bleeding occurs rarely, particularly with type 3 von Willebrand disease. Von Willebrand disease is often discussed in reviews of conditions mistaken for child abuse, and we have encountered this difficulty in our practice, but case reports of this confusion are fewer than we would expect.[62] Differentiation can actually be difficult as the PTT may be normal or only mildly prolonged. Clinical penetrance is variable, so a family history may be misleading. Finally, the levels of factor VIII antigen, von Willebrand factor, and ristocetin-associated cofactor may vary as acute phase reactants, requiring repeat measurements to demonstrate abnormal levels. The bleeding time and platelet function tests have been promoted as screening tests, but both have limitations. A careful history, screening with a panel of tests for von Willebrand disease, and careful follow-up of abnormal or even low normal levels is necessary to avoid missing this disorder. As with all bleeding disorders, and particularly with a disorder this common, identifying the presence of von Willebrand disease does not rule out abuse, but must be carefully weighed when making a diagnosis.

Thrombocytopenia is the other common coagulopathy that may be confused with child abuse. Three out of the 50 children reported by Wheeler and Hobbs[1] with mistakes in diagnosis had thrombocytopenia, and other cases have been reported. The cause in each of those children was the most common cause of childhood thrombocytopenia, immune thrombocytopenic purpura, also known as idiopathic thrombocytopenic purpura or ITP. This condition is often preceded by a viral illness, which triggers an immunoglobulin response that binds to antigens on the surface of circulating platelets. Platelets are sequestered in the spleen and liver and destroyed, producing thrombocytopenia. As the platelet count drops, exaggerated traumatic bruising, seemingly spontaneous bruising, and the appearance of petechiae are noted. Epistaxis, mucous membrane hemor-

rhage, and menorrhagia may occur, and serious internal bleeding is an uncommon complication. Excess bruising may prompt consideration of child abuse, but the presence of petechiae may suggest an underlying platelet problem. Differentiation will not be difficult if a complete blood count (CBC) is obtained. Abnormal bleeding is uncommon unless platelets are below 50,000/μL, and serious bleeding typically occurs at counts below 20,000/μL.

Vitamin K deficiency was mentioned previously, principally in the context of infancy. In older children, fat malabsorption and malnutrition may result in coagulopathy leading to consideration of abuse.[2,63] Ingestion of warfarin inhibits vitamin K–dependent activation of clotting factors, inducing a coagulopathy. The literature principally links warfarin ingestion to child abuse, primarily in cases of Munchausen syndrome by proxy.[64,65] Toddlers, however, may discover rat poison and ingest the pellets, leading to anticoagulation, bruising, and internal bleeding. Leukemia was mentioned earlier in this chapter as a cause of subperiosteal new bone. Leukemia may have many manifestations including bruising, internal hemorrhage, pathologic skeletal fractures, and sudden unexpected death. In some cases this may lead to suspicion of child abuse.[66]

Other, rarer, coagulopathies may result in easy bruising or bleeding.[67,68] Nonspecific tests of clotting have been suggested to evaluate for these. The bleeding time is often recommended when evaluating children for child abuse. Unfortunately, bleeding times are difficult to standardize, particularly in centers with limited experience. For this reason some pediatric hematologists recommend against them. The PFA-100, an automated test of platelet aggregation, has been suggested by some. There is some question about the sensitivity of this test for identifying von Willebrand disease, and we have been involved in a case where von Willebrand disease was dismissed based on a normal PFA-100 only to be diagnosed months later based on an abnormal von Willebrand panel and family history. Most coagulopathies, however, can be ruled out by scrupulously adhering to a policy of checking the platelet count with a CBC, and measuring the PT and PTT. Recommendations for screening with a thrombin time, fibrinogen, factor XIII, von Willebrand panel, and other tests vary. A broader panel would seem to be indicated when the injury is serious, bruising lacks an identifiable pattern, and other manifestations of child abuse are absent.

Bone Fragility

Skeletal fragility is a commonly discussed confounder when diagnosing child abuse, and there is a good deal of literature discussing confusion between OI and child abuse. Osteogenesis imperfecta is the prototype disease for skeletal fragility, and perhaps for the entire issue of misdiagnosis of child abuse.[69-74] For all this attention in the literature, reports by Wardinsky and Vizcarrondo,[3] Kaplan,[2] and Wheeler and Hobbs[1] revealed only one child who suffered from OI in 81 cases

misdiagnosed with abuse. Some authors have strenuously argued that OI is much more common and is often confused with child abuse.[75-77] At times this argument has been taken too far, and its proponents criticized.[78]

Osteogenesis imperfecta is a congenital disorder of collagen synthesis leading to bone fragility and accompanying signs.[79,80] Clinically, the disorder is divided into 4 types. Type I is the mildest type. Patients have distinctly blue sclerae, relatively normal growth and stature, a mild propensity to wormian bones of the skull, and variable problems with early adult hearing loss. About half have soft, fragile teeth as well. Type II is the severest, and is nearly always fatal in the perinatal period or early infancy. Type III is a severe type, with neonatal fractures and deformities, poor growth and short stature, progressive bony deformity, variably blue sclerae, many wormian bones of the skull, fragile teeth, and early adult hearing loss. Type IV presents the most diagnostic difficulty, as it is the most variable type. Some reports indicate normal neonatal size, followed by significant growth delay and short stature, but some individuals may approach normal stature. Sclerae may be light blue or gray at birth, but become whiter with age, and distinctly blue sclerae are absent. Wormian bones are generally present, but there may be only a few in half of patients, and only half display fragility of the teeth. Hearing loss is an inconsistent sign. Type IV patients average one fracture per year throughout childhood, but there is great variability, with 5% of patients having as many as 10 fractures per year.[79] Type I patients generally suffer fewer fractures, and Type III patients suffer more. This classification scheme, based on clinical signs, may be supplanted because it does not directly correlate to either the genotype or the collagen synthetic phenotype. A further challenge to the nosology of OI is the description of types V, VI, and VII, none of which have collagen mutations. Type V was defined in a family with moderate to severe skeletal fragility and calcification of the intraosseous membrane of the radius and ulna.[81] Type VI was defined in a group of patients with moderate to severe skeletal fragility, vertebral compression fractures, low bone mineral density, and high alkaline phosphatase.[82] Type VII demonstrates moderate to severe skeletal fragility, fractures at birth, blue sclerae, early skeletal deformity, and rhizomelia.[83] While OI types I through V are typically described as autosomal-dominant, a negative family history may be of limited value. Almost 100% of severe cases represent new mutations, and up to 60% of milder cases represent new mutations. The presence of multiple cases in a single generation, with unaffected parents, probably represents somatic or germline mosaicism in the parent, rather than an autosomal-recessive pattern.

The occurrence of a fracture with poor explanatory history should prompt a consideration of OI. A family history should be taken, though its limitations must be remembered. The skeletal x-ray survey should be scrutinized for demineralization, thinning of the cortices of long bones, bowing deformity, and the presence of wormian bones. Much has been made of normal bone mineralization. Early in life, at the time of the first fracture, bone mineral density is likely to be normal, though with repeated fracture, immobilization, and age the bone mineral density will drop. Because this sign may not develop until later in life, normal bone mineralization does not effectively exclude OI in infancy. Other signs, such as blue sclerae, short stature, and dentinogenesis imperfecta, should be looked for in both the child and any family members present for examination.

At some point it may be desirable to have a collagen synthetic phenotype or a genotype determined. Steiner et al[84] initially suggested that clinical evaluation by an experienced physician is usually adequate for assessment. Marlowe et al's[85] further study did identify OI in children evaluated for child abuse with no clinical suspicion of OI. The only clinical profile that safely excluded OI was the presence of additional nonskeletal evidence of child abuse. Universal laboratory testing for OI in children with suspicion of abuse based on skeletal injuries alone has not yet become the standard of care. Decisions on testing must be made on a case-by-case basis. When concern for OI is clinically based, when clinical experience to exclude OI is lacking, when skeletal injuries are the only basis for considering abuse, or when legal situations mandate, 2 diagnostic laboratory tests are available. A collagen synthetic phenotype involves culturing fibroblasts from a skin biopsy, having them secrete collagen, and studying the collagen by electrophoresis. This test is 87% sensitive to the forms of OI that can possibly be confused with child abuse. Sequencing of the *COL1A1* and *COL1A2* genes may be performed on blood or fibroblasts from skin biopsy. This test is 100% sensitive for type I but only 70% to 80% sensitive for type IV, the type of OI that causes the most diagnostic confusion.

When fractures in different stages of healing are found, the possibility that some are birth-related must be considered, as birth fractures are well described in OI. Newly recognized, healing fractures that are inconsistent with birth injury present a particular problem. Because children with severe OI sustain frequent fractures following limited trauma, identifying occult fractures in these children is common. The occurrence of occult healing fractures in children with mild fragility is likely to indicate a painful injury that was not attended to and cause concern for abuse. Intermediate variants may defy obvious assumption. When clinical indications suggest that caretakers have overlooked painful or disabling injuries, inflicted trauma must be considered, even in the presence of OI. The comorbidity of OI and child abuse has been reported.[86]

Other conditions lead to osseous fragility. Nutritional rickets is a condition that is still seen in developed countries. It is most common in breastfed infants with dark skin who are infrequently exposed to direct sunlight. Fractures are sometimes associated with rickets, and

rickets-associated fractures have led to suspicion of child abuse.[87-89] A review of these reports illustrates that this is not always a case of one diagnosis or the other. Rickets, especially in combination with a compromised family environment, can lead to the false diagnosis of child abuse, but sometimes a compromised family environment leads to abuse, and perhaps rickets. The presence of frayed, moth-eaten metaphyses on skeletal survey should prompt a consideration of rickets. On physical examination, children with rickets can manifest flaring of the distal radius and ulna or a rachitic rosary (ie, prominence of the costochondral junctions on the chest). Laboratory evidence of rickets includes low 25-OH vitamin D levels, elevated parathyroid hormone and alkaline phosphatase, and sometimes low serum calcium and phosphate.

Calcium phosphate metabolism is affected by a number of chronic disease states. Renal tubular disorders, including familial hypophosphatasia, idiopathic hypercalciuria, and renal rickets associated with chronic renal failure can all leach skeletal mineral deposits. Drugs, including immunosuppressive medications used in organ transplant and anticonvulsants that affect carbonic anhydrase type II, can lead to renal calcium wasting. Corticosteroids are a well-known cause of skeletal mineral loss. Gastrointestinal diseases affecting vitamin D and calcium absorption include celiac disease, inflammatory bowel disease, and biliary atresia. Endocrine disorders associated with polyostotic fibrous dysplasia, or McCune Albright syndrome, and primary hyperparathyroidism result in demineralization. Both leukemia and sickle cell disease have been shown to reduce bone mineral content. Copper deficiency associated with parenteral nutrition and Menkes disease affect bone strength through their effect on collagen synthesis. Each of these diseases has an increased incidence of fracture, and confusion with child abuse has been reported despite obvious chronic disease.[90]

Osteopenia associated with spastic cerebral palsy is an instructive example. These children often fail to bear weight normally, decreasing the mechanostat stimulus for bone mineralization. They may be malnourished, and fad therapeutic diets are common in this population. Many of these children are prescribed anticonvulsant drugs that can affect renal calcium handling and vitamin D metabolism in the liver and kidneys. Disordered calcium metabolism, demineralization of the skeleton, and increased risk of skeletal fracture can result. Laboratory findings are inconsistent, and calcium and phosphate levels are likely to be normal. The earliest laboratory test to demonstrate a problem is the 25-OH vitamin D level. Two case reports illustrate the complex relationship between skeletal fragility and child abuse. Torwalt and colleagues[91] reported a 4-year-old with spasticity secondary to earlier traumatic brain injury. The child died of pneumonia at age 4, and multiple fractures were discovered at autopsy. Child abuse was initially suspected, but ultimately spontaneous fractures related to spastic cerebral palsy were diagnosed. Conradi

and Brisie[92] reported a 4-year-old who developed severe spastic encephalopathy as a consequence of Reye syndrome. Seven weeks after presentation, and 3 weeks after discharge, multiple acute and healing fractures were attributed to accidental trauma possibly complicated by the neurologic state and recent illness. Four months later the child died in the home and was diagnosed with fatal battered child syndrome.

Premature infants are known to suffer fractures from routine handling and therapy in the neonatal intensive care unit (NICU). Infants at particular risk are those with a history of birth before 28 weeks weighing less than 1,000 g, and those with glucocorticoid exposure, the use of calcium-wasting diuretics, extended use of total parenteral nutrition (TPN), TPN-associated liver disease, necrotizing enterocolitis, and sustained acidosis or immobilization. The failure to fortify human milk fed to the infant or to use calcium phosphate–modified infant formula until 40 weeks' gestational age further increases risk. Elevated alkaline phosphatase levels confirm osteopenia of prematurity in infants at risk. When neonatal fractures are not recognized before hospital discharge, they may be identified as healing fractures at a later time, creating concern for child abuse. There is also concern that these infants may be more prone to fracture at a later time. Studies of bone mineralization have shown that the skeletons of premature infants are less mineralized than age- or weight-matched term infants for a variable time after birth, in different skeletal locations, extending to 2 years of age. Despite this,

Dahlenburg and colleagues[93] found no overrepresentation of premature birth among children younger than 5 years with skeletal fractures. Bowden et al[94] studied 46 children born at less than 32 weeks' gestation and compared them with age-matched, term-born controls at age 8 years. The children born prematurely were actually significantly less likely to sustain an accidental skeletal fracture. This experience suggests that while we must be aware of the possibility that healing fractures occurred in the nursery due to bone fragility, new fractures in NICU graduates are not very likely to be the result of ongoing skeletal fragility and normal handling.

Nutritional rickets and preterm birth both produce bone fragility that tends to reverse with age and advances in diet. As such they are temporary conditions producing brittle bones. Two authors have argued for a temporary brittle bone disease that renders infants susceptible to fracture during the first year of life, then resolves.[76,95] One author has attributed the condition to copper deficiency. The other has attributed the condition to intrauterine confinement and deficient bone mineralization from a decreased mechanostat signal in utero. Both hypotheses have been rejected by other authors and neither has gained wide acceptance.[73,96] There is concern that both authors' research and practice studied abused children who sustained multiple inflicted fractures that resolved after protective placement, provision of remedial services, or family monitoring. Until further data emerge, and these entities become proven, viable diagnoses, confusion between child abuse and a "temporary brittle bone disease" (other than those discussed previously) need not be considered, although physicians caring for abused children need to remain aware of developments in this area.

Ehlers-Danlos syndrome (EDS) is a group of collagen disorders primarily affecting soft tissues rather than bones. Multiple typing schemes have been proposed, but 3 named types predominate. Classical, hypermobility, and vascular types are all inherited in an autosomal-dominant pattern. Incidence is approximately 1 in 5,000 for these types taken together, with classical and hypermobility predominating and vascular type occurring in 1 in 100,000 to 200,000 births.[97] Classical and hypermobility types of EDS have a soft, velvety feel to the skin, which is unusually distensible. Joints are highly flexible in these conditions, providing a diagnostic clue. Suspicion of child abuse may arise because of easy bruising, laceration from minor trauma, and the tendency to form hypertrophic or papyraceous scars. Each will tend to suggest frequent or severe trauma, though only common childhood trauma has occurred. Vascular EDS adds the possibility of major blood vessel and hollow viscus rupture either spontaneously or following minor trauma. The occurrence of ruptured hollow viscus in early childhood is highly associated with child abuse. Mistaking signs and symptoms of EDS as resulting from child abuse has been reported.[3,98,99] Examination findings of unusual joint mobility with loose and elastic skin should raise the possibility of EDS. Genetic testing is available if laboratory confirmation is required.

A thorough medical history, including a family history for pertinent disorders; a complete physical examination, searching for cardinal findings; and a willingness to consider underlying fragility form the basis for excluding most disorders resulting in the misdiagnosis of abuse. A few of these conditions must be screened for with readily available laboratory testing: the CBC, PT, PTT, and von Willebrand panel. Other laboratory tests, including genetic and collagen phenotype testing, should be individualized. If a physiological susceptibility to easy injury is identified, the premise for considering child abuse must be reexamined. This will not, in all cases, eliminate child abuse from consideration. The possibility of an abused, brittle child presents additional diagnostic difficulty but must be considered.

Final Considerations

Cultural Practices

Once the possibilities of a non-traumatic condition that simulates trauma or an underlying fragility have been excluded, presumptions about injury and its necessary traumatic causes are valid. If unusual accidental causes do not apply, and genuine patterns are present, presumptions about infliction are likely to be correct. Sometimes, however, inflicted trauma does not constitute child abuse. A range of cultural practices produces cutaneous trauma in distinct patterns. While some of these, such as female circumcision, are treated as child abuse in Western cultures, others are non-painful and nondestructive, and thus treated as acceptable treatment of children. The

healing practices of coin rubbing, cupping, and moxibustion are commonly discussed examples.

Coin rubbing is practiced widely throughout Southeast Asia and southern China. Warm oil or a balm is applied to the skin, and then a coin is vigorously rubbed against the warmed and lubricated skin. Stripes of petechial bruising may appear. These are usually produced in a regular geometric pattern on the body. The result is, literally, inflicted bruising, but the motive is healing, and neither harm nor pain is intended. People subject to coin rubbing may report moderate discomfort or no discomfort at all. While bruising certainly represents tissue damage in the form of capillary rupture, it is not permanently destructive, and resolution within weeks can be expected. For these reasons, many communities have chosen to accept this practice as non-abusive. Consequently, coin rubbing, Cao Gio, and other synonymous practices have been reported as conditions mistaken for child abuse.[1,2,100–102]

Cupping is even more widely distributed and is practiced by both European and Asian peoples throughout the world. In cupping, a heated cup is placed against the skin and held until the trapped air cools and contracts, forming a vacuum. The attached cup is then left in place for some time. The suction may create a confluence of petechiae in the shape of the cup. Once again this is inflicted injury but with the intention to heal not harm. The resulting lesions are temporary and non-painful. Again, cultural sensitivity has led many communities to accept this practice as non-abusive.[103]

Moxibustion is the Chinese medical practice of burning small amounts of the herb *Artemisia vulgaris* near acupuncture points. While it is described as non-harmful and non-painful, burn marks on the skin have been recognized and interpreted as child abuse. Again this practice is sometimes accepted as non-abusive, but the injury, a burn, is more significant than the production of petechiae. This then sets the stage for consideration of other practices, such as ritual scarification and female circumcision, often referred to as female genital mutilation. Each is perceived as beneficial or even essential in the culture of origin. When brought into another society, a value judgment must be made about what is acceptable, and what is not. Even the most acceptable practices sometimes have unintended harmful outcomes. Severe accidental burns have been described when burning alcohol, used to heat cups, is spilled on the skin, or heated balm, used in coin rubbing, catches fire. Each of these practices also may substitute for modern Western medical practices. The ultimate determination of what is abuse, what is medical neglect, and what is acceptable, and how to handle practices that are culturally appropriate in the culture of origin but unacceptable in current society remains a difficult one.

Conclusion

Familiarity with each of the conditions discussed here is likely to be helpful, but incomplete, in identifying child abuse because there are sure to be others we have missed, and new differential diagnoses may be reported. The general principles we sought to illustrate within this discussion are equally important. When child abuse is suspected, the examiner should consider both traumatic and non-traumatic causes. Epidemiological data must be applied cautiously, known exceptions identified, and new exceptions considered. Injury patterns suggestive of inflicted trauma must be scrutinized to see if they represent a clear match for their proposed cause or may have arisen by chance. Where real trauma has occurred, an assessment of the severity of that trauma must consider the possibility of a vulnerable or fragile child. Finally, where inflicted trauma results from a folk medical practice, the community standard and presumptions about harm must be examined. Such cautious consideration requires data that can only be obtained through a thorough, far-reaching medical history and physical examination. Medical professionals often diagnose child abuse when a given history is not consistent with the injuries found and reject differential diagnoses because they are not classical or not common. The onus is on the professional to be sure that the proposed abuse is as consistent, common, or classical as the history and diagnoses they have rejected in their diagnostic considerations. Only the correct diagnosis, and an accurate statement of abuse probability, will allow the child protection system to properly pursue their task of putting children in the safest, most nurturing environment available.

References

1. Wheeler DM, Hobbs CJ. Mistakes in diagnosing non-accidental injury: 10 years' experience. *Br Med J.* 1988;296:1233–1236

2. Kaplan MJ. Pseudoabuse—the misdiagnosis of child abuse. *J Forensic Sci.* 1986;31:1420–1428

3. Wardinsky TD, Vizcarrondo FE. The mistaken diagnosis of child abuse: a three-year USAF medical center analysis and literature review. *Mil Med.* 1995;160:15–19

4. Johnson CF, Coury DL. Bruising and hemophilia: accident or child abuse? *Child Abuse Negl.* 1988;12:409–415

5. Cordova A. The Mongolian spot: a study of ethnic differences and a literature review. *Clin Pediatr.* 1981;20:714–719

6. Leung AK. Mongolian spots in Chinese children. *Int J Dermatol.* 1988;27:106–108

7. Tsai FJ, Tsai CH. Birthmarks and congenital skin lesions in Chinese newborns. *J Formos Med Assoc.* 1993;92:838–841

8. Oates RK. Overturning the diagnosis of child abuse. *Arch Dis Child.* 1984;59:665–666

9. Sekula SA, Tschen JA, Duffy JO. Epidermal nevus misinterpreted as child abuse. *Cutis.* 1986;37:276–278

10. Grieg AV, Harris DL. A study of perceptions of facial hemangiomas in professionals involved in child abuse surveillance. *Pediatr Dermatol.* 2003;20:1–4

11. Levin AV, Selbst SM. Vulvar hemangioma simulating child abuse. *Clin Pediatr.* 1988;27:213–215

12. Robinson AL, Koester GA, Kaufman A. Striae vs scars of ritual abuse in a male adolescent. *Arch Fam Med.* 1996;3:398–399

13. Heller D. Lumbar physiological striae in adolescence suspected to be non-accidental injury. *Br Med J.* 1995;311:738

14. Cohen HA, Matalon A, Mezger A, Ben Amitai D, Barzilai A. Striae in adolescents mistaken for physical abuse. *J Fam Pract.* 1997;45:84–85

15. Leventhal JM, Griffin D, Duncan KO, Starling S, Christian CW, Kutz T. Laxative induced dermatitis of the buttocks incorrectly suspected to be abusive burns. *Pediatrics.* 2001;107:178–179

16. Coffman K, Boyce WT, Hansen RC. Phytophotodermatitis simulating child abuse. *Am J Dis Child.* 1985;139:239–240

17. Barradell R, Addo A, McDonagh AJ, Cork MJ, Wales JK. Phytophotodermatitis mimicking child abuse. *Eur J Pediatr.* 1993;15:291–292

18. Goskowicz MO, Friedlander SF, Eichenfield LF. Endemic "lime" disease: phytophotodermatitis in San Diego County. *Pediatrics.* 1994;9:828–830

19. Hill PF, Pickford M, Parkhouse N. Phytophotodermatitis mimicking child abuse. *J R Soc Med.* 1997;90:560–561

20. Heider TR, Priolo D, Hultman CS, Peck MD, Cairns BA. Eczema mimicking child abuse: a case of mistaken identity. *J Burn Care Rehabil.* 2002;23:357–359

21. Brown J, Melinkovich P. Shonlein-Henoch purpura misdiagnosed as suspected child abuse. A case report and literature review. *JAMA.* 1989;256:617–618

22. Daly KC, Siegel RM. Henoch-Schonlein purpura in a child at risk of abuse. *Arch Pediatr Adolesc Med.* 1998;152:96–98

23. Plunkett J, Plunkett M. Physiologic periosteal changes in infancy. *Am J Forensic Med Pathol.* 2000;21:213–216

24. Ved N, Haller JO. Periosteal reaction with normal-appearing underlying bone: a child abuse mimicker. *Emerg Radiol.* 2002;9:278–282

25. Kwon DS, Spevak MR, Fletcher K, Kleinman PK. Physiologic subperiosteal new bone formation: prevalence, distribution, and thickness in neonates and infants. *AJR Am J Roentgenol.* 2002;179:985–988

26. Pergolizzi R Jr, Oestreich AE. Child abuse fracture through physiologic periosteal reaction. *Pediatr Radiol.* 1995;25:566–567

27. Tien R, Barron BJ, Dhekne RD. Caffey's disease: nuclear medicine and radiologic correlation: a case of mistaken identity. *Clin Nucl Med.* 1988;13:583–585

28. Lim HK, Smith WL, Sato Y, Choi J. Congenital syphilis mimicking child abuse. *Pediatr Radiol.* 1995;25:560–561

29. Hart BL, Dudley MH, Zumwalt RE. Postmortem cranial MRI and autopsy correlation in suspected child abuse. *Am J Forensic Med Pathol.* 1996;17:217–224

30. Oestreich AE, Ahmad BS. The periphysis and its effect on the metaphysis: I. Definition and normal radiographic pattern. *Skeletal Radiol.* 1992;21:283–286

31. Curto TL. Variations in acromial ossification simulating infant abuse in victims of sudden infant death syndrome. *J Emerg Med.* 1992;10:206

32. Kleinman PK, Spevak MR. Variations in acromial ossification simulating infant abuse in victims of sudden infant death syndrome. *Radiology.* 1991;180:185–187

33. Bulloch B, Schubert CJ, Brophy PD, Johnson N, Reed MH, Shapiro RA. Cause and clinical characteristics of rib fractures in infants. *Pediatrics.* 2000;105:e48

34. Cadzow SP, Armstrong KL. Rib fractures in infants: red alert! The clinical features, investigations and child protection outcomes. *J Paediatr Child Health.* 2000;36:322–326

35. Thomas PS. Rib fractures in infancy. *Ann Radiol.* 1977;20:115–122

36. Landman L, Homburg R, Sirota L, Dulizky F. Rib fractures as a cause of immediate neonatal tachypnoea. *Eur J Pediatr.* 1986;144:487–488

37. Rizzolo PJ, Coleman PR. Neonatal rib fracture: birth trauma or child abuse? *J Fam Pract.* 1989;29:561–563

38. Barry PW, Hocking MD. Infant rib fracture—birth trauma or non-accidental injury. *Arch Dis Child.* 1993;68:250

39. Hartmann RW. Radiological case of the month. *Arch Pediatr Adolesc Med.* 1997;151:947–948

40. Lysack JT. Classic metaphyseal lesion following external cephalic version and cesarean section. *Pediatr Radiol.* 2003;33:422–424

41. Papp S, Dhaliwal G, Davies G, Borschneck D. Fetal femur fracture and external cephalic version. *Obstet Gynecol.* 2004;104:1154–1156

42. Thodurou SD, Ierodiaconou MN, Mitsou A. Obstetrical fracture separation of the upper femoral epiphysis. *Acta Orthop Scand.* 1982;53:239–243

43. McCollough FL, McCarthy RE. Bilateral distal femoral epiphyseal fracture following home delivery: a case report. *J Ark Med Soc.* 1988;84:364–366

44. Grayev AM, Boal DKB, Wallach DM, Segal LS. Metaphyseal fractures mimicking abuse during treatment for clubfoot. *Pediatr Radiol.* 2001;31:559–563

45. Grant P, Mata MB, Tidwell M. Femur fracture in infants: a possible accidental etiology. *Pediatrics.* 2001;108:1009–1012

46. Strait RT, Siegal RM, Shapiro RA. Humeral fractures without obvious etiologies in children less than 3 years of age: when is it abuse? *Pediatrics.* 1995;96:667–671

47. Shaw BA, Murphy KM, Shaw A, Oppenheim WL, Myracle MR. Humerus shaft fractures in young children: accident or abuse. *J Pediatr Orthop.* 1997;17:293–297

48. Hymel KP, Jenny C. Abusive spiral fractures of the humerus: a videotaped exception. *Arch Pediatr Adolesc Med.* 1996;150:226–227

49. Li L, Fowler D, Liu L, Ripple MG, Lambros G, Smialek JE. Investigation of sudden infant deaths in Maryland (1990–2000). *Forensic Sci Int.* 2005;148:85–92

50. Centers for Disease Control and Prevention. Contribution of selected metabolic diseases to early childhood deaths—Virginia, 1996–2001. *MMWR Morb Mortal Wkly Rep.* 2003;52:677–679

51. Opdal SH, Rognum TO. The sudden infant death syndrome gene: does it exist? *Pediatrics.* 2004;114:e506–e512

52. Hunt AC. Ring-resolution of bruises—a little recognised phenomenon. *J Clin Forensic Med.* 2006;Mar 30

53. Feldman KW. Patterned abusive bruises of the buttocks and the pinna. *Pediatrics.* 1992;90:633–636

54. Rutty GN, Smith CM, Malia RG. Late-form hemorrhagic disease of the newborn: a fatal case report with illustration of investigations that may assist in avoiding the mistaken diagnosis of child abuse. *Am J Forensic Med Pathol.* 1999;21:48–51

55. Brousseau TJ, Kissoon N, McIntosh B. Vitamin K deficiency mimicking child abuse. *J Emerg Med.* 2005;29:283–288

56. Fenton LZ, Sirotnak AP, Handler MH. Parietal pseudofracture and spontaneous intracranial hemorrhage suggesting nonaccidental trauma: report of 2 cases. *Pediatr Neurosurg.* 2000;33:318–322

57. Wetzel RC, Slater AJ, Dover GJ. Fatal intramuscular bleeding misdiagnosed as suspected nonaccidental injury. *Pediatrics.* 1995;95:771–773

58. Rutty GN, Woolley A, Brookfield C, Shepherd F, Kitchen S. The PIVKA II test: the first reliable coagulation test for autopsy investigations. *Int J Legal Med.* 2003;117:143–148

59. Hadley JR. Disorders of coagulation misdiagnosed as nonaccidental bruising. *Pediatr Emerg Care.* 1997;13:347–349

60. Hazewinkel MH, Hoogerwerf JJ, Hesseling PB, et al. Haemophilia patients aged 0–18 years in the Western Cape. *S Afr Med J.* 2003;93:793–796

61. Pinto FC, Porro FF, Suganuma L, Fontes RB, deAndrade AF, Marino R Jr. Hemophilia and child abuse as possible causes of epidural hematoma. *Arq Neuropsiquiatr.* 2003;61:1023–1025

62. Falaki NN. Index of suspicion: case 3. *Pediatr Rev.* 1998;19:245–248

63. Carpentieri U, Gustavson LP, Haggard ME. Misdiagnosis of neglect in a child with bleeding disorder and cystic fibrosis. *South Med J.* 1978;71:854–855

64. Babcock J, Hartman K, Pedersen A, Murphy M, Alving B. Rodenticide-induced coagulopathy in a young child. A case of Munchausen syndrome by proxy. *Am J Pediatr Hematol Oncol.* 1993;15:126–130

65. White ST, Voter K, Perry J. Surreptitious warfarin ingestion. *Child Abuse Negl.* 1985;9:349–352

66. McClain JL, Clark MA, Sandusky GE. Undiagnosed, untreated acute lymphoblastic leukemia presenting as suspected child abuse. *J Forensic Sci.* 1990;35:735–739

67. Vora A, Makris M. Personal practice: an approach to investigation of easy bruising. *Arch Dis Child.* 2001;84:488–491

68. Thomas AE. The bleeding child; is it NAI? *Arch Dis Child.* 2004;89:1163–1167

69. Ablin DS, Greenspan A, Reihart M, Grix A. Differentiation of a child abuse from osteogenesis imperfecta. *AJR Am J Roentgenol.* 1990;154:1035–1045

70. Kleinman PK. Differentiation of child abuse and osteogenesis imperfecta: medical and legal implications. *AJR Am J Roentgenol.* 1990;154:1047–1048

71. Gahagan S, Rimsza ME. Child abuse or osteogenesis imperfecta: how can we tell? *Pediatrics.* 1991;88:987–992

72. Smith R. Osteogenesis imperfecta, non-accidental injury, and temporary brittle bone disease. *Arch Dis Child.* 1995;72:169–171

73. Ablin DS, Sane SM. Non-accidental injury: confusion with temporary brittle bone disease and mild osteogenesis imperfecta. *Pediatr Radiol.* 1997;27:111–113

74. Chapman S, Hall CM. Non-accidental injury or brittle bones. *Pediatr Radiol.* 1997;27:106–110

75. Patterson CR, McAllion SJ. Osteogenesis imperfecta in the differential diagnosis of child abuse. *Br Med J.* 1989;299:1451–1454

76. Patterson CR. Osteogenesis imperfecta and other bone disorders in the differential diagnosis of unexplained fractures. *J Soc Med.* 1990;83:72–74

77. Patterson CR, Burns J, McAllion SJ. Osteogenesis imperfecta: the distinction from child abuse and the recognition of a variant form. *Am J Med Genet.* 1993;45:187–192

78. Williams C. A controversial expert witness. *Fam Law.* 2000:175–180

79. Vetter U, Pontz B, Zauner E, Brenner RE, Spranger J. Osteogenesis imperfecta: a clinical study of the first ten years of life. *Calcif Tissue Int.* 1992;50:36–41

80. Steiner RD, Pepin MG, Byers PH. Osteogenesis Imperfecta. http://www.genetests.org/query?dz=oi. Accessed January 28, 2005

81. Glorieux FH, Rauch F, Plotkin H, et al. Type V osteogenesis imperfecta: a new form of brittle bone disease. *J Bone Miner Res.* 2000;15:1650–1658

82. Glorieux FH, Ward LM, Rauch F, Lalic L, Roughley PJ, Travers R. Osteogenesis imperfecta type VI: a form of brittle bone disease with a mineralization defect. *J Bone Miner Res.* 2002;17:30–38

83. Ward LM, Rauch F, Travers R, et al. Osteogenesis imperfecta type VII: an autosomal recessive form of brittle bone disease. *Bone.* 2002;31:12–18

84. Steiner RD, Pepin M, Byers PH. Studies of collagen synthesis and structure in the differentiation of child abuse from osteogenesis imperfecta. *J Pediatr.* 1996;128:542–547

85. Marlowe A, Pepin MG, Byers PH. Testing for osteogenesis imperfecta in cases of suspected non-accidental injury. *J Med Genet.* 2002;39:382–386

86. Knight DJ, Bennet GC. Nonaccidental injury in osteogenesis imperfecta: a case report. *J Pediatr Orthop.* 1990;10:542–544

87. Duncan AA, Chandy J. Case report: multiple neonatal fractures—dietary or deliberate? *Clin Radiol.* 1993;48:137–139

88. Sergi C, Linderkamp O. Pathological case of the month: classic rickets in a setting of significant psychosocial deprivation. *Arch Pediatr Adolesc Med.* 2001;155:967–968

89. Bloom E, Klein EJ, Shushan D, Feldman KW. Variable presentations of rickets in children in the emergency department. *Pediatr Emerg Care.* 2004;20:126–130

90. DeRusso PA, Spevak MR, Schwarz KB. Fractures in biliary atresia misinterpreted as child abuse. *Pediatrics.* 2003;112:185–188

91. Torwalt CR, Balachandra AT, Youngson C, de Nanassy J. Spontaneous fractures in the differential diagnosis of fractures in children. *J Forensic Sci.* 2002;47:1340–1344

92. Conradi S, Brisie R. Battered child syndrome in a four year old with previous diagnosis of Reye's syndrome. *Forensic Sci Int.* 1986;30:195–203

93. Dahlenburg SL, Bishop NJ, Lucas A. Are preterm infants at risk for subsequent fractures? *Arch Dis Child.* 1989;64:1384–1385

94. Bowden LS, Jones CJ, Ryan SW. Bone mineralization in ex-preterm infants aged 8 years. *Eur J Pediatr.* 1999;158:658–661

95. Miller ME, Hangartner TN. Temporary brittle bone disease: association with decreased fetal movement and osteopenia. *Calcif Tissue Int.* 1999;64:137–143

96. Hicks R. Relating to methodological shortcomings and the concept of temporary brittle bone disease. *Calcif Tissue Int.* 2001;68:316–319

97. Ehlers Danlos Syndrome. Genetics Home Reference, National Institutes of Health. http://ghr.nlm.nih.gov/condition=ehlersdanlossyndrome;jsessionid=FE0CD5 4FDC485FAC2FFA9C17847D9FE9. Accessed May 2006

98. Owen SM, Durst RD. Ehlers-Danlos syndrome simulating child abuse. *Arch Dermatol.* 1984;120:97–101

99. Roberts DL, Pope FM, Nicholls AC, Narcisi P. Ehlers-Danlos syndrome type IV mimicking non-accidental injury in a child. *Br J Dermatol.* 1984;111:341–345

100. Rosenblat H, Hong P. Coin rolling misdiagnosed as child abuse. *CMAJ.* 1989;140:417

101. Hulewicz BS. Coin rubbing injuries. *Am J Forensic Med Pathol.* 1994;15:257–260

102. Look KM, Look RM. Skin scraping, cupping, and moxibustion that may mimic physical abuse. *J Forensic Sci.* 1997;42:103–105

103. Asnes RS, Wisotsky DH. Cupping lesions simulating child abuse. *J Pediatr.* 1981;99:267–268

Interviewing the Prepubertal Child for Possible Sexual Abuse

Kathleen Coulborn Faller

Family Assessment Clinic
School of Social Work
University of Michigan

Introduction

In this chapter, the following topics are covered: the extent of the problem of sexual abuse, whether the health care professional should question the child when there are concerns about sexual abuse, research about the process of sexual abuse disclosure, general guidelines for questioning children, record keeping, interview structure, the use of demonstrative communication, gathering information about the extent of abuse, a rationale for following the advice about questioning, and reporting interview findings. The purpose of this chapter is to provide health care professionals with the skills they need to effectively interview a prepubertal child for possible sexual abuse.

The Extent of the Problem of Child Sexual Abuse

How common is child sexual abuse? Professionals understand the extent of the sexual abuse problem primarily from prevalence and incidence studies. Knowledge about sexual abuse preva-lence (how many people experience sexual abuse during childhood) comes, for the most part, from studies involving adults who report sexual victimization as children. There are sufficient numbers of studies of general population samples[1] (eg, stratified samples), community-based samples,[2] special populations (eg, psychiatric patients),[3] and college students[4,5] to permit meta-analyses of these studies.[6,7] The most recent meta-analysis was conducted by Bolen and Scannapieco.[6] They reviewed 22 studies with random samples and concluded that sexual abuse preva-lence rate for women is between 30% and 40%. Fewer researchers have exam-ined prevalence among men, but Bolen and Scannapieco[6] conclude at least 13% of men are sexually abused during childhood.

The other strategy for understanding the extent of sexual abuse is through reported incidences of sexual abuse. Data from the National Child Abuse and Neglect Data System are the most commonly used to estimate annual rates of sexual abuse.[8] The number of reports varies by year, but is usually about 300,000 cases, approximately one third of which are substantiated after investigation by child protection agencies. But one study suggests these officially substantiated cases of sexual abuse represent only the tip of the iceberg. The Gallup Organization conducted a survey of a representative sample of 1,000 American parents in 1995.[9] One of the questions these parents were asked was whether their child had been sexually abused over the past year. The responses to this question yielded an estimate of 1 million children having been sexually abused in 1995, not the 100,000 cases substantiated by child protection agencies, thus 10 times the number of substantiated cases. Even the Gallup survey projection is probably an underestimate. Parents are not always aware of their children's sexual abuse and, no doubt in some instances, decline to report abuse because they are the perpetrators or are close to the perpetrators.

Why should health care professionals be cognizant of prevalence and incidence rates of sexual abuse? These rates tell us sexual abuse is a common problem in our society, not a rare occurrence. Child victims regularly present in medical practices. These children may see health care professionals because they have physical sequelae of sexual abuse, although physical symptoms are not common; behavioral or emotional manifestations of sexual victimization; or for reasons unrelated to concerns about sexual abuse.[10]

Whether Health Care Professionals Should Question Children About Possible Sexual Abuse

Should health care professionals question a prepubertal child suspected of being sexually victimized? Many factors influence this decision.

First, health care professionals need to consider local policy. In many communities, multidisciplinary and multiagency teams develop policies about how mandated reporters should respond to possible sexual victimization on their caseloads, including whether reporters should question children.

Second, in many cases, there is a window of opportunity, that is, a time when the child is willing to talk to someone about abuse and/or the caretaker is willing to allow the child to be interviewed. Once this window closes, the opportunity to protect the child may vanish.

Third, the health care professional may or may not have the facilities and the skills for interviewing young children. Many specialized child interview programs are based in health care settings and receive referrals from child protective services and law enforcement for medical examinations and interviews.[11-13] Professionals who staff such programs usually are well-trained and qualified to question prepubertal children about possible sexual abuse.

Understanding the Disclosure Process

Although some children tell immediately when they have been sexually abused,[14] most children do not.[15-19] Failure to report sexual victimization, even when asked, is common.[20-23] For example, Lyon[21] recently reviewed studies dating from 1965 through 1993 of 529 children with gonorrhea. He found that only 43% of children gave some indication of their sexual abuse.

Similarly, many children delay disclosure of their victimization.[24-28] For instance, Elliott and Briere[24] studied 336 children aged 8 to 15 years who received forensic evaluations at the Harbor-University of California at Los Angeles Sexual Abuse Crisis Center. Among their findings were that 75% of children had failed to disclose their sexual victimization within the year after it occurred.

Finally, retraction of the allegation after the child begins to experience the consequences of disclosure is characteristic of the disclosure process.[26,28-30] Illustrative is the case record review by Malloy and colleagues[30] of 217 randomly selected substantiated sexual abuse cases from the Los Angeles County dependency court. The children in those cases were interviewed on average 12 times. Over the course of the interviews, 23% of the children fully recanted their sexual abuse allegations and 11% partially recanted. Predictors of full recantation were younger victim age, closer relationship to the offender, and lack of maternal support. The predictor of partial recantation (minimization of the abuse) was more severe sexual abuse. Thus health care professionals should not be surprised if prepubertal children are not forthcoming when asked about sexual abuse.

Conversely, the available research suggests that false allegations of sexual abuse are uncommon.[31-34] Rates vary somewhat depending on the source of the report and the context in which the allegation is made, but range from 0%[34] to 10%[31] of reports made by children. Research suggests that of the small number of false reports, most are made by older children.[25,31,32]

Despite the body of research indicating that it is difficult for children to tell about sexual abuse and that false allegations are rare, especially in prepubertal children, the direction of advice for health care professionals is to employ questioning techniques that guard against eliciting false allegations from children about possible sexual abuse.

General Guidelines for Questioning Children

The following are some generally agreed on guidelines or principles for questioning children about possible sexual abuse.[11,35-37] These guidelines take into account concerns about false allegations, but also provide professionals with strategies to use when children have difficulty disclosing.

1. Gather information from the child rather than asking the child to confirm information from the caretaker or other sources.
2. Use as many open-ended questions as possible.
3. Attempt to obtain a narrative account of what happened from the child.
4. If open-ended questions are not effective, don't give up; use a more closed-ended question.

5. If you use a more closed-ended question, place less confidence in the information obtained.
6. A closed-ended question, which elicits a positive response, should be followed by a more open-ended one (eg, "Tell me everything about that.").
7. Explore alternative explanations for the concern about sexual abuse (eg, no sexual abuse occurred, child care behavior mistaken for sexual behavior, advanced sexual knowledge from an experience other than sexual abuse).

Record Keeping

Accurate and complete records are important when health care professionals question children about sexual abuse. Videotaping interviews may not be feasible in health care settings because facilities lack this capacity, but videotapes provide the best record. If videotaping is not possible, audiotaping is a good substitute. Taped interviews are superior to notes, which have been shown in research to be incomplete.[38,39] If the professional must rely on notes, it is essential that notes include the child's verbatim statements about the sexual abuse and the questions the professional employed to gather information. Any reports should include the professional's questions and the child's verbatim responses.[38,40,41]

Interview Structure

There is a substantial body of writing about how to structure and what to include in an interview about possible sexual abuse.[35,37,42-44] Presently interview protocols advise 3[36,45,46] to 9[43,44,46] phases,

but simplicity is probably best with the prepubertal child. Professionals should expect an interview about possible sexual abuse to have a beginning (rapport-building and child assessment), a middle (abuse-related), and an end (closure). Professionals should also follow the child's lead, which may limit the ability of the professional to impose structure.

Beginning Phase

In the beginning phase, health care professionals should develop rapport with the child and assess the child's capacity to communicate. A good practice is to use open-ended questions during the rapport-building stage, such as, "Tell me all about school," which will inform the professional about the child's ability to respond to open-ended questions and may build the child's capacity to answer such questions.[47] If the child cannot provide responses to open-ended questions, the professional should employ more closed-ended questions during rapport building, such as, "Who are your friends?" to learn what kinds of questions the child can understand. Children's ability to report events that happened to them in the past and their knowledge of their environment (eg, who lives at their house) are other capacities to assess during the beginning phase of the interview.

Middle or Abuse-Related Phase

The literature provides numerous strategies for transitioning to the middle or abuse-related phase of the interview, but the strategies are not designed specifically for medical settings.[37,44,47-50] A useful approach for health care professionals is to state, in as open-ended a manner as possible, why there are concerns about sexual abuse and ask the child to respond. For example, "When I looked at your privates, I saw that someone or something had hurt you. Tell me what happened," or "Your mom said something happened to you at child care. Tell me about what happened."

Much has also been written about the appropriate types of questions to employ when inquiring about sexual abuse. Table 8.1 provides a continuum of 10 types of questions. The table divides questions into 3 categories: preferred, less preferred, and least preferred. Writers differ in the terms they use for types of questions (hence the different terms appearing under the heading, question/probe type) and, to some extent, in their views about the most appropriate types of questions.[36,37,47] Table 8.1 provides terms for the different types of questions/probes found in the literature, definitions for the question/probe types, and examples. The table lists questions from more open-ended to more closed-ended and indicates that professionals should have greater confidence in information elicited using more open-ended questions and prompts.

Although best practice is to begin with open-ended questions and probes (general questions, open abuse-related questions, and invitational probes) when questioning children, these types of questions usually will be insufficient for obtaining a complete history. Indeed, prepubertal children, if they are forthcoming with answers to these types of questions, will probably only provide a small amount of information. Sometimes facilitative cues (question type 4) such as, "Anything else?" and "Then what happened?" will be useful, but most prepubertal children are unaccustomed to being asked to provide narratives to open-ended questions. Thus usually the professional will need to ask focused questions (question type 5), such as, "Tell me what happened to your peepee?"[51] and "wh" questions (question type 6). "Wh" questions prompt children do describe "who" abused them and "what" exactly the person did, as well as contextual information, for example, "where" the abuse happened, "who" else was there, and "when" the abuse happened. It is also helpful to gather sensorimotor details about the sexual acts, such as what the sexual act felt like.

Multiple choice (question type 7) and direct (question type 8) questions are less preferred and some writers are more opposed to them than others.[36] Professionals are advised to avoid leading (question type 9) or coercive (question type 10) questions when asking children about sexual abuse.

However, the appropriateness of a question depends a great deal on its context, particularly the amount of evidence there is supporting sexual abuse (eg, medical evidence) and what the child has disclosed earlier in the interview or said to others prior to the interview. For example, if a child has already disclosed sexual victimization in the interview, and the professional is gathering details, a leading question (ie, "Now earlier you said your grandpa was in your bed, didn't you?") is quite appropriate.

TABLE 8.1
A Continuum of Questions to Be Used When Interviewing Children

Open-ended	More Confidence in Child's Response	
Question/Probe Type	Definition	Examples
Preferred Questions/Probes		
1. General question	Open-ended inquiry about the child's well-being or salient issues; does not assume abuse may have occurred	1. How are you doing today? 2. How have you been feeling?
2. Open abuse-related question Directive question	Open-ended inquiry that assumes there may be abuse or trauma	1. Do you know why I am talking to you? 2. I see from your medical examination that something may have happened to you. Tell me about it as best you can.
3. Invitation or invitational question	Utterances that invite free recall and a narrative	1. Can you tell me everything you can remember? 2. Tell me all about what happened, from the beginning to the end.
4. Facilitative cue Narrative cue Facilitators	Interviewer gesture or utterance aimed at encouraging more narration	1. Uh huh (affirmative). 2. Okay. 3. Anything else? 4. What happened next?
5. Focused question Focused probe	A probe that focuses the child on a particular topic, place, or person, but refrains from providing information about the subject[57]	1. Tell me what your mom is worried about. 2. Can you tell me about what happened to your privates?
6. "Wh" questions Cued invitations	Inquiry to gather contextual and specific detail about the child's experience: who, what, when, where	1. When did this happen? 2. Where were you? 3. Where was your mom?
Less Preferred Questions/Probes		
7. Multiple-choice question Option-posing question Forced choice question Restricted choice question (Walker, 1999)	A question that presents the child with a number of alternative responses from which to choose	1. Did he do it one time or more than one time? 2. Did the abuse happen during the day, at night, or both?
8. Direct question Specific question Option-posing question Yes/no question	A direct inquiry about abuse or abuse-related details	1. Did John hurt your peepee? 2. Did he put his finger inside you? 3. Was he wearing his pajamas too?

TABLE 8.1

A Continuum of Questions to Be Used When Interviewing Children, *continued*

Open-ended	More Confidence in Child's Response	
Question/Probe Type	Definition	Examples
Less Preferred Questions/Probes		
9. Leading question Tag question	A statement the child is asked to affirm	1. Isn't it true that your brother put his penis in your mouth? 2. Your stepfather is the one who hurt you, isn't he?
10. Coercion Coercive question	Use of inappropriate inducements to gain cooperation or to elicit information from the child	1. If you tell me what happened, then I'll stop questioning you. 2. You can't leave this room until we are finished talking.
Closed-ended	Less Confidence in Child's Response	

Ending or Closure Phase

Closure is important for the professional and the child. When the professional thinks all information related to the abuse has been gathered, he or she may ask, "Is there anything else you think I should know about what happened?" Closure should include calming the child, if the child is upset, and letting the child know what will happen next. With regard to what will happen next, professionals need only describe next steps (eg, that a child protection worker will talk to the child) not long-term outcomes. Some professionals provide the child with contact information if the child is old enough to use it.

Use of Demonstrative Communication

Because children may lack verbal communication skills or may be reluctant or distressed when asked to respond verbally to questions about sexual abuse, health care professionals may employ demonstrative communication modes. These can include having the child draw, write responses, or use body maps—for instance, anatomical drawings, anatomical dolls, or a "gingerbread" body outline. These modes of communication are also very useful in gathering details about the sexual abuse and its context (eg, getting the child to draw a picture of the place where the abuse occurred, if the child is able) and for pacing the interview so the child does not feel pressured. When these communication modes are employed, the professional is not interpreting play or drawings, but rather asking the child to demonstrate. For example, the professional might say, "Can you mark on the drawing the part or parts that Mr Jones used to hurt you?"

Extent of the Child's Abuse

Many children experience multiple acts and forms of sexual victimization, especially in intrafamilial situations.

Moreover, children may experience multiple types of maltreatment. In such circumstances, professionals must decide how much questioning the child can tolerate in an interview and structure their inquiry accordingly. Additional factors to consider include the capacity of the professional setting to conduct several interviews and community practice related to interviewing children about maltreatment.

It is useful to learn about the scope of a child's sexual abuse for assessing safety issues and trauma, but prepubertal children will have difficulty describing frequency and duration of sexual abuse. Current advice is to ask children, "Did the abuse happen one time or more than one time?" Sometimes children can recall their age when the abuse started, which will allow an estimate of duration. When there have been multiple instances of sexual abuse and details are required to determine the report's validity, professionals can ask, "Tell me about the last time the abuse happened." Another good question is, "Tell me about the time you remember the most." After disclosure about one offender, the professional may ask if anyone else has sexually abused the child.

Sometimes it is appropriate to ask about other types of maltreatment (eg, neglect and physical abuse) and parental problems (eg, substance abuse and domestic violence). Professionals should be guided by the child's level of distress, the child's willingness to continue talking, and community practice regarding child abuse investigations in determining whether to question about other types of maltreatment and endangerment.

Why Should the Health Care Professional Adhere to This Advice?

Health care professionals may wonder why they should follow the questioning and interview strategies that have been described. These are very different from the typical questioning strategies health care professionals use, such as taking a medical history, which ordinarily involves direct questions. There are at least 2 reasons for following the advised strategies. Children's free recall memory is the most accurate, even though with prepubertal children the information may be sparse. This recall is best tapped by open-ended questions. Consequently it is advisable to begin inquiry with open-ended questions and rely on more closed-ended ones when the child has exhausted free recall.

Second, if only closed-ended probes are employed (eg, direct, leading, and coercive questions), the child's disclosures may be doubted by professionals mandated to investigate sexual abuse and by other interested parties (eg, attorneys, the person accused of sexual abuse). If the content of the interview and the child's statements are challenged, the child may not be protected.

Reporting by Mandated Professionals

As with other types of child maltreatment, health care professionals must report cases where they have reasonable cause to suspect sexual abuse. When the abuser is a caretaker or a caretaker has not protected the child from sexual abuse, the case is reportable to child protective services.[52]

Sexual abuse differs from other types of child maltreatment in that a substantial proportion of sexual abuse is committed by unrelated offenders.[53] These cases usually fall within the mandate of law enforcement. Although reporting statutes vary by state and reporting policies vary by locality, health care professionals generally are not required to report extrafamilial child sexual abuse.[53]

Nevertheless, professionals should develop a policy, which probably should be written, about how to handle reporting of extrafamilial sexual abuse. Such a policy could include instructing the caretaker to report, reporting to the appropriate law enforcement agency, alerting other agencies or professionals, and contacting a court. Regardless of the policy adopted, child safety is paramount. Health care professionals should ensure that children's well-being is not being jeopardized by their lack of action or policy.

Conclusion

Health care professionals are challenged to develop skills for interviewing prepubertal children who may have been sexually abused. Advice about interview strategies and questions envisions ideal interviews. In reality, many prepubertal children cannot provide a narrative and need to be asked focused, direct, and sometimes even leading questions.[54-56] The "Memorandum of Good Practice," which provides an interview structure used by law enforcement in England, proposes the concept of a "good enough interview."[54,55] This concept can also be adopted by health care professionals.

Health care professionals may be in a unique position to help children who have been sexually abused. Because of their central role in the lives and well-being of their patients, they are likely to be sought out by caretakers and trusted by children. Health care professionals can use their window of opportunity to improve the lives and futures of their patients by questioning children in a sensitive and appropriate way so that they can disclose their sexual victimization.

References

1. Russell DEH, Bolen R. *The Epidemic of Rape and Child Sexual Abuse in the United States.* Thousand Oaks, CA: Sage; 2000
2. Saunders B, Villeponteaux L, Lipovsky J, Kilpatrick D. Child sexual assault and a risk factor for mental disorders among women: a community survey. *J Interpersonal Violence.* 1992;7:189–204
3. Boudreau E, Kilpatrick D, Resnick H, Best C, Saunders B. Criminal victimization, posttraumatic stress disorder, and comorbid psychopathology in a community sample. *J Trauma Stress.* 1998;11:665–678
4. Finkelhor D. *Sexually Victimized Children.* New York, NY: The Free Press; 1979
5. Finkelhor D. *Sourcebook on Child Sexual Abuse.* Newbury Park, CA: Sage; 1986
6. Bolen R, Scannapieco M. Prevalence of child sexual abuse: a corrective meta-analysis. *Soc Serv Rev.* 1999;73:281–313
7. Gorey K, Leslie D. Prevalence of child sexual abuse: integrative review and adjustment for potential response and measurement bias. *Child Abuse Negl.* 1997;21:391–398
8. National Child Abuse and Neglect Data System. *Summary of Key Findings From Calendar Year 2004.* Washington, DC: National Clearinghouse on Child Abuse and Neglect; 2006. http://www.acf.hhs.gov/programs/cb/pubs/cm04/index.htm. Accessed August 9, 2007

9. Moore D, Gallup G, Schussel R. *Disciplining America's Children: A Gallup Poll Report*. Princeton, NJ: The Gallup Organization; 1995

10. Bays J, Chadwick D. Medical diagnosis of the sexually abused child. *Child Abuse Negl*. 1993;17:91–110

11. Davies D, Cole J, Albertella G, McCulloch L, Allen K, Kekevian L. A model for conducting forensic interviews with child victims of abuse. *Child Maltreatment*. 1996;1:189–199

12. Drach K, Wientzen J, Ricci L. The diagnostic utility of sexual behavior problems in diagnosing sexual abuse evaluation clinic. *Child Abuse Negl*. 2001;25:289–503

13. Giardino A, Finkel MA. Evaluating child sexual abuse. *Pediatr Ann*. 2005;34:382–394

14. Sas L, Cunningham A, Hurley P. *Tipping the Balance to Tell the Secret: The Public Discovery of Child Sexual Abuse*. London, Ontario, Canada: London Family Court Clinic; 1995

15. London K, Bruck M, Ceci S, Shuman D. Disclosure of child sexual abuse: what does the research tell us about how children tell? *Psychol Public Policy Law*. 2005;11:194–226

16. Olafson E. When paradigms collide: Roland Summit and the rediscovery of child sexual abuse. In: Conte J, ed. *Critical Issues in Child Sexual Abuse*. Thousand Oaks, CA: Sage; 2002:71–106

17. Olafson E, Corwin D, Summit RC. Modern history of child sexual abuse awareness: cycles of discovery and suppression. *Child Abuse Negl*. 1993;17:7–24

18. Summit R. The child sexual abuse accommodation syndrome. *Child Abuse Negl*. 1983;7:177–193

19. Summit R. Abuse of the child sexual abuse accommodation syndrome. *J Child Sex Abuse*. 1992;1:153–163

20. Lawson L, Chaffin M. False negatives in sexual abuse disclosure interviews. *J Interpers Violence*. 1992;7:532–542

21. Lyon TD. False denials: overcoming methodological biases in abuse disclosure research. In: Pipe M, Lamb M, Orbach Y, Cederborg A, eds. *Disclosing Abuse: Delays, Denials, Retractions, and Incomplete Accounts*. Mahway, NJ: Earlbaum; 2007

22. Muram D. Child sexual abuse: relationship between sexual acts and genital findings. *Child Abuse Negl*. 1989;13:211–216

23. Muram D, Speck P, Gold S. Genital abnormalities in female siblings and friends of child victims of sexual abuse. *Child Abuse Negl*. 1991;15:105–110

24. Elliott DM, Briere, J. Forensic sexual abuse evaluations of older children: disclosures and symptomatology. *Behav Sci Law*. 1994;12:261–277

25. Faller KC. *Child Sexual Abuse: An Interdisciplinary Manual for Diagnosis, Case Management, and Treatment*. New York, NY: Columbia University Press; 1988

26. Paine ML, Hansen D. Factors influencing children to self-disclose sexual abuse. *Clin Psychol Rev*. 2002;22:271–295

27. Sauzier M. Disclosure of sexual abuse: for better or for worse. *Pediatr Clin North Am*. 1989;12:455–469

28. Sorenson T, Snow B. How children tell: the process of disclosure of sexual abuse. *Child Welfare*. 1991;70:3–15

29. Lyon TD. Scientific support for expert testimony on child sexual abuse accommodation. In: Conte J, ed. *Critical Issues in Child Sexual Abuse*. Thousand Oaks, CA: Sage; 2002:107–138

30. Malloy L, Lyon T, Quas J, Forman J. Factors affecting children's sexual abuse disclosure patterns in a social services sample. Paper presented at: San Diego Conference on Child and Family Maltreatment; January 2005; San Diego, CA

31. Tufts-New England Medical Center, Division of Child Psychiatry. *Sexually Exploited Children: Service and Research Project. Final Report for the Office of Juvenile Justice and Delinquency Prevention*. Washington, DC: US Department of Justice; 1984

32. Jones DPH, McGraw EM. Reliable and fictitious accounts of sexual abuse to children. *J Interpersonal Violence.* 1987;2:27–45

33. Oates RK, Jones DPH, Denson A, Sirotnak A, Gary N, Krugman R. Erroneous concerns about child sexual abuse. *Child Abuse Negl.* 2000;24:149–157

34. Trocme N, Bala N. False allegations of abuse and neglect when parents separate. *Child Abuse Negl.* 2005;29:1333–1346

35. Bourg W, Broderick R, Flagor R, Kelly D, Ervin D, Butler J. *A Child Interviewer's Guidebook.* Thousand Oaks, CA: Sage; 1999

36. Faller KC. *Understanding and Assessing Child Sexual Maltreatment.* 2nd ed. Thousand Oaks, CA: Sage; 2003

37. Merchant L, Toth P. *Child Interview Guide.* Seattle, WA: Harborview Center for Sexual Assault and Traumatic Stress; 2001

38. Berliner L, Lieb R. *Child Sexual Abuse Investigations: Testing Documentation Methods.* Olympia, WA: Washington State Institute for Public Policy. Document No. 01-01-4102

39. Lamb M, Orbach Y, Sternberg K, Hershkowitz I, Horowitz D. Accuracy of investigators' verbatim notes of their forensic interviews with alleged child abuse victims. *Law Human Behav.* 2000;24:699–708

40. American Professional Society on the Abuse of Children. *Guidelines for Psychosocial Evaluation of Suspected Sexual Abuse in Children.* 2nd ed. http://www.APSAC.org. Accessed August 23, 2007

41. American Professional Society on the Abuse of Children. *Guidelines on Investigative Interviewing in Cases of Alleged Child Abuse.* http://www.APSAC.org. Accessed August 23, 2007

42. Morgan M, Edwards V. *How to Interview Sexual Abuse Victims, Including the Use of Anatomical Dolls.* Thousand Oaks, CA: Sage; 1995

43. Poole D, Lamb M. *Investigative Interviews of Children.* Washington, DC: American Psychological Association; 1998

44. State of Michigan. *Forensic Interview Protocol.* Lansing, MI: Governor's Task Force on Children's Justice, Michigan Department of Human Services; 2005. DHS Pub 779

45. McDermott-Steinmetz-Lane M. *Interviewing for Child Sexual Abuse: Strategies for Balancing Forensic and Therapeutic Factors.* Notre Dame, IN: Jalice; 1997

46. Yuille JC, Hunter R, Joffe R, Zaparniuk J. Interviewing children in sexual abuse cases. In: Goodman GS, Bottoms BL, eds. *Child Victims, Child Witnesses: Understanding and Improving Children's Testimony.* New York, NY: Guilford Press; 1993:95–115

47. Sternberg K, Lamb M, Hershkovitz I, et al. Effects of introductory style on children's abilities to describe experiences of sexual abuse. *Child Abuse Negl.* 1997;21:1133–1146

48. Lamb M, Sternberg K. *Eliciting Accurate Investigative Statements From Children.* Presented at: 15th National Symposium on Child Sexual Abuse; March 1999; Huntsville, AL; 1999

49. Stellar M, Boychuk T. Children as witnesses in sexual abuse cases: investigative interview and assessment techniques. In: Dent H, Flin R, eds. *Children as Witnesses.* Chichester, UK: J. Wiley; 1992:47–72

50. Sternberg K, Lamb M, Orbach Y, Esplin P, Mitchell S. Use of a structured investigative protocol enhances young children's responses to free-recall prompts in the course of forensic interviews. *J Applied Psych.* 2000;86:997–1005

51. Walker AG. *Handbook on Questioning Children.* 2nd ed. Washington, DC: American Bar Association Center on Children and the Law; 1999

52. National Center for the Prosecution of Child Abuse. *Child Abuse and Neglect State Statute Series.* Washington, DC: National Clearinghouse on Child Abuse and Neglect Information; 1997

53. Faller KC. Extrafamilial sexual abuse. *Child Adolesc Clin North Am.* 1994:713–727

54. Home Office. *Memorandum of Good Practice on Video Recorded Interviews With Child Witnesses in Criminal Proceedings.* London, UK: Her Majesty's Stationery Office; 1992

55. Home Office. *Achieving the Best Evidence in Criminal Proceedings: Guidance for Vulnerable and Intimidated Witnesses, Including Children.* London, UK: Her Majesty's Stationery Office; 2002

56. Sjoberg R, Lindblad F. Limited disclosure of sexual abuse in children whose experiences were documented by videotape. *Am J Psych.* 2002;159:312–314

57. Myers JEB, Goodman G, Saywitz K. Psychological research in children as witnesses: practical applications for forensic interviews and courtroom testimony. *Pacific Law J.* 1996;27:1–82

Chapter 9

Medical Aspects of Prepubertal Sexual Abuse

Martin A. Finkel

CARES (Child Abuse Research Education & Service) Institute
University of Medicine and Dentistry of New Jersey
School of Osteopathic Medicine

Diagnostic Considerations

The medical diagnosis and treatment of residua secondary to inappropriate sexual contact is only one of the many aspects of the evaluation of child sexual abuse. The collective insights of many disciplines interacting with mutual respect and understanding is essential to ensure an understanding of what a child may have experienced if abuse has occurred.

The field of medical diagnosis and treatment of child sexual abuse has evolved over the last 25 years.[1-14] During this period, physicians have enhanced their knowledge and skills in evaluating children alleged to be abused.[15] Most of the literature has been focused on responding to the challenges of diagnosing sexual abuse in girls, with significantly less attention to male victims. Much of the assessment is the same whether the victim is a boy or a girl.

Physicians define their role in child sexual abuse in terms of recognition, treatment, prevention, and interaction with the child protection system. Some clinicians see their role limited only to referring suspected sexual abuse cases to a local or regional diagnostic center that has been developed to serve the needs of these children. Others see an opportunity to participate actively in evaluating children and have learned much from the child protection, law enforcement, and mental health communities regarding the needs of abused children.

A successful medical evaluation requires an understanding of the clinical presentation of child sexual abuse and the technical skills to conduct an examination. The physician who understands the dynamics of how children are engaged in sexually inappropriate contact, the progression of the activities over time, the use of threats, the types of disclosure, and why children might recant is best prepared to obtain a complete medical history of the events surrounding the abuse. This knowledge and the requisite skills necessary to obtain the history of the alleged inappropriate contact are essential. Clinicians must be as adept at obtaining the history and documenting the history as they are at obtaining cultures for sexually transmitted infections (STIs).

Children will come for an examination in a variety of ways. A parent may call after a clear disclosure, seeing changes in the behavior of the child, or after having been told of behavioral signs by a relative, friend, or schoolteacher. The presentation of a sexually abused child is unlike that involving other acute pediatric diseases. Sexually abused children do not typically disclose their experiences or demonstrate behavioral signs and symptoms immediately after an episode of sexual contact.[16-21] Children who disclose shortly after a sexually inappropriate contact are more likely to have experienced their abuse by an extra-familial perpetrator. Extra-familial perpetrators are more likely to use force and restraint when engaging children in sexual activities and, thus, these children are more likely to demonstrate acute signs of injury. Children presenting with acute injuries involving extra-genital and anogenital sites are the least difficult to diagnose. But because most sexual contact with children does not follow the rape model, few children will present with acute injuries immediately following sexual contact.

Most children are sexually abused by individuals who have ready access to them and are known, loved, and trusted by the child.[20-22] Consequently, when children are engaged in sexual activities, the individual initiating the contact tends not to have a desire to harm the child physically, differentiating sexual abuse of prepubertal children from classic rape. By contrast, when children experience physical abuse, there may have been some intent to harm the child physically.[20] Most children who are physically maltreated have cutaneous or other manifestations of their abuse that suggest a non-accidental etiology. In sexual abuse, the perpetrator's pathologic but effective strategy is to engage the child with as little discomfort as possible, which increases the likelihood of engaging the child again in the inappropriate contact. Although most children are not physically injured during sexual abuse, the individual engaging the child in the activities demonstrates a callous indifference to the emotional impact of the activities. Thus it is essential to understand the contextual framework in which children are engaged and maintained in sexual activities.[9,20,21,23] The clinician's diagnostic assessment is based on historical and behavioral details that at times are supported by confirmatory physical findings, forensic evidence, and/or STIs.

Medical History

The cornerstone of evaluating any medical problem is the medical history. The medical history determines how the physician will proceed with the examination and the scope of testing required. Few physicians would examine an adult patient without obtaining a history. It would be equally inappropriate to proceed with an examination of a child capable of talking without attempting to hear about the experience from the child directly. The child's history helps the physician to understand the child's experience, its context, and time frames of the events. Physicians are more likely to be able to diagnose a medical disorder if they understand not only the signs and symptoms of the disorder but also its evolution. To obtain a complete history, the physician should be familiar with the relevant mental health and social work literature on child sexual abuse. With this knowledge, physicians will understand how children are engaged and maintained in sexually inappropriate activities and begin to appreciate the clinical expression of their experience.[20,21,24–30]

A complete medical history should be obtained from the child's non-offending caretaker and should include a birth, family, surgical, developmental, hospitalization, and medication history. It is important to recognize that the adult providing the history may have been unaware of the specific symptoms that the child may have had related to the sexual contact. Therefore the gastrointestinal (GI) and genitourinary (GU) review of systems may not be complete until the child is spoken to independently.

Statements made by the child either spontaneously or elicited through non-leading questions must be preserved verbatim. The idiosyncratic statements of children provide the best insight into the child's experience and add context to the concern. The medical history obtained from the child may provide great insight into the spectrum of a child's experience and the potential for diagnosing either residual to an injury or STI. Child protection and/or law enforcement may have conducted an initial interview of the child before referring the child for diagnosis and treatment of any physical residua to the alleged sexual contact. The physician should focus the medical history on whether the child has been injured as a result of the alleged contact and obtain historical details concerning signs and symptoms specific to the contact. Some of these details are obtained from the review of systems and medical history given by the accompanying parent.

The medical record should include verbatim documentation of questions asked and the exact responses of the child. Observations concerning the child's affect and behavior during the medical history are extremely important and may assist in formulating a clinical assessment. Mental health professionals are best equipped to interpret subtle changes in affect and behavior.

At times it may be difficult to take a history from a child regarding sexually inappropriate experiences. The ability to listen to children talk about their experiences is not intuitive but rather a developed skill. The physician must appear empathic but neutral when obtaining a history. As children talk, they also observe the physician's reaction to what they have to say. If the physician appears uncomfortable listening or is insensitive to the child's needs, the child may simply stop talking. Therefore it is critical that the physician is nonjudgmental and facilitating while keeping in mind that the questions posed must be presented in a non-leading manner.

Although physicians consider the sexual abuse of children abhorrent, a child experiencing inappropriate contact by someone they love and trust may view the activity quite differently, particularly when the activity is presented in a "playful" or "loving" context. Children's responses to these experiences may be neutral, positive, or negative, depending on how the activities were represented to the child.[31] Therefore the physician should not automatically presume that the child was psychologically damaged, embarrassed, or hurt by the experience.[20,31] Young children are most likely to express confusion, excitement, or ambivalence and may be less likely to understand the inappropriateness and implications of the experiences.

When obtaining a history, it is important to understand that children who experience abuse have special emotional needs. Because of their abuse, they may have some difficulty developing rapport and trust with the examining physician. If the examiner is unhurried, nonjudgmental, and empathic, the child will be more likely to view the clinician as understanding and will, therefore, be more likely to share both the details of the events and the accompanying affective associations.

The purpose of the medical history is to gather information as well as impart information in the form of therapeutic messages. These messages also assist in relaying to the child that the physician understands what the child has experienced. For example, it is important for children to understand that they were incapable of consenting in an informed manner to the sexual contact that they have experienced. Many children who have been repeatedly engaged in an activity and receive rewards for participating have difficulty in accepting that they are not responsible for having "allowed" the contact to happen. Unfortunately, such feelings may be reinforced when the child discloses abuse and the non-offending parent responds by saying, "Why did you let him do it?" "Why didn't you stop him?" or "Why didn't you tell sooner?" Such responses make the child feel responsible for what has happened. When children are engaged in sexual activities, they are not given choices and are incapable of consenting to sexual activities. Children also are not empowered to stop the activities in which they are engaged.

Another extremely important message to impart is that the child did the right thing by telling and that he or she did not do anything wrong. This concept, coupled with a statement that this type of thing happens to a lot of children, helps decrease the sense of stigmatization, embarrassment, and isolation commonly seen after sexually inappropriate contact.

Abused children have experienced the abuse of power and authority.[20,21] As a result, they may continue to behave, even after disclosure, in a manner reflective of their sense of powerlessness and remain at high risk for future abuse.[25,32] Thus it is important to begin to empower children after their disclosure. This process can begin by simply asking a child what he or she wants to happen now that they have disclosed their abuse. Children must be given the opportunity to begin to make choices that are in their best interests. Most children who purposefully disclose do so simply because they want the abuse to stop. Children frequently are fearful of the consequences of disclosure because of the overt or implicit threats used by the perpetrator to maintain secrecy. Secrecy facilitates repetition and removes accountability by the perpetrator.[20,21,32] Children generally cannot conceive of the cascade of events that is precipitated by their disclosures. They cannot anticipate that the consequences of their disclosure may result in the prosecution of a family member, foster care placement for themselves, and possible abandonment by their non-offending parent. Children should be encouraged to ask questions and be assured that they will be supported through the ensuing process.

Before proceeding with the history, the clinician should review with child protection workers and law enforcement all previously conducted interviews. These interviews should be assessed for their thoroughness, which will assist in determining the scope of the medical history to be conducted. Children should be spoken to as soon after disclosure as possible because early statements are generally more spontaneous.[33]

In addition to reviewing the details of all prior interviews with the child, it is equally important to address the parental response since disclosure and to record any observations that the non-offending caretaker may have made. The non-offending parent can provide a wealth of information concerning the child's medical history and change in daily habits, as well as any behavioral changes and the child's statements that contributed to the suspicion that the child may have been abused. At the onset of the history taking, the child and parent may be seen together, but then each should be seen independently to address individual concerns or worries. Many times, children and adolescents have unanticipated and unrealistic worries or concerns about their bodies as a result of what they have experienced. Addressing these issues is essential in identifying the possibility of an altered body image resulting from abuse. Prepubertal children frequently express idiosyncratic concerns about their bodies and may worry that they could have a disease or be pregnant in the absence of a rational explanation for their concern.[20,32] It is important to let children know that no worry or question is too silly or uninformed.

The young child must view the clinician as both nonthreatening and empathic if he or she is to separate from the parent. Every effort must be made by the clinician to create an environment in which the child will feel safe and understood. The clinician's history-taking style must be modified to meet the needs of the varying ages and developmental levels of children.

The history should focus primarily on the specifics of what the child experienced and the context in which the alleged contact occurred. The child's history of the experience sets the stage to diagnose any residua to the alleged contact, whether it be acute or chronic injury, seminal products, or an STI.

Children are told that the purpose of the examination is to make sure they are physically OK and to address any worries or concerns they may have about their bodies because of what happened.

Some children find it difficult to verbalize their experiences. Using anatomical drawings, paper and crayons, or anatomically detailed dolls may facilitate articulating or demonstrating the child's experience.[34-36] Children use a variety of terms to describe their private parts. The terms a particular child uses for genital and anal anatomy need to be determined. If the child appears embarrassed, give the child permission to use his or her own words by telling the child that you have heard all kinds of names, some of which are silly and some of which are embarrassing to say. Some children prefer writing the name down or whispering the name of their private parts.

Box 9.1 lists elements the medical history should address.

Depending on the child's developmental level and emotional preparedness to discuss what he or she has experienced, the level of detail of the experience will vary. The physician should view the child's experience as a puzzle, gathering as many pieces as possible to glean the most accurate and complete picture. When questions are posed, they should be simple, unambiguous, and non-leading. Questions are of value only when they are not suggestive of the answer.

BOX 9.1
Elements of the Medical History Related to Sexual Abuse[a]

The health care professional responsible for taking the medical history should obtain information from the patient or caregiver about
a. How access to the child was achieved
b. How the sexual interaction was represented to the child to engage the child in the activity(s)
c. Progression of the activity(s) over time
d. What rewards, threats, bribery, coercion, and/or intimidation was used to maintain the child in the activity(s) over time
e. Where the contact occurred
f. The frequency of contact
g. The child's description of how he or she felt when engaged in the contact
h. Specific details of what the child experienced and any discomfort associated with the events, including observations by the child in regard to bleeding, bruises, or ejaculate
i. Circumstances surrounding either accidental or purposeful disclosure
j. To whom the disclosure was made and the response of that individual
k. Whether any liquids or pills were provided to the child that altered the child's state of consciousness
l. What the child would like to happen now that the disclosure has occurred

[a]Adapted with permission from Sgroi SM. *Handbook of Clinical Intervention in Child Sexual Abuse.* Books L, ed. Lexington, MA: DC Heath and Co; 1982 and MacFarlane K, Kerbs S. Techniques for interviewing and evidence gathering. In: MacFarlane K, ed. *Sexual Abuse of Young Children.* New York, NY: The Guilford Press; 1987.

Complex questions have the potential to confuse the child and, thus, the child's response will be more difficult to interpret. Make sure the child understands the questions and feels free to ask for clarification if he or she does not understand. By using an open-ended style that progresses from the more general questioning to more specific areas, it is easier for the child to talk about the experience.[20,37–40]

To achieve effective communication with child victims, the clinician must (a) identify and overcome the child's fears and perceived consequences of the experience and subsequent disclosure; (b) understand the coping strategies children use as a defense pattern; (c) appreciate that children provide the details of their experience in a fragmentary manner and may repress specific memories of their experience; (d) recognize that depending on developmental age, children will have varying abilities to communicate the frequency or time frame in which they experience the contact; and (e) become adept at providing options for children to answer questions in the most truthful and least-threatening manner.[37,41–43]

Sexual Victimization of Boys

Surprisingly little literature exists on medical aspects of sexual victimization of males. Numerous studies have described the prevalence rates of male victimization as between 4% and 76%.[44–46] Some researchers believe that the prevalence of sexual abuse of males is similar to that of females, but males are less likely to disclose their abuse. Males seem to be less likely to disclose because of anxiety related to possible homosexuality, perceived threat to "manliness" by inability to stop abuse, and fear. The frequently cited prevalence of victimization for females is 1 in 4 and for males approximately 1 in 6. There is little doubt that male victimization is underrecognized and underreported, and males are less likely to receive services.

Males are most commonly victimized by males. Male perpetrators are likely to use threats and force to engage males in sexual acts if coercion and deceit are insufficient. Boys younger than 13 years are most vulnerable to abuse by extrafamilial perpetrators and strangers, whereas children aged 6 years and younger are more likely to experience abuse by family members. Regardless of the child's age, vulnerability increases with any physical or developmental disability. There is an increased vulnerability for boys whose family circumstances involve one parent, separation, divorce, remarriage with blended families, and parental substance abuse. Although less common, males may be abused by females. Perpetrators often include family members such as mothers, adolescent siblings, and female caretakers. Males who experience sexually inappropriate contact frequently act out their victimization by engaging other children in sexual activities as well.[47] With ready access to the Internet, young adolescents are being exposed to pornography that, when combined with curiosity regarding emerging sexuality, results in many boys acting out with younger siblings whom they have easy access to and control over.[14,48] Male victims, just as female victims, are likely to try to push out of their minds these kinds of experiences and fail to disclose in part because of fear but also to protect the perpetrator when the perpetrator is a family member.

Young male victims are frequently identified because they sexually act out, which not uncommonly includes engaging other age mates in reciprocal genital touching, oral-genital activities, and genital to anal contact. Parents tend to minimize these behaviors when discovered and may intuitively respond in a punitive manner, thinking that admonition will cease the behaviors. When the age differential between the actors is less than 5 years, the concern is focused on who initiated the activity and where the behavior was learned. Parents and some professionals may view these interactions among age mates as normal and curious interactions. The more intrusive and adult-like the sexual interactions are, the more likely that they emanate from exposure to sexually inappropriate materials, sexual contact, or both.

Just as in female victimization, the medical history is key to understanding the context in which the child was engaged in the activities, the progression of the interactions, the use of threats, and insight into whether the child experienced physical discomfort associated with the activities and the reasons for disclosure. Two factors that increase the likelihood of physical residua to the sexual contact are a significant age differential between the victim and perpetrator and the use of force and restraint. When children experience anal trauma there is the potential to develop a fecal retentive disorder, but this disorder on its own is not diagnostic of sexual abuse.

If there are signs or symptoms present referable to either the GU or GI systems, there should be an attempt to determine whether those signs and symptoms have any temporal relationship to the alleged contact.

Descriptive studies regarding diagnostic findings generally are found in limited case report publications.[49-51] The literature on anal findings in males is quite limited, and the earlier studies that describe findings reflect considerable variability from study to study regarding frequency. There is not one published series of cases that attempts to systematically correlate the presence of physical findings with the medical history of anal penetration or interpret findings in a manner that correlates with the timing of anal injuries. The anal sphincter by design dilates to allow passage of large-diameter objects on a routine basis without injury to the anoderm or verge. Thus it is not surprising that objects such as a penis or digit could readily pass into the anorectal canal without significant residua if the perpetrator uses lubrication and avoids the use of force, and when the activities occur in the context of a "cooperative" victim. When injuries occur they will typically be superficial, such as fissures that heal rapidly. Genital injuries occur most commonly as the result of rubbing, pinching, sucking, and biting, and these injuries also are generally superficial and heal without residua. Males are less likely to disclose their victimization than girls and, thus, they present generally long after the last contact, when any injuries they may have incurred have healed. There are no published studies on the frequency of genital trauma in males. Sporadic case reports generally describe unusual injuries to the penis such as degloving, amputation, and lacerations secondary to an object. Males can acquire STIs and may have stigmata of such on examination. Occasionally oral findings of trauma may be observed secondary to forced fellatio as tears of the labial frenulum and petechiae on the soft and hard palate.

The dynamics of sexual abuse of boys is not dissimilar to that of females. They too experience engagement generally by someone they know and trust and the progression of victimization follows the classic sequence of engagement, sexual interaction, secrecy, disclosure, and recantation. The long-term impact of sexual victimization is potentially significant. Victims are at risk of running away and of developing posttraumatic stress disorder (PTSD); major depression; anxiety disorders; dissociation; bulimia; sexual dysfunction; and high-risk behaviors such as prostitution, suicide, and substance abuse among others.[5,52–54] It is incumbent on the pediatrician to refer all children who have experienced sexual abuse to a psychologist for a comprehensive psychological evaluation to determine the impact of their victimization. The treatment plan prepared by the psychologist should include trauma-focused cognitive behavior therapy because it is the treatment of choice for children experiencing sexual victimization and has been demonstrated to effectively treat PTSD and many of the behavioral problems that sexually abused children experience. Treatment also reduces the potential for revictimization and sexually reactive behaviors.

Physical Examination

Setting and Timing

All children alleged to have been sexually abused should have a complete head-to-toe examination, even if the last alleged contact was months or years before and the child feels fine. The history may reveal that the child has an altered body image or feels that his or her body may have been injured in some nondescript way. If these concerns are present and addressed, the examination has the potential to have considerable therapeutic value, even if acute or chronic signs of injury or STIs are not identified. The purpose of the physical examination is not only to diagnose and treat any "abnormality" as a result of the contact but, of equal importance, to reassure "normality," which may help the child achieve a sense of physical intactness.

The disclosure of abuse precipitates a crisis for the family. Non-offending parents frequently want an immediate answer as to whether the child's statements are true. Child protective services (CPS), law enforcement, and parents may believe that the physical examination will confirm the contact and, thus, they seek an immediate examination, usually by visiting their primary care physician. They also may decide to go to their local emergency department (ED) on their own or per the primary care physician's instructions.

Unfortunately, the ED generally is the least appropriate environment for the first encounter, unless the hospital has appropriate personnel and equipment to serve the needs of sexually abused children.[55,56] Physicians with knowledge of child sexual abuse should help determine the most appropriate time and place for an examination. It is of paramount importance to establish the timing of the last abusive encounter so the physician can determine the urgency of conducting the medical examination.

Because most children do not disclose their abuse immediately, the need for a rape kit, the diagnosis of acute GU infections, STIs, and/or trauma are not usually the primary consideration. Consequently, most examinations can be scheduled for an outpatient assessment after the initial CPS or law enforcement intervention.

Acute genital and anal injuries are infrequent, but when they do occur, an immediate examination is indicated.[57] When there is a need to use a rape kit, each component must be performed by personnel who are skilled in the collection and preservation of each component. (See Chapter 12.) Under most circumstances, the child victim can identify the perpetrator. Information derived from performing forensic evaluation can be helpful in confirming contact and an individual's identity.

Typically, when children present for examination after an alleged inappropriate sexual experience, either nonspecific findings or no residua of the contact are evident. When no acute signs of injury are present, the clinician must determine whether any chronic changes in genital or anal anatomy are present. Chronic residua to genital or anal

trauma by definition will be evident long after the last sexual contact. The retrospective interpretation of changes in anal and genital anatomy and the inherent difficulties of such an assessment are discussed later in this chapter.[58]

As a rule, if the last episode of alleged contact occurred within 72 hours, an examination should be done immediately to identify and treat residua of the contact. Every effort should be made to see that the acute examination is conducted by someone with the appropriate skills and photodocumentation capabilities to avoid the child being subjected to a repeat examination.

When more than 72 hours have passed since the last contact, the primary focus of CPS and law enforcement should be the initial coordinated interview. Once this is completed, the child can be referred for a medical examination followed by an assessment of the mental health impact of the contact and the development of a therapeutic plan. Concurrently, the child protection agency will be assessing the non-offending parent and/or caretaker to determine if the safety of the child can be ensured.

Preparation of the Child

Sexually abused children have been deceived, betrayed, and coerced into sexual contact and may have considerable difficulty in developing trust. Completion of a thorough examination depends on the ability of the physician to anticipate and address the child's anxiety and fears. Because abused children have already experienced the abuse of power and authority, they should never experience the same by coercion and deceit, or the forced abduction of their legs by a "helping physician." A forced examination of an uncooperative child is universally unsuccessful and results only in a more frightened and less trusting child who is more difficult to examine in the future. If it appears that the child is unlikely to cooperate and there is no medically urgent indication for the examination, the examination should be rescheduled to a time when the child may be more receptive. When the presenting signs and symptoms suggest a need for an immediate examination and the child cannot cooperate, sedation and/or examination under anesthesia is appropriate.[59]

When children are fearful, there is usually an underlying basis that can be readily identified. Young children are most fearful of needles, being hurt, or the unknown. Each of these issues is addressed differently depending on the child's age.[31] The purpose of the examination should be explained, telling the child how the examination will proceed and reassuring them that they can ask questions at any point if there is something that they do not understand. Wherever appropriate, the child is given choices, which assists the child in achieving a sense of control. Young children may prefer sitting in their caregiver's lap rather than being positioned on the examination table.

It also is important to address parental anxiety. The most common fear that parents express about the genital examination is that their young child will undergo an adult speculum and bimanual examination. Reassuring the parent that the prepubertal child will not have

this type of examination relieves parental anxiety and enables the parent to be supportive, comforting, and attentive to the child's needs during the examination. If possible written material should be provided to the caretaker before the examination that anticipates and explains frequently asked questions about the medical examination. This information also may decrease anticipatory anxiety on the part of the parent and, in turn, reduce the child's anxiety.[60]

Examination of the anogenital region should occur only in the context of a complete physical examination. When children are engaged in sexual activities, the contact is focused on their anogenital region. Implicitly, the message to the child who undergoes a head-to-toe examination is that all parts of his or her body are important. The examination of the genitalia and anus requires a significant amount of time. The anogenital examination should not be the first component of the physical but, rather, as a part of the natural progression of the head-to-toe examination.

Extra-genital signs of trauma, although less frequently present, are detected during a complete examination. Abused children may have had their general medical needs neglected, and the examination along with a complete review of systems and medical history serve to address overall health needs and identify previously unsuspected medical problems.

Female Examination Positions
Over the last 25 years there has been a profusion of medical literature describing the optimal manner in which to

conduct a genital examination of the prepubertal child in a way that is both child sensitive and ensures complete visualization.[61–66] The optimal examination position(s), combined with a variety of techniques, allows a full appreciation of the nuances of normal genital anatomy and the tissue changes that may reflect residua to trauma.

The position in which a child is most comfortable, most cooperative, and least embarrassed is the position that should be used initially. Frequently, a combination of the supine frog-leg and knee-chest positions maximizes observation of the hymenal membrane and structures of the vaginal vestibule.[62] Small children are most likely to be comfortable when examined in the supine frog-leg position on the examination table or while being held in the caretaker's lap (Figure 9.1). All children should wear a gown and be draped to protect their sense of privacy. Very young children are curious and may prefer not to be encumbered by a gown.

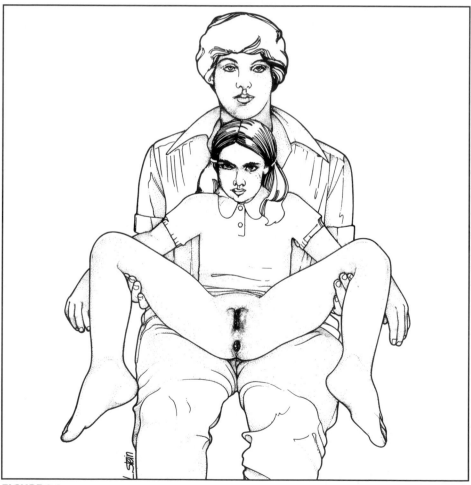

FIGURE 9.1
Prepubertal child positioned in the lap of accompanying adult for genital and anal examination.

In the recumbent supine position, the child sits like a frog with her legs in full abduction and the feet in apposition. When using the separation technique,

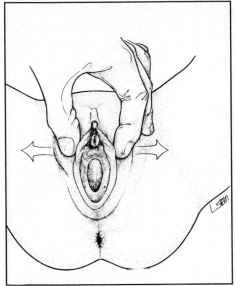

FIGURE 9.2
Visualization of the structures of the vaginal vestibule assisted by placement of the fingers to separate labia, in the supine frog-leg position.

place the first and second fingers at the 10 and 2 o'clock positions, exerting gentle pressure until the labia separate and the hymenal membrane is visualized. With this technique, little or no tension is placed on the hymenal membrane (Figure 9.2).

With the child in the frog-leg position, visualization of the structures of the vaginal vestibule is achieved with the use of labial separation with or without traction. The traction technique affords improved visualization of the hymenal orifice.[65] Traction is most valuable in children who have redundant hymenal membrane tissue because the mucosal surface's cohesive forces tend to obscure full visualization of the orifice. When using labial traction (Figure 9.3), grasp the labia between the thumb and index finger of each hand and exert gentle traction in the posterolateral direction. Steady tension may be necessary to overcome cohesive forces of a moist hymenal membrane, allowing the orifice to pop open. When a child is examined in the knee-chest position, the appearance of the hymen may be quite different. For example a membrane edge that appears as folded over, narrow, and rounded in the frog-leg position may appear wider, thinner, and more delineated than previously observed in the knee-chest position. This change in appearance can be attributed to

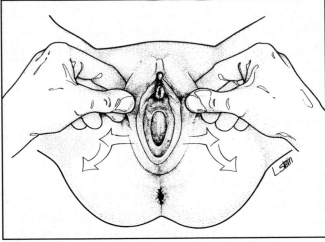

FIGURE 9.3
Lateral and posterior traction of labia further facilitates visualization of structures of the vaginal vestibule, in the supine frog-leg position.

the effect of gravity, which allows the anterior vaginal wall to fall forward and any redundant tissue in the inferior quadrants of the hymen to thin out. The prone knee-chest position does have the advantage of facilitating visualization of the cervix if the hymenal orifice is of sufficient diameter and the patient is relaxed.[63]

The prone knee-chest position (Figure 9.4) is somewhat awkward for all but the youngest children. One approach to preparing the child for a knee-chest examination is to ask the child if they have seen how babies sleep on their tummies with their behinds up in the air. Explain to the child that this is the position that you want them to be in, and have the accompanying adult assist in positioning the child. While the child is in this position, the clinician places the thumbs on the buttocks at the 10 and 2 o'clock positions and gently elevates the buttocks in a lateral and superior direction (Figure 9.5). The prone knee-chest position may not be necessary if the examiner is confident that complete visualization of all of the tissues has been achieved in the supine frog-leg position. One caveat is that if there seems to be an abnormal finding observed when the child is in the frog-leg position, it should be confirmed in the knee-chest position as well.

Other variables that may account for a changing appearance of the hymenal orifice are the state of relaxation and degree of labial traction and separation.[62,65,67] McCann et al[65] observed that the prone knee-chest position and the supine traction technique proved superior to the supine separation technique for visualizing the hymenal membrane

and its orifice. Maximal anteroposterior hymenal orifice diameters were obtained in the prone knee-chest position. Maximal transverse horizontal diameters were obtained in the supine position with traction. Variability in measurements due to differences in the state of relaxation occur because the hymenal membrane is attached laterally to the vaginal wall. When the pubococcygeal muscles are tense, the vestibule is contracted, and the orifice may appear small; when relaxed, the orifice appears more dilated. The addition of labial traction provides another variable in measuring the maximal orifice diameter. The greater the traction, the larger the orifice might appear.

The lithotomy position also can be used for examining the older prepubertal female child. Once the patient is in the appropriate position for the examination, every effort must be made to minimize any discomfort. Children may be fearful of being touched by a cotton swab because of a previous experience with throat cultures. A few simple steps can minimize the potential for causing discomfort. All visualization should be done before attempting any touching with cotton swabs. The unestrogenized hymenal membrane is very sensitive, and if touched directly, will cause discomfort. Therefore, when attempting to collect vaginal secretions for cultures, use urethral swabs (mini-culturette), which easily pass through a hymenal orifice of 2.5 mm or greater without touching the edge of the membrane or the external surface. A urethral swab moistened with sterile non-bacteriostatic saline before use will further reduce the chances of

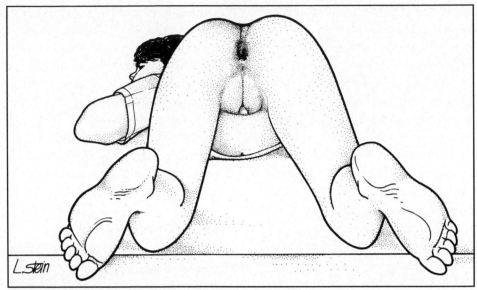

FIGURE 9.4
Knee-chest position for genital examination of the prepubertal child to supplement the supine frog-leg position.

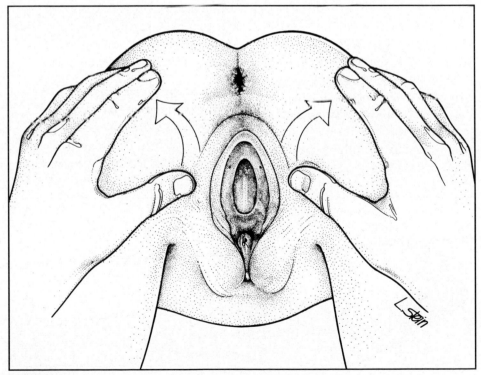

FIGURE 9.5
Visualization of the structures of the vaginal vestibule while in the knee-chest position is facilitated by superior and lateral traction, as noted by hand placement.

discomfort if the hymen is touched. Large cotton swabs are more likely to cause discomfort and should be avoided in prepubertal children. Before introducing the mini-culturette, separate the labia by applying pressure points with the second and third fingers of the left hand on each buttock lateral to the fourchette. The downward and lateral pressure opens the vestibule for visualization. The pressure sensation of the index fingers on the buttocks will distract the child, and the swab can be introduced through the orifice to collect the specimen without touching the hymen under most circumstances. Alternatively, the clinician can pass a urethral catheter through the orifice and irrigate the posterior portion of the vagina with a few milliliters of saline. The vaginal wash is then plated on an appropriate culture medium. Generally, the examination of the prepubertal child is principally an external visualization facilitated by varying techniques of separation, traction, and positioning. Instrumentation of prepubertal children is rarely necessary. Use of a nasal speculum, as

described in standard texts, is awkward and of limited value.[68] Vaginal specula are reserved for prepubertal children who require an examination under anesthesia when there is a concern for internal injuries following an acute assault. Even removal of the most commonly found foreign body (toilet paper) can generally be achieved without a speculum or anesthesia using a simple irrigation technique.

Examination of the Anus

The anus can be readily visualized in the prone or supine knee-chest position. The prone knee-chest position may be uncomfortable for any child who has experienced anal penetration. Thus the left lateral decubitus (lateral knee-chest) or supine frog-leg with legs flexed onto the abdomen (supine knee-chest) is the best position for examining either the male or female anus (Figure 9.6).

The anal and perianal tissues are carefully examined for both acute and healed signs of trauma. Acute signs of trauma may be evident as superficial abrasions and chafing of the anal verge

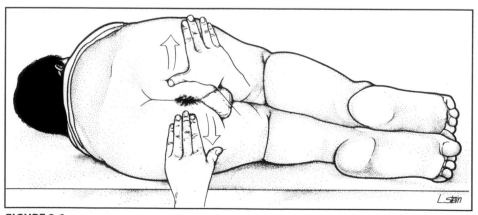

FIGURE 9.6
Hand placement for separation of the buttocks to view external anal tissues with the child in the left lateral decubitus position.

and the tissues that form the gluteal cleft. Perianal redness is frequently observed in non-abused and abused children and, thus, it is a nonspecific finding. The specificity of erythema increases when associated with other signs of trauma and confirms that there is a timely relationship between the alleged contact and the observed finding. When examining the anal verge tissues with the anus in a dependent position, it should be anticipated that the longer the tissues are examined in this position the greater the likelihood that there will be dependent pooling of blood in the hemorrhoidal veins, creating a bluish coloration to the tissue that can be quite dramatic and may be misinterpreted as bruising. If this is observed the examiner simply touches the anal verge, resulting in contraction of the sphincter, which should then result in the disappearance of the "bruising."

The anal sphincter is anatomically designed to contract and pass stool on a routine basis. Children can pass, by parental description, surprisingly large-diameter stools without problems. Anal fissures can be seen following passage of a large-diameter stool, as commonly associated with constipation. Fissures can also be the result of the introduction of a foreign body, such as a finger, penis, or other object. Anal fissures are a non-specific finding of superficial mucosal trauma. The specificity of a fissure increases with a corroborating history.

An anoscope can be introduced into the most distal portion of the rectosigmoid for visualization of the pectin line. If there is a concern for internal blunt force trauma beyond the rectosigmoid, then the examination should be completed with sigmoidoscopy under anesthesia. The probability of finding extensive internal injuries when there are no external anal verge signs of trauma is minimal and, thus, sigmoidoscopy is rarely indicated, except when acute blunt force anal penetrating trauma is suspected.

Examination of Male Genitalia

Male children benefit from a genital examination conducted in the context of a head-to-toe physical as female children do. The potentially embarrassing nature of a genital examination should be acknowledged and the examination should proceed with patience and sensitivity, affording the male child the same level of personal privacy as female children. Following the examination, male children will find knowing that their body is fine beneficial in spite of what they may have either experienced or had to do. This reassurance can only be accomplished if the child experiences a thorough examination that provides an opportunity for the child to express any concerns they have about their body. Male and female children share similar concerns of whether their body could have been damaged or changed, that people can tell, or that they could have acquired an STI as a result of the activities. Male children may also be concerned, whether expressed directly or not, that because of their experience they may be homosexual. This issue should be discussed routinely to provide assurance that just because they were coerced into an activity they could not consent to does not mean that they should be worried about their sexual identity.

Improving Visualization and Documentation

Once a child is comfortable and positioned for the examination, supplemental lighting, filters, and magnification can assist in optimizing visualization of all the details of the genital and anal tissues. Adequate lighting is a prerequisite to a thorough examination and any photographic or video documentation that should follow. Several inexpensive light sources, such as a goose-neck lamp, halogen procedure lights, and handheld devices can be used, although they are usually inadequate to ensure the consistent results that can be achieved by a light source attached to a colposcope or a fiberoptic scope with video capabilities. Moreover, the light created by inexpensive sources is insufficient for adequate photodocumentation.[69]

The genital and anal tissues of prepubertal children are best examined with the use of magnification. Although this task can be achieved with a handheld lens or the magnifying capabilities of an otoscope or ophthalmoscope, none of these methods are satisfactory. The least optimal choice is the otoscope or ophthalmoscope, in part because of a limited angle of view, a small lens, and a short working distance required between the child's genitalia and the examiner.

The colposcope is an instrument that provides an excellent light source with multiple or variable magnification capabilities, and for most examiners it is the instrument of choice. An alternative to the traditional colposcope is the fiberoptic scope that incorporates an excellent light source, variable magnification, and a wide angle of view. Most fiberoptic scopes are a far less expensive alternative to the traditional colposcope.

The traditional colposcope, outfitted with a 35-mm or digital camera attachment, affords consistent and easy documentation of physical findings in either a digital or film format. Digital cameras provide some advantages over traditional film in that they allow immediate viewing of images and can be easily downloaded into a computer database or printed. Polaroid systems produce immediate images; however, they are generally of poor resolution and inadequate for reproduction. When a colposcope is not available, a macro-focusing lens with 1:1 magnification capabilities and a ring flash can be used to document physical findings.[69]

A colposcope with video capabilities has many advantages over still photography in the documentation of examination findings. Still images provide only a moment in time, 2-dimensional record of a given finding. The genital and anal tissues are dynamic, and video colposcopy assists in observing and recording the variable appearance of the tissues from moment to moment. Video colposcopy has the added advantage, particularly in prepubertal children, of allowing the child to observe exactly what the examiner is doing on the video monitor. For most children, this helps demystify the examination. Having a sense of control and participation throughout the examination at times comforts children who watch. Before a view of the child's genitalia, young children might find it fascinating to see their belly button or fingernail on the television monitor. The child is then instructed to watch the monitor and observe the examiner's approaching finger before actually being touched. Children who are fearful of being touched by a cotton swab can be handed one and shown on the monitor where the examiner would like the swab placed. In this way, fearful children can collect their own specimens.

Video colposcopy is particularly advantageous for clinicians in a teaching institution. A teaching library is invaluable in demonstrating examination techniques and the full spectrum of genital and anal anatomy to residents and visiting clinicians. Residents participating in the examination of a child can review the tape in an unhurried manner out of the child's presence. Video colposcopy also allows instant replay for further study and interpretation. The examination can be recorded on either videotape or on DVD, which provides advantages over tape in regard to archiving and image capture.

A colposcope generally provides between 4- and 30-fold magnification, depending on the manufacturer.[70] The most useful range is between 4× and 15× magnification. Above 15× magnifications, both the angle of view and depth of the field are minimal. A colposcope equipped with an intraocular scale assists in obtaining an accurate measurement of the hymenal orifice diameter or the dimensions of specific abnormal findings. Colposcopes have built-in, red-free filters that cast a green light, enhancing the appearance of the vascular pattern and the mucosa. A filter assists in the recognition of superficial abrasions of the mucosa of the vestibule and interruptions in the vascular pattern. Scar tissue also may be more apparent because its avascular appearance contrasts with the surrounding vascularized tissues.

Digital or film documentation of all abnormal findings should accompany every examination.[71] Because of limitations of substantiating allegations of sexual abuse in the young child, establishing baseline documentation of anogenital anatomy may serve as a useful reference for those children who remain at risk. The adage, "A picture is worth a thousand words," applies to documenting findings that may be difficult to describe. The photograph memorializes findings of residual tissue damage from the alleged contact. Photographs also can be used to obtain a second opinion; demonstrate healing; show the presence of STIs; teach; and, where appropriate, demonstrate physical findings in court. From a practical perspective, digital images are replacing 35-mm film. Digital imaging provides a more convenient format for viewing and storing images than film. Digital imprinting provides identifying information on the image, leaving no question as to the identity of the person represented in the image. A system that logs images is important as a way of maintaining a chain of custody. Digital images can be electronically altered and, thus, it remains the responsibility of the individual who obtained the images to ensure the image integrity and be able to testify that the image represents what was observed and has not been altered.

When extra-genital signs of trauma are photographed, an accompanying ridged millimeter rule and gray scale (ABFO no. 2) should be included with the identifying name and date. This is critically important when bite marks are present. With a standard reference scale, an odontologist can determine whether the arch of a bite mark is that of a child or an adult.[72] Before photographing a child, explain that the only person who can take a picture of them with their clothing off is a doctor, with their mother or another trusted adult present. Reassure the child that the photograph will represent only a small part of his or her body, and that no one can identify them from the photograph. Ask the children if anyone has ever taken a picture of them with their clothing off. This question may uncover previously unsuspected pornography. Further questioning may include, "Have you ever seen any pictures of people with their clothing off?"; "Were any of the people in the photograph children"? Show the children the camera, whether handheld or attached to a colposcope, and allow them to take a picture of their names and identifying information, such as date of birth and visit, if they so desire. Always respect the child's desire not to be photographed if expressed or sensed. With the advent of the Internet, there has been unfortunate and unprecedented access to pornography by young children and adolescents. When young adolescents are exposed to pornography, there is the potential that they will act out what they have seen with younger children who they have ready access to, commonly siblings, cousins, or sibling playmates.

Anatomy and Terminology

Familiarity with genital and anal anatomy and knowledge of descriptive terminology assists clinicians in enhancing their level of comfort in examining the sexually abused child and providing documentation in the medical record. The medical record must accurately reflect all of the nuances of the child's genital and anal anatomy in clear and descriptive terms. Before the American Professional Society on the Abuse of Children consensus statement on terminology in the medical evaluation of sexual abuse, there was some inconsistency in the manner in which findings were interpreted and described. It is important that clinicians involved in examining children speak the same language and describe normal and abnormal anatomical variations that exist from one child to the next by using the same terminology (Figures 9.7 and 9.8). When documenting findings, the description should be as specific as possible, and a term such as *normal genitalia* is of little descriptive value. The term *normal* does not take into account that the genitalia have many components, and the appearance of normal varies from child to child. Vulva, pudenda, and perineum also lack specificity and are of limited value. For example, *vulva* or *pudendum feminum* is a term that includes all of the components of the external visible genital structures, encompassing the mons pubis, labia majora and minora, clitoris, vestibule of the vagina, bulb of the vestibule, Skene and Bartholin glands, and vaginal orifice. The perineum is the area between the thighs bounded by the vulva and anus in girls and scrotum and anus in boys.[73–77]

When the labia are separated, the vaginal vestibule can be visualized.

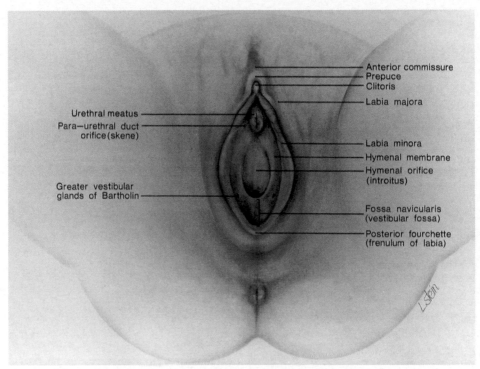

FIGURE 9.7
Genital anatomy of the normal prepubertal female child.

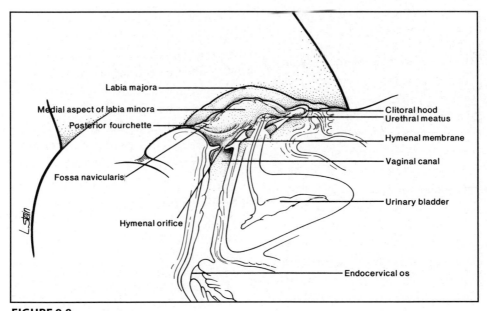

FIGURE 9.8
Cross-section of the female pelvis illustrating recessed position of the hymenal membrane at the entrance of the vaginal canal.

The vestibule of the vagina encompasses the area bordered laterally by the labia minora, the clitoris superiorly, and the fourchette posteriorly. Within the vestibule there are 6 perforations: urethra, periurethral ducts or Skene glands, vaginal orifice, and greater vestibular ducts or Bartholin glands.[75,76] The vaginal orifice is the perforation of the hymenal membrane.

The hymenal membrane is recessed in the vestibule, protecting it from direct trauma; hence the implausibility of injury to the membrane from athletic activity such as bicycling, horseback riding, or gymnastics. The common misconception that athletic activities result in injuries to the hymen has no scientific support. The rare impaling injury, when it occurs, is readily differentiated from trauma resulting from the direct and premeditated introduction of a foreign body such as a digit or a penis into the vagina.

The internal surface of the hymenal membrane marks the beginning of the vagina. The hymenal membrane is attached laterally to the walls of the vagina and posteriorly to the floor of the vagina. The concave area between the posterior attachment of the hymen and the fourchette is the fossa navicularis. The posterior joining of the labia minora forms the fourchette. The labia majora are described in most texts as joining posteriorly to form the posterior commissure; however, other authors describe them as not joining but tapering off anterolaterally into the perineum.[73-75]

Another anatomically vague term is *introitus*. Introitus is a generic term defined as the entrance to a canal or space.[77] The term *introital diameter* has been used as a synonym for the opening in the hymen typically referred to as the *vaginal orifice*.[78] To avoid confusion of terms, the opening in the hymenal membrane should be referred to as the *hymenal membrane orifice* or *vaginal orifice* rather than introitus.

Hymenal Membrane

"The most insignificant anatomical structure of the female without an analog in the male has assumed a social importance at variance with its almost neutral physiologic value or its potential influence upon health."[79] This vestigial remnant has merited mythological, psychological, sociological, and now an amazing degree of medical notoriety as clinicians begin to take a twenty-first century look at this tissue.

Much of the assessment of child sexual abuse has been focused on the appearance of the hymenal membrane orifice. Law enforcement, social workers, and parents may want to know if the hymen is intact or broken, as if it were either impenetrable or a piece of china. Many professionals believe that the determination as to whether a child has been sexually abused will be answered by the mere examination of the hymen alone. In support of this desire to know, there is a volume of literature describing the appearance of the hymenal membrane in terms of both its normative state and changes due to injury.[21,64,80-82]

Embryologically, "the hymen develops as a result of the advancement of mesenchyme into the epithelial mass at the junction of the pelvic part of the urogenital sinus and the vaginal plate."[83] The external surface of the hymen is covered by urogenital sinus epithelium. Cells derived from the vagina cover the inner aspect of the hymen. The degree of vascularity and the amount of connective tissue between the epithelial layers vary considerably. The membrane is innervated and, in the prepubertal child, the hymen can be exquisitely sensitive to touch.

Many misconceptions concerning the hymen have developed over the years. The origin of these misconceptions is difficult to trace. One misconception is the existence of an entity known as congenital absence of the hymen. Children may occasionally be referred because the child "does not appear to have a hymen" or is thought to have been "born without a hymen." Absence of the hymen cannot and does not exist on an embryologic basis as a sole congenital anomaly. It may be absent in the presence of other major urogenital anomalies, of which the least significant concern is the presence or absence of the hymen. If the genitourinary tract is normally developed, the hymen is present. In a 1904 discussion concerning malformations of the hymen, Gelhor[84] noted, "Total absence of hymen, reports of which are found in older literature, have not been observed by modern authors, while not denying the possibility, consider this phenomenon exceedingly rare." Jenny et al[80] examined 1,311 female newborns, all of whom had hymens.

Genital trauma can alter the appearance of the prepubertal and pubertal child's hymen in a variety of ways. In adult women, remnants of the hymenal membrane are referred to as carunculae hymenales. Microscopically, these carunculae are compact mounds of elastic and connective tissue that have lost their papillae.[84] Carunculae hymenales do not exist in prepubertal children.

Over the last 25 years, there has been a limited but developing body of literature describing changes to the hymen in the prepubertal child resulting from trauma.[58,66,85–87]

The appearance of the hymenal membrane is quite variable. Some aspects of the membrane, such as the orifice configuration and the transverse and horizontal diameters, are easily described and measured. Other characteristics, such as thickness and the degree of elasticity or distensibility, which also are quite variable, present problems for objective quantification. Whenever the hymen and the hymenal tissues are described in the medical record, it is important to be as specific as possible concerning the character of the hymen and to avoid inaccurate and nondescriptive terms, such as *marital, broken, virginal,* or *intact.*

Many nonmedical professionals have the perception that the hymen is an impermeable membrane, and any opening is abnormal. An imperforate hymen is the only anatomical variant of hymenal configurations in which no opening is present. Distal vaginal atresia can be confused with imperforate hymen. Classically the imperforate hymen is diagnosed in puberty when the amenorrheic female presents with a midline abdominal mass and blue-domed appearance of the hymen.[88] Before puberty, the imperforate hymen results in the formation of a mucocolpos. Other configurations of the hymenal membrane orifice are annular, crescentic, fimbriated, septate, or cribriform. Each of these types merits a brief discussion and is illustrated in the accompanying colpophotographic case slides. For an annular orifice to exist, hymenal membrane tissue must be present circumferentially. The orifice itself can be placed either centrally or ventrally. When the orifice appears crescentic, hymenal membrane tissue is not evident between approximately the 11 and 1 o'clock positions; the superior edge of the hymenal membrane interdigitates with the vaginal walls laterally, leaving a posterior rim of tissue that is variable in its width. When a band of hymenal membrane traverses an annular orifice, creating 2 openings, it is referred to as *septate*. This configuration is much different, however, from a septum of the vagina that extends posteriorly and divides the vaginal canal and may be associated with other congenital anomalies. When multiple openings are present in the membrane, the term *cribriform* is used, which means "like a sieve."[77] A hymenal membrane orifice with multiple finger-like projections on the edge of the membrane is referred to as *fimbriated*. These fingers most likely represent papillary excrescences.[83,84] Suffice it to say that these projections frequently overlap, obscuring the orifice itself unless considerable labial separation and traction are applied. The degree of tautness of the membrane bridging the vaginal canal is variable and is dependent on the degree of relaxation of the patient when the membrane is examined. The terms *redundant* or *folded* also have been used to describe the membrane when it is not taut. The membrane's edge may have congenital clefts, external hymenal ridges, tags, bumps, or cysts. Supporting structures called *pubourethral, pubovaginal,* or *pubococcygeal* ligaments may be visible. Pubourethral ligaments, sometimes referred to as *periurethral supporting bands,* are most commonly seen and become more apparent with labial traction.[89] Hymenal tags, which project from the margin of the hymen and prolapse over the edge of the membrane, were observed in 5.75% of 56 infants studied.[81] Longitudinal intravaginal columns (columnae rugarum) are present on the anterior and posterior vaginal walls.[73] These columns are traversed by smaller columns, creating the rugae vaginalis.[73] Berenson et al[89] described longitudinal external and intravaginal ridges in their study of the hymenal configuration of 468 neonates. They noted that the hymen in 80% of the newborns was annular, and in 19% it was fimbriated; the remaining variations accounted for 1%. They also described the presence of anterior clefts in 34% of neonates with annular hymens. No posterior clefts were observed, further supporting concerns of most experts that interruptions in the integrity of the membrane's edge observed posteriorly are of posttraumatic etiology. The unestrogenized tissues of the hymenal membrane and the vestibular aspects of the labia minora and fossa are vascular and can appear diffusely reddened. Redness is nonspecific and, without knowledge of the premorbid appearance of the genitalia, it is difficult to determine whether the redness is due to increased vascularity and secondary to trauma unless it is accompanied by signs of injury. Retrospective interpretation of changes in vascular patterns of the vestibular tissues without other stigmata and/or a history of genital trauma should be approached with caution. Traction can create midline blanching. Thus, before interpreting a midline avascular area as scar tissue, the examiner must be sure that traction is not creating the observed finding. The frequency of congenital midline avascular interruptions of the external surface of the membrane or fossa is unknown. The vascular pattern of the external surface of the hymenal membrane and fossa is most commonly described as reticular, fine lacy, and symmetrical. An interruption in the vascular pattern of the fossa that is interpreted as scar tissue should be accompanied by a history of significant trauma. Small 1- to 2-mm, ovoid translucent elevations that may be observed in the fossa generally represent lymphoid follicles and should be readily differentiated from vesicles or cysts.[90] The study by McCann et al[65] of genital findings in non-abused prepubertal children further elucidated a spectrum of normal variants.[91]

Another characteristic of the hymenal membrane that has resulted in much interpretive debate is the hymenal orifice's transverse diameter measurement.[2,61,77,92–94] Early reference to the significance of a specific hymenal orifice diameter that, if exceeded, was strongly suggestive of sexual abuse, has been problematic. One author noted, "The findings presented indicate that in the absence of known perineal injury, the discovery of an enlarged vaginal opening (greater than 4 mm) correlates 3 out of 4 incidents to positive sexual abuse history given by the child."[2] This criterion alone cannot be considered evidence of sexual abuse. Subsequent commentary by Paradise[94] on the predictive accuracy of interpreting orifice diameters illustrates the limitations of a single measurement: "Most physicians would be relieved to have a single specific test for sexual abuse. Until we have this test, an overemphasis on minute changes in the diameter of the hymenal opening will result in a number of children being identified as victims of sexual abuse, whereas a majority of sexual abuse victims with normal hymenal measurements will remain unidentified."

Clinicians are frequently asked to make a statement as to whether an object has been placed through a given hymenal orifice into the vagina. Measurements obtained during an examination have low predictive value and may not be helpful in determining whether penetration has occurred. Clinically the routine measurement of the anteroposterior and transhymenal orifice diameter may be of limited value.

Obtaining a maximal transverse and vertical diameter can be difficult because of the significant variability of the diameter depending on the examination position, degree of traction, and state of relaxation of the child (Figures 9.9–9.11). The most accurate way to measure these dimensions is through the use of a computerized digital image that has software providing measuring capability. An alternative is through the

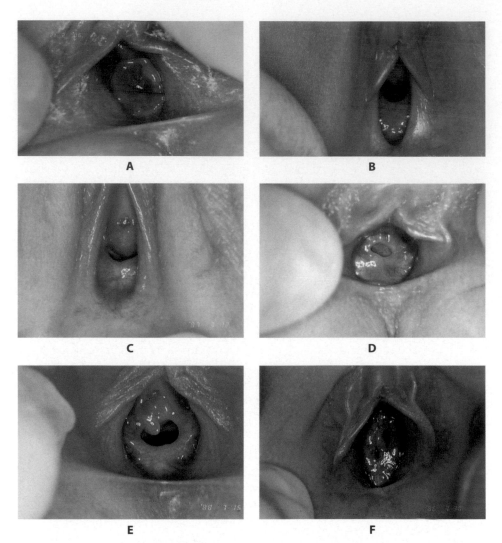

FIGURE 9.9
Normal prepubertal anatomical variations.

A: Fifteen-month-old girl has flared configuration to the annular orifice. Note thickened normal variation of the membrane.

B: A 4-year-old girl has a crescentic orifice with thin, sharply demarcated edge. External surface of the membrane has a lacy vascular pattern. Slight blanching in the fourchette results from traction.

C: A 7 1/2-year-old girl with a crescentic orifice. The membrane has a less translucent and thicker appearance. Urethral meatus is apparent.

D: A 2-year-old girl has a superior and eccentrically oriented annular orifice. External surface of the membrane is translucent. Labial traction is necessary to visualize the orifice.

E: A 9-year-old girl has a prominent hymenal membrane projection of tissue at 11 o'clock with a small bump at 5 o'clock. Projection and bump may have been previously attached, forming a septum.

F: A 5-year-old girl has a septum of the hymen, resulting in 2 orifices. Cohesive characteristics of moist tissue might obscure the presence of 2 orifices if traction is not used.

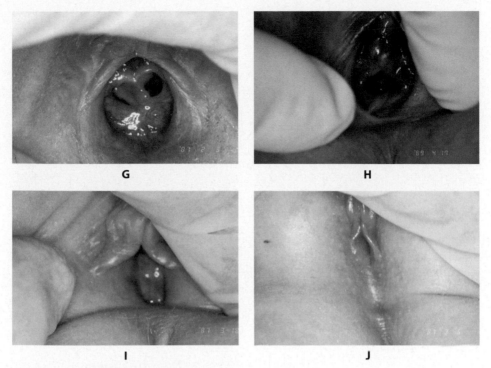

FIGURE 9.9, *continued*

Normal prepubertal anatomical variations.

G: A 5-year-old girl has a vaginal septum that bisects the annular orifice. Associated upper genital tract anomalies must be considered.

H: A 6-year-old girl has a prominent hymenal tag prolapsing from the vagina through the orifice and onto the external surface of the membrane.

I: A 2-year-old girl has no observable hymenal orifice with labial separation, traction, or positioning.

J: A 4 1/2-year-old girl has acquired labial agglutination that obscures examination of structures of the vaginal vestibule. Small anterior separation of labia minora allows urine to escape.

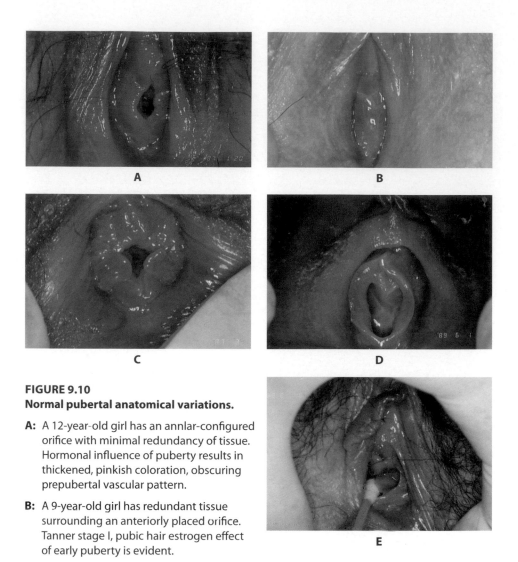

FIGURE 9.10
Normal pubertal anatomical variations.

A: A 12-year-old girl has an annlar-configured orifice with minimal redundancy of tissue. Hormonal influence of puberty results in thickened, pinkish coloration, obscuring prepubertal vascular pattern.

B: A 9-year-old girl has redundant tissue surrounding an anteriorly placed orifice. Tanner stage I, pubic hair estrogen effect of early puberty is evident.

C: A 12-year-old girl with Tanner stage III anatomy. Multiple congenital clefts circumferentially lead to fimbriated or "frilly" appearance of hymen. Note that clefts do not extend to the vaginal wall.

D: An 11-year-old with Tanner stage III anatomy. Note the flared appearance of the annular orifice, but no interruptions in the edge circumferentially. Elasticity of tissues is sufficient to admit a foreign body, such as a digit, without residua as alleged.

E: A 14-year-old girl with Tanner stage IV anatomy. Prominent intravaginal longitudinal ridge (columnae rugarum) is attached to the internal surface of the membrane. When ridge attaches to membrane, it may result in the appearance of a bump on the external surface. Intravaginal ridges and small transverse ridges (rugae vaginalis) are normal anatomical structures. (Note: All pubertal children were examined in lithotomy position unless otherwise noted).

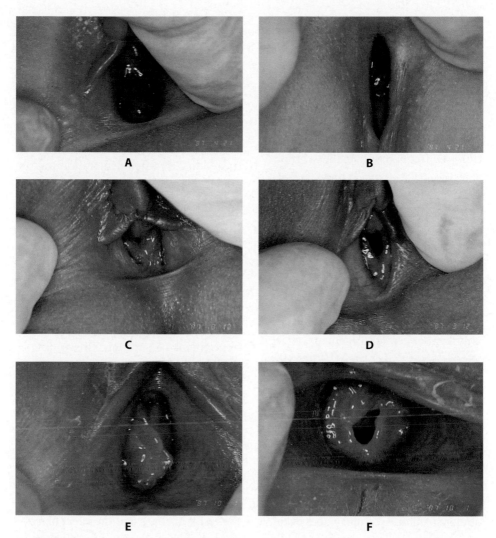

FIGURE 9.11
Variability of appearance of genital tissues because of positional changes and relaxation.

A: A 4-year-old girl in whom the hymenal orifice was not visualized with labial separation and traction in the supine frog-leg position because of redundant hymenal membrane tissue surrounding the orifice. This observation requires examination in the prone knee-chest position for improved visualization.

B: Same patient as in 9.11A, examined in the knee-chest position. Note how gravity has resulted in redundant anterior tissue falling forward, allowing visualization of the annular orifice.

C: A 4-year-old with a minute orifice visualized with labial separation.

D: Same patient as in 9.11C, but note the different appearance of the orifice now that the child is relaxed. Relaxation is particularly important when attempting to assess the maximal transverse hymenal orifice diameter.

E: A 9-year-old with Tanner stage II anatomy. With redundant estrogenized tissue, labial separation alone is insufficient to visualize hymenal orifice.

F: Same patient as in 9.11E viewed with labial traction, which affords complete visualization of the hymenal orifice edge circumferentially. When labial traction is exerted, superficial tears of the fourchette may occur, particularly in prepubertal children.

calibrated intraocular scale of a colposcope eyepiece. Calipers, millimeter rulers, and Glassier rods are less useful alternatives for obtaining these measurements. Measurements alone are of limited value, however, because of the wide variability of normal.

Children frequently state that a given object was placed inside them, and yet there may be no confirmatory physical findings. The ability to differentiate "in" from "on" is a developmental task for which limited normative data exist. Children feeling pressure between the labia and over the fourchette and the periurethral/clitoral hood region may perceive a penis as being placed inside. This form of genital-to-genital contact is referred to as *vulvar coitus*. When vulvar coitus occurs, trauma to the fourchette, medial aspects of the labia, and the periurethral area may be obvious without signs of injury to the hymen, which is recessed and located at the entrance to the vagina. Genital-to-genital contact in the context of vulvar coitus does not necessarily result in trauma to the vestibular structures. If injury does occur, it is most likely to be superficial and heal without residua. A digit placed between the labia also may be perceived as being inside without findings of penetration through the orifice. In genital fondling, penetration of a finger is generally limited to the vestibule itself.

In prepubertal children, the hymen can vary in appearance from thick and presumably elastic or thin and nonelastic. The extent to which the hymen is distensible in the prepubertal child is difficult to quantify clinically. Muram[95] studied the relation between specific sexual acts and genital findings in cases in which all of the perpetrators admitted to the sexual contact. Specific findings of hymenal vaginal tears were found in 60% of the girls when the offender had admitted to vaginal penetration, contrasted to 23% when penetration was denied. Normal-appearing genital tissues or nonspecific findings were present in 39% of victims when penetration was admitted. A hymenal vaginal tear is defined as a laceration of the hymen extending to the posterior vaginal wall. An interruption in the integrity of the edge of the hymenal membrane extending to the floor of the vagina is specific to traumatic penetration. This finding is most commonly observed at the posterior rim of the hymen in the midline.

McCann et al[65] studied the genital anatomy of 114 carefully selected, non-abused girls ranging in age from 10 months to 10 years. This study emphasized the frequency of normal or acquired genital findings that are not the result of abuse and the effect of examination technique and position on the varying appearance of a particular finding (Figure 9.12).

Findings of erythema of the vestibular tissues, periurethral bands, lymphoid follicles, urethral dilatation, labial adhesions, posterior fourchette midline avascular areas, friability of the fourchette, tags, notches, mounds and projections, and intravaginal columns and transverse ridges are common normal variants. When an intravaginal column buttresses against the hymenal membrane edge, it may appear as a bump or mound on the edge of the hymen. Some examiners have interpreted bumps and mounds as a posttraumatic finding.

In 1989 White et al[78] evaluated 242 children to ascertain whether the vaginal introital diameter (hymenal orifice) was useful in evaluating a child for sexual abuse. These clinicians concluded that a hymenal orifice diameter greater than 4 mm is highly associated with sexual contact in children younger than 13 years. In their non-abused subgroup of 23 children with a median age of 6 years, none was found to have a transverse diameter of greater than 4 mm. They also observed that "introital dilation may not always occur with fondling or penile penetration: 27% of children who gave a history of sexual contact with penetration had a vaginal introital diameter of less than or equal to 4 mm."

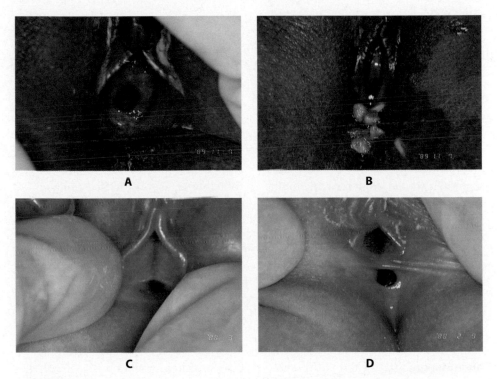

FIGURE 9.12
Miscellaneous.

A: A 5-year-old girl has erythema of the tissues of the vestibule. She had persistent vaginal discharge for 4 months and intermittent vaginal bleeding.

B: Same patient as in 9.12A after irrigation of vagina with sterile water removed the tissue paper that was the nidus for persistent infection.

C: A 4-year-old girl in whom the labial agglutination line is translucent. Agglutination obscures the appearance of the vaginal vestibule.

D: A 4-year-old girl with labial agglutination that is thickened and was present longer than that in the patient in 9.12C. This child experienced genital fondling, and this agglutination may be the postinflammatory residual to this contact.

This finding raises a question as to whether these children had an accurate perception of penetration because it is unlikely that an object could penetrate an orifice less than 4 mm without residua. For a digit or penis to penetrate through a hymenal orifice, a minimal transverse diameter is necessary. The diameter of a digit and a penis is many times the 4 mm proposed in this study. In the non-abused group, which ranged from ages 1 to 12 years, none had a transverse diameter greater than 4 mm. This fact also raises the question as to whether the measurements cited in this study were maximal diameters. A millimeter rule alone cannot be used to determine whether a child has been vaginally penetrated.

If the posterior rim of the hymen is narrow without signs of trauma, the examiner should avoid referring to this finding as attenuated. The definition of attenuation is "to make thin."[77] To apply this term correctly, the examiner must know that the posterior rim of the hymen was wider at some previous point in time and has since been narrowed. If the pre-morbid state is unknown, then the examiner should describe the observed finding as a narrow posterior rim and dispense with the term *attenuated*.

The 2005 guidelines of the American Academy of Pediatrics (AAP) Committee on Child Abuse and Neglect note the following: "The diagnosis of child sexual abuse often can be made on a child's history. Sexual abuse is rarely diagnosed on the basis of physical examination or laboratory findings. Physical findings are often absent even when the perpetrator admits to penetration of the child's genitalia."[96]

Diagnostic findings in the AAP statement deemed concerning are: "(1) abrasions or bruising of the genitalia; (2) an acute or healed tear in the posterior aspect of the hymen that extends to or nearly to the base of the hymen; (3) a markedly decreased amount of hymenal tissue or absent hymenal tissue in the posterior aspect; (4) injury to or scarring of the posterior fourchette, fossa navicularis, or hymen; and (5) anal bruising or lacerations." The guidelines further state: "...the presence of semen, sperm or acid phosphatase; a positive culture for *N gonorrhoeae* or *C trachomatis;* or a positive serologic test for syphilis or HIV infection make the diagnosis of sexual abuse a near medical certainty, even in the absence of a positive history, if perinatal transmission has been excluded for the STDs."

Whether an acute or healed genital or anal injury is identified, it is incumbent on the clinician to obtain a complete history regarding the nature of the injury. When inflicted trauma is suspected, the essential components of the history include (a) the size and type of penetrating object, (b) the degree of discomfort associated with the event, (c) the number of episodes of contact, (d) associated symptoms (eg, bleeding, dysuria), (e) whether treatment was sought and received, and (f) the interval of time between the last alleged contact and the time of examination. Key differences in the history of accidental trauma, such as a straddle injury, are that accidental injuries are more commonly observed by a third party, medical attention is sought immediately after the injury, a scene-of-injury visit confirms the plausibility of the injuries and the accompanying history, and the pattern of injury is consistent with the history.[50,97] Of 161 accidental genital injuries reported in the literature, 3.7% involved the hymen. Impaling injuries do not always present with dramatic histories, and the resulting injuries can mimic those of sexual abuse.[98] There is no support for the supposition that hymenal injuries are the direct result of either masturbation or the use of tampons.[99] Again, the history remains paramount in differentiating the cause of an injury.

Anal Anatomy

When documenting anal findings it is important to be as specific as possible when describing both normal and abnormal observations (Figure 9.13). The tissue overlying the subcutaneous external anal sphincter is the anal verge. The anal verge begins at the most distal portion of the anoderm and extends to the exterior margin of the anal skin. Within the loose connective tissue surrounding the external anal orifice is the external hemorrhoidal plexus of the perianal space. The anoderm extends from the anal verge to the pectinate or dentate line. There is a scalloped appearance to the anoderm at the point in which it interdigitates with the ampulla of the rectum because of the alternating rectal sinuses and columns. The external anal tissue generally has symmetrical, circumferentially radiating folds known as *rugae,* formed by the corrugator cutis ani muscle.[73]

Anal and Perianal Findings

Despite a consensus as to the appropriate descriptive terminology of anal anatomy, disagreement remains regarding the interpretation of anal findings and the frequency with which anal signs are

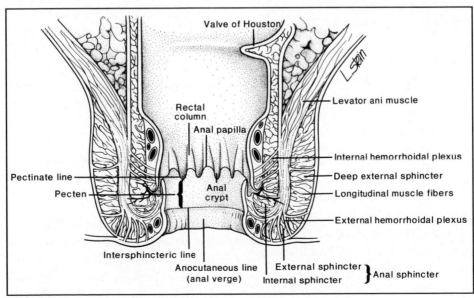

FIGURE 9.13
Cross-section of clinically significant structures of the rectosigmoid and anus.

observed. Contributing to the difficulty of interpreting the residua of anal trauma is the unquestionable ability of the external anal sphincter to dilate to accommodate a large bolus of fecal matter without injury to the tissues. Therefore, depending on the presence or absence of the following variables, a child may or may not have any residua to the introduction of a foreign body into the anus (Figure 9.14). These variables are (a) size of object introduced, (b) presence or absence of force, (c) use of lubricants, (d) degree of "cooperativeness" of victim, (e) number of episodes of penetration, and (f) time interval since last alleged contact.

Hobbs and Wynne[7] reported that 40% to 50% of boys and girls with a history of anal penetration have abnormalities identified on examination. In the only article in the American literature specific to findings after anal abuse, 66% of 310 prepubertal children had normal-appearing perianal tissues.[100] There has been a paucity of recent medical literature on the residua of anal abuse, with a trend suggesting that just as in other forms of sexual abuse diagnostic findings are infrequent. Acute anal injuries are easily recognizable and must be considered in light of the presenting history.

The adult literature concerning descriptive reports of anal injuries in the consenting male homosexual population is limited. No description of chronic sequelae could be found, except an anecdotal notation that "colleagues in genitourinary medicine tell me that even in adults admitting to regular anal intercourse, the anus may appear entirely normal."[101]

Of the physical findings considered to result from chronic anal penetration, the most controversial is the reflexive dilatation of the buttocks with separation. Hobbs and Wynne[102] have confidence in this particular sign and state, "Dilatation over 0.5 cm without the passage of wind does not, in our experience, occur in normal children examined as described. The presence of stool visible in the rectum should not discount the significance of the finding." Hobbs and Wynne[102] reported this finding in 42% of sexually abused children with anal signs. Other authors have not found reflexive dilatation as prevalent in their series.[66,101,103] In a non-abused population, McCann and Voris[66] observed that anal sphincter dilation occurred in 49% of children, and the mean antero-posterior diameter of the orifice was 1 cm, with a range of 0.1 to 2.5 cm. On its own, this sign should not be interpreted as abnormal. In the population of children specifically evaluated by Hobbs and Wynne[7] for anal abuse, 86% showed anal dilations, 61% fissures, 25% venous congestions, 16% scars, 16% funneling, 7% laxity, and 32% other nonspecific signs. Hobbs and Wynne[102] noted, "Interestingly, few anally abused children (or their parents) communicated anal complaints to the doctor even when there was obvious physical abnormality."

McCann and Voris[66] observed that a variety of perianal findings seen in abused children also may be seen in non-abused children, thus highlighting problems with the sensitivity and specificity of soft tissue findings. Nonspecific findings noted by McCann and Voris

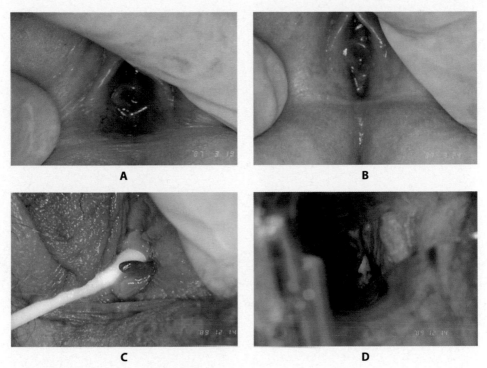

FIGURE 9.14
Acute genital and anal trauma and healed residua.

A: A 10-month-old girl has acute hemorrhage into the hymenal membrane and perihymenal tissues after attempted penetration.

B: Same patient as in 9.14A, 5 days after acute injury. No residua are apparent because of healing of superficial injuries by regeneration of labile cells.

C: A 13-year-old girl has acute hemorrhage into the fimbria of the hymenal membrane after penile penetration of the vagina.

D: Same patient as in 9.14C, examined intravaginally with a speculum. Note the acute laceration of the vaginal canal (from 3 to 5 o'clock).

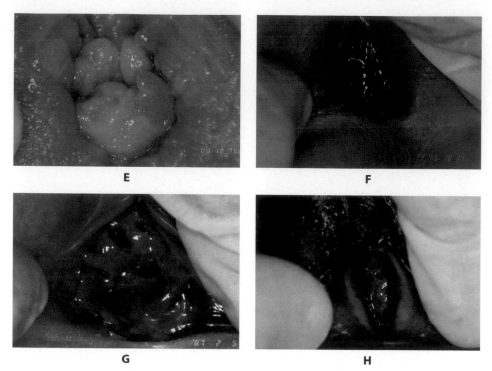

E

F

G

H

FIGURE 9.14, *continued*
Acute genital and anal trauma and healed residual.

E: Same patient as in 9.14C and 9.14D, 5 days later. Examination demonstrates complete healing of the injury to the membrane as well as the intravaginal mucosal laceration (not illustrated).

F: A 19-month-old girl with prominent lacerations to the vaginal wall, membrane, and fourchette on post-assault day 4 after penile vaginal penetration. Tissue edema and hemorrhage into tissues are evident.

G: Same patient as in 9.14F. Follow-up examination demonstrates healed residual to acute genital trauma, illustrating a marked difference from the appearance of acute injuries. Lacerated hymenal membrane remnants and scar tissue distort appearance in an unanticipated manner. Also evident are 2 condylomata at 7 o'clock position, emphasizing the need for continued follow-up of children at risk for contracting sexually transmitted infections with long incubation periods.

H: A 5-year-old girl with erythema and superficial abrasions to the medial aspect of the labia minora after vulvar coitus. Note the lack of signs of penetration through the hymenal orifice.

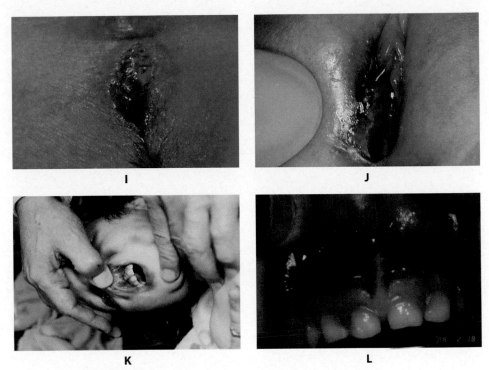

FIGURE 9.14, *continued*
Acute genital and anal trauma and healed residual.

I: A 2-year-old girl with acute laceration of the perineum and anal verge tissue at the 12 o'clock position after attempted penile anal penetration.

J: A 6-year-old girl with an acute crush injury to the labia minora and majora after falling on a metal bar of a jungle gym. Note that the injury does not involve the hymenal membrane recessed in the vaginal canal.

K: A 2-year-old girl has complete avulsion of the labial frenulum after physical and sexual assault.

L: Same patient as in 9.14K, with the mother's fingers elevating the upper lip to reveal residual to the avulsion. The minimal amount of scar tissue demonstrates the difficulty in appreciating how extensive the initial injuries may have been by observing only healed residua.

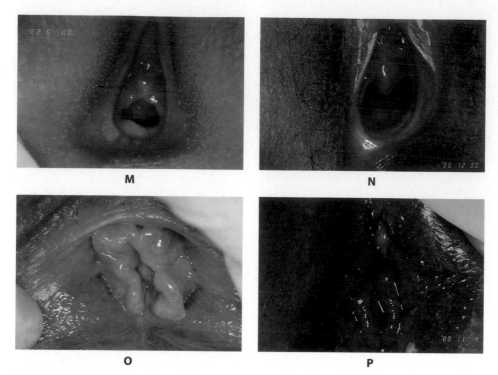

FIGURE 9.14, *continued*
Acute genital and anal trauma and healed residual.

M: A 4-year-old girl has healed interruption in the integrity of the hymenal membrane between 8 and 10 o'clock positions after painful digital penetration through the orifice. Lymphoid follicles are present in the fossa between 6 and 7 o'clock positions.

N: A 12-year-old girl with Tanner stage II anatomy. Extremely narrowed posterior ring appears contiguous with the floor of the vagina. The child experienced repeated penile vaginal penetration. Premorbid appearance of the posterior rim is not observed.

O: A 13-year-old girl with Tanner stage III anatomy. Healed residual to complete transection of the hymenal membrane at the 6 o'clock position. Scar tissue is evident at the base of the transection in the fossa.

P: A 10-month-old girl after surgical repair of complete transection of the external anal sphincter after penile anal penetration. Rectal mucosa prolapsed because of tissue edema and decreased rectal tone.

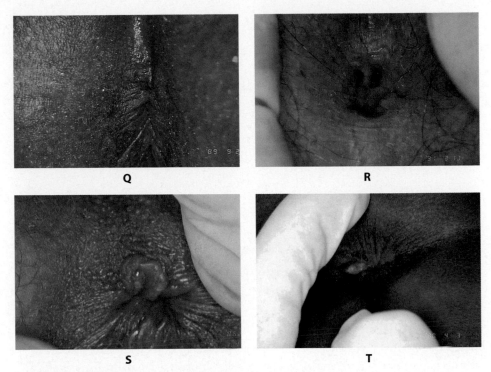

FIGURE 9.14, *continued*
Acute genital and anal trauma and healed residual.

Q: Same patient as in 9.14P at final follow-up examination 10 months after acute injury. Note minimal distortion of the rugal pattern. With traction and flattening of verge tissues, a small avascular area remains.

R: A 12 1/2-year-old girl has healed laceration of the anal sphincter at 10, 5, and 7 o'clock positions. Anus remains open without traction. Rectal tone is dramatically diminished, and no reflex constriction occurs.

S: A 14-year-old girl has a posttraumatic anal tag, the result of resorbed hematoma of anal verge tissue after penile anal penetration.

T: A 4-year-old boy has a hypopigmented area in the anal verge with neovascularity apparent as granulation tissue continues to mature.

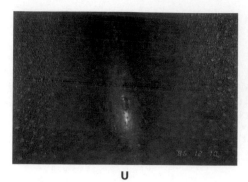
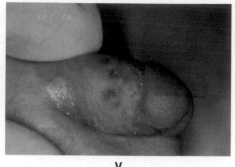

U   V

FIGURE 9.14, *continued*
Acute genital and anal trauma and healed residual.

U: A 3-year-old boy has superficial ulceration of the gluteal crease, which represents residual to the rubbing of the ventral side of a penis between the buttocks.

V: A 3-year-old boy has circumferential bite marks to the shaft of the penis.

included perianal erythema (41%), increased perianal pigmentation (30%), venous congestion (73%), anal dilatation (49%), skin tags (11%), and scars (2%). Also described were congenital smooth areas in 26% of the children. These "smooth fan-shaped areas in the midline of the verge, either with or without depressions, appeared to be a congenital anomaly of the superficial division of external sphincter muscle fibers." This particular finding has the potential to be misinterpreted as scar tissue. Once more, a history of injury must be obtained before concluding that scar tissue is present.

Trauma to the anal verge may result in a localized collection of blood distorting the anal verge. After resorption of the hematoma, a small tag of loose skin may remain.[104] The most commonly observed perianal tags are congenital. A prominent extension of the median raphe, a normal variation of anatomy, may extend into the anal verge and appear similar to a tag.

Children have difficulty in determining whether an object has been placed "in" their anorectal canal. Pressure over the external anal verge tissues may cause a slight dilation of the anus and thus be perceived as "in" when, in fact, penetration into the canal per se did not occur. Therefore reliance on the child's perception of the experience as confirmatory of penetration should be approached with caution until further studies address the accuracy of a child's ability to differentiate "in" from "on" at varying developmental stages.

The most common object to penetrate the anus of a child is a digit. A digit can be readily introduced into the anus repeatedly without discomfort or residua. When reviewing a history of penetration, it is important to determine whether the child had any discomfort associated with the contact, whether there was discomfort following the event, and any associated observations. A simple question to ask the child is

"What did it feel like when it happened?" If the child responds that it hurt, clarify whether it was his feelings or his body that hurt. If the child complained of physical discomfort or pain following anal penetration, the child should be asked to explain how he experienced the discomfort and whether he observed anything that made him know he was hurt. The child might respond that he observed blood when wiping self or on stool with passage of a bowel movement. When there has been trauma to the anoderm the child may express experiencing a burning sensation with passage of a bowel movement.

When examining the anus for residua to penetration, male patients are best examined in the left lateral decubitus position, a position in which they have not experienced the alleged abuse (Figure 9.6). If a child has a history of chronic abuse, and no acute abnormalities are observed externally, anoscopy will provide little additional information and is not recommended. The digital rectal examination also provides little information to assist the examiner in determining if a child has been anally assaulted. If, however, on anoscopy or digital rectal examination the child provides a spontaneous utterance likening the experience to that of the penetrating event, this valuable disclosure information should be recorded as the child's verbatim statement. If the anus dilates, the presence or absence of stool should be noted. Reflex dilation of the anus with stool in the rectal ampulla is a normal response.

When acute signs of injury to the anal verge tissue are observed, anoscopy is then important to identify the presence of lacerations, petechiae, bruising of the anorectal canal, and seminal products. Surprisingly, external signs of trauma may be minimal in patients with significant acute internal injuries to the anorectal canal. Accidental impaling injuries involving the anus and perineum are readily differentiated from sexual assault both in their pattern and the history of their presentation.

Male Genitalia

When examining the male genitalia the medical record should document the following: (a) Tanner stage, (b) circumcision status, (c) retractability of foreskin if uncircumcised, (d) appearance of glans and frenulum, (e) urethral discharge, (f) any signs of injury to the glans or shaft of the penis, (g) the location of testes, (h) signs of scrotal trauma, (i) presence of hernias, and (j) inguinal adenopathy.

Injury to the male genitalia may include superficial abrasions to the shaft, petechiae, tears of the frenulum of the glans, bruising, and bite marks. When superficial injuries are present, an accompanying history of fondling, masturbation, and/or oral-genital contact is frequently present. Under most circumstances, there are no residua to these activities. Occasionally the male genitalia may have evidence of a patterned injury that was the result of physical discipline striking the genitalia but without the genitalia being the target organ from a sexual perspective.

Residua of Sexual Contact

Patterns of Trauma

The difficulties associated with the retrospective interpretation of the residua of sexual contact are numerous. Few physical findings represent definitive evidence of sexual assault.[105] When a child presents with acute injuries, the pattern and extent of the trauma should be documented. The spectrum of acute injury is variable, involving superficial mucosal abrasions and scratches to clear transecting lacerations of genital and anal structures.[106] Superficial injuries and signs of irritation may be subtle and nonspecific. The extent of injury depends on many variables, most significant of which is the degree of force, the object used to inflict the injury, and the nature of the contact, with particular reference to whether penetration occurred.

The legal and medical definitions of penetration differ. The medical definition of penetration is "the passing into the deeper tissues or into a cavity."[77] From a strictly medical perspective, penetration in regard to the female genitalia implies the introduction of an object between the labia, through the hymenal orifice, and into the posterior portion of the vagina. As previously cited, children frequently state that an object was placed inside of them when corroborating evidence is not present. Most penetration of children is akin to the legal definition, which is "the insertion of the male part into the female parts to however slight an extent; and by which insertion the offense is complete without proof of an emission."[107] Certainly, any genital-to-genital or genital-to-anal contact is inappropriate, regardless of the depth of penetration.

In genital fondling of the female, the hand is usually placed over the mons pubis and the index and third finger separate the labia and enter the vaginal vestibule. Rubbing of the tissues bordering the vaginal vestibule may acutely demonstrate evidence of erythema, superficially denuded mucosa, abrasions/scratches, and edema of the inner aspects of the labia minora and the periurethral area. Generally, fondling/ penetration between the labia results in injuries between the 9 and 3 o'clock positions, with the child supine, and less likely to involve the fourchette or fossa. Most fondling/digital penetration contact does not result in serious trauma, but the forceful introduction of a finger into the vagina can result in significant trauma due to the limited elasticity of the prepubertal hymen.

Depending on the differential between the hymenal orifice size and the penetrating digit, the child may have either no residua from introduction through the orifice or a laceration of the membrane edge. Acute injuries to the hymen should be readily apparent, although injury to the hymenal membrane or fossa as a result of fondling is infrequent.

Children who are fondled and experience trauma to the periurethral area may complain of dysuria after the alleged event. This symptom is specific to irritation/inflammation of the distal urethra. If a history of dysuria is obtained in a non-leading and non-suggestive manner, it is valuable corroborating history of sexual contact and may be admissible in court. In a review of 105 cases meeting inclusion criteria, 23% of fondled children provided a history of post-fondling dysuria. All of these children answered standard questions that were non-leading and non-suggestive.

Dysuria also can be a posttraumatic event, occurring during vulvar coitus. This form of genital-to-genital contact also may be perceived by the child as penetrating. In vulvar coitus, the shaft of the penis is rubbed between the labia and can result in abrasions and bruising of the inner aspects of the labia minora. The penis can cause trauma to the periurethral/clitoral hood region and the fourchette as well. Because the hymenal membrane is recessed in the vaginal canal, vulvar coitus is not likely to result in injury to the hymenal orifice. Berkowitz et al[108] reported that trauma to the external surface of the hymenal membrane occurring within the context of vulvar coitus resulted in scar tissue, presumably creating a stenosis of a previously larger orifice, creating the appearance of an acquired imperforate hymen. Dysuria also may follow coitus. Dysuria associated with coitus is commonly referred to as *honeymoon cystitis.*[109]

When genital-to-anal contact occurs frequently, the dorsal side of the shaft of the penis is rubbed over the external anal verge tissues, causing pressure on the external sphincter, which may be perceived as penetration in the anorectal canal. When the shaft is rubbed between the buttocks over the natal cleft, it may result in superficial abrasions. This

activity is commonly referred to by boys as "freaking." When either vulvar coitus or natal cleft rubbing occurs, the individual may ejaculate, and seminal products may be collected from the abdomen, inner thighs, buttocks, and back.

When an object forcefully penetrates the vagina through the hymenal orifice in a young child, residual signs are generally obvious when examined acutely. This type of penetration will most likely result in a laceration to the edge of the membrane that extends to the vaginal floor. Most lacerations are seen between the 5 and 7 o'clock positions with the child supine but can be seen anywhere between the 3 and 9 o'clock positions. Forceful penetration also may result in lacerations to the fossa navicularis, the lateral walls of the vagina, and possible perforation of the posterior fornix into the peritoneum.[104,110] Although most lacerations of the hymen stop at the floor of the vagina, some extend through the fossa and fourchette and into the perineal body. This type of injury is readily recognizable, and its full extent must be assessed with the child under anesthesia.

Accidental injuries to the genitalia do occur, and the pattern of trauma and the accompanying history are usually suggestive of its etiology.[111,112] Most accidental injuries are the result of a child falling on a horizontal bar of a bicycle, jungle gym, or the classic picket fence. The horizontal bar usually results in a crush injury of the clitoral hood/labia minora between the bar and the inner aspect of the thigh. This injury is usually unilateral. Picket injuries are more likely to be impaling. Occasionally, the forceful abduction of thighs results in a superficial laceration of the perineum. One report of injury to the genitalia occurred as a result of a seat belt.[113] Masturbation is unlikely to result in any injuries to the genitalia other than localized erythema or superficial abrasions as the result of rubbing. Children do insert objects between the labia, but they rarely do so in a forceful way that would result in injury because of the exquisite sensitivity of the hymenal tissue.

Rubbing of the inner aspects of the labia occurring either in the context of vulvar coitus, genital fondling, or possibly masturbation can result in inflammation. Because of the close proximity of the inner aspects of the inflamed labia minora in prepubertal children, the mucosal surfaces may agglutinate. Labial agglutination is an acquired postinflammatory condition seen only in the prepubertal child and involves the thin, unestrogenized vascular tissues of the inner aspect of the labia minora. The ability to examine the hymenal membrane may be compromised depending on the degree of fusion. The agglutination may extend from the fourchette to the clitoral hood with only a minute opening for urine to escape, creating the appearance of an "absent" vagina. Although labial agglutination is a common finding in young children, its association as a residual to sexual abuse was described only recently.[114–116] Caution should be exercised if agglutination is the only abnormal finding on examination. When agglutination is present, it can be medically dehisced by estrogen cream. "Gentle traction," as described in standard texts, should not be used because it results only in denuded edges that are painful and quickly re-adhere, making reexamination even more difficult.

Extra-genital signs of trauma are infrequent in most cases of child sexual abuse. When they do occur, they usually occur within the context of rape. If a child is forced to perform fellatio on an individual, tears to the labial frenulum and petechiae of the palate may be noted. Injuries reflective of force and restraint may be seen as ligature marks around the wrists and ankles. Bruising of the extremities may appear as grasp marks. Bite marks may be present on the neck, breast, buttocks, or inner thighs.

Retrospective Interpretation

Most children do not present for an examination immediately after their alleged sexual abuse; therefore, few children will have acute signs of injury or evidence to collect.[57] Thus the clinician is required to examine tissues that have healed. Without knowledge of the premorbid appearance of the genital tissues, it is difficult to judge whether a particular finding is the direct result of sexual abuse. Several clinical scenarios can occur. First, the child may be seen long after the last episode of alleged contact, and thus only healed residua can be observed. Second, the child may have experienced genital or anal trauma resulting in residua and is being examined during the period of formation of granulation tissue and no obvious acute injury. Third, the child may present when nonspecific findings are present, and the physician must correlate the history of the alleged contact and the findings as residual to that contact. Finally, the child may present with acute signs of injury, the least problematic situation to evaluate. The pathology of healing is well understood.[117] These principles of healing have only recently been applied to genital and anal injuries for a prospective look at how acute injuries heal.[58,118] Observations by Finkel[58] on the healing chronology of genital and anal injuries have laid the foundation for our understanding of the retrospective interpretation of changes in genital and anal anatomy. Studies by McCann et al[118] and Heppenstall-Heger et al[119] have continued to elucidate the residua to genital and anal trauma.

Formulating a Conclusion

In formulating a diagnostic assessment, the clinician must consider (a) historical details and behavioral indicators reflective of the contact, (b) symptoms that result from the contact, (c) acute genital/anal injuries and/or chronic residua, (d) forensic evidence, and (e) STIs. The medical assessment only rarely can stand on its own because of the relative infrequency of findings that are diagnostic. The diagnosis will reflect a combination of disclosure evidence, behaviors, medical history, physical examination, and laboratory/evidentiary results.

The following are examples of these common scenarios:

1. Medical history/behaviors are clear and descriptive of inappropriate sexual contact but no physical examination findings present.
2. Medical history/behaviors are clear and descriptive of inappropriate sexual contact with symptom-specific complaints reflective of genital and/or anal trauma.
3. Medical history/behaviors are clear and descriptive of inappropriate sexual contact and physical examination findings are present (ie, acute/healed injuries, STI, other physical forensic evidence).
4. Medical history/behaviors are suspicious and/or concerning that the child either experienced something inappropriate and/or was exposed to something inappropriate and the examination is without physical examination findings.
5. Medical findings that mimic sexual abuse but on evaluation are associated with medical conditions and not the result of abuse.
6. Observed inappropriate sexual interactions without physical examination findings. (Common scenario with young children with sexually reactive behaviors.)
7. Insufficient historical, behavioral, or physical examination findings to support suspicion that the child experienced anything of a sexually inappropriate nature.
8. Physical examination and/or laboratory studies diagnostic of sexual contact without supporting history.

The evaluation of a child alleged to have been sexually abused is a challenging and emotionally charged issue. The need for a balanced objective and defensible opinion could not be more evident than when addressing this issue. As the medical profession and society at large has increased its awareness of and ability to respond to the issue of sexual victimization and exploitation of children, fewer children will be victimized. The pediatrician can play an extremely important role in education about and the prevention of sexual abuse as well as recognition, evaluation, and referral. Children and parents would be well served if pediatricians routinely as a part of the annual health maintenance assessments spoke to children and parents beginning at age 3 years about the importance of personal space and privacy. Four simple messages to children and parents may reduce the potential for victimization and increase the likelihood of disclosure. These suggestions are (1) Teach children about "OK and not OK" touching. Although this knowledge may not prevent sexual abuse it can increase a child's awareness of the issue and the likelihood of disclosure. (2) Teach children who can and under what circumstances someone can touch their private parts. (3) Teach children the appropriate names for their private parts so they have the language to communicate if something happens. (4) Teach children that secrets are never OK because it is the secrecy of sexual abuse that allows the activities to occur and continue over time. Teach children that surprises are OK but if anyone tells them to keep something secret or they think they should keep it secret, they must tell a parent or trusted adult.

Sexual victimization has the potential for profound life long adverse effects on a developing child. With education and primary prevention the pediatrician can help to reduce the potential for victimization.[120,121]

References

1. Bach CM, Anderson SC. Adolescent sexual abuse and assault. *J Curr Adolesc Med.* 1980;1:285-293
2. Cantwell H. Vaginal inspection as it relates to child sexual abuse in girls under thirteen. *Child Abuse Negl.* 1981;7:171
3. DeJong AR, Emment GA, Hervada AR. Sexual abuse of children: sex-race and age dependent variations. *Am J Dis Child.* 1982;136:129–134
4. Ellerstein NS, Canavan JW. Sexual abuse of boys. *Am J Dis Child.* 1980;134:255–257
5. Elliott DM, Briere J. Posttraumatic stress associated with delayed recall of sexual abuse: a general population study. *J Trauma Stress.* 1995;8:629–647
6. Giardino A, Finkel MA. *A Practical Guide to the Evaluation of Sexual Abuse in the Prepubertal Child.* Newbury Park, CA: Sage Publications; 1992
7. Hobbs CJ, Wynne JM. Buggery in childhood—a common syndrome of child abuse. *Lancet.* 1986;2510:792–796
8. Jaffee AC, Dynneson L, TenBensel RW. Sexual abuse of children: an epidemiologic study. *Am J Dis Child.* 1975;129:689–692
9. Kempe CH. Sexual abuse, another hidden pediatric problem: the 1977 C Anderson Aldrich lecture. *Pediatrics.* 1978;62:382–389
10. Paul DM. The medical examination in sexual offenses. *Med Sci Law.* 1975;15:154
11. Rimsza ME, Niggeman MS. Medical evaluation of sexually abused children: a review of 311 cases. *Pediatrics.* 1982;69:8–14
12. Spencer MJ, Dunklee P. Sexual abuse of boys. *Pediatrics.* 1986;78:133–138
13. Tilleli JA, Turek D, Jaffee AC. Sexual abuse in children. *N Engl J Med.* 1980;302:319–323

14. Wolak J, Finkelhor D, Mitchell K. Internet-initiated sex crimes against minors: implications for prevention based on findings of a national study. *J Adolesc Health*. 2004;35:e11–e20

15. Finkel MA. Technical conduct of the child sexual abuse medical examination. *Child Abuse Negl*. 1998;22:555–566

16. Burgess AW, Holmstrom LL. Sexual trauma of children and adolescents. *Nurs Clin North Am*. 1975;10:551–563

17. Burgess AW, Holmstrom LL. Coping behavior of the rape victim. *Am Psychiatry*. 1976;133:413–418

18. Finkelhor DH. *Sexually Victimized Children*. New York, NY: The Free Press; 1979

19. Green AH. True and false allegations of sexual abuse in child custody disputes. *J Am Acad Child Psychiatry*. 1986;25:449–456

20. Sgroi SM. *Handbook of Clinical Intervention in Child Sexual Abuse*. Books I., ed. Lexington, MA: DC Heath and Co; 1982

21. Summit RC. The child sexual abuse accommodation syndrome. *Child Abuse Negl*. 1983;7:177–193

22. Centers for Disease Control and Prevention. Youth risk behavior surveillance—United States. *MMWR Morb Mortal Wkly Rep*. 1996;45:1–3

23. Finkelhor DH, ed. *Child Sexual Abuse New Theory and Research*. New York, NY: The Free Press; 1984

24. Finkelhor D, Hotaling GT. Sexual abuse in the National Incidence Study of Child Abuse and Neglect: an appraisal. *Child Abuse Negl*. 1984;8:23–32

25. Finkelhor DH, Browne A. Assessing the long term impact on child sexual abuse: a review and conceptualization. In: Walker LEA, ed. *Handbook on Sexual Abuse of Children—Assessment and Treatment Issues*. New York, NY: Springer; 1988

26. Finkelhor D, Hotaling G, Lewis IA, Smith C. Sexual abuse in a national survey of adult men and women: prevalence, characteristics, and risk factors. *Child Abuse Negl*. 1990;14:19–28

27. Krugman RD. Recognition of sexual abuse in children. *Pediatr Rev*. 1986;8:25–30

28. National Center on Child Abuse and Neglect. *Study Findings—Study of National Incidence and Prevalence of Child Abuse and Neglect, 1988*. Washington, DC: US Department of Health and Human Services; 1988

29. Rosenfeld AA, ed. Sexual abuse of children: personal and professional responses. In: Newberger EH, ed. *Child Abuse*. Boston, MA: Little Brown; 1982

30. Vander Mey BJ. The sexual victimization of male children: a review of previous research. *Child Abuse Negl*. 1988;12:61–72

31. Lynch L, Faust J. Reduction of distress in children undergoing sexual abuse medical examination. *J Pediatr*. 1998;133:296–299

32. Finkelhor D, Browne A. The traumatic impact of child sexual abuse: a conceptualization. *Am J Orthopsychiatry*. 1985;55:530–541

33. Cronch LE, Viljoen JL, Hansen DJ. Forensic interviewing in child sexual abuse cases: current techniques and future directions. *Aggress Violent Behav*. 2006;11:195–207

34. Boat BW, Everson MD. Use of anatomical dolls among professionals in sexual abuse evaluations. *Child Abuse Negl*. 1988;12:171–179

35. Goodwin J. Evaluation and treatment for incest victims and their families: a problem-oriented approach. In: Goodwin J, ed. *Sexual Abuse*. Chicago, IL: Yearbook; 1989

36. White S, Strom GA, Santilli G, Halpin BM. Interviewing young sexual abuse victims with anatomically correct dolls. *Child Abuse Negl*. 1986;10:519–529

37. MacFarlane K, Kerbs S. Techniques for interviewing and evidence gathering. In: MacFarlane K, ed. *Sexual Abuse of Young Children*. New York, NY: The Guilford Press; 1987

38. Green HA, ed. Overview of normal psychosexual development. In: Green AH, Schetky DH, eds. *Child Sexual Abuse: A Handbook for Health Care and Legal Professionals.* New York, NY: Brunner Mazel Publishers; 1988

39. Jampole L, Weber MK. An assessment of the behavior of sexually abused and nonsexually abused children with anatomically correct dolls. *Child Abuse Negl.* 1987;11:187–192

40. Long S. Guidelines for treating young children. In: MacFarlane K, ed. *Sexual Abuse of Young Children.* New York, NY: The Guilford Press; 1987

41. Jones DPH, McQuiston M. *Interviewing the Sexually Abused Child.* 2nd ed. Denver, CO: C. Henry Kempe National Center for the Prevention and Treatment of Child Abuse and Neglect; 1986

42. Myers JEB. Role of physician in preserving verbal evidence of child abuse. *J Pediatr.* 1986;109:409–411

43. Myers JEB. *Legal Issues in Child Abuse and Neglect Practice.* 2nd ed. Thousand Oaks, CA: Sage; 1998:102–152

44. Finkelhor D. *Child Sexual Abuse: New Theory and Research.* New York, NY: The Free Press; 1984:150–170

45. Holmes WC, Slap GB. Sexual abuse of boys: definition, prevalence, correlates, sequelae, and management [see comments]. *JAMA.* 1998;2801:1855–1862

46. West DJ. Boys and sexual abuse: an English opinion. *Arch Sex Behav.* 1998;27:539–559

47. Friedrich WN, Beilke RL, Urquiza AJ. Behavior problems in young sexually abused boys: a comparison study. *J Interpers Violence.* 1988;3:21–28

48. Mitchell KJ, Finkelhor D, Wolak J. Protecting youth online: family use of filtering and blocking software. *Child Abuse Negl.* 2005;29:749–752

49. Donald TG. Pediatric male rectal and genital trauma: accidental and nonaccidental injuries. *Pediatr Emerg Care.* 1998;14:452–453

50. Kadish HA, Schunk JE, Britton H. Pediatric male rectal and genital trauma: accidental and nonaccidental injuries. *Pediatr Emerg Care.* 1998;14:95–98

51. Reinhart MA. Sexually abused boys. *Child Abuse Negl.* 1987;11:229–235

52. Boudewyn AC, Liem JH. Childhood sexual abuse as a precursor to depression and self-destructive behavior in adulthood. *J Trauma Stress.* 1995;8:445–459

53. Brown LK, Kessel SM, Lourie KJ, Ford HH, Lipsitt L. Influence of sexual abuse on HIV-related attitudes and behaviors in adolescent psychiatric inpatients. *J Am Acad Child Adolesc Psychiatry.* 1997;36:316–322

54. Wolfe DA, Sas L, Wekerle C. Factors associated with the development of posttraumatic stress disorder among child victims of sexual abuse. *Child Abuse Negl.* 1994;18:37–50

55. Makoroff KL, Brauley JL, Brander AM, Myers A, Shapiro RA. Genital examinations for alleged sexual abuse of prepubertal girls: findings by pediatric emergency medicine physicians compared with child abuse trained physicians. *Child Abuse Negl.* 2002;262:1235–1242

56. Wright RJ, Wright RO, Farnan L, Isaac NE. Response to child abuse in the pediatric emergency department: need for continued education. *Pediatr Emerg Care.* 1999;15:376–382

57. Heger A, Ticson L, Velasquez O, Bernier R. Children referred for possible sexual abuse: a comparison of clinical history and medical findings in 2384 children. *Child Abuse Negl.* 2002;26:645–659

58. Finkel MA. Anogenital trauma in sexually abused children. *Pediatrics.* 1989;84:317–322

59. Parker RI, Mahan RA, Giugliano D, Parker MM. Efficacy and safety of intravenous midazolam and ketamine as sedation for therapeutic and diagnostic procedures in children [see comments]. *Pediatrics.* 1997;99:427–431

60. Finkel MA, Giardino A. *Medical Evaluation of Child Sexual Abuse: A Practical Guide*. Newbury Park, CA: Sage Publications; 2002:81–84

61. Adams JA, Ahmad M, Philips P. Anogenital findings and hymenal diameter in children referred for sexual abuse examination. *Adolesc Pediatr Gynecol*. 1988;1:123

62. Bays J, Chewning M, Kelter L, Sewell R, Steinberg B, Thomas P. Changes in hymenal anatomy during examination of prepubertal girls for possible sexual abuse. *Adolesc Pediatr Gynecol*. 1990;3:42

63. Emans SJ, Goldstein D. The gynecologic examination of the prepubertal child with vulvovaginitis: use of the knee-chest position. *Pediatrics*. 1980;65:758–760

64. Herman-Giddens ME, Frothingham TE. Prepubertal female genitalia: examination for evidence of sexual abuse. *Pediatrics*. 1987;80:203–208

65. McCann J, Wells R, Simon M, Voris J. Genital findings in prepubertal girls selected for nonabuse: a descriptive study. *Pediatrics*. 1990;86:428–439

66. McCann J, Voris J. Perianal injuries resulting from sexual abuse: a longitudinal study. *Pediatrics*. 1993;91:390–397

67. Paradise JE. The medical evaluation of the sexually abused child. *Pediatr Clin North Am*. 1990;37:839–862

68. Davies J. Anatomy of the female genital tract. In: Danforth D, ed. *Danforth's Obstetrics and Gynecology*. 6th ed. Philadelphia, PA: Lippincott; 1990

69. Ricci LR. Medical forensic photography of the sexually abused child. *Child Abuse Negl*. 1988;12:305–310

70. Ferris DG, Willner WA, Ho JJ. Colpophotography systems: a review [erratum in J Fam Pract. 1992;34:25]. *J Fam Pract*. 1991;33:633–639

71. Finkel MA, Ricci LR. Documentation and preservation of visual evidence in child abuse. *Child Maltreat*. 1997;2:322–330

72. American Board of Forensic Odontology. Guidelines for bite mark analysis. *J Am Dent Assoc*. 1986;112:383–386

73. Gray H. *Anatomy of the Human Body*. Philadelphia, PA: Lea & Febiger; 1985

74. MacNaulty AS. *British Medical Dictionary*. Philadelphia, PA: Lippincott; 1961

75. Pritchard JA, ed. Anatomy of the reproductive tract of woman. In: Cunningham FG, MacDonald C, Grant NC, eds. *Williams Obstetrics*. Norwalk, CT: Appleton-Century-Crofts; 1985

76. Sloane E. *Biology of Women*. New York, NY: Wiley and Sons; 1985

77. *Stedman's Medical Dictionary*. Baltimore, MD: Williams and Wilkins; 1990

78. White ST, Ingram DL, Lyna R. Vaginal introital diameter in the evaluation of sexual abuse. *Child Abuse Negl*. 1989;13:217–224

79. Wile IS. The psychology of the hymen. *J Nerv Ment Dis*. 1937(February):143–156

80. Jenny C, Kuhns ML, Arakawa F. Hymens in newborn female infants. *Pediatrics*. 1987;80:399–400

81. Mor N, Merlob P, Reisner SH. Tags and bands of the female external genitalia in the newborn infant. *Clin Pediatr (Phila)*. 1983;22:122–124

82. Pokorny SF. Configuration of the prepubertal hymen. *Am J Obstet Gynecol*. 1987;157:950–956

83. Mahran M, Saleh AM. The microscopic anatomy of hymen. *Anat Rec*. 1964;149:313–318

84. Gelhor G. Anatomy, pathology and development of the hymen. *Am J Obstet Dis Women Child*. 1904;50:161

85. Emans SJ, Woods ER, Flagg NT, Freeman A. Genital findings in sexually abused, symptomatic and asymptomatic, girls. *Pediatrics*. 1987;79:778–785

86. Lauber AA, Souma ML. Use of toluidine blue for documentation of traumatic intercourse. *Obstet Gynecol*. 1982;60:644–648

87. McCann J. The appearance of acute, healing, and healed anogenital trauma. *Child Abuse Negl*. 1998;22:605–615; discussion 617–622

88. Deuterman JL, Gabby SL. Imperforate hymen. *Illinois Med J*. 1942;82:161

89. Berenson A, Heger A, Andrews S. Appearance of the hymen in newborns. *Pediatrics.* 1991;87:458–465

90. Merlob P, Bahari C, Liban E, Reisner SH. Cysts of the female external genitalia in the newborn infant. *Am J Obstet Gynecol.* 1978;132:607–610

91. Myhre AK, Berntzen K, Bratlid D. Genital anatomy in non-abused preschool girls. *Acta Paediatr.* 2003;922:1378–1380

92. Goff CW, Burke KR, Rickenback C, Buebendorf DP. Vaginal opening measurement in prepubertal girls. *Am J Dis Child.* 1989;143:1366–1368

93. Heger A, Emans SJ. Introital diameter as the criterion for sexual abuse [comment]. *Pediatrics.* 1990;85:222–223

94. Paradise JE. Predictive accuracy and the diagnosis of sexual abuse: a big issue about a little tissue. *Child Abuse Negl.* 1989;13:169–176

95. Muram D. Child sexual abuse: relationship between sexual acts and genital findings. *Child Abuse Negl.* 1989;13:211–216

96. Kellogg N, American Academy of Pediatrics Committee on Child Abuse and Neglect. Evaluation of sexual abuse in children. *Pediatrics.* 2005;116:506–512

97. Bond GR, Dowd MD, Landsman I, Rimsza M. Unintentional perineal injury in prepubescent girls: a multicenter, prospective report of 56 girls. *Pediatrics.* 1995;95:628–631

98. Boos SC. Accidental hymenal injury mimicking sexual trauma. *Pediatrics.* 1999;103:1287–1290

99. Emans SJ, Woods ER, Allred EN, Grace E. Hymenal findings in adolescent women: impact of tampon use and consensual sexual activity. *J Pediatr.* 1994;125:153–160

100. Muram D. Anal and perianal abnormalities in prepubertal victims of sexual abuse. *Am J Obstet Gynecol.* 1989;161:278–281

101. Clayden GS. Reflex anal dilatation associated with severe chronic constipation in children [see comments]. *Arch Dis Child.* 1988;63:832–836

102. Hobbs CJ, Wynne JM. Sexual abuse of English boys and girls: the importance of anal examination. *Child Abuse Negl.* 1989;13:195–210

103. Stanton A, Sunderland R. Prevalence of reflex anal dilatation in 200 children [see comments]. *BMJ.* 1989;298:802–803

104. Paul DM. The medical examination in sexual offenses against children. *Med Sci Law.* 1977;17:251–258

105. Biggs M, Stermac LE, Divinsky M. Genital injuries following sexual assault of women with and without prior sexual intercourse experience. *CMAJ.* 1998;159:33–37

106. Norrel MK, Benrub GI, Thompson RJ. Investigation of the microtrauma after sexual intercourse. *J Reprod Med.* 1984;29:269–271

107. *Blacks Law Dictionary.* 5th ed. St Paul, MN: West Publishing; 1979

108. Berkowitz CD, Elvik SL, Logan M. A simulated "acquired" imperforate hymen following the genital trauma of sexual abuse. *Clin Pediatr.* 1987;26:307–309

109. Macklin M. Honeymoon cystitis [letter]. *N Engl J Med.* 1978;2988:1035

110. Paul DM. What really happened to baby Jane? The medical aspects of the investigation of alleged sexual abuse of children. *Med Sci Law.* 1986;26:85–102

111. Dowd MD, Fitzmaurice L, Knapp JF, Mooney D. The interpretation of urogenital findings in children with straddle injuries. *J Pediatr Surg.* 1994;29:7–10

112. Waltzman ML, Shannon M, Bowen AP, Bailey MC. Monkeybar injuries: complications of play. *Pediatrics.* 1999;103:e58

113. Baker RB. Seat belt injury masquerading as sexual abuse [letter]. *Pediatrics.* 1986;77:435

114. Berkowitz CD. Sexual abuse of children and adolescents. *Adv Pediatr.* 1987;34:275–312

115. Berkowitz CD, Elvik SL, Logan MK. Labial fusion in prepubescent girls: a marker for sexual abuse? *Am J Obstet Gynecol.* 1987;156:16–20

116. McCann J, Voris J, Simon M. Labial adhesions and posterior fourchette injuries in childhood sexual abuse. *Am J Dis Child.* 1988;142:659–663

117. Kissane JM, ed. Inflammation and healing. In: Kissane JM, ed. *Anderson's Pathology.* 8th ed. St Louis, MO: CV Mosby; 1985

118. McCann J, Voris J, Simon M. Genital injuries resulting from sexual abuse: a longitudinal study. *Pediatrics.* 1992;89:307–317

119. Heppenstall-Heger A, McConnell G, Ticson L, Guerra L, Lister J, Zaggagoza T. Healing patterns in anogenital injuries: a longitudinal study of injuries associated with sexual abuse, accidental injuries, or genital surgery in the preadolescent child. *Pediatrics.* 2003;112:829–837

120. Dube SR, Felitti VJ, Dong M, Giles WH, Anda RF. The impact of adverse childhood experiences on health problems: evidence from four birth cohorts dating back to 1900. *Prev Med.* 2003;37:268–277

121. Felitti VJ, Anda RF, Nordenberg D, et al. Relationship of childhood abuse and household dysfunction to many of the leading causes of death in adults. The Adverse Childhood Experiences (ACE) Study. *Am J Prev Med.* 1998;14:245–258

Chapter 10

Medical Management of the Adolescent Sexual Abuse/ Assault Victim

Heather Littleton

Department of Psychology
Sam Houston State University

Abbey Berenson

Center for Interdisciplinary Research in Women's Health,
University of Texas Medical Branch

Sexual Abuse and Sexual Assault of Adolescents

Sexual abuse is "the employment, use, persuasion, inducement, enticement, or coercion of any child to engage in sexually explicit conduct or any simulation of such conduct" by an individual who could function as a parent or caretaker.[1] Like prepubertal children, adolescents can be victims of sexual abuse. In addition, many adolescents who were abused before puberty still are experiencing the adverse effects of their earlier experiences.

Data on the prevalence of sexual abuse of adolescents vary considerably across studies, in part due to varying techniques used to assess sexual abuse. For example, some studies evaluated the prevalence of sexual abuse by asking adolescents whether they had been sexually abused and, thus, relied on the adolescents' subjective interpretation of the term *sexual abuse*.[2] In contrast, other studies assessed the prevalence of sexual abuse through the provision of clear descriptions of incidents that would qualify as sexual abuse, with the degree of restrictiveness regarding what incidents would qualify as sexual abuse varying (eg, whether coercion or force was used, whether physical contact occurred).[2] In addition, studies vary in the method in which data were obtained (eg, interview vs self-report), with at least one study suggesting that computerized assessments were more likely to lead to honest reporting compared with a face-to-face interview or paper-and-pencil self-report.[2,3]

Studies of school-based and community samples of adolescents in the United States and other developed countries have found that the prevalence of sexual abuse ranges from 2% to 10% in boys and from 3% to 34% in girls.[4-12] Studies that provided an objective definition of sexual abuse generally reported a higher prevalence of abuse as did studies that included noncontact forms of abuse (eg, exhibitionism). Generally, studies examining the age of the youngster when the abuse began have found the mean age of onset to be between the ages of 9 and 10 years, suggesting that a sizable proportion of victims were sexually abused in adolescence.[13,14] Indeed, a national telephone survey of adults found that 39% of male sexual abuse victims were 12 years or older when the abuse occurred, as were 34% of female victims.[15] Similarly, a study of adult female twins in one US state found that most women reported that their sexual abuse occurred when they were between the ages of 12 and 15 years.[16] In addition, a birth cohort study of New Zealand residents interviewed when they were 18 years old found that 57% of sexual abuse incidents occurred when the individual was between the ages of 11 and 16 years.[17]

Sexual assault is "any genital, anal, or oral penetration, by a part of an individual's body or by an object, using force or without the person's consent," including someone who is unable to consent due to impairment from alcohol or drugs, sleep, or unconsciousness.[18] Adolescents are at much greater risk than prepubertal children of experiencing sexual assault by a peer or acquaintance; however, the prevalence of sexual assault among adolescents has been studied much less frequently than the prevalence of sexual abuse, and has been studied primarily in adolescent girls.

The prevalence of sexual assault among adolescents in community and school samples has ranged from 3% to 16% of females and from 2% to 3% of males.[19-23] Again, studies that used objective criteria to assess the prevalence of sexual assault generally reported a higher prevalence than those that relied on subjective criteria (eg, Have you ever been date raped?). Also, these studies rarely assessed the prevalence of instances of nonconsensual sex that occurred when the adolescent was incapacitated or unconscious. Thus the findings of these studies likely are an underrepresentation of the actual prevalence of sexual assault among adolescents.

Risk Factors

Prior research has not examined adolescent sexual abuse risk factors. General risk factors include growing up in a home where one caregiver is absent[7,15,24] or living in a home in which there is a change in caregivers.[12] In addition, growing up in a home in which there is a high level of marital conflict[12,24] or where one or both parents have substance use problems is associated with an increased risk of being the victim of sexual abuse.[24] Victims of sexual abuse often come from homes in which they are physically abused or in which domestic violence occurs.[7,25] Children who come from these homes typically receive less parental monitoring than their peers, placing them at risk of being targeted by perpetrators.[26,27] In addition, if the adolescent has had multiple caregivers, the likelihood that the child or adolescent is exposed to a sexually abusive caregiver increases. Finally, for some, sexual abuse may occur within a constellation of abusive behaviors perpetrated by a violent family member.[25]

Given that the prevalence of peer sexual assault among adolescent girls is much higher than among boys, it is not surprising that research examining risk factors for peer sexual assault has focused almost exclusively on girls. One of the most consistently found risk factors for sexual assault in adolescence is a history of childhood abuse, especially sexual abuse.[12,21,28–31] In addition, the greater the severity of prior sexual abuse (eg, abuse involved penetration, abuse of longer duration) as well as the more recent the sexual abuse, the stronger the association with risk of sexual assault.[12,28] Early initiation of dating or sexual activity and having multiple sexual partners also have been found to be associated with increased risk of sexual assault in adolescence.[30–33] Substance use, particularly potentially problematic drinking or drug use, is associated with an increased risk of sexual assault during adolescence as well.[21,29,34] Finally, adolescents who have previously experienced sexual assault are more likely to experience a subsequent assault.[34]

Evaluation of the Adolescent Patient for Experiences of Sexual Abuse or Assault

It is important for health care providers who work with adolescents to understand that many adolescents will not spontaneously disclose sexual abuse or assault and, indeed, many will never have discussed their sexual abuse or assault with anyone prior to the health care visit. Adolescents often report being afraid of the effects disclosing the abuse will have on family members and may view themselves as partly responsible for the abuse.[35] Other reasons adolescents do not disclose sexual abuse or assault include instability in the family and fears that disclosure will lead to further family disruption, concerns about being blamed for the abuse, concerns regarding the consequences of having the abuse brought to the attention of authorities, and concerns about loss of privileges (eg, dating, late curfew), particularly in the case of peer sexual assault.[36]

Another reason that adolescents do not disclose abuse is because they do not consider the experience as abuse or assault. Many instances of sexual abuse do not involve the use of overt violence on the part of the perpetrator. Instead, victims are progressively "groomed" through use of punishment and rewards and a gradual escalation in abusive behavior. In addition, perpetrators often report that they select victims on the basis of their perceived vulnerability, such as low self-esteem or loneliness.[37] As a result, many adolescents are unsure if their experience was really abuse.[36] In addition, many victims have ambivalent feelings toward the abuser, such as feelings of love or dependency, as well as feelings of hatred.[37] Similarly, many instances of peer sexual assault do not involve severe violence and occur within the context of a friendship or romantic relationship. As a result, more than half of victims of sexual assault do not consider their experience as a rape or sexual assault, and instead give the experience a more benign label such as a miscommunication.[38]

Given these impediments to disclosure, it is imperative that health care providers routinely screen for sexual violence among their adolescent patients. This screening should be conducted using behaviorally specific questions. Box 10.1 provides screening questions that could be used with adolescents.[39,40] In evaluating adolescents for a history of sexual abuse or assault, it is important to establish a trusting and nonjudgmental atmosphere. This can be done by expressing concern about the adolescent's sexual, as well as general, health and not responding in a judgmental manner to disclosures by the adolescent regarding behaviors such as substance use and consensual sexual activity.[18] In addition, discussion about the adolescent's experiences of sexual violence should be done when parents or caregivers are not present and should be conducted in private. Introducing the topic of sexual violence after discussion of more general topics with the adolescent is also recommended to increase his or her comfort level.

If an adolescent reports having experienced sexual abuse or sexual assault, the provider needs to first ascertain how long ago the abuse or assault occurred, or in the case of multiple abusive experiences, how long ago the most recent abuse occurred. If the adolescent reports having experienced sexual abuse or assault within the past 72 hours, a forensic examination should be performed.[41,42] Often, these examinations are conducted in a hospital setting or a specialized clinic. The adolescent should be assisted with setting up an appointment for this evaluation, and transportation to the forensic examination should be provided to increase the likelihood that the adolescent will attend the appointment.[42]

The provider also needs to determine whether the abuse/assault experience has been previously reported and, if not, whether he or she is legally obligated to make a report. All states require reporting of sexual relationships between a child and an individual in a caretaking role.[1] In contrast, most states

BOX 10.1
Example of Screening Questions for Sexual Abuse and Sexual Assault Experiences

- Has anyone, male or female, ever tried or succeeded in touching you in a sexual way or having any kind of sexual contact with you that you did not want?
- Have you ever had a sexual experience with someone older or someone who had authority over you such as a doctor, teacher, minister, therapist, babysitter, or any other older person?
- Have you ever had sexual contact with a relative such as an uncle, brother, father, grandfather, mother, stepparent, or sister?
- Have you ever had any kind of sexual contact with someone that you did not want because you were asleep, unconscious, or "out of it," such as from using alcohol or drugs?
- Have you ever had someone threaten to hurt you or actually use physical force to make you have any kind of sexual contact with them?
- Have you had any other upsetting sexual experiences that you haven't mentioned yet?

do not require reporting of peer sexual assaults, provided the victim is older than a certain age[1]; however, it should be noted that some states increasingly are requiring reporting of instances of statutory rape (ie, intercourse between an individual considered to be a minor and an adult) and, thus, certain incidents of peer sexual assault may need to be reported under statutory rape laws.[1]

In addition, the provider needs to obtain a comprehensive sexual history from the adolescent, including information about consensual sexual experiences, prior menstrual history, and use of contraceptives.[43] Similarly, the provider needs to inquire about potential physical health sequelae of experiencing sexual abuse, including pain or signs of pregnancy

in females and symptoms of sexually transmitted infections.[18,44] Finally, the provider needs to obtain information about the general nature of the abuse so that he or she will know how best to help the patient. Other important information includes the patient's relationship with the assailant, whether the abuse is ongoing, the exact nature of the abuse, if others know about the abuse, whether the adolescent noticed any injuries as a result of the sexual abuse, and if the adolescent patient is experiencing other types of violence. An example of a form that could be used when working with an adolescent who reports experiencing sexual abuse or assault is provided in Box 10.2.

BOX 10.2
Types of Questions to Be Asked of an Adolescent Patient Who Screens Positive for an Experience of Sexual Abuse or Assault

- How many times have you had this type of unwanted sexual contact? Was it only once or more than one time?

- When was the first time this happened? When was the last time?

- Who was the person who did this to you?

- What did the person do to you? Did he/she touch your private parts or other parts of your body? Did he/she put anything in your mouth? Your vagina? Your butt?

- Did he put his penis in your mouth? Your vagina? Your butt?

- Did he/she do anything to make you have sexual contact with him/her? Offer you something if you agreed? Threaten to hurt you or someone you loved? Force you by holding you down or hitting or slapping you?

- Were you drinking alcohol or using any other drugs when this happened?

- Has this person hurt you in any other way, such as slapping you or punching you?

- After this experience, did you have any pain or other physical symptoms?

- Does any other person hurt you in any way?

- Have you told anyone else about this experience?

- Have the police or child protective services been told about this experience?

Examination of the Adolescent Who Has Been Sexually Abused or Sexually Assaulted

In most cases, examining an adolescent who has been sexually abused or assaulted does not involve collecting of forensic evidence, given that most providers will not be conducting an evaluation of the patient within 72 hours of an abuse or assault incident. However, in all cases, a careful examination of the patient should occur. It is important to bear in mind that most victims will not have any obvious signs that sexual abuse or assault has occurred. In addition, if the adolescent is sexually active, it will likely be difficult to definitively determine if any positive findings (eg, genital injury, positive sexually transmitted infection [STI] test) occurred as a result of consensual sexual intercourse or as a result of the abusive experience.

Examination of the adolescent abuse or assault victim should be conducted in a careful and sensitive manner. It is common for an adolescent victim to experience fear or embarrassment. A study of adolescent girls evaluated for suspected sexual abuse found that more than 40% believed that the examination would be scary and more than 50% believed that the examination would be embarrassing.[45] To lessen these fears and anxieties, the provider can allow the patient to bring a friend or family member into the examination room. The provider also should give the patient a verbal description of each aspect of the examination and what the adolescent can expect. In addition, the patient should have control over when a particular procedure is started and the

option to halt the procedure.[18] Modifications also should be made to make the examination as comfortable as possible (eg, use of a smaller speculum with an adolescent girl).

Recent research supports that rates of physical findings suggestive of abuse are rare, particularly if the adolescent is not evaluated in the immediate aftermath of the abuse, although it should be noted that research evaluating adolescent victims of sexual abuse or assault is still in its infancy.[46] Studies clearly indicate that genital injuries as a result of sexual abuse or other trauma in prepubertal children heal quickly with residua occurring rarely, with the exception of cases where a complete transection of the hymen occurs.[47] Indeed, a study conducted by Berenson and colleagues[48] comparing genital findings of prepubertal girls with and without histories of sexual abuse concluded that only deep notches in the hymen, transections, and perforations should be taken as definitive evidence of sexual abuse. In addition, given the increased elasticity of the hymen among adolescents due to the influence of estrogen, the likelihood of a positive hymenal finding may be even more rare among adolescents not abused before puberty as well.[49,50] Studies have reported these findings in only 4% to 6% of female adolescent victims of sexual abuse or assault.[51,52] Studies of male victims are even less common, although one recent investigation found clear evidence of sexual abuse in only 1% of primarily prepubertal male victims reporting penetrative abuse.[53] Similarly, another study of healing following anal trauma (due to abuse or other trauma) found that only 6% of anal injuries did not heal completely.[47] Among victims evaluated immediately after an assault, tears to the posterior fourchette and fossa navicularis, abrasions to the labia minora, and ecchymosis of the hymen are the most commonly noted injuries, although most do not have any injuries.[46,54]

Medical Management of the Sexual Abuse or Sexual Assault Patient

All adolescent sexual abuse or assault patients should receive comprehensive STI testing and all female adolescents should receive pregnancy testing. Research suggests that STIs are common among adolescent victims. For example, one British study of adolescent sexual abuse victims found that 24% of girls who denied consensual sexual activity tested positive for one or more STIs as did 39% of girls who reported consensual sexual activity in addition to abuse.[55] A comprehensive study of STIs among adolescent girls in the United States evaluated for suspected sexual abuse found that 4.6% tested positive for gonorrhea, 9.4% for chlamydia, and 5% for trichomoniasis. The prevalence of STIs among male victims of sexual abuse is not well studied. One study found that 7% of male chronic sexual abuse victims tested positive for gonorrhea.[2] Average rates of common STIs among adolescent and adult sexual assault victims are 3% for gonorrhea, 3% for chlamydia, 9% for trichomoniasis, 18% for bacterial vaginosis, and 6% for condylomata acuminata.[56]

Due to these high prevalence rates, the Centers for Disease Control and Prevention (CDC) recommends that cultures for gonorrhea and chlamydia be taken from all sites of penetration or attempted penetration, including the throat or anus. In addition, it is recommended that a wet mount and culture be taken for trichomoniasis. If symptoms are present, the wet mount also should be examined for evidence of bacterial vaginosis and candidiasis. Finally, a serum sample should be taken for evaluation for human immunodeficiency virus (HIV), hepatitis B, and syphilis.[57] A follow-up visit should be scheduled in 1 to 2 weeks for repeat STI testing if treatment is not provided. Serologic tests for HIV and syphilis should be repeated at 6, 12, and 24 weeks.[57] The CDC recommended treatments for some of the more commonly encountered STIs are in Table 10.1.[57]

For adolescents evaluated within 72 hours of a sexual assault, prophylactic treatment for STIs should be provided. The STI prophylactic treatment recommended by the CDC for adolescent and adult sexual assault victims is provided in Table 10.2.[57] The CDC does not make definitive recommendations for HIV prophylaxis; however, it is stated that HIV prophylaxis should be considered when the risk of transmission is high (eg, multiple penetrative assaults, known HIV-positive offender).[57] Studies of the use of HIV prophylaxis generally have found low treatment adherence because of the treatment expense and side effects. Indeed, one study found that only 2 of the 8 child and adolescent

TABLE 10.1
CDC Recommendations for Treatment of STIs

STI	Treatment Regimen	Notes
Gonorrhea (*Neisseria gonorrhoeae*) and chlamydia (*Chlamydia trachomatis*)	***Recommended Regimens*** **Azithromycin** 1 g orally in a single dose OR **Doxycycline** 100 mg orally twice a day for 7 days ***Alternative Regimens*** **Erythromycin base** 500 mg orally 4 times a day for 7 days OR **Erythromycin ethylsuccinate** 800 mg orally 4 times a day for 7 days OR **Ofloxacin** 300 mg orally twice a day for 7 days OR **Levofloxacin** 500 mg orally once daily for 7 days	No follow-up necessary, except for pregnant patients. Partners should be treated. Pregnancy: should be treated with a cephalosporin or spectinomycin IM along with erythromycin or amoxicillin for chlamydia.
Trichomoniasis (*Trichomonas vaginalis*)	**Metronidazole** 2 g orally, single dose OR **Tinidazole** 2 g orally in a single dose ***Alternative Regimen*** **Metronidazole** 500 mg orally twice a day for 7 days	No follow-up necessary. Partners should be treated.
Bacterial vaginosis	**Metronidazole** 500 mg orally twice a day for 7 days OR **Metronidazole** gel 0.75% 5 g intravaginally once a day for 5 days OR **Clindamycin** cream 5% 5 g intravaginally once a day for 7 days	No follow-up necessary. Treatment of partners not necessary. Pregnancy: topical agents not recommended.
Herpes simplex virus infections	**Acyclovir** (400 mg orally, 3 times a day for 7–10 days OR **Acyclovir** 200 mg orally 5 times a day for 7–10 days OR **Famciclovir** 250 mg orally 3 times a day for 7–10 days OR **Valacyclovir** 1 g orally twice a day for 7–10 days	Counseling is recommended regarding risk of transmission to partners. Partners should be tested. Pregnancy: insufficient data regarding safety of treatment.

Abbreviations: CDC, Centers for Disease Control and Prevention; STI, sexually transmitted infection, IM, intramuscularly.

TABLE 10.2
CDC Recommended Prophylactic Treatment for Adolescent and Adult Victims of Sexual Assault Who Have Been Assaulted Within the Past 72 Hours

Drug	Dosage	Effect
Ceftriaxone	25 mg IM in a single dose	Targets gonorrhea and incubating syphilis
Metronidazole	2 g orally in a single dose	Targets trichomoniasis and gastrointestinal parasites
Azithromycin OR Doxycycline	1 g orally in a single dose (DO NOT ADMINISTER TO PREGNANT WOMEN.) 100 mg orally twice a day for 7 days	Targets chlamydia
Hepatitis B vaccination	One dose at acute visit, follow-up doses 1–2 months and 4–6 months after first dose	If not previously vaccinated, HBIG not necessary

Abbreviations: CDC, Centers for Disease Control and Prevention; IM, intramuscularly; HBIG, hepatitis B immune globulin.

patients who initiated HIV prophylaxis completed a 4-week regimen.[58] Therefore, the provider should carefully explain the risks, benefits, and costs to any patient being considered for HIV prophylaxis.

Because approximately 5% of sexual assaults of adolescent or adult women result in pregnancy,[59] the option of pregnancy prophylaxis should be provided to female patients.[18,42] There are currently 2 Federal Drug Administration–approved emergency contraception formulations. Plan B is a progestin-only regimen containing a total of 1.5 mg of levonorgestrel in 2 pills.[21] Preven is an estrogen-progestin regimen containing 200 µg of ethinyl estradiol and 1 mg levonorgestrel in 4 pills.[21,60] Research supports that a progestin-only regimen (Plan B) is associated with a lower incidence of nausea and vomiting as well as lower pregnancy rates than the combined regimen.[21,60] Use of Plan B is estimated to prevent approximately 85% of pregnancies.[60] There is evidence for the effectiveness of Plan B when used within 72 hours of unprotected intercourse, although it may be moderately effective up to 120 hours after unprotected intercourse.[21] The first dose should be given as soon as possible after unprotected intercourse and a second dose 12 hours after the first dose, although recent data suggest that both doses can be given at the same time without affecting the risk of side effects or efficacy.[21] It also should be noted that many pharmacies do not routinely stock emergency contraception and some pharmacists have denied women prescriptions for emergency contraception on moral grounds.[60–63] Therefore, it is recommended that providers be aware of pharmacies that routinely provide prescriptions for emergency contraception, or that they keep samples available to provide

TABLE 10.3
Combination Oral Contraceptives and Recommended Pills per Dose for Pregnancy Prophylaxis

Brand	Company	Pills per Dose
Ovral	Wyeth-Ayerst	2 white pills
Lo/Ovral	Wyeth-Ayerst	4 white pills
Nordette	Wyeth-Ayerst	4 light orange pills
Enpresse	Barr	4 orange pills
Triphasil	Wyeth-Ayerst	4 yellow pills
Seasonale	Barr	4 pink pills
Ogestrel	Watson	2 white pills

to patients. Alternatively, a 2-dose regimen of a number of combination oral contraceptives can be used as emergency contraception.[60] A partial list of these medications and necessary dosages can be found in Table 10.3.

The provider should make it a priority to ensure that prophylactic treatment is provided to the patient if she is referred for forensic evaluation because research suggests that provision of prophylaxis is not standard practice in many emergency departments (EDs). For example, a recent study of sexual assault victims treated in EDs found that only 28% were given pregnancy prophylaxis and only 69% received STI prophylaxis.[64] Similarly, a recent survey of EDs in one US state found that only 42% routinely offered emergency contraception to victims of sexual assault.[65]

The provider should conduct the forensic examination of a recently assaulted patient (ie, assaulted within the past 72 hours) if no hospital or specialty clinic is available. Forensic examination kits (rape kits) that contain tools to collect

forensic evidence including bags/envelopes for hair samples and clothing, combs to collect hair samples, a cuticle stick, plastic pipettes, and collection tubes generally can be obtained from local law enforcement.[43] Law enforcement officials also should be contacted immediately to ensure that the evaluation is conducted efficiently.[43]

Before the examination begins, the patient should be asked to disrobe over sheets or heavy paper and then place his or her clothing in a large paper bag.[42] Undergarments should be placed in a separate bag.[43] After the patient has disrobed, any visible physical injuries should be documented.[42] Photographs of any visible injuries should be taken when possible. The patient's identification card or name should be photographed at the beginning and end of the series of photographs to establish identity. Scalp and pubic hair samples should be collected first using the included comb. Loose hairs should be distinguished from the patient's hair and placed in a separate envelope.[43] A saliva specimen should be taken using a piece of filter paper.[42] Nail scrapings or clippings should be taken as well if the patient scratched his or her assailant.[43] The patient's abdomen also should be examined for any signs of trauma (eg, tenderness, rebound signs).[42]

When conducting the pelvic examination with female patients, the method of visualization should be noted and only water used for lubrication.[42,43] A swab of the vulva will increase the likelihood of finding the presence of semen.[42] Vaginal aspirates should be collected using pipettes, and a vaginal wash is recommended to increase the likelihood that evidence of any semen present is obtained.[42,43] After the examination is completed, a small drop of any vaginal secretions obtained should be placed on a slide and viewed with a microscope to detect any motile sperm.[42] A Pap smear also is recommended to increase the likelihood that evidence of the presence of semen is obtained.[42] In contrast to prepubertal victims, where seminal evidence is unlikely to be detected if the examination is not conducted within 9 hours, seminal evidence has been detected on the cervix of adolescents and adults up to 70 hours after an assault.[43,66] Use of colposcopy should be considered to detect subtle vaginal and cervical injuries.[47] The colposcope also can be used to photograph other injuries, although it should be noted that such photographs also can be taken with a handheld camera. An inspection of the anal area also is recommended to identify signs of injury; swabs should be taken particularly if anal penetration was reported by the patient.[42] Similarly, oral swabs should be taken, particularly if the patient reports oral penetration. All swabs should be placed in containers with saline solution to be tested for the presence of semen.[42] Finally, a blood sample should be taken.[42]

The provider must follow proper procedures regarding the evidence "chain of custody." All personnel obtaining specimens need to be identified on the specimen label or seal. In addition, specimens should be stored in a secure (locked) location until they are transferred to the police. Finally, release forms need to be signed transferring the evidence to the police.[43]

Charting

The provider should take careful notes when speaking to the patient about the sexual abuse or assault and should carefully document any injuries, their exact location and nature, and the patient's explanation for how they occurred. The provider should consider including photographs of any injuries and results of any positive STI cultures. It is important for the health care provider to remember that he or she is not to act as a detective when evaluating patients who report sexual abuse or assault and that his or her first priority is to provide care to the patient. Probing for minute details of the circumstances of the abuse or assault may lead to discrepancies between the patient's medical record and any report made to the police or child protective services.[18]

The provider also should be careful in the language he or she uses when discussing the adolescent's abuse or assault. For example, phrases such as "alleges" or "claims" should be avoided. Instead, matter of fact language should be used, such as, "patient reports that her boyfriend forced her to have vaginal intercourse 2 weeks ago." Evaluative statements regarding the veracity of the patient's report should also be generally avoided. The provider should not assume that the absence of an emotional response when discussing the abuse or assault suggests that the assault did not occur. Similarly, the presence of delinquent or other problem behaviors by an adolescent does not negate the possibility that he or she experienced sexual abuse or assault. Indeed, these behaviors often are a response to sexual abuse or assault.[67]

Appropriate Referrals and Follow-up

Adolescent patients who have experienced sexual abuse or assault should be screened for depression, post-traumatic stress disorder (PTSD), and other anxiety disorders. While only limited research has examined the prevalence of these disorders among sexually abused youngsters, data suggest that a sizable portion of victims experience significant psychological distress. For example, the prevalence of PTSD among child and adolescent victims of sexual abuse has ranged from 15% to 35%.[3,68] In addition, a study of young adult victims of child sexual abuse found that 30% to 60% retrospectively reported experiencing major depressive disorder as an adolescent and 40% to 44% retrospectively reported experiencing one or more anxiety disorders as an adolescent.[69] Sample screening questions are presented in Box 10.3. If a patient's response suggests that he or she may be experiencing significant psychological

---

BOX 10.3

Screening Questions to Assess Psychological Distress in Victims of Sexual Abuse or Assault

- Have you been sad or blue a lot lately? How long have you been feeling this way? Would you say that you feel down more days than you feel good?

- Do you find yourself less interested in things you used to enjoy?

- Do you have a hard time concentrating on things like schoolwork, conversations, things on television?

- Have things gotten so bad that you have thought about hurting yourself? Have you ever tried to hurt yourself or end your life?

- Do you find yourself having thoughts, feelings, or dreams about your experience with unwanted sex that you do not want to have?

- Do you find yourself avoiding things because they remind you somehow of your experience with unwanted sex?

- Do you feel like you always have to be on guard or on the lookout for danger?

- How has your sleep been? How many hours of sleep do you get most nights?

- Do you often find yourself worrying about things like schoolwork, being on time, doing things perfectly?

- Do you have panic attacks, that is, do you ever suddenly feel really anxious for no apparent reason (your heart is beating fast, you are breathing quickly, you are sweating, you feel dizzy)?

- Do you ever feel really anxious in certain social situations like having to talk in school or talking with other teenagers? Would you say that you feel more anxious in these situations than most teenagers your age?

distress, a referral for psychological treatment should be made and a referral for psychiatric treatment should be considered. All patients who have experienced sexual violence should be provided information about community resources for sexual abuse and assault victims.

The type of treatment that shows the most promise for adolescents who have experienced sexual abuse or assault is cognitive behavioral therapy (CBT).[70–73] Cognitive behavioral therapy interventions involve several treatment components, often including psychoeducation about trauma and its effects, exposure to the trauma memory or reminders of the trauma, and cognitive restructuring of distorted cognitions associated with the trauma (eg, "It is my fault that I was abused.").[73] These interventions also often include some type of anxiety management intervention such as relaxation training, as well as parent training to enable parents or caregivers to be actively involved in facilitating the child or adolescent's treatment.[73] Cognitive behavioral therapy has been shown to be effective at reducing PTSD symptoms, depressive symptoms, adjustment problems, and increasing social competence in child and adolescent victims of sexual abuse.[70–72]

Research on psychopharmacologic interventions for children and adolescents with significant trauma histories is clearly in its infancy. Selective serotonin reuptake inhibitors (SSRIs) have shown the most promise in reducing PTSD symptoms in adults.[74] In contrast, no controlled trials of SSRIs have been conducted with children or adolescents,

although open-label trials suggest that they may be effective in reducing PTSD symptoms.[75,76] Clonidine also has been studied in open label trials for treatment of childhood PTSD, as has carbamazepine.[75] Both trials suggested that the medications were effective at reducing PTSD symptoms, although it should be noted that there was no control group in either of these studies and both had very small sample sizes.[75] Thus current recommendations are that CBT should be the first-line treatment, with pharmacotherapy potentially a useful adjunct, particularly if CBT does not provide total symptom relief.[75]

Legal Issues

There are 2 primary legal issues involved in providing services to adolescents who have experienced sexual abuse or assault: mandatory reporting and consent for treatment. Mandatory reporting laws require health care providers, among other certain professionals, to report instances of childhood sexual abuse involving any type of sexual contact with a person in a caretaking or custodial role, such as a parent, neighbor, babysitter, or coach.[1] In general, there is no obligation for health care providers to report instances of sexual assault not perpetrated by someone in a caretaking role (eg, sexual assault by a peer).[1] However, with the expansion of some statutory rape laws as well as the increased push for mandatory reporting of rape involving young adolescents, this is changing.[77] For example, Tennessee requires reporting of any instance of intercourse with a child younger than 13 years. Thus instances of peer assault involving a victim who was 12 years or younger would need to be reported in this state.[1] In another example, California requires reporting of instances of intercourse when one of the individuals is younger than 14 years and the other is older than 14 years.[1] Health care providers are immune from prosecution if they make a report of suspected child sexual abuse in good faith.[78] Reciprocally, states can impose criminal penalties on providers who do not make reports of suspected sexual abuse.[78] Providers are strongly encouraged to become familiar with the laws in their states.

The second legal issue regarding adolescent victims of sexual abuse or assault concerns consent for treatment. In nearly all states adolescents may consent to the diagnosis and treatment of STIs, and medical care can be provided to them without parent or guardian knowledge.[57] Similarly, adolescents in many states may consent to HIV testing as well as to vaccination services[57]; however, the health care provider is urged to consult the laws in his or her state regarding consent to treatment for adolescents.

Other Key Issues Involving Adolescent Sexual Abuse or Assault Patients

In addition to often experiencing significant psychological distress, there are a number of other issues that the health care provider may have to confront when working with adolescents who have experienced sexual abuse or assault. One primary issue concerns the development of the abused adolescent's sexuality. The ways in which sexual

abuse victims' sexuality is shaped has been termed traumatic sexualization.[79] Victims of sexual abuse learn about sexuality in a developmentally inappropriate manner and, further, learn to view sex as a means to an end (eg, to receive rewards or to avoid punishment). Some also have hypothesized that chronic sexual abuse may lead to hyperarousal[80] and that abused adolescents may have more difficulties with sexual decision-making,[80] perhaps due to holding distorted beliefs about sex. A history of sexual abuse or adolescent sexual assault has been associated with a number of sexual risk behaviors among adolescents, including having multiple sexual partners, inconsistent use of condoms, early age of sexual debut, adolescent pregnancy, and use of substances before sex.[7,12,13,81–84] Thus it may be particularly important to discuss issues with abused or assaulted adolescents regarding the importance of use of contraception, to prevent pregnancy as well as to reduce the likelihood of contracting an STI. In addition, the provider should express concern if an adolescent reports engaging in risky sexual behavior and discuss the possibility that the adolescent's behavior may be a response to his or her abusive experiences.

Many male victims assaulted by male perpetrators may become concerned about their sexual identity and orientation.[2,85] For example, male victims may believe that because they experienced physiological arousal during the abuse, they are potentially homosexual.[85] Similarly, abused boys may be concerned that they were targeted for the abuse because they were perceived as feminine or homosexual.[85] Some adolescents will attempt to overcome these concerns through engaging in excessive sexual activity or by being sexually aggressive.[2,85] Thus providers working with male adolescent victims should carefully probe for these concerns and reassure the patient that his physiological response to the abuse is not an indicator that he wanted the abuse. In addition, providers should discuss appropriate sexual behavior with male victims and refer victims engaging in aggressive sexual behavior for further treatment.

The adolescent patient also may have a number of concerns regarding legal involvement in his or her case, and some adolescents may not want their sexual abuse to be reported to the authorities. Victims of sexual abuse, and sexual assault victims who choose to press charges, may find the need to provide details of their experience multiple times to be distressing and embarrassing.[86] If the adolescent has experienced intra-familial abuse, he or she may be concerned about being removed from the home or having the perpetrator removed from the home. Finally, the adolescent may feel embarrassed or anxious about having to potentially testify in court. It is possible that the adolescent may express some or all of these concerns when discussing his or her abusive experience. The provider should respond to these concerns by reassuring the adolescent that the abuse or assault was not his or her fault and that the only person who should feel embarrassed is the perpetrator. In addition, many rape crisis centers offer assistance to victims who are going through the legal process, and so such a referral may be appropriate.

Adolescents who have experienced sexual abuse or assault also have been found to be more likely to engage in a number of other risky behaviors. Adolescents with a history of sexual abuse or assault report having more suicidal thoughts, are more likely to engage in self-mutilation, and are more likely to have made one or multiple suicide attempts, compared with adolescents without such a history.[8,9,14,81,87] A sexual abuse history also has been associated with an increased risk of engaging in a number of substance use behaviors among adolescents, including binge drinking,[81,07,88] heavy smoking,[81] and marijuana use.[88] There are a number of potential reasons for these associations. First, adolescents who experience sexual violence may come from homes where there are high levels of parental conflict and low levels of parental monitoring.[87] Second, adolescents with sexual abuse histories may have poor interpersonal skills, increasing the likelihood that they associate with deviant peers.[67] Finally, adolescents who have experienced sexual abuse or assault may be experiencing high levels of distress and, thus, could engage in risky behaviors in an attempt to reduce this distress. Therefore, providers should carefully assess if abused adolescents are engaging in risky behaviors and discuss treatment options with them for these problems. This type of discussion is particularly important for adolescents who come from chaotic homes or who are experiencing significant distress.

Finally, studies of adolescent girls suggest that those who have experienced sexual abuse are more likely to experience further sexual assaults in adolescence.[12,28,30] The mechanisms for this association are not fully understood but likely include increased substance use, early onset of sexual activity, and difficulties in recognizing sexual risk in interpersonal situations.[12,28] Given this risk, providers' discussion with adolescent victims, particularly female victims, should include discussion of the possibility that engaging in risky behaviors (eg, binge drinking, having sex with multiple partners) also places them at risk for experiencing further sexual victimization. In addition, the provider should emphasize to the adolescent the need for treatment for these behaviors and that stopping these behaviors will likely reduce their risk of experiencing further sexual violence.

Conclusion

A sizable percentage of adolescents are victims of sexual abuse or have had prepubertal sexual abuse experiences, with estimates ranging from 3% to 34% of girls and from 2% to 10% of boys. In addition, many adolescent girls are victims of peer sexual assault, with estimates ranging from 3% to 16% of girls. Approximately 2% to 3% of boys also are victims of peer sexual assault. Risk factors for sexual abuse include growing up in a home with high levels of marital conflict, parental substance abuse, change in caregivers, or lack of a caregiver. Risk factors for peer sexual assault include a history of childhood abuse, early initiation of sexual activity,

substance use, and a prior history of peer sexual assault.

Many adolescents will not spontaneously disclose incidents of sexual abuse or assault to health care providers because of fears of being blamed for the abuse, family instability, or fear of the consequences of disclosure (eg, removal from home, having to disclose the abuse to authorities). In addition, many adolescent victims may not consider their experience as abuse or have ambivalent feelings toward the perpetrator. Thus health care providers should routinely screen adolescents for these experiences using behaviorally specific questions. Adolescent sexual abuse or assault victims should be offered testing and treatment for STIs as well as pregnancy testing. If the adolescent has been assaulted within 72 hours, a forensic evaluation should be conducted and STI and pregnancy prophylaxis should be offered. Many adolescents will experience significant psychological sequelae following sexual abuse or assault, such as the development of depression and PTSD. Thus providers should screen for the presence of significant psychological distress in all patients who have experienced sexual abuse or assault and make appropriate referrals for further mental health treatment.

Providers also should be aware of the legal issues in working with adolescent victims. First, health care providers are mandatory reporters of all suspected incidents of childhood sexual abuse. In addition, in most states, adolescents are able to consent for testing and treatment of STIs and HIV and, thus, providers do not need parental permission to provide these services to adolescents. Finally, providers should be aware of potential difficult issues that may arise when working with adolescent victims of sexual abuse or assault. First, abused adolescents engage in more sexual risk behaviors such as having multiple partners, inconsistent use of condoms, and use of substances before sex. In addition, abused adolescents often engage in other risky behaviors, such as self-mutilation, suicide attempts, binge drinking, heavy smoking, and marijuana use. Finally, adolescents who experience sexual abuse or assault are at elevated risk for experiencing further sexual assaults.

References

1. Mitchell CW, Rogers RE. Rape, statutory rape, and child abuse: legal distinctions and counselor duties. *Prof School Couns.* 2003;6:332–338
2. Holmes WC, Slap GB. Sexual abuse of boys: definition, prevalence, correlates, sequelae, and management. *JAMA.* 1998;280:1855–1862
3. Walker JL, Carey PD, Mohr N, Stein DJ, Seedat S. Gender differences in the prevalence of childhood sexual abuse and in the development of pediatric PTSD. *Arch Womens Ment Health.* 2004;7:111–121
4. Saewyc EM, Pettingell S, Magee LL. The prevalence of sexual abuse among adolescents in school. *J School Nurs.* 2003;19:266–272
5. Lodico MA, Gruber E, DiClemente RJ. Childhood sexual abuse and coercive sex among school-based adolescents in a Midwestern state. *J Adolesc Health.* 1996;18:211–217
6. Gagne MH, Lavoie F, Hebert M. Victimization during childhood and revictimization in dating relationships in adolescent girls. *Child Abuse Negl.* 2005;29:1155–1172

7. Luster T, Small SA. Sexual abuse history and number of sex partners among female adolescents. *Fam Plan Perspect.* 1997;29:204–212
8. Bensley LS, Van Eenwyk J, Spieker SJ, Schoder J. Self-reported abuse history and adolescent problem behaviors I: antisocial and suicidal behaviors. *J Adolesc Health.* 1999;24:163–172
9. Martin G, Bergen HA, Richardson AS, Roeger L, Allison S. Sexual abuse and suicidality: gender differences in a large community sample of adolescents. *Child Abuse Negl.* 2004;28:491–503
10. Bouvier P, Halperin D, Rey H, et al. Typology and correlates of sexual abuse in children and youth: multivariate analyses in a prevalence study in Geneva. *Child Abuse Negl.* 1999;23:779–790
11. Costello EJ, Erkanli A, Fairbank JA, Angold A. The prevalence of potentially traumatic events in childhood and adolescence. *J Trauma Stress.* 2002;15:99–112
12. Fergusson DM, Horwood LJ, Lynskey MT. Childhood sexual abuse, adolescent sexual behaviors and sexual revictimization. *Child Abuse Negl.* 1997;2:789–803
13. Cinq-Mars C, Wright J, Cyr M, McDuff P. Sexual at-risk behaviors of sexually abused adolescent girls. *J Child Sex Abuse.* 2003;12:1–18
14. Wright J, Friedrich W, Cinq-Mars C, Cyr M, McDuff P. Self-destructive and delinquent behaviors of adolescent female victims of child sexual abuse: rates and covariates in clinical and nonclinical samples. *Violence Victims.* 2004;19:627–643
15. Finkelhor D, Hotaling G, Lewis IA, Smith C. Sexual abuse in a national survey of adult men and women: prevalence, characteristics, and risk factors. *Child Abuse Negl.* 1990;14:19–28
16. Bulik CM, Prescott CA, Kendler KS. Features of childhood sexual abuse and the development of psychiatric and substance use disorders. *Br J Psychiatry.* 2001;179:444–449

17. Lynskey MT, Fergusson DM. Factors protecting against the development of adjustment difficulties in young adults exposed to childhood sexual abuse. *Child Abuse Negl.* 1997;21:1177–1190

18. American Medical Association. Strategies for the treatment and prevention of sexual assault. American Medical Association Web site. http://www.ama-assn.org/ama1/pub/upload/mm/386/childsexabuse.pdf

19. Ackard DM, Neumark-Sztainer D. Date violence and date rape among adolescents: associations with disordered eating behaviors and psychological health. *Child Abuse Negl.* 2002;26:455–473

20. Hall ER, Flannery RB. Prevalence and correlates of sexual assault experiences in adolescents. *Victimology Int J.* 1984;9:398–406

21. ACOG Committee on Practice Bulletins—Gynecology. Clinical management guidelines for Obstetrician-Gynecologists, Number 69, December 2005: Emergency contraception. *Obstet Gynecol.* 2005;106:1443–1452

22. Raghavan R, Bogart LM, Elliott MN, Vestal KD, Schuster MA. Sexual victimization among a national probability sample of adolescent women. *Perspect Sex Reprod Health.* 2004;36:225–232

23. Ackard DM, Neumark-Sztainer D. Multiple sexual victimization among adolescent boys and girls: prevalence and association with eating behaviors and psychological health. *J Child Sex Abuse.* 2003;12:17–37

24. Putnam F. Ten-year research update review: child sexual abuse. *J Am Acad Child Adolesc Psychiatry.* 2003;42:269–278

25. Kellogg ND, Menard SW. Violence among family members of children and adolescents evaluated for sexual abuse. *Child Abuse Negl.* 2003;27:1367–1376

26. Hilton MR, Mezey GC. Victims and perpetrators of child sexual abuse. *Br J Psychiatry.* 1996;169:408–421

27. Kuhn JA, Arellano CM, Chavez EL. Correlates of sexual assault in Mexican American and White non-Hispanic adolescent males. *Violence Victims.* 1998;13:11–20

28. Classen CC, Palesh OG, Aggarwal R. Sexual revictimization: a review of the empirical literature. *Trauma Violence Abuse.* 2005;6:103–129

29. Collins ME. Factors influencing sexual victimization and revictimization in a sample of adolescent mothers. *J Interpers Violence.* 1998;13:3–24

30. Krahé B, Scheinberger-Olwig R, Waizenhofer E, Kolpin S. Childhood sexual abuse and revictimization in adolescence. *Child Abuse Negl.* 1999;22:383–394

31. Himelein MJ, Vogel RE, Wachowiak DG. Nonconsensual sexual experiences in precollege women: prevalence and risk factors. *J Couns Dev.* 1994;72:411–415

32. Rickert VI, Wiemann CM. Date rape among adolescents and young adults. *J Pediatr Adolesc Gynecol.* 1998;11:167–175

33. Maxwell CD, Robinson AL, Post LA. The nature and predictors of sexual victimization and offending among adolescents. *J Youth Adolesc.* 2003;32:465–477

34. Rickert VI, Wiemann CM, Vaughan RD, White JW. Rates and risk factors for sexual violence among an ethnically diverse sample of adolescents. *Arch Pediatr Adolesc Med.* 2004;158:1132–1139

35. Goodman-Brown TB, Edelstein RS, Goodman GS, Jones DPH, Gordon DS. Why children tell: a model of children's disclosure of sexual abuse. *Child Abuse Negl.* 2003;27:525–540

36. Crisma M, Bascelli E, Paci D, Romito P. Adolescents who experienced sexual abuse: fears, needs and impediments to disclosure. *Child Abuse Negl.* 2004;28:1035–1048

37. Paine ML, Hansen DJ. Factors influencing children to self-disclose sexual abuse. *Clin Psychol Rev.* 2002;22:271–295

38. Littleton HL, Rhatigan D, Axsom D. Unacknowledged rape: how much do we know about the hidden rape victim? *J Aggress Maltreat Trauma.* 2007;14:57–74

39. Williams LM, Siegel JA, Pomeroy JJ. Validity of women's self-reports of documented child sexual abuse. In: Stone AA, Turkkan JS, Bachrach CA, Jobe JB, Kurtzman HS, eds. *The Science of Self-Report: Implications for Research and Practice.* Mahwah, NJ: Lawrence Erlbaum Associates; 2000:211–226

40. Koss MP, Gidycz CA, Wisniewski N. The scope of rape: incidence and prevalence of sexual aggression and victimization in a national sample of higher education students. *J Consult Clin Psychol.* 1987;55:162–170

41. Sinal SH. Sexual abuse of children and adolescents. *S Med J.* 1994;87:1242–1258

42. Bechtel K, Podrazik M. Evaluation of the adolescent rape victim. *Pediatr Clin North Am.* 1999;46:809–823

43. Poirier MP. Care of the female adolescent rape victim. *Pediatr Emerg Care.* 2002;18:53–59

44. Holmes MM, Resnick HS, Frampton D. Follow-up of sexual assault victims. *Am J Obstet Gynecol.* 1998;179:336–342

45. Mears CJ, Heflin AH, Finkel MA, Deblinger E, Steer RA. Adolescents' responses to sexual abuse evaluation including the use of video colposcopy. *J Adolesc Health.* 2006;33:18–24

46. Grossin C, Sibille I, de la Grandmaison GL, Banasr A, Brion F, Durigon M. Analysis of 418 cases of sexual assault. *Forensic Sci Int.* 2003;131:125–130

47. Heppenstall-Heger A, McConnell G, Ticson L, Guerra L, Lister J, Zaragoza T. Healing patterns in anogenital injuries: a longitudinal study of injuries associated with sexual abuse, accidental injuries, or genital surgery in the preadolescent child. *Pediatrics.* 2003;112:829–837

48. Berenson AB, Chacko MR, Wiemann CM, Mishaw CO, Friedrich W, Grady JJ. A case-control study of anatomic changes resulting from sexual abuse. *Am J Obstet Gynecol.* 2000;182:820–834

49. Giardino AP, Finkel MA. Evaluating child sexual abuse. *Pediatr Ann.* 2005;34:382–394

50. Edgardh K, Ormstad K. The adolescent hymen. *J Reprod Med.* 2002;47:710–714

51. Adams JA, Knudson S. Genital findings in adolescent girls referred for suspected sexual abuse. *Arch Pediatr Adolesc Med.* 1996;150:850–857

52. Kellogg ND, Menard SW, Santos A. Genital anatomy in pregnant adolescents: "normal" does not mean "nothing happened." *Pediatrics.* 2004;113:e67–e69

53. Heger A, Ticson L, Velasquez O, Bernier R. Children referred for possible sexual abuse: medical findings in 2384 children. *Child Abuse Negl.* 2002;26:645–659

54. Slaughter L, Brown CRV, Crowley S, Peck R. Patterns of genital injury in female sexual assault victims. *Am J Obstet Gynecol.* 1997;176:609–616

55. Kawsar M, Walters E, McCabe S, Forster GE. Prevalence of sexually transmitted infections and mental health needs of female child and adolescent survivors of rape and sexual assault attending a specialist clinic. *Sex Transm Infect.* 2004;80:138–141

56. Beck-Sague CM, Solomon F. Sexually transmitted diseases in abused children and adolescent and adult victims of rape: review of selected literature. *Clin Infect Dis.* 2001;28:s74–s83

57. Centers for Disease Control and Prevention. Sexually transmitted diseases treatment guidelines. *MMWR Recomm Rep.* 2006;55(RR-11):1–100

58. Babl FE, Cooper ER, Damon B, Louie T, Kharasch S, Harris J. HIV postexposure prophylaxis for children. *Am J Emerg Med.* 2000;18:282–287

59. Holmes MM, Resnick HS, Kilpatrick DG, Best CL. Rape-related pregnancy: estimates and descriptive characteristics from a national sample of women. *Am J Obstet Gynecol.* 1996;175:320–324

60. American Academy of Pediatrics. Emergency contraception. *Pediatrics.* 2005;116:1026–1035

61. Tanne JH. Emergency contraception is under attack by US pharmacists. *Br Med J.* 2005;330:983

62. Zwillich T. US pharmacies vow to withhold emergency contraception. *Lancet.* 2005;365:1677–1678

63. Fielder JH. Pharmacists refuse to fill emergency contraception prescriptions. *IEEE Eng Med Biol Mag.* 2005;24:88–91

64. Campbell R. What really happened? A validation study of rape survivors' help-seeking experiences with the legal and medical systems. *Viol Victims.* 2005;20:55–68

65. Patel A, Simons R, Piotrowski ZH, Shulman L, Petraitis C. Under-use of emergency contraception for victims of sexual assault. *Int J Fertil Womens Med.* 2004;49:269–273

66. Christian CW, Lavelle JM, De Jong AR, Loiselle J, Brenner L, Joffe M. Forensic evidence findings in prepubertal victims of sexual assault. *Pediatrics.* 2000;106:100–104

67. Tyler KA. Social and emotional outcomes of childhood sexual abuse: a review of recent research. *Aggress Viol Behav.* 2002;7:567–589

68. Cuffe SP, Addy CL, Garrison CZ, et al. Prevalence of PTSD in a community sample of older adolescents. *J Am Acad Child Adolesc Psychiatry.* 1998;37:147–154

69. Fergusson DM, Horwood LJ, Lynskey MT. Childhood sexual abuse and psychiatric disorder in young adulthood: II. Psychiatric outcomes of childhood sexual abuse. *J Am Acad Child Adolesc Psychiatry.* 1996;35:1365–1374

70. Cohen JA. Early mental health interventions for trauma and traumatic loss in children and adolescents. In: Litz BT, ed. *Early Interventions for Trauma and Traumatic Loss.* New York, NY: Guilford Press; 2004:131–146

71. Carr A. Interventions for post-traumatic stress disorder in children and adolescents. *Pediatr Rehab.* 2004;7:231–244

72. Cohen J, Mannarino AP, Berliner L, Deblinger E. Trauma-focused cognitive behavioral therapy for children and adolescents. *J Interpers Viol.* 2000;15:1202–1223

73. Dalgleish T, Meiser-Stedman R, Smith P. Cognitive aspects of posttraumatic stress reactions and their treatment in children and adolescents: an empirical review and some recommendations. *Behav Cognit Psychother.* 2005;33:459–486

74. Marmar CR, Neylan TC, Schoenfeld FB. New directions in the pharmacotherapy of posttraumatic stress disorder. *Psychiatry Q.* 2002;73:259–270

75. Donnelly CL. Pharmacologic treatment approaches for children and adolescents with posttraumatic stress disorder. *Child Adolesc Psychiatry Clin North Am.* 2003;12:251–269

76. Brown EJ. Efficacious treatment of stress disorder in children and adolescents. *Pediatr Ann.* 2005;34:139–146

77. Kmett Danielson C, Holmes MM. Adolescent sexual assault: an update of the literature. *Curr Opin Obstet Gynecol.* 2004;16:383–388

78. American Medical Association. Diagnostic and treatment guidelines on child sexual abuse. American Medical Association Web site. http://www.ama-assn.org/ama1/pub/upload/mm/386/sexualassault.pdf

79. Wyatt GE. Child sexual abuse and its effects on sexual functioning. *Ann Rev Sex Res.* 1991;2:249–266

80. Loeb T, Williams JK, Carmona JV, et al. Child sexual abuse: associations with the sexual functioning of adolescents and adults. *Ann Rev Sex Res.* 2002;13:307–345

81. Howard DE, Wang MQ. Psychosocial correlates of US adolescents who report a history of forced sexual intercourse. *J Adolesc Health.* 2005;36:372–379

82. Lodico MA, DiClemente RJ. The association between childhood sexual abuse and prevalence of HIV-related risk behaviors. *Clin Pediatr.* 1994;33:498–502

83. Ohene SA, Halcon L, Ireland M, Carr P, McNeely C. Sexual abuse history, risk behavior, and sexually transmitted diseases: the impact of age at abuse. *Sex Transm Dis.* 2005;32:358–363

84. Raj A, Silverman JG, Amaro H. The relationship between sexual abuse and sexual risk among high school students: findings from the 1997 Massachusetts Youth Risk Behavior Survey. *Mat Child Health J.* 2000;4:125–134

85. Romano E, De Luca RV. Male sexual abuse: a review of effects, abuse characteristics, and links with later psychological functioning. *Aggress Viol Behav.* 2001;6:55–78

86. Ghetti S, Alexander KW, Goodman GS. Legal involvement in child sexual abuse cases: consequences and interventions. *Int J Law Psychiatry.* 2002;25:235–251

87. Luster T, Small SA. Sexual abuse history and problems in adolescence: exploring the effects of moderating variables. *J Marriage Fam.* 1997;59:131–142

88. Champion HLO, Foley KL, DuRant RH, Hensberry R, Altman D, Wolfson M. Adolescent sexual victimization, use of alcohol and other substances, and other health risk behaviors. *J Adolesc Health.* 2004;35:321–328

Chapter 11

Sexually Transmitted Infections in Child Sexual Abuse

Allan R. DeJong

Children At Risk Evaluation (CARE) Program
Alfred I Du Pont Hospital for Children

Introduction

Sexually abused children and adolescents are at risk for acquiring infections prevalent among sexually active adolescents and adults. The infection or colonization may be symptomatic or asymptomatic. Sexually transmitted infections (STIs) are not commonly identified in prepubertal children. Therefore, the presence of an STI in a child should raise concerns of sexual abuse. Some children, however, acquire some STIs through vertical transmission at birth and through nonsexual contact. Discovery of an STI in a child may prompt an evaluation for child sexual abuse and may be the only physical evidence of sexual abuse in some cases.[1-7]

Sexually active adolescents and young adults have the highest rates of STIs, and STIs are more commonly identified in pubertal adolescents than in prepubertal children evaluated for suspected sexual assault or abuse. The presence of an STI in the pubertal adolescent may represent an infection acquired through abuse or prior sexual activity. The risk of acquiring an STI through sexual assault or abuse is directly related to the prevalence of STIs found in the adult and adolescent population.[8-13] One study showed that 43% of the adult and adolescent sexual assault victims had at least one preexisting STI, but relatively few developed new chlamydial (2%) or gonococcal (4%) disease. However, 12% developed trichomoniasis and 19% bacterial vaginosis as a result of their assault.[8]

Sexually transmitted infections have been detected in approximately 1% to 30% of children and adolescents examined for sexual abuse. The actual risk of acquiring STIs by child sexual abuse victims is unknown. Several studies suggest approximately 5% of prepubertal children evaluated for sexual abuse have an STI.[1,14] The differences in observed frequency of STIs in the children studied may be related to many variables: type of sexual contact, age of the child, frequency of the abuse, types of testing performed, regional differences in the prevalence of STI, and percentage of children referred because of their symptoms of STI. The incubation periods for the organisms and the timing of the examination after the abuse are critically important in detecting infections.[15-18]

The Centers for Disease Control and Prevention (CDC) suggests a general rule that, "The identification of a sexually transmissible agent from a child beyond the neonatal period suggests sexual abuse."[2] This general rule has some merit, but the strength of the association between STI and child sexual abuse varies from disease to disease (Table 11.1). Several factors must be considered when evaluating the strength of association between an STI and child sexual abuse, particularly the age of the child and the specific disease identified. One needs to consider the possibilities that the identified organism represents a perinatally acquired infection or an infection spread by fomites or nonsexual contact.

TABLE 11.1
Significance of Sexually Transmitted Infections in Children

Sexually Transmitted Infection	Persistence Following Perinatal Transmission	Significance of Relationship to Sexual Contact
Gonorrhea	Up to 1 y	Definitive[a]
Chlamydia trachomatis	Up to 3 y	Definitive[a]
Syphilis	Months to years	Definitive[a]
Human immunodeficiency virus	Asymptomatic for years	Definitive[b]
Trichomonas vaginalis	Up to 1 y	Very likely[a]
Chancroid	Unlikely to be asymptomatic	Very likely[c]
Granuloma inguinale	Unlikely to be asymptomatic	Very likely[c]
Human papillomavirus	Asymptomatic up to 3 y	Possible[d]
Herpes simplex virus (types 1 and 2)	Symptomatic by 6 wk	Possible[e]
Hepatitis B virus	Asymptomatic for years	Possible
Pubic lice	Symptomatic within 3 wk	Possible
Head/body lice	Symptomatic within 3 wk	Inconclusive
Hepatitis C	Asymptomatic for years	Inconclusive
Molluscum contagiosum	Unknown	Inconclusive
Bacterial vaginosis	Unknown	Inconclusive
Group B streptococci	Unknown	Inconclusive

[a]Unless acquired perinatally.
[b]Unless acquired perinatally or through blood transfusion or contaminated needle.
[c]Rare infection with little data available on children.
[d]Longer asymptomatic time frames in laryngeal papillomas.
[e]Genital location of lesions increase likelihood of abuse.

However, the explanation that perinatal or nonsexual transmission for a specific disease is plausible does not mean it is correct. Children with STIs may be unable or unwilling to disclose sexual abuse. When no source of the organism is identified, it is not acceptable to conclude that the transmission must have been perinatal or nonsexual. Likewise, the inability to document a specific STI in a possible or suspected perpetrator does not exclude the possibility that this individual was the source of the child's infection.[7]

This chapter will review the prevalence, clinical features, likelihood of sexual transmission, and appropriate diagnostic evaluation and treatment of STIs in children. The diagnosis of an STI in a child with suspected sexual abuse has social and legal implications. The disease must be diagnosed by using tests that have a very high degree of specificity in children. Missing evidence of an STI in a child may place that child at risk of continued abuse. A mistaken diagnosis or mistaken interpretation, however, could lead to inappropriate child protection and criminal interventions.

Infections and Organisms

Children can acquire a variety of STIs through sexual and nonsexual transmission. These infections and organisms are discussed in detail in the following pages and in a summary of incubation period, symptoms, and appropriate diagnostic tests in Table 11.2.

Gonorrhea

Neisseria gonorrhoeae is the small gram-negative, oxidase-positive, diplococcal bacterium that causes gonorrhea or gonococcal infections. The incubation period is 2 to 7 days. Infections may be associated with symptoms including vaginal discharge (vaginitis), rectal pain, pruritus and discharge (proctitis), and exudative tonsillopharyngitis (pharyngitis). Gonococcal infections of the pharynx and of the rectum, however, are typically asymptomatic. If symptoms do occur, they almost always develop within a week of exposure. Vaginal discharge, if left untreated, may turn from purulent to serous and disappear in 2 months. Within 28 weeks of incubation, 90% of infected children are free of infection.[19] Prepubertal genital infections are commonly associated with perineal pain, pruritus, dysuria, or a purulent penile or vaginal discharge, but symptoms may decrease or even resolve within several weeks without treatment. Adolescents may present with cervical or urethral discharge, but up to one-half of infections in adolescents and adults are asymptomatic. In prepubertal boys the infection may present as asymptomatic pyuria, but symptomatic urethritis is more typical as it is in adult males.[15,19,20]

Reported rates of gonococcal infection range from 1% to 30% among sexually abused children.[15] The prevalence in prepubertal children is probably less than 2%, and probably less than 7% among pubertal children routinely cultured because of suspected sexual

TABLE 11.2

Incubation, Symptoms, and Diagnostic Tests for Sexually Transmitted Infections in Children

Sexually Transmitted Infection	Incubation	Symptoms	Diagnostic Tests
Gonorrhea	2–7 d	Vaginal discharge in pre-pubertal girls. Cervical, throat, and rectal infections are typically asymptomatic.	Culture on selective media with confirmation by 2 or more tests
Chlamydia trachomatis (except LGV)	Usually 5–7 d	Vaginal discharge in some prepubertal girls but most infections of vagina, cervix, throat, and rectum are asymptomatic.	Tissue culture with confirmatory staining with fluorescein-conjugated species-specific antibody
LGV	Usually 10–14 d	Usually single ulcer, papule, pustule, or vesicle with tender inguinal adenopathy.	Tissue culture
Syphilis	Range 10–90 d; usually 2–4 wk	Primary—usually painless typically single ulcer with slightly raised borders. Secondary—fever and rash, particularly palms and soles, condyloma latum.	Non-treponemal test (RPR or VDRL) confirmed by a positive treponemal test (FTA-ABS or MHA-TP) Dark field exam of primary lesion
Human immunodeficiency virus	6 wk– 6 mo	Lymphadenopathy, wasting, opportunistic infections asymptomatic for many years.	ELISA screening antibody testing with confirmation by IFA or Western blot (PCR for viral RNA is not appropriate.)
Trichomonas vaginalis	4–28 d	Vaginal discharge, but often asymptomatic.	Microscopy of fresh wet mount secretions, culture on special culture media
Chancroid	1–35 d; usually 3–7 d	Single or few shallow, painful ulcers with irregular edges.	Culture
Granuloma inguinale	Several days to several months	Irregular typically painless ulcers and granulomas, with subcutaneous inguinal swelling.	Tissue smears or biopsy showing "Donovan bodies"
Human papilloma-virus	1 mo–2 y (or longer)	Irregular raised lesions of variable sizes, but infections may be asymptomatic.	Clinical diagnosis, biopsy may be helpful in atypical lesions Subclinical infection– viral typing by PCR

TABLE 11.2
Incubation, Symptoms, and Diagnostic Tests for Sexually Transmitted Infections in Children,
continued

Sexually Transmitted Infection	Incubation	Symptoms	Diagnostic Tests
Herpes simplex virus (types 1 and 2)	2–14 d; usually 2–7 d	Painful vesicles and ulcers. Systemic symptoms common in primary infection.	Tissue culture followed by viral typing
Hepatitis B virus	45–160 d	Anorexia, abdominal pain, and jaundice, but sometimes asymptomatic.	Hepatitis B serology
Pubic lice	2–3 wk to mature	Pruritus, visible lice and nits on pubic hair or eyelashes.	Microscopic identification of lice
Head/body lice	2–3 wk to mature	Pruritus, visible lice and nits never on eyelashes.	Microscopic identification of lice
Hepatitis C	2 mo–6 mo	Asymptomatic for years.	Hepatitis C serology
Molluscum contagiosum	2 wk– 6 mo	Small skin-colored papules with central depressed core.	Visual identification of lesions
Bacterial vaginosis	Variable 7–14 d	Vaginal discharge but may be asymptomatic.	Microscopy showing "clue cells," with pH of secretions >4.5 and positive "whiff test" = fishy odor following addition of 10% potassium hydroxide
Group B streptococci	Variable, but typically <1 wk	Typically asymptomatic but may cause vaginal discharge.	Culture

Abbreviations: LGV, lymphogranuloma venereum; RPR, rapid plasma reagin; VDRL, Venereal Disease Research Laboratories; FTA-ABS, fluorescent treponemal antibody; MHA-TP, microhemagglutination-*Treponema pallidum*; ELISA, enzyme-linked immunosorbent assay; IFA, immunofluorescence assay; PCR, polymerase chain reaction; RNA, ribonucleic acid.

abuse.[3,8,14,17,21–25] Accurate diagnosis of a gonococcal infection can only be made by cultures using a modified Thayer-Martin, Martin-Lewis, or chocolate blood agar-based media. The predictive value of Gram stains alone is not known in children. The laboratory must perform appropriate confirmatory tests because similar bacteria, including *Moraxella catarrhalis, Kingella dentrificans, Neisseria meningitidis, Neisseria lactamica,* and *Neisseria cinerea,* can be misidentified as *N gonorrhoeae.*[26] Positive cultures should be confirmed by 2 of the following methods: biochemical (carbohydrate utilization), enzyme substrate, serologic, or nucleic acid testing.[2,26]

Culture results in suspected victims and suspected perpetrators require careful interpretation. Untreated asymptomatic gonococcal infection may persist for as long as 6 months in untreated adults, and pharyngeal infections may persist despite treatment. Therefore, repeatedly positive cultures do not necessarily mean repeated exposure and repeated abuse. Conversely, perpetrators who have taken commonly prescribed antibiotics for another infection may eradicate the gonococci and have negative cultures when they are subsequently screened as possible sources of the child's infection.

Spontaneous resolution of gonococcal infection without any antibiotic therapy commonly occurs within weeks to months of onset, and about 95% of all untreated infections in adults resolve within 6 months. Blood tests for the presence of antibody to the organism are unreliable because of a high false-negative rate among recently infected individuals.[27,28]

Routine cultures of the throat, rectum, and genital areas have been suggested for all sexually abused children regardless of history or symptoms.[2,3] Routine cultures may detect clinically unsuspected infections. In one study, 532 sexually abused children younger than 14 years had routine cultures taken from all 3 body sites.[3] Eight of the 25 cases of gonorrhea were discovered at sites that had not been involved in the sexual contact according to the child's initial history. Eleven infections detected were in children who had no symptoms of infection, including 3 of 12 prepubertal girls with vaginal infections. The 3 girls without symptoms all had reported genital contact. Recent research has focused on using selective criteria for STI screening. These studies have found rates of gonococcal infection in abused children to be less than 3%, and found low rates of asymptomatic vaginal infections.[21,22,25,29] One study showed that vaginal infections in 6 prepubertal girls were symptomatic, and no isolated pharyngeal or rectal infections were identified.[25] In another study, only 5% of prepubertal girls with vaginal infections (4 of 84) did not have vaginal discharge. The girls with asymptomatic infections would have been identified using selective criteria for increased risk of STI.[29] Selective criteria are useful in girls, but there are limited data on boys who have typically asymptomatic pharyngeal and rectal infections.[15]

N gonorrhoeae is not part of the normal genital flora.[24,30,31] The mode of transmission of gonorrhea is sexual in adolescents and adults.[32] Sexual transmission is not always documented in children, with reported rates ranging from 36% to 100 %.[24,28,33–39] Some cases represent perinatal transmission, and variable proportions with an unknown mode of transmission including children evaluated before 1970 and young children likely to have minimal verbal skills. One study of children with gonorrhea reported 100% of the children older than 4 years experienced sexual transmission, while only 35% of 1- to 4-year-olds had documented sexual transmission.[39] Additional studies have shown significant risk of gonorrhea in child and adult household contacts of sexually abused children, but the mode of transmission was not uniformly addressed.[27,40]

Gonococci can survive up to 24 hours on fomites (toilet seats, towels) in moist purulent secretions. This fact raises the possibility of nonsexual transmission in some cases, although clear documentation of cases of nonsexual transmission is not available.[4] Supportive evidence for nonsexual transmission was suggested by the authors of a study in 1927, who reported a hospital outbreak of 67 infants infected in the nursery over a 1-month period by an unknown source.[19] Inadvertent prepubertal spread of *N gonorrhoeae* by nonsexual contact or by sexual play has frequently been suggested, rarely described, and never rigorously documented.

Children with positive culture results may not be ready or able to disclose abuse, so it is not appropriate to conclude that infection resulted from nonsexual contact. The health care professional should assume that prepubertal children with gonorrhea have acquired it by sexual contact and that these contacts were abusive. The ease of transmission of gonorrhea to children is unknown. In adults, the infection may be transmitted in as few as 1 of 3 sexual contacts with an infected individual. Mucosal contact with infected genital secretions is required for transmission. Actual penile penetration is not required.[15,16, 27,28]

Chlamydial Infections

Chlamydia trachomatis is a gram-negative, obligate intracellular bacteria. The species includes the biologic variants: the oculogenital biovars and the lymphogranuloma venereum (LGV) biovars. The oculogenital biovars cause most urogenital infections as well as perinatal conjunctivitis and pneumonia. The LGV biovars are responsible for lymphogranuloma venereum. *C trachomatis* or chlamydial infections are the most frequently recognized STI in adolescents and adults.[15] Rectogenital infection rates of 1% to 8% are reported among sexually abused children.[9, 22,25,41–43] The prevalence in prepubertal girls has been found to approach the lower end of this range (0.8%), while the prevalence in pubertal girls approaches the upper end of the range (7.0%).[22,25] Some infected prepubertal girls have a vaginal discharge; but most chlamydial infections do not produce symptoms. The time between sexual contact and onset of vaginal symptoms in children is unknown. The question of whether infections can relapse and how long infections may persist have not been answered. For these reasons, it is difficult to determine when an infection was acquired.[19]

Chlamydial infections are difficult to detect in children for several reasons. The estimated sensitivity of a single cervical swab culture ranges from 50% to 90%; isolation from vaginal pool swabs is lower. Recovery of the organism also depends on specimen handling before inoculation of the culture, and culture confirmation depends on the techniques that are used. Dacron- or rayon-tipped plastic or metal shaft swabs should be used because cotton or calcium alginate tips or wooden shafts may kill the organisms. Cellular material must be collected because chlamydiae are obligate intracellular organisms.[44] Diagnosis in sexually abused children must be made using a culture technique rather than the more commonly available rapid detection methods. Enzyme immunoassay (EIA) and direct fluorescence antibody (DFA) tests are extremely unreliable for vaginal or rectal specimens in children because cross-reactivity with many common bacteria including *N gonorrhoeae, Gardnerella vaginalis, Escherichia coli,* as well as other gram-negative enteric organisms and group A and B streptococci, may occur.[45] DNA probe tests have limited specificity at anogenital sites in children and they should not be used for any sexual abuse victims. False-positive cultures have been associated with the use

of EIA to confirm tissue cultures.[2,23,46] Because of the legal implications, only tissue cultures for chlamydia, confirmed by microscopic identification of inclusion by fluorescein-conjugated, species-specific antibody staining, should be used in evaluating sexual abuse in children.[2,6,23,44,46]

Perinatal maternal-infant transmission is common. As many as 50% to 60% of infants born to infected mothers acquire the infection or colonization, including 14% with subclinical rectal and vaginal colonization. Neonatal infections have been documented to persist for 12 months in 35% of colonized infants, and one infant still had a positive oropharyngeal culture at 28.5 months after birth, but was subsequently negative at 3 years.[47,48] Therefore, positive cultures in children 3 years of age or younger may occasionally represent persistent perinatal infections. The mode of transmission is sexual in chlamydial infections in adolescents and adults. A study comparing adolescent females who were sexually active to adolescent females who were virgins found 13 of 68 sexually active females had positive cultures and only 1 of 52 virginal females had positive cultures.[32] Positive cultures in adolescents are also difficult to interpret. *C trachomatis* was isolated from 18 of 127 female adolescent victims of sexual abuse; however, 16 of the 18 positive cultures were from previously sexually active adolescents.[49] Therefore, it may be correct to attribute many of the infections in this study to the prior consenting activity.

Sexual transmission has been documented in 11% to 100% of children with chlamydial genital infections.[33,43,50] Of the studies reporting low rates of sexual transmission, one reported unknown mode of transmission for 8 of 9 children with combined gonococcal and chlamydial infections[43] and another used DFA testing to test for chlamydia and determined only 5 of 12 cases were attributable to sexual transmission.[33] The first study seems to have had inadequate evaluation for abuse and the second study is likely to have had a high false-positive rate using DFA testing. Chlamydial vaginal infections beyond the first year of life are strongly associated with sexual contact when proper methods are used for detecting the infection and sexual abuse. Some infections in preschool children, however, may represent persistence of perinatal infection, and many infections detected in adolescents may actually be the result of previous consensual sexual activity. The number of children with reported pharyngeal or rectal infections is too small to draw any conclusions about infections at these sites.[15,19,45,50]

Nucleic acid amplification tests for C trachomatis *and* N gonorrhoeae

Nucleic acid amplification tests (NAATs) have revolutionized testing for STIs in adolescents and adults, especially in the diagnosis of *C trachomatis* and *N gonorrhoeae*. Nucleic acid amplification tests are very sensitive, highly specific, and can allow noninvasive testing (urine) with only a small decrease in sensitivity. Studies in adults have suggested they are marginally more sensitive than cultures for *N gonorrhoeae* but 10% to 30% more sensitive than cultures

for *C trachomatis*. Test specificity is very high in adults, but there may be some cross-reactivity of NAATs for gonorrhea with some non-gonococcal *Neisseria* species. Nucleic acid amplification tests theoretically are able to detect a single gene sequence in a sample and can be positive because of organisms in the ejaculate in acute assault cases, and can remain positive for up to 3 weeks after treatment.[23,51] Commercially available NAATs for chlamydia and gonorrhea include polymerase chain reaction (PCR), COBAS AMPLICOR CT/NG (Roche Molecular Systems); strand displacement assay, Probe Tec ET CT/NG (Becton, Dickinson); and transcription-mediated amplification (TMA), Aptima Combo 2 (Gen-Probe). Ligase chain reaction (LCR) tests for chlamydia and gonorrhea are no longer available due to excessive variability of results. Strand displacement assay and TMA can be used to detect chlamydia and gonorrhea in urethral and urine specimens in males, and cervical, urethral, and urine specimens in females. Polymerase chain reaction can be used on specimens from the same sites except for gonorrhea testing in urine specimens in females. Transcription-mediated amplification is the only test available for use on vaginal specimens. None of these tests have been standardized or approved for rectal specimens from adults, or rectogenital specimens in children.[23,52]

Most studies comparing the performance of NAATs with cultures have used adolescent and adult subjects, but several series have included small groups of prepubertal children. As might be expected, they found NAATs to be more sensitive than chlamydia cultures, but specificity was less certain.[51, 53-55] In addition, some studies in children included pubertal and postpubertal adolescents, and some used LCR, limiting their interpretation regarding prepubertal children.

One practical problem addressed by the use of NAATS is the limited access to laboratories that still perform gonorrhea and chlamydia cultures. The CDC suggests that NAATs can be used for detection of chlamydia when evaluating a prepubertal child if culture is not available, and the positive test can be confirmed by a second NAAT that targets another genetic sequence.[2]

One major problem inherent in the use of NAATS in prepubertal children is the low prevalence of gonorrhea and chlamydia among sexually abused children. If very few tested patients have the disease, even a highly specific test will yield a substantial number of false positives. The positive predictive value of a test is dependent on the specificity of the test and the prevalence of the disease in the population studied. If the prevalence of gonorrhea or chlamydia in prepubertal children evaluated for sexual abuse is 1%, even if the test has a specificity of 99%, about half of the positive tests will be false positives. If the prevalence of either infection is 2%, about a third of the tests will be false positives. However, clinicians face a dilemma because the false-negative rate is likely to be high for chlamydia cultures, and cultures may not be available in many localities, which leads to concerns about underdiagnosing and undertreating infections in children. This dilemma forces clinicians to consider options. If the major

goal is to identify and treat the highest number of prepubertal children who are at risk of having gonorrhea or chlamydia, using NAATs achieves this goal. It also allows testing with minimally invasive urine tests. If the major goal is to identify the child with either infection, using the gold standard tests that are accepted proof of sexual contact, cultures are appropriate. If the goal is to have the best assessment of risk of infection and the best evidence, a dual or serial approach is best. The clinician can obtain both NAATs and cultures at the same time, or initially "screen" with a NAAT and obtain a culture to confirm the presence of the organism. The serial approach requires getting the child to return for confirmatory testing, which may be difficult in some settings. Data on adults suggest a confirmatory test using a second NAAT that targets a different genetic sequence may be acceptable.[2]

Despite the logic behind the above alternatives, the use of NAATs in the diagnosis of chlamydia and gonorrhea in prepubertal children remains controversial at this time.[1,2,23,56] The diagnosis of child sexual abuse is based on the history. When the history confirms sexual abuse, the purpose of the examination is to diagnose and treat conditions that may result from the abuse. The use of the most sensitive tests would be justified in this situation. If a child is suspected to be abused based on physical or behavioral signs and symptoms, but no history of abuse is available, only the use of the most specific test is justified.

Syphilis

Abused children may present with asymptomatic disease, or symptomatic primary or secondary syphilis. Primary lesions or chancres are moist ulcerations with raised borders that may be mistaken for anal fissures or perianal cellulitis; secondary syphilis may be mistaken for a viral exanthem with a variable skin rash, classic lesions of the palms and soles, or flat-surfaced, raised perineal lesions known as *condylomata lata.*[57-59]

Treponema pallidum, the causative organism, is a thin, motile spirochete that is capable of surviving only briefly outside a host and cannot grow on any known media. Non-treponemal reagin tests, such as the Venereal Disease Research Laboratories test and the rapid plasma reagin, are commonly used for screening victims. Specific antibody tests for *T pallidum,* such as the fluorescent treponemal antibody or the microhemagglutination-*T pallidum,* must be done to confirm the screening test. The false-positive rate for both treponemal and non-treponemal tests in the general population is 1% to 2%. False-positive non-treponemal tests are the result of cross-reactivity with 1 of more than 200 non-treponemal antigens. False positives can occur in numerous conditions, including other spirochetal infections, infectious mononucleosis, measles, varicella, hepatitis, autoimmune diseases, pregnancy, lymphoma, intravenous drug use, atopic dermatitis, bacterial pneumonias, bacterial endocarditis, rickettsial infections, and after immunizations. False-negative results can occur when very high antibody concentrations inhibit agglutination, known as the

prozone effect. False-positive treponemal tests can occur in patients with elevated globulins, lyme disease, leprosy, malaria, infectious mononucleosis, relapsing fever, leptospirosis, and autoimmune disease. False-negative treponemal and non-treponemal tests can occur in human immunodeficiency virus infections. Repeat testing is often required because of the long, variable incubation period (10–90 days).[7,57,60]

Syphilis is detected in 0.0% to 1.8% of reported victims of sexual abuse.[3-5,15,21,25,60-63] Although routine testing of all victims is usually recommended, the apparently low risk in abused children may support the practice of screening all adolescents but testing only children with a history of genital or perianal lesions, an exanthem, the presence of another STI, with known syphilis infection in the perpetrator, or patients who live in high-risk areas for syphilis.[15,21,25,60] Non-treponemal tests may yield negative results within months of treatment, and all are negative within 2 years. Treponemal tests usually remain positive for life, but up to one-quarter of individuals with treated primary syphilis will have negative treponemal tests.

There is extensive literature on syphilis in adults, but information on children, except for perinatal transmission, is limited to case reports or small case series. Acquiring syphilis through blood transfusions is rare, and a few cases of facial lesions resulting from nonsexual transmission in children have been reported.[17] Two case reports attribute transmission by kissing from adult relatives with oral syphilis lesions to a 6-year-old girl and a 2 1/2-year-old boy in the absence of disclosure of abuse.[64,65] Infections occurring in infancy may have resulted from prenatal exposure. Primary disease presenting after 4 months of age or secondary disease presenting after the first year of life should not be considered congenitally acquired. Evaluation of the mode of transmission of syphilis in preschool-aged children is difficult, however.[66] Prepubertal children with primary or secondary stages of syphilis occurring beyond early infancy should be presumed to be victims of sexual abuse.[6,33,59,60,61]

Human Papillomavirus

Human papillomavirus (HPV) is a DNA virus that can cause infections of skin and mucous membranes. More than 130 types of HPV have been identified, and different HPV types exhibit trophism for anogenital, oropharyngeal, or cutaneous sites. Anogenital warts are most commonly caused by types 6 and 11, but types 16, 18, 31, and 35 are also relatively common; at least another 2-dozen types have been implicated. Human papillomavirus types 16, 18, 31, and 45 have the highest oncogenic potential, but others present a moderately high risk of cancer. Oral and pharyngeal warts (laryngeal papilloma) are also most commonly associated with types 6 and 11, with 16 and 18 involved in most of the other cases. Cutaneous warts are usually caused by types 1 and 2, but types 3, 4, 7, and 10 are also common. The trophism exhibited by the different types is not absolute; cutaneous HPV types have been documented to occur at anogenital sites.[67]

An average incubation period of 2 to 3 months in both non-sexually or sexually acquired HPV infections has been suggested, but the interval from exposure to development of the lesions is extremely variable, possibly ranging from several weeks to several years.[67,68] Most infections are subclinical or latent, distorting the concept of incubation period. The classic visible lesions characterizing HPV infection, condylomata acuminata or anogenital warts, are soft, irregular, multidigitate wartlike growths. Other common appearances of the lesions include small, flat, red, violaceous, or pigmented papules on the penile shaft, flat cervical growths, and fine irregularities of the vulvar tissues called *papillomatosis labialis*. Most lesions occur in the perineal area, although they can be found on any moist skin areas or mucous membranes. Several levels of the genitourinary tract may be involved simultaneously, and some lesions may be entirely internal, located inside the urethra, vagina, or rectum.[68,69] Oral lesions may also occur in children, having a similar appearance to the lesions on mucous membranes in the anogenital area. Laryngeal papillomas or juvenile onset recurrent respiratory papillomatosis is another presentation of HPV infection in children. National data suggest that two-thirds of cases are diagnosed by age 4 years and more than three-quarters of cases are diagnosed before age 7 years.[67]

Diagnosis is usually made by the typical clinical wart-like appearance of the lesions and occasionally by biopsy, although specific viral typing techniques can be used. Commercially available tests such as Hybrid Capture 2 Assay (HC2, Digene Corporation) detect a number of common anogenital types, but do not identify cutaneous types.[52] Some wart-like lesions in the anogenital area are not caused by HPV.[70]

Human papillomavirus infections are probably the most common STI in adolescents and young adults but have been considered an uncommon STI in children. The prevalence of HPV among sexually active young women as demonstrated by PCR testing ranges from 13% to 80%, depending on both the population studied and on the total number of HPV types for which screening was done.[67] Most HPV infections in adolescents and adults are subclinical or latent infections, and the typical infection is both asymptomatic and transient. Most visible anogenital warts are caused by only 6 HPV types. Therefore, screening for HPV infection using PCR testing incorporating a large number of HPV types is the most sensitive method. Visualization of cellular changes associated with HPV infection on Pap smears has significantly lower sensitivity because many infected women have normal Pap smears, and observation for visible anogenital warts has the lowest sensitivity.[52] Clearly there is a large reservoir of HPV among sexually active women of child-bearing and child-caring age, and most do not know they are infected.

Prenatal transmission, presumably through hematogenous spread, has been reported in a few cases presenting within the first week of life.[67,71] The role of perinatal transmission remains unclear. The presence of HPV DNA in infants born to infected mothers ranges from 1% to 77% and in uninfected mothers ranges from 1% to 50%, suggesting the possibility of nonsexual transmission from caretakers being important in the children of both HPV-positive and HPV-negative mothers.[15] The most comprehensive prospective study of infants and toddlers presents a strong argument against perinatal transmission; 74% of the mothers were HPV positive, but less than 3% of the infants were positive. Women who were HPV DNA positive were just as likely as HPV DNA–negative women to have HPV DNA–positive infants and toddlers, and the HPV subtypes in infant-mother pairs were not concordant.[72] Additional studies have found discordance between infants and their mothers and fathers,[73] as well as evidence that persistent cervical HPV and subclinical oral HPV in the mothers are significant risk factors for persistent HPV in infants.[74] Although these studies do not exclude the possibility of vertical perinatal transmission, they suggest that exposure of an infant to HPV during vaginal delivery may be associated with only a low risk of acquiring HPV infection, and nonsexual transmission may occur during activities of normal infant care.[67]

Nonsexual transmission of common warts (usually HPV type 2) has been implicated in some of the typical perineal lesions in young children.[71,75-77] DNA typing has demonstrated that 10% to 42% of children have anogenital lesions by skin HPV types.[15,75] It cannot be assumed, however, that all perineal lesions caused by HPV type 2 or type 3 are acquired by non-abusive contact because no consistent correlation is found between the frequency of hand and genital warts. In addition, the common wart virus also could be spread from the infected hands of an individual through inappropriate genital fondling. The risk of acquiring HPV infection from cobathing and sexual play is unknown. Nonsexual transmission might have occurred in 4 of 15 cases in one case series because of a positive maternal history of genital warts or exposure to skin warts. Social and medical evaluation revealed sexual abuse in the 4 cases, emphasizing the need for thorough investigation of sexual abuse in children with genital warts.[78]

Human papillomavirus type 6 and type 11 are the predominant types found in laryngeal papillomas, and perinatal transmission is considered the etiology. Sexual transmission is rarely considered in children, although sexual transmission is considered the etiology of laryngeal papillomas in adults.[67] The actual proportion of genital warts in children resulting from sexual transmission and other modes of transmission is also unknown. Some case series of children treated for genital warts have not evaluated or reported the mode of transmission,[79] others have documented low rates of suspected sexual transmission.[78,80–84] Some reports document sexual transmission in half of the cases, with differences in proportion on sexual transmission partially explained by referral patterns, the thoroughness of the evaluation for possible sexual abuse, and the age of the children included. In one study a confirmed history of sexual abuse was obtained from 7 of 9 children older than 3 years; no history could be obtained from any of the 9 children 3 years and younger.[85] In another study, none of the infected children younger than 3 years were determined to be sexually abused; however, 50% of children 4 years and older had proven sexual transmission.[76] The likelihood of sexual transmission seems to increase with the age of the children studied.

Subclinical HPV infection has been demonstrated by DNA probes and antibody techniques in up to 24% of oral mucosal samples in preschool children[82] and in 52% of oral samples in children 3 to 11 years of age.[86] Human papillomavirus DNA has been found in 8% of girls with lichen sclerosus[87] and in the anal area in 1.2% and genital area in 3% of 5- to 6-year-old children who were reported to have not been abused.[88] Subclinical infection has also been demonstrated in 5% to 33% of sexually abused children.[84,89,90] The virus can remain latent in normal-appearing areas adjacent to the skin lesions. Therefore, a positive test for HPV DNA or the appearance of new lesions months after sexual contact or treatment of lesions may or may not be attributable to reexposure through continuing sexual contact. Viral transmission may occur from an individual without obvious mucosal or cutaneous lesions, so considering the potential role of subclinical infections is essential. The long and variable incubation period of HPV, the contradictory data on perinatal transmission, and general prevalence of subclinical infection make it difficult to identify the source and mode of transmission in many cases of childhood HPV infection.

Viral typing could allow comparison of the child's lesions and lesions from individuals with possible contact with the child.[91] However, HPV types 6 and 11 are commonly found in both adults and children, and the same HPV type in a child and an adult contact neither proves the adult was the source nor specifies whether the transmission was sexual or nonsexual. Multiple HPV types may coexist in the same individual, further complicating this analysis. The high prevalence of subclinical infection limits the detection of HPV by usual detection methods in males.[92] Human papillomavirus typing does provide some information as to whether the infection originates from a cutaneous or mucosal site, but cutaneous warts could be transferred by autoinoculation or by common acts of sexual abuse such as fondling and digital penetration. Therefore, HPV typing but does not provide practical evidence for determining if a child has been sexually abused.

Every child with anogenital or oral HPV infection should have a complete medical evaluation for sexual abuse. This should include taking a history from the child's caretaker regarding possible sexual abuse and nonsexual exposures, age-appropriate interviewing of the child, a thorough physical examination, and an evaluation for other STIs on the basis of risk factors from the history and examination.[7] If the history, the child's interview, the physical examination, and the tests for other STIs do not support a diagnosis of sexual abuse, the conclusion should be that there was no clear evidence of sexual abuse, and the case might represent nonsexual transmis-sion. Although some authors may suggest a referral to child protective services in all cases for children older than a certain age at first presentation (eg, 2 years, 3 years, 4 years), one should consider not reporting a case in which there are no other reasons to suspect sexual abuse. Children with laryngeal papillomas should have similar evaluation for sexual abuse if they present when they are older than 5 years.

Trichomoniasis

Trichomonas vaginalis is 1 of 5 *Tricho-monas* species of flagellated protozoans that infect humans. *T vaginalis* is the only clinically important species; the other 4 are nonpathogenic species: *Trichomonas tenax* is normal mouth flora; *T faecalis, Trichomonas ardin delteili,* and *Trichomonas hominis* are normal fecal flora. *T hominis* can survive and multiply at room temperature and survive in feces up to 24 hours. Skilled technicians can differentiate *T vaginalis* from the other species found in fresh vaginal secretions or urine through morphological differences, including the number and location of flagella, the appearance of the undulating membrane, and the characteristic motility pattern. *T vaginalis* must be differentiated from the other species that occasionally will be found in contaminated urine or vaginal secretions.[15] *T vaginalis* infections are characterized by a purulent vaginal discharge, although asymptomatic infections can occur. It is not known how long children can be infected before developing symptoms.[20] Infected mothers may transmit the infection to their infants during birth, and these infections can persist for up to 1 year. However, the prevalence of *T vaginalis* in vaginally delivered infants of mothers with documented infection is not known.[15] The organism may be detected in a urine sample, but the diagnosis is usually made by microscopic examination of a wet mount of the vaginal discharge that reveals the causative protozoan in motion. Wet mount preparations identify only 50% to 75% of cases detectable using specific culture techniques. The sensitivity of culture methods using Diamond's media, Trichosel media, and InPouch TV (BioMed Diagnostics) approach 90%. Additional tests are available, but these have not been standardized for use in children. A rapid, commercially available antibody-based test, OSOM Trichomonas Rapid Test (Genzyme Diagnostics), reports a sensitivity of 83% and specificity of 99%. An automated DNA probe, Affirm VPIII Microbial Identification Test (Becton, Dickinson), reports a sensitivity of 89.5% and specificity of 99.8%.[52]

Trichomoniasis and bacterial vaginosis (BV) are the most frequently acquired infections following sexual assault in adult and adolescent females.[8,15,17] *T vaginalis* infection is uncommon in prepubertal girls beyond infancy and strongly suggests sexual abuse. Trichomoniasis is a common STI in sexually active adolescents and adults, and infected males are typically asymptomatic.

Four studies evaluating the etiology of vulvovaginitis in premenarcheal girls found no cases of *T vaginalis* infection.[31,93–95] Prevalence studies of trichomoniasis in children either have not specifically addressed sexual abuse or have not addressed the mode of transmission at all.[21] Furthermore, a vaginal wet mount is not routinely performed during the evaluation for suspected sexual abuse of prepubertal children. Two studies employing routine testing found no cases of *T vaginalis*. One study found no positives among 160 cases and 95 controls younger than 10 years using *T vaginalis* cultures[24] and the other found no positives using microscopic analysis of urine and vaginal secretions to evaluate 119 prepubertal girls with suspected sexual abuse.[25]

Nonsexual transmission is theoretically possible because the organism can survive up to several hours on objects, wet clothing, mud baths, and warm mineral water, although no cases of proven fomite transmission have been reported in either adults or children.[4,7] Therefore, trichomoniasis infections in prepubertal children beyond the first months of life are strongly suggestive of sexual abuse.[1,96] Evaluation of a child with *T vaginalis* infection should include an appropriate interview of the child, physical examination, and appropriate testing for other STIs.

Herpes Simplex Virus Infection

Herpes simplex viruses (HSVs) are enveloped, double-stranded DNA viruses that are neurotrophic and capable of establishing latent and recurrent infections. Herpes simplex virus infection is characterized by painful vesicular or ulcerated lesions involving skin and mucous membranes, but primary infection can be asymptomatic. The lesions in primary infections, often accompanied by fever, appear after an incubation period of 2 to 20 days (mean 6 days) after exposure. Nonsexual transmission is not well studied, but HSV type 1 (HSV-1) infections are a fairly common childhood infection usually involving only the mouth but occasionally the mouth and genital area simultaneously.[97–101] Herpes simplex virus type 1 infections usually cause oral, labial, ocular, and brain infections, and most HSV type 2 (HSV-2) infections occur in the genital area or in cutaneous and disseminated neonatal infections. Herpes simplex virus type 1 is more likely to produce recurrent disease in the mouth or lips and HSV-2 is more likely to produce recurrent disease in the genital area. A genital infection with HSV-1 is usually a primary infection because recurrent genital HSV-1 is uncommon. However, HSV-1 or HSV-2 can be found at either location. Historically, less than 20% of herpes genital infections were due to HSV-1, but multiple studies from around the world have documented HSV-1 as the cause of 33% to 71% of all herpes infections in the genital area. This increasing proportion of genital herpes caused by HSV-1 may be in part due to increased condom use during penile-anal and penile-genital intercourse, but lack of condom use in orogenital sex.[102]

Primary herpes genital infection is seen most frequently among sexually active adolescents and young adults. Genital herpes infections are uncommon in prepubertal children, and sexual abuse has been documented to be the cause in many cases.[4,18,19] In one study of 1,583 children younger than 13 years evaluated for suspected sexual abuse, 2 children (0.1%) had HSV-2 infection, but only 1 gave a history of sexual abuse.[21] However, most of the data on HSV-1 and HSV-2 genital infections in children come from case reports or small case series.[24,97–99,103–106] These cases include isolated genital infections with either HSV-1 or HSV-2, simultaneous infection of the oral and genital areas with HSV-1 and HSV-2, and one case of isolated perianal HSV-2 infection. A history of sexual contact was present in some cases and absent in others. The actual risk of acquiring the infection through sexual abuse is unknown.[15]

Although asymptomatic viral shedding is frequent in adults, routine HSV cultures are of little value in asymptomatic children. Cultures of active lesions may be positive in approximately 95% from vesicles, but only 70% from ulcerations and 30% from crusted lesions. Suspicious lesions (vesicles or ulcerations) must be cultured and can be subtyped to distinguish HSV-1 from HSV-2 infections. Polymerase chain reaction testing has high sensitivity and specificity, but may be subject to contamination. Varicella-zoster infection may mimic genital or perianal infection but viral culture or DFA testing can be used to differentiate between the viruses.[107,108] Similar lesions can be caused by Epstein-Barr virus, influenza, and coxsackievirus infections. Many commercially available serologic tests for HSV antibody can document seronegativity but cannot consistently differentiate between HSV-2 and HSV-1 antibody. Commercially available type-specific serologic tests based on glycoprotein G, including Herpes Select 1 and 2

(Focus Technology, Inc.) and POCkit HSV2 (Dianology), may have acceptable accuracy in distinguishing HSV-1 from HSV-2 with sensitivities of 80% to 98% and specificity of 96% or higher in adults. Even these tests cannot be considered to be completely accurate in determining whether an individual has been infected with HSV. Data on the performance of these tests in children are lacking at this time.[52,109,110] Epidemiological studies in Nigeria and India have shown that 8.5% to 50% of children aged 1 to 10 years were seropositive for HSV-2, raising the possibility of but not proving contamination as the source of infection.[19] No cases of fomite transmission have been documented, but HSV can survive for up to 4 hours on plastic, rubber, and metal surfaces.[4] When a child has simultaneous oral and genital infection, or when an infant or toddler has a caretaker with oral lesions, it may be reasonable to conclude that nonsexual transmission of genital lesions due to HSV-1 is the cause. The evidence suggests that except for transmission at birth, most HSV-2 genital infections are sexually transmitted.[97,98] However, either HSV-1 or HSV-2 infections in the genital area of a child or adolescent documented by viral culture should be considered possible evidence of sexual abuse or sexual contact considering both the changing epidemiology of HSV infection in the genital area in adolescents and adults.

Bacterial Vaginosis

Bacterial vaginosis seems to be a marker of sexual activity in adults, but children may acquire the infection through sexual and nonsexual means. Bacterial vaginosis (or nonspecific vaginitis) is a polymicrobial infection resulting from the replacement of *Lactobacillus* species with *Gardnerella vaginalis* (GV), *Mycoplasma hominis,* and various anaerobic organisms. Although GV is one bacterium that may be involved in this infection, the presence or absence of this organism in a vaginal culture does not prove or disprove the diagnosis. Diagnosis requires both a microscopic examination of the discharge and simple chemical tests. The characteristic thin, gray-white to yellow vaginal discharge is examined microscopically for the presence of "clue cells," which are epithelial cells with clusters of bacteria adhering to the surface. A "whiff test" is performed by the addition of 10% KOH to the vaginal secretions, which results in a fishy or amine aroma in the presence of BV. Bacterial vaginosis has been defined as "definite" when both clue cells and a positive whiff test are found, and "possible" when one of the 2 tests is positive.[7,17] A vaginal pH greater than 4.5 is present in postpubertal females with the infection, but vaginal pH is not a reliable criterion in younger girls. Gram-stained vaginal smears showing no lactobacilli and predominant gram-negative and gram-variable rods are sensitive and specific for BV in adults.[15]

The infection rate is increased following sexual contact, but this entity may be the most common cause of nonsexually transmitted vaginitis in children and adolescents.[15,111] In a study of 26 girls younger than 14 years with symptomatic vulvovaginitis, the vaginal washings of 9 (35%) had diagnostic tests positive for BV. Only 3 of these girls had a history of sexual abuse.[20,112] The development of a new vaginal discharge following sexual abuse has been associated with BV, but the presence of this infection in a child may be attributed to either sexual or nonsexual transmission.[15,111,112] There is extensive literature on GV and BV in adults. Both the organism and the clinical infection are more prevalent among sexually active individuals, but both are also found in nonsexually active individuals.

Several studies have compared the prevalence of GV in predominantly premenarcheal girls with and without vaginitis. Two studies of premenarcheal girls with vaginitis reported no positive cultures for GV among 54 and 200 girls respectively.[31,94] One study found 2 of 50 cases were positive and 0 of 21 controls were positive for GV,[95] and another had no positive cultures for GV in either the 50 cases or 50 controls. Of 59 children cultured for GV, 3 of 8 positives had vaginitis and 8 of 51 negatives had vaginitis. The rate of positive cultures varied by age: 18% in children younger than 3 years, 2.5% in children 3 to 10 years old, and 63% in children 11 to 15 years old.[30]

Some studies have compared the prevalence of GV in cases of sexual abuse and in controls. One study found definite BV in 4 vaginal washings from 31 children, obtained 2 or more weeks after sexual abuse, whose initial test results were negative.[112] None of 23 specimens from non-abused girls were positive. Another study evaluated girls 1 to 11 years of age for GV. Of 137 with highly suspected or known sexual abuse 14.6% were positive; of 48 girls with genital symptoms but no history of abuse 4.2%

were positive. Of 71 girls with neither a history of abuse or genital symptoms 4.2% were positive.[113] A study involving girls 1 to 12 years of age found similar prevalence of GV in 3 groups of girls: 191 girls giving a history of sexual abuse or having another STI (5.3% positive), 144 girls evaluated for possible abuse but who gave no history of sexual contact and had no STI (4.9% positive), and 31 controls (6.4%).[114] Another study found GV in 24 of 209 sexually abused girls, but in only 1 of 101 controls whose parents denied they were sexually active or sexually abused.[24] Two studies in post-menarcheal adolescents show higher rates of GV in girls who are sexually active (34% and 60%) compared with girls denying sexual activity (17% and 33%). Clinical BV was equally prevalent among those reporting or denying sexual contact in the one study[111] and was slightly more common among girls with GV than those without GV.[115] Only 2 studies provide data on prepubertal asymptomatic boys: one study found no anogenital cultures positive for GV in 99 boys while the other found 2 positive anal cultures but no positive genital cultures in 99 boys.[116,117] Review of the literature on children and adolescents with GV and BV suggests the following: both are found in girls with and without a history of sexual abuse or sexual contact, both are more prevalent in sexually abused or sexually active individuals than in controls, both are more prevalent in post-menarcheal than in premenarcheal girls, the GV organism is inconsistently associated with either genital symptoms or clinical BV, and the GV organism is rarely (but occasionally) found in asymptomatic, "non-abused" boys. Therefore, despite an association with sexual contact in children and adolescents, both GV and BV have limited or indeterminate specificity for sexual contact or sexual abuse.

Human Immunodeficiency Virus Infection

Human immunodeficiency virus (HIV) infection in children and adolescents is a complex, variable disease. Infected adults and children develop serum antibodies to this human RNA retrovirus within 6 to 12 weeks after exposure. When testing is done within 2 weeks of exposure, a negative test provides information of prior HIV status only.[118] The median interval from percutaneous or transfusion exposure is 3 weeks. If the initial test is negative, testing should be repeated at 6 weeks. Follow-up testing must be done at least 3 to 6 months after exposure because, rarely, more than 6 weeks may elapse between exposure and seroconversion.[17] The actual timing of follow-up specimens is not clear because no data are available on the incubation period following sexual assault in children. Screening for HIV infections is typically done using EIA for HIV antibody. The predictive value of a positive screening test is low in a low-prevalence population. In the last few years the US Food and Drug Administration approved 4 "rapid" HIV antibody screening tests: OraQuick Rapid HIV-1 Antibody Test (OraSure Technologies, Inc.), Reveal Rapid HIV-1 Antibody Test (Med Mira Laboratories, Inc.), Uni-Gold Recombigen HIV Test (Trinity Biotech Plc., Co.), and Murex-SUDS-Single Use Diagnostic System

Rapid HIV-1 Antibody Test (Abbott Laboratories). If the standard or rapid EIA test is positive, it should be repeated, followed by an immunofluorescence assay or a Western blot test to distinguish between true and false positives.[2]

The potential long-term risk of HIV infection among child sexual abuse victims is unknown, but it would be extremely unlikely for HIV infection to follow a single episode of sexual abuse. Screening of victims for HIV infection seems most reasonable if the child gives a history of vaginal or rectal penetration by multiple perpetrators or an unknown perpetrator or is symptomatic for HIV or any STI or if the perpetrator is known to have HIV infection, is a known homosexual or bisexual, or is a known intravenous drug abuser.[15] High prevalence of HIV infection regionally may also be considered a risk factor. Some experts recommend that all sexually abused children be screened for HIV, recognizing that many positive tests will result because of previously undocumented neonatal transmission. Screening of the perpetrator first, and then screening only a child whose perpetrator was positive for HIV is ideal, but this may not be a legal option in many states. The issue of HIV infection should be addressed with every victim and his or her family, and regardless of the decision about testing, appropriate counseling support and follow-up should be provided.[15,102,118] Sexual abuse has been implicated in cases of HIV infection.[119–121] Human immunodeficiency virus infection in children should be considered sexually transmitted unless transmission perinatally or through transfusion is documented.

Other Sexually Transmitted Infections

Anogenital signs and symptoms can be the result of sexual abuse, but these are common in nonabused children as well. Most children presenting with anogenital signs and symptoms in the absence of a verbal disclosure of abuse are unlikely to be diagnosed with either STIs or sexual abuse even after a thorough assessment.[122] Symptoms suggesting urinary tract infections (UTIs) are much more common than actual UTIs in sexually abused children.[123,124]

Information is limited about other STIs and their association with sexual abuse of children. This lack of information is attributed to several factors: many have primarily nonsexual modes of transmission in children, some have a low prevalence among adults, and some are extremely rare in children.[7,13,15]

Mycoplasma hominis, Mycoplasma genitalium, and *Ureaplasma urealyticum* are small pleomorphic bacteria that lack a cell wall. Colonization or asymptomatic infections with the genital mycoplasmas, *M hominis, M genitalium,* and *U urealyticum,* strongly correlate with sexual activity in adults. Symptomatic infections are not common. Neither organism is clearly linked to vaginal infections, but *U urealyticum* has been shown to be the cause of at least 10% of nonspecific urethritis in males.[20] Two controlled studies of pharyngeal, anorectal, and vaginal colonization rates

in abused and non-abused children with genital mycoplasmas have been reported.[125,126] One study showed no significant difference in colonization with genital mycoplasmas between abused children and controls.[126] In the other, *M hominis* was isolated from the anorectal and vaginal cultures of 23% and 34% of the 47 abused girls compared with 8% and 17% respectively, of the 36 controls. *U urealyticum* was isolated from the anorectal and vaginal cultures of 19% and 30% of the abused girls compared with 3% and 8% of 36 controls.[125] No association was found between colonization with either organism and the presence of a discharge in these children. In summary, increased colonization has been demonstrated among sexually abused children for both *M genitalium* and *U urealyticum.* These organisms should not be considered significant markers for sexual abuse, however, because asymptomatic colonization is also common among non-abused children.

Ectoparasites including *Sarcoptes scabiei* (scabies), *Phthirus pubis* (pubic or "crab" lice), *Pediculus humanus humanus* (body lice), and *Pediculus humanus capitis* (head lice) can be sexually transmitted, but close nonsexual body contact is the predominant mode of transmission in children. Pubic lice is the only species of lice to infest the eyelashes, and in addition to the pubic and perianal hair, it can infest the beard, eyebrows, and axillary hair. Scabies, body lice, and head lice are primarily spread by close body contact in all age groups. Sexual contact is the primary mode of transmission for pubic lice in adolescents and adults, and the possibility of sexual abuse should be considered in children with this ectoparasite.[2,7]

Molluscum contagiosum, a poxvirus infection, is transmitted through close body contact. The lesions are dome-shaped, skin-colored papules that often have umbilicated white centers. Occasionally they form larger, clustered lesions that may have multiple umbilications and mimic the appearance of warts. The lesions are typically found on the extremities and trunk in children, but the virus may be self-inoculated through scratching and touching of the perineal skin. It has been linked to sexual activity in adolescents and adults, but nonsexual transmission is common in both children and adults.[7,70]

Shigellosis, salmonellosis, amebiasis, giardiasis, and infections with *Campylobacter* species are predominantly caused by nonsexual transmission. These enteric pathogens are also known to be sexually transmitted, primarily among males having sexual contact with males.[2,7]

Sexual transmission accounts for most cases of hepatitis B virus (HBV) infections in the United States. Hepatitis B virus infections are increased in homosexuals, bisexuals, and heterosexuals with multiple partners. Infants can acquire the infection through vertical transmission, and older children develop HBV primarily through nonsexual contact with infected individuals. Sexual transmission is possible for hepatitis C virus (HCV), but the very low prevalence of infection among sexual partners of individuals with chronic

HCV infection suggests the risk of sexual transmission is limited. Most cases of HCV infections in children result from vertical transmission, and in adults result from exposure to infected blood.[2]

Lymphogranuloma venereum, chancroid, and granuloma inguinale are uncommon STIs in the United States. In 2004 the CDC received reports for only 27 cases of LGV and 30 cases of chancroid. Granuloma inguinale is considered rare, and no current data are available.[13] All 3 diseases are likely to be underdiagnosed and underreported. Children can acquire LGV through sexual contact, but accidental inoculation may occur through contact with drainage from ulcers or buboes (abscesses). Lymphogranuloma venereum, caused by *C trachomatis* biovars or serotypes L1, L2, and L3, is a systemic infection that is associated with ulcers and granulomas, inguinal and perianal abscesses, and proctocolitis. It either seems to be increasing in frequency or becoming better recognized among adults. Chancroid is caused by *Haemophilus ducreyi*, a gram-negative coccobacillus, with sexual contact its only known route of transmission. Granuloma inguinale is caused by *Calymmatobacterium granulomatis (Donovania granulomatis)*, a gram-negative bacillus, and is rare outside of the tropics.[20] This organism is not highly contagious; however, it can be transmitted sexually, through close nonsexual contact, and through fomites.

Group B beta-hemolytic streptococci (GBS) colonize the genital tract of between 5% and 40% of postpubertal women, and neonates may develop severe infections through vertical transmission. The organism is also a known colonizer of the anogenital area of children and a possible pathogen for vulvovaginitis in children, adolescents, and adults.[127] In a study of the normal vaginal flora of girls 2 months to 15 years of age, colonization with GBS was found in 23% of girls 2 to 35 months of age, 16% of girls 3 to 10 years of age, and 20% of girls 11 to 15 years of age. Multiple site colonization (vaginal, anal, pharyngeal) was common in the youngest group, and 2-site colonization (vaginal, anal) was common in the oldest group. In girls 3 to 10 years of age, vaginal and anal colonization were 4% each, and pharyngeal colonization was 14%.[128] One study of childhood vulvovaginitis showed that 5% of controls but no symptomatic girls had GBS, and in another study, 2% of both cases and controls had GBS.[93,95] Group B streptococci commonly colonize the anogenital tract of females of all ages, and occasionally are found in symptomatic females with vulvovaginitis. There are clear data to link either symptomatic or asymptomatic GBS with sexual abuse considering the significant rate of colonization in all age groups.

Recommended STI Testing of Suspected Sexual Abuse or Assault Victims

Prepubertal Children
Routine STI testing of all children who are suspected of being sexually abused is not recommended. The decision to test for STIs should be made on an individual basis, weighing the risk of infection against the additional discomfort of obtaining specimens from a young child. Criteria for screening for STI include historical and physical parameters associated with increased risk of infection (Box 11.1). The CDC recommends selected, high-risk child sexual abuse victims be tested for gonorrhea, chlamydia, syphilis, HIV, and hepatitis B. In girls, vaginal secretions should be evaluated for trichomoniasis and BV. Children should be assessed for warts or lesions and any ulcers or vesicles cultured for herpes. Follow-up testing is also recommended (Box 11.2)

Pubertal Adolescents and Adults
Routine STI testing of pubertal adolescents and adults who are suspected of being sexually abused is generally recommended (Box 11.3). Among sexually active adolescents and adults who have high prevalence of STIs, post-assault STI testing may identify previously acquired STIs, incubating STI infection from the assault, or in some cases pathogens in the ejaculate that may or may not result in infection. Some evaluators do not routinely test adolescents and adults whom they are routinely treating with prophylactic antibiotics because of concerns that information about a previously acquired STI may undermine the credibility of the victim. This approach may undermine the public health response to reporting and assessing or treating sexual contacts for infection, while ignoring the fact that identification and treatment of STIs following an assault in adolescents and adults is more important from a psychological and medical standpoint rather than an evidentiary perspective.

BOX 11.1

Selection Criteria for Testing Sexually Abused Children and Adolescents for Sexually Transmitted Infections (STIs)[a]

Historical
Perpetrator has known STI or has high risk for STI
Sibling or other child in household has known STI
Abuse by multiple perpetrators
Prior consenting sexual contact
History of genital discharge

Physical
Sexual maturity rating/Tanner Stage 3 or greater
Genital discharge present
Genital injury present
Presence of specific STI lesions (ulcers, warts)

General
Child or parent requests STI testing
High prevalence of STIs in child's community

---

[a]Data supporting criteria from girls primarily; limited data available from boys. Criteria adapted from CDC STI guidelines 2006; Siegel RM, Schubert CJ, Myers PA, Shapiro RA. The prevalence of sexually transmitted diseases in children and adolescents evaluated for sexual abuse in Cincinnati: rationale for limited STD testing in prepubertal girls. *Pediatrics*. 1995;96:1090–1094; Ingram DL, Everett VD, Flick LAR, Russell TA, White-Sims ST. Vaginal gonococcal cultures in sexual abuse evaluations: evaluation of selective criteria for preteenage girls. *Pediatrics*. 1997;99:e8. Atabaki S, Paradise JE. The medical evaluation of the sexually abused child: lessons from a decade of research. *Pediatrics*. 1999;104:178–186.

BOX 11.2

CDC-Recommended STI Testing for Prepubertal Children Evaluated for Suspected Sexual Abuse

---

Routine testing is not recommended. The following tests for STI be performed on selected, high-risk child sexual abuse victims.

1. Gonococcal (gonorrhea) cultures from pharyngeal, anal, and urethral (boys) or vaginal (girls) sites

2. Chlamydial cultures from vaginal and anal sites in girls and anal and urethral sites in symptomatic boys

3. Blood sample for immediate serology for syphilis, HIV, hepatitis B (hepatitis B surface antigen), and for retention for any subsequent testing

4. Examination for anogenital warts or ulcerative lesions and cultures sent for herpes if ulcers are present

5. For females, culture or wet mount of vaginal secretions for microscopic examination for trichomonas and tests for bacterial vaginosis

6. Two weeks later recommend repeating all these tests

7. Twelve weeks later recommend repeating all the serologic tests

8. Six months later recommend HIV testing

9. For prepubertal girls presenting with vaginal discharge, routine bacterial cultures because may have nonsexually transmitted rather than sexually transmitted pathogens

---

Abbreviations: CDC, Centers for Disease Control and Prevention; STI, sexually transmitted infection; HIV, human immunodeficiency virus.

BOX 11.3
CDC-Recommended STI Evaluation for Adolescent and Adult Victims of Acute Sexual Assault

1. Cultures for gonorrhea and chlamydia from all sites of penetration or attempted penetration.

2. FDA-approved NAAT can be substituted for gonorrhea and chlamydia cultures in adolescents and adults, but positive tests should be confirmed with a second NAAT that targets a different nucleotide sequence or uses a different amplification technique than the initial test.

3. Wet mount and culture of vaginal specimen for *Trichomonas vaginalis*.

4. If vaginal discharge or odor is present, wet mount for BV and candida.

5. Blood sample for serologic testing for syphilis, HIV, and hepatitis B.

6. Repeat testing should be considered at a 2-week follow-up.

7. Six weeks later repeat serologic testing for syphilis and HIV.

8. Three months later repeat serologic testing for syphilis and HIV.

9. Six months later repeat serologic testing for syphilis and HIV.

Abbreviations: CDC, Centers for Disease Control and Prevention; FDA, Food and Drug Administration; NAAT, nucleic acid amplification tests; BV, bacterial vaginosis; HIV, human immunodeficiency virus.

STI Treatment

Prophylactic Antibiotic Therapy

Prophylactic antibiotic therapy for sexually abused children is a controversial subject, but routine prophylaxis is not generally recommended.[1,2,7,14,17,19,20,25] Routine prophylaxis with an antibiotic that covers chlamydia, gonorrhea, trichomoniasis, and BV is commonly offered to adolescents and adults presenting with recent sexual contact (Table 11.3). If the individual was not immunized for hepatitis B, a first dose of vaccine is recommended, with follow-up doses to be given 1 to 2 months and 4 to 6 months after the initial dose. Postexposure prophylaxis (PEP) for HIV is controversial in suspected sexual abuse victims of all ages. Human immunodeficiency virus prophylaxis has been shown to be effective for perinatal transmission and occupational needle-stick exposures, but there are little data on the efficacy of HIV prophylaxis for nonoccupational exposures. The CDC recommends considering the use of PEP for HIV in sexual abuse or assault cases when the perpetrator is known to be HIV infected, the exposure event presents a substantial risk of transmission, and treatment can be initiated within 72 hours.[129] If the perpetrator's HIV status is unknown, PEP should be considered on a case-by-case basis. If there is "negligible exposure risk," HIV PEP is not recommended. Health care providers should discuss the risk of acquiring HIV; the potential benefits of PEP, yet unknown efficacy in this setting; and known toxicity with the victim and his or her parents in the case of children. Many clinicians prefer a 3-drug combination of 2 nucleoside analog reverse transcriptase inhibitors (NRTIs), zidovudine and lamivudine for example, and one protease inhibitor, such as nelfinavir for child and adolescent PEP.[130] The 3-drug regimens have been shown

TABLE 11.3

CDC-Recommended Prophylaxis for Adolescent and Adult Victims of Acute Sexual Assault[a]

Drug	Dosage
Ceftriaxone	125 mg intramuscularly in a single dose
	Plus
Metronidazole	2 g orally in a single dose
	Plus
Azithromycin	1 g orally in a single dose
OR	
Doxycycline	100 mg orally twice a day for 7 days
Hepatitis B vaccine	If not previously immunized, give initial dose and schedule follow-up doses 1–2 months and 4–6 months after first dose.

Abbreviation: CDC, Centers for Disease Control and Prevention.

[a]This is empiric therapy for gonorrhea, *Chlamydia*, incubating syphilis, trichomoniasis, and bacterial vaginosis. Routine prophylaxis is not recommended for prepubertal children.

Human immunodeficiency virus (HIV) prophylaxis is controversial. Discuss risk of HIV, discuss HIV prophylaxis, including toxicity and unknown efficacy. Consultation with HIV specialist is recommended if prophylaxis is to be given.

to be more likely to suppress virus replication, but multiple drug regimens are likely to increase potential toxicity and decrease compliance with the required 28-day PEP course. Therefore, some clinicians recommend using only 2 NRTI drugs for PEP. Clinicians involved in acute sexual abuse evaluations of children and adolescents should establish a protocol that includes the approach to PEP discussion, immediate availability of a 3-day starter kit of the PEP drugs, and a follow-up in consultation with a pediatric infectious diseases specialist.[130]

Specific Therapy for Documented Infections

Selective testing should be done for STIs in children as outlined previously. Specific therapy should be initiated if testing reveals specific infections.[2] Appropriate treatment regimens are shown in Table 11.4. Ceftriaxone is the preferred treatment for proctitis, pharyngitis, and vaginal or urethral gonococcal infections, and is effective in treating gonorrhea and incubating syphilis. Cefixime 400 mg orally as a single dose has been recommended for uncomplicated gonorrhea infections in adults, where it is slightly less effective than ceftriaxone (97.1% vs 99.1%). Therapy of anogenital warts is complicated, and some clinicians often recommend waiting for spontaneous resolution of the lesions. Each therapeutic method is directed toward symptomatic warts. These methods, however, often do not eradicate the infection, prevent recurrences, or decrease infectivity. Most therapeutic methods require administration by a health care provider. Two options are available for patient-applied treatment of HPV lesions: podofilox 0.5% solution or gel, an antimitotic drug, and imiquimod 5% cream, an immune enhancer that stimulates production of interferon and other cytokines. Inflammatory reactions are common, but often milder than with other agents. There are no data on the efficacy of cimetidine in genital warts

TABLE 11.4

Guidelines for Treatment of Sexually Transmitted Infections in Children and Adolescents According to Syndrome

Preferred regimens are listed. For further information concerning other acceptable regimens and diseases not included. In addition, revised recommendations on the treatment of sexually transmitted infections have been issued by the Centers for Disease Control and Prevention in 2006.

Syndrome	Organisms/Diagnoses	Treatment of Adolescent	Treatment of Infant/Child
Urethritis and cervicitis Urethritis: Inflammation of urethra with mucoid, mucopurulent, or purulent discharge Cervicitis: Inflammation of cervix with mucopurulent or purulent cervical discharge. Cervicitis occurs rarely in prepubertal girls	*Neisseria gonorrhoeae, Chlamydia trachomatis* Other causes of urethritis and cervicitis include *Ureaplasma urealyticum*, possibly *Mycoplasma genitalium*, and sometimes *Trichomonas vaginalis* and herpes simplex virus	Cefixime, 400 mg, orally, in a single dose OR Ceftriaxone, 125 mg, IM, in a single dose OR Ciprofloxacin, 500 mg, orally, in a single dose OR Ofloxacin, 400 mg, orally, in a single dose OR Levofloxacin, 250 mg, orally, in single dose **If chlamydial infection not ruled out, PLUS EITHER** Azithromycin, 1 g, orally, in a single dose OR Doxycycline, 100 mg, orally, twice a day for 7 days	**Children <45 kg** Ceftriaxone, 125 mg, IM, in a single dose OR Spectinomycin, 40 mg/kg (maximum 2 g) IM in a single dose **If chlamydial infection not ruled out, PLUS** Erythromycin base or ethylsuccinate, 50 mg/kg per day, orally, in 4 divided doses (maximum 2 g/d) for 14 days **Children ≥45 kg but younger than 8 years** Azithromycin, 1 g, orally, in a single dose **Children 8 years of age or older** Azithromycin, 1 g, orally, in a single dose OR Doxycycline, 100 mg, orally, twice a day for 7 days

Abbreviation: IM, intramuscularly.

in children. Oral antiviral agents seem to shorten the duration of symptoms and reduce viral shedding in primary HSV infections but have no effect on the risk, frequency, or severity of recurrences. These agents also can be effective in reducing the severity and duration of symptoms when used to treat recurrent episodes.[2,20]

Summary

Sexually abused children and adolescents are at risk for acquiring STIs. Sexually transmitted infections are common among sexually active adolescents but are not commonly identified in prepubertal children. Therefore, the presence of an STI in a child should raise concerns of sexual abuse, and an appropriate evaluation for child sexual abuse should be initiated. Several studies suggest approximately 5% of prepubertal children evaluated for sexual abuse will have an STI. Sexually transmitted infections are more commonly identified in pubertal adolescents than in prepubertal children being evaluated for suspected sexual assault or abuse. The presence of an STI in the pubertal adolescent may represent an infection acquired through the abuse or prior sexual activity. Selective testing and specific treatment of STIs are often recommended in prepubertal children, while routine testing and prophylaxis are typically recommended in adolescents.

Although any STI could be acquired through abusive contact, the strength of the association between STI and child sexual abuse varies from disease to disease. Several factors must be considered when evaluating the strength of associa-

tion between an STI and child sexual abuse, particularly the age of the child and the specific disease identified. The disease must be diagnosed by using tests that have an acceptable degree of specificity in children. The diagnosis of an STI in a child with suspected sexual abuse has social and legal implications. Missing evidence of an STI in a child may place the child at risk for continued abuse; however, a mistaken diagnosis or mistaken interpretation could lead to inappropriate child protection and criminal interventions.

References

1. Kellogg N, American Academy of Pediatrics Committee on Child Abuse and Neglect. The evaluation of sexual abuse in children. *Pediatrics.* 2005;116:506–512

2. Centers for Disease Control and Prevention. Sexually transmitted diseases treatment guidelines 2006. *MMWR Recomm Rep.* 2006;55(RR-11):1–100

3. De Jong AR. Sexually transmitted diseases in sexually abused children. *Sex Transm Dis.* 1986;13:123–126

4. Neinstein LS, Goldenring J, Carpenter S. Nonsexual transmission of sexually transmitted diseases: an infrequent occurrence. *Pediatrics.* 1984;74:67–76

5. White ST, Loda FA, Ingram DL, Pearson A. Sexually transmitted diseases in sexually abused children. *Pediatrics.* 1983;72:16–21

6. Hammerschlag MR. Sexually transmitted diseases in sexually abused children: medical and legal implications. *Sex Transm Infect.* 1998;74:167–174

7. Finkel MA, De Jong AR. Medical findings in child sexual abuse. In: Reece R, Ludwig S, eds. *Child Abuse: Medical Diagnosis and Management.* 2nd ed. Philadelphia, PA: Lippincott Williams & Wilkins; 2001:207–286

8. Jenny C, Hooton PM, Bowers A, et al. Sexually transmitted diseases in victims of rape. *N Engl J Med.* 1990;322:713–716

9. Schwarcz SK, Whittington WL. Sexual assault and sexually transmitted diseases: detection and management in adults and children. *Rev Infect Dis.* 1990;12(suppl 6):S682–S690

10. American Academy of Pediatrics Committee on Adolescence. Care of the adolescent sexual assault victim. *Pediatrics.* 2001;107:1476–1479

11. Renolds MW, Peipert JF, Collins B. Epidemiologic issues of sexually trans-mitted diseases in sexual assault victims. *Obstet Gynecol Surv.* 2000;55:51

12. Risser WL, Bortot AT, Benjamins LJ, et al. The epidemiology of sexually transmitted infections in adolescents. *Semin Pediatr Infect Dis.* 2005;16:160–167

13. Centers for Disease Control and Prevention. *Sexually Transmitted Diseases Surveillance, 2004.* Atlanta, GA: Department of Health and Human Services, 2005:41–44

14. Atabaki S, Paradise JE. The medical evaluation of the sexually abused child: lessons from a decade of research. *Pediatrics.* 1990;104(suppl):S178–S186

15. Hammerschlag MR. The transmissibility of sexually transmitted diseases in sexually abused children. *Child Abuse Negl.* 1998;22:623–635

16. Ingram DL. The transmissibility of sexually transmitted diseases in sexually abused children: response to recommen-dations for a medical research agenda. *Child Abuse Negl.* 1998;22:637–639

17. Beck-Sague CM, Solomon F. Sexually transmitted diseases in abused children and adolescent and adult victims of rape: review of selected literature. *Clin Infect Dis.* 1999;28(suppl 1)S74–S83

18. Woods CR. Sexually transmitted diseases in prepubertal children: mechanisms of transmission, evaluation of sexually abused children, and exclusion of chronic perinatal viral infections. *Semin Pediatr Infect Dis.* 2005;16:317–325

19. Ingram, DL. Controversies about the sexual and nonsexual transmission of adult STDs to children. In: Krugman RD, Leventhal JM, eds. *Child Sexual Abuse. Report of the Twenty Second Ross Roundtable on Critical Approaches to Common Pediatric Problems.* Columbus, OH: Ross Laboratories; 1991:14–28

20. Hammerschlag MR. Sexually transmitted diseases in sexually abused children. *Adv Pediatr Infect Dis.* 1988;3:1–18

21. Ingram DL, Everett VD, Lyna PR, White ST, Rockwell LA. Epidemiology of adult sexually transmitted disease agents in children being evaluated for sexual abuse. *Pediatr Infect Dis J.* 1992;11:945–950

22. Ingram DM, Miller WC, Schoenbeck VJ, Everett VD, Ingram DL. Risk assessment of gonococcal and chlamydia infections in young children undergoing evaluation for sexual abuse. *Pediatrics.* 2001;107:e73

23. Hammerschlag MR. Appropriate use of nonculture tests for the detection of sexually transmitted diseases in children and adolescents. *Semin Pediatr Infect Dis.* 2003;14:54–59

24. Gardner JJ. Comparison of the vaginal flora in sexually abused and nonabused girls. *J Pediatrics.* 1992;120:872–877

25. Siegel RM, Schubert CJ, Meyers PA, Shapiro RA. The prevalence of sexually transmitted diseases in children and adolescents evaluated for sexual abuse in Cincinnati: rationale for limited STD testing in prepubertal girls. *Pediatrics.* 1995;96:1091–1094

26. Whittington WL, Rice RJ, Biddle JW, Knapp JS. Incorrect identification of *Neisseria gonorrhoeae* from infants and children. *Pediatr Infect Dis.* 1988;7:3–10

27. Alexander JW, Griffith H, Housch JG, Holmes JR. Infections in sexual contacts and associates of children with gonorrhea. *Sex Transm Dis.* 1984;11:156–158

28. Folland DS, Burke RE, Hinman AR, Schiffner W. Gonorrhea in preadolescent children: an inquiry into the source of infection and mode of transmission. *Pediatrics.* 1977;60:153–156

29. Ingram DL, Everett VD, Flick LAR, Russell TA, White-Simms ST. Vaginal gonococcal cultures in sexual abuse evaluations: evaluation of selective criteria for preteenaged girls. *Pediatrics.* 1997;99:e8

30. Hammerschlag MR, Alpert S, Rosner I, et al. Microbiology of the vagina in children: normal and potentially pathogenic organisms. *Pediatrics.* 1978;62:57–62

31. Paradise JE, Campos JM, Friedman HM, Frishmuth G. Vulvovaginitis in premenarcheal girls: clinical features and diagnostic evaluation. *Pediatrics.* 1982;70:193–198

32. Bump RC, Sachs LA, Buesching WJ. Sexually transmissible infectious agents in sexually active and virginal asymptomatic adolescent girls. *Pediatrics.* 1986;77:488–494

33. Argent AC, Lachman PI, Hanslo D, Bass D. Sexually transmitted diseases in children and evidence of sexual abuse. *Child Abuse Negl.* 1995;19:1303–1310

34. Sgroi SM. Pediatric gonorrhea beyond infancy. *Pediatr Ann.* 1979;8:326–336

35. Branch GB, Paxton R. A study of gonococcal infections among infants and children. *Public Health Rep.* 1965;80:347–352

36. Shore WB, Winkelstein JA. Nonvenereal transmission of gonococcal infections to children. *J Pediatr.* 1971;79:661–663

37. Shapiro RA, Schubert CJ, Siegel RM. *Neisseria gonorrhea* infections in girls younger than 12 years of age evaluated for vaginitis. *Pediatrics.* 1999;104:e72

38. Farrel MK, Billmire ME, Shamroy JA, Hammond JG. Prepubertal gonorrhea: a multidisciplinary approach. *Pediatrics.* 1981;67:151–153

39. Ingram DL, White ST, Durfee MF, Pearson AW. Sexual contact in children with gonorrhea. *Am J Dis Child.* 1982;136:994–996

40. Nair P, Glazer-Semmel E, Gould C, Ruff E. *Neisseria gonorrhoeae* in asymptomatic prepubertal household contacts of children with gonococcal infection. *Clin Pediatr (Phila).* 1986;25:160–163

41. Hammerschlag MR, Doraiswamy B, Alexander ER, Cox P, Price W, Gleyzer A. Are rectovaginal chlamydial infections a marker of sexual abuse in children? *Pediatr Infect Dis.* 1984;3:100–104

42. Ingram DL, White ST, Occhiuti AR, Lyna PR. Childhood vaginal infections: association of *Chlamydia trachomatis* with sexual contact. *Pediatr Infect Dis.* 1986;5:226–229

43. Rettig PJ, Nelson JD. Genital tract infection with *Chlamydia trachomatis* in prepubertal children. *J Pediatr.* 1981;99:206–210

44. Hammerschlag MR. Chlamydial infections. *J Pediatr.* 1989;114:727–734

45. Hammerschlag MR, Rettig PJ, Shields ME. False-positive results with the use of chlamydial antigen detection tests in the evaluation of suspected sexual abuse in children. *Pediatr Infect Dis.* 1988;7:11–14

46. Hammerschlag MR, Ajl S, Laroque D. Inappropriate use of nonculture tests for the detection of *Chlamydia trachomatis* in suspected victims of child sexual abuse: a continuing problem. *Pediatrics.* 1999;104:1137–1139

47. Schacter J, Grossman M, Sweet RL, Holt J, Jordan C, Bishop E. Prospective study of perinatal transmission of *Chlamydia trachomatis. JAMA.* 1986;255:3374–3377

48. Bell TA, Stamm WE, Wang SP, Kuo CC, Holmes KK, Grayston JT. Chronic *Chlamydia trachomatis* infections in infants. *JAMA.* 1992;267:400–402

49. Bump RC. *Chlamydia trachomatis* as a cause of prepubertal vaginitis. *Obstet Gynecol.* 1985;65:384–388

50. Ingram DL, Runyan DK, Collins AD, et al. Vaginal *Chlamydia trachomatis* infection in children with sexual contact. *Pediatr Infect Dis.* 1984;3:97–99

51. Kellogg ND, Baillergeon J, Lukefahr JL, Lawless K, Menard SW. Comparison of nucleic acid amplification tests and culture techniques in the detection of *Neisseria gonorrhoeae* and *Chlamydia trachomatis* in victims of suspected child sexual abuse. *J Pediatr Adolesc Gynecol.* 2004;17:331–339

52. Spigarelli MG, Biro FM. An update on diagnosing STIs and HIV. *Contemp Ob Gyn.* 2005;50:76–90

53. Embree JE, Lindsay D, Williams T, Peeling RW, Woods S, Morris M. Acceptability and usefulness of vaginal washes in premenarcheal girls as a diagnostic procedure for sexually transmitted diseases. The Child Protection Center at the Winnipeg Children's Hospital. *Pediatr Infect Dis J.* 1996;15:662–667

54. Mathews-Greer J, Sloop G, Springer A, McRae K, LaHaye E, Jamison R. Comparison of detection methods for *Chlamydia trachomatis* and *Neisseria gonorrhoeae* in pediatric sexual abuse victims. *Pediatric Infect Dis J.* 1999;18:165–167

55. Girardet RG, McClain N, Lahoti S, Cheung K, Hartwell B, McNeese M. Comparison of the urine-based ligase chain reaction test to culture for detection of *Chlamydia trachomatis* and *Neiserria gonorrhoeae* in pediatric sexual abuse victims. *Pediatr Infect Dis J.* 2001;20:144–147

56. Hammerschlag MR. Use of nucleic acid amplification tests in investigating child sexual abuse. *Sex Transm Infect.* 2001;77:153–157

57. Ginsberg CM. Acquired syphilis in prepubertal children. *Pediatr Infect Dis J.* 1983;2:232–234

58. Goldenring JM. Secondary syphilis in a prepubertal child: differentiating condylomata lata from condylomata acuminata. *NY State J Med.* 1989;March:180–181

59. Connors JM, Schubert C, Shapiro R. Syphilis or abuse: making the diagnosis and understanding the implications. *Pediatr Emerg Care.* 1998;14:139–142

60. Lande MB, Richardson AC, White KC. The role of syphilis serology on the evaluation of suspected sexual abuse. *Pediatr Infect Dis J.* 1992;11:125–127

61. Horowitz S, Chadwick DL. Syphilis as a sole indicator of sexual abuse: two cases with no intervention. *Child Abuse Negl.* 1990;14:129–132

62. deVilliers FP, Prentice MA, Bergh AM, Miller SD. Sexually transmitted disease surveillance in a child abuse clinic. *S Afr Med J.* 1992;81:84–86

63. Pandhi D, Kumar S, Reddy BS. Sexually transmitted diseases in children. *J Dermatol.* 2003;30:314–332

64. Ozturk F, Gurses N, Sancak R, Bay A, Baris S. Acquired secondary syphilis in a 6-year-old girl with no history of sexual abuse. *Cutis.* 1998;62:150–151

65. Williams J, Radha S, Sundararai AS. Nonvenereal transmission of venereal syphilis in a child. *Indian J Sex Transm Dis.* 1990;11:27–28

66. Christian CW, Lavalle J, Bell LM. Preschoolers with syphilis. *Pediatrics.* 1999;103:e4

67. Sinclair KA, Woods CR, Kirse DJ, Sinal SH. Anogenital and respiratory tract human papillomavirus infections among children: age, gender and potential transmission through sexual abuse. *Pediatrics.* 2005;116:815–825

68. De Jong AR, Weiss JW, Brent RL. Condyloma acuminata in children. *Am J Dis Child.* 1982;136:704–706

69. American Academy of Dermatology Task Force on Pediatric Dermatology. Genital warts and sexual abuse in children. *J Am Acad Dermatol.* 1984;11:529–530

70. Smith YR, Haefner HK, Lieberman RW, Quint EH. Comparison of microscopic examination and human papillomavirus DNA subtyping in vulvar lesions of premenarchal girls. *J Pediatr Adolesc Gynecol.* 2001;14:81–84

71. Obalek S, Missiewicz J, Jablonska S, Favre M, Orth G. Childhood condyloma acuminatum: association with genital and cutaneous human papillomaviruses. *Pediatr Dermatol.* 1993;10:101–106

72. Watts DH, Koutsky LA, Holmes KK, Goldman D, Kuypers J, Kiviat NB. Low risk of perinatal transmission of human papillomavirus: results from a prospective cohort study. *Am J Obstet Gynecol.* 1998;178:365–373

73. Smith EM, Richie JM, Yankowitz J, et al. Human papillomavirus prevalence and types in newborns and parents: concordance and modes of transmission. *Sex Transm Dis.* 2004;31:63–64

74. Rintala MAM, Grenman SE, Puranen MH, et al. Transmission of high-risk human papillomavirus (HPV) between parents and infant: a prospective study of HPV in families in Finland. *J Clin Microbiol.* 2005;43:376–381

75. Handley J, Armstrong K, Bingham A, et al. Common association of HPV-2 with anogenital warts in children. *Pediatr Dermatol.* 1997;14:339–334

76. Cohen BA, Honig P, Androphy E. Anogenital warts in children. *Arch Dermatol.* 1990;126:1575–1580

77. Boyd AS. Condylomata acuminata in the pediatric population. *Am J Dis Child.* 1990;144:817–824

78. Hanson RM, Glasson M, McCrossin I, Rogers M, Rose B, Thompson C. Anogenital warts in childhood. *Child Abuse Negl.* 1989;13:225–233

79. Allen AL, Siefried EC. The natural history of condyloma in children. *J Am Acad Dermatol.* 1998;39:951–955

80. Weinberg R, Sybert VP, Feldman KW, Neville J. Outcome of CPS referral for sexual abuse in children with condylomata acuminata. *Adolesc Pediatr Gynecol.* 1994;7:19–24

81. Davis AJ, Evans S. Human papilloma virus infection in the pediatric and adolescent patient. *J Pediatr.* 1989;115:1–9

82. Jenison SA, Yu XP, Valentine JM, et al. Evidence of prevalent genital type human papillomavirus infections in adults and children. *J Infect Dis.* 1990;162:60–69

83. Smith-McCune K, Horbach N, Dattel B. Incidence and clinical correlates of human papillomavirus infection in a pediatric population referred for evaluation of sexual abuse. *Adolesc Pediatr Gynecol.* 1993;6:20–24

84. Stevens-Simon C, Nelligan D, Breese P, Jenny C, Douglas JM. The prevalence of genital human papillomavirus infections in abused and nonabused preadolescent girls. *Pediatrics.* 2000;106:645–649

85. Gutman LT, St Clair KK, Everett VD, et al. Cervical-vaginal and intraanal human papillomavirus infection in young girls with external genital warts. *J Infect Dis.* 1994;170:339–344

86. Rice PS, Mant C, Cason J, et al. High prevalence of human papillomavirus type 16 among children. *J Med Virol.* 2000;61:70–75

87. Powell J, Strauss S, Gray J, Wojnarowska F. Genital carriage of human papilloma virus (HPV) DNA in prepubertal girls with and without vulval disease. *Pediatr Dermatol.* 2003;20:191–194

88. Myhre AK, Dalen A, Berntzen K, Bratlid D. Anogenital human papillomavirus in non-abused preschool children. *Acta Paediatr.* 2004;92:1445–1452

89. Gutman LT, St. Claire K, Herman-Giddens ME, Johnston WW, Phelps WC. Evaluation of sexually abused and non-abused young girls for intravaginal human papillomavirus infection. *Am J Dis Child.* 1992;146:694–699

90. Siegfried E, Rasnick-Conley J, Cook S, Leonardi C, Monteleone J. Human papillomavirus screening in pediatric victims of sexual abuse. *Pediatrics.* 1998;101:43–47

91. Rock B, Naghashfar MS, Barnett N, Buscema J, Woodruff JD, Shah K. Genital tract papillomavirus infection in children. *Arch Dermatol.* 1986;122:1129–1132

92. Weaver BA, Feng Q, Holmes KK, et al. Evaluation of genital sites and sampling techniques for detection of human papillomavirus DNA in men. *J Infect Dis.* 2004;189:677–685

93. Heller RH, Joseph JM, Davis HJ. Vulvovaginitis in the premenarcheal child. *J Pediatr.* 1969;74:370–377

94. Pierce AM, Hart CA. Vulvovaginitis: causes and management. *Arch Dis Child.* 1991;67:509–512

95. Jaquiery A, Hogg G, Grover S. Vulvovaginitis: clinical features, aetiology, and microbiology of the genital tract. *Arch Dis Child.* 1999;81:64–67

96. Jones JG, Yamauchi T, Lambert B. *Trichomonas vaginalis* infestation in sexually abused girls. *Am J Dis Child.* 1985;139:846–847

97. Gardner M, Jones JG. Genital herpes acquired by sexual abuse of children. *J Pediatr.* 1984;104:243–244

98. Kaplan KM, Fleisher GR, Paradise JE, Friedman HN. Social relevance of genital herpes simplex in children. *Am J Dis Child.* 1984;138:872–874

99. Taieb A, Body S, Astar I, du Pasquier P, Maleville J. Clinical epidemiology of symptomatic primary herpetic infection in children. A study of 50 cases. *Acta Paediatr Scand.* 1987;76:128–132

100. Becker TM, Magder L, Harrison HR, et al. The epidemiology of infection with the human herpesviruses in Navajo children. *Am J Epidemiol.* 1988;127:1071–1078

101. Schmitt DL, Johnson DW, Henderson FW. Herpes simplex type 1 infections in group day care. *Pediatr Infect Dis J.* 1991;10:729–734

102. Roberts CM. Genital herpes in young adults: changing sexual behaviours, epidemiology and management. *Herpes.* 2005;12:10–14

103. Nahmias AJ, Dowdle WR, Naib ZM, Josey WE, Luce CF. Genital infection with *Herpesvirus hominis* types 1 and 2 in children. *Pediatrics.* 1968;42:659–666

104. Krugman S. Primary herpetic vulvovaginitis: report of a case; isolation and identification of herpes simplex virus. *Pediatrics.* 1952;9:585–588

105. McCann J, Voris J. Perianal injuries resulting from sexual abuse: a longitudinal study. *Pediatrics.* 1993;91:390–397

106. Dershwitz RA, Levitsky LL, Feingold M. Picture of the month. Vulvovaginitis: a cause of clitoromegaly. *Am J Dis Child.* 1984;138:887–888

107. Christian CW, Singer ML, Crawford JE, Durbin D. Perianal herpes zoster presenting as suspected child abuse. *Pediatrics.* 1997;99:608–610

108. Simon HK, Steele DW. Varicella: pediatric genital/rectal vesicular lesions of unclear origin. *Ann Emerg Med.* 1995;25:111–114

109. Ashley RL. Sorting out the new HSV type specific antibody tests. *Sex Transm Infect.* 2001;77:232–237

110. Strick L, Wald A. Type-specific testing for herpes simplex virus. *Expert Rev Mol Diagn.* 2004;4:443–453

111. Bump RC, Buesching WJ. Bacterial vaginosis in virginal and sexually active adolescent females: evidence against exclusive sexual transmission. *Am J Obstet Gynecol.* 1988;158:935–939

112. Hammerschlag MR, Cummings M, Doraiswamy B, Cox P, McCormack WM. Nonspecific vaginitis following sexual abuse in children. *Pediatrics.* 1985;75:1028–1031

113. Bartley DL, Morgan L, Rimsa ME. *Gardnerella vaginalis* in prepubertal girls. *Am J Dis Child.* 1987;141:1014–1017

114. Ingram DL, White ST, Lyna PR. *Gardnerella vaginalis* infection and sexual contact in female children. *Child Abuse Negl.* 1992;16:847–853

115. Shafer MA, Sweet RL, Ohm-Smith MS, Shalwitz J, Beck A, Schacter J. Microbiology of the lower genital tract in postmenarchal adolescent girls: differences by sexual activity, contraception, and presence of nonspecific vaginitis. *J Pediatr.* 1985;107:974–981

116. Myhre AK, Bevanger LS, Berntzen K, Bratlid D. Anogenital bacteriology in non-abused preschool children: a descriptive study of the aerobic genital flora and the isolation of anogenital *Gardnerella vaginalis. Acta Pediatr.* 2002;91:885–891

117. Wahl NG, Castilla MA, Lewis-Abney K. Prevalence of *Gardnerella vaginalis* in prepubertal males. *Arch Pediatr Adolesc Med.* 1998;152:1095–109

118. Jason JM. Abuse, neglect, and the HIV-infected child. *Child Abuse Negl.* 1991;15(suppl):79–88

119. Gutman LT, St Clair KK, Weedy C, et al. Human immunodeficiency virus transmission by child sexual abuse. *Am J Dis Child.* 1991;145:137–141

120. Gellert GA, Durfee MA, Berkowitz CD, Higgins KV, Tubiolio VC. Situational and sociodemographic characteristics of children infected with human immunodeficiency virus from pediatric sexual abuse. *Pediatrics.* 1993;91:39–44

121. Lindegren ML, Hanson IC, Hammett TA, et al. Sexual abuse of children: intersection with the HIV epidemic. *Pediatrics.* 1998;102:e46

122. Kellogg ND, Parra JM, Menard S. Children with anogenital symptoms and signs referred for sexual abuse evaluations. *Arch Pediatr Adolesc Med.* 1998;152:634–641

123. Reinhart MA. Urinary tract infection in sexually abused children. *Clin Pediatr.* 1987;26:470–472

124. Klevan J, De Jong AR. Urinary tract symptoms and urinary tract infections in sexually abused children. *Am J Dis Child.* 1990;144:242–244

125. Hammerschlag MR, Doraiswamy B, Cox P, Cummings M, McCormack WM. Colonization of sexually abused children with genital mycoplasmas. *Sex Transm Dis.* 1987;14:23–25

126. Ingram DL, White ST, Lyna P, Schmid JE, Koch GG, Everett VD. Ureaplasma urealyticum and large colony mycoplasma colonization in female children and its relationship to sexual contact, age, and race. *Child Abuse Negl.* 1992;16:265–272

127. Clark LR, Atendido M. Group B streptococcal vaginitis in postpubertal adolescent girls. *J Adolesc Health.* 2005;36:437–440

128. Hammerschlag MR, Baker CJ, Alpert S, et al. Colonization with group B streptococci in girls under 16 years of age. *Pediatrics.* 1977;60:473–476

129. Smith DK, Grohskopf LA, Black RJ, et al. Antiretroviral postexposure prophylaxis after sexual, injection-drug use, or other nonoccupational exposure to HIV in the United States: recommendations from the US Department of Health and Human Services. *MMWR Recomm Rep.* 2005;54(RR-2):1–20

130. American Academy of Pediatrics Committee on Pediatric AIDS. Postexposure prophylaxis in children and adolescents for non-occupational exposure to human immunodeficiency virus. *Pediatrics.* 2003;111:1475–1489

Chapter 12

The Role of Forensic Materials in Sexual Abuse and Assault

Kathi Makoroff

Mayerson Center for Safe and Healthy Children, Cincinnati Children's Hospital Medical Center, University of Cincinnati College of Medicine

Melissa Desai

The Children's Hospital of Philadelphia

Elizabeth Benzinger

Ohio Bureau of Criminal Identification and Investigation

Definition and Importance of Forensic Material

In the context of child abuse, the term *forensic* refers to evidence or information that is used by the legal system in courts of law. Forensic evaluation in cases of child abuse can include injury pattern recognition, timing of visceral or head injuries, thermal injury determination, and analysis of materials following sexual abuse. Forensic evidence collection may include materials from skin, mucosal membranes, saliva, hair samples, blood samples, and any material found on clothing or linens. Evidence analysis involves the detection, collection, preservation, and analysis of evidence. Although verbal and physical examination findings are important in courts of law, this chapter will focus on the collection of materials from the body or potential crime scene that can be analyzed in the course of a child abuse investigation.

The Impact of Forensic Evidence in Child Abuse Cases

The need to collect forensic evidence and its importance in criminal prosecutions is limited in cases of child abuse, in large part because of the dynamics and nature of child sexual abuse. Few pediatric victims disclose their sexual abuse during the first hours after an assault, when the yield from forensic evidence collection would be greatest. For those who are identified shortly after an assault, some are not brought for medical evaluation immediately. Others have already bathed and changed their clothing, which decreases the likelihood of obtaining evidence from physical examination. Furthermore, the abuse may not have involved any exchange of body tissues or secretions, limiting the yield from evidence collection. The identification of forensic evidence in a series of child sexual abuse varies from approximately 3% to 25%, depending on the population studied and laboratory methods used.[1-4] In a review of 500 victims of sexual assault, Dahlke et al[2] reported forensic evidence identification in only 3% of children younger than 11 years, compared with 36% of young adolescents who were sexually assaulted. Adolescent victims, whose sexual assault may be more characteristic of adult rape crimes, may be better able to disclose their abuse and are more likely than prepubertal children to have forensic evidence identified after sexual assault.

The collection of forensic samples in adult victims of sexual assault has been associated with charges being filed against an assailant.[5] However, there is evidence that for child and adolescent victims, the finding of forensic evidence may not predict successful prosecution. In a study of 355 sexual assault cases, successful prosecution was associated with younger age (adolescent vs adult), the presence of trauma on examination, and weapon use by the assailant.[6] Forensic evidence identification (sperm detection) was not associated with conviction. De Jong and Rose[7] reviewed prosecution results for 137 sexually abused children, ages 1 to 16, and found that physical or forensic evidence was neither predictive nor essential for conviction. Young children had lower rates of felony conviction, despite higher frequencies of physical findings, in part because they were less able than older children to testify about their experiences.

Timing Considerations

Time since assault is an important factor when collecting forensic evidence. For adolescent assaults, forensic evidence should be collected within 72 hours of sexual abuse/assault and when the history of the event indicates contact with the alleged perpetrator's genitalia, semen, blood, or saliva.[8] Cases where the history indicates a struggle that may have left skin cells or blood from the alleged perpetrator on the victim, or cases where other trace evidence (debris, fibers) may be left on the victim, should be evaluated within 72 hours as well. Forensic evidence should also be collected within 72 hours if the history of contact with the perpetrator is unclear (due to the child's age) or if the history is unavailable but there is reason to believe that sexual abuse did occur.

In cases of acute sexual abuse, physical evidence is lost with time. Eating, drinking, cleansing after defecation and urination, douching, and bathing reduce the amount of evidence material present. Evidence present in the form of semen or saliva is lost through gross physical action as well as microbial action. Microbial action and cellular breakdown processes rapidly degrade DNA present in foreign body fluids, and the rate of breakdown varies by specimen and from one body part to another. Finally, the constant turnover of cells on mucous membranes serves to add new DNA from the patient to the mix, overwhelming the smaller amount of DNA present from the perpetrator.

Understanding that forensic specimen recovery may not be possible or optimal at a later time, however, must be balanced against the patient's comfort at the time of the evaluation.

There is evidence that the guideline of 72 hours for forensic evidence collection may not be fitting in cases of prepubertal sexual assault. The 72-hour recommendation is, in part, based on the amount of time that motile and non-motile sperm can be identified in the vagina following sexual intercourse or sexual assault in adults.[9] In a study of 273 prepubertal children who underwent forensic evidence collection, no swabs taken from the child's body were positive for spermatozoa or blood more than 13 hours following the assault.[1] More than 90% of children with positive forensic evidence findings were evaluated within 24 hours of assault. Most forensic evidence was found on clothing and linens, although it was collected in only 35% of cases. In a second study of 190 children younger than 13 years who were evaluated within 72 hours of sexual assault, no child younger than 10 years had a positive body swab for semen or sperm.[10] Another study examined 80 children and adolescents who presented to an emergency department within 72 hours of a reported episode of sexual abuse or assault.[11] Only 3 children (aged <12 years) had semen recovered from forensic testing. All 3 presented within 24 hours after the reported abuse or assault, and all 3 children had semen recovered from clothing or linen only. These studies highlight the importance of forensic evidence from clothing and linens, and the limitations of forensic evidence in the evaluation of prepubertal sexual assault.

Forensic Evidence Collection

Evidence Collection in Cases of Acute Sexual Assault

Although protocols for evidence collection vary in different jurisdictions, general guidelines do exist. Using a standardized protocol with specific instructions for proper specimen collection, packaging, labeling, storing, and processing is essential to preserve the physical evidence in suspected cases of sexual or physical abuse. Standardized collection kits with detailed instructions, checklists, collection devices, and containers should be provided. In addition, chain of evidence procedures in which each person handling the evidence documents receipt and delivery of specimens should be followed to ensure that the evidence will be admissible in legal proceedings.

A medical examination and evidence collection should begin as soon as the patient is medically stable. Examiners should wear gloves at all times, both when collecting and handling specimens, in order to prevent contamination. Specimens should be obtained from all orifices and other areas believed to have been in contact with the perpetrator including genitals, anus, mouth, and fingers.

Assault histories may not correspond to forensic laboratory findings. For example, the patient may not recall important details due to the effects of drugs and/or alcohol or trauma. Certain acts may not be discussed due to embarrassment.

Very young children may not understand the relationship between the sexual abuse act and the need for the medical evaluation. Thus evidence collection protocols that advise specimen collection only at the site of the assault may cause key evidence to be missed. Rather, the best evidence collection strategy uses a thorough basic collection protocol that is expanded, rather than limited, by the patient's history.

Collecting Samples From the Victim and Perpetrator

Cotton-tipped swabs are the best collection medium. Calcium alginate culture swabs are not used because the calcium alginate interferes with DNA extraction procedures and renders the collection unusable. Although gauze squares or other wipes are the most efficient way to swab a large area, recovering the DNA from such large pieces of material is technically difficult. In most cases, 2 to 3 swabs are taken from each body site: oral, genital, and anal. Dry swabs are used for wet secretions and saline moistened swabs are used for dry sites. All swabs should be completely air-dried for at least 1 hour before labeling and placing in a tube or envelope. Swabs should not touch one another to prevent cross-contamination.

Some forensic laboratories request dry smears of the samples. If so, one of the collected swabs should be used to make a smear by rolling the swab back and forth across a slide in non-overlapping strokes. The smear is then allowed to dry; it is not stained or fixed, and a cover slip is not used. The forensic laboratory examines the smear for spermatozoa.

The swab that is used for the smear is retained. In prepubertal children who may have vaginal openings that do not permit insertion of a cotton swab, all swabs are collected from the external genitalia. In adolescent patients, separate swabs should be collected from the vagina and the cervix. Saliva and DNA left by the perpetrator during any oral-genital contact can be collected from the external genitalia using 2 to 3 additional swabs. Oral swabs should be obtained by swabbing the buccal mucosa and under the tongue.

Anal samples are important to collect in all cases. Due to drainage and/or external deposition of semen, anal swabs are frequently positive in cases of reported vaginal assault. In addition, less DNA from the female is present on the swabs, which assists in interpreting mixed DNA profiles. If the patient is unable to cooperate with the collection of internal anal samples, the swabs are collected only from the external anal area. In males, the external surface of the penis is swabbed; swabs should not be inserted into the urethra.

The underwear that the patient wears to the examination is collected in all cases. If underwear has been changed since the assault, advise law enforcement to obtain those garments worn at the time of the assault and include them in the forensic analysis. Underwear frequently contains better semen or saliva evidence than body cavity swabs. When no underwear is worn, the garment closest to the body is treated as underwear. Each item of clothing should be placed in its own brown paper bag. If any of the collected garments are wet, they should be allowed to air-dry prior to placing in a brown paper bag. Plastic bags should not be used because they may lock in moisture and promote the degradation of evidence.

Fingernail scrapings can be obtained by collecting material from under the victim's nails onto a clean piece of paper. A fingernail scraper should be used to scrape the underside of all fingers of one hand with the debris collected onto a paper. The paper should be folded and labeled and the same procedure should be repeated for the other hand.

Foreign hairs are collected by gently combing head and pubic hair over a sheet of paper or an envelope. Pubic hairs found on genitalia of prepubertal children should be packaged separately and labeled with the exact location from which they were obtained. Standards should also be obtained by cutting pubic and head hair from the patient and marking it as a control. Because root hair can contribute specific information to the hair analysis, previous recommendations advised plucking of pubic hair from the victim so as to include the root hair. However, hair transfer has been found in less than 20% of sexual intercourse cases and less than 5% of sexual assaults, thus routine plucking of hair is no longer recommended.[12,13] Currently hair standards are collected using clean scissors to cut approximately 25 head hairs at the skin surface from a variety of areas all over the scalp. Hair morphology varies within individuals, and this procedure serves to collect hairs of many variations.

If dried blood is present, there are several ways to collect the sample as evidence. An attempt can be made to scrape it onto a clean piece of paper with a tongue depressor or scalpel blade. Alternatively, a slightly moistened swab can be rubbed over the dried blood to collect the sample and then allowed to air-dry as is procedure for the rest of the evidence swabs.

In certain cases, evidence from the perpetrator's body should also be collected without delay. An act that involves digital or penile penetration leaves DNA from the victim on the body of the perpetrator, while digital penetration frequently leaves no evidence on the victim. The suspect may carry DNA from the victim on his or her body or clothing. Whenever an incident is reported within approximately 2 days of occurrence, the suspect should undergo physical evidence collection including finger and fingernail swabbings, external penile swabbings, and clothing collection. This information should be communicated and coordinated with law enforcement.

Specimen Preservation

Warm, moist conditions promote microbial destruction of human DNA. All swabs and clothing items should be thoroughly air-dried for at least 1 hour before packaging. It is important that chain of evidence procedures are maintained while the samples are air-drying. Culture tubes are not to be used to store the swabs because the medium in the tubes is designed to promote the growth of microorganisms, which will destroy the DNA. All packaging should be made of paper or light cardboard to permit additional drying. All samples must be labeled with the patient's information, including the collection site, when applicable.

Detecting Foreign Materials on Skin

Light sources may help identify foreign materials on a victim's skin. Traditionally, a Wood lamp, which emits wavelengths of approximately 365 nm, has been used to detect specimens not clearly visible to the eye. A Wood lamp can illuminate semen as well as other substances such as milk, petroleum, lubricating jelly, lotions, and contraceptive foams, but does not adequately differentiate between these various substances. Thus it may actually make it more difficult to identify semen amongst the nonbiological fluids.[14,15] One study examined pediatric emergency medicine physicians' use of a Wood lamp to differentiate between semen applied to skin and other substances typically found on a child's perineal area, such as diaper cream.[15] Physicians had difficulty identifying semen from the other specimens. This further supports the fact that if a Wood lamp is used for substance detection, interpretation of the results should be viewed with caution because the sensitivity and specificity of findings are not very high.

Because different specimens including biological fluids, hairs, and fibers illuminate under distinct wavelengths, having the ability to vary the wavelength of light emitted can increase the yield and differentiation of material detection. Therefore, contemporary alternative light sources are now recommended alternatives to Wood lamps because they can emit light of wavelengths ranging from 365 nm to 700 nm and are thus more successful at identifying foreign materials on a victim's body.

Semen, for example, hydrolyzes to a clear residue when it dries and may not be readily visible on physical examination. Its peak fluorescence is at a smaller wavelength (approximately 450 nm) than a Wood lamp, thus an alternative light source that could identify semen at its peak fluorescence would better detect semen residue. Alternative light sources also help differentiate biological fluids by their illumination pattern. For instance, while semen and urine both fluoresce at approximately 450 nm, urine fluoresces homogenously and semen fluoresces irregularly.[14] Additionally, the intensity of the fluorescence of semen diminishes dramatically by 28 hours after application to the skin, yet the fluorescence of urine lasts up to 80 hours.[14]

Besides examining the skin with a Wood lamp or alternative light source, the skin should also be examined under normal white light. Any area of the skin that fluoresces, or any area that appears suspicious as a forensic substance, should be swabbed with a lightly moistened cotton-tipped swab. A gauze pad should not be used because DNA from such large pieces of material is difficult to extract. Because saliva does not fluoresce, it is recommended to do blind swabbing of the skin with damp swabs based on the patient's history of oral contact by the perpetrator.

Role of the Crime Laboratory

Specimen Analysis

Forensic scientists use various protocols and have different capabilities and resources for scientific analysis of submitted samples. Specimens collected may be analyzed immediately or stored for later analysis as needed by the forensic investigator. Clothing and bedding items are surveyed for semen stains with the use of a high-intensity ultraviolet light source. Areas of fluorescence are then subjected to chemical testing. A rapid presumptive test for semen consists of a color indicator test for the presence of acid phosphatase (AP) activity. Stains and swabs showing positive AP results are then subject to confirmatory testing. Microscopic identification of spermatozoa or antibody-based tests for the prostate-specific antigen (PSA) serve as confirmatory tests.

Seminal Fluid Analysis

The presence of seminal fluid is usually identified by the presence of either AP or PSA (P-30 antigen). Seminal products may be present without the identification of sperm cells.

Acid phosphatase is an enzyme found in low concentrations (<50 IU/L) in vaginal fluid and is also secreted by the prostate gland, achieving high concentrations (130–1,800 IU/L) within seminal fluid. The presence of AP is not affected by vasectomy. Acid phosphatase persists longer than sperm after sexual assault,[16] and levels typically return to normal between 18 and 24 hours after ejaculation. Acid phosphatase is usually undetectable in the vagina after 48 hours.[17] The enzyme is stable in dried secretions and clothing and, in some instances, it can be detected after months or even years.

P-30 antigen (PSA) is a glycoprotein present in seminal fluid and adult male urine but is not found in prepubertal male urine or female body fluids. It is thus a more specific marker for ejaculation than AP. It is also a more sensitive test for seminal fluid, lasting in the vagina for up to 48 hours.

Sperm Analysis

Spermatozoa can be identified by microscopic evaluation of either a wet mount preparation from a swab sample, preferably after Gram staining or Christmas tree staining, or of a Pap smear from an adolescent victim. In the appropriate context, the identification of sperm is sufficient for diagnosis of sexual abuse. Motile sperm is the best indicator of recent ejaculation but is uncommonly recovered in child sexual abuse cases. Motile sperm survive longer in the adolescent cervix than in the vagina, so that samples should be taken from both locations in adolescent patients. Although sperm motility is lost within 24 hours in the vagina, nonmotile sperm can be identified in the vagina for up to 72 hours, and up to a week in the cervix. Sperm may also be found on dried secretions from clothing or bedding for months.

Samples containing spermatozoa can be subject to a differential DNA extraction procedure where the DNA from non-sperm cells is isolated and removed from the sample. Subsequently, an extraction procedure that removes the DNA from the sperm cells produces a concentrated sample that is used for DNA typing.

Saliva, Hair, and Fibers

Saliva is detected using tests for amylase activity. Amylase is present in highest concentrations in saliva but can be found in other body fluids as well. In practice, there is a poor correlation between the presence of amylase activity and typeable human DNA. Therefore, skin stain swabs testing negative for amylase may still contain useful DNA information.

Hairs and fibers are ubiquitous in the environment, and the presence of hairs or fabric fibers from a perpetrator who has legitimate contact with the patient is expected and has limited investigatory potential. An exception, however, is if a pubic hair is found in the vaginal cavity of a prepubertal child. In cases involving strangers or individuals who have no legitimate or recent contact with the patient, careful collection and packaging of outer clothing is appropriate to preserve hair, fiber, and other trace evidence. Since the advent of DNA technology, trace evidence has been de-emphasized. However, trace findings such as vegetation residue, sawdust, metal filings, paint or paint chips, and fibers have been used to determine the occupation of an unknown perpetrator, location of an assault, and the type of vehicle used. Databases of fibers may be used to identify a particular type of carpet installed in certain types of vehicles. The first step in analyzing hair specimens is to identify those that may be foreign to the patient. This is done through microscopic comparison of collected hair with a set of cut hair standards to look at the morphological characteristics of the hair samples. The hair determined to be of possible foreign origin may then be subject to DNA extraction and typing.

Genetic Profiling

A modern forensic laboratory has the ability to detect trace quantities of blood, semen, sperm, saliva, and hair and to develop DNA profiles from the remnants of as little as 300 nucleated cells or a half-inch hair fragment (Table 12.1). If the alleged perpetrator is male, fluorescence in situ hybridization analysis uses a Y-chromosome–specific DNA probe to identify male cells in the collected sample and thus requires a smaller amount of specimen.[18] Furthermore, Y-chromosome–directed short tandem repeats also target male DNA, and there are preliminary data that this type of analysis can detect perpetrator

TABLE 12.1
Specimen Analysis Based on Collection Site

Swab	Typical Body Fluid Testing
Vaginal	Semen
Cervical os	Spermatozoa
External penile	Semen, saliva
External female genitalia	Semen, saliva
Anal or perianal	Semen
Bite mark	Saliva
Other skin stain	Semen, saliva

DNA in cases of acute (<72 hours) pediatric sexual assault.[19] One study from the Philippines evaluated 26 child assault victims who were examined from 6 to 72 hours after the reported assault. Y-chromosome–directed short tandem repeat DNA was detected in 24 of the 26 cases (92%), while microscopic examination revealed the presence of spermatozoa in only 19% of cases.[19]

If sufficient DNA is obtained from extraction, sequence-based analyses are conducted on restriction fragment length polymorphisms or variable tandem repeats. If only a small amount of DNA is collected, it may be subjected to polymerase chain reaction amplification to allow for additional analysis. This technique can be used on as little as 1 ng of material. The Federal Bureau of Investigation analyzes the collected DNA at 13 specific locations (loci) and compares it with existing databases of genetic profiles.[20] If a match is found, statistical analysis determines the likelihood of finding the particular DNA sequence in the general population.

Perpetrator Identification

The widespread development of all-felon DNA databasing legislation has made it possible to compare unknown DNA profiles against millions of other forensic, felon, and arrestee case profiles. DNA identification provides the most specific information about the perpetrator of abuse and is considered an extremely valid and reliable method of perpetrator identification.[20-22] A comprehensive review of DNA profiling technology can be found in *Forensic DNA Typing, Biology, Technology and*

Genetics of STR Markers.[23]

The ability of forensic DNA laboratories to develop profiles from trace amounts of body fluids as well as blind swabbings increases the frequency of finding evidence beyond what was previously possible based only on the identification of motile sperm. These advanced techniques have not been reported in child sexual abuse research, and further study may influence previously published conclusions. Although modern techniques may increase the possibility of recovering forensic evidence in acute cases of sexual abuse/assault, the fact that physical or forensic evidence may not be recovered must be communicated to the patient, family, law enforcement, and child protective services professionals.

Forensic Toxicology

There are an increasing number of drug-facilitated sexual assault (DFSA) cases in which drugs are being given to victims as part of a sexual assault. These drugs include flunitrazepam (Rohypnol), gamma hydroxybutyrate (GHB), lorazepam, alprazolam, diphenhydramine, and chloral hydrate. These drugs impair the victim's memory, and they are usually given in a drink or administered in some way without the victim's knowledge. The victim may present with only nonspecific symptoms such as confusion, drowsiness, or nausea.[24] Therefore, medical and forensic providers must have a high index of suspicion for toxicological testing in cases of abuse.

Even when DFSA is suspected, the drugs can be difficult to detect. The amount of time that the drugs remain in the urine or the blood depends on the drug ingested; the amount ingested; and the patient's weight, size, and metabolism. Urine samples are preferable to blood samples because drug metabolites remain in the urine for a longer time than they remain in circulation. For example, Rohypnol can be detected in the blood for 4 to 12 hours but it remains in the urine for up to 48 hours. Similarly, GHB may only remain in the blood for 4 to 8 hours but can be identified in the urine for up to 12 hours. The first postexposure urine void is typically the one most likely to be positive.[24]

Because many hospitals and even some crime laboratories do not have the capability to adequately test for the specific drugs of concern, it is important to send samples to a laboratory equipped to detect trace amounts of a wide variety of these drugs. Protocols and procedures should be in place to ensure that the correct specimens are properly collected and are sent to laboratories that specialize in forensic toxicology. It is also important to discuss with the patient, family, and law enforcement investigators that there is a chance that a substance will not be detected even after testing is performed.

Conclusion

A revolution in forensic science has been driven by the advent of DNA technology. Whereas in the late 1980s the available protein-based typing methods for blood and semen were insensitive and lacked the ability to determine identity, the methods available today are so sensitive as to foster debate as to whether trace amounts of DNA and

various body fluids have been transferred in the course of casual contact or in the act of a criminal offense. Changes in technology, legal requirements, and our understanding of sexual abuse require frequent updating of evidence collection strategies. Evidence collection procedures that were state of the art 10 years ago may be inadequate today.

Investigation of a child sexual abuse case is a complicated task that requires collaboration between the victim, health care professionals, and forensic investigators. The paramount concern is the welfare of the child, and a comprehensive medical and forensic examination should be performed only after stabilization of the child's health. Evidence collection protocols have been established to delineate appropriate chain of evidence specimen collection techniques, and it is imperative that providers are familiar and proficient in specimen identification, collection, and handling. It is also important to remember that the likelihood of identifying a perpetrator can be maximized not only with a thorough and timely examination but, more importantly, with a comprehensive event history.

References

1. Christian CW, Lavelle JM, De Jong AR, Loiselle J, Brenner L, Joffe M. Forensic evidence findings in prepubertal victims of sexual assault. *Pediatrics.* 2000;106:100–104
2. Dahlke MB, Cooke C, Cunnane M, Chawla P, Lau P. Identification of semen in 500 patients seen because of rape. *Am J Clin Path.* 1977;68:740–746

3. Enos WF, Conrath TB, Byer JC. Forensic evaluation of the sexually abused child. *Pediatrics.* 1986;78:385–398

4. De Jong AR, Rose M. Legal proof of child sexual abuse in the absence of physical evidence. *Pediatrics.* 1991;88:506–511

5. Willott GM, Allard JE. Spermatozoa— their persistence after sexual intercourse. *Forensic Sci Int.* 1982;19:135–154

6. Gray-Eurom K, Seaberg DC, Wears RL. The prosecution of sexual assault cases: correlation with forensic evidence. *Ann Emerg Med.* 2002;39:39–46

7. De Jong AR, Rose M. Frequency and significance of physical evidence in legally proven cases of child sexual abuse. *Pediatrics.* 1981;84:1022–1026

8. Kellogg N, American Academy of Pediatrics Committee on Child Abuse and Neglect. The evaluation of sexual abuse in children. *Pediatrics.* 2005;116:506–512

9. McGregor MJ, DuMont J, Myhr TL. Sexual assault forensic medical examination: is evidence related to successful prosecution? *Ann Emerg Med.* 2002;39:639–647

10. Palusci VJ, Cox EO, Shatz EM, Schultze JM. Urgent medical assessment after child sexual abuse. *Child Abuse Negl.* 2006;30:367–380

11. Young KL, Jones JG, Worthington T, Simpson P, Casey PH. Forensic laboratory evidence in sexually abused children and adolescents. *Arch Pediatr Adolesc Med.* 2006;160:585–588

12. Exeline DL, Smith FP, Drexler SG. Frequency of pubic hair transfer during sexual intercourse. *J Forensic Sci.* 1998;43:505–508

13. Young KL, Jones JG, Worthington T, Simpson P, Casey PH. Forensic laboratory evidence in sexually abused children and adolescents. *Arch Pediatric Adolescent Med.* 2006;160:585–588

14. Gabby T, Winkleby MA, Boyce WT, Fisher DL, Lancaster A, Sensabaugh GF. Sexual abuse of children. The detection of semen on skin. *Am J Dis Child.* 1992;146:700–703

15. Santucci KA, Nelson DG, McQuillen KK, Duffy SJ, Linakis JG. Wood's lamp utility in the identification of semen. *Pediatrics.* 1999;104:1342–1344

16. Soules MR, Pollard AA, Brown KM, Verma M. The forensic laboratory evaluation of evidence in alleged rape. *Am J Obstet Gynecol.* 1978;130:142–147

17. Graves HCB, Sensabaugh GF, Blake ET. Post-coital detection of a male-specific semen protein: application to the investigation of rape. *N Engl J Med.* 1985;312:338–343

18. Palusci VJ, Christian CW. Forensic evidence in child sexual abuse. In: Finkel MA, Giardino AP, eds. *Medical Evaluation of Child Sexual Abuse.* 3rd ed. Elk Grove Village, IL: American Academy of Pediatrics. In press

19. Delfin FC, Madrid BJ, Tan MP, De Ungria MC. Y-STR analysis for detection and objective confirmation of child sexual abuse. *Int J Legal Med.* 2005;119:158–163

20. Turman KM. Understanding DNA evidence: a guide for victim service providers. *OVC Bull.* April 2001:1 11. http://www.ojp.usdoj.gov/ovc/publications/bulletins/dna_4_2001/NCJ185690.pdf

21. Annas GJ. Setting standards for the use of DNA-typing results in the courtroom— the state of the art. *N Engl J Med.* 1992;107:1476–1479

22. Nishimi RY. Forensic DNA analysis: scientific, legal, and social issues. *Cancer Invest.* 1992;10:553–563

23. Butler J. *Forensic DNA Typing Biology, Technology and Genetics of STR Markers.* 2nd ed. Burlington, MA: Elsevier Academic Press; 2005

24. LeBeau M, Andollo W, Hearn WL, et al. Recommendations for toxicological investigations of drug-facilitated sexual assaults. *J Forensic Sci.* 1999;44:227–230

Chapter 13

Conditions Mistaken for Child Sexual Abuse

Nancy D. Kellogg

Child Safe
University of Texas Health Sciences Center

Lori Frasier

Medical Director, Child Protection Team
Center for Safe and Healthy Children
Primary Children's Hospital

The anogenital examination has become an important component of the investigation of suspected sexual abuse. The results of the medical examination may have significant child protection and legal repercussions because they carry the weight of evidence in the legal outcome of the case. Most children who present with possible sexual abuse have reported some type of sexual contact, exhibit disturbing behaviors, or have physical signs or symptoms such as genital irritation or bleeding. Anogenital findings diagnostic of blunt force or penetrating anal or genital injury are found only in the minority of cases, even when penetration is alleged.[1-5] It is not uncommon, however, for a child to present with a specific anal or genital complaint, or a possible physical finding that raises the suspicion of sexual abuse. Many anogenital conditions have been observed and reported that "mimic" sexual abuse. In one study of children referred for sexual abuse evaluations based only on anogenital symptoms and signs, 85% had normal or nonspecific examination findings.[6] This chapter will focus on those conditions and an approach to the evaluation of anogenital problems.

The clinical evaluation of a child with anogenital symptoms presents unique challenges for the general practitioner. Clinicians acknowledge that sexual abuse is a diagnosis that is important not to miss and may feel it is better to report to child protective services, even when clinical indicators are nonspecific or confusing. A particular conundrum occurs when the parent presents with a preverbal child, who has an anogenital complaint, and has voiced concern that an individual has sexually abused the child. The possibility of sexual abuse must be adequately addressed and the parent's degree of concern, more than objective findings, may drive the clinician's consideration of sexual abuse in the diagnosis. Even when there is no suspicion for sexual abuse, the clinician may feel "safer" reporting a child with anogenital symptoms for suspected abuse. Reporting such cases may result in unnecessary investigations, intrusive questioning, and strained family relationships. General practitioners are encouraged to become familiar with anogenital conditions that may mimic trauma resulting from sexual abuse and to consider referring children who present with only anogenital symptoms for further evaluation by physicians specializing in child sexual abuse assessments before reporting to child protective services.

Behavioral Conditions

Diverse symptoms and behavioral changes have been linked with child sexual abuse,[7] including difficulty sleeping, nightmares, unusual fears, sudden change in school performance, secondary enuresis[8] or encopresis,[9] and sexualized behavior. Clinicians should be aware that sexual abuse is only one of many explanations for such behaviors. For example, children may exhibit sexualized behaviors after exposure to nudity, sexually explicit media, or adult sexual activity within their home.

Caretakers and health care providers are sometimes challenged to determine whether a child's sexual behavior is normal or suggestive of abuse. Information found in the Child Sexual Behavior Inventory can provide reassurance that certain behaviors are common in a child of a particular age.[10] A child who exhibits sexual behaviors that are uncommon for the age and gender (eg, putting their

mouth on another's genitalia or asking others to engage in sexual acts) or who engages in sexual behavior with an individual who is significantly older or younger, or more or less knowledgeable, should be referred for further evaluation.[11] Coercive sexual behavior by a child also warrants further evaluation for possible sexual abuse.

Parental issues can cause confusion about possible child sexual abuse. Mental illness, substance abuse, parental history of sexual abuse, unusual genital care practices, and hostile custody disputes[12–15] may result in misinterpretation of behavioral or physical signs as indicators of abuse. A clinician evaluating a child for possible abuse should take a careful history to detect these confounding factors.

Bleeding

In a study of 157 children presenting with only physical signs or symptoms suspicious for abuse, and no behavioral concerns or disclosure of sexual abuse, half had presenting complaints of anogenital bleeding, bruising, irritation, or redness; approximately 60% of those who presented with bleeding or bruising had evidence of such on examination.[6] Fecal stains and foods or dyes may simulate blood stains on underwear, or blood may be transferred from a nongenital site to the underwear during toileting or changing clothes. The clinician should first attempt to identify the source of bleeding, keeping in mind that minor trauma can heal rapidly and active bleeding may not be identified during the examination. In addition to sexual abuse, etiologies for anogenital bleeding include estrogen withdrawal in female neonates, menses, maceration due to irritative substances such as diapers and feces, vaginal foreign bodies, *Shigella* vaginitis, and acquired skin disorders that mimic trauma (Table 13.1).

Anogenital injuries that result in bleeding can be iatrogenic, accidental, intentional due to physical abuse, or intentional due to sexual abuse. Small fissures of the posterior fourchette can occur when the examining physician

TABLE 13.1
Anogenital Symptoms and Signs That May Mimic Sexual Abuse

Sign or Symptom	Differential Diagnosis

Bleeding	Trauma
	   -Iatrogenic
	   -Accidental
	   -Physical
	   -Sexual
	Superficial excoriations due to irritants, hygiene, diaper dermatitis
	Anal fissures
	Dehisced labial adhesions
	Urethral prolapse
	Infection
	   -*Shigella enterocolitica*
	   -Group A beta-hemolytic streptococcus
	   -Candidiasis
	Menstruation
	Vaginal foreign body
	Precocious puberty
	Tumor-ovarian, vaginal

Bruising	Trauma
	   -Accidental
	   -Physical
	   -Sexual
	Lichen sclerosus et atrophicus
	Hemangiomas/varicosities
	Urethral prolapse
	Coagulaopathy
	Prominent or superficial blood vessels
	Dye from clothing
	Nevi/mongolian spots

Genital erythema	Normal prepubertal vascularity Irritation due to diarrhea/constipation Nonspecific vulvitis related to poor hygiene Use of irritating products, including soaps, bleach Diaper dermatitis Minor trauma Insect bites, including fleas, chiggers, scabies Folliculitis Psoriasis Masturbation

TABLE 13.1
Anogenital Symptoms and Signs That May Mimic Sexual Abuse, *continued*

Sign or Symptom	Differential Diagnosis
Scarring/healed trauma	Trauma 　　-Accidental 　　-Physical 　　-Sexual Normal variations in anatomy Anal dilation due to 　　-Presence of stool 　　-Encopresis 　　-Neurologic deficit 　　-Examination position Labial adhesion Linea vestibularis Diastasis ani Partial or complete failure of midline fusion Perihymenal or periurethral bands
Vaginal discharge	Common pathogens 　　-Group A beta-hemolytic streptococcus 　　-Group B streptococcus 　　-*Candida* vaginitis 　　-Bacterial vaginosis 　　-*Haemophilus influenzae* 　　-Gram-negative enterics/bowel contamination 　　-Respiratory pathogens 　　-Overgrowth of "usual or normal genital flora" Sexually transmitted infections Physiological leukorrhea Poor hygiene Smegma Semen Healing trauma Vaginal foreign body Pinworms
Vesicles or ulcers	Herpes simplex virus 1 or 2 Varicella-zoster virus 　　-Chicken pox 　　-Shingles Epstein-Barr virus Nonspecific viral infections Behçet syndrome Contact dermatitis-allergic/irritant (nickel, products, perfumes, latex) Partial or complete failure of midline fusion defects Contact/irritant dermatitis Impetigo Blister beetle (black or gray insect up to 1 inch found in the Southwest)

TABLE 13.1
Anogenital Symptoms and Signs That May Mimic Sexual Abuse, *continued*

Sign or Symptom	Differential Diagnosis
Papules/nodules	Human papillomavirus (condylomata acuminata) Molluscum contagiosum Skin tags Folliculitis/ingrown hair Nevi Urethral/periurethral cysts Benign papillomatosis Fordyce granules Perianal pseudo-verrucous papules and nodules Pink pearly papules of the penis Inclusion cysts Crohn disease Condyloma latum Linear epidermal nevus Scrotal raphe Spermatocele Syringoma Darier disease Langerhans cell histiocytosis

exerts traction on the labia[16]; similarly, labial adhesions may dehisce during the course of the examination. One physician describes watching as a mother caused an anal fissure by "violently opposing the child's buttocks" in an effort to demonstrate how other physicians had examined the child for possible abuse.[17]

Splitting injury to the midline anogenital structures can occur with sudden, violent abduction of the legs.[18–21] A history of possible abuse should be taken; however, in one report of such injury, the cause was forced abduction of the legs during sexual abuse.[22] In a series of 56 prepubertal girls with unintentional perineal injury, only one had hymenal involvement. She had fallen at a park, abducting her legs. There was a pinpoint abraded area on the hymen.[23] The

author saw a 5-year-old girl with persistent genital bleeding after she fell "doing a split," on railroad ties on a school playground. She had been playing under adult supervision and denied sexual abuse. The child was examined under anesthesia and found to have a small laceration in the fossa navicularis.

Penetrating genital or anal injury can occur when children fall astride sharp objects.[24] A Texas study of 16 cases of anorectal trauma in children younger than 16 years revealed that 80% of cases involved sexual abuse.[25] Documented causes of rectal injury or perforation include falls with impalement on broom or toilet-brush handles, pogo sticks, chair legs, bicycle seat poles, sprinklers, high-jump bars, and tree branches (Figure 13.1). Anal injuries in children also are reported from gunshot wounds, stabbings, motor vehicle crashes, coat hangers inserted by family members (for reasons not documented), and a swallowed fish bone that lacerated the rectal mucosa.[25-27]

Motor vehicle crashes can cause injuries to the genitalia.[28,29] A 5-year-old girl was referred for possible sexual abuse when an emergency department (ED) physician noted bloody vaginal discharge after a motor vehicle crash. Her father, who was the driver of the car and had weekend custody, was referred to local authorities for investigation. Her injuries included a hematoma of the mons, abrasions of the labia, and a tear in the perineal body. The hymen was undamaged. The child denied sexual abuse. The injuries were attributed to an

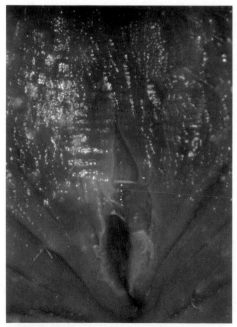

FIGURE 13.1
Perianal laceration. This could be caused by penetrating sexual assault or an accidental penetrating injury.

improperly worn seat belt, and the investigation was closed.[28]

Water under high pressure, from activities such as water or jet skiing or from water slides, can cause serious penetrating injury to the vagina with little external evidence of trauma. These injuries are more common in parous women, but have been reported in prepubertal girls. Persistent vaginal bleeding after such activities requires an examination under anesthesia, which may reveal injuries requiring surgical repair.[30]

A review of rectal and genital trauma in boys compared physical findings in boys examined in the ED for accidental injury with the abnormal findings in a group of boys who were seen for suspected sexual abuse. The injuries were caused by falling or being caught on an object, being kicked, being shot, or being hurt by a toilet seat or bicycle. Accidental trauma resulted in lacerations or perforations of the scrotum or penis. No patient had isolated anal injuries. In contrast, the sexually abused group all had rectal lesions, none had scrotal injuries, and penile injuries were rare.[31]

Some dermatologic conditions that may produce bleeding can simulate abusive injuries. Anal fissures and vulvar or perihymenal maceration due to infectious or noninfectious causes are common. Labial adhesion or fusion is a common condition in prepubertal children. Labial adhesions resemble a scar and may bleed when dehiscence occurs, usually during normal activities (Figure 13.2). A few millimeters of labial fusion posteriorly is a common finding, observed in 39% of non-abused girls in one study.[7] Extensive labial adhesion, with fusion leaving only an opening of a few millimeters under the clitoris, occurs in fewer than 1% of girls[32] (Figure 13.3). Labial fusion may be secondary to atrophic or inflammatory conditions such as lichen sclerosus, vulvovaginitis, atopic or seborrheic dermatitis, varicella,[33] or herpes.[34] In one study, labial adhesions were found more commonly in non-Hispanic white girls with a history of sexual abuse involving penetration than girls without a history of penetration.[35]

Patients with urethral prolapse can present with genital bleeding, dysuria, urinary frequency, or introital pain. Physical examination reveals eversion of the urethral mucosa in a rosette surrounding the meatus. The friable mass of tissue may ulcerate, necrose, or become infected. It may obscure the anatomy of the hymen and be mistaken for abusive injury[36-38] (Figure 13.4).

Urethral prolapse occurs only in female patients and most commonly in prepubescent black girls. Other reported causes or associated findings include burns, urinary tract infection, straddle injury, and strangury.[38,39] Treatment options include both nonsurgical and surgical approaches. In mild cases, antibiotics and topical steroids, or a short course of estrogen, are curative. Reduction of the prolapse and insertion of a catheter, or primary excision of the prolapse, occasionally are warranted.[36] In addition, treatment of underlying predisposing factors, such as constipation, also is recommended.

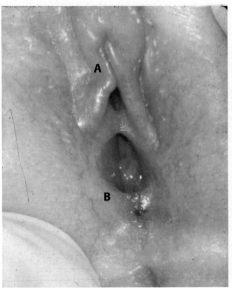

FIGURE 13.2
This child has 2 labial adhesions, an anterior one **(A)** and a small posterior adhesion **(B)**. The posterior adhesion has dehisced slightly and may bleed.

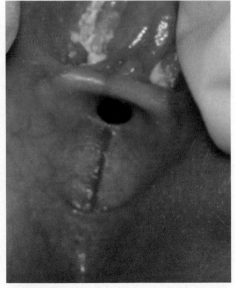

FIGURE 13.3
Extensive labial adhesion.

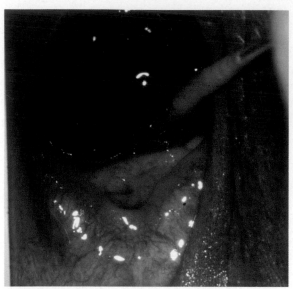

FIGURE 13.4
Urethral prolapse; the swab is elevating the
prolapsed urethra to expose the hymen
beneath it.

Hemangioma of the hymen, vulva, vagina, or perineal body can bleed and be confused with trauma resulting from sexual abuse.[40,41] Hemangiomata may bleed or ulcerate, heightening concerns about possible molestation.[42]

Case Examples

A 5-year-old girl was brought to the ED after blood was found in the bathtub, in her underwear, and in her vaginal area. Physical examination showed vulvar erythema, a blood clot in the introitus, and a laceration of the hymen. The child was placed in foster care. Three days later, she was seen at a sexual abuse clinic and found to have a normal hymen with urethral prolapse and a tear in the urethral mucosa rather than the hymen. The child was treated and returned home.

A 5-week-old girl was treated for denuded erythematous areas of the labia and mons and diagnosed with candida diaper dermatitis. Three days later, apparent healing of second- and third-degree burns of the labia were noted and confirmed by surgical consultation. The mother stated that the rash had appeared after the infant was left in the care of her father. A report of suspected abuse was filed, listing the father as the suspected perpetrator. One month later, the child was found to have a capillary-cavernous hemangioma of the vulva corresponding to the original denuded area. Although the mother denied the previous existence of this lesion, old records indicted that a hemangioma of the labia majora with some denuded areas had been noted at the 3-week visit (Figure 13.5). The child abuse report was rescinded.[43]

Bruising

Causes for anogenital bruising include accidental injuries, abusive injuries, and conditions that simulate bruising. Injuries to the perineum can be classified as penetrating and non-penetrating. Straddle injuries, the most common injury to the genitalia, seldom involve penetration. Straddle injuries usually are associated with a history of an acute and dramatic fall onto an object such as a furniture arm or bar on a bicycle or play equipment (Figures 13.6 and 13.7). These injuries usually crush the soft tissue between the hard external object and a firm internal base, such as the pubic symphysis, the ischiopubic ramus, or the adductor longus tendon. Compared with injuries caused by abuse, straddle injuries are more often unilateral and anterior, causing damage to the external genitalia rather than the hymen or vagina.

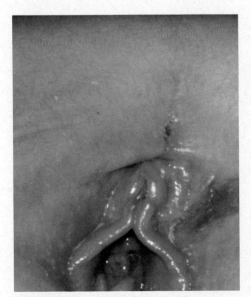

FIGURE 13.5
Hemangioma of labia majora, which can mimic a bruise or abrasion.

Typically bruising and swelling are noted of the anterior labia, clitoris, and periurethral tissue. Accidental injury to the internal genital structures or anus is rare, because the bones of the pelvis and the soft tissue of the buttocks and labia protect internal structures.[42,44-46]

In 2 reported cases, genital injury occurred in boys who were injured while break dancing. One had a hematocele of the scrotum, and the other had a partial rupture of the bulbar urethra after a fall onto the corner of a coffee table.[47]

Masturbation rarely causes genital injury.[48-50] Masturbation tends to involve the clitoris and labia, rather than internal structures. No genital or anal injuries were reported in a study of self-injurious behavior in 97 mentally retarded children aged 11 months to 21 years.[51]

Bruises often occur in conjunction with bleeding due to abrasions or lacerations. In a series of 100 children examined in an ED for straddle injuries, most had minor lacerations and abrasions of the genitalia. Among 72 girls, the injury was to the labia majora or minora in 79%; in 16%, the injury was to the posterior fourchette; and 11% had hematoma of the vulva. Seven girls had injuries to the vagina and 2 had injuries to the hymen. Three girls had unintentional penetrating injuries caused by falls onto a plunger handle, a sharp fence post, and the exposed steering column of a bike. Five girls with injuries not accounted for by their histories eventually revealed sexual abuse. Among 28 boys, the most common injury was ecchymosis or minor laceration of the scrotum or penis. The authors listed factors that require investigation for sexual abuse. These include straddle injuries in non-ambulatory children (<9 months), extensive trauma, coexisting nongenital trauma, and lack of correlation between history and physical findings (more specifically, perianal, vaginal, or hymenal injury without a history of penetrating trauma).[52]

Jones and Bass[53] reviewed perineal injuries in 463 children aged 13 years or younger seen over a 12-year period at a South African hospital. Accidental trauma accounted for 57% of injuries. The leading cause was straddle injury

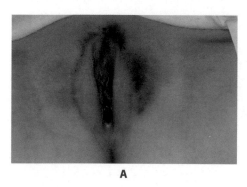
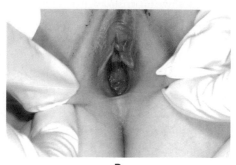

A   B

FIGURE 13.6
Straddle injury to the right labium. The hymen was undamaged.

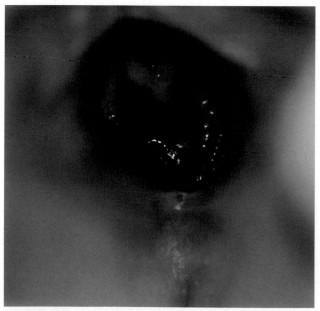

FIGURE 13.7
Midline straddle injury that occurred when the child fell on the handle of a wagon. Soft tissues of the hymen are bruised.

on such objects as bicycle bars, beds, fences, concrete walls, and playground equipment. Other causes of accidental perineal injury were impalement, motor vehicle crashes, zipper injuries, and animal bites. Sexual or physical abuse accounted for 38% of perineal injuries. The most common genital injuries resulting from abuse were tears of the posterior fourchette and tears of the hymen. Four children were injured by forceful enemas, a highly regarded tribal treatment. Three had enemas administered by hosepipes, and one by a goat's horn. Two had third-degree perineal tears. Five percent of injuries could not be classified because the history was vague or unavailable.

Suction-drain injury occurs when children sit directly on uncovered swimming pool suction-drain vents capable of forming a strong vacuum. The child's perineum forms a firm seal, with relaxation of the anal sphincter and evisceration of the small intestine through tears in the anterior bowel wall. Associated injuries include perianal bruising and rectal prolapse.[54,55] Less severe forms of anogenital suction injury might be mistaken for abusive trauma.

Injuries suspicious for physical abuse sometimes occur in the genital or anal area (Figure 13.8). Lesions may be actual bruises or a finding that simulates bruises. Patterns of inflicted physical abuse injuries are described in Chapter 7 and are typically distinguishable from patterns of inflicted sexual abuse injuries (Figure 13.8). Any of the conditions described in Chapter 9 as causing apparent bruises that may be mistaken for physical abuse could also lead to mistaken diagnosis of sexual abuse if the lesions occurred in the anogenital area. These include mongolian spots, hemangiomas, Ehlers-Danlos syndrome, meningococcemia, erythema multiforme, and bleeding disorders such as idiopathic thrombocytopenic purpura.[42] Patients with Henoch-Schönlein

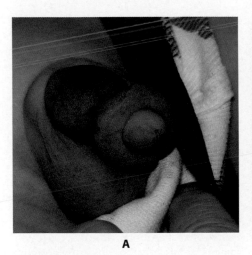

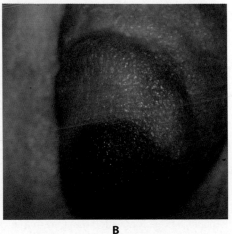

A   B

FIGURES 13.8
A. Bruise of penis caused when a caregiver "pinched" the child in an effort to toilet train him. **B.** Henoch-Schönlein purpura of the penis.

purpura can present with pain, swelling, and hematoma of the penis or scrotum. In 2 reported cases, scrotal involvement preceded the characteristic rash by 36 hours[56] (Figure 13.8B).

Other conditions that may simulate bruising include perianal venous congestion (Figure 13.9), lichen sclerosus, and partial or complete failure of midline fusion (Figure 13.10). A skin condition that is commonly mistaken for sexual abuse is lichen sclerosus (Figures 13.11 and 13.12). The initial lesions may be whitish or yellow papules that fuse to form white plaques. The skin becomes atrophic and thin, with fissuring and alarming subepidermal hemorrhages after such minor trauma to the anogenital area as wiping with toilet paper. Lichen sclerosus usually occurs on the vulva and perianal region, producing a characteristic "hourglass" area of decreased pigmentation (Figure 13.13). It also can occur at the urethral opening and cause phimosis in boys.[57] Less often, it appears on the trunk, extremities, axilla, face, and neck. Despite its distressing appearance, lichen sclerosus is more often accompanied by itching or soreness than by actual pain, except when fissures cause pain with micturition or defecation, or if lesions become infected. It may cause labial fusion or, in severe forms, atrophic genital scarring. Lichen sclerosus resolves spontaneously, usually during adolescence, in about one half of the cases. If the diagnosis is in doubt, a skin biopsy may be done.[38,58–63]

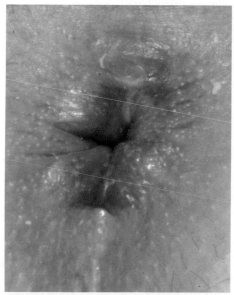

FIGURE 13.9
Perianal venous congestion that may mimic bruising.

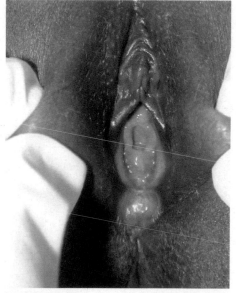

FIGURE 13.10
Failure of midline fusion. Note that the fusion failure extends from the anus to the posterior fourchette.

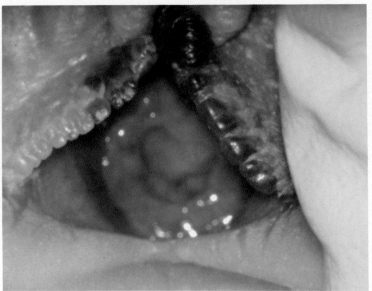

FIGURE 13.11
Hemorrhagic bullae of the labia minora are an indicator of lichen sclerosus, the mucosa is generally not involved.

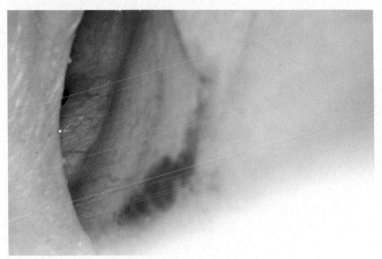

Figure 13.12
Hemorrhage of the inner labia minora seen in lichen sclerosus.

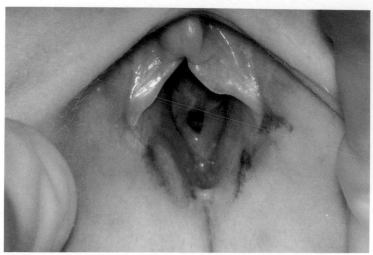

FIGURE 13.13
Lichen sclerosus, demonstrating involvement of the keratinized epithelium and sparing of the mucosa. Note the normal hymen.

Authors of a retrospective review of 42 confirmed cases of lichen sclerosus in girls aged 3 to 15 years reported that the onset of the disease was associated with prior accidental injury in 6 cases and with sexual abuse in 12 (29%) cases. Two of the latter were "new" cases, uncovered by careful history and physical examination at the time of consultation. Five girls had evidence of autoimmune disease, arthritis, or serum autoantibodies.[64]

Infrequently, dyes may simulate bruising. A 9-month-old child referred for genital bruising was found to have purple stains from gentian violet applied to treat *Candida*. Dye "bleeding" from new black or blue clothing has also stained children's skin and caused consternation over abuse as well as other serious medical conditions. The dye may not wash off with water but will wipe off with alcohol. In one case, numerous diagnoses were considered over a 2-day period by the parents (a dermatologist and an allergist) of a 10-year-old boy with blue discoloration of his hands and face. As his mother was observing his respiratory status as he slept, she realized that the color came from his new blue sheets.[65]

Eversion of the anal canal, or rectal prolapse, has been described as a result of anal sodomy.[66] This sign is not diagnostic of abuse, however, because it is associated with numerous conditions in children, including chronic constipation, acute diarrhea, cystic fibrosis, neurologic abnormalities, repaired imperforate anus, and rectal polyps.[67]

Genital Erythema

Many young children are brought to their physician's office because of a "red bottom" and a concern for sexual abuse. Because anogenital erythema is a benign and common finding with a myriad of traumatic and non-traumatic causes, it is important for the clinician to establish why the parent is concerned about sexual abuse. While some parents' concerns are driven by the belief that an ex-spouse or partner is abusive to their child, other parents' concerns may stem from vague suspicions of certain individuals or from their own sexually abusive experience. For some parents, reassurance regarding the medical findings is a relief, but for parents who are convinced their child has been abused, reassurance may not be welcomed information. If the clinician is concerned that the parent may subject their child to numerous additional examinations in an effort to solicit support for their unfounded beliefs, a report to child protective services for subjecting the child to unnecessary examinations may be warranted.

Erythema of the anogenital area is a common but nonspecific sign with numerous causes (poor hygiene, diaper dermatitis, sensitivity to natural or artificial substances, pinworms, enhanced vascularity of the hymen or vestibule, chronic vaginal discharge, and candidal infection). In addition to various food substances that may be transmitted from the child's hand to the genital area, contact dermatitis can be triggered by soaps, fabric softener, bubble bath, toilet paper, dyes or sizing in clothing, or topical medication.[38,68] Allergy to latex rubber products can manifest as dermatitis in areas in contact with underwear elastic (and also tires, scuba gear, windsurfing boards, squash balls, rubber fingerstalls, elastic stocking tops, and rubber spectacle chains).[69] Among female and male adolescents, shaving the pubic area may produce erythema or folliculitis (Figure 13.14). Among young children, a shift in caretakers may result in varying routines in bathing, diapering, laundering, and toilet assistance that, in turn, may result

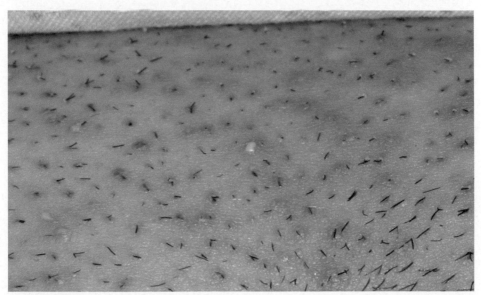

FIGURE 13.14
Pustulosis after shaving of pubic hair.

in mild anogenital irritation in the child. Such symptoms do not imply neglect unless they are chronic and result in a need for medical intervention.

Streptococcal infection of the anus, vagina, and urethra may cause clinical findings that result in a concern about abuse. Perianal streptococcal disease manifests as a painful or itchy rash sometimes associated with fissures, painful defecation, and blood-streaked stools (Figure 13.15). The rash can be pink, red, or beefy red with mucoid discharge or crusting, mucosal edema, and denuded tissue. Fever is not present.[70,71] In one study, 60% of children had positive throat cultures as well as positive anal cultures for group A beta-hemolytic streptococci (GABHS).[70] The culture request must specify that GABHS is suspected, because rectal swabs are routinely plated on media hostile to streptococci. Intrafamilial spread may occur if bathwater is shared.[70]

Any condition that causes anogenital irritation or pruritus can cause a behavioral response in the child that may simulate masturbation and create a concern

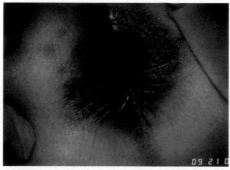

FIGURE 13.15
Perianal streptococcal infection.

for sexual abuse in the parent or caretaker. Insect bites can cause intense pruritus, resulting in acute swelling and erythema of the genitals. One example is chiggers, which are insects that are active during summer months in the southern and midwestern United States. Their bites may be confined to the penis, vulva, scrotum, or groin.[72] Scabies also can infect the genitals, producing similar findings. Other conditions that may cause genital and anal pruritus include pinworms, atopic dermatitis, and contact dermatitis.

Perianal erythema and increased pigmentation are nonspecific findings that are not diagnostic of sexual abuse.[73] Several reports exist of diseases producing perianal skin changes mistaken for sexual abuse trauma, including lichen sclerosus, Crohn disease,[74] and hemolytic uremic syndrome.[75]

Case Examples

A 2-year-old boy told his mother that his "bottom hurt" on returning from child care. His physician diagnosed anal trauma, and a child care worker was interviewed by the police after the child said, "Mark hurt me." After the child was examined at a child abuse center, the diagnosis of perianal streptococcal cellulitis was made. On further questioning, the child said the child care worker had hurt him when he was wiping after toileting. The pain apparently occurred because of preexisting anal irritation from the infection.[42] Other conditions that may cause pain when the child is wiped after toileting include diaper dermatitis, candidiasis, and urethral prolapse.

Three children younger than 3 years were seen with reddening of the anus, venous dilation, and alternating contraction and relaxation of the anal sphincter after several days of bloody diarrhea. Sexual abuse was considered until signs of hemolytic-uremic syndrome developed. In retrospect, the anal changes were thought to be due to *Escherichia coli* colitis.[75]

Scarring/Healed Trauma

There are many variations of normal genitalia, and some may be misdiagnosed as residua of genital or anal trauma. These types of findings are more typically reported by physicians who conduct detailed anogenital examinations but are sometimes reported by caretakers as well. A presenting complaint of "she has no hymen" or "her opening appears stretched" should be evaluated carefully by a physician with extensive experience and knowledge of normal variations of anatomy. Kellogg et al[6] found that all 38 children who were referred for a sexual abuse examination because of abnormal anatomy (such as "no hymen") had normal anatomy.

Common variations include hymens with narrow rims, hymenal notches, vestibular grooves, anterior hymenal clefts, and anal skin tags. Other congenital structures that have been confused with scar tissue resulting from trauma include periurethral bands, hymenal tags, hymenal septa, septal remnants, intravaginal ridges, and tissue bridges or "tethers" between the hymen and perihymenal tissues (Table 13.1).[7,16,76] Clefts, or defects in the hymenal rim that extend to the base, may be congenital or related to trauma. Anterior and lateral concavities and hymenal clefts have been demonstrated in newborns.[76] Deep concavities, notches, and clefts in the posterior rim of the hymen are uncommon and have been attributed to penetrating trauma,[76,77] but have also been demonstrated in adolescents who denied sexual activity but confirmed painful tampon insertion.[78] Other hymenal findings that have previously been attributed to sexual abuse include a large horizontal opening and a narrow hymenal rim of 1 to 2 mm. However, one study of prepubertal children with a history of penetration found that such measurements were insufficiently sensitive or specific for penetrative trauma.[79] Sometimes the examiner may not visualize the hymen because of inadequate examination techniques or because a labial adhesion obscures the hymen and may erroneously report an abnormality. Specialized examination techniques used in the assessment of suspected victims of sexual abuse are described elsewhere in Chapter 9.

Caution is advised in interpreting anogenital abnormalities that are found in the midline; several midline congenital abnormalities have been recognized since clinicians began scrutinizing children's genitalia for signs of abuse. Anal skin tags have been seen after trauma from anal sodomy,[20] but midline tags are a common congenital finding (Table 13.2). Anterior midline anal skin tags were found in 11% of non-abused children in one study.[73] A median raphe, particularly in a girl, may be confused with scar tissue. In boys, the raphe is

TABLE 13.2
Anal Findings in Normal, Constipated, and Abused Children

	McCann et al[7]	Stanton and Sunderland[90]	Agnarsson et al[85]	Clayden[86]	Hobbs and Wynne[66]
Subject number and type	N = 267, non-abused	N = 200, no abuse history	N = 136, referred for constipation	N = 129, referred for constipation	N = 337, evidence of abuse
Examination method	Knee chest	Unk	Supine or left lateral	Unk	Left lateral
Anal dilation	12%[a] 49%[b]	14%	19%[c]	15%	18%
Anal fissure	0%	2%	26%	NR	22%
Anal tag	11% (all but one in midline)	NR	5%	NR	3% (scars or tags)

Abbreviations: NR, not reported; Unk, unknown, probably left lateral position.

[a]Observed for 1 minute (knee–chest position).

[b]Observed up to 4 minutes (knee–chest position).

[c]Observed for 1 minute (left lateral position).

more obvious, as it runs without interruption along the underside of the penis, over the scrotum, and along the perineal body, tucking into the anus anteriorly (Figure 13.16).

Another finding to interpret with caution is pale midline avascular streaks of the posterior vestibule, particularly if all other genital findings are normal. In one study of 123 female newborns, 14% had white spots in the posterior vestibule, and 10% had white streaks extending from the posterior commissure into the posterior vestibule. The authors termed these structures *linea vestibularis*[80] (Figure 13.17). Midline avascular areas were found in one quarter of prepubertal girls selected for non-abuse in 2 separate studies from Australia[16] and the United States.[7] Other causes of avascular streaks in the posterior vestibule are scarring after trauma and partially resolved labial adhesions. It is difficult to differentiate linea vestibularis from scarring; if a laceration has been previously documented in the same location or the midline streak is raised, contracted, or irregular, then scarring is more likely.

Failure of midline fusion is a term currently used for a congenital midline lesion that has been mistaken for scarring due to abuse.[81] The genitalia are normal except for a midline defect that may extend from the fossa navicularis to the anus; partial defects may involve only the anal verge. The tissue at the base of the defect is pale and vascular, and the skin edges bordering the defect are smooth. Some with failure of midline fusion may have an anteriorly located anus. This is a congenital anomaly in which the anus is located anterior to the midpoint between the posterior commissure and the coccyx. When associated with refractory constipation and pain with defecation, it may require surgical correction[82] (Figures 13.10 and 13.18).

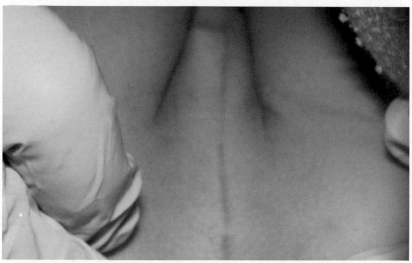

FIGURE 13.16
Median raphe of a male. Midline raphes can also be seen in females.

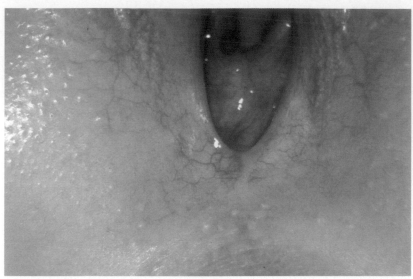

FIGURE 13.17
Linea vestibularis in the midline is often mistaken for a scar.

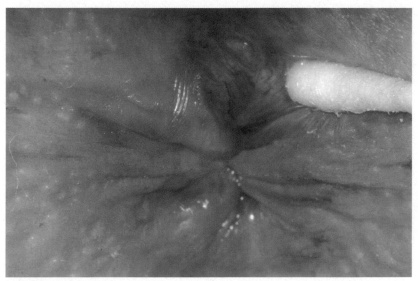

FIGURE 13.18
Failure of midline fusion at 12 o'clock on the anus. This finding appears inflamed in this patient.

McCann et al[73] noted a common congenital anomaly of the external anal sphincter that results in smooth, fan-shaped areas, with or without depressions, in the midline at the anal verge. In this study of 81 children, 26% had these smooth areas, which have been mistaken for anal scars, funneling, or thumbprints characteristic of abuse

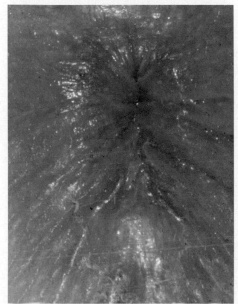

FIGURE 13.19
Diastasis ani at 6 o'clock is a common and normal finding.

(Figure 13.19). McCann and colleagues termed this structure *diastasis ani.*

Anal dilation may be physiological, trauma-induced, drug-induced, or related to neurologic conditions.[73,83] McCann's group[73] observed anal dilation in 49% of non-abused children after they had spent several minutes in the prone knee-chest position (Figures 13.20A and 13.20B). Anal dilation more than 20 mm in diameter without stool in the ampulla may indicate anal sodomy, particularly if dilation recurs in different examining positions. Both external and internal sphincters should dilate. Causes of anal dilation mistaken for abuse include postmortem changes,[84] sedation, severe constipation,[66,85,86] and neurogenic patulous anus.[87] A study of postmortem perianal findings in children revealed that anal dilation is common (77% of 50 cases). In other case reports, anal dilation has led to a suspicion of sexual abuse in developmentally delayed children with myotonic dystrophy sometimes in association with arthrogryposis.[87,88] In one study, an exposed pectinate line,

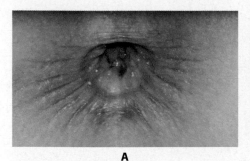

A

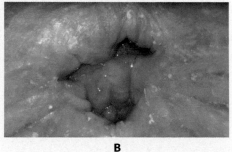

B

FIGURE 13.20

A. Physiological anal dilation in a symmetrical fashion. **B.** Somewhat more asymmetrical anal dilation exposing the pectinate line and slightly prolapsing the rectal mucosa. This was a transient but normal finding in this child.

which can be confused with tears or fissures of the anal verge, was seen in almost 50% of postmortem examinations[89] (Figure 13.21). Debate continues as to the types and frequency of anal findings attributable to chronic constipation. Table 13.2 summarizes studies on the frequency of anal dilation, fissures, and tags in non-abused children, abused children, and children referred to specialists for constipation.[85,86,66,73,90]

Masturbation and use of tampons are often cited in the courtroom as causes of genital trauma. Tampons do not usually traumatize the hymen.[50,91] Some authors state that tampon use may increase the distensibility of the hymen from slight stretching,[92] but Stewart[93] found no differences in the genital examinations of girls who did or did not use tampons. In another study of adolescents screened for sexual activity, posterior hymenal clefts were documented in 2 girls who denied sexual activity but reported painful tampon insertion.[78]

Because children with mental retardation or developmental delay are at higher risk of child abuse, their caretakers are understandably alert to potential signs of abuse. However, these children also may have congenital abnormalities or behaviors that are easily confused with signs and symptoms of abuse. For example, multiple perianal nodules are seen in infants with systemic hyalinosis,[94] the labia majora are absent in Escobar syndrome, and vaginal strictures are seen in dyskeratosis congenital syndrome.[95] Clinicians evaluating children with congenital anomalies for possible sexual abuse may need to consult references describing the many syndromes associated with anogenital anomalies.[95]

Case Example

A physician was summoned by a nurse practitioner who was performing a well-child examination on a healthy infant. As the baby's legs were lifted, an alarming degree of dilation of the external anal sphincter was observed. As the clinician puzzled over how to interpret this finding, the internal sphincter opened, and the baby passed a large stool. The anal examination was subsequently normal.

Vaginal/Genital Discharge

Many children present to medical facilities with a chief complaint of vaginal discharge. The concern

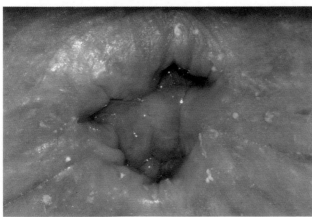

FIGURE 13.21
Exposed Pectinate line which is sometimes confused with anal lacerations.

for sexual abuse usually arises from the perception that it is abnormal for prepubertal girls to have a discharge, or "an odor," and that such findings may indicate a sexually transmitted infection (STI). The discharge may have been observed directly on the child's genitals or as a stain on the underpants. Causes for vaginal discharge include the accumulation of smegma between the labia majora and minora, hormone-related changes (leukorrhea), retained foreign bodies, and infectious causes, including both sexually and non–sexually transmitted pathogens. In cases of significant genital trauma, a discharge may result from granulation tissue and serous secretions.

Most vaginitis in children is not caused by STIs. Jenny[96] reviewed 22 non-venereal causes of vulvovaginitis in children. *Shigella* vaginitis has been confused with gonorrhea and also with

discharge resulting from a vaginal foreign body. Among 32 girls with *Shigella* vaginitis in one report, 8 were suspected of having gonorrhea, and 6 had been treated erroneously for gonorrhea. Foreign body was considered in 22 girls, pelvic radiographs were obtained in 13, and 3 were examined under anesthesia (Figure 13.22). Vaginal discharge from *Shigella* is often bloody but can also be watery, purulent, and any color from white to green (Figure 13.23). Diarrhea is not a common associated finding.[97]

Sexually Transmitted Infections

Most STIs can be transmitted in nonsexual ways; the child's history is important in determining the likelihood of sexual or nonsexual transmission. Diseases that may result in vaginal or urethral discharge through sexual contact

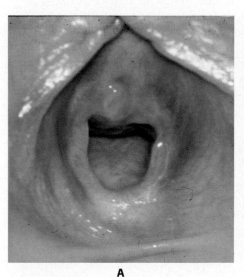

A

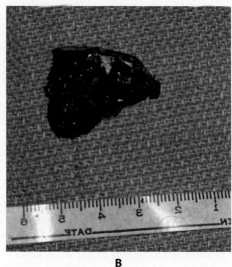

B

FIGURE 13.22
This child was seen for a vaginal discharge and treated with antibiotics. After the discharge recurred, a foreign body **(B)** was removed from her vagina under anesthesia.

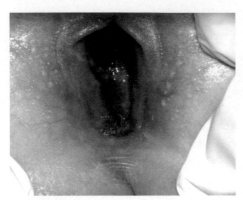

FIGURE 13.23
Shigella vaginitis causing bleeding.

include gonorrhea, *Chlamydia,* and *Trichomonas.* Children and adolescents who are infected with an STI but who are without a history of sexual abuse or contact require careful assessment of the diagnostic test used and possible nonsexual modes of transmission. When there are no other indicators of sexual abuse or activity, the diagnostic test used should be the gold standard, or the most specific test, so that the probability of false-positives is minimized. Clinicians should also ensure that a second confirmatory test is done whenever feasible.

A positive culture for *Neisseria gonorrhoeae* should be verified by at least 2 confirmatory tests. Whittington et al[98] wrote that 14 of 40 specimens submitted to the Centers for Disease Control and Prevention for confirmation as *N gonorrhoeae* had been misidentified by the referring laboratory. These mistakes resulted in initiation of sexual abuse investigations in 8 cases and referral of 14 additional children for unnecessary examination or treatment. The organisms were correctly identified as

Branhamella catarrhalis, Kingella denitrificans, and 3 species of nonpathogenic *Neisseria* commonly found in the eye, pharynx, and rectum. DNA probes are also sometimes used to confirm *N gonorrhoeae* recovered from culture techniques.

Currently the gold standard test for *Chlamydia trachomatis* is cell culture; in a child without a history or other findings of sexual abuse, a *Chlamydia* infection should be confirmed by culture. Other diagnostic tests, such as nucleic acid amplification tests, are significantly more sensitive than, and as specific as, culture,[99] but are not yet acceptable as diagnostic tests in children without other signs of sexual contact or abuse. In adolescents and adults with a history of abusive or consensual sexual contact, nucleic acid amplification tests are generally preferred to culture for diagnostic purposes. Among prepubertal children with credible sexual abuse histories, nucleic acid amplification tests may be used for initial identification and treatment purposes, and a second nucleic acid amplification test targeted to a different genome may serve to confirm the diagnosis of gonorrhea or *Chlamydia* infection. Culture is the only approved test for oral and rectal samples. Persistent carriage of perinatally acquired *Chlamydia* has been documented for more than 1 year in the infant vagina and rectum and for more than 2 years in the eye and pharynx.[96]

Trichomonas vaginalis may be identified by wet mount examination, rapid immunochromatographic testing, or culture. Wet mount examination of spun urine may reveal *Pentatrichomonas*

hominis, which colonizes the gastrointestinal tract and is not sexually transmitted; this organism is difficult to differentiate from *Trichomonas,* which differs only in the number of flagellum (5 and 3, respectively).

The most common pathogen found in bacterial vaginosis is *Gardnerella vaginalis. Gardnerella* has been found to be as common in non-abused prepubertal girls as in abused prepubertal girls, so is not considered to be specific for sexual transmission or contact.[100]

Non–Sexually Transmitted Infections

Non–sexually transmitted pathogens such as respiratory and gastrointestinal organisms may produce genital or vaginal discharge through contiguous spread or by autoinoculation with infective secretions, typically by manual transfer. Pinworms can traverse from anus to vagina and produce discharge. *Candida* vaginitis may occur after antibiotic therapy or in association with other medical conditions. Culture or wet mount examination will help distinguish between pathogens and STIs. Sometimes a culture will yield "usual genital flora," which consists of one or more of the following organisms: *Lactobacillus* species, alpha streptococci, gamma streptococci, diphtheroids, and *Neisseria* species other than gonorrhea.[6]

Autoinoculation by contaminated nasopharyngeal secretions via manual transfer is the postulated mode of infection in most cases of GABHS anogenital infection.[101] Identical streptococcal types have been isolated from pharyngeal and anogenital sites when both were infected.[70,102] While there is a possibility of transmission during oral sodomy by a perpetrator with GABHS pharyngitis, sexual transmission cannot be reliably determined or differentiated from nonsexual transmission.[68,103] In addition, impetigo can be transmitted to the anogenital areas through nonsexual means (Figure 13.24).

Streptococcal vaginitis causes erythema of the mucosal tissues and many types of discharge: thin, thick, serous, blood tinged, creamy, white, yellow, or green. The introitus and vaginal mucosa may be fiery red, edematous, and tender[104,105] (Figures 13.25 and 13.26). A study in 1948 of vaginal cultures from 286 children from infancy to 14 years found that 13% grew hemolytic strains of streptococci (primarily group A), and 12% grew gonococci. Streptococcal vaginitis was sometimes associated with fever, pharyngitis, or scarlet fever.[102]

Patients with streptococcal balanitis can present with urethral discharge and/or erythema and swelling of the foreskin. The discharge may be thin and serous or thick and purulent. Sexual abuse was suspected in a 6-year-old boy who presented with symptoms due to streptococcal balanitis.[101]

Vesicles or Ulcers

Genital ulceration has a variety of causes, only some of which are related to sexual contact. Adler[106] categorizes genital ulcers by whether the ulcers are multiple or solitary, and painful or painless (Table 13.3). Multiple painful ulcers are usually associated with herpes

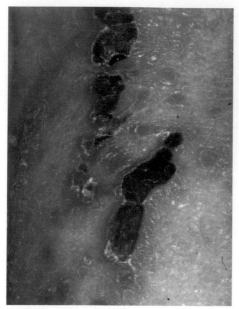

FIGURE 13.24
Genital impetigo.

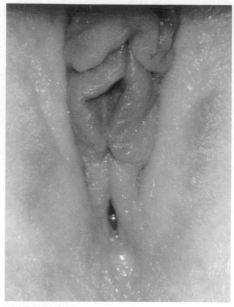

FIGURE 13.25
This child with streptococcal vaginitis had significant genital irriation and bleeding.

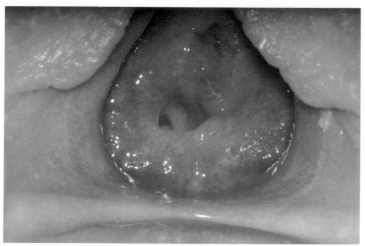

FIGURE 13.26
Same child as in Figure 13.26. Intense hymenal erythema and bleeding led to a culture diagnosis of group A beta-hemolytic streptococcal infection.

TABLE 13.3
Conditions Causing Genital Ulcers[a]

Multiple	Solitary
Painful	
Herpes simplex (type 1 or 2)	Tuberculosis
Herpes zoster	Trauma
Behçet syndrome	Ulcerated hemangioma
Haemophilus ducreyi (chancroid)	
Yaws	
Stevens-Johnson syndrome	
Drug eruption	
Erythema multiforme	
Impetigo	
Folliculitis	
Furuncle[b] ←――――――――――――――→	
Scabies (secondary infection)	
Candida	
Vincent organism	
Jacquet erosive diaper dermatitis	
Granuloma gluteale infantum	
Balanitis/vulvitis	
Painless	
Secondary syphilis	Crohn disease[c]
	Carcinoma[c]
	Lymphogranuloma venereum[c]
←――――――――――――――→	Primary syphilis[b]
	Tertiary syphilis (gamma)
	Tertiary syphilis (gamma)
	Reiter disease
←――――――――――――――→	Granuloma inguinale[b]
←――――――――――――――→	Leukoplakia[b]
←――――――――――――――→	Lichen sclerosus[b]
←――――――――――――――→	Carcinoma[b]
	(Trauma)

[a]Adapted with permission from Adler MW. ABC of sexually transmitted diseases. Genital ulceration. *Br Med J (Clin Res Ed).* 1983;287:1780.

[b]May be multiple or solitary lesions.

[c]May be painless or painful lesions.

simplex. Herpes infection that is manifested during the perinatal period may have been acquired at birth. Both types 1 and 2 can be transmitted through sexual abuse or contact, but type 1 infection can be transmitted in nonsexual ways such as autoinoculation from oral lesions or from herpetic lesions on a caretaker's hand to the genitals of a child via diapering.[107,108] Varicella manifesting on the vulva can cause confusion with genital herpes. Tzanck smears do not distinguish herpes varicella from herpes zoster[68,96,109]; the most accurate and reliable test is the herpes culture. Herpes zoster rarely occurs in the genital area. Group A beta-hemolytic streptococci vulvitis or proctitis can present as painful vesicles or ulcers; whenever herpes is suspected, a routine culture should also be submitted to differentiate herpes from GABHS (Figure 13.24).

Primary syphilis produces painless genital ulceration. Because serological tests for syphilis are not always positive when the ulcers of primary syphilis manifest, negative serological tests should be repeated in 3 or 4 weeks if syphilis is suspected. A positive non-treponemal test for syphilis (rapid plasma reagin [RPR] or Venereal Disease Research Laboratories) should be confirmed by a treponemal test (fluorescent treponemal antibody). Some laboratories conduct an enzyme-linked immunosorbent assay test for syphilis first, followed by an RPR to differentiate past treated disease from active or inadequately treated disease. Other causes of painless genital ulcers include lichen sclerosus, Crohn disease, lymphogranuloma venereum, and granuloma inguinale.

Clinicians treating patients from tropical countries should be aware that yaws may be confused with syphilis. Endemic to tropical areas, yaws is caused by *Treponema pallidum pertenue*, a microorganism that cannot be distinguished serologically or microscopically from *Treponema pallidum pallidum*, the organism causing syphilis, and is also treated with intramuscular penicillin. Yaws is transmitted by skin-to-skin contact, with early lesions occurring in extragenital sites, most often the lower limbs. The genital lesions of yaws have been confused with venereal syphilis.

Reiter disease and Behçet syndrome are multisystem diseases that rarely afflict prepubertal children. Both are characterized by painful oral and genital ulcers, arthritis, and ocular inflammation. Conjunctivitis is seen in Reiter disease. Because Reiter disease can follow both STIs such as *Chlamydia*, and non–STI infection such as *Shigella*, clinicians should be aware of the possibility of sexual abuse.[110,111] Pediatric Behçet syndrome is more common in the preadolescent and adolescent age groups and may also produce erythema nodosum; ocular disease may progress to glaucoma and cataracts.[110] Other diseases producing multiple painful geni-tal ulcers or debrided areas include Stevens-Johnson syndrome, erythema multiforme, folliculitis, impetigo, drug eruptions, and *Candida*.[106]

Ulcerations from Jacquet erosive diaper dermatitis are now rare because of the availability of good-quality cloth and disposable diapers. The disease is characterized by small, centrally ulcerated erythematous nodules on the concave surfaces in the diaper area (Figure 13.27). Hara et al[112] reported a case in an 8-year-old girl with urinary incontinence because of ectopic ureters; she used toilet paper as an absorptive replacement for diapers. Granuloma gluteale infantum manifests with relatively large, firm nodules on the convex portion of the diaper area. It may be related to use of topical steroids.[112]

Oral ulcers and mucosal lesions can be caused by accidental trauma, infectious agents such as herpes and coxsackievirus, or oral sodomy. A South African study of 660 boys in reform schools, ages 14 to 22 years, found 19 boys with palatal lesions thought to be related to oral fellatio. The lesions were single or multiple red atrophic patches on the central posterior palate. Seven boys were missing the front incisors, probably to facilitate oral sex. No lesions were seen in 600 control subjects from state schools.[113]

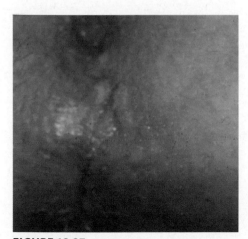

FIGURE 13.27
Jacquet diaper dermatitis, a nodular or ulceronodular condition caused by irritation with urine and feces. Sometimes it is called pseudo-overrucous papules and nodules.

Case Examples

An 8-year-old girl presented with a 16-month history of painless, nonpruritic vulvar erythema and edema. She had been examined by several physicians and treated unsuccessfully for contact dermatitis and candidiasis. An extensive evaluation for sexual abuse was unrevealing. Her perianal examination was reportedly normal. One month before admission, she developed bloody purulent perianal discharge. A 3.6-kg weight loss was associated with decreased oral intake because of fear of stimulating painful defecation. She had no growth retardation or other systemic symptoms. Examination under anesthesia revealed a non-tender red, firm, edematous vulva; a firm edematous clitoris; friable vaginal mucosa; and 5 fistulous openings in the perianal area. Cultures of the vagina and peri-rectum revealed no pathogens. Biopsies of the colon, rectum, and vulva showed many non-caseating granulomas and other features of Crohn disease. Treatment with parenteral alimentation, prednisone, and metronidazole resulted in resolution of the vulvar and perianal abnormalities.[114]

A 3.5-year-old Indonesian boy presented with a 3-month history of ulcerated, crusted papillomatous lesions on the chin, neck, extremities, and prepuce of the penis. Dark-field examination of exudate from the skin lesions revealed many treponemes. He was diagnosed with yaws. His 8-year-old brother and his mother also had yaws.[115]

Papules/Nodules

Anogenital papules and nodules may occur from infectious, irritative, or accidental causes. The most common anogenital papule or growth that results in concerns for sexual abuse is venereal warts. *Venereal* refers only to the location of the verrucous lesion and not to the mode of transmission. Anogenital warts in children may be transmitted sexually, vertically from mother to child through birth, hematogenously from mother to fetus,[116] and through postnatal nonsexual contact. Evidence of autoinoculation of hand warts to the anal area has been provided by DNA typing.[117,118] Transmission within families also seems possible when bathwater, towels, bathing suits, or underwear is shared.[117,119,120] In a study[121] of 76 families consisting of a mother, father, and infant, several oral and genital swabs were analyzed from all members of the family; the sampling interval was from the prenatal period up to the infant's age of 24 months. Samples were submitted for polymerase chain reaction, followed by subtyping. In only 2.6% of the families were all members negative during the entire sample period; the study did not indicate how many of the family members with human papillomavirus (HPV) had clinical disease. In this study, the infant's risk of acquiring genital HPV correlated with the mother's oral HPV positivity 6 months after the infant's birth. This study raised numerous questions regarding the modes of transmission for HPV. As the incidence of HPV infection in adults has increased, a parallel increase has occurred among children and may be attributable to perinatal transmission.[117]

Infection before birth, presumably bloodborne, also has occurred.[122]

In one study of anogenital warts in children aged 10 months to 12 years, the etiology was reported to be unknown in 42%, vertical transmission in 42%, sexual abuse in 10%, and autoinoculation in 5%. How the authors placed patients in these categories is not clear, however, other than by examining the child and other family members for warts and by culturing for other STIs. No HPV typing was done.[123]

Other authors have reported incidences of sexual abuse in children with anogenital warts of 10%,[117] 27%,[124] 50%,[125] and 91%.[126] Higher incidence is found when the evaluation includes a family investigation and interviews of the children. Nonsexual transmission is more likely when HPV is present in children younger than 4 years; sexual transmission is more likely in older children.[127] Condylomata acuminata, caused by HPV, have been confused with condylomata lata, caused by syphilis.[128–130] Perianal lesions of eosinophilic granuloma were mistaken for condylomata lata in a 2-year-old boy[131] (Figure 13.28). A test for syphilis should be considered in children with atypical anogenital growths. Benign papillomatosis is a common finding in the fossa navicularis in adolescents and can be confused with HPV lesions (Figure 13.29). Molluscum contagiosum, flesh-colored raised papules, sometimes associated with umbilicated centers, may be seen on the buttocks, thighs, or genitals; this infection is usually not sexually transmitted in children (Figure 13.30).

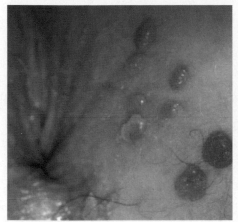

FIGURE 13.28
Other conditions such as eosinophilic granuloma have been reported to be confused with genital warts. This image demonstrates perianal genital warts caused by human papillomavirus.

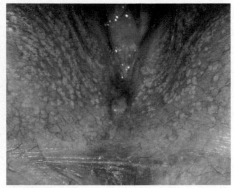

FIGURE 13.29
Benign papillomatosis of the fossa navicularis of an adolescent.

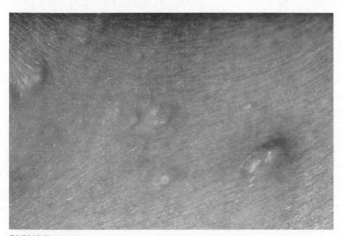

FIGURE 13.30
Molluscum contagiosum. Typical pearly papules with a central umbilication. Molluscum contagiosum is not considered to be sexually transmitted in young children.

Shaving the pubic hair is a trend noted with increasing frequency among adolescent females and males in the United States. This practice sometimes results in folliculitis, abscesses, and ingrown hairs, presenting as flesh-colored papules or pustules. These lesions are sometimes confused with herpes or molluscum contagiosum. While molluscum and folliculitis are restricted to the vulva, inguinal, and perineal areas, herpes may involve the vestibule and other glabrous surfaces. Strangulation of the penis or clitoris by hair or fibers usually occurs accidentally.[132–136] Careful inquiry should be made, however, as tourniquet injuries of the genitalia and digits have occurred as a result of physical or sexual abuse.[137,138] One 6-year-old boy with apparent paraphimosis began voiding through a fistula on the undersurface of the penis at the coronal sulcus. Under general anesthesia, a fine nylon thread was found encircling the penis, tied in a knot that was buried by the healed skin on the dorsal surface.[139]

Conclusion

As parents become better educated about the risks of sexual abuse, they are seeking consultation, education, and reassurance from their health care providers when their children have anogenital symptoms. Clinicians should be aware that the presenting symptoms may not correlate with the examination findings (eg, a "vaginal laceration" may in fact be vulvar excoriation from candidiasis). If the child is preverbal, or verbal and has not disclosed sexual abuse, a careful and comprehensive evaluation should include considering conditions confused with abuse in addition to injuries and infections specific to sexual abuse. A mistaken diagnosis of sexual abuse can be traumatic to all concerned. Consultation with specialists in gynecology, dermatology, surgery, urology, genetics, pathology, infectious diseases, or child abuse may be prudent when the diagnosis is in doubt.

References

1. Adams JA, Knudson S. Genital findings in adolescent girls referred for suspected sexual abuse. *Arch Pediatr Adolesc Med.* 1996;150:850–857

2. Berenson AB, Chacko MR, Wiemann CM, Mishaw CO, Friedrich WN, Grady JJ. A case-control study of anatomic changes resulting from sexual abuse. *Am J Obstet Gynecol.* 2000;182:820–831; discussion 831–834

3. Heger A, Ticson L, Velasquez O, Bernier R. Children referred for possible sexual abuse: medical findings in 2384 children. *Child Abuse Negl.* 2002;26:645–659

4. Heger AH, Ticson L, Guerra L, et al. Appearance of the genitalia in girls selected for nonabuse: review of hymenal morphology and nonspecific findings. *J Pediatr Adolesc Gynecol.* 2002;15:27–35

5. Kellogg ND, Menard SW, Santos A. Genital anatomy in pregnant adolescents: "normal" does not mean "nothing happened." *Pediatrics.* 2004;113:e67–e69

6. Kellogg ND, Parra JM, Menard S. Children with anogenital symptoms and signs referred for sexual abuse evaluations. *Arch Pediatr Adolesc Med.* 1998;152:634–641

7. McCann J, Wells R, Simon M, Voris J. Genital findings in prepubertal girls selected for nonabuse: a descriptive study. *Pediatrics.* 1990;86:428–439

8. Klevan JL, De Jong AR. Urinary tract symptoms and urinary tract infection following sexual abuse. *Am J Dis Child.* 1990;144:242–244

9. Clark AF, Tayler PJ, Bhatc SR. Nocturnal fecal soiling and anal masturbation. *Arch Dis Child.* 1990;65:1367–1368

10. Friedrich WN, Fisher JL, Dittner CA, et al. Child sexual behavior inventory: normative, psychiatric, and sexual abuse comparisons. *Child Maltreat.* 2001;6:37–49

11. Friedrich WN, Fisher J, Broughton D, Houston M, Shafran CR. Normative sexual behavior in children. *Pediatrics.* 1991;88:456–464

12. Cobbs LW. A paranoid accusation of child molestation. *Hosp Pract (Off Ed)*. 1982;17:76A–B, 76F, 76H

13. Goodwin J, Sahd D, Rada RT. Incest hoax: false accusations, false denials. *Bull Am Acad Psychiatry Law*. 1978;6:269–276

14. Herman-Giddens ME, Berson NL. Harmful genital care practices in children. A type of child abuse. *JAMA*. 1989;261:577–579

15. Jones DPH, McGraw JM. Reliable and fictitious accounts of sexual abuse to children. *J Interpers Violence*. 1987;2:27–43

16. Gardner JJ. Descriptive study of genital variation in healthy, nonabused premenarchal girls. *J Pediatr*. 1992;120:251–257

17. Baker RB. Anal fissure produced by examination for sexual abuse. *Am J Dis Child*. 1991;145:848–849

18. Hobbs CJ, Wynne JM. Child sexual abuse—an increasing rate of diagnosis. *Lancet*. 1987;2:837–841

19. Kohr RM. Elevator surfing: a deadly new form of joyriding. *J Forensic Sci*. 1992;37:640–645

20. Paul DM. The medical examination in sexual offences against children. *Med Sci Law*. 1977;17:251–258

21. West R, Davies A, Fenton T. Accidental vulval injuries in childhood. *BMJ*. 1989;298:1002–1003

22. Finkel MA. Anogenital trauma in sexually abused children. *Pediatrics*. 1989;84:317–322

23. Bond GR, Dowd MD, Landsman I, Rimsza M. Unintentional perineal injury in prepubescent girls: a multicenter, prospective report of 56 girls. *Pediatrics*. 1995;95:628–631

24. Unuigbe JA, Giwa-Osagie AW. Pediatric and adolescent gynecological disorders in Benin City, Nigeria. *Adolesc Pediatric Gynecol*. 1988;1:257–261

25. Black CT, Pokorny WJ, McGill CW, Harberg FJ. Ano-rectal trauma in children. *J Pediatr Surg*. 1982;17:501–504

26. Jona JZ. Accidental anorectal impalement in children. *Pediatr Emerg Care*. 1997;13:40–43

27. Press S, Grant P, Thompson VT, Milles KL. Small bowel evisceration: unusual manifestation of child abuse. *Pediatrics*. 1991;88:807–809

28. Baker RB. Seat belt injury masquerading as sexual abuse. *Pediatrics*. 1986;77:435

29. Wynne JM. Injuries to the genitalia in female children. *S Afr Med J*. 1980;57:47–50

30. Kunkel NC. Vaginal injury from a water slide in a premenarcheal patient. *Pediatr Emerg Care*. 1998;14:210–211

31. Kadish HA, Schunk JE, Britton H. Pediatric male rectal and genital trauma: accidental and nonaccidental injuries. *Pediatr Emerg Care*. 1998;14:95–98

32. Christensen EH, Oster J. Adhesions of labia minora (synechia vulvae) in childhood. A review and report of fourteen cases. *Acta Paediatr Scand*. 1971;60:709–715

33. Berkowitz CD, Elvik SL, Logan MK. Labial fusion in prepubescent girls: a marker for sexual abuse? *Am J Obstet Gynecol*. 1987;156:16–20

34. DeMarco BJ, Crandal RS, Hreshchyshyn MM. Labial agglutination secondary to a herpes simplex II infection. *Am J Obstet Gynecol*. 1987;157:296–297

35. Berenson AB, Chacko MR, Wiemann CM, Mishaw CO, Friedrich WN, Grady JJ. A case-control study of anatomic changes resulting from sexual abuse. *Am J Obstet Gynecol*. 2000;182:820–31; discussion 820–834

36. Jerkins GR, Verheeck K, Noe HN. Treatment of girls with urethral prolapse. *J Urol*. 1984;132:732–733

37. Johnson CF. Prolapse of the urethra: confusion of clinical and anatomic characteristics with sexual abuse. *Pediatrics*. 1991;87:722–725

38. Williams TS, Callen JP, Owen LG. Vulvar disorders in the prepubertal female. *Pediatr Ann*. 1986;15:588–589, 592–601, 604–605

39. Lowe FC, Hill GS, Jeffs RD, Brendler CB. Urethral prolapse in children: insights into etiology and management. *J Urol*. 1986;135:100–103

40. French G, Johnson CF. Genital bleeding: two uncommon causes in patients referred to a sexual abuse clinic. *Clin Pediatr.* 1994;33:38–41

41. Hostetler BR, Jones CE, Muram D. Capillary hemangiomas of the vulva mistaken for sexual abuse. *Adolesc Pediatr Gynecol.* 1994;7:44–46

42. Bays J, Jenny C. Genital and anal conditions confused with child sexual abuse trauma. *Am J Dis Child.* 1990;144:1319–1322

43. Levin AV, Selbst SM. Vulvar hemangioma simulating child abuse. *Clin Pediatr (Phila).* 1988;27:213–215

44. Jones LW, Bass DH. Perineal injuries in children. *Br J Surg.* 1991;78:1105–1107

45. Muram D. Genital tract injuries in the prepubertal child. *Pediatr Ann.* 1986;15:616–620

46. West R, Davies A, Fenton T. Accidental vulval injuries in childhood. *BMJ.* 1989;298:1002–1003

47. Gearhart JP, Lowe FC. Genitourinary injuries secondary to break dancing in children and adolescents. *Pediatrics.* 1986;77:922–924

48. Hobbs CJ, Wynne JM. Child sexual abuse—an increasing rate of diagnosis. *Lancet.* 1987;2:837–884

49. Huffman JW, Dewhurst CJ, Capraro VJ. *The Gynecology of Childhood and Adolescence.* 2nd ed. Philadelphia, PA: WB Saunders; 1981

50. Woodling BA, Kossoris PD. Sexual misuse: rape, molestation, and incest. *Pediatr Clin North Am.* 1981;28:481–499

51. Hyman SL, Fisher W, Mercugliano M, Cataldo MF. Children with self-injurious behavior. *Pediatrics.* 1990;85:437–441

52. Dowd MD, Fitzmaurice L, Knapp JF, Mooney D. The interpretation of urogenital findings in children with straddle injuries. *J Pediatr Surg.* 1994;29:7–10

53. Jones LW, Bass DH. Perineal injuries in children. *Br J Surg.* 1991;78:1105–1107

54. Cain WS, Howell CG, Ziegler MM, Finley AJ, Asch MJ, Grant JP. Rectosigmoid perforation and intestinal evisceration from transanal suction. *J Pediatr Surg.* 1983;18:10–13

55. From the Centers for Disease Control. Suction-drain injury in a public wading pool—North Carolina, 1991. *JAMA.* 1992;267:2868

56. Chamberlain RS, Greenberg LW. Scrotal involvement in Henoch-Schönlein purpura: a case report and review of the literature. *Pediatr Emerg Care.* 1992;8:213–215

57. Chalmers RJ, Burton PA, Bennett RF, Goring CC, Smith PJ. Lichen sclerosus et atrophicus. A common and distinctive cause of phimosis in boys. *Arch Dermatol.* 1984;120:1025–1027

58. Berth-Jones J, Graham-Brown RA, Burns DA. Lichen sclerosus. *Arch Dis Child.* 1989;64:1204–1206

59. Handfield-Jones SE, Hinde FR, Kennedy CT. Lichen sclerosus et atrophicus in children misdiagnosed as sexual abuse. *Br Med J (Clin Res Ed).* 1987;294:1404–1405

60. Harrington CI. Lichen sclerosus. *Arch Dis Child.* 1990;65:335

61. Helm KF, Gibson LE, Muller SA. Lichen sclerosus et atrophicus in children and young adults. *Pediatr Dermatol.* 1991;8:97–101

62. Jenny C, Kirby P, Fuquay D. Genital lichen sclerosus mistaken for child sexual abuse. *Pediatrics.* 1989;83:597–599

63. Priestly BL, Bleehen SS. Lichen sclerosus et atrophicus in children misdiagnosed as sexual abuse. *Br Med J (Clin Res Ed).* 1987;295:211

64. Warrington SA, de San Lazaro C. Lichen sclerosus et atrophicus and sexual abuse. *Arch Dis Child.* 1996;75:512–516

65. Leiferman KM, Gleich GJ. The case of the blue boy. *Pediatr Dermatol.* 1991;8:354

66. Hobbs CJ, Wynne JM. Sexual abuse of English boys and girls: the importance of anal examination. *Child Abuse Negl.* 1989;13:195–210

67. Zempsky WT, Rosenstein BJ. The cause of rectal prolapse in children. *Am J Dis Child.* 1988;142:338–339

68. Herman-Giddens ME, Berson NL. Dermatologic conditions misdiagnosed as evidence of child abuse. *JAMA.* 1989;261:3547–3548

69. Fisher AA. Nonoccupational dermatitis to "black" rubber mix: part II. *Cutis.* 1992;49:229–230

70. Kokx NP, Comstock JA, Facklam RR. Streptococcal perianal disease in children. *Pediatrics.* 1987;80:659–663

71. Krol AL. Perianal streptococcal dermatitis. *Pediatr Dermatol.* 1990;7:97–100

72. Smith GA, Sharma V, Knapp JF, Shields BJ. The summer penile syndrome: seasonal acute hypersensitivity reaction caused by chigger bites on the penis. *Pediatr Emerg Care.* 1998;14:116–118

73. McCann J, Voris J, Simon M, et al. Perianal finding in prepubertal children selected for non-abuse: a descriptive study. *Child Abuse Negl.* 1989;13:179–193

74. Hey F, Buchan PC, Littlewood JM, Hall RI. Differential diagnosis in child sexual abuse. *Lancet.* 1987;1:283

75. Vickers D, Morris K, Coulthard MG, Eastham EJ. Anal signs in haemolytic uraemic syndrome. *Lancet.* 1988;1:998

76. Berenson A, Heger A, Andrews S. Appearance of the hymen in newborns. *Pediatrics.* 1991;87:458–465

77. Kerns DL, Ritter ML, Thomas RG. Concave hymenal variations in suspected child sexual abuse victims. *Pediatrics.* 1992;90:265–272

78. Adams JA, Botash AS, Kellogg N. Differences in hymenal morphology between adolescent girls with and without a history of consensual sexual contact. *Arch Pediatr Adolesc Med.* 2004;158:280–285

79. Berenson AB, Chacko MR, Wiemann CM, Mishaw CO, Friedrich WN, Grady JJ. Use of hymenal measurements in the diagnosis of previous penetration. *Pediatrics.* 2002;109:228–235

80. Kellogg ND, Parra JM. Linea vestibularis: a previously undescribed normal genital structure in female neonates. *Pediatrics.* 1991;87:926–929

81. Adams JA, Horton M. Is it sexual abuse? Confusion caused by a congenital anomaly of the genitalia. *Clin Pediatr (Phila).* 1989;28:146–148

82. Fukunaga K, Kimura K, Lawrence JP, et al. Anteriorly located anus: is constipation caused by abnormal location of the anus? *J Pediatr Surg.* 1996;31:245–246

83. Bays J, Chadwick D. Medical diagnosis of the sexually abused child. *Child Abuse Negl.* 1993;17:91–110

84. Kirschner RH, Stein RJ. The mistaken diagnosis of child abuse. A form of medical abuse? *Am J Dis Child.* 1985;139:873–875

85. Agnarsson U, Warde C, McCarthy G, Evans N. Perianal appearances associated with constipation. *Arch Dis Child.* 1990;65:1231–1234

86. Clayden GS. Reflex anal dilatation associated with severe chronic constipation in children. *Arch Dis Child.* 1988;63:832–836

87. Reardon W, Hughes HE, Green SH, Lloyd Woolley V, Harper PS. Anal abnormalities in childhood myotonic dystrophy—a possible source of confusion in child sexual abuse. *Arch Dis Child.* 1992;67:527–528

88. Suarez L, Belanger-Quintana A, Escobar H, et al. Suspected sexual abuse: an unusual presentation form of congenital myotonic dystrophy. *Eur J Pediatr.* 2000;159:539–541

89. McCann J, Reay D, Siebert J, Stephens BG, Wirtz S. Postmortem perianal findings in children. *Am J Forensic Med Pathol.* 1996;17:289–298

90. Stanton A, Sunderland R. Prevalence of reflex anal dilatation in 200 children. *BMJ.* 1989;298:802–803

91. Dickenson RL. Tampons as menstrual guards. *JAMA.* 1945;128:490–494

92. Cowell CA. The gynecologic examination of infants, children, and young adolescents. *Pediatr Clin North Am.* 1981;28:247–266

93. Stewart D. Tampon use and physical findings in sexually abused adolescents. Paper presented at: Fourth Annual Meeting of the North American Society for Pediatric and Adolescent Gynecology; 1990; Costa Mesa, CA

94. Glover MT, Lake BD, Atherton DJ. Infantile systemic hyalinosis: newly recognized disorder of collagen? *Pediatrics.* 1991;87:228–234

95. Jones KL. *Smith's Recognizable Patterns of Human Malformation.* 4th ed. Philadelphia, PA: WB Saunders; 1988

96. Jenny C. Sexually transmitted diseases and child abuse. *Pediatr Ann.* 1992;21:497–503

97. Murphy TV, Nelson JD. *Shigella* vaginitis: report of 38 patients and review of the literature. *Pediatrics.* 1979;63:511–516

98. Whittington WL, Rice RJ, Biddle JW, Knapp JS. Incorrect identification of *Neisseria gonorrhoeae* from infants and children. *Pediatr Infect Dis J.* 1988;7:3–10

99. Kellogg ND, Baillargeon J, Lukefahr J, Lawless K, Menard S. Comparison of nucleic acid amplification tests and culture techniques in the detection of *Neisseria gonorrhoeae* and *Chlamydia trachomatis* in victims of suspected child sexual abuse. *J Pediatr Adolesc Gynecol.* 2004;17:331–339

100. Bartley DL, Morgan L, Rimsza ME. *Gardnerella vaginalis* in prepubertal girls. *Am J Dis Child.* 1987;141:1014–1017

101. Kyriazi NC, Costenbader CL. Group A beta-hemolytic streptococcal balanitis: it may be more common than you think. *Pediatrics.* 1991;88:154–155

102. Boisvert PL, Walcher DN. Hemolytic streptococcal vaginitis in children. *Pediatrics.* 1948;2:24–29

103. Palmer WM. Streptococcal vaginitis and sexual abuse. *Pediatr Infect Dis J.* 1982;1:374–375

104. Ginsberg CM. Group A streptococcal vaginitis in children. *Pediatr Infect Dis J.* 1982;1:36–37

105. O'Connor PA, Oliver WJ. Group A beta-hemolytic streptococcal vulvovaginitis: a recurring problem. *Pediatr Emerg Care.* 1985;1:94–95

106. Adler MW. ABC of sexually transmitted diseases. Genital ulceration. *Br Med J (Clin Res Ed).* 1983;287:1780–1781

107. Kaplan KM, Fleisher GR, Paradise JE, Friedman HN. Social relevance of genital herpes simplex in children. *Am J Dis Child.* 1984;138:872–874

108. Nahmias AJ, Dowdle WR, Naib ZM, Josey WE, Luce CF. Genital infection with herpesvirus hominis types 1 and 2 in children. *Pediatrics.* 1968;42:659–666

109. Boyd M, Jordan SW. Unusual presentation of varicella suggestive of sexual abuse. *Am J Dis Child.* 1987;141:940

110. Eldem B, Onur C, Ozen S. Clinical features of pediatric Behçet's disease. *J Pediatr Ophthalmol Strabismus.* 1998;35:159–161

111. Zivony D, Nocton J, Wortmann D, Esterly N. Juvenile Reiter's syndrome: a report of four cases. *J Am Acad Dermatol.* 1998;38:32–37

112. Hara M, Watanabe M, Tagami H. Jacquet erosive diaper dermatitis in a young girl with urinary incontinence. *Pediatr Dermatol.* 1991;8:160–161

113. van Wyk CW. The oral lesion caused by fellatio. *Am J Forensic Med Pathol.* 1981;2:217–219

114. Lally MR, Orenstein SR, Cohen BA. Crohn's disease of the vulva in an 8-year-old girl. *Pediatr Dermatol.* 1988;5:103–106

115. Engelkens HJ, Judanarso J, van der Sluis JJ, van der Stek J, Stolz E. Disseminated early yaws: report of a child with a remarkable genital lesion mimicking venereal syphilis. *Pediatr Dermatol.* 1990;7:60–62

116. Smith EM, Ritchie JM, Yankowitz J, et al. Human papillomavirus prevalence and types in newborns and parents: concordance and modes of transmission. *Sex Transm Dis.* 2004;31:57–62

117. Cohen BA, Honig P, Androphy E. Anogenital warts in children. Clinical and virologic evaluation for sexual abuse. *Arch Dermatol.* 1990;126:1575–1580

118. Fleming KA, Venning V, Evans M. DNA typing of genital warts and diagnosis of sexual abuse of children. *Lancet.* 1987;2:454

119. Bergeron C, Ferenczy A, Richart R. Underwear: contamination by human papillomaviruses. *Am J Obstet Gynecol.* 1990;162:25–29

120. Pacheco B, Paola G, Ribas J, Vighi S, Rueda N. Vulvar infection caused by human papillomavirus in children and adolescents without sexual contact. *Adolesc Pediatr Gynecol.* 1991;4:136–142

121. Rintala MA, Grenman SE, Puranen MH, et al. Transmission of high-risk human papillomavirus (HPV) between parents and infant: a prospective study of HPV in families in Finland. *J Clin Microbiol.* 2005;43:376–381

122. Tang CK, Shermeta DW, Wood C. Congenital condylomata acuminata. *Am J Obstet Gynecol.* 1978;131:912–913

123. Handley JM, Maw RD, Horner T, Lawther H, Bingham EA, Dinsmore WW. Scissor excision plus electrocautery of anogenital warts in prepubertal children. *Pediatr Dermatol.* 1991;8:243–245, 248–249

124. Boyd AS. Condylomata acuminata in the pediatric population. *Am J Dis Child.* 1990;144:817–824

125. Roussey M, Dabadie A, Chevrant-Breton O, et al. Condylomes acumines chez l'enfant. *Arch Fr Pediatr.* 1988;45:29–34

126. Herman-Giddens ME, Gutman LT, Berson NL. Association of coexisting vaginal infections and multiple abusers in female children with genital warts. *Sex Transm Dis.* 1988;15:63–67

127. Sinclair KA, Woods CR, Kirse DJ, Sinal SH. Anogenital and respiratory tract human papillomavirus infections among children: age, gender, and potential transmission through sexual abuse. *Pediatrics,* 2005;116:815–825

128. Connors JM, Schubert C, Shapiro R. Syphilis or abuse: making the diagnosis and understanding the implications. *Pediatr Emerg Care.* 1998;14:139–142

129. Goldenring JM. Secondary syphilis in a prepubertal child. Differentiating condylomata lata from condylomata acuminata. *N Y State J Med.* 1989;89:180–181

130. Horowitz S, Chadwick DL. Syphilis as a sole indicator of sexual abuse: two cases with no intervention. *Child Abuse Negl.* 1990;14:129–132

131. Cavender PA, Bennett RG. Perianal eosinophilic granuloma resembling condyloma latum. *Pediatr Dermatol.* 1988;5:50–55

132. Barton DJ, Sloan GM, Nichter LS, Reinisch JF. Hair-thread tourniquet syndrome. *Pediatrics.* 1988;82:925–928

133. Chapman HL. Digital strangulation by hair wrapping. *Can Med Assoc J.* 1968;98:125

134. Morgenstern J. Retention of urine, and edema of the penis from constriction of hairs. *Pediatrics.* 1988;5:248–249

135. Pantuck AJ, Kraus SL, Barone JG. Hair strangulation injury of the penis. *Pediatr Emerg Care.* 1997;13:423–424

136. Press S, Schachner L, Paul P. Clitoris tourniquet syndrome. *Pediatrics.* 1980;66:781–782

137. Dr G. Ligature of the penis. *Lancet.* 1832;2:136

138. Narkewicz RM. Distal digital occlusion. *Pediatrics.* 1978;61:922–923

139. Harrow BR. Strangulation of penis by a hidden thread. *JAMA.* 1967;199:171

Chapter 14

Child Neglect

Howard Dubowitz

Department of Pediatrics, University of Maryland School of Medicine
Division of Child Protection, University of Maryland Hospital

Maureen M. Black

Department of Pediatrics, University of Maryland School of Medicine
Growth and Nutrition, University of Maryland Medical System

The neglect of neglect is well documented.[1-3] Public and professional attention focuses largely on physical and sexual abuse, with little emphasis on child neglect. Yet neglect is the most prevalent form of child maltreatment and is associated with substantial morbidity and mortality. Our goal in this chapter is to integrate the literature on child neglect to provide useful information for health professionals.

Definition

Child neglect is difficult to define.[1,4] Definitions vary across disciplines, agencies, and states, with a spectrum of goals and thresholds.[5] For example, although health care providers might view repeated non-adherence with medications as neglectful, this would not generally meet the more stringent criteria of child protective services (CPS) unless serious harm resulted. All disciplines concerned with children share a primary purpose in defining child neglect: to ensure the adequate health and safety of children.[4] Thus a single definition of neglect might focus on this broad goal, while recognizing that the heterogeneity of neglect requires varied responses. Neglect is generally defined in state laws and the child welfare system as parental or caregiver acts of omission, such as inadequate supervision of a child, that result in actual or potential harm.[6] Alternatively, others have proposed a broader, child-centered definition including all circumstances where the basic needs of children are not adequately met, regardless of the contributor(s).[7-9] Basic needs include adequate food, supervision, and protection; clothing; health care; education; a stable home; and the emotional needs for love and nurturance. In this view of neglect, the focus is on the child's basic needs, not on parental behavior.

A child-focused definition of neglect offers several advantages. First, it draws attention to factors other than parental inaction that may harm or endanger children, such as inadequate access to health care. Distinct from defining when a child's basic needs are not adequately met, identifying the contributors is important for guiding appropriate responses. While parents are primarily responsible for their children's care, professionals, the community, society, and even youth themselves have a shared responsibility to meet the needs of children and adolescents.[7,9] Different forms of neglect, of varying severity and chronicity and within differing contexts, require a variety of responses. For example, a parent's ignorance of a child's nutritional needs requires a very different approach than protecting children from lead in the environment.

The framework of "is this neglect, or not?" is often simplistic. The degree to which children's needs are met falls on a spectrum ranging from optimal to grossly inadequate. At what threshold is a condition (eg, lack of health care) endangering or harmful? It is often difficult to determine, for example, whether being a "latchkey child" endangers or harms a child. Extreme situations are clear, but the gray zone is vast. One approach is to limit the definition of neglect to those circumstances where there is reasonable evidence indicating likely harm to children. A child with severe asthma exposed to passive smoke at home is an example. Research has found that professionals and laypersons, people from different socioeconomic groups, and those in urban and rural settings hold generally similar views concerning adequate child care and neglect.[10–12]

It also is important to recognize the variability among children. Being a latchkey child might be satisfactory for a mature child in one neighborhood,

but dangerous for another.[13] In clinical practice, it is necessary to consider each child's specific situation to determine whether basic needs are being adequately met. In considering neglect, several factors should be evaluated: whether actual or potential harm has occurred, the severity of harm involved, and the frequency/chronicity of the circumstances.

Actual or Potential Harm

In current practice, neglect is often considered only when actual harm has occurred. However, in some situations, the potential for moderate to serious harm also is construed as neglect, such as when a young child is poorly supervised and incurs repeated non-inflicted injuries ("accidents"). Laws in most states include the risk of harm in their neglect definitions.[6] Some argue, however, that "clear and identifiable harm or injury" is central to a definition of neglect,[14] and professionals have been reluctant to judge a situation as neglect without actual harm.[15]

The potential for harm is an important consideration in neglect. Many forms of neglect have no immediate physical consequences, although there may be substantial and long-term psychological harm.[16–19] But the potential for harm can be difficult to predict. How does one estimate the risks of not keeping follow-up appointments? For most medical conditions, little information is available to estimate the risks; in the realm of mental health, predicting outcomes is even more difficult. Epidemiological data can be helpful (eg, in estimating the risk of not wearing a seatbelt).

Knowledge of a child's specific condition also can be informative, such as a child with severe asthma who is repeatedly hospitalized after running out of medications.

Potential harm has 2 elements: (1) the likelihood of harm and (2) the nature or severity of the harm. For example, an 80% risk may be more worrisome than a 10% risk, but some risks entail only minor harm; others might be life-threatening. Another consideration is that taking risks and experiencing mishaps are important for learning and development. Think of an infant learning to walk. Nevertheless, helping families minimize the likelihood of moderate to serious harm to their children is an important concern in providing services to children and families (eg, anticipatory guidance or injury prevention).

Severity

The severity of neglect is typically based on the degree of harm involved and the likelihood of sequelae. A serious injury is apt to be seen as more severe neglect than a minor injury; any injury is likely to be seen as more severe than a potential injury. Such thinking may be simplistic. The correlation between the neglect and the apparent outcome(s), especially in the short term, is often modest.

The impact of neglect can be very serious. Approximately one half of the estimated 1,500 annual fatalities attributed to child maltreatment involve neglect.[20,21] The psychosocial sequelae of neglect may be serious and should be considered in assessing severity.[22,23]

There is also increasing evidence of the long-term harm associated with neglect.

Frequency/Chronicity

A pattern of omissions in care has been important in determining neglect. Single or occasional lapses in care are often considered "only human" and are not regarded as neglect. A single lapse in care can, however, have devastating results, such as an unattended toddler drowning in a pool. In contrast, other circumstances are unlikely to be harmful unless they recur. For example, a child occasionally missing asthma medications may involve little risk, but that risk increases if medications are missed repeatedly. The term *neglect* quickly brings to mind the child welfare system and legal definitions. However, a broad view of neglect means that many circumstances may be better addressed using less intrusive community resources. In summary, we suggest that child neglect be defined as a condition in which a child's basic need(s) is not adequately met, regardless of cause. Child neglect is a heterogeneous phenomenon, varying in type, severity, and chronicity. Both actual and potential harm are of concern. A pattern of basic needs not being met characterizes neglect, but single, momentary lapses in care or exposure to harm may also constitute neglect, particularly when serious risks are involved. Finally, the context in which the neglect occurs must be understood to tailor interventions to the specific needs of individual children and families.

Incidence

In 2004, 62.4% of the 872,000 substantiated CPS reports were for neglect, 2.1% for medical neglect, 17.5% for physical abuse, 9.7% for sexual abuse, and 7.0% for psychological maltreatment.[21] This translates to a rate of 7.7 per 1,000 children identified as neglected, a rate that has been steady over the past 5 years. Medical personnel made 7.9% of all reports.

Child abuse and neglect, however, are often not observed, detected, or reported to CPS,[24] making it difficult to estimate their incidence or prevalence. The Third National Incidence Study of Child Abuse and Neglect was conducted in 42 counties representative of the United States.[24] Community professionals, including pediatricians, were trained as "sentinels" to document instances meeting the study definitions of child maltreatment, regardless of whether they were reported to CPS. The definitions included potential and actual harm. It was not possible, however, to include laypersons as sentinels, the source of almost half of CPS reports.

The incidence of different types of maltreatment is shown in Table 14.1. It is noteworthy that 70% of cases involved neglect, especially physical neglect. Seven forms of physical neglect were examined, including (1) refusal of health care; (2) delay in health care; (3) abandonment; (4) expulsion of a child from the home; (5) other custody issues, such as repeatedly leaving a child with others for days or weeks at a time; (6) inadequate supervision, such as leaving a young child unsupervised for extended periods; and (7) other physical neglect, which included inadequate nutrition, clothing, or hygiene. Delay in health care was defined as "failure to seek timely and appropriate medical care for a serious health problem which any reasonable layman would have recognized as needing professional medical attention."

TABLE 14.1
Incidence of Child Abuse and Neglect in the United States in 1993

Category	No. of children[a]	Rate per 1,000 Children
Physical abuse	311,500	4.9
Sexual abuse	133,600	2.1
Emotional abuse	188,100	3.0
Total Abuse	**590,800**	**9.4**
Physical neglect	507,700	8.1
Emotional neglect	203,000	3.2
Educational neglect	285,900	4.5
Total Neglect	**917,200**	**14.6**

[a] Children were classified in each category that applied, so the rows are not additive.

Seven forms of emotional neglect were examined, including (1) inadequate nurturance/affection; (2) chronic/extreme spouse abuse; (3) permitted drug/alcohol abuse (if the parent had been informed of the problem and had not attempted to intervene); (4) permitted other maladaptive behavior, such as chronic delinquency; (5) refusal of psychological care; (6) delay in psychological care; and (7) other emotional neglect, such as chronically applying expectations clearly inappropriate in relation to the child's age or developmental level.

Children's mental health needs are often not met.[25] One study of youth between ages 9 and 17 years found that only 38% to 44% of children meeting stringent criteria for a psychiatric diagnosis in the prior 6 months had had a mental health contact in the previous year.[26] Neglected dental care is widespread. For example, a study of preschoolers found that 49% of 4-year-olds had dental caries, and fewer than 10% were fully treated.[27] Neglected health care is not rare, and if access to health care and health insurance is a basic need in the United States today, 8.3 million (11.2%) children experienced this form of neglect in 2004.[28]

In the last National Incidence Study, educational neglect included 3 types: (1) permitted chronic truancy (if the parent had been informed of the problem and had not tried to intervene); (2) failure to enroll/other truancy, such as causing a child to miss at least 1 month of school; and (3) inattention to special educational need. The special educational need criterion was defined as "refusal to allow or failure to obtain recommended remedial educational services, or neglect in obtaining or following through with treatment for a child's diagnosed learning disorder or other special education need without reasonable cause."

Etiology

Belsky[29] has provided a theoretic framework for understanding the etiology of child maltreatment, including neglect. There is no single cause of child neglect. Developmental-ecological theory posits that multiple and interacting factors at the individual (parent and child), familial, community, and societal levels contribute to child maltreatment. For example, although maternal depression is often associated with child neglect, maternal depression does not necessarily lead to neglect. However, the likelihood of neglect increases when maternal depression occurs together with other risks, such as poverty and lack of social support.

Individual Level

Parental Characteristics
Maternal problems in emotional health, intellectual abilities, and substance abuse have been associated with child neglect. Emotional disturbances, including depression, have been a major finding among mothers of neglected children.[17,30,31] Polansky et al[30] described the apathy-futility syndrome in mothers of neglected children, characterized by an emotional numbness, loneliness, interpersonal relationships that involve desperate clinging, a lack of competence in many areas of living, a reluctance to

talk about feelings, the expression of anger through passive aggression and hostile compliance, poor problem-solving skills, a pervasive conviction that nothing is worth doing, and an ability to evoke a sense of futility in others. Mothers of neglected children have been described as more bored, depressed, restless, lonely, and less satisfied with life than mothers of non-neglected children[32] and more hostile, impulsive, stressed, and less socialized than mothers of either abused or non-maltreated children.[33] Intellectual impairment, including mental retardation and a lack of education, have also been associated with neglect.[32,34–36]

Maternal drug use during pregnancy has become a pervasive problem. Results from the 2005 National Survey on Drug Use and Health conducted by the Substance Abuse and Mental Health Services Administration (SAMHSA), Office of Applied Studies[37] found that 3.9% of pregnant women (ages 15–44 years) reported illicit drug use in the past month, compared with 9.9% among nonpregnant women in the same age range. These rates did not differ from rates obtained in 2002 and 2003, but the rates were higher in low-income women and women with other risk behaviors. Although most illicit drugs pose risks to the fetus and child, the magnitude of these risks and the long-term sequelae of drug exposure are unclear.[38,39] It is often difficult to separate the drug effects from the environmental effects of being raised in a drug-using household or community. The compromised caregiving abilities of drug-abusing parents are a major concern. It has

been proposed, mostly unsuccessfully, in legislatures of several states that maternal drug use be considered a form of child, or fetal, neglect (or abuse), with grounds for CPS involvement and even criminal prosecution. Many professionals prefer a therapeutic approach, offering appropriate services to mothers and babies.[40] Only when such a plan fails and the child remains at significant risk is neglect considered with possible CPS involvement.[35] High rates of drug addiction[32] have been found among families of neglected children.[41] Jones[42] reported rates of 28% and 25% for alcohol and drug abuse, respectively, in families of children who had been neglected.

Child Characteristics

Theories of child development and child maltreatment emphasize the importance of considering children's characteristics, because caregivers respond differently to these characteristics. For example, parents of children who are temperamentally difficult report more stress in providing care than parents of easygoing children. Situations that lead to parental stress may contribute to child maltreatment.[43] This association is supported by research that has, for example, found increased depression and stress in parents of chronically disabled children.[44]

Several studies have found low birth weight or prematurity to be significant risk factors for abuse and neglect.[45,46] Because these babies usually receive close pediatric follow-up as well as other interventions, however, it is difficult to discern whether their increased rates of reported maltreatment reflect greater surveillance. In addition, medical neglect might be expected to occur more often among children who require frequent health care[16] because their increased needs place them at risk for these needs not being met.

Other studies have found increased rates of abuse and neglect among children with chronic disabilities. Diamond and Jaudes[47] found cerebral palsy to be a risk factor for neglect. Increased neglect, but not abuse, also was found among a group of disabled children who had been hospitalized.[48] Conversely, Benedict et al[49] found no increase in maltreatment among 500 moderately to profoundly retarded children, 82% of whom also had cerebral palsy.

In summary, although child factors should be considered in evaluations of child neglect, the preponderance of the evidence suggests that child factors do not cause neglect, but may place difficult demands on parents that, in turn, increase the likelihood of neglect. Families of children with chronic illness or behavior problems may benefit from services, such as support, education, and respite care, to enable them to meet their children's needs. Further research is needed to identify the characteristics and conditions that influence children's vulnerability to neglect.

Family Level

Problems in parent-child relationships have been found among families of neglected children. Research on dyadic interactions indicates less mutual engagement by both mother and child[50] and frequent disturbances in attachment between mother and infant.[51,52] Several

other studies revealed poor nurturing qualities of mothers of neglected children. In comparison with parents of abused and non-maltreated children, parents of neglected children had the most negative interactions with their children.[53] Those parents made more requests of their children, while being least responsive to requests from them. One study noted the negative and controlling behavior of mothers of neglected children during child-directed play.[54] Bousha and Twentyman[55] found that mothers of neglected children interacted least with their children compared with mothers of abused and non-maltreated children.

Although mothers of neglected children may have unrealistic expectations of their young children compared with matched controls,[41] a lack of knowledge concerning child developmental milestones (eg, age at which an infant is able to sit unsupported) has not been clearly associated with child neglect.[56] Deficient parental problem-solving skills, poor parenting skills, and inadequate knowledge of children's developmental needs have been associated with child neglect.[41,57,58]

In his work with neglected children, Kadushin[34] described chaotic families with impulsive mothers who repeatedly demonstrated poor planning and judgment, coupled with either father absence (often abandonment or incarceration) or negative mother-father relationships. Although most of the research on child neglect and high-risk families focuses on mothers and ignores fathers,[59] there is evidence that father involvement in low-income families of 5-year-olds can protect children against neglect.[60] Neglect has been associated with social isolation.[32,61] Single parenthood without support from a spouse, family members, or friends poses a risk for neglect. In one large controlled study, mothers of neglected children perceived themselves as isolated and as living in unfriendly neighborhoods.[62] Indeed, their neighbors saw them as deviant and avoided social contact with them. Mothers of neglected children in another study had less help with child care and fewer enjoyable social contacts compared with mothers of children who had not been neglected.[58]

Several other studies have found an association between social isolation and child neglect. Wolock and Horowitz[32] found that "participation in a social network offers a family entry into a system of interpersonal and emotional exchanges," something that was lacking for many families of neglected children. Giovannoni and Billingsley[63] described a pattern of estrangement from kin among mothers of neglected children that included a lack of supportive relationships. Summarizing the literature on social support and child maltreatment, Seagull[64] asked whether social isolation is a contributory factor to neglect or a symptom of underlying dysfunction. In either case, social isolation seems to be strongly associated with child maltreatment, and particularly with neglect.

Stress also has been strongly associated with child maltreatment. In one study, the highest level of stress, reflecting concerns about unemployment, illness, eviction, and arrest, was noted among families of neglected children compared with abusive and control families.[65] Lapp[66] found stress was frequent among parents reported to CPS for neglect, particularly regarding family, financial, and health problems.

Crittenden[67] described how distortions in information processing can lead to neglect. She described 3 types of neglect associated with deficits in cognitive processing, affective processing, or both: (1) disorganized, (2) emotionally neglecting, and (3) depressed. The first type, "disorganized," is characterized by families who respond impulsively and emotionally, with little regard for the cognitive demands. The family operates in a crisis mode and seems chaotic and disorganized. Children may be caught in the midst of this crisis, and their needs are not met. The second type, emotionally neglecting, includes families in which there is minimal attention to the emotional needs of the child. Parents may handle the demands of daily living (eg, ensure that children receive food and clothing), but pay little or no attention to how the child feels. The third type, depressed, is the classic presentation of neglect. Parents are depressed and therefore unable to process either cognitive or affective information. Children may be left to fend for themselves emotionally and physically. Although the interventions for these 3 different family patterns differ, they all require addressing the problematic family dynamics and parent-child relationship.

Community/Neighborhood Level

The community context and its resources influence parent-child relationships and are strongly associated with child maltreatment.[68] A community with a rich array of services, such as family-centered activities, high-quality and affordable child care, and a good transportation system, enhances the ability of families to nurture and protect their children. Informal support networks, safety, and recreational facilities also are important in supporting healthy family functioning. Garbarino and Crouter[68] described the feedback process whereby neighbors may monitor each other's behavior, recognize difficulties, and intervene. This feedback can be supportive and diminish social isolation, and may help families obtain services.

A comparison of neighborhoods with low and high rates for child maltreatment showed that families with the most needs tended to cluster together in areas, often those with the least social services.[69] In addition to the role of personal histories, the authors attribute the formation of high-risk neighborhoods to political and economic forces. Families in a high-risk environment are less able to give and share and might be mistrustful of neighborly exchanges. In this way, a family's problems may be compounded rather than ameliorated by the neighborhood context, dominated as it is by other needy families.

Socioeconomic factors (ie, poverty) seem to be strongly associated with child maltreatment.[24,69] In addition, Garbarino and Crouter[68] found that parents' negative perceptions of the quality of life in the neighborhood were related to increased child maltreatment. In summary, communities can serve as valuable sources of support to families, or they may add to the stresses that families are experiencing.

Societal Level

Many factors at the broader level of the community or society compromise the ability of families to care adequately for their children. In addition, these societal or institutional problems can be directly neglectful of children. "More than a dozen blue-ribbon commissions and task forces over the past decade have warned of the inadequacy of America's educational system and urged reform."[70] Approximately 4 million (12.6%) young people aged 16 to 24 years have not completed high school and are not enrolled in school.[71] This translates to a dropout rate of 10.7% for youth in this age group, a rate that has been stable over the past decade. In a national study, 70% of children with learning disabilities received special education services according to their parents; only 25% of those with serious emotional or behavior problems received special services.[72] The SAMHSA National Mental Health Information Center includes information on resources for children, such as the National Child Traumatic Stress Network, which is designed to raise the standard of care and improve access to services for traumatized children, their families, and communities nationwide.[73]

The harmful effects of poverty on the health and development of children are pervasive.[43] In addition to its influence on family functioning, poverty directly threatens and harms the well-being of children.[74-77] A recent report from Child Trends indicates that children in poor families lag behind children in wealthier families in health insurance and academic performance.[78] For many children, living in poverty means exposure to environmental hazards (eg, lead, violence), hunger, few recreational opportunities, and inferior health and health care. A 2005 UNICEF study[79] found that 21.7% of US children live below the national poverty line. Of all the risk factors known to impair the health and well-being of children, poverty is clearly important.

Poverty has been directly associated with neglect[32]: "These families are the poorest of the poor."[63] Although poverty has been associated with all forms of child maltreatment, the contribution to neglect is particularly striking.[80] It should be noted, however, that most low-income families are not neglectful of their children.

The child welfare system,[81] the very system intended to assist children in need of care and protection, is another example of societal neglect. "If the nation had deliberately designed a system that would frustrate the professionals who staff it, anger the public who finance it, and abandon the children who depend on it, it could not have done a better job than the present child welfare system."[70] Inadequately financed, with staff who are generally under trained and overwhelmed, and with poorly coordinated services, CPS is often unable to fulfill its mandate of protecting children. Not surprisingly, reports by the National Commission on Child Welfare and Family Preservation,[82] the National Advisory Board to the National Center on Child Abuse and Neglect,[83] and the National Center for Children in Poverty[84] have called for a drastic overhaul of the child welfare system. The quest for reform has continued in recent years.[85,86]

Manifestations of Child Neglect

Different types of neglect have been described, reflecting various basic needs of children that are not adequately met. We focus on the main types likely to be encountered by health care providers (Box 14.1). Specific suggestions for addressing these types of neglect are offered; more general principles are provided in later sections.

Non-Adherence (Noncompliance) With Health Care Recommendations

This form of neglect occurs when recommendations for health care or further evaluation are not implemented, resulting in actual or potential harm. The term *non-adherence* is preferred because it avoids the blaming connotation of *noncompliance,* recognizing the many potential contributors to health care recommendations not being implemented.[87] It is important to ascertain that the child's condition is clearly attributable to the lack of care. For example, a child with brittle diabetes might be out of control despite good care. It also is helpful to acknowledge that some recommended care may not be important (eg, a follow-up appointment for an ear infection in a child with no symptoms), so that such lapses in care should not be labeled neglectful. Similarly, lapses in primary care in a healthy child are

BOX 14.1
Manifestations of Possible Neglect Encountered by Pediatricians

- Noncompliance (non-adherence) with health care recommendations
- Delay or failure in obtaining health care
- Refusal of medical treatment
- Hunger, failure to thrive and, perhaps, unmanaged morbid obesity
- Drug-exposed newborns, older children
- Ingestions; injuries; exposure to secondhand smoke, guns, domestic violence; failure to use car safety seats/seat belts (may reflect inadequate protection from environmental hazards)
- Emotional affect (eg, excessive quietness or apathy in a toddler); behavior (eg, repetitive movements) and learning problems, especially if not being addressed; extreme risk-taking behavior (may reflect inadequate nurturance, affection, or supervision)
- Inadequate hygiene, perhaps contributing to medical problems
- Inadequate clothing, perhaps contributing to medical problems
- Educational needs not being met
- Abandoned children
- Homelessness

unlikely to result in harm and should probably not be considered neglect, although encouraging adherence to the health maintenance schedule would be reasonable.

A few issues are specific to the assessment and management of non-adherence.[87] Identifying and addressing the barrier(s) to care is the key, including careful consideration of the provider-family relationship and communication. Management strategies include making the treatment as practical as possible, ensuring clear communication, and following up to help ensure that the plan is successfully implemented.

Delay or Failure in Obtaining Health Care

Another form of medical neglect occurs when health care is needed but not obtained in a timely manner, or at all, resulting in actual or potential harm.[88] Parents (or primary caregivers) are responsible for recognizing health problems in their children and for taking care of minor needs, such as cleaning a wound. They are also responsible for recognizing the need for professional care and helping their child obtain such care.

Current child welfare practice typically considers neglect when a child has a significant health problem that a parent (or "average layperson") can reasonably be expected to recognize and respond to but fails to do so in a timely manner. For example, severe respiratory distress in a child with asthma should be obvious; in contrast, asymptomatic lead poisoning is rarely apparent. In addition, there is a need to show that the lack of care has harmed the child, or jeopardized his or her health.

In assessing these situations, there is a need to consider whether the delay in care was significant. For example, an infant may have had gastroenteritis for days but appeared well before abruptly decompensating with dehydration. Caution is needed before concluding, "if the child had been brought in earlier, this intensive care unit admission would have been avoided."

As with other types of neglect, there may be multiple and interacting reasons why care was not obtained; identifying and understanding those reasons is the guide to appropriate intervention. Failure or delay in seeking care may be related to maternal factors such as depression, to family factors such as a lack of transportation, and to community factors such as limited access to health care. Health care providers may unknowingly contribute to medical neglect.[87] In many instances, parents depend on health care providers to explain a child's condition and plan for treatment. If the explanation is rushed or explained in "medicalese," parents may not understand the recommendations, resulting in errors and omissions in care. Health care providers share in the responsibility to ensure that children receive adequate health care. Families with children who have chronic diseases need to be educated regarding when to seek professional help.

A different circumstance involves various cultural practices, such as the Southeast Asian folkloric remedy of cao gio (coin rubbing). Used for a wide variety of symptoms, cao gio describes the vigorous rubbing of a coin up and down the body to heal the body. Bruising and welts commonly result. Aside from questions of abuse, concerns of neglect arise when alternative (to mainstream medicine) remedies are used and complications ensue, especially if there is effective medical treatment available (eg, for bacterial meningitis). The threshold for intervention is guided by the level of certainty that a given treatment is harmful, as well as whether a distinctly preferable alternative exists.[88]

Sensitivity and humility are essential in broaching cultural differences, and often a satisfactory compromise can be found. Sensitive health care providers avoid an ethnocentric approach (ie, believing one's own way is best). While it is important to respect different cultural practices, one needs to recognize that there are cultural practices that harm children (eg, female genital mutilation) and should not be accepted. It is often effective to intervene with elder family members or leaders of the cultural group, encouraging them to modify their practice, thereby protecting children, increasing adherence, and minimizing the risk of the individual family member (the child or parent who deviates from their community norm) being ostracized.

From the child's standpoint, not receiving necessary health care constitutes neglect, regardless of the cause(s);

however, identifying the contributory factors is crucial for planning an appropriate intervention. If a parent does not know how to mix infant formula, parent education is recommended. When a child is exposed to lead in the environment, in addition to the individual and family measures, a public health strategy is needed to remove the lead from the environment. When a lack of health insurance causes families to avoid health care expenses, changes in social policies are needed.

Refusal of Medical Treatment

A different manifestation of medical neglect may occur when parents actively refuse medical treatment based on their belief that an alternative treatment is preferable and/or because the prescribed approach is prohibited by their religion. At one end of this spectrum are the cases in which a child is thought to be in need of treatment for a serious condition and the parents refuse permission to treat the child. Jehovah's Witnesses, for example, with their prohibition of blood transfusions, routinely refuse surgery when the need for blood transfusions is anticipated. Another example is the Christian Scientist Church, with its own faith healers and its rejection of Western medicine. Asser and Swan[89] reviewed information from 172 child deaths between 1975 and 1995 that were attributed to a lack of medical care due to religious reasons. Almost all of these deaths were deemed preventable judging from the general state of medical treatment for the specific condition at the time of death. Deaths represent the "tip of the iceberg"; the morbidity is

likely far greater. Less dramatic examples of differing values might be the rejection of mental health interventions or of dietary recommendations for obesity.

At what point should alternative approaches and beliefs be challenged? At what point does one declare that a child's basic health care needs are not being adequately met and that a neglectful situation exists? How do we balance our concern with civil liberties and respect for different beliefs in a pluralistic society with an interest in protecting children? The principle of *parens patria* establishes the state's duty to protect the rights of its younger citizens.

Thirty-nine states and the District of Columbia have religious exemptions in their civil codes on child abuse or neglect that exempt parents who do not provide or seek medical care for sick children, stating for example "that a child is not to be deemed abused or neglected merely because he or she is receiving treatment by spiritual means, through prayer according to the tenets of a recognized religion."[90] These exemptions have largely been based on the arguments of various religious groups that the US Constitution guarantees the protection of religious practice. This interpretation of the Constitution is contradicted by court rulings prohibiting parents from martyring their children based on parental beliefs[91] and from denying them essential medical care.[92] Many states allow religious exemptions for preventive pediatric care. For example, 48 states have such exemptions for immunizations, 2 for bicycle helmets.[89] The American Academy of Pediatrics (AAP) strongly opposes the religious exemptions, advocating that the opportunity to grow and develop safe from physical harm with the protection of our society is a fundamental right of every child and the basic moral principles of justice and of protection of children as vulnerable citizens require that all parents and caretakers must be treated equally by the laws and regulations that have been enacted by state and federal governments to protect children.[90]

As with cultural differences, assessment of these situations requires respect and humility, as well as some knowledge of the religion. Working with religious leaders and seeking compromise are important. Sometimes a satisfactory compromise cannot be reached and the child is harmed or at risk of harm. Bross[93] presented criteria for legal involvement in this form of medical neglect. First, the treatment refused by the parents should have definite and substantial benefits over the alternative. Therefore, if the treatment has only a modest chance of success or if it carries a risk of major complications, the basis for advocating legal intervention is questionable and neglect is probably not an issue. Second, not receiving the recommended treatment should result in serious harm. Most cases that have been settled in court have involved the risk of death or severe impairment, although some court decisions have mandated treatment for less serious conditions. Third, with treatment, the child is likely to enjoy a "high-quality" or "normal" life. This criterion reflects the court's reluctance to mandate treatment for severely handicapped and terminally ill children. Of note, the Baby Doe laws concerning treatment of severely impaired newborns seem to have had little impact on how these cases are managed. Fourth, in the case of older children (eg, teenagers), youth should consent to treatment. When these conditions are met, there is a legal basis for intervening. If efforts to provide treatment and reach a satisfactory compromise are not successful, legal intervention on behalf of the child may be necessary. Ridgway[94] reviewed published judicial opinions on cases involving 66 children where there were parent-physician disputes over the care of sick children. Physicians prevailed in 80% of disputes and in 90% of those that were religion based. The court acknowledged the adolescent's view in only half of 19 cases. In most cases, the petitioning physician was the only source of medical information.

Failure to Thrive, Food Insecurity, Hunger, and Overweight

Failure to thrive (FTT) is addressed in Chapter 15; only a few points will be raised here. Caution is needed in identifying children who are proportional and growing at an expected rate, even if their weight for age and height for age are low. Tracking weight for length for children younger than 3 years and body mass index (BMI) for children older than 2 years provides an indicator of body fat. Growth parameters are a crude reflection of nutritional status. The classic dichotomy of "organic and nonorganic" is no longer used because most growth problems involve both nutritional and psychosocial factors.[95]

Although neglect plays an important role in many cases of FTT, there are many other reasons for a child's growth to falter. Thus inferences of neglect should be based on a firm understanding of contributors to the child's condition and not automatically assumed in cases of FTT.

Food insecurity refers to limited or uncertain access to enough food to meet the basic needs of household members at all times and may result in hunger.[96,97] Young children in food-insecure households may experience health risks and iron deficiency,[98,99] and school-aged children and adolescents may experience less physical activity, poor academic performance, and overweight.[100–102] The seemingly paradoxical relationship between food insecurity and overweight may be partially explained by families' reliance on low-quality, high-energy foods to avoid hunger.

Pediatric overweight is a serious problem that has increased in prevalence over the past 30 years; more than 17% of children have a BMI greater than the 95th percentile, more than 3 times the expected rate of 5%.[103] Morbidity associated with adult obesity includes cardiovascular problems, hypertension, diabetes, psychosocial problems, and premature mortality. Analyses have shown the continuity of overweight from preschool years through adulthood,[104] particularly when parents also are obese,[105] emphasizing the importance of early prevention. In a 10-year follow-up investigation of 1,258 students (originally aged 9–10 years) in Copenhagen, Lissau, and Sorensen[106]

reported that after controlling for age, demographics, and childhood BMI, children who were neglected (received little parent support) were 7-fold more likely to become obese as young adults than were children who were not neglected. Children who experienced multiple forms of neglect (lack of support and lack of hygiene) were 9.8 times more likely to become obese adults. The mechanisms linking neglect and overweight were not examined, but one possibility is that the children who experienced neglect looked to food for gratification.

Analogous to FTT, there should be a thorough assessment to understand the basis for overweight. Again, multiple and interacting factors may be involved. Whatever the causes, overweight that is not being addressed may be a form of neglect deserving intervention. Being overweight is an example of a problem that clearly has multiple contributors, with parents likely to contribute only partly. It is also challenging in that effective interventions are limited and often difficult to access.

Drug-Exposed Newborns and Older Children

Use of illegal drugs during pregnancy has been identified as a public health problem.[107] Associations linking prenatal substance exposure with negative behavioral, cognitive, and academic consequences for children are controversial,[39,108,109] often due to the associated risk factors (eg, poverty, poor nutrition, legal drug use, cigarettes, alcohol, family problems) that frequently coexist with substance abuse.[110] Children who are exposed to illegal substances are often at risk for behavioral and developmental problems, though the mechanisms remain under investigation.

The pervasive use of legal drugs (ie, tobacco, alcohol) during pregnancy raises an important issue, given our knowledge of the risks involved. It is probably not helpful to label any use of these drugs as neglect; however, their use should be discouraged during pregnancy. Regarding older children, the risks of secondhand smoke, especially to vulnerable children with underlying lung disease, is clear. The same principle applies: behaviors that counter children's basic needs and harm them are forms of neglect. Approaches to prenatal substance exposure have varied greatly. Chasnoff and Lowder[111] offer an algorithm beginning with inducements to engage in drug treatment but leading to CPS and court involvement if therapeutic efforts fail.

Inadequate Protection From Environmental Hazards

A basic need of children is to be protected from environmental hazards, inside and outside of the home. Ingestions, injuries, exposure to guns, domestic violence, and failure to use car safety seats/seat belts may represent inadequate protection that threatens children's health. In addition, elevated lead exposure has been associated with small decrements in children's IQ (2–5 points).[112,113] Through brief screening and anticipatory guidance, health care professionals can play important roles in helping caregivers recognize and prevent potential threats in their household. It is beyond the scope of

this chapter to discuss each of these issues; practical guidance on their assessment and management is offered in the AAP *TIPP (The Injury Prevention Program) and Connected Kids: Safe, Strong, Secure* resources.[114]

Inadequate Nurturance and Affection

Emotional (eg, excessive quietness or apathy in a toddler), behavioral (eg, repetitive movements), and learning problems, especially if not being addressed, as well as extreme risk-taking behavior, may reflect inadequate nurturance and affection. Emotional, behavioral, and learning problems occur for many reasons. In assessing such problems, health care providers need to consider an array of potential contributors, as described under Etiology. Another concern may be the nature of the family's response to an identified problem, or the lack of any response. Of all forms of neglect, inadequate nurturance and affection may be especially harmful.[115]

Inadequate Supervision, Abandonment

Neglect occurs when children are not supervised in accordance with their developmental needs, resulting in significant risks to their health and well-being (eg, an infant left unattended in a bathtub, a preschooler left home alone, a teenager out overnight without parental approval). Children's emotional and behavioral status need to be considered; it would be reckless to leave a child with a history of fire setting unattended. Some risk-taking is inevitable and necessary for healthy development (eg, an infant falling while learning to walk), but the potential harm should be minor at most. Abandonment is the extreme form and has been arbitrarily defined as occurring when children are not "claimed" within 2 days. Another form of abandonment occurs when teenagers are forced to leave the home.

Inadequate Hygiene

This form of neglect occurs when a child repeatedly does not meet basic standards of hygiene (eg, child obviously smelly or filthy, not just scruffy). Poor hygiene can contribute to medical problems (eg, wound infection), as well as psychological problems, if the child is teased or ostracized by peers. One study of the risk of infection to neonates in intensive care found room for staff improvement regarding their hand-washing practices.[116]

The assessment should establish whether there has been a pattern of poor hygiene, what family members think about hygiene, what barriers they face, and what the consequences have been. Is the family amenable to improving their hygiene? Management includes kindly but forthrightly conveying one's concern and, with a social worker if possible, exploring ways to remedy the situation.

Inadequate Clothing

This form of neglect also involves a pattern in which a child repeatedly wears clothing that is obviously unsuitable for the weather or poorly fitting, while recognizing the fashion of the day (eg, lack of jacket in very cold weather, painfully

small shoes). In extreme situations, inadequate clothing may contribute to health problems; more often it causes discomfort and possible ridicule. The general approach is similar to that for inadequate hygiene.

Educational Neglect

A child's educational needs are neglected when the child is not enrolled in school, when a child fails to attend without a satisfactory reason (>2 d/mo), and when a child's special educational needs are not adequately met. Homeschooling that is appropriately regulated seems to be an acceptable alternative. Health care providers are in a position to know about school attendance and possible barriers, especially those pertaining to the child's health. For children with learning and other disabilities, pediatric providers often play a valuable role in helping to ensure that children's special educational needs are met. School problems may result from abuse or neglect[117]; children are especially vulnerable to school failure if their families are not advocating on their behalf.

Impact of Neglect on Children

Neglect has substantial and potentially long-term effects on children's physical and mental health and their psychosocial and cognitive development. Children who have been neglected perform worse academically than do non-neglected children, especially when neglect occurs in combination with other forms of maltreatment.[117] Two factors have hindered research on the consequences of child neglect, however. First, children who are neglected often also experience abuse, making it difficult to discern specific consequences of neglect. Second, neglect often occurs in the context of poverty, making it difficult to differentiate outcomes related to neglect from the consequences of poverty. Elmer's[117] early study among children from very low-income families, for example, found that maltreatment had little impact beyond the detrimental effects of poverty. Others have found that neglect exacerbates the negative aspects of poverty.[118] As suggested earlier, another view is that given the harmful effect of poverty on children's health and development, poverty per se can be seen as a form of societal neglect. It is also important to note that although poverty correlates with neglect, most children in low-income families are not neglected by their families.

The mechanisms linking neglect with children's behavior and development are unclear. One recent avenue of investigation is through psychobiology, primarily through chronic stress associated with the absence of adequate caregiving.[119] One possibility is that neglect creates chronic psychological stress, which activates a biological stress response through deregulation of the limbic-hypothalamic-pituitary-adrenal (LHPA) axis, particularly when it occurs during periods of rapid brain development. Deregulated LHPA, as indicated by increased salivary cortisol secretion, has been found among maltreated children[120] and children raised under deprived conditions in Romanian orphanages.[121] Recent advances in noninvasive measurement techniques, such as structural and functional magnetic resonance imaging, have enabled investigators to begin to examine the neurobiological consequences of neglect. Researchers have also found that when comparing different forms of maltreatment to controls, neglect was most strongly associated with smaller regions 3, 4, 5, and 7 of the corpus callosum.[122] Data from animal studies are promising, and ongoing research examining the psychobiological consequences of neglect may make major contributions to our understanding of early child development.

Physical Outcomes

Physical needs involve health, including the basic needs of food, shelter, and medical care, as well as protection from threats (eg, poisons, environmental hazards). Unmet physical needs can lead to significant long-term morbidity and premature death. Inadequate food prenatally can lead to diminished birth weight[123] and to FTT.[124] Inadequate health care can result in injuries not being treated,[125] health problems not being identified or treated,[126] untreated dental problems[127] or, in the extreme, death.[25]

Exposure to household hazards can have health consequences. Inadequate supervision is associated with exposure to toxins[128] and injuries due to falls.[129] Problematic supervision can also contribute to children accessing firearms[130] or being trapped in house fires,[131] both potentially deadly. Exposure to intimate partner (or domestic) violence has also been found to impair children's health.[132,133]

Longitudinal research has found correlations between child neglect and adult health decades later. There seems to be an increased risk of liver disease, possibly mediated by increased sexual activity.[134] Dong and colleagues[135] also found a link with later ischemic heart disease, and a connection with asthma and lung cancer was recently reported out of the same Adverse Childhood Experiences (ACEs) study. Widom and Brzustowicz[19] have also reported neglect to be associated with an increased risk of elevated hemoglobin A1c, a marker for diabetes mellitus. In the ACEs study, the researchers investigated several experiences aside from physical and emotional neglect, such as physical and sexual abuse, living with a drug-addicted parent, living in a home where a household member is incarcerated, and exposure to intimate partner violence. In general, they have not found any one of these experiences to be especially more predictive of adverse health outcomes than the others.

Physical neglect signals that a child may be in need of protection and intervention. Inadequate growth may be a marker of family dysfunction.[136] Children who do not grow adequately may experience permanent deficits in growth, school performance, and work capacity.[137-139] Risk factors accumulate, such that children experiencing multiple forms of neglect are at increased risk for negative sequelae.[140,141] In a cross-sectional evaluation of infants and toddlers, the cognitive performance of children with both FTT and neglect was significantly below that of children with neither risk factor, neglect only, or FTT only.[142] A longitudinal investigation of the same children at age 6 years examined the impact of early FTT and/or maltreatment on children's well-being reported by mothers, teachers, and standardized testing.[143] The children who experienced both neglect and FTT as infants had more behavior problems at home and school, fewer cognitive skills, and less success at school than their peers with neither risk. Children who experienced only one risk had intermediate scores, supporting the accumulation of risk model.[144,145] These results are consistent with findings from other investigators who have examined the accumulation of risk and found that multiple risks are much more detrimental than a single risk.[50,140,141,145] Thus neglect is particularly serious when it occurs with other risk factors such as FTT.

Psychosocial Outcomes

The impact of neglect on children's psychological development is best understood when evaluated with respect to general theories of child development. Children proceed through a series of developmental tasks from infancy through adolescence,[146] beginning with attachment during the first year of life. Autonomy and self-regulation are the primary tasks of the second and third years as toddlers acquire skills that contribute to their independence in both functional areas (eating, toileting) and interpersonal relationships (language). Peer relationships, the tasks of early childhood, become increasingly important as children attend preschool and elementary school. Finally, during middle childhood, children must integrate the earlier tasks to develop the interpersonal skills necessary for satisfying relationships during adolescence.[147,148] Although each task is associated with a specific age range, the tasks are not limited to that period and extend throughout childhood from infancy through adolescence.

Infancy

Most of the maltreatment that occurs during infancy is neglect, given the dependency needs of infants. The interdependence between infants and their primary caregivers is well documented.[149] As infants and caregivers look to one another for affective cues, they develop a synchrony in which responses stimulate expectations for subsequent interactions.[149] Under ideal conditions, infants and caregivers develop a mutually satisfying pattern of interactions that facilitates healthy physical and psychological development in the infant. Infants learn that their needs will be met according to predictable cues, and they learn to trust their caregivers. When caregivers are not consistent in their responses, infants may be denied models to imitate feedback. Without satisfying interactions, infants may have difficulty developing trust and a secure attachment with their primary caregivers; they are also at risk for subsequent emotional and relational problems.

In a recent application of developmental-ecological theory among very low-income inner-city families of infants and toddlers, the relationships between neglect and child and family functioning differed by the type of neglect.[150] There were no direct links from family functioning, support, or life events to emotional neglect, but mothers who were involved in well-functioning families were more likely to regard their child as having an easy temperament, and children who were perceived as being relatively easy were less likely to experience emotional neglect. These findings illustrate the importance of conceptualizing neglect from a developmental-ecological perspective that incorporates the family and the child's contribution through their temperament. The link between mothers' perceptions of their children's temperament and child neglect suggests that maternal perceptions of children's temperament are an important component of neglect that should be incorporated into intervention strategies. In contrast, when physical neglect was considered, there were no associations with child temperament and family context. Thus different factors may be associated with physical and emotional neglect.

School-Aged Children

Several investigators have shown that neglected children are more likely to exhibit developmental, emotional, and behavioral problems than are non-neglected children.[50,54,151,152] However, there is variation in the specific behavior problems shown by neglected children. Several investigators have noted that at times neglected children are passive and withdrawn and at other times are aggressive.[55,153] Thus children who have been neglected may have dysfunctional working models of social interactions, and in response to routine peer play they may display both withdrawn and aggressive behavior.

Egeland et al[152,154] followed 4 groups of mother-child pairs (abusive, neglectful, psychologically unavailable, and non-maltreating controls) and reported that children of neglectful and psychologically unavailable mothers were more likely to be anxiously attached when compared with non-maltreated children. Without a secure attachment relationship with the primary caregiver, the tasks of autonomy and self-development and the ability to form trusting relationships with peers are threatened.[155] Neglected children have fewer positive social interactions with peers than do non-neglected peers and are often less self-assured.[156]

The vulnerability of neglected children is well described in a longitudinal follow-up study.[153] By early school age, neglected children had deficits in cognitive performance, academic achievement, classroom behavior, and personal social interactions with peers and adults. The neglected children rarely expressed positive affect and demonstrated more developmental problems than any other subgroup of maltreated children. Several authors have found that children with a history of neglect have more school absences,[157] more retentions, and lower grades than do non-neglected children.[117]

Risk and compensatory factors also influence children's adjustment to neglect. For example, a child who is intelligent, attractive, or talented may be more able to withstand neglectful situations than one who is not intelligent, not attractive, and has low self-esteem.[158] Although protective factors may militate against some of the negative sequelae associated with neglect, Farber and Egeland[158] argued that the environmental challenges associated with maltreatment, and particularly with neglect or psychological unavailability, tend to overpower these protective factors, thereby increasing children's vulnerability.

Adolescents

Adolescence is marked by transition as the dependency of childhood evolves into the independence (or interdependence) of adulthood. The primary tasks of adolescence are the ability to form multiple attachment relationships, internalize standards of morality, and assume responsibility for personal actions.[159,160] Adolescents who have experienced prior neglect are at risk for emotional and behavioral problems if they have not mastered earlier developmental tasks successfully.

Neglect during adolescence can be particularly difficult to define because the boundaries between adolescent independence and parental responsibility are unclear. As children age, the influence of parents is supplemented and sometimes replaced by the influence of peers and other forces in the community. Although adolescents do not require the close supervision required by younger children, they continue to require parental guidance and monitoring.[159] Adolescents benefit from parents who adopt a democratic and respectful approach and at the same time establish clear demands and are warm and accepting.[160] Without access to parents who provide both supervision and nurturance, adolescents may be at increased

risk for behavioral and emotional problems, such as engaging in high-risk
behaviors (eg, early initiation of sexual
activity, substance abuse).

Principles of Evaluation

The following are some generic principles for evaluating possible child neglect.
They are based on developmental-
ecological theory, in which children
are evaluated in the context of their
family and community.

1. Determine whether a child is ex-
    periencing neglect. This diagnosis
    or formulation should be based on
    whether a child's basic needs are not
    being adequately met, resulting in
    actual or potential harm.
2. Ensure the child's safety. This is a pri-
    ority and hinges on an assessment
    of the likelihood, immediacy, and
    severity of future harm. Estimating
    the likelihood is often guided by
    knowledge of the child or children
    in similar circumstances. Epidemio-
    logical data are sometimes useful, for
    example, in estimating the risks of
    not being immunized. The imme-
    diacy of harm depends on the par-
    ticular circumstances. An abandoned
    infant faces obvious and immediate
    risks, whereas an inadequate diet in
    an older child poses longer-term risks.

    The assessment of severity is based
    on the frequency and nature of prior
    incidents and their effect on the child,
    in addition to possible future harm.
    For example, a child with mild asthma
    might experience little harm if medi-
    cations are frequently unavailable; a
    child with severe disease might be
    seriously harmed. In some instances,
    scientific data are useful (eg, in
    appreciating the risks of high lead
    levels).[113]
3. Develop a comprehensive under-
    standing of what is contributing to
    the neglectful situation. An accurate
    understanding of factors contribut-
    ing to the neglectful situation is key
    to help tailor the intervention to the
    specific needs of a child and family.
    Individual parent and child, familial,
    community, and societal factors, dis-
    cussed under Etiology, all need to be
    considered.
4. Use an interdisciplinary approach.
    This is optimal because it is difficult
    for a single professional to adequately
    evaluate and manage child neglect.
    A social work assessment addresses
    resources within the family and the
    community. For hospitalized chil-
    dren, a primary care nurse may have
    helpful observations of the family
    and their relationships. Psychological
    evaluations can assess a child's devel-
    opmental and emotional status and
    parents' abilities to nurture and pro-
    tect their children. Teachers can
    provide valuable information on
    children's school behavior and per-
    formance. Health care providers
    can review the medical record for
    conditions and observations as well
    as adherence to appointments and
    recommendations. In summary, pro-
    fessionals must share information
    and work collaboratively to reach
    a comprehensive understanding of
    the situation and plan accordingly.

Principles of Prevention and Intervention

Mrazek and Haggerty[161] categorized prevention programs along 3 dimensions: universal, selected, and indicated. Universal or population-based interventions are designed to prevent neglect for an entire population of children and are mass distributed. Examples include mass media campaigns to draw public attention to the importance of protecting children and promoting their optimal development. Selected interventions are directed toward families who are at high risk for child neglect. Selected interventions often target families who are socially isolated, highly stressed, have alcohol and/or substance abuse problems, or who have few resources. Indicated interventions are directed toward families in which child neglect has already occurred. The goal of this type of intervention is to minimize the negative effects of neglect on the child and to prevent further neglect.

In a review of prevention strategies for neglect, Holden and Nabors[162] noted the paucity of prevention programs and recommended the need for theory-driven, longitudinal programs that extend beyond the prevention of neglect to the promotion of healthy caregiving practices. Although there is a lack of specificity in the determinants of child neglect, there are multiple avenues for intervention. Home intervention has attracted national attention as an effective strategy in promoting the health and development of young children. The long-term successes noted by Olds et al[163,164] in a home-visitation program among high-risk families in Elmira, NY, many of whom were adolescent mothers, are encouraging. In our own work among low-income children who were born healthy but experienced FTT in their first 2 years of life, we have found that early home intervention is effective in preventing neglect by promoting a nurturant home environment and reducing the developmental delays often experienced by low-income, urban children.[165] Family Connections is another prevention program where social work students provided home-based services to families at risk for neglect.[166] Both the 3- and 9-month interventions resulted in enhanced parenting attitudes, parenting competence, and social support; diminished parental depressive symptoms and stress; improved physical and psychological care of the children; and fewer child behavior problems.

1. Interventions should be based on existing knowledge and theory. Interventions proven to be effective should be favored whenever possible. For example, because neglectful families often need basic parenting skills, a behavioral approach is usually preferable to insight-oriented psychotherapy.[167]
2. Maternal mental health problems, particularly depression, occur commonly among families of neglected children. Effective treatment for depressive symptoms,[168,169] often based on cognitive-behavioral therapy, can reduce maternal depression among mothers of neglected children. Brief screens for depression can be incorporated into health care settings for children and women.[170–172]

3. Developmental-ecological theory provides an understanding of the etiology of neglect and guides prevention and intervention. Interventions should be targeted to many of the underlying contributory factors, including parenting limitations and environmental stresses, while using available strengths and resources. Project 12 Ways[173] is an example of a multimodal program providing an array of services tailored to the needs of individual families. Serving mainly neglectful families in rural Illinois, this program includes training in parenting skills, stress reduction, self-control (impulse control), money management, job-finding services, weight reduction and smoking cessation, marital counseling, and teaching parents how to play with their children. Of note, the weight-control program has been very popular with parents and has served as an inducement to become involved with other aspects of the program. Evaluations of Project 12 Ways have found short-term improvements in family functioning and diminished rates of child maltreatment.[173]

4. Encourage the use of the family's natural and informal supports. Professionals must keep in mind the availability of support from family and friends, and encourage their involvement. For example, by inviting fathers to participate in health care visits, health care providers can convey to families the importance of fathers, and can facilitate fathers' involvement in child care, either directly or through support for the mother.[60] If a mother needs time for herself, she might request help with babysitting from extended family members. A variety of other community resources, such as church or peer support groups (eg, Family Support Centers, Parents Anonymous), can address the social isolation that is often associated with child neglect.

5. Begin with the least intrusive approach, using more intrusive approaches only if necessary. Successful intervention requires working with a family, and good rapport between professionals and the family is critical to effective help. Therefore intrusive approaches, or interventions that are perceived as punitive, should not be the first- or second-line strategies, unless the risk to the child is sufficiently serious to justify such measures. For example, if an infant has not been fed and is found alone and filthy, a report to CPS is clearly indicated.

A useful first approach is to enhance the parents' child-rearing skills through anticipatory guidance. For example, non-inflicted injuries may be prevented by discussing a toddler's emerging mobility and curiosity, and the need to clear the home of potential hazards. Specific advice (eg, "Remove small, hard objects that could cause a baby to choke.") is more likely to be remembered than is more general guidance (eg, "Safety-proof your house."). Helping parents resolve a problem they identify as important can help establish rapport and trust.

6. Child protective services should be contacted when necessary. Child

protective services is charged with ensuring that children are adequately protected. When clinicians suspect child abuse or neglect, they are obligated to contact CPS to investigate the situation and to determine what services the family may need to ensure that the child is adequately protected. Child protective services should not be regarded as a punitive agency or a threat to families; the CPS report should be presented as an effort to clarify the situation and to obtain help if needed. The professionals who work for CPS often have expertise and resources to help families protect and nurture their children. Although they have the power to petition the courts to remove children from the care of their parents, they are guided by principles of first ensuring a child's safety and keeping families together if possible.

7. Structured interventions should be used. Videka-Sherman[174] emphasized the importance of structure in an intervention. This structure pertains to clear guidelines as to which families receive what services; how interventions should be implemented; and the development of short-term, intermediate, and long-term goals. Parents should participate in establishing goals, and goals should be reasonable and clearly identified, and measurable, in writing.

8. Home-based intervention enables an appreciation of the family's circumstances, facilitates a rapport and connectedness between the interventionist and the family, and allows direct guidance in the setting in which recommendations need to be implemented. A randomized trial of nurse home visitors for high-risk mothers (low income, single, or adolescent) having their first babies improved the functioning of those families and reduced the incidence of child maltreatment.[175] The most comprehensive package of services (ie, prenatal and postnatal nurse home visitor, transportation to health care visits, and developmental screening of the children) yielded significant improvements, but only among the highest-risk families (ie, mothers who were low income, single, primigravida, and adolescent). Although several evaluations of parent-aid or home-visitor programs suggest that home intervention might be a particularly effective strategy, additional research is needed to refine our understanding of home visiting.[176] For example, uncertainty persists regarding the optimal professional background of the home visitor, and the content, frequency, and duration of the intervention. Home visiting might be most effective when combined with other services in a comprehensive program. Despite limitations in our current knowledge, home visiting seems to be a promising strategy for families at risk for child maltreatment. One recommended approach is to make home visitors universally available, but optional, for all families with a new baby.[83] Most of the research has been conducted in relatively well-controlled efficacy trials. A recent evaluation of a scaled-up system in Hawaii showed no significant impact on parental risk factors

for maltreatment and on rates of maltreatment.[177] There was substantial variability in agency program implementation and family participation, with some positive agency-specific program effects on child development and parent-child interaction, suggesting a need for close agency monitoring and supervision.

9. Interventions often must be long term. Brief crisis services, such as respite care, are cost-effective means of decreasing parent stress and providing immediate support to families, thereby reducing the likelihood of neglect. However, these types of services do not necessarily change underlying conditions that may lead to neglect. Comprehensive, long-term programs, including center-based and home-visiting programs, have demonstrated effects on children's cognitive, academic, behavioral, and emotional adjustment, as well as parents' responsiveness with their children. Long-term programs are necessary to alter maladaptive patterns of family interaction, enhance problem-solving and coping abilities, and address the broader conditions that may lead to poverty (eg, poor educational attainment and unemployment) and possibly to neglect. Continuity of care and case coordination are important ingredients of effective programs. The problems in many families of neglected children are often multiple, deeply rooted, and chronic. It is helpful at the outset for both professionals and families to recognize that long-term intervention may be necessary; in most instances, perhaps 12 to 18

months, and for some families, years. This time commitment raises the dilemma for public policy of how best to allocate limited resources. Some have suggested that if good efforts are made for 18 months, yet little progress is achieved and the family remains at high risk, an alternative long-term plan for the child should be made.[178]

10. The specific type of program most appropriate for the prevention of child neglect depends on families' specific needs (eg, parents with severe emotional difficulties are better served by mental health services). Programs with a narrow focus (eg, targeting individual family members without attention to the broader context) tend to be less effective than multilevel programs because parent, child, family, community, and societal factors are associated with child neglect. Because neglect takes several forms, it is difficult to define a specific set of program components that characterizes an effective prevention program; programs with the flexibility to tailor services to the specific needs of families have been found to be most effective. Finally, effective programs build on family competencies and use strengths to improve families' functioning.

Promising Interventions

Specific therapeutic interventions have been helpful to families of neglected children. For example, several programs have documented the effectiveness of behavioral management techniques (ie, alternatives to hitting) with maltreating parents.[178,179] The most effective programs focus on basic problem-solving skills and concrete family needs,[180] provide positive behavior-management strategies, and address environmental factors.[181]

Parents may benefit from a therapeutic relationship that includes nurturance, support, empathy, encouragement to express feelings, and motivation to change behavior. Parents of neglected children often require attention to their own emotional or interpersonal needs to nurture their children adequately. Insight-oriented therapy that is abstract, verbal, time-consuming, and expensive, however, is often thought to be inappropriate for most parents of neglected children. An evaluation of 19 demonstration programs for maltreating families concluded that individual therapy was less effective than family or group therapy.[182]

Although a family-level approach is generally needed, neglected children may require individual attention. The focus of CPS has largely been on parents, and few maltreated children have received direct services.[182] Treatment of neglected children is needed to reduce the likelihood of psychological harm and of the possible intergenerational transmission of neglectful parenting. Preschool programs, for example, can provide stimulation and nurturance while offering parents respite. It is important, however, that parents be included in any treatment of their children so that the therapeutic approach also can be implemented at home.

Few treatment programs are available specifically for neglected or maltreated children, and little evaluation research has been done in this area. Nevertheless, some specific interventions seem to be useful, including therapeutic day care programs for younger children and group therapy for older children and adolescents.[183]

In a review of the empiric knowledge base for intervening in child neglect, Videka-Sherman[174] described the need to focus on building positive family experiences, "not just controlling or decreasing negative interaction." For example, parents of neglected children need to learn how to play with their children. One approach involves teaching mothers how to teach their children in a cognitive stimulation program.[184] Children who had gone through the program had a higher IQ at age 6 years and were more likely to be in the appropriate grade at age 8 years compared with controls. Videka-Sherman also noted the need to be innovative and to look for resources in the homes of families of neglected children. Pots and pans can be used for play, and basic play materials, such as paper and crayons, might need to be provided.

Prevention by Pediatric Primary Care Providers

There is a need to screen for risk factors for neglect and also to screen for neglect that may not be apparent. For example, without direct questioning, a mother's depression or a child's hunger may go undetected. Some of these problems are sufficiently prevalent (eg, maternal depression, substance abuse) to justify universal and systematic screening during pediatric health maintenance visits. Safety and injury prevention have long been concerns in pediatrics. We can build on this work, broadening our interest to consider additional hazards in children's environments, such as intimate partner (or domestic) violence.

One challenge is to educate and support health care providers who may have received little training in these areas and who feel understandably uncomfortable broaching such topics. Another challenge involves the time constraints in practice. There is a need to set priorities, identify ways to screen briefly for these problems, and then briefly assess and intervene. Health professionals can be important gatekeepers to needed services. In addition to screening, health care providers should be astute observers of risk factors or actual problems they may confront. For example, a parent may appear high on drugs, or cold and angry toward the child. Such behaviors serve as "red flags" for providers to clarify the situation sensitively and to intervene as appropriate. Aside from problems, it is as important to identify strengths[167]; these are valuable in engaging parents (eg, "I see how much you care about Johnny."). For example, a parent's wish to be a good parent might be the impetus to seek drug treatment. A teen's wish to play sports may motivate him to adhere to his asthma treatment plan. An understanding of both the risks and strengths in the family is critical for estimating risks and for intervening successfully.

For children with chronic diseases, targeted health education and support help ensure adequate care. For other children, anticipatory guidance,[185]

whether it be about wearing a bike helmet or having a smoke alarm, is an effort to prevent harm and to ensure children's protection from environmental hazards. Health care providers' support, monitoring, and counseling are useful ways of helping families take adequate care of their children. At times, referrals to other professionals and agencies are necessary for services such as developmental evaluations, Special Supplemental Nutrition Program for Women, Infants, and Children (WIC), Head Start, or psychotherapy. Helping a family obtain appropriate services is another valuable role that health care providers can play.

Principles of Advocacy

The developmental-ecological model suggests that family and community factors contribute to child neglect.[29,186] Health care providers can be effective advocates on behalf of children and families in a variety of ways. Explaining to a parent the safety needs of an increasingly mobile and curious toddler is one form of advocacy. Helping a family obtain services in the community is another form of advocacy, as is remaining involved with a family after a report to CPS is made. Finally, efforts to develop programs in a community and to improve social policies and institutional practices concerning children and families also are important forms of advocacy.

If poverty is a major contributor to child neglect (and other forms of child maltreatment), the treatment plan should help the family access services to reduce the negative consequences of poverty (eg, emergency food, housing subsidies). Health professionals may encourage parents to consider opportunities such as job training or further education.

Health professionals may work in their communities in a variety of ways to develop and support programs that nurture families and children. Although improving the health, development, and safety of children can be a challenge, much is known about children's needs, and health care providers can be effective advocates for children's protection and well-being.

References

1. Black MM. The roots of child neglect. In: Reece RM, ed. *The Treatment of Child Abuse.* Baltimore, MD: Johns Hopkins University Press; 2000

2. Black MM. Long-term psychosocial management of neglect. In. Reece RM, ed. *The Treatment of Child Abuse.* Baltimore, MD: Johns Hopkins University Press; 2000

3. Wolock I, Horowitz B. Child maltreatment as a social problem: the neglect of neglect. *Am J Orthopsychiatry.* 1984;54:530

4. Giovannoni JM, Becerra RM. *Defining Child Abuse.* New York, NY: The Free Press; 1979

5. Zuravin SJ. Child neglect: a review of definitions and measurements research. In: Dubowitz H, ed. *Neglected Children: Research, Practice and Policy.* Thousand Oaks, CA: Sage Publications; 1999:24–26

6. Title 45: Public Welfare, *CFR S1340.2: Definitions.* Washington, DC: US Department of Health and Human Services; 1983

7. Dubowitz H, Black MM, Starr RH, Zuravin S. A conceptual definition of child neglect. *Crim Justice Behav.* 1993;20:8

8. Helfer RE. The neglect of our children. *Pediatr Clin North Am.* 1990;37:923–942

9. Lally JR. Three views of child neglect: expanding visions of preventive definitions. *Child Abuse Negl.* 1984;8:243–254

10. Dubowitz H, Klockmer A, Starr RH, et al. Community and professional definitions of neglect. *Child Maltreat.* 1998;3:243

11. Polansky NA, Williams DP. Class orientations to child neglect. *Soc Work.* 1978;23:397–401

12. Polansky NA, Chalmer MA, Williams DP. Assessing adequacy of child rearing; an urban scale. *Child Welfare.* 1978;57:439–449

13. Berman BD, Winkleby M, Chesterman E, et al. After-school child care and self-esteem in school-age children. *Pediatrics.* 1992;89:654–659

14. Valentine DP, Acuff DS, Freeman ML, et al. Defining child maltreatment: a multidisciplinary overview. *Child Welfare.* 1984;58:497

15. Gelles R. Problem in the defining and labeling of child abuse. In: Starr RH, ed. *Child Abuse Prediction: Policy Implications.* Cambridge, MA: Ballenger Publishing; 1982

16. Jaudes PK, Diamond LJ. Neglect of chronically ill children. *Am J Dis Child.* 1986;140:655–658

17. Zuravin S. *Child Abuse, Child Neglect and Maternal Depression: Is There a Connection?* National Center on Child Abuse and Neglect. Washington, DC: Clearinghouse on Child Abuse and Neglect Information; 1988

18. Chapman DP, Whitfield CL, Felitti VJ, Dube SR, Edwards VJ, Anda RF. Adverse childhood experience and the risk of depressive disorders in adulthood. *J Affect Disord.* 2004;82:217–225

19. Widom CS, Brzustowicz LM. MAOA and the "cycle of violence": childhood abuse and neglect, MAOA genotype, and risk for violent and antisocial behavior. *Biol Psychiatry.* 2006;60:684–689

20. Daro D, McCurdy K. *Current Trends in Child Abuse Fatalities and Reporting: The Results of the 1991 50-State Survey.* Chicago, IL: National Center for the Prevention of Child Abuse; 1992

21. US Department of Health and Human Services, Administration on Children, Youth and Families. *Child Maltreatment—2004.* Washington, DC: US Government Printing Office; 2006

22. Gaudin JM. Child neglect: short-term and long-term outcomes. In: Dubowitz H, ed. *Neglected Children: Research, Practice and Policy.* Thousand Oaks, CA: Sage Publications; 1999:89–108

23. Hildyard KL, Wolfe DA. Child neglect: developmental issues and outcomes. *Child Abuse Negl.* 2002;26:679–695

24. Sedlack AJ, Broadhurst DD. *Third National Incidence Study of Child Abuse and Neglect: Final Report.* Washington, DC: US Department of Health and Human Services; 1996

25. US Department of Health and Human Services. *Mental Health: A Report of the Surgeon General—Executive Summary.* Rockville, MD: US Department of Health and Human Services, Substance Abuse and Mental Health Services Administration, Center for Mental Health Services, National Institutes of Health, National Institute of Mental Health; 1999

26. Leaf P, Alegria M, Cohen P, et al. Mental health service use in the community and schools: results from the four-community MACA study. *J Am Acad Child Adolesc Psychiatry.* 1996;35:889–897

27. Tang J, Altman D, Robertson D, et al. Dental caries: prevalence and treatment levels in Arizona preschool children. *Public Health Rep.* 1997;112:319–331

28. The National Coalition on Health Care Insurance Coverage. http://www.nchc.org/facts/coverage.shtml. Accessed September 10, 2007

29. Belsky J. Child maltreatment: an ecological integration. *Am Psychol.* 1980;35:320–335

30. Polansky N, Chalmers MA, Buttenwieser EW, Williams DP. *Damaged Parents: An Anatomy of Child Neglect.* Chicago, IL: University of Chicago; 1981

31. Wolock I, Horowitz H. Child maltreatment and maternal deprivation among AFDC recipient families. *J Soc Serv Res.* 1981;8:83

32. Wolock I, Horowitz H. Child maltreatment and maternal deprivation among AFDC recipient families. *J Soc Serv Res.* 1979;53:175

33. Friedrich WN, Tyler JA, Clark JA. Personality and psychophysiological variables: its abusive, neglectful, and low-income control mothers. *J Nerv Ment Dis.* 1985;173:449–460

34. Kadushin A. Neglect in families. In: Nunnally EW, Chilman CS, Cox FM, eds. *Mental Illness, Delinquency, Addictions, and Neglect.* Newbury Park, CA: Sage; 1988

35. Martin M, Walters S. Familial correlates of selected types of child abuse and neglect. *J Marriage Family.* 1982;44:267

36. Ory N, Earp J. Child maltreatment and the use of social services. *Public Health Rep.* 1981;96:238

37. Substance Abuse and Mental Health Services Administration, Office of Applied Studies. http://www.oas.samhsa.gov/nsduh/2k6nsduh/2k6Results.cfm#2.6. Accessed September 10, 2007

38. Accornero VH, Morrow CE, Bandstra ES, Johnson AL, Anthony JC. Behavioral outcome of preschoolers exposed prenatally to cocaine: role of maternal behavioral health. *J Pediatr Psychol.* 2002;27:259–269

39. Hurt H, Brodsky NL, Roth H, Malmud E, Giannetta JM. School performance of children with gestational cocaine exposure. *Neurotoxicol Teratol.* 2005;27:203–211

40. Larson CS. Overview of state legislative and judicial responses. In: *The Future of Children: Drug Exposed Infants.* Los Altos, CA: Center for the Future of Children; 1991

41. Azar ST, Robinson DR, Hekimian E, Twentyman CT. Unrealistic expectations and problem solving ability in maltreating and comparison mothers. *J Consult Clin Psychol.* 1984;52:687–691

42. Jones MA. *Parental Lack of Supervision: Nature and Consequence of a Major Child Neglect Problem.* Washington, DC: Child Welfare League of America; 1987

43. National Center for Children in Poverty. *Alive and Well? A Research and Policy Review of Health Programs for Poor Young Children.* New York, NY: Columbia University School of Public Health; 1991

44. Shapiro J. Family reactions and coping strategies in response to the physically ill or handicapped child. *Soc Sci Med.* 1983;17:913–931

45. Benedict MI, White RB. Selected perinatal factors and child abuse. *Am J Public Health.* 1985;75:780–781

46. Herrenkohl EC, Herrenkohl RC. Some antecedents and developmental consequences of child maltreatment. In: Rizley R, Cicchetti D, eds. *Developmental Perspectives on Child Maltreatment.* San Francisco, CA: Jossey-Bass; 1981

47. Diamond LJ, Jaudes PK. Child abuse and the cerebral palsied patient. *Dev Med Child Neurol.* 1983;25:169–174

48. Glaser D, Bentovim A. Abuse and risk to handicapped and chronically ill children. *Child Abuse Negl.* 1979;3:565

49. Benedict MI, White RB, Wulff LM, Hall BJ. Reported maltreatment in children with multiple disabilities. *Child Abuse Negl.* 1990;14:207–217

50. Dietrich KN, Starr RH Jr, Weisfeld GE. Infant maltreatment: caretaker-infant interaction and developmental consequences at different levels of parenting failure. *Pediatrics.* 1983;72:532–540

51. Crittenden PM. Maltreated infants: vulnerability and resilience. *J Child Psychol Psychiatry.* 1985;26:85–96

52. Egeland B, Brunquell D. An at-risk approach to the studies of child abuse and neglect. *J Am Acad Child Adolesc Psychiatry.* 1979;18:219

53. Burgess RL, Conger RD. Family interaction in abusive, neglectful, and normal families. *Child Dev.* 1978;49:1163–1173

54. Aragona JA, Eyberg SM. Neglected children: mothers' report of child behavior problems and observed verbal behavior. *Child Dev.* 1981;52:596–602

55. Bousha DM, Twentyman CT. Mother-child interactional style in abuse, neglect, and control groups: naturalistic observations in the home. *J Abnorm Psychol.* 1984;93:106–114

56. Twentyman CT, Plotkin RC. Unrealistic expectations of parents who maltreat their children: an educational deficit that pertains to child development. *J Clin Psychol.* 1982;38:497–503

57. Herrenkohl RC, Herrenkohl EC, Egolf BP. Circumstances surrounding the occurrence of child maltreatment. *J Consult Clin Psychol.* 1983;51:424–431

58. Jones JM, McNeely RL. Mothers who neglect and those who do not: a comparative study. *Soc Casework.* 1980;61:559

59. Gutterman NB, Lee Y. The role of fathers in risk for physical child abuse and neglect: possible pathways and unanswered questions. *Child Maltreat.* 2005;10:136–149

60. Dubowitz H, Black MM, Kerr MA, Starr RH Jr, Harrington D. Fathers and child neglect. *Arch Pediatr Adolesc Med.* 2000;154:135–141

61. Polansky NA, Ammons PW, Gaudin JM Jr. Loneliness and isolation in child neglect. *Soc Casework.* 1985;66:3–12

62. Polansky NA, Gaudin JM Jr, Ammons PW, Davis KB. The psychological ecology of the neglectful mother. *Child Abuse Negl.* 1985;9:265–275

63. Giovannoni JM, Billingsley A. Child neglect among the poor: a study of parental adequacy in families of three ethnic groups. *Child Welfare.* 1970;49

64. Seagull EA. Social support and child maltreatment: a review of the evidence. *Child Abuse Negl.* 1987;11:41–52

65. Gaines R, Sangrund A, Green AH, Power E. Etiological factors in child maltreatment: a multivariate study of abusing, neglecting, and normal mothers. *J Abnorm Psychol.* 1978;87:531–540

66. Lapp J. A profile of officially reported child neglect. In: Trainer CNI, ed. *The Dilemma of Child Neglect: Identification and Treatment.* Denver, CO: The American Humane Association; 1983

67. Crittenden PM. Child neglect: causes and contributors. In: Dubowitz H, ed. *Neglected Children: Research, Practice and Policy.* Thousand Oaks, CA: Sage Publications; 1999:47–68

68. Garbarino J, Crouter A. Defining the community context of parent-child relations. *Child Dev.* 1978;49:604–616

69. Garbarino J, Sherman D. High-risk neighborhoods and high-risk families: the human ecology of child maltreatment. *Child Dev.* 1980;51:188–198

70. National Commission on Children. *Beyond Rhetoric: A New American Agenda for Children and Families: Final Report of the National Commission on Children.* Washington DC: Government Printing Office; 1991

71. US Department of Health and Human Services, Health Resources and Services Administration, Maternal and Child Health Bureau. *Child Health USA 2004.* Rockville, MD: US Department of Health and Human Services; 2004

72. Zill M, Schoenborn CA. *Developmental, Learning and Emotional Problems: Health of Our Nation's Children, United States, 1988. Advance Data From Vital and Health Statistics, No. 190.* Hyattsville, MD: National Center for Health Statistics; 1990

73. The National Child Traumatic Stress Network. http://www.nctsnet.org/nccts/nav.do?pid=abt_mv. Accessed September 10, 2007

74. Klerman LV. The health of poor children: problems and programs. In: Huston AC, ed. *Children in Poverty: Child Development and Public Policy.* New York, NY: Cambridge University Press; 1991

75. Parker S, Greer S, Zuckerman B. Double jeopardy: the impact of poverty on early child development. *Pediatr Clin North Am.* 1988;35:1227–1240

76. Wise PH, Meyers A. Poverty and child health. *Pediatr Clin North Am.* 1988;35:1169–1186

77. National Institute of Child Health & Human Development. Duration and development timing of poverty and children's cognitive and social development. *Child Dev.* 2005;76:795–810

78. Wertheimer R. *Poor Families in 2001: Parents Working Less and Children Continue to Lag Behind.* Washington DC: Child Trends; 2006

79. UNICEF. *Child Poverty in Rich Countries.* Florence, Italy: UNICEF Innocenti Research Centre; 2005

80. American Humane Association. *Highlights of Official Child Abuse and Neglect Reporting, 1983.* Denver, CO: American Humane Association; 1985

81. Child Welfare Information Gateway. How does the child welfare system work? [factsheet]. http://www.childwelfare.gov/pubs/factsheets/cpswork.cfm

82. National Commission on Child Welfare and Family Preservation. *A Commitment to Change.* Washington, DC: American Public Welfare Association; 1990

83. National Advisory Board on Child Abuse and Neglect. *Creating Caring Communities: Blueprint for Effective Federal Policy on Child Abuse and Neglect.* Washington, DC: US Department of Health and Human Services; 1991

84. National Center for Children in Poverty. *Child Welfare Reform.* New York, NY: Columbia University School of Public Health; 1991

85. Center for Study of Social Policy, Center for Community Partnerships in Child Welfare. *Child Welfare Summit: Looking to the Future: An Examination of the State of Child Welfare and Recommendations for Action.* Washington, DC: Center for Study of Social Policy; 2003

86. Cohen BJ. Reforming the child welfare system: competing paradigms of change. *Child Youth Serv Rev.* 2005;27:653–666

87. Liptak GS. Enhancing patient compliance in pediatrics. *Pediatr Rev.* 1996;17:128–134

88. Dubowitz H. Neglect of children's health care. In: Dubowitz H, ed. *Neglected Children: Research, Practice and Policy.* Thousand Oaks, CA: Sage Publications; 1999:109–131

89. Asser SM, Swan R. Child fatalities from religion-motivated medical neglect. *Pediatrics.* 1998;101:625–629

90. American Academy of Pediatrics Committee on Bioethics. Religious objections to medical care. *Pediatrics.* 1997;99:279–281

91. *Prince v Commonwealth of Massachusetts,* 321 US 158 (1944)

92. *Jehovah's Witnesses in the State of Washington v King County Hospital.* 278 F Supp 488, aff'd, 390 US 598 (1968)

93. Bross DC. Medical care neglect. *Child Abuse Negl.* 1982;6:375–381

94. Ridgway D. Court-mediated disputes between physicians and families over the medical care of children. *Arch Pediatr Adolesc Med.* 2004;158:891-896

95. Black MM, Feigelman S, Cureton P. Evaluation and treatment of children with failure to thrive: an interdisciplinary perspective. *J Clin Outcomes Manage.* 1999;6:60

96. Nord M, Bickel G. *Measuring Children's Food Security in US Households, 1995-1999.* Washington, DC: US Department of Agriculture, Food and Economic Division; 2002. Economic Research Report No. 25

97. Nord M, Andrews M, Carlson S. *Household Food Security in the United States, 2004.* Washington, DC: US Department of Agriculture, Economic Research Service; 2005:1–57. Food Assistance and Nutrition Research Report No. 25

98. Cook JT, Frank DA, Levenson SM, et al. Child food insecurity increases risks posed by household food insecurity to young children's health. *J Nutr.* 2006;136:1073–1076

99. Skalicky A, Meyers AF, Adams WG, Yang Z, Cook JT, Frank DA. Child food insecurity and iron deficiency anemia in low-income infants and toddlers in the United States. *Matern Child Health J.* 2006;2:177–185

100. Alaimo K, Olson CM, Frongillo EA. Food insufficiency and American school-aged children's cognitive, academic, and psychosocial development. *Pediatrics.* 2001;108:44–53

101. Casey PH, Szeto K, Lensing S, Bogle M, Weber J. Children in food-insufficient, low-income families: prevalence, health, and nutrition status. *Arch Pediatr Adolesc Med.* 2001;155:508–514

102. Casey PH, Simpson PM, Gossett JM, et al. The association of child and household food insecurity with childhood overweight status. *Pediatrics.* 2006;118:e1406–e1413

103. Ogden CL, Carroll MD, Curtin LR, McDowell MA, Tabak CJ, Flegal KM. Prevalence of overweight and obesity in the United States, 1999–2004. *JAMA.* 2006;295:1549–1555

104. Serdula MK, Ivery D, Coates RJ, et al. Do obese children become obese adults? A review of the literature. *Prev Med.* 1993;22:167–177

105. Whitaker RC, Wright JA, Pepe MS, Seidel KD, Dietz WH. Predicting obesity in young adulthood from childhood and parental obesity. *N Engl J Med.* 1997;337:869–873

106. Lissau I, Sorensen TI. Parental neglect during childhood and increased risk of obesity in young adulthood. *Lancet.* 1994;343:324–327

107. Gomby DS, Shiono PH. Estimating the number of substance-exposed infants. In: *Future of Children: Drug Exposed Infants.* Los Altos, CA: Center for the Future of Children; 1991

108. Chasnoff IJ, Anson A, Hatcher R, Stenson H, Laukea K, Randolph LA. Prenatal exposure to cocaine and other drugs: outcome at four to six years. *Ann N Y Acad Sci.* 1998;846:314–328

109. Linares TJ, Singer LT, Kirchner HL, et al. Mental health outcomes of cocaine-exposed children at 6 years of age. *J Pediatr Psychol.* 2006;31:85–97

110. Frank DA, Augustyn M, Knight WG, Pell T, Zuckerman B. Growth, development, and behavior in early childhood following prenatal cocaine exposure: a systematic review. *JAMA.* 2001;285:1613–1625

111. Chasnoff IJ, Lowder LA. Prenatal alcohol and drug use and risk for child maltreatment: a timely approach to intervention. In: Dubowitz H, ed. *Neglected Children: Research, Practice and Policy.* Thousand Oaks, CA: Sage Publications, 1999;132–155

112. Factor-Litvak P, Wasserman G, Kline JK, Graziano J. The Yugoslavia Prospective Study of environmental lead exposure. *Environ Health Perspect.* 1999;107:9–15

113. Lanphear BP, Hornung R, Khoury J, et al. Low-level environmental lead exposure and children's intellectual function: an international pooled analysis. *Environ Health Perspect.* 2005;113:894–899

114. Brassard MR, Hart SN, Hardy DB. The Psychological Maltreatment Rating Scales. *Child Abuse Negl.* 1993;17:715–729

115. Lam BC, Lee J, Lau YL. Hand hygiene practices in a neonatal intensive care unit: a multimodal intervention and impact on nosocomial infection. *Pediatrics.* 2004;114:e565–e571

116. Eckenrode J, Laird M, Doris J. School performance and disciplinary problems among abused and neglected children. *Dev Psychol.* 1998;29:53

117. Elmer E. A follow-up study of traumatized children. *Pediatrics.* 1977;59:273–279

118. Herrenkohl RC, Herrenkohl EC, Egolf BP, et al. The developmental consequences of abuse: the Lehigh Longitudinal Study. In: Starr RL, Wolfe DA, eds. *The Effects of Child Abuse and Neglect: Issue and Research.* New York, NY: Guilford Press; 1991:57–85

119. DeBellis MD. The psychobiology of neglect. *Child Maltreat.* 2005;2:150–172

120. DeBellis MD. Developmental traumatology: the psychobiological development of maltreated children and its implication for research, treatment, and policy. *Dev Psychopath.* 2001;13:537–561

121. Gunnar MR, Morison SJ, Chisolm K, Schuder M. Salivary cortisol levels in children adopted from Romanian orphanages. *Dev Psychopathol.* 2001;13:611–628

122. Teicher MH, Dumont NL, Ito Y, Vaituzis C, Giedd JN, Andersen SL. Childhood neglect is associated with reduced corpus callosum area. *Biol Psychiatry.* 2004;56:80–85

123. Martorell R, Gonzalez-Cossio T. Maternal nutrition and birth weight. *Yearb Phys Anthropol.* 1987;30:195–220

124. Krugman SD, Dubowitz H. Failure to thrive. *Am Fam Physician.* 2003;68:879–884

125. Overpeck MD, Kotch JB. The effect of US children's access to care on medical attention for injuries. *Am J Public Health.* 1995;85:402–404

126. Dubowitz H, Giardino A, Gustavson E. Child neglect: a concern for pediatricians. *Pediatr Rev.* 2000;21:111–116

127. Edelstein BL. External forces impacting US health care: implications for future of dental practice. *J Am Coll Dent.* 2002;69:39–43

128. Leibelt EL, DeAngelis CD. Evolving trends and treatment advances in pediatric poisoning. *JAMA.* 1999:282:1113–1115

129. American Academy of Pediatrics Committee on Injury and Poison Prevention. Falls from heights: windows, roofs, and balconies. *Pediatrics.* 2001;107:1188–1191

130. Farah MM, Simon HK, Kellermann AL. Firearms in the home: parental perceptions. *Pediatrics.* 1999;104:1059–1063

131. Squires T, Busuttil A. Child fatalities in Scottish house fires 1980–1990: a case of child neglect? *Child Abuse Negl.* 1995;19:865–873

132. Dubowitz H, Kerr M, Hussey J, Black M, Starr R, Morrel T. Type and timing of mothers' victimization: effects on mothers and children. *Pediatrics.* 2001;107:728–735

133. Morrel T, Dubowitz H, Kerr M, Black M, The effect of maternal victimization on children: a cross-informant study. *J Fam Violence.* 2003;18:29–41

134. Dong M, Dube SR, Felitti VJ, Giles WH, Anda RF. Adverse childhood experiences and self-reported liver disease: new insights into a causal pathway. *Arch Intern Med.* 2003;163:1949–1956

135. Dong M, Giles WH, Felitti VJ, et al. Insights into causal pathways for ischemic heart disease: Adverse Childhood Experiences Study. *Circulation.* 2004;110:1761–1766

136. Ammaniti M, Ambruzzi AM, Lucarelli L, Cimino S, D'Olimpio F. Malnutrition and dysfunctional mother-child feeding interactions: clinical assessment and research implications. *J Am Coll Nutr.* 2004;23:259–271

137. Drotar D. The family context of non-organic failure to thrive. *Am J Orthopsychiatry.* 1991;61:23–34

138. Galler JR. The behavioral consequences of malnutrition in early life. In: *Nutrition and Behavior.* New York, NY: Plenum Press; 1984

139. Martorell R, Rivera J, Kaplowitz H. Consequences of stunting in early childhood for adult body size in rural Guatemala. *Ann Nestle.* 1990;48:85

140. Sameroff AJ, Seifer R. Familial risk and child competence. *Child Dev.* 1983;54:1254–1268

141. Dube SR, Anda RF, Felitti VJ, Chapman DP, Giles WH. Childhood abuse, neglect, and household dysfunction and the risk of illicit drug use: the Adverse Childhood Experiences Study. *Pediatrics.* 2003;111:564–572

142. Mackner LM, Starr RH, Black MM. The cumulative effect of neglect and failure to thrive on cognitive functioning. *Child Abuse Negl.* 1997;21:691–700

143. Kerr M, Black MM, Krishnakumar A. Failure-to-thrive, maltreatment and the behavior and development of 6-year-old children from low-income urban families: a cumulative risk model. *Child Abuse Negl.* 2000;24:587–598

144. Rutter M. Psychosocial resilience and protective mechanisms. *Am J Orthopsychiatry.* 1987;57:316–331

145. Sameroff AJ, Seifer R, Barocas R, Zax M, Greenspan S. Intelligence quotient scores of 4-year-old children: social-environmental risk factors. *Pediatrics.* 1987;79:343–350

146. Steinberg L. Cognitive and affective development in adolescence. *Trends Cogn Sci.* 2005;9:69–74

147. Cicchetti D. How research on child maltreatment has informed the study of child development: perspectives from developmental psychopathology. In: Cicchetti D, Carlson V, eds. *Child Maltreatment.* New York, NY: Cambridge University Press; 1984

148. Sroufe LA. The coherence of individual development: early care, attachment and subsequent developmental issues. *Am Psychol.* 1979;34:834

149. Belsky J, Rovine M, Taylor D. The Pennsylvania Infant and Family Development Project: the origins of individual differences in infant-mother attachment: maternal and infant contributions. *Child Dev.* 1984;55:718–728

150. Harrington D, Black MM, Starr RH Jr, Dubowitz H. Child neglect: a model of temperament and family context. *Am J Orthopsychiatry.* 1998;68:108–116

151. Drotar D, Nowak M, Malone CA, Eckerle D, Negray J. Early psychological outcomes in failure to thrive: predictions from an interactional model. *J Clin Child Psychol.* 1985;14:105

152. Egeland B, Sroufe A. Developmental sequelae of maltreatment in infancy. In: Rizley K, Cicchetti D, eds. *New Directions for Child Development: Developmental Perspectives in Child Maltreatment.* San Francisco, CA: Jossey-Bass; 1981

153. Erikson MF, Egeland B, Pianta R. The effects of maltreatment on the development of young children. In: Cicchetti D, Carlson V, eds. *Child Maltreatment.* Cambridge University Press; 1989:579–619

154. Egeland B, Stroule LA, Erickson M. The developmental consequences of different patterns of maltreatment. *Child Abuse Negl.* 1984;7:459

155. Sroufe A, Waters O. Attachment as an organizational construct. *Child Dev.* 1977;48:1184

156. Hoffman-Plotkin D, Twentyman CT. A multimode assessment of behavioral and cognitive deficits in abused and neglected preschoolers. *Child Dev.* 1984;55:794–802

157. Wodarski JS, Kurtz PD, Gaudin JM, et al. Maltreatment and the school-age child: major academic, socioemotional, and adaptive outcomes. *Soc Work.* 1990;35:460–467

158. Farber FA, Egeland B. Invulnerability among abused and neglected children. In: Anthony EJ, Cohler BJ, eds. *The Invulnerable Child.* New York, NY: Guilford; 1987

159. Lamborn SD, Mounts NS, Steinberg L, Dornbusch SM. Patterns of competence and adjustment among adolescents from authoritative, authoritarian, indulgent and neglectful families. *Child Dev.* 1991;62:1049–1065

160. Steinberg L, Dornbusch S, Brown BB. Ethnic differences in adolescent achievement: an ecological perspective. *Am Psychol.* 1992;47:723–729

161. Mrazek PJ, Haggerty RJ. *Reducing Risks for Mental Disorders: Frontiers for Preventive Intervention Research.* Washington, DC: National Academy Press; 1994

162. Holden EW, Nabors L. The prevention of child neglect. In: Dubowitz H, ed. *Neglected Children: Research, Practice and Policy.* Thousand Oaks, CA: Sage Publications; 1999:174–190

163. Olds D, Eckenrode J, Henderson CR, et al. Long-term effects of home visitation on maternal life course and child abuse and neglect. *JAMA.* 1997;278:637–643

164. Olds D, Henderson CR Jr, Cole R, et al. Long-term effects of nurse home visitation on children's criminal and antisocial behavior: 15-year follow-up of a randomized controlled trial. *JAMA.* 1998;280:1238–1234

165. Black MM, Dubowitz H, Hutcheson J, Berenson-Howard J, Starr RH Jr. A randomized clinical trial of home intervention among children with failure to thrive. *Pediatrics.* 1995;95:807–814

166. DePanfilis D, Dubowitz H. Family Connections: a program for preventing child neglect. *Child Maltreat.* 2005;10:108–123

167. DePanfilis D. Intervening with families when children are neglected. In: Dubowitz H, ed. *Neglected Children: Research, Practice and Policy.* Thousand Oaks, CA: Sage Publications; 1999:211–236

168. Kaslow NJ, Thompson MP. Applying the criteria for empirically supported treatments to studies of psychosocial intervention for child and adolescent depression. *J Clin Child Psychol.* 1998;27:146–155

169. Lewinsohn PM, Clarke GN, Rhode P, et al. A course in coping: a cognitive-behavioral approach to the treatment of adolescent depression. In: Hibbs ED, Jensen PS, eds. *Psychosocial Treatments for Child and Adolescent Disorders: Empirically Based Strategies for Clinical Practice.* Washington, DC: American Psychological Association; 1996:109–135

170. Roberts RE, Lewinsohn PM, Seeley JR. Screening for adolescent depression: a comparison of depression scales. *J Am Acad Child Adolesc Psychiatry.* 1991;30:58–66

171. Whooley MA, Avins AL, Miranda J, et al. Case-finding instrument for depression: two questions are as good as many. *J Gen Intern Med.* 1997;12:439–445

172. Dubowitz H, Feigelman S, Lane W, et al. Screening for depression in an urban pediatric primary care clinic. *Pediatrics.* 2007;119:435–443

173. Lutzker JR, Rice JN. Project 12-Ways: measuring outcome of a large in-home service for treatment and prevention of child abuse. *Child Abuse Negl.* 1984;8:519–524

174. Videka-Sherman L. Intervention for child neglect: the empirical knowledge base. In: Cowan A, ed. *Current Research on Child Neglect.* Rockville, MD: Aspen Systems Corporation; 1988

175. Olds DL, Henderson CR Jr, Chamberlin R, Tatelbaum R. Preventing child abuse and neglect: a randomized trial of nurse home visitation. *Pediatrics.* 1986;78:65–78

176. US General Accounting Office. *Home Visiting: A Promising Early Intervention Strategy for At Risk Families.* Washington DC: US Government Printing Office; 1990

177. Duggan A, Fuddy L, Burrell L, et al. Randomized trial of a statewide home visiting program to prevent child abuse: impact in reducing parental risk factors. *Child Abuse Negl.* 2005;29:209–213

178. Crimmins DB, Bradlyn AS, Lawrence JS, et al. A training technique for improving the parent-child interaction skills of an abusive neglectful mother. *Child Abuse Negl.* 1984;8:533–539

179. Szykula SPA, Fleischman MJ. Reducing out-of-home placements of abused children: two controlled field studies. *Child Abuse Negl.* 1985;9:277–283

180. Sudia C. What services do abusive families need? In: Pelton L, ed. *The Social Context of Child Abuse and Neglect.* New York, NY: Human Sciences Press; 1981

181. Gambrill ED. Behavioral interventions with child abuse and neglect. *Prog Behav Modif.* 1983;15:1–56

182. Daro D. *Confronting Child Abuse: Research Official Child Abuse and Neglect Reporting, 1983, Denver: American Humane Association, Neglect for Effective Program Design.* New York, NY: The Free Press; 1988

183. Howing PT, Wodarski JS, Gaudin JM Jr, Kurtz PD. Effective interventions to ameliorate the incidence of child maltreatment: the empirical base. *Soc Work.* 1989;34:330–338

184. Yahraes H. Teaching mother's mothering. In: Videka-Sherman L, ed. *Intervention for Child Neglect: Perinatal Knowledge Base: Child Neglect Monograph: Proceedings From a Symposium.* Washington, DC: US Department of Health and Human Services; 1988

185. Dubowitz H. Preventing Child neglect and physical abuse: a role for pediatricians. *Pediatr Rev.* 2002;23:191–196

186. Belsky J. Etiology of child maltreatment: a developmental-ecological analysis. *Psychol Bull.* 1993;114:413–434

Chapter 15

Failure to Thrive

Deborah A. Frank

Grow Clinic, Department of Pediatrics, Boston Medical Center
Department of Pediatrics, Boston University School of Medicine

Stephanie Blenner

Grow Clinic, Department of Pediatrics, Boston Medical Center

MaryAnn B. Wilbur

Grow Clinic, Department of Pediatrics, Boston Medical Center

Maureen M. Black

Department of Pediatrics, University of Maryland School of Medicine

Dennis Drotar

Department of Pediatrics, Case Western Reserve University School of Medicine

Failure to thrive (FTT) refers to children whose weight is significantly lower than the norms for their age and gender.[1] Chronic FTT may lead to a slowdown in linear growth, resulting in low height for age. In a survey conducted among 1,429 children from low-income families in Massachusetts, 10.4% had height for age below the fifth percentile, twice as many as would be expected.[2] Up to 50% of children with FTT are never identified[3] by clinicians, suggesting an even higher prevalence. Although FTT is more common among infants from low-income families with limited resources, it can be found in all segments of the population.[4]

This chapter addresses the growth deficiencies that occur in industrialized countries, not the severe malnutrition that occurs in developing countries. Nevertheless, clinicians should be aware that micronutrient deficiencies, such as iodine, iron, zinc, and vitamin B_{12}, have been associated with behavioral and developmental problems in children.[5] Reviews of malnutrition in developing countries have reported significant long-term deficits in growth, intelligence, academic performance, and work capacity.[6] Several recent follow-up evaluations have found that by school age, most children with a history of FTT have experienced growth recovery.[7-10]

Although many children with a history of FTT continue to be shorter than age-matched peers, they rarely experience growth deficits severe enough to be classified as wasted or stunted, which are indicators of severe malnutrition.[7,8] When cognitive and academic performance have been considered by school-aged children with FTT recruited from primary care or community sites, achieved IQ scores that were approximately 4.2 points lower than children with a history of adequate growth.[8,10,11] These findings suggest early FTT may result in a small, though potentially important, impact on cognitive performance, but not the severe deficits implied by earlier studies that evaluated primarily hospitalized children.

Evolution of the Diagnosis of FTT

Some clinicians base their diagnosis on a single measure of weight for age or weight for height below the fifth or third percentile, with little attention to the child's growth history; others base their diagnosis on a deceleration in growth over time.[3] A child who is proportional (weight for height approximates the 50th percentile) and gaining weight along the fifth percentile with respect to weight and height for age, and has no health or nutritional problems, may be small but normal. In contrast, a child whose rate of growth is below expectations may be of concern, even if none of the growth indices have dropped below the fifth percentile. Deceleration in the rate of growth is a good indicator of growth problems but requires multiple measures over time and relatively

sophisticated interpretation.[12] Thus FTT can be an imprecise diagnosis.[13]

Traditionally, FTT was dichotomized into "organic FTT," in which the child's growth failure was ascribed to a major medical illness, and "nonorganic FTT," which was attributed primarily to psychological neglect or "maternal deprivation."[14-17] This simplistic dichotomous conceptualization of FTT is obsolete.[18] We now recognize that in all cases of nonorganic FTT, and in many cases of organic FTT, the cause of growth failure is malnutrition, whether primary or secondary.[16,18-22] Malnutrition not only jeopardizes the child's growth, but may also impair immunocompetence and undermine cognitive and socioaffective competence.[1,23-28] The modern diagnosis and treatment of FTT focus on the assessment of and therapy for malnutrition and its complications.[1,18,19,22,27,29,30] The needs of each child and family that are not thriving should be assessed along 4 parameters: medical, nutritional, developmental, and social.

Until recently, many investigators relied on hospitalized or referred samples of children with FTT.[31] However, most children with FTT are not hospitalized, but are treated as outpatients, consistent with recommendations from the American Academy of Pediatrics (AAP) Committee on Nutrition, published in the *Pediatric Nutrition Handbook*.[32-35] Failure to thrive is often managed successfully in specialized, interdisciplinary clinics.[36] Thus much of the existing literature, which was based on hospitalized children, may represent the most extreme and complex cases of FTT, rather than most children with FTT.

Ecological Context

Although FTT may occur in all segments of the population, it most often occurs in the context of poverty.[37,38] In some samples, as many as 10% of young, low-income American children meet criteria for FTT.[39] By definition, the federal poverty level ($20,000 for an average family of 4 in 2005), defined as 3 times the cost of a minimally nutritious diet, implies an income level inadequate for meeting children's needs for shelter, clothing, and food.[38,40] Indeed, children living in families with incomes up to 185% of poverty are considered at nutritional risk.[41,42] In addition to an insufficient budget for food purchases, economically disadvantaged families often lack access to supermarkets and live in homes lacking adequate food storage and preparation facilities.[43-45] A recent study has shown that food stamp benefits are inadequate for purchasing even a marginally healthful diet, even if the family is receiving the maximum allotment.[46]

National programs designed to protect the health and nutritional status of low-income children have not been adequately funded to meet the needs of American children. Food stamps provide maximal benefits of approximately $1.40 per meal per person on average only to families who have no other cash income, and most families do not receive even this maximum benefit, so that many families relying on the program routinely run out of food near the end of the month.[47,48] The highly successful Special Supplemental Nutrition Program for Women, Infants, and Children (WIC) is estimated by the US Department of Agriculture to reach only 81% of all eligible women, infants, and children, whereas school breakfast is available to only about 1 in 4 children who receive school lunch.[49-51] Although the WIC program food packages have been updated and improved over recent years, they are intended as only a supplement to the other food provided in the household. At $38 per month per recipient, they provide less than 100% of the recommended daily allowances (RDAs) for a number of nutrients.[52,53] For some children in certain age groups receiving WIC, and many pregnant and postpartum mothers, the combination of WIC food and other food available in the household is insufficient to provide adequate nutrients.[52,53] Even with simultaneous participation in multiple programs (food stamps, WIC, school meals), many low-income families are unable to obtain enough food to avoid frequent episodes of food insecurity and hunger, and the chronic mild to moderate undernutrition that ensues.[48,51,54]

There are several mechanisms whereby poverty may increase children's vulnerability to FTT. Poverty can affect children directly through lack of food, health care, and adequate educational opportunities, and indirectly through increased family stress, which may interfere with parents' ability to provide nutritious meals on a regular basis or in a responsive style. Food insecurity has been associated with increased hospitalizations and parental perceptions of poor health among infants,[55] and with developmental, academic, and learning problems among school-aged children.[56] To minimize the temptation to scapegoat families in clinical assessment and intervention, it is important to recognize that FTT often reflects economic conditions and changes in social policy that are far beyond the control of individual parents or health care providers.[57,58] Children also fail to thrive in homes of any social class in cases of parent-child interactive disorders, parental psychopathology, family dysfunction, or organic pathology. The impact of such problems on children's health increases dramatically in the context of poverty.

Family Risk Factors

Multiple family risk factors may interact with poverty to disrupt the child's caloric intake and trigger growth deficiency. Belsky's model of parental competence[59,60] provides a useful framework in which to consider family influences on growth deficiency. In this model, parental competence is influenced by 3 sets of factors: (a) parental resources, especially early developmental experiences and personality; (b) child characteristics, such as temperament, physical health, and illness; and (c) the family and social context of parent-child relations, including the parents' relationship, family social networks and resources, employment, and community resources.[54,59–63]

Parental Personal Resources

Although early clinical studies reported that mothers of children with FTT often had serious psychopathology,[64] controlled studies that have compared mothers of children with FTT and mothers of adequately growing children, adjusting for socioeconomic status, have found either no differences in psychopa-

thology[65,66] or no higher rates of affective and personality disorders.[67–70] However, in individual cases, parental mood disturbances and/or adjustment problems that do not meet the criteria for a formal psychiatric diagnosis may affect the quality of parent-child interactions and interfere with the effectiveness of early intervention on the behavior and development of children who fail to thrive.[71] In a prospective study, Altemeier et al[72] found that mothers of children who eventually developed FTT reported more problematic childhoods than did mothers whose children grew adequately. Maternal reports of being abused as a child correlated positively with subsequent FTT in their offspring. Conversely, maternal perceptions of a happy childhood, that they were loved as a child, and that their parents were pleased with them correlated negatively with their child's development of FTT.[72] Benoit et al[66] found that more mothers of infants with FTT were classified as insecure in their attachment relationships to their own mothers compared with mothers of infants who grew at an average rate. Lack of resolution of mourning over the loss of a loved one was found in more mothers in the FTT group compared with controls. Mothers of children with FTT have reported high rates of physical abuse as children and as adults.[66,73] Such psychological vulnerabilities in parental emotional resources could contribute to the development of less adaptive parent-child relationship patterns.[31,67,70,74–76]

Child Characteristics

Children's physical and temperamental characteristics may contribute to the development of FTT by presenting parents with child-rearing challenges that exceed their economic and psychosocial resources.[1,18,77] Among some children, the behavior problems associated with feeding are part of their overall temperament, including irritability, apathy, and generalized inactivity or overactivity.[65,78,79] Pollitt and Leibel[80] suggested that lethargic, listless infant behavior might evoke less responsive behavior from parents and contribute to FTT.[81-83] Prematurity, low birth weight, and early childhood illness impose additional caregiving burdens on parents and may heighten the risk for FTT.[84]

Hunger and satiety are guided by internal regulatory processes. Poor appetite, observed sometimes as early as the first 6 weeks of life[85]; delayed or dysfunctional oral-motor development[81]; and deficient signaling of needs during mealtimes may contribute to FTT. Once a child begins to demonstrate deficient growth and nutrition, whatever the specific cause, the child's irritability and inconsistent social responsiveness may engender feelings of helplessness among parents as well as beliefs that the child is physically deficient or ill.

Parent-Child Interactions

Families help children build expectations around food and mealtimes. If there is a disruption in the communication between parents and children, mealtimes may become a setting for battles over food. Feeding styles refer to behavioral patterns between parents and children that occur during meals: responsive, controlling, indulgent, and uninvolved.[86] Low maternal responsivity, insensitivity to cues, and poor problem-solving skills have been reported between children with FTT and their mothers observed during mealtime and playtime.[87-89] Under optimal circumstances, the communication between parents and children is clear because each adapts to the signals of the other and to the demands of the situation. Having a child who does not grow can be stressful and threaten parents' sense of competence and ability to communicate with their child. Parent-child interaction breaks down if communication is distorted and marked by signals that lack clarity, misperceptions of signals, inconsistent responses, or responses that are not in keeping with the signals.

Family and Social Context

Families of infants with FTT have been identified as having lower economic levels, higher family stress, less available extended family for help with child-rearing, and greater social isolation than have comparison groups.[68,69,90-92] All of these factors could affect the family members' capacities to mobilize caretaking resources on behalf of the child. Relationship patterns also may be strained in some families of infants with FTT.[22] Drotar and Eckerle[93] found that mothers of infants with FTT reported less supportive and cohesive family relationships than did families of adequately growing infants. The quality of family relationships and organization may affect the timing, frequency, and consistency of reinforcement for feeding patterns and ultimately is reflected in the child's growth and health.[60]

Medical Issues in Evaluation and Treatment

Family History

The assessment of FTT begins with a family history, focusing on issues such as consanguinity, recurrent miscarriage or stillbirth, developmental delay, atopy, human immunodeficiency virus (HIV) risk, alcoholism and other substance use, psychiatric diagnoses, and potentially growth-retarding familial illnesses such as cystic fibrosis, celiac disease, inflammatory bowel disease, or lactose intolerance. Height of both parents should be ascertained, as well as parents' history of growth delay in childhood and timing of puberty. A familial pattern of short stature, or constitutional delay of growth, may relieve the clinician and the family of the need for extensive workup if the child is short but not underweight for height.[94,95] Norms exist for correcting height percentiles for midparental height by using the National Center for Health Statistics (NCHS) grids.[96] It is critical, however, to assess whether the parents themselves were malnourished as children, as is often the case among immigrant and low-income families. In such cases, the parents' short stature does not provide an accurate indication of the child's genetic growth potential.[97] Moreover, an experience of severe childhood deprivation may influence the parents' caretaking practices.[98]

In addition to identifying biological constraints on growth, a detailed family medical history may uncover significant psychosocial stressors. A chronically ill grandparent or sibling may divert the family's caretaking energies from the child who fails to thrive; FTT has been described in siblings of children with leukemia.[99] A family history of serious mental illness, intergenerational substance abuse, or developmental impairment also may be present.[15] In our clinical experience, it is not unusual for a parent of a child who fails to thrive to have a history of an eating disorder in childhood or adolescence, occasionally carrying the actual diagnosis of anorexia nervosa.[100,101]

Perinatal Factors

After ascertaining family history, the medical assessment of a child who is not thriving should proceed to a detailed assessment of the child's prenatal and perinatal history by interview and, when possible, by review of neonatal records. This approach not only elucidates potential biological risks to growth, but also may be helpful in identifying ongoing psychosocial risk factors that are concurrently influencing postnatal growth. Low birth weight is a major predictor of later referral for FTT. In several clinical series, 10% to 40% of children hospitalized for FTT without a major medical diagnosis had a birth weight less than 2,500 g, compared with 7% of the general population at the time those studies were done.[14,18,30,102,103] In controlled studies of FTT that excluded infants with birth weights less than 2,500 g from their definition of FTT, infants later diagnosed with FTT still had lower birth weights than those who grew normally.[80]

To evaluate accurately the impact of perinatal risk factors on later growth, a detailed history should be obtained covering the issues summarized in Box 15.1. It is critical to ascertain not only the child's birth weight, but also gestational age, length, and head

BOX 15.1
Pregnancy and Delivery

Mother's Reproductive History
Age Gravidity/parity/abortions (spontaneous or induced), stillbirths History of pregnancy with identified patient

Conception planned or unplanned
  Difficulties with fertility
  Conceived while mother using contraception
  Abortion considered
Mother's nutritional status during pregnancy
  Weight at conception
  Pregnancy weight gain
  WIC
  Hyperemesis
Mother's health habits during pregnancy
  Cigarette packs per day
  Alcohol
  Prescribed drug use (particularly anticonvulsants)
  Illicit drug use
  X-rays
  Occupational exposure
Complications of pregnancy
  Infections/high fevers
  Bleeding
  Toxemia
  Violence or trauma
Labor and delivery

Vaginal or cesarean Anesthesia Maternal complications Neonatal status
Gestational age Apgar scores Birth weight, length, head circumference (parameters and percentiles for gestational age) Neonatal course

Mother and child separation
  Need for special care
  Duration of hospitalization for mother and child
Complications: jaundice, respiratory, CNS, sepsis, necrotizing enterocolitis
Early feeding difficulties
Transfusions
Eye examination
Hearing examination

Abbreviations: WIC, Special Supplemental Nutrition Program for Women, Infants, and Children; CNS, central nervous system.

circumference at birth. Such data will identify prematurity as well as various patterns of intrauterine growth retardation that have prognostic implications for later growth.

Prematurity

Children born prematurely may be inappropriately labeled as FTT if the percentiles used for assessing growth parameters are not corrected for gestational age by subtracting the number of weeks that the child was premature from the child's postnatal age at time of assessment. A statistically significant difference in growth percentiles will be found without such correction in head circumference until 18 months postnatal age, in weight until 24 months postnatal age, and in length until 40 months postnatal age.[104] Even after such correction, infants with very low birth weights (<1,501 g) may remain smaller than infants born at term for at least the first 3 years of life.[105] In these children, the distribution of mean height, weight, and head circumference corrected for gestational age is shifted downward relative to the NCHS norms so that the proportion of children with attained weight or height below the NCHS fifth percentile is increased.[105] The rate of growth of such infants, however, should be the same as that of term infants of the same corrected age.[105,106] Moreover, weight for length should be proportional despite somewhat lower fat stores.[107] Although the field lacks clear guidelines, preterm infants born before 34 weeks generally should be fed a formula for preterm infants until they weigh at least 2,000 g, and then an enriched "post-discharge formula" that is higher in calories and

micronutrients per ounce than that designed for term infants. Such enriched formulas are more expensive than term formula and may be difficult for economically stressed families to afford unless the family receives a physician's prescription to WIC. In general, these post-discharge formulas should be continued until 9 to 12 months corrected age or minimally until the baby's weight for length is maintained above the 25th percentile.[108]

Formerly premature children who show depressed weight for height or whose growth progressively deviates from a channel parallel to the NCHS norms should be assessed carefully for potentially correctable (and sometimes iatrogenic) causes of growth failure. These causes may include inappropriate feeding practices for corrected age, such as early discontinuation of post-discharge formula or initiation of solid feedings at 6 months postnatal age for an infant born at 28 weeks whose corrected age is only 3 months. In addition, the neurologic, gastrointestinal, and cardiorespiratory sequelae of prematurity, as well as the behavioral disorganization characteristic of some premature infants, may all contribute to postnatal malnutrition. Growth difficulties should not be discounted in such children on the grounds that they were "born small." In addition to affecting the infant's behavior or physical growth potential directly, prematurity and low birth weight also may act indirectly to increase the risk of growth failure by intensifying family stress and requiring early separation between parents and child for neonatal intensive care.

Intrauterine Growth Retardation

Size at birth reflects both the duration and the rate of growth during gestation. Infants whose rate of intrauterine growth is depressed are at risk for postnatal growth failure, regardless of gestational age. Intrauterine growth retardation (IUGR) is conventionally defined as birth weight less than the 10th percentile for gestational age. The degree of risk for postnatal growth failure after IUGR is not uniform, varying with both the cause of the IUGR and the pattern of relative deficit in length, weight, or head circumference at birth.

The best prognosis for postnatal growth pertains to infants with asymmetrical IUGR, whose weight at birth is disproportionately more depressed than their length or head circumference. Such infants are at risk for FTT because they are often behaviorally difficult.[109] With enhanced postnatal nutrition, however, they can manifest significant catch-up growth in the first 6 to 8 months of life so that later growth trajectories may be within the normal range.[109,110] For such infants, early identification of growth failure and intensive nutritional and environmental intervention are critical because the potential for catch-up growth to repair the intrauterine deficit is maximal in the first 6 months of life.[111,112]

Infants with symmetrical IUGR, whose weight, length, and head circumference are proportionately depressed at birth, carry a relatively poor prognosis for later growth and development. A symmetrical pattern of IUGR should alert the clinician to the possibility of chromosomal abnormalities, intrauterine infections, or prenatal teratogen exposure. For this reason, symmetrically growth-retarded children should be carefully scrutinized for dysmorphic features that may provide clues to syndrome diagnosis. Exposure to anticonvulsants, including hydantoin and valproate sodium, may be associated with symmetrical IUGR and dysmorphic features.[113] Prenatal exposure to legal and illegal psychoactive substances during pregnancy often contributes to symmetrical IUGR, but the prognostic implications for later growth, particularly somatic growth, are variable.[114] Because the issue of prenatal substance exposure and later growth potential is often raised in protective service cases, it warrants discussion in some detail.

Prenatal Exposure to Legal Psychoactive Substances and Later Growth

Although heavy use of caffeine prenatally is associated in some studies with depressed intrauterine growth, such use has no detectable effects on the later size of exposed infants.[115] Some investigators, but not all, have noted correlations between heavy cigarette exposure during pregnancy and statistically significant decrements in stature at school age, but the magnitude of the deficit (1–2 cm) is usually not large enough to trigger referral for FTT.[116–118] Postnatal use of fluoxetine in breastfeeding women was associated with some reduction in infant weight gain between 2 weeks and 6 months.[119] The effects of prenatal alcohol exposure are variable. Growth deficits persist from infancy to school age in children with dysmorphic features consistent with fetal alcohol syndrome, and in lower (but not higher) income children who were exposed to alcohol in the womb yet are not dysmorphic.[118,120–122] Length and head circumference are more depressed than weight in such cases.[118,123]

Although fetal alcohol syndrome, and perhaps fetal alcohol spectrum disorder, constrains postneonatal growth, clinicians also must remain alert to potentially treatable postneonatal medical and psychosocial factors that may prevent children with fetal alcohol syndrome or other intrauterine exposures from attaining their limited growth potential. As with very low birth weight infants, children with fetal alcohol syndrome in whom rate of growth deviates from their own previously established patterns should be evaluated meticulously.[124] Neurologically based oral-motor difficulties are often associated with fetal alcohol syndrome and may limit caloric intake, unless gastrostomy tubes are placed.[125] Even more commonly, the growth of children with fetal alcohol syndrome who remain in the care of mothers with active untreated alcoholism shows effects of inadequate care and nutrition. Such children should not remain in conditions of profound deprivation on the grounds that they have fetal alcohol syndrome and "can't grow." Our clinical experience shows that with appropriate nutritional, neurodevelopmental, and psychosocial intervention, children with fetal alcohol syndrome and fetal alcohol spectrum disorder can be brought into the normal range of weight for height, but may remain short and microcephalic despite intervention.

Prenatal Exposure to Illicit Psychoactive Substances and Later Growth

Until recently, the 3 most frequently used illicit drugs during pregnancy were marijuana, cocaine, and opiates. Increasing concern is now focusing on methamphetamine exposure during pregnancy. Unfortunately, few follow-up studies of the growth of infants exposed to marijuana, cocaine, or opiates beyond the neonatal period have been performed, and none, to our knowledge, have been published regarding children with intrauterine exposure to methamphetamines. Infants exposed to marijuana during pregnancy have been reported as having a decreased weight and length, and sometimes a decreased head circumference, compared with unexposed newborns, presumably because smoking marijuana, like smoking tobacco, increases maternal carbon monoxide levels, and decreases fetal oxygenation.[126–128] In one long-term follow-up study, children at age 6 years were found to have decreased heights correlated with prenatal marijuana exposure.[127] However, in a similar study of prenatal marijuana exposure, children with a history of prenatal marijuana exposure had weights and lengths significantly greater than their non-exposed peers, even after controlling for confounding variables.[97,129] Therefore, it is unclear if prenatal marijuana exposure is a biological risk factor for later FTT, and clinicians should not dismiss FTT in these children by attributing it to prenatal marijuana exposure.

Prenatal cocaine exposure is independently associated with decrements in gestational age, and with consistently lower birth weight, length, and head circumference.[127,130–133] At age 7 to 16 weeks, no difference was found in feeding behaviors between infants who were exposed prenatally to cocaine and those who were not exposed.[134] If levels of exposure to cigarettes and alcohol are not controlled statistically, researchers have noted small but statistically significant decrements in head circumference and, in one cohort, in weight, among prenatally cocaine-exposed children followed up until age 3 years.[130,135] However, in 2 studies that controlled statistically for the level of prenatal exposure to tobacco and alcohol, no negative effect of prenatal cocaine exposure was noted on weight, height, or head circumference.[131,136] Accelerated rates of postneonatal weight gain have been noted after prenatal cocaine exposure.[130–133] Therefore, clinicians should not accept prenatal exposure to cocaine as a sufficient explanation for postnatal failure to gain weight.

Prenatal exposure to heroin or methadone also has been linked to depressed birth weight, length, and head circumference, but follow-up studies of the growth patterns of these infants are not entirely consistent. Wilson et al[137] reported that 3- to 6-year-old children prenatally exposed to heroin were smaller in all growth parameters than were nonexposed social class controls. In most studies, however, smaller head circumference but few differences in somatic growth were noted when prenatally opiate-exposed infants were compared with children of the same social class without intrauterine opiate exposure.[138]

Growth failure in any child of a mother with a history of illicit substance use, particularly intravenous use, mandates assessment to rule out HIV infection because FTT is a common symptom in infected children.[139,140] The quality of care the child is receiving at the time of referral also must be evaluated because continued parental substance abuse may be contributing to concurrent nutritional deprivation of the child. Even though prenatal exposure to psychoactive substances may cause a decrease in birth weight, length, and head circumference, most such substances do not inhibit a child from showing postnatal somatic catch-up growth in response to adequate nutrition.[114] Heavy prenatal exposure to alcohol or opiates may be associated with relative microcephaly, and fetal alcohol syndrome is characterized by persistent short stature. However, prenatal exposure to the most commonly used psychoactive substances does not adequately explain a child who is underweight for height or one whose growth progressively deviates from a previously established trajectory.

Postnatal Medical Issues

Almost all severe and chronic childhood illnesses can cause growth failure. The mechanisms of such failure are multiple enzymatic, metabolic, and endocrine in some cases, but also nutritional and psychosocial.[141, 142] Chronic physical problems that necessitate procedures such as gastrostomy or nasogastric feedings may impede the development of normal feeding patterns.

Hospitalization should not be regarded as a diagnostic test for chronic illness.[143]

According to an old myth, environmentally deprived children (nonorganic FTT) grow in the hospital, whereas children with serious medical illnesses (organic FTT) will not. In fact, a positive growth response to hospitalization poorly differentiates major organic illness from environmental risk because children with such illness and children with primary malnutrition will grow if given adequate caloric intake.[144] Chronically ill children who do well in the hospital usually have complex technical, psychosocial, and nutritional needs that can be met by multiple shifts of highly trained medical personnel, but overwhelm parents who are not receiving adequate caretaking support at home. Conversely, unless the hospital provides specialized milieu therapy, usually not available on acute care wards, children with severe interactive feeding disorders or depression may deteriorate nutritionally in the hospital because separation from primary attachment figures and multiple caretakers may exacerbate their affective and behavioral feeding difficulties. Children who are simply underfed do well either in the hospital or in any setting when adequate calories are offered. Thus response to hospitalization in itself does not necessarily contribute to identifying the cause of FTT.

Whether in inpatient or outpatient settings, chronic illnesses severe enough to jeopardize growth usually can be ascertained from a meticulous history and physical examination (Boxes 15.2 and 15.3). The list of occult medical conditions presenting as FTT is relatively circumscribed, and often these are identified during the review of systems (Box 15.2), focusing on infections and conditions that interfere with caloric intake or use. In a series of children hospitalized for FTT of unknown origin, the most common previously undiagnosed illnesses were gastrointestinal, including chronic nonspecific diarrhea, celiac disease, food allergies, gastroesophageal reflux, cystic fibrosis, and lactose intolerance.[17,145–149] Immigrant children and children attending congregate child care or living in homeless shelters should be evaluated for giardiasis and enteric pathogens if they have gastrointestinal symptoms such as

BOX 15.2
Child's Family and Postneonatal Health History

Midparental height

Consanguinity

Heritable conditions

Immunizations

Allergies

Surgeries

Hospitalizations

Current medications

Review of systems

Timing of onset of growth faltering
  Weight loss
  Diarrhea/vomiting
  Dysphagia
  Snoring, difficulty with tonsils or
    adenoids
  Recurring pneumonia, otitis, or sinusitis
  Painful teeth
  Loss of previously acquired milestones,
    seizures
  Thrush/recurrent monilial rash
  Atopic dermatitis, hives

Pets

Travel

Passive tobacco exposure

diarrhea or abdominal pain, because these are common causes of malabsorption and growth failure.[149,150] Outside the gastrointestinal system, clinicians should consider urinary tract infections and renal tubular acidosis as potentially clinically silent contributors to FTT. Subtle neurologic dysfunction manifested as fine and oral-motor dysfunction also should

be considered and evaluated by direct observation.[82]

Both overdiagnosis and underdiagnosis of "food allergy" can contribute to FTT.[151] In 1995 the European Academy of Allergy and Clinical Immunology created a standard terminology by which to assign a patient's reaction to a food.[152,153] Only those reactions that are the consequence of an immune response (immunoglobulin [Ig] E mediated) to a food or food additive are formally considered to be food allergies,[153,154] whereas a non–IgE-mediated immune reaction is classified as *adverse food reactions* or *food sensitivity*.[153,155] An exceedingly restrictive diet based on an imprecise or factitious diagnosis of food allergy may present as FTT.[151] It is crucial that the cause of an apparent adverse reaction to a food be aggressively sought. Whereas negative skin tests are 95% accurate, positive tests are only 50% accurate and must be confirmed by history or a food challenge.[153] It may take as long as 14 days to see a clinical response to an elimination diet. A double-blind, placebo-controlled food challenge is the gold standard for food allergy diagnosis, but may not always be practical in primary care settings.[156] Alternative or additional methods such as radioallergosorbent (RAST) tests may be easier to obtain.[147,156] The physician should be aware that *Helicobacter pylori*, other infections, and celiac disease may be manifested by the same symptoms as food allergies.[147,153,155,157,158] Conversely, 30% of atopic dermatitis in young children is triggered by food allergy, so that evaluation for food allergy should be considered in any child with FTT and

BOX 15.3
Physical Examination

Vital signs: blood pressure if older than 2, temperature, pulse, respirations

Anthropometry (See Table 15.1.)

General appearance: activity, affect, posture

Skin: hygiene, rashes, trauma (bruises, burns, scars)

Head: hair whorls, color and pluckability of hair, occipital alopecia, fontanel size and patency, frontal bossing, sutures, shape, facial dysmorphisms

Eyes: ptosis, strabismus, funduscopic where possible, palpebral fissures, conjunctival pallor

Ears: external form, rotation, tympanic membranes

Mouth, nose, throat: hydration, dental eruption and hygiene caries, glossitis, cheilosis, gum bleeding

Neck: hairline, masses, lymphadenopathy

Abdomen: protuberance, hepatosplenomegaly, masses

Genitalia: malformations, hygiene, trauma

Rectum: fissures, trauma, hemorrhoids

Extremities: edema, dysmorphisms, rachitic changes, nails and nail beds

Neurologic: cranial nerves, reflexes, tone, retention of primitive reflexes, quality of voluntary movement eczema. Because children often "outgrow" their adverse reaction to a food by age 3 years, such evaluations should be repeated periodically so that the child's diet does not remain unnecessarily restricted.[153,156,159]

In recent years the differential diagnosis of FTT has expanded to include HIV infection. This diagnosis should be considered particularly in children whose mothers have a history of illicit psychoactive substance use, have had multiple sexual partners, or are sexual partners of substance-abusing or bisexual men. The diagnosis also must be ruled out in children of immigrants from areas where heterosexual transmission of HIV is endemic and when the child or mother, or her sexual partner, has had a blood transfusion.[140]

In addition to primary illnesses that may be associated with secondary malnutrition and growth failure, the clinician must be alert to the medical complications of primary malnutrition, particularly recurring infections and lead poisoning. Malnutrition severe enough to produce growth failure also impairs immunocompetence, particularly cell-mediated immunity and the production of complement and secretory IgA.[160-162] Recurring otitis media and gastrointestinal and respiratory illnesses are more common among children who fail to thrive than among well-nourished children of the same age.[30,163-165] Children who fail to thrive are often trapped in an infection-malnutrition cycle. With each illness, the child's appetite and nutrient intake decrease while nutrient requirements

increase as a result of fever, diarrhea, and vomiting. In settings in which nutrient intake is already marginal, even when the child is well, cumulative nutritional deficits occur, leaving the child increasingly vulnerable to more severe and prolonged infections and even less adequate growth. Commonly in developing countries and occasionally in developed countries, malnourished children succumb to fulminating infections.

Elevated lead levels correlate with impaired growth, even in the 5- to 35-mg/dL range.[166] Here, too, a negative cycle develops. Nutritional deficiencies of iron and calcium enhance the absorption of lead and other heavy metals.[167] As lead levels rise, constipation, abdominal pain, and anorexia occur, leading to even less adequate dietary intake.[168] In one study, 16% of children with FTT had lead levels high enough to warrant chelation.[169]

Physical Examination and Laboratory Evaluation

The physical examination of the child who fails to thrive (Box 15.3) has 3 goals: (a) identification of chronic illness, (b) recognition of syndromes that alter growth, and (c) documentation of the effects of malnutrition. Some findings may be nonspecific and require elucidation by laboratory assessment. For example, hepatic enlargement may be seen with primary malnutrition, acquired immunodeficiency syndrome, or underlying liver disease.

Laboratory evaluation should be restrained and guided by history and the findings of the physical examination. For example, a child who has no symptoms of cardiorespiratory distress or heart murmur does not need an electrocardiogram. Basic laboratory studies should be used to identify derangements caused by malnutrition and to rule out the potentially occult diseases just described.[102] All children should have a complete blood count, assessment of lead and free erythrocyte protoporphyrin levels, urinalysis, and a tuberculin test. Iron deficiency is a common finding. If the child does not respond promptly to nutritional intervention, blood urea nitrogen, creatinine, and serum electrolytes should be measured. These tests also are mandatory in children with vomiting or diarrhea, clinically obvious dehydration, or third-degree malnutrition, which is often associated with hypokalemia. In children with severe anthropometric deficits, it is useful to obtain an albumin level to assess protein status and to determine alkaline phosphatase, calcium, and phosphorus levels. A depressed alkaline phosphatase value suggests zinc deficiency; an elevated level, especially if associated with a depressed phosphorous value, is suggestive of rickets.[170] Human immunodeficiency virus testing, sweat test, and stool assessments for *Giardia* or other parasites should be performed in epidemiologically at-risk populations, including children with recent travel to or emigration from endemic areas.[139,140,160] Serum IgA and antitransglutaminase antibodies screen for celiac disease[171] can identify a potentially occult cause of poor growth. RAST or skin testing for food allergies should be considered in children with

FTT and atopic dermatitis, as well as for those with a history of rash, urticaria, or recurring vomiting and diarrhea after ingestion of selected foods. In a child with FTT and vomiting not explained by food allergies and unresponsive to empiric management, radiographic, pH probe, or endoscopic studies may be indicated to rule out anatomical abnormalities, gastroesophageal reflux, and esophagitis, particularly among children with neurologic impairments and unexplained respiratory symptoms.[96] For short children with weight proportionate to height, bone-age radiographic studies of the wrists and knees are helpful in discriminating those who are constitutionally short (bone age equals chronological age and is greater than height age) from those with growth hormone or thyroid deficiencies or chronic malnutrition (bone age equals height age and is less than chronological age).[142,172] Children with enlarged livers should have liver functions evaluated. Careful physical examination will usually identify untreated dental cavities and abscesses that make eating and chewing painful and lead to inadequate caloric intake.[173,174] Large tonsils or chronic snoring warrant ear, nose, and throat evaluation and possibly a sleep study because tonsilloadenohypertrophy and sleep-disordered breathing may contribute to growth failure.[108] Furthermore, it is important to observe a feeding because subtle oral-motor difficulties may interfere with dietary intake in children with otherwise subclinical neurologic abnormalities.[81,82]

Medical Management

The pediatric health care provider should play an ongoing role in the management of children with FTT. Children must be seen more frequently than is dictated by routine health management schedules to monitor their growth and development in response to interventions. Weekly visits often may be necessary at the beginning of diagnosis and treatment. Meticulous management of concurrent chronic illness is essential, enlisting and coordinating assessments in as many disciplines as necessary. Lead poisoning, if identified, should be treated according to standard protocols.[125]

The health care provider must take an aggressive stance to interrupt the infection-malnutrition cycle. In addition to all immunizations routinely recommended by the AAP, the influenza vaccine is indicated in children with FTT even after the age of 5 years because of their nutritional depletion.[160] Families should be instructed to seek care at the first signs of infection so that immediate workup and treatment are provided. Recurring otitis media or sinusitis is an indication for otolaryngologic referral. In addition, for each episode of acute illness, the clinician should provide specific instruction about appropriate diet during and after the illness to try to maintain and repair nutritional status. A child should never receive a clear liquid diet for more than 24 hours.[149]

Hospitalization is indicated for severely malnourished children, for children with serious intercurrent infections, for those whose safety is in question, or if the specialized coordination of disciplines or diagnostic procedures is necessary and can be assembled most efficiently inside the hospital. In many centers, the availability of interdisciplinary outpatient clinics for the diagnosis and management of FTT has greatly reduced the need for hospitalization.[175] Referral for specialized, interdisciplinary outpatient assessment should be considered, however, for any child who has not responded to 2 or 3 months of intensive management in a primary care setting.

Nutritional/Behavioral Evaluation and Treatment

The major components of a nutritional history for a child who is failing to thrive are summarized in Box 15.4. The assessment should focus not only on current feeding practices, but also on the development of feeding since birth. Often a child's growth failure is triggered by a shift in feeding practices. For example, the shift from soy formula to whole milk at age 12 months, as mandated by the WIC program, may trigger FTT in a severely lactose-intolerant or milk protein–allergic child.[176] In many children, feeding struggles and growth failure begin with the introduction of solid foods at age 5 to 7 months. In rare instances, the introduction of gluten-containing cereals triggers celiac disease and growth failure. Thus comparison of the lifelong feeding history with the growth curve can provide diagnostic clues to the nutritional risk factors in FTT.

In assessing current feeding practices of the child who fails to thrive, the

BOX 15.4
Nutritional Evaluation Protocol

Interview

Feeding history adjusted for age
    Breast or formula
    Age solids introduced
    Age switched to whole milk
    Food allergy or intolerance
    Vitamin or mineral supplements
    Complementary or alternative supplements

Current feeding behaviors
    Difficulties with sucking, chewing, or swallowing
    Frequency of feeding
    Who feeds
    Where fed (alone or held, with or separate from family, lap or high chair)
    Finickiness, negativism
    Perceived appetite
    Pica

Caretaker's nutrition knowledge
    Difficulties with English or literacy
    Religious or cultural beliefs influencing feeding
    Adequacy of developmentally appropriate nutrition information
    Unusual dietary belief (food fad constraints on permitted foods): Are some foods perceived
        as dangerous?

Adequacy of financial resources for food purchase
    Food stamps: How much/month for how many people?
    WIC
    Adequacy of earned income
    Benefits: TANF, SSI
    Recent change in food budget (cuts or increases in benefits, new mouths to feed, job gain
        or loss)
    Family's knowledge of how to budget food purchasing

Material resources for food preparation and storage
    Refrigeration
    Cooking facilities
    Running water
    24-hour dietary recall: Was yesterday typical?

Food frequency

Abbreviations: WIC, Special Supplemental Nutrition Program for Women, Infants, and Children; TANF, Transitional Aid to Needy Families; SSI, Supplemental Security Income.

clinician should ascertain when, where, how, and by whom the child is fed, as well as what the child is fed and why. Comprehensive assessment of feeding problems requires a combination of methods such as structured interviews with primary caregivers and direct observation of the child's response to feeding in multiple situations. Caregivers should be asked to complete an oral or written checklist of possible behavioral feeding problems (eg, spitting out food, tantrums during meals, food refusal), to supply a few days of food-intake records, and to indicate how the parents have tried to manage the child's problems.[177-179] Parental interactions with and response to their children during mealtimes should be assessed to determine the interrelationship among specific child problem behaviors, parental responses, and antecedent cues. Ideally, history should be supplemented by a home-based feeding observation that will elucidate not only interactive or mechanical feeding difficulties but also the material conditions of the home and family routines.[180]

Heptinstall et al[181] found that inconsistent timing of the presentation of meals and dysfunctional mealtime procedures, such as solitary meals without supervision, occurred more frequently in growth-deficient children than in normal controls. Common sources of difficulty in the timing of feedings include infrequent feedings (restricting a toddler to 3 meals a day), constant feedings (grazing), and lack of a consistent feeding schedule. Children are often fed in inappropriate settings, which may or may not be under the parents' control. For example, children from very low-income families may have to be fed sitting on the floor or the bed because there is nowhere else to sit. Conversely, many parents can be encouraged to put the child in a high chair or booster seat, when one is available, and not to position the child in front of the television or other distractions during feeding. A hammer-lock hold in a parent's lap is usually ineffective and uncomfortable for both parent and child. A home observation also will elucidate the affective tone of the feeding process and identify dysfunctional interactions, such as interrupting the feeding too often to clean the child, struggles over the child's efforts to feed independently, or inappropriate coaxing or threatening of the child. Efforts should be made to identify all the different caretakers (relatives, neighbors, siblings, child care providers, etc) involved in feeding the child and to enlist these individuals in improving the child's nutritional intake.

Serious deficits in age-appropriate feeding behavior, such as chewing, self-feeding, use of utensils, swallowing, or sucking, may benefit from intensive behavioral training or occupational therapy programs using procedures such as shaping, fading, and modeling to teach novel behaviors (eg, chewing for a child who has had prolonged pureed feedings) or to enhance adaptive feeding responses.[177,178,181] Disruptive behaviors such as tantrums, expelling food, selective food refusal, attempting to leave the table or high chair, throwing food, whining, or crying may improve after application of learning-treatment methods such as extinction, time-out, and the contingent application of reinforcers, such as parental attention.[182] Inappropriate parental responses such as coaxing, threatening, or "giving in" to the child's demands by terminating the meal or allowing the child to eat only preferred items reinforce these maladaptive behaviors and should be modified.[183]

In addition to how the child is fed, the clinician must ascertain what the child is fed and why. The family's level of nutritional knowledge and dietary beliefs should be assessed. American parents and children are continually bombarded with nutritional misinformation from television and other commercial sources urging them to spend their scant food resources on expensive heavily sweetened or salted foods of low nutritional quality.[184–186] Certain groups of parents, particularly adolescents and those who are intellectually limited, illiterate, or unable to speak English, are particularly likely to lack adequate information regarding nutritionally sound feeding practices. Immigrants are at risk unless they are able to obtain culturally appropriate foods. Most ethnic diets are adequate, but when traditional foods are unavailable, immigrants may not know what to select from the foods available in American markets. Parents also may offer children an inadequate, strictly vegetarian diet because of adherence to unusual dietary practices prescribed by a nontraditional religion or food fads, such as macrobiotics.[187] Parents seeking to prevent obesity or cardiovascular disease also may inadvertently cause their toddlers to fail to thrive by overzealous enforcement of a low-fat, "prudent diet" appropriate for adults, but not for growing children.[188] Restricted diets imposed because of actual or presumed food allergies often are not adequately supplemented with alternate sources of calories and micronutrients, with consequent nutritional deficiencies.[153]

The family's economic resources for food purchase, food storage, and food preparation must be tactfully ascertained. A 24-hour dietary recall and 7-day food frequency are essential in determining the quality and quantity of the child's diet. Common findings among children with FTT include excessive intake of juice, water, tea, or carbonated and sweetened beverages, which depress appetite but provide few nutrients. In addition, fruit juices high in fructose or sorbitol have been associated with malabsorption and osmotic diarrhea in some cases of FTT.[189,190] Low-income families may have particular difficulties in meeting the needs of children with increased nutritional needs (such as children born prematurely or children with significant heart or lung disease) or those with restricted and, therefore, more expensive diets, as in the cases of multiple food allergies, lactose intolerance, or gluten-sensitive enteropathy.[155,191]

Anthropometric Assessment

Serial anthropometric assessments are critical to the management of FTT. Initial measurements of the growth trajectory form the basis for triage and calculation of caloric needs, as well as providing some prognostic information for later developmental potential. Frequent follow-up assessments also provide the clearest indication of the effectiveness of intervention.

Children referred for FTT must be measured in a standard fashion by trained personnel using the same scale at each measurement, according to published protocols for obtaining accurate and reproducible anthropometric measurements.[1,12,192,193] Infants should be weighed naked, and young children should wear underwear only.

Weight for age is commonly used in pediatric clinics to track children's growth and is an excellent indicator of changes in weight over time.[194] However, weight for age is difficult to interpret because it does not account for variations in height.[195] When a child's weight for age is low, it is not clear whether the primary problem is low weight, short stature, or a combination. Weight for height (weight plotted by height regardless of age) reflects body proportionality. The update of the growth charts by the NCHS in 2000 included body mass index (BMI) for children older than 2 years (BMI = weight in kilograms/height in centimeters squared). These growth charts are available online at www.cdc.gov/growthcharts. By international consensus, the NCHS growth charts serve currently as the references for evaluating growth in young children regardless of ethnic or racial background.[39] These recently revised growth charts eliminate the discontinuity between recumbent length and standing height and provide percentile lines above and beyond the fifth and 95th percentiles.[196] It is important to note that despite their accepted use, these references include an unknown number of ill and deprived children and thus may be imprecise tools for identifying aberrant growth.[39] The World Health Organization has recently developed standards for expected growth from a multiethnic, multinational sample restricted to healthy, initially breastfed children, and growth charts are now available at www.who.int/childgrowth/software/en/. As of this writing they are not yet approved for clinical use in the United States.

Low weight for height, or wasting, is often an early sign of malnutrition and may reflect low caloric intake. Chronic malnutrition may result in decelerated skeletal growth, indicated by low height for age, or stunting. Thus weight for height and height for age provide a nonredundant, comprehensive picture of growth.[195,197] When constitutional, endocrine, and genetic factors can be ruled out, depressed height for age is considered a manifestation of the cumulative effects of chronic malnutrition.[165] Children at highest risk are those for whom both weight for height and height for age are depressed, indicating acute malnutrition superimposed on a chronic problem.

There are special growth charts for very premature infants.[105] Another option is to use standard growth charts and correct for prematurity. Recommendations are to adjust for gestational age up to 24 months on weight, 40 months on height, and 18 months on head circumference.[198]

Weight for age, weight for height, and height for age can be expressed as percentile scores, SD scores, or percentage of median scores. Percentile scores are commonly used clinically because they are relatively easy to interpret, but are less useful when describing variations at the extremes (eg, less than fifth percentile). SD scores (Z-scores) are commonly used for analyses because they can be used to characterize extremes and facilitate comparisons across ages.[195] Percentage of median scores are often used to describe change and are calculated by dividing the child's weight (or height) by the median expected weight (or height) (50th percentile) based on the child's chronological (or corrected for prematurity) age. A useful clinical technique, initially devised by Kaplowitz and Webb,[195] Waterlow,[165] and Gomez[189] is to categorize the child's malnutrition as first (mild), second (moderate), or third (severe) degree based on their weight for age, height for age, and weight for height percentage of median (Table 15.1). Children with third-degree malnutrition (weight for age <60% of median, or weight for height <70% of median) are in acute danger of severe morbidity and possible mortality from their malnutrition and should usually be hospitalized. At present, the standard NCHS growth charts are cross-sectional for monitoring weight gain over time, and therefore do not fully illustrate the magnitude of changes in a child's weight relative to height.[12]

The goal of nutritional intervention in FTT is to achieve catch-up growth (ie, growth at a faster than normal rate for age so that the child's relative deficit of body size is restored). If the child with an established growth deficit simply resumes growth at the normal rate for age, relative deficits persist compared with children of the same age who have always grown normally. To assess whether catch-up growth is occurring, the clinician must be aware of age-specific changes in normal growth rates, as summarized by Guo et al[196]; these are not altered by the new edition of the NCHS norms.[196] In the first 3 months of life, median weight gain averages 26 to 31 g/d; from 3 to 6 months, 17 to 18 g/d; from 6 to 9 months, 12 to 13 g/d; from 9 to 12 months, 9 g/d; and from 12 months onward, 7 to 9 g/d. A goal for catch-up growth may be as much as 2 to 3 times the average rate of weight gain for corrected age. Thus a 1-year-old child who is gaining 30 g/d is showing excellent catch-up growth, whereas a 1-month-old child who also is gaining 30 g/d is growing at only the normal rate for age and will not repair existing deficits. The goal for catch-up growth must be continually revised as the child matures and gradually decreases as the child's weight for height approaches the target level.

TABLE 15.1
Percentage Medial as Indicator of Severity of Nutritional Deficit

Grade of Malnutrition	Weight for Age	Height for Age	Weight for Height
Normal	90–110	>95	>90
First degree (mild)	75–89	90–94	80–90
Second degree (moderate)	60–74	85–89	70–79
Third degree (severe)	<60	<85	<70

Principles of Nutritional Treatment

To achieve catch-up growth, the underweight child must receive nutrients in excess of the normal age-specific requirements of the RDAs.[200] Daily caloric needs for catch-up growth in calories per kilogram can be estimated as follows: kilocalories per kilogram = 120 kcal/kg × median weight for current height divided by current weight (kg).[201] In most cases, according to this calculation, children require 1.5 to 2 times the expected intake for their age to achieve optimal catch-up growth.[20,182,201] Protein intake should be enhanced in similar proportions to permit maximal growth.[201]

Nutritional rehabilitation must address the child's needs for micronutrients as well as calories and protein. Iron deficiency, with or without associated anemia, may be seen in children presenting with FTT.[1] Vitamin D–deficiency rickets also has been described.[170] Even among children whose micronutrient stores are adequate at initial presentation with FTT, the demand of rapid tissue synthesis during catch-up growth may produce nutritional deficiencies. Even if zinc status cannot be measured, zinc supplementation should be provided to meet the RDA because such supplementation has been shown to decrease the energy cost of weight gain.[19,202,203] A multivitamin supplement containing the RDA for all vitamins and for iron and zinc should, therefore, be prescribed routinely for children with FTT during nutritional rehabilitation, with additional supplementation of iron or vitamin D to therapeutic levels in children with iron deficiency or rickets.[204] Use of a once-a-day vitamin supplement also is useful to reduce pressure on caretakers to ensure that their child is receiving a completely balanced diet. Caretakers will no longer have to worry about whether their child is eating green beans or other low-calorie vegetables as a source of vitamins and can focus on ensuring adequate intake of minerals, fiber, calories, and protein.

In general it is not possible for a child to eat twice the normal volume of food to obtain the nutrient levels necessary for catch-up growth. Instead the child's usual diet must be fortified to increase nutrient density (eg, providing formula of 24–30 cal/oz rather than the standard 20 cal/oz). There are at least 2 supplementation options for children aged 1 to 6 years. Two prepackaged 30 cal/oz preparations, one milk-based and one soy-based, are now commercially available. Like investigators in developing countries, we have found such preparations to be well accepted, well tolerated for rapid weight gain, and effective when its cost can be subsidized by health insurance or other mechanisms.[200] Because these formulas do not require parental preparation and are often perceived by families as "medicine" exclusively for the use of the child with FTT, it can be used effectively in high-risk families who otherwise have difficulties in preparing appropriately enriched diets for their child. However, 2 issues complicate the use of the product. First, it is very expensive for families who do not qualify for insurance or public assistance. Second, WIC will provide the special preparation or the food package, not both, although this problem may be alleviated by anticipated change in the WIC regulations in 2007 or 2008. For children who tolerate lactose and milk protein, there is another commercially available instant breakfast product, sold in the cereal section of grocery stores, that provides the same number of calories, vitamins, and minerals when mixed with whole milk as the prepackaged preparation. Some families find it more economical to purchase this product and continue to receive the food package from WIC. Detailed protocols for other methods of dietary supplementation have been published elsewhere.[182] The participation of an experienced pediatric nutritionist is critical in developing a dietary regimen appropriate for each child.

The process of refeeding to promote catch-up growth must be undertaken with some circumspection in children with third- degree and severe second-degree malnutrition. If high food intakes are provided at the beginning of nutritional resuscitation, these children may develop vomiting, diarrhea, and circulatory decompensation.[201,205] To minimize these complications, such children should, for the first 7 to 10 days of treatment, be restricted to the normal dietary intake for age, offered as frequent small feedings. In severe cases requiring hospitalization, clinicians need to be aware that this may not coincide with cafeteria schedules and may require scheduling of additional feedings. Intake may then be gradually advanced over the next week to a diet that meets the calculated requirements for catch-up growth. Moderately and mildly malnourished children may be

offered food ad libitum while calorie counts are maintained. Once a baseline of spontaneous intake is established, preferred foods may be enriched to bring dietary intake to catch-up levels.

Depending on the severity of initial deficit, 2 days to 2 weeks may be required to initiate catch-up growth.[20] Less severely malnourished children should be monitored frequently as outpatients during this phase. Accelerated growth must then be maintained for 4 to 9 months to restore a child's weight for height.[20,200] Biweekly to monthly outpatient visits for weight checks, adjustment of diet, monitoring of feeding practices and behavior, and treatment of intercurrent medical problems are essential during this period. Intake and rates of growth spontaneously decelerate toward normal levels for age as deficits are replenished. Because weight is restored more rapidly than height, caretakers may become alarmed that the child is becoming overweight. They should be reassured that the catch-up growth in height lags behind that in weight by several months, but balance will occur if dietary treatment is not prematurely terminated.[7,144,175] However, growth and feeding patterns should be monitored closely to ensure that families are not adopting maladaptive patterns that may lead to overweight. In our programs, the anthropometric criterion for discharge from a specialized outpatient program is when the child is able to maintain weight for height above the 10th percentile and a normal rate of weight gain for age on at least 2 assessments, 1 month apart, on a normal diet for age (ie, the weight for height deficit is repaired, and the child no longer requires an especially enriched diet to sustain normal growth).

Psychosocial Issues in Evaluation and Treatment

Psychological Assessment

As shown in Table 15.2, a wide range of psychological functions, including intellectual and socioemotional development, may be affected by growth deficiency, malnutrition, and associated risk factors and should be documented in a comprehensive assessment approach.[62,206] Psychological assessment is best construed as a continuing process that begins with an initial or baseline assessment at the time the child's growth deficiency is first noticed and includes sequential assessments of the child's short- and longer-term responses to intervention.[62] One important purpose of assessment is to document the functional impact of the child's FTT, malnutrition, and associated risk factors on cognitive, motor, and socioemotional development and behavior. The second is to monitor the effects of treatment.

TABLE 15.2

Comprehensive Psychosocial Assessment of FTT

Area of Assessment	Method of Assessment	Information Obtained
Psychological status, cognitive development	Bayley Scales of Infant Development	Intellectual strengths and deficits relative to age norms
Social and affective-responsiveness	Behavioral observations and rating scales	Child's degree of social withdrawal: response to objects
Behavior during feeding	Behavioral observations and rating scales	Presence of behavioral feeding problems and skill deficits
Parent-child relationship	Observations of mother-child interaction	Strengths and deficits in parent-child relationship
Family environment Stimulation provided by family members	Observation of interaction with child; Home Scale	Level of stimulation provided
Family structure	Interview about family tree	Quality of family functioning and stability
Family resources	Interview about finances	Level of family resources and depletion
Family stress: relationships and support	Interview	Level of family stress: strengths and problems in family functioning
Parental beliefs about FTT	Interview	Parental beliefs about causes and consequences of FTT

Abbreviation: FTT, failure to thrive.

Intellectual and Motor Development

Children who experience prolonged malnutrition and/or chronic FTT seem to be at risk for intellectual and motor deficits severe enough to affect their learning potential.[31,42,93,207,208] The severity of developmental impairments varies substantially, however, among preschool and school-aged children with histories of early FTT.[8,25,207,209–215] Studies have underscored the central importance of a history of serious malnutrition as well as the quality of the home environment and compensatory educational experience in predicting the intellectual development of affected children in later life.[87,93,207,211,212,216–222]

Standardized infant assessment tests provide objective information concerning the child's strengths and weaknesses in intellectual and motor functioning.[61,62,223,224] Assessments are useful to determine children's eligibility for early intervention services. In addition, cognitive assessment data can be used to develop a program of stimulation that can be incorporated into a plan for home intervention. In addition, sequential assessments of cognitive and motor development are especially helpful to document progress in test performance after initial nutritional or psychological intervention and to plan additional interventions.[183]

Intellectual assessment can be a productive means of involving the parents of children with FTT in their child's treatment planning.[183] Observing their child's assessment helps parents appreciate the nature of their children's developmental strengths and weaknesses. When parents have observed developmental testing, it is also easier and more productive to discuss the pattern of their child's intellectual strengths and deficits with them. If parents are invited to discuss their child's development and participate in the evaluation, they are less defensive about the overall evaluative process.

In evaluating the child's development, the clinician should pay careful attention to the potential effects of the child's nutritional state on his or her response to test items. Infants who have experienced nutritional and/or stimulus deprivation are often withdrawn, which may severely limit their capacity to respond, at least initially.[26] Intellectual tests given shortly after referral may underestimate intellectual potential.

Socioemotional Development

Children with FTT are at risk for deficits in their socioemotional development. Although no one pattern of behavioral disturbance is associated with FTT, deficits in social responsiveness, affect, activity level, and avoidance of social contact have been noted by many observers.[31,70,213,225–230] Polan et al[67] found that children with FTT consistently demonstrated less positive affect in a range of situations than did normally growing children, and that acute and chronic malnutrition were associated with heightened negative affect.

Children with early histories of FTT have a higher incidence of insecure attachments characterized by anxious, avoidant, or disorganized behavior than do children with normal patterns of growth.[29,63,231] Valenzuela[232] suggested that the combination of the negative effects of malnutrition on children's reactivity to stress, coupled with the impact of such behaviors on the responsiveness of caregivers, might result in a vicious cycle that could eventually culminate in the development of a behavioral disorder. Controlled studies of children with early histories of FTT are consistent with this hypothesis, in that they suggest a continuing risk to socioemotional development beyond the point of initial diagnosis of FTT.[233] Areas of particular vulnerability among children with early histories of FTT and malnutrition include the ability to contain impulses and to organize their behavior.[21,23,24,76,207,211,216–218,225]

Because multiple areas of psychological development may be affected, a comprehensive assessment of several behavioral domains, including social responsiveness, affect, and response to feeding, is generally necessary for children with FTT. Structured instruments can be used to guide such observations. Rating scales such as the Bayley Behavioral Rating Scale assess the child's affective responsiveness and response to tasks during testing. Parent report scales, such as the Brief Infant Toddler Social Emotional Assessment (BITSEA)[234] assess clinically relevant aspects of children's behavioral style (eg, persistence, social responsiveness) during multiple situations. A comprehensive assessment of the child's behavior and emotional development can be used to generate a profile of behavioral strengths and deficits to guide treatment planning and evaluation of the child's progress. Ordinarily one would expect improvement in the child's social responsiveness and affect after nutritional treatment. Some children with FTT, however, continue to demonstrate significant deficits in responsiveness and/or problems in feeding that pose a salient burden to their caregivers and, hence, should be addressed in specialized intervention.

Assessment of the Family Environment

In addition to assessing the impact of FTT and associated risk factors on the child's psychological development, it also is necessary to assess aspects of the family environment (relationships, resources, and parent-child interaction) that would be expected to influence the child's response to medical and psychological intervention (Table 15.2). Given the impact of parent-child relationships on child development, observations of the parents' interactions with the child in a range of situations (feeding, teaching the child a skill, or free play) provides a useful method of assessment.[235,236] The patterns of parent-child relationships associated with FTT are complex and heterogeneous.[19,76,177,178,235,237] Deficient stimulation is one typical pattern; conflict and parental reinforcement of deviant behavior is another.[76,177,178] Several methods of assessment are available.[19,177,178] The Home Observation for Measurement of the Environment (HOME) Inventory is a reliable and valid measure of the level of stimulation provided to the child in the family environment.[19] Short questionnaire forms of the HOME Inventory are used in pediatric practice to assess the quality of the home environment.

One method of evaluating children's feeding skills and the parent-child relationship is to videotape parents and children having a meal. Parents may bring food or the clinic may provide food (eg, baby food, microwavable meals, applesauce, pudding, crackers, and milk). Feeding occurs in a room equipped with a high chair, child's table and chair, and adult chairs. Rating systems, such as the Behavioral Pediatrics Mealtime Observation Scale, are useful in characterizing the interaction between the parent and child.[238] Videotaping parents and children having a meal is an excellent way to identify family strengths and weaknesses and to enable families to use themselves as models in working toward behavior change.

The quality of relationships within the family, including the relationships and interactions of other family members with the child, can have an important influence on the child who fails to thrive. For this reason, focused and sensitive clinical assessments are needed to assess family feeding and cultural practices; routines and organization; finances; the quality of maternal relationships with other family members; and family members' perceptions of the causes, influences, and consequences of the child's FTT.[93,183] Clinical interviews are especially useful in helping family members share their ideas about what may be influencing the child's feeding, physical growth, and development, and to provide a context in which to observe fathers' and other family members' interactions with their children.[93,183] Because parents' appraisal of their child as "physically ill," "quiet," or "demanding" may influence their interactions with the child, it also is instructive to assess parents' perceptions of the child's need for interaction and nurturance.

Parental beliefs about food, children's size and health, nutritional needs, and family mealtime patterns may contribute to children's growth by influencing the availability of foods and the feeding atmosphere.[239] Approximately one-third of families of children with FTT do not recognize that their child has a growth problem.[240] Parents who do not believe that their child is experiencing a problem are unlikely to adhere to recommendations regarding behavior change. Participation in the process of constructing a genogram, a detailed and expanded family tree, is a useful way to help family members share their beliefs and impressions of family history and current relationships, and their child's growth and feeding patterns.

Intervention

The clinical management of FTT should be approached as a chronic condition requiring long-term multidisciplinary follow-up, with exacerbations and remissions expected. Successful intervention requires active team involvement of a pediatric health care provider, a pediatric nutritionist, a pediatric psychologist, and a social worker, with other professionals available as needed. The initial focus of interdisciplinary management is assessment of the child and family for purposes of planning treatment. Subsequently, the focus concerns intervention and ongoing monitoring of the child's progress. In an optimal team approach, professionals interact frequently and directly with the family and with each other, ideally in the context of scheduled clinic visits and case conferences. In addition, regular home visits by one or several of these professionals are effective to gather diagnostic information and provide ongoing support and guidance for the family.[18,241]

The first priority is to stabilize the child's acute medical problems and nutritional deficits, and to enhance as much as possible the material conditions of the home and family resources by helping parents to use federal feeding programs, referring them to local emergency relief programs, and providing advocacy around housing, heat, and other survival issues. Intervention includes attention to the family context, including mealtime routines and developmentally appropriate expectations and opportunities for children. For example, as children acquire the ability to pick up food (during the second 6 months of life), encouraging them to self-feed keeps their attention during meals and builds both confidence and competence. Because children learn to eat by modeling from others, family members should eat with children. Routines regarding meal and snack times enable children to anticipate when they will be eating and to avoid anxiety associated with hunger. Children need to eat frequently, but should not graze or eat continuously throughout the day. Parents are responsible for establishing mealtime routines and determining what and when food will be offered.[242] Children are responsible for determining how much they will eat. When children refuse to eat,

parents should calmly terminate the meal, rather than engaging in conflict, bribery, or force-feeding, and offer another feeding at the next scheduled time (during the day, usually no more than 2.5 hours from the previous feeding).

Eligibility and referral to early intervention or Head Start programs is often indicated to enhance the child's level of cognitive, motor, and social development and to reduce the risk for developmental problems in later life.[243] Children who have developmental disabilities in addition to FTT may be eligible for Supplemental Security Income (SSI) payments, which are frequently higher than those usually provided by Transitional Assistance to Needy Families. However, SSI standards for disability are strict and can be difficult to meet. Impoverished families should receive help in applying for these benefits. Moreover, whenever possible, services that supplement and structure the efforts of the primary caretaker, such as visiting nurses, trained homemakers, or respite day care, can be helpful and should be used. Various forms of mental health intervention, ranging from behavior modification of feeding problems to medication for a severely depressed parent to multigenerational family therapy, should be provided as indicated by the clinical assessment. Even after nutritional resuscitation has been achieved, families and children should be offered periodic reassessment as the child reaches school age to ensure early identification of behavioral or psychoeducational problems, which may require specialized educational services.

Long-term Follow-up

Bithoney et al[144] evaluated a multidisciplinary team-treatment approach including comprehensive assessment and treatment planning. This team included pediatricians, a pediatric nurse practitioner, a child development specialist, a pediatric gastroenterologist, and a social worker who delivered treatments including intensive case management and follow-up use of calorie-dense formulas and, when appropriate, referral for developmental stimulation, behavior modification (for eating disorders), visiting nurse, or homemaker services. Analysis of physical growth outcomes over a 6-month follow-up indicated that children with FTT who received the comprehensive, multidisciplinary team approach grew better than children with comparable physical growth deficits who received a typical management approach in a pediatric primary care clinic.[144]

Treatment is challenging. We identified 6 home visitation trials of various intensity and duration conducted among children with FTT; with most reporting marginal impact of this intervention on children's growth and development. Development seems to be more positively affected than growth. Haynes and colleagues[244] studied 50 hospitalized children with FTT and 26 adequately growing children and found no effect of short-term home visitation on the children's growth, development, or parent-child interaction patterns. Drotar and Eckerle[93] used a randomization procedure to assign children into 1 of 3 home intervention programs and found no difference in growth or cognitive performance at 3 years of age. The Infant Health and Development Project, a randomized clinical trial of home- and center-based intervention among infants who were either born preterm or had low birth weight (<2,500 g), provided the opportunity for an assessment of the outcomes of 180 children with FTT. Casey et al[105] found that children in the intervention and control groups were just as likely to experience FTT. Intervention was associated with better IQ scores and scores on the HOME Inventory at 36 months. In addition, intensity of intervention seemed to make a difference. Children with FTT who attended the child development center for more than 250 days had more optimal cognitive development, behavior, and linear growth than did children who attended for fewer than 250 days. Wright and colleagues[35] studied 229 children with FTT identified through community screening and showed that children assigned to the intervention group who received home health visitors as part of a multidisciplinary primary care practice were heavier and taller at age 3 years than children assigned to the control group.[35] Raynor and colleagues[245] enrolled 83 children with FTT and provided home visiting to 42. After 12 months, both groups experienced a significant increase in weight, but there were no differential effects of home visiting. Black and colleagues[87] conducted a weekly home-based intervention among 130 infants and toddlers with FTT recruited from primary care. After 1 year of intervention, there were no differences in height or weight, but the infants in the intervention group had better cognitive performance and caregivers who were more responsive and child-focused than infants in the control group.[241] Two years after the home intervention ended, when the children were 4 years of age, children in the intervention group had better cognitive scores and were more socially interactive than children in the control group, but only if their mothers were not depressed.[71] At age 8 years, children in the intervention group did not differ from a comparison group of adequately growing children from a similar socio-economic group,[246] both of whom were performing better than children with FTT in the control group.

Special Issues in Implementation

Parental Understanding of FTT and Acceptance of Clinical Management

To avoid overburdening families, practitioners set treatment priorities in collaboration with parents. Whenever possible, it is most useful to begin management with a problem that is salient to parents. In addition, goals for intervention should fit with the family's resources and understanding of the child's problem. Parents of infants with FTT may have difficulty participating actively and productively in their child's clinical management for several reasons. The suspicion that they may have contributed, however unwittingly, to their child's growth deficiency is threatening to most parents. In addition, parents may be so preoccupied with personal, family, or financial stresses that they fail to adhere to recommendations for treatment.[93]

Another reason that parents may have difficulty participating is that their

concepts of the etiology and appropriate treatment of their child's growth deficiency may differ substantially from those of professionals. For example, in contrast to professional concepts that FTT may relate to parental underfeeding or interactional problems, parents often focus on physical or biological explanations of this problem.[69] Sturm and Drotar[247] noted that maternal attributions of the FTT diagnosis included unspecified physical problems or illnesses (47%), specific physical problems (37% [eg, colitis, family problems]), constitutional (10% [eg, "meant to be small"]), and child behavior (7% [eg, food refusal]). Maternal perceptions of the physician's diagnosis most often included specific physical problems or growth difficulty rather than family or interactional problems. These findings suggested that mothers understood FTT predominantly as a physical or medical condition and had difficulty acknowledging the potential role of environmental factors. Parental perceptions that their child's FTT reflects physical rather than environmental problems may help to preserve their self-esteem. In addition, the co-occurrence of FTT with other physical symptoms and parental experiences with their child's hospitalization and extensive medical workup would be expected to reinforce their perceptions of the physical origins of FTT.

Differences in parent-practitioner concepts of the etiology and treatment of FTT may engender conflict and frustration and disrupt adherence to psychosocial treatment recommendations.[247] For example, parents who believe strongly that their child's growth deficiency is a physical problem may expect a physical rather than psychosocial treatment for this problem, and may require more explanation and support than parents who are able or willing to acknowledge the relevant environmental factors. For this reason, practitioners should provide comprehensive, integrated, interdisciplinary treatment to families, rather than segmented treatment that focuses on singular aspects of the problem, such as medical or nutritional, without attention to family or parent-child interactions.[248]

Enhancing Parental Participation in Assessment and Treatment Planning

Asking parents about their specific concerns regarding their child's problems may enhance their acceptance of assessment and eventually of an intervention plan. In addition, parents are more likely to accept a psychological or behavioral explanation of FTT if it is linked to their child's temperament, behavior, or sensitivities. For example, management of meals, food selection, or caloric requirements can be interpreted as ways that parents can meet their child's special needs.[183] Informing parents that their child may be especially sensitive to stress or events in family life also provides a rationale to evaluate the impact of family routines or parental relationships on the child's growth and nutrition.

Our experience suggests that the Katon and Kleinman[58] model of clinical negotiation is a useful framework in which to conduct clinical management with parents of children who fail to thrive.

To establish a more informed basis of negotiation with parents, practitioners may find it helpful to assess parental beliefs about the etiology, consequences, and treatment of their child's condition. Specific questions that are useful in this assessment are listed in Box 15.5.

Open discussion of alternatives for treatment is usually more productive than engaging in debates about what may have caused FTT. Focusing on what parents can do to help the child in the future (rather than what they may have done in the past) emphasizes the positive opportunity parents now have to help their child.[247] Parents are more likely to accept recommendations for treatment if they feel that their opinions concerning their child's condition and treatment are respected and understood. For this reason, involving parents in the treatment process by asking their opinions, listening to their concerns, and providing opportunity for expression of anger and frustration can be effective. Involving other family members (eg, fathers, grandparents, child care providers) in the assessment and discussion of treatment recommendations can ensure that the recommendations are sensitive to family issues and help to mobilize support within the family.

Individualizing Intervention

Videotapes made by families during mealtimes are often an effective part of the intervention. By watching themselves with their children, parents serve as their own models and identify strategies that promote better feeding. They practice newly acquired skills through repeated videotaped observations,

BOX 15.5
Questions to Elicit Parental Attributions Concerning Failure to Thrive

1. How tall is your child compared with other children of the same age?
    a. Taller   b. About the same   c. Shorter

2. How concerned are you about your child's height?
    a. Not concerned   b. Somewhat concerned   c. Very concerned

3. How heavy is your child compared with other children of the same age?
    a. Heavier   b. About the same   c. Thinner

4. How concerned are you about your child's weight?
    a. Not concerned   b. Somewhat concerned   c. Very concerned

5. How much does your child eat compared with other children of the same age?
    a. More than others   b. About the same   c. Less than others

7. How concerned are you about the amount your child eats?
    a. Not concerned   b. Somewhat concerned   c. Very concerned

8. How does the variety of your child's diet compare with the diet of other children of the same age?
    a. Wider variety than   b. About the same   c. More restricted than others
        others

9. How concerned are you about the variety of your child's diet?
    a. Not concerned   b. Somewhat concerned   c. Very concerned

10. How is your child's behavior at meals compared with other children of the same age?
    a. Behaves better than   b. About the same   c. Behaves worse than others
        others

11. How concerned are you about your child's behavior?
    a. Not concerned   b. Somewhat concerned   c. Very concerned

12. For each concern
    a. When did you first become concerned?
    b. Do other people (family, friends) share your concern?
    c. What advice have you received?
    d. What solutions have you tried? What was the result?
    e. What do you think will help your child's condition?

analyze interaction patterns, and identify aspects of their own behavior that contribute to feeding problems or success in their children. The therapeutic use of videotaped interactions has been effective in promoting interactive behavior with adolescent mothers[249] and caregivers who are intellectually limited or burdened with multiple stressors.[250–253] Repeated videotaping becomes familiar to families if it is incorporated into routine clinical evaluation and intervention procedures. One objective of incorporating the videotape into intervention is to help parents recognize how important they are to their child and to enhance the value of the child to them. Parents of children with FTT may feel frustrated, guilty, and disappointed with their child's poor growth. These feelings can be exacerbated by clinicians who either encourage parents to get more calories into their children without addressing the problems associated with low weight gain or blame parents when their children do not gain weight. Effective clinicians look for examples of strengths in the parent-child relationship, including parental responsivity, such as acknowledging the child who looks to the parent for guidance, cues, or reactions. This strategy emphasizes the parent's importance in the partnership and helps the parent develop a sense of efficacy in improving the relationship. Screening for common mental health problems, such as depression, can identify parents who may benefit from a therapeutic intervention that addresses their own mental health needs.

Viewing interaction on videotape also helps parents see the relationship from the child's perspective. They see how the child communicates internal signals of hunger and satiety and reacts to a smile or to a criticism from the parent. For example, some children signal satiety by throwing food or turning the bowl upside down. Recognizing the child's perspective is a critical step in intervention because it helps parents understand that children are influenced not only by internal regulatory processes, but also by the behavior of others. By watching themselves interacting with their child, parents learn to differentiate successful from unsuccessful strategies. Parents serve as their own models and are empowered by identifying strategies that work for them and their child. By practicing newly acquired skills through repeated videotaped observations, parents learn to analyze interaction patterns and identify aspects of their own behavior that contribute to feeding problems

or success in their children. The clinician does not instruct or teach the parent how to interact with her child, but through the use of videotapes, the clinician helps the parent gain a better understanding of the feeding partnership and how behavior in one partner influences the entire interaction. Parents practice responsive feeding styles with their child with the goal of improving and clarifying their communication so it is not based on feeding problems.

Dysfunctional Families

When the efficacy of parent-centered intervention is limited by chronic family problems, such as conflicts between parents, family-centered intervention may be necessary. Family-centered intervention involves multiple family members in achieving the following goals: (a) improvement in the organization and planning concerning allocation of family resources (attention and nutrition to the child), (b) reduction of family conflict, (c) provision of emotional support to the child's primary caretaker to enhance the quality of nurturing and caretaking, and (d) management of acute family crises.[93]

Indications for Protective Services Involvement

The AAP published a clinical report titled, "Failure to Thrive as a Manifestation of Child Neglect."[254] However, many of the risk factors for neglect as the cause of FTT listed in the AAP statement, including social isolation, lack of knowledge of normal growth and development, and parental psychopathology, are common psychosocial correlates of living in poverty. Although these factors put children at higher risk for developing FTT, they do not necessarily suggest neglect or abuse on the part of the child's caregivers. Nonetheless, practitioners inevitably encounter families of children with FTT who are both highly dysfunctional and resistant to recommended interventions. In a minority of children, FTT may result from diagnosable neglect by caregivers. When FTT and abuse or neglect co-occur, the behavior and developmental consequences for children are more severe than if either condition occurs separately.[255, 256] One study found increased risk of subsequent involvement with protective services in children diagnosed with FTT in the first year of life.[257] Documenting the family's response to intervention, as well as the child's physical, nutritional, and developmental progress, is helpful in decisions regarding the need to engage protective services.

Children with FTT who are referred to protective services agencies fall into 2 broad categories: those whose safety, in the judgment of clinical personnel, requires placement away from their current caretakers, and those in less severe jeopardy, whose current caretakers require protective monitoring and support to obtain or adhere with necessary services for the health and growth of the child. Placement of a child with FTT outside of the home should not be considered a routine diagnostic strategy, but is the only safe intervention in certain situations, particularly when caretakers are out-of-control substance abusers, have inflicted injury on the child, have intentionally withheld available food from the child, or are profoundly psychiatrically or cognitively impaired, and when no other competent caretakers are available within the existing family system.[14,255,258,259] School-aged children with psychosocial dwarfism (more recently termed *hyperphagic short stature*) who are from such abusive situations often require intensive services, including removal from the home.[229,231,257,260]

Placement must be undertaken with great care because suboptimal foster care only worsens FTT.[261] Because children who fail to thrive usually have multiple special needs requiring visits to many different professionals as well as specialized dietary, developmental, and medical management at home, foster parents must not be overburdened with the care of many other young children or children with special needs. Foster parents (whether professional or kinship) require the same intensive multidisciplinary support as biological parents to provide adequate care for a child who is failing to thrive. To avoid deterioration of the child with FTT who is placed in foster care, clinicians should meet face to face with prospective alternate caregivers and educate them regarding the child's dietary and behavioral regimen, medical problems, and emotional needs. Foster parents and kinship caregivers should have a WIC referral, appropriate nutritional supplements, child care equipment, and health insurance before children are placed in their homes. The professional or kinship foster family must be willing to commit to close cooperation with clinic visits and home-based treatment for the child who fails to thrive. Having a protective services worker bring the child to medical care without the foster/kinship caregivers is ineffective because clinical change can be effected only when clinicians work directly and closely with the child's primary caregivers. Extra payment to the foster families caring for children with FTT is warranted because of the child's increased dietary needs as well as frequent visits to health care and mental health/developmental professionals. Although expensive, well-supported foster care is far more cost-effective in restoring normal growth and development in children from high-risk homes than is extended institutionalization, which is associated with a poor developmental prognosis.[257,262,263]

Protective services intervention may in some settings be a necessary strategy to obtain needed multidisciplinary services, such as home visits or developmentally appropriate day care, for a child who is failing to thrive. Close communication between the protective services agency and the health care providers usually enhances parental adherence. Ideally, such services should be available through other community agencies without the stigma of protective services involvement, but in today's budget climate, this is often not the case. In our clinical experience in a municipal hospital with intensive multidisciplinary management, more than two-thirds of all cases involving FTT in deprived urban families can be managed without any protective services involvement. For children from families with more

material resources and greater access to private medical and mental health care, rates of required protective services referral are probably lower.

Conclusion

Failure to thrive is a chronic condition that is the final common pathway of the interaction of diverse medical, nutritional, developmental, and social stresses. Effective care is interdisciplinary, respectful of parents, and sustained beyond the time of acute nutritional and medical crises. Ultimately, the goal of sustained interdisciplinary management is a thriving child in a thriving family.

References

1. Bithoney WG, Rathbun JM. *Developmental-Behavioral Pediatrics.* Philadelphia, PA: WB Saunders; 1983

2. Guyer B, Wehler CA, Anderka MT, et al. Anthropometric evidence of malnutrition among low income children in Massachusetts. *Mass J Community Health.* 1986;1:3–9

3. Wright CM. Identification and management of failure to thrive: a community perspective. *Arch Dis Child.* 2000;82:5–9

4. Karp RJ. *Malnourished Children in the United States: Caught in the Cycle of Poverty.* New York, NY: Springer Publishing Company; 1993

5. Lozoff B, Black M. Impact of micronutrient deficiencies on behavior and development. In: Pettifor J, Zlotkin S, eds. *Nutrition-Micronutrient Deficiencies during the Weaning Period and the First Years of Life.* Basel, Switzerland: Karger; 2003:119–135

6. Grantham-McGregor S. A review of studies of the effect of severe malnutrition on mental development. *J Nutr.* 1995;125(suppl 8):2233S–2238S

7. Black MM, Krishnakumar A. Predicting longitudinal growth curves of height and weight using ecological factors for children with and without early growth deficiency. *J Nutr.* 1999;129(suppl 2):539S–543S

8. Drewett RF, Corbett SS, Wright CM. Cognitive and educational attainments at school age of children who failed to thrive in infancy: a population-based study. *J Child Psychol Psychiatry.* 1999;40:551–561

9. Corbett SS, Drewett FR. To what extent is failure to thrive in infancy associated with poorer cognitive development? A review and meta-analysis. *J Child Psychol Psychiatry.* 2004;45:641–654

10. Rudolf MC, Logan S. What is the long term outcome for children who fail to thrive? A systematic review. *Arch Dis Child.* 2005;90:925–931

11. Mackner L, Black M, Starr RJ. Cognitive development of children in poverty with failure to thrive: a prospective study through age 6. *Assoc Child Psychol Psychiatry.* 2003;44:743–751

12. Wright CM, Matthews JNS, Waterson A, Aynsley-Green A. What is a normal rate of weight gain in infancy? *Acta Paediatr.* 1994;83:351–356

13. Casey PH. Failure to thrive. In: Levine M, Carey W, Crocker A, eds. *Developmental Behavioral Pediatrics.* Vol 2. Philadelphia, PA: WB Saunders; 1992:375–383

14. Bullard DM Jr, Glaser HH, Hegarty MC. Failure to thrive in the "neglected" child. *Am J Orthopsychiatry.* 1966;37:680–690

15. Coleman RW, Provence S. Environmental retardation in infants living in families. *Pediatrics.* 1957;19:285–291

16. Goldbloom RB. Failure to thrive. *Pediatr Clin North Am.* 1982;29:151–166

17. Sills RH. Failure to thrive: the role of clinical and laboratory evaluation. *Am J Dis Child.* 1978;32:967–969

18. Frank DA, Zeisel SH. Failure to thrive. *Pediatr Clin North Am.* 1988;35:1187–1206

19. Casey PH. Failure to thrive: a reconceptualization. *J Dev Behav Pediatr.* 1983;4:63–66

20. Casey PH, Arnold WC. Compensatory growth in infants with severe failure to thrive. *South Med J.* 1985;78:1057–1060

21. Frank DA. Malnutrition and child behavior: a view from the bedside. In: Brozek P, ed. *Malnutrition and Behavior.* Lausanne, Switzerland: Nestle Foundation; 1984

22. Whitten CF, Pettit MG, Fischoff J. Evidence that growth failure from maternal deprivation is secondary to under-eating. *JAMA.* 1969;209:1675–1682

23. Barrett DE, Radke-Yarrow M, Klein RE. Chronic malnutrition and child behavior: effects of early caloric supplementation on social and emotional functioning at school age. *Dev Psychol.* 1982;10:541–552

24. Barrett DE, Frank DA. *The Effects of Undernutrition on Children's Behavior.* New York, NY: Gordon Breach; 1987

25. Chase HP, Martin HP. Undernutrition and child development. *N Engl J Med.* 1970;282:933–939

26. Dobbing J. Infant nutrition and later achievement. *Nutr Rev.* 1984;42:1–7

27. Drotar D. *Failure to Thrive.* New York, NY: Guilford; 1988

28. Frank DA, Allen D, Brown JL. Primary prevention of failure to thrive: social policy and implications. In: Drotar D, ed. *New Directions in Failure to Thrive.* New York, NY: Plenum Press; 1985

29. Crittenden PM. Nonorganic failure to thrive: deprivation or distortion. *Int Ment Health J.* 1987;8:51–64

30. Shaheen E, Alexander D, Truskowsky M, Barber GJ. Failure to thrive: a retrospective profile. *Clin Pediatr.* 1968;7:255–261

31. Drotar D, Eckerle D, Satola J, Pallota J, Wyatt B. Maternal interactional behavior with nonorganic failure to thrive infants: a case comparison study. *Child Abuse Negl.* 1990;14:41–51

32. American Academy of Pediatrics Committee on Nutrition. *Pediatric Nutrition Handbook.* 5th ed. Elk Grove Village, IL: American Academy of Pediatrics; 2004

33. Kessler DB. Failure to thrive and pediatric undernutrition: historical and theoretical context. In: Kessler D, Dawson P, eds. *Failure to Thrive and Pediatric Undernutrition*. Baltimore, MD: Paul H. Brookes Publishing Company; 1999:3–18

34. Black MM. Failure to thrive: strategies for evaluation and intervention. *School Psychol Rev.* 1995;24:171–185

35. Wright CM, Callum J, Birks E, Jarvis S. Effect of community based management in failure to thrive: randomized controlled trial. *Br Med J.* 1998;317:571–574

36. Bithoney WG, McJunkin J, Michalek J, Snyder J, Egan H, Epstein D. The effect of a multidisciplinary team approach on weight gain in nonorganic failure-to-thrive children. *J Dev Behav Pediatr.* 1991;12:254–258

37. Jones YD, Nesheim MC, Habicht JP. Influence on child growth associated with poverty in the 1970s: an examination of HANES I and HANES II, cross-sectional US national surveys. *Am J Clin Nutr.* 1985;42:714–724

38. Brown JL, Pizer HF. *Living Hungry in America*. New York, NY: Macmillan; 1987

39. Garza C, deOnis M. Rationale for developing a new international growth reference. *Food Nutr Bull.* 2004;25:S5–S14

40. *Poverty Threshold, 2005*. Washington, DC: US Bureau of Census; 2006. http://www.census.gov/hhes/www/poverty/threshld/thresh05.html. Accessed May 30, 2007

41. Dalaker J, Naifeh M. *Poverty in the United States: 1997*. Washington, DC: US Bureau of Census; 1998. Current Population Reports, Series P60-201

42. Silver J, DiLorenzo P, Zukoski M. Starting young: improving the health and developmental outcomes of infants and toddlers in the child welfare system. *Child Welfare.* 1999;78:148–165

43. Blumberg SJ, Bialostosky K, Hamilton WL. The effectivenes of a short form of the Household Food Security Scale. *Am J Public Health.* 1999;89:1231–1234

44. Bickel G, Carlson S, Nord M. *Household Food Security in the United States, 1995–1998*. Washington, DC: US Department of Agriculture Food and Nutrition Services and Economic Research Service; 1999

45. Wehler C. *Community Childhood Hunger Identification Project: A Survey of Childhood Hunger in the United States*. Washington, DC: Food Action Research Center; 1991

46. Neault N, Cook JT, Morris V, Frank DA. *The Real Cost of a Healthy Diet: Healthful Foods Are Out of Reach for Low-Income Families in Boston, Massachusetts*. Boston, MA: Boston Medical Center; 2005. http://dcc2.bumc.bu.edu/csnappublic/HealthyDiet_Aug2005.pdf

47. Dalaker J. *Poverty in the United States: 1998*. Washington, DC: US Bureau of Census; 1999. Current Population Reports, Series P60-207

48. Castner L, Rosso R. *Characteristics of Food Stamp Households: Fiscal Year 1998*. Report submitted to the USDA. Princeton NJ: Mathematical Policy Research, Inc; 2000

49. Center on Budget and Policy Priorities. *WIC Newsletter 1991*. 1992; Vol. 12

50. Garbarino J. The stress of being a poor child in America. *Child Adolesc Psychiatric Clin North Am.* 1998;7:105–119

51. Wiecha J, Palombo R. Multiple program participation: comparison of nutrition and food assistance program benefits with food costs in Boston, Massachusetts. *Am J Public Health.* 1989;9:591–594

52. Primus W, Rawlings L, Larin K. *The Initial Impacts of Welfare Reform on the Incomes of Single-Mother Families*. Washington, DC: Center on Budget and Policy Priorities; 1999

53. Kramer-LeBlanc CS, Mardis A, Gerrior S. *Review of the Nutritional Status of WIC Participants*. Washington, DC: USDA Center for Nutrition Policy and Promotion; 1999

54. Garbarino J, Sherman D. High risk neighborhoods and high risk families: the human ecology of child maltreatment. *Child Dev.* 1990;51:188–198

55. Cook JT, Frank DA, Levenson SM, et al. Child food insecurity increases risks posed by household food insecurity to young children's health. *J Nutr.* 2005;136:1073–1076

56. Jyoti DF, Frongillo EA, Jones SJ. Food insecurity affects children's academic performance, weight gain, and social skills. *J Nutr.* 2005;135:2831–2839

57. Huston A, McLoyd V, Cull C. Children and poverty: issues in contemporary research. *Child Dev.* 1991;65:275–282

58. Katon W, Kleinman A. Doctor-patient negotiation and other social science strategies in patient care. In: Eisenberg L, Kleinman A, eds. *The Relevance of Social Science for Medicine.* Dordrecht, Holland: Reidel Press; 1981

59. Belsky J. The determinants of parenting: a process model. *Child Dev.* 1984;55:83–96

60. Drotar D, Sturm LA. Parental influences in nonorganic failure to thrive: implications for management. *Int Ment Health J.* 1987;8:37–45

61. Drotar D, Malone CA, Negray J. Environmentally based failure to thrive and children's intellectual development. *J Child Psychol Psychiatry.* 1980;10:236–247

62. Drotar D, Malone CA, Negray J. Intellectual assessment of young children with environmentally based failure to thrive. *Child Abuse Negl.* 1980;6:23–29

63. Gordon AH, Jameson JC. Infant-mother attachment in parents with non-organic failure to thrive syndrome. *J Am Acad Child Psychiatry.* 1979;18:251–259

64. Elmer E. Failure to thrive: role of the mother. *Pediatrics.* 1960;25:717–725

65. Singer LT, Song L, Hill BP, Jaffee AC. Stress and depression in mothers of failure to thrive children. *J Pediatr Psychol.* 1990;15:711–720

66. Benoit D, Zeanah CH, Barton ML. Maternal attachment disturbance in failure to thrive. *Int Ment Health J.* 1989;10:185–191

67. Polan HJ, Leon A, Kaplan MD, Kessler DB, Stern D, Ward MJ. Disturbances of affect expression in failure to thrive. *J Am Acad Child Adolesc Psychiatry.* 1991;30:897–903

68. Kotelchuck M. Nonorganic failure to thrive: the status of interactional and environmental theories. In: Camp B, ed. *Advances in Behavioral Pediatrics.* Greenwich, UK: Jai Press; 1980

69. Kotelchuck M, Newberger EH. Failure to thrive: a controlled study of family characteristics. *J Am Acad Child Psychiatry.* 1983;22:322–328

70. Pollitt E, Eichler A, Chan CK. Psychosocial development and behavior of mothers of failure to thrive children. *Am J Orthopsychiatry.* 1975;45:525–537

71. Hutcheson JJ, Black MM, Talley M, et al. Risk status and home intervention among children with failure to thrive: follow up at age 4. *J Pediatr Psychol.* 1997;22:651–668

72. Altemeier WA III, O'Conner SM, Sherrod KB, Vietze PM. Prospective study of antecedents for non-organic failure to thrive. *J Pediatr.* 1985;106:360–365

73. Weston JA, Colloton M, Halsey S. A legacy of violence in nonorganic failure to thrive. *Child Abuse Negl.* 1993;17:709–714

74. Drotar D, Sturm LA. The role of parent-practitioner communication in the management of non-organic failure to thrive. *Fam Syst Med.* 1988;6:42–51

75. Powell GF, Low J, Speers MA. Behavior as a diagnostic aid in failure to thrive. *J Dev Behav Pediatr.* 1987;8:18–24

76. Ramey CT. Nutrition, response-contingent stimulation and the maternal deprivation syndrome: results of an early intervention program. *Mer Palm Q.* 1975;21:45–53

77. Kelly C, Ricciardelli LA, Clarke JD. Problem eating attitudes and behaviors in young children. *Int J Eat Disord.* 1999;25:281–286

78. Black MM, Hutcheson J, Dubowitz H, Berenson-Howard J, Starr RH. The roots of competence: mother-infant interaction among low-income, African-American families. *Appl Dev Psychol.* 1996;17:367–391

79. Wolke D, Skuse D, Mathisen B. Behavioral style in failure to thrive: a preliminary communication. *J Pediatr Pscyhol.* 1990;15:237–243

80. Pollitt E, Leibel R. Biological and social correlates of failure to thrive. In: Greene L, Johnson E, eds. *Social and Biological Predictions of Nutritional Status, Physical Growth, and Neurological Development.* New York, NY: Academic Press; 1980

81. Mathisen B, Skuse D, Wolke D. Oral-motor dysfunction and failure to thrive among inner-city infants. *Dev Med Child Neurol.* 1989;31:293–302

82. Reilly S, Skuse DH, Wolke D. Oral-motor dysfunction in children who fail to thrive: organic or non-organic? *Dev Med Child Neurol.* 1999;41:115–122

83. Riordan MM, Iwata BA, Wohl MK. Behavioral treatment of food refusal and selectivity in developmentally disabled children. *Appl Res Ment Retard.* 1980;1:95–112

84. Shapiro V, Fraiberg S, Adelson E. Infant-parent psychotherapy on behalf of a child in a critical nutritional state. *Psychoanal Study Child.* 1976;31:461–491

85. Wright CM, Parkinson KN, Drewett DF. How does maternal and child feeding behavior relate to weight gain and failure to thrive? *Pediatrics.* 2006;117:1262–1269

86. Faith MS, Scanlon KS, Birch LL, Francis LA, Sherry B. Parent-child feeding strategies and their relationships to child eating and weight status. *Obesity Res.* 2004;12:1711–1722

87. Black MM, Hutchenson JJ, Dubowitz H, Berenson-Howard J. Parenting style and developmental status among children with nonorganic failure to thrive. *J Pediatr Pscyhol.* 1994;19:689–707

88. Hutcheson J, Black MM, Starr R. Developmental changes in interactional characteristics of mothers and their children with failure to thrive. *J Pediatr Psychol.* 1993;18:453–466

89. Robinson JR, Drotar D, Boutry M. Problem-solving abilities among mothers of infants with failure to thrive. *J Pediatr Psychol.* 2001;26:21–32

90. Bithoney WG, Newberger EH. Child and family attributes of failure to thrive. *J Dev Behav Pediatr.* 1987;8:32–36

91. Kanawati AA, McClaren DS. Failure to thrive in Lebanon II: an investigation of the causes. *Acta Pediatr Scand.* 1973;62:571

92. Skuse DH, Reilly S, Wolke D. Psychosocial adversity and growth during infancy. *Am J Clin Nutr.* 1994;48:S113–S130

93. Drotar D, Eckerle D. Family environment in nonorganic failure to thrive. a controlled study. *J Pediatr Pscyhol.* 1989;14:245–257

94. James WP, Ferro-Luzzi A, Sette S. The potential use of maternal size in priority setting when combating childhood malnutrition. *Eur J Clin Nutr.* 1999;53:112–119

95. Kaplowitz P, Webb J. Diagnostic evaluation of short children with height 3SD or more below the mean. *Clin Pediatr.* 1994;33:530–535

96. Hillemeier AC. Gastroesophageal reflux: diagnostic and therapeutic approaches. *Pediatr Clin North Am.* 1996;43:197–212

97. Frisancho AR, Cole PE, Klayman JE. Greater contribution to secular trend among offspring of short parents. *Hum Biol.* 1977;49:51–60

98. Fraiberg S, Adelson E, Shapiro B. Ghosts in the nursery. *J Am Acad Child Psychiatry.* 1975;14:387–421

99. Lansky SB, Stephenson L, Weller E. Failure to thrive during infancy in sibling of pediatric cancer patients. *Am J Pediatr Hematol Oncol.* 1982;4:361–366

100. Agras S, Hammer L, McNicolas F. A prospective study of the influence of eating-disordered mothers on their children. *Int J Eat Disord.* 1999;25:253–262

101. Russell GF, Treasure J, Eisler I. Mothers with anorexia nervosa who underfeed their children: their recognition and management. *Psychol Med.* 1998;28:93–108

102. Hawford JT. Growth problems in children: an approach to evaluation and therapy. In: Moss A, ed. *Pediatric Update.* New York, NY: Elsevier; 1979

103. Oates RK, Yu JS. Children with non-organic failure to thrive: a community problem. *Med J Aust.* 1971;2:199–203

104. Brandt I. Growth dynamics of low birthweight infants with emphasis on the prenatal period. In: Falkner F, Tanner J, eds. *Human Growth, Neurobiology and Nutrition.* New York, NY: Plenum Press; 1979

105. Casey PH, Kraemer HC, Bernbaum J, Yogman MW, Sells JC. Growth status and growth rates of a varied sample of low birth weight preterm infants: a longitudinal cohort from birth to three years of age. *J Pediatr.* 1991;119:559–605

106. Karniski W, Blair C, Vitucci J. The illusion of catch-up growth in premature infants. *Am J Dis Child.* 1987;1414:520–526

107. Georgieff MK, Mills MM, Zempel CE. Catch-up growth, muscle and fat accretion and body proportionality of infants one year after neonatal intensive care. *J Pediatr.* 1989;114:288–292

108. Nieman L. Follow up nutrition after discharge from the neonatal intensive care unit. *Building Block for Life.* 2006;29:1–8

109. Als H, Tronic E, Adamson L. The behavior of full-term but underweight infants. *Dev Med Child Neurol.* 1976;18:590–602

110. Villar J, Smeriglio V, Martorell R. Heterogeneous growth and mental development in intrauterine growth-retarded infants during the first 3 years of life. *Pediatrics.* 1984;74:783–791

111. Hediger M, Overpeck MD, Mauer KR, Kuczmarski RJ, McGlynn A, Davis WW. Growth of infants and young children born small or large for gestational age: findings from the Third National Health and Nutrition Examination Survey. *Arch Pediatr Adolesc Med.* 1998;152:1225–1231

112. Ounstead M, Moar V, Scott A. Growth in the first four years II: diversity with groups of small-for-dates and large-for-dates babies. *Early Hum Dev.* 1982;7:29–39

113. Hanson J, Smith D. The fetal hydantoin syndrome. *J Pediatr.* 1975;87:285–290

114. Frank DA, Wong F. Effects of prenatal exposures to alcohol, tobacco, and other drugs. In: Kessler D, Dawson P, eds. *Failure to Thrive and Pediatric Under-nutrition: A Transdisciplinary Approach.* Baltimore, MD: Paul H. Brookes Publishing; 1999

115. Fried PA, O'Connell CM. A comparison of the effects of prenatal exposure to tobacco, alcohol, cannabis and caffeine on birth size and subsequent growth. *Neurotoxicol Teratol.* 1987;9:79–85

116. Lassen K, Oei TPS. Effects of maternal cigarette smoking during pregnancy on long-term physical and cognitive parameters of child development. *Addict Behav.* 1998;23:635–653

117. Rush D, Callahan KR. Exposure to passive cigarette smoking and child development. *Ann N Y Acad Sci.* 1989;148:1150–1155

118. Nordstrom-Klee B, Delaney-Black V, Covington C, Ager J, Sokol R. Growth from birth onwards of children prenatally exposed to drugs: a literature review. *Neurotoxicol Teratol.* 2002;24:481–488

119. Chambers CD, Anderson PO, Thomas RG, Dick LM, Felix RJ, Johnson KA. Weight gain in infants breastfed by mothers who take fluoxetine. *Pediatrics.* 1999;104:e61

120. Coles CD. Effects of prenatal alcohol exposure at school age I: physical and cognitive development. *Neurotoxicol Teratol.* 1991;13:357–367

121. Day N, Richardson G, Robles N. Effect of prenatal alcohol exposure on growth and morphology of offspring at 8 months of age. *Pediatrics.* 1990;85:748–752

122. Fried PA, Watkinson B. 36- and 48-month neurobehavioral follow-up on children prenatally exposed to marijuana, cigarettes, and alcohol. *J Dev Behav Pediatr.* 1990;11:49–58

123. Shaywitz S, Cohen D, Shaywitz B. Behavior and learning difficulties in children of normal intelligence born to alcoholic mothers. *J Pediatr.* 1980;96:978–985

124. Hanson J, Jones K, Smith D. Fetal alcohol syndrome. *JAMA.* 1976;235:1458–1460

125. VanDyke DC, MacKay L, Ziaylek E. Management of severe feeding dysfunction in children with fetal alcohol syndrome. *Clin Pediatr.* 1981;21:336–339

126. Frank DA, Bauchner H, Parker S. Neonatal body proportionality and body composition following in utero exposure to cocaine and marijuana. *J Pediatr.* 1990;116:622–626

127. Zuckerman B, Frank DA, Hingson R. Effects of maternal marijuana and cocaine use on fetal growth. *N Engl J Med.* 1989;320:762–768

128. Cornelius MD, Goldschmidt L, Day NL, Larkby C. Alcohol, tobacco and marijuana use among pregnant teenagers: 6-year follow-up of offspring growth effects. *Neurotoxicol Teratol.* 2002;24:703–710

129. Fried PA, Watkinson B, Gray R. Differential effects on cognitive functioning in 9- to 12-year olds prenatally exposed to cigarettes and marijuana. *Neurotoxicol Teratol.* 1998;20:293–306

130. Chasnoff IJ, Griffith DR, Friar C. Cocaine/polydrug use in pregnancy: two year follow-up. *Pediatrics.* 1992;89:284–289

131. Jacobson JL, Jacobson SW, Sokol RJ. Effects of prenatal exposure to alcohol, smoking, and illicit drugs on postpartum somatic growth. *Alcohol Clin Exp Res.* 1994;18:317–323

132. Weathers WT, Crane MM, Sauvain KJ. Cocaine use in women from a defined population: prevalence at delivery and effects on growth in infants. *Pediatrics.* 1993;91:350–354

133. Lumeng JC, Cabral HJ, Gannon K, Heeren T, Frank DA. Pre-natal exposures to cocaine and alcohol and physical growth patterns to age 8 years. *Neurotoxicol Teratol.* 2007;29:446–457

134. Neuspiel DR, Hamel C, Hochberg E. Maternal cocaine use and infant behavior. *Neurotoxicol Teratol.* 1991;13:229–233

135. Hurt H, Brodsky NL, Betancourt L. Cocaine-exposed children: follow-up through 30 months. *J Dev Behav Pediatr.* 1995;16:29–35

136. Richardson GA, Conroy ML, Day NL. Prenatal cocaine exposure: effects on the development of school-age children. *Neurotoxicol Teratol.* 1996;18:627–634

137. Wilson GS, McCreary R, Kean J, Baxter JC. The development of preschool children of heroin-addicted mothers: a controlled study. *Pediatrics.* 1979;63:135–141

138. Deren S. Children of substance abusers: a review of the literature. *J Subst Abuse Treat.* 1986;3:77–94

139. Atwood WJ, Berger JR, Kaderman R. Human immunodeficiency virus type I infection of the brain. *Clin Microbiol Rev.* 1993;6:339–366

140. Barbour SD. Acquired immune deficiency syndrome of childhood. *Pediatr Clin North Am.* 1987;34:247–268

141. Kappy MS. Regulation of growth in children with chronic illness: therapeutic implications for the year 2000. *Am J Dis Child.* 1987;141:489–493

142. Phillip M, Hershkovitz E, Rosenblum H. Serum insulin-like growth factors I and II are not affected by undernutrition in children with nonorganic failure to thrive. *Horm Res.* 1998;49:76–79

143. Fryer GE Jr. The efficacy of hospitalization of nonorganic failure-to-thrive children: a meta-analysis. *Child Abuse Negl.* 1988;12:375–381

144. Bithoney WG, McJunkin J, Michalek J. Prospective evaluation of weight gain in both nonorganic and organic failure to thrive children: an outpatient trial of a multidisciplinary team strategy. *J Dev Behav Pediatr.* 1989;10:27–31

145. Berwick DM, Levy JC, Kleinerman R. Failure to thrive: diagnostic yield of hospitalization. *Arch Dis Child.* 1982;57:347–351

146. Fleisher DR. Comprehensive management of infants with gastroesophageal reflux and failure to thrive. *Curr Probl Pediatr.* 1995;25:247–253

147. Herr T, Cook PR, Highfill G. In vitro testing in pediatric food allergy. *Otolaryngol Head Neck Surg.* 1999;120:233–237

148. Homer C, Ludwig S. Categorization of etiology of failure to thrive. *Am J Dis Child.* 1980;133:848–851

149. Sullivan PB. Nutritional management of acute diarrhea. *Nutrition.* 1998;14:758–762

150. Gupta MC, Urrutia JJ. Effect of periodic antiascaris and antigiardia treatment on nutritional status of preschool children. *Am J Clin Nutr.* 1982;36:79–86

151. Roesler TA, Barry P, Bock SA. Exposure to passive cigarette smoking and child development. *Ann N Y Acad Sci.* 1994;148:1150–1155

152. Hattevig G, Sigurs N, Kiellman B. Effects of maternal dietary avoidance during lactation on allergy in children at 10 years of age. *Acta Paediatr.* 1999;88:7–12

153. James JM, Burks AW. Food hypersensitivity in children. *Curr Opin Pediatr.* 1994;6:661–667

154. Kulig M, Bergmann R, Niggemann B, Burow G, Wahn U. Prediction of sensitization to inhalant allergens in childhood: evaluating family history, atopic dermatitis, and sensitization to food allergens. *Clin Exp Allergy.* 1998;28:1397–1403

155. Kaila M, Salo MK, Isolauri E. Fatty acids in substitute formulas for cow's milk allergy. *Allergy.* 1999;54:74–77

156. Niggemann B, Sielaff B, Beyer K. Outcome of double-blind, placebo controlled food challenge tests in 107 children with atopic dermatitis. *Clin Exp Allergy.* 1999;29:91–96

157. Jarvinen K, Juntunen-Backman K, Suomalainen H. Relation between HLA-DR expression on human breast milk macrophages and cow milk allergy (CMA) in suckling infants. *Pediatr Res.* 1999;45:76–81

158. Kramer V, Heinrich J, Wist M. Age of entry to day nursery and allergy in later childhood. *Lancet.* 1999;353:450–454

159. Salvioli G, Faldella G, Alessandroni R. Prevention of allergies of infants: breast-feeding and special formulas: influence on the response to immunization. *Acta Biomed Ateneo Parmense.* 1997;68(suppl 1):21–27

160. American Academy of Pediatrics Committee on Infectious Diseases. *Red Book: Report of the Committee on Infectious Diseases.* 27th ed. Elk Grove Village, IL: American Academy of Pediatrics; 2006:405–410

161. Chevalier P, Sevilla R, Sejas R. Immune recovery of malnourished children takes longer than nutritional recovery: implications for treatment and discharge. *J Trop Pediatr.* 1998;44:304

162. McLaren DS. Vitamin A and the immune response. *J Indian Med Assoc.* 1999;97:320–323

163. Mitchell WG, Gorrell RW, Greenberg RA. Failure to thrive: a study in a primary care setting: epidemiology and follow-up. *Pediatrics.* 1980;65:971–977

164. Suskind RM. Malnutrition and the immune response. In: Suskind R, ed. *Textbook of Pediatric Nutrition.* New York, NY: Raven Press; 1981

165. Waterlow JC. Classification and definition of protein-calorie malnutrition. *Br Med J.* 1972;3:530–555

166. Schwartz J, Angle C, Pitcher H. Relationship between childhood blood levels and stature. *Pediatrics.* 1986;77:281–288

167. Mahaffey KR, Amnest JL, Roberts J. National estimates of blood lead levels: United States, 1976–1980: associated with selected demographic and socioeconomic factors. *N Engl J Med.* 1982;307:573–579

168. *Preventing Lead Poisoning in Young Children: A Statement by the Centers for Disease Control and Prevention.* Atlanta, GA: US Department of Health and Human Services; 1991

169. Bithoney WG. Elevated lead levels in children with nonorganic failure to thrive. *Pediatrics.* 1986;78:891–895

170. Bergstrom WH. Twenty ways to get rickets in the 1990s. *Contemp Pediatr.* 1991;December:88–93

171. Catassi C, Farsano A. Celiac disease as a cause of growth retardation in childhood. *Curr Opin Pediatr.* 2004;16:445–449

172. Orbak Z, Akin Y, Varoglu E, Tan H. Serum thyroid hormone and thyroid gland weight measurements in protein-energy malnutrition. *J Pediatr Endocrinol Metab.* 1998;11:719–724

173. Acs G, Shulman R, Ng MW. The effect of dental rehabilitation on the body weight of children with early childhood caries. *Pediatr Dent.* 1999;21:109–113

174. Boyd LD, Palmer C, Dwyer JT. Managing oral health related nutrition issues of high risk infants and children. *J Clin Pediatr Dent.* 1998;23:31–36

175. Peterson KE, Washington J, Rathbun JM. Team management of failure to thrive. *J Am Diet Assoc.* 1984;84:810–815

176. Zeiger RS, Sampson HA, Bock SA. Soy allergy in infants and children with IgE-associated cow's milk allergy. *J Pediatr.* 1999;134:614–622

177. Linscheid TR. Disturbances of eating and feeding. In: Magrab P, ed. *Psychological Management of Pediatric Problems.* Baltimore, MD: University Park Press; 1978

178. Linscheid TR, Rasnake LK. Behavioral approaches to the treatment of failure to thrive. In: Drotar D, ed. *New Directions in Failure to Thrive: Implications for Research and Practice.* New York, NY: Plenum Press; 1985

179. McJunkin JE, Bithoney WG, McCormick C. Errors in formula concentration in an outpatient population. *J Pediatr.* 1987;111:848–850

180. Pollitt E. Failure to thrive: socioeconomic, dietary intake and mother-child interaction. *Fed Proc.* 1975;34:1593–1597

181. Heptinstall G, Puckering C, Skuse D, Start K, Zur-Szpiro S, Dowdney L. Nutrition and meal-time behavior in families of growth retarded children. *Hum Nutr Appl Nutr.* 1987;41:390–402

182. Rathbun JM, Peterson KE. Nutrition in failure to thrive. In: Grank R, ed. *Pediatric Nutrition.* Boston, MA: Butterworth; 1987

183. Drotar D, Wilson F, Sturm LA. Parent intervention in failure to thrive. In: Schaefer C, Briesmeister J, eds. *Handbook of Parent Training: Parents as Cotherapists for Children's Behavioral Problems.* New York, NY: Wiley; 1989

184. Faine MP, Oberg D. Snacking and oral health habits of Washington state WIC children and their caregivers. *ASDC J Dent Child.* 1994;61:350–355

185. Siener K, Rothman D, Farrar J. Soft drink logos on baby bottles: do they influence what is fed to children? *ASDC J Dent Child.* 1997;64:55–60

186. Sherman A. *Extreme Child Poverty Rises Sharply in 1997.* Washington, DC: Children's Defense Fund; 1999

187. Zmora E, Gorodicher R, Bar-Ziv J. Multiple nutritional deficiencies in infants from a strict vegetarian community. *Am J Dis Child.* 1979;133:141–144

188. Pugliese MT, Weyman-Daum M, Moses N. Parental health beliefs as a cause of nonorganic failure to thrive. *Pediatrics.* 1987;80:175–182

189. Cole CR. Should infants avoid apple and pear juices? *Arch Pediatr Adolesc Med.* 1999;153:1098–1102

190. Smith MM, Lifshitz F. Excess fruit juice consumption as a contributing factor in nonorganic failure to thrive. *Pediatrics.* 1994;93:438–443

191. Maldonado J, Gil A, Narbona E. Special formulas in infant nutrition: a review. *Early Hum Dev.* 1998;53(suppl):S23–S32

192. Solomons NW. Assessment of nutritional status: functional indicators of pediatric nutrition. *Pediatr Clin North Am.* 1985;32:319–324

193. Graitcer PL, Gentry EM. Measuring children: one reference for all. *Lancet.* 1981;2:297–299

194. Kielman A, McCord C. Weight-for-age as an index of risk of death in children. *Lancet.* 1978;1:1247–1250

195. Waterlow JC, Buzina R, Keller W, Lane JM, Nichaman MZ, Tanner JM. The presentation and use of height and weight data for comparing the nutritional status of groups of children under the age of 10 years. *Bull World Health Org.* 1977;55:489–498

196. Guo S, Roche AF, Fomon SJ. Reference data on gains in weight and length during the first two years of life. *J Pediatr.* 1991;119:355–362

197. Sherry B. Epidemiology of inadequate growth. In: Kessler D, Dawson P, eds. *Failure to Thrive and Pediatric Under-nutrition.* Baltimore, MD: Paul H. Brookes Publishing Company; 1999:19–36

198. Cunningham CE, McLaughlin M. Nutrition. In: Kessler D, Dawson P, eds. *Failure to Thrive and Pediatric Under-nutrition.* Baltimore, MD: Paul H. Brookes Publishing Company; 1999:99–119

199. Gomez F. Mortality in second and third degree malnutrition. *J Trop Pediatr.* 1956;2:77–83

200. Morales E, Craig LD, MacLean WC. Dietary management of malnourished children with a new enteral feeding. *J Am Diet Assoc.* 1991;91:1233–1238

201. MacLean WC. Protein-energy malnutrition. In: Grand R, Sutphen J, Dietz W, eds. *Pediatric Nutrition.* Boston, MA: Butterworth; 1987

202. Black MM. Zinc deficiency and child development. *Am J Clin Nutr.* 1998;68:464S–469S

203. Walravens P, Hambridge M, Koepfer D. Zinc supplementation in infants with a nutritional pattern of failure to thrive: a double-blind, controlled study. *Pediatrics.* 1989;83:532–538

204. Doherty CP. Zinc and rehabilitation from severe protein-energy malnutrition: higher-dose regimens are associated with increased mortality. *Am J Clin Nutr.* 1998;68:742–748

205. Viteri F. Primary protein-calorie malnutrition. In: Suskind R, ed. *Textbook of Pediatric Nutrition.* New York, NY: Raven Press; 1981

206. Glaser HH, Heagarty MC, Bullard DJ, Pivchik E. Physical and psychological development of children with early failure to thrive. *J Pediatr Pscyhol.* 1968;73:690–698

207. Galler JR, Ramsey F, Solimano G. The influence of early malnutrition on subsequent behavioral development III: learning disabilities as a sequelae to malnutrition. *Pediatr Res.* 1984;18:309–313

208. Singer LT, Fagan JF. Cognitive development in the failure to thrive infant: a three year longitudinal study. *J Pediatr Pscyhol.* 1984;9:363–383

209. Ashem B, Jones M. Deleterious effects of chronic undernutrition on cognitive abilities. *J Child Psychol Psychiatry.* 1978;19:23–31

210. Dowdney L, Skues D, Morris K. Short normal children and environmental disadvantage: a longitudinal study of growth and cognitive development. *J Child Psychol Psychiatry.* 1998;39:1017–1029

211. Galler JR, Ramsey F, Solimano G. A follow-up study of the effects of early malnutrition on subsequent development II: fine motor skills in adolescence. *Pediatr Res.* 1985;19:524–527

212. Mendez MA, Adair LS. Severity and timing of stunting in the first two years of life affect performance on cognitive tests in late childhood. *J Nutr.* 1999;129:1555–1562

213. Ramey CT, Yeates KO, Short EJ. The plasticity of intellectual development: insights from preventive intervention. *Child Dev.* 1985;55:1913–1925

214. Skuse DH, Pickles A, Wolke D. Postnatal growth and mental development evidence for a "sensitive period." *J Child Psychol Psychiatry.* 1994;35:521–545

215. Skuse DH. Non-organic failure to thrive: a reappraisal. *Arch Dis Child.* 1985;60:173–178

216. Galler JR, Ramsey F, Solimano G. The influence of early malnutrition on subsequent behavioral development I: degree of impairment in intellectual performance. *J Am Acad Child Psychiatry.* 1983;22:8–15

217. Galler JR, Ramsey F, Solimano G. The influence of early malnutrition on subsequent behavioral development II: classroom behavior. *J Am Acad Child Psychiatry.* 1983;22:16–22

218. Galler JR, Ramsey F, Solimano G. The influence of early malnutrition on subsequent behavioral development V: child's behavior at home. *J Am Acad Child Psychiatry.* 1985;24:58–64

219. Evans SL, Reinhart JB, Succop RA. Failure to thrive: a study of delayed cognitive development in 45 infants at risk for later mental retardation. *Pediatrics.* 1972;2:440–457

220. Horwood L, Mogridge N, Darlow BA. Cognitive, educational, and behavioral outcomes at 7 and 8 years in a national very low birthweight cohort. *Arch Dis Child.* 1998;79:F12–F20

221. McKay H, Sinisterra L, McKay A. Improving cognitive ability in chronically deprived children. *Science.* 1978;200:270–278

222. Zeskind PS, Ramey CT. Fetal malnutrition: an experimental study of its consequences on infant development in the caregiving environments. *Child Dev.* 1978;49:1155–1162

223. Bayley N. *Bayley Scales of Infant Development Manual.* New York, NY: Psychological Corporation; 1969

224. Bayley N. *Bayley Scales of Infant Development Manual.* 2nd ed. San Antonio, TX: Psychological Corporation; 1993

225. Drotar D. Behavioral diagnosis in nonorganic failure to thrive: a critique and suggested approach to psychological assessment. *J Dev Behav Pediatr.* 1989;10:48–55

226. Chavez A, Martinez C. Consequences of insufficient nutrition on child character and behavior. In: Levitsky D, ed. *Malnutrition, Environment, and Behavior.* New York, NY: Cornell University Press; 1979

227. Drotar D, Sturm LA. Behavioral symptoms, problem solving, and personality development of preschool children with early histories of nonorganic failure to thrive. *J Dev Behav Pediatr.* 1992;13:226–273

228. Gaensbauer TJ, Sands K. Distorted affective communications in abused/neglected infants and their potential impact on character. *J Am Acad Child Psychiatry.* 1979;18:236–250

229. Powell GF, Brasel JA, Blizzard RM. Emotional deprivation and growth retardation stimulating idiopathic hypopituitarism: clinical evaluation of the syndrome. *N Engl J Med.* 1967;276:1271–1283

230. Powell GF, Low JL. Behavior in nonorganic failure to thrive. *J Dev Behav Pediatr.* 1983;8:18–24

231. Gilmour J, Skuse D. A case-comparison study of the characteristics of children with a short stature syndrome induced by stress (hyperphagic short stature) and a consecutive series of unaffected "stressed" children. *J Child Psychol Psychiatry.* 1999;40:969–978

232. Valenzuela M. Attachment in chronically underweight young children. *Child Dev.* 1990;61:1984–1996

233. Drotar D, Sturm LA. Prediction of intellectual development in young children with early histories of nonorganic failure to thrive. *J Pediatr Psychol.* 1988;13:281–296

234. Briggs-Gowan MJ, Carter AS, Irwin JR, Watchel K, Cicchetti DV. The brief infant-toddler social and emotional assessment: screening for social emotional problems and delays in competence. *J Pediatr Psychol.* 2004;29:143–155

235. Alfasi G. A failure-to-thrive infant at play: applications of microanalysis. *J Pediatr Psychol.* 1982;7:111–123

236. Richards CA, Andrews PL, Spitz L. Role of the mother's touch in failure to thrive: a preliminary investigation. *J Am Acad Child Adolesc Psychiatry.* 1994;33:1098–1105

237. Ramey CT, Heiger L, Klisz D. Synchronous reinforcement of vocal responses in failure to thrive in infants. *Child Dev.* 1972;43:1449–1455

238. Crist W, Napier-Phillips A. Mealtime behaviors of young children: a comparison of normative and clinical data. *J Dev Behav Pediatr.* 2001;22:279–286

239. Costanzo PR, Woody EZ. Domain-specific parenting styles and their impact on child's development of particular deviance: the example of obesity. *J Soc Clin Psychol.* 1985;4:425–445

240. Ayoub C, Milner J. Failure to thrive: parental indicators, types, and outcomes. *Child Abuse Negl.* 1985;9:491–499

241. Black MM, Dubowitz H, Hutcheson J, Berenson-Howard J, Starr RJ. A randomized clinical trial of home intervention for children with failure to thrive. *Pediatrics.* 1995;95:807–814

242. Satter E. *How to Get Your Kid to Eat... But Not Too Much.* New York, NY: Bull Publishing; 1987

243. Grantham-McGregor S, Schofield W, Powell C. Development of severely malnourished children who received psychosocial stimulation: six-year follow-up. *Pediatrics.* 1987;79:247–254

244. Haynes C, Cutler C, Gray J, Kempe R. Hospitalized cases of nonorganic failure to thrive: the scope of the problem and short-term lay health visitor intervention. *Child Abuse Negl.* 1984;8:229–242

245. Raynor P, Rudolf MC, Cooper K, Marchant P, Cottrell D. A randomized controlled trial of specialist health visitor intervention for failure to thrive. *Arch Dis Child.* 1999;80:500–505

246. Black MM, Dubowitz H, Krishnakumar A, Starr RH. Early intervention and recovery among children with failure to thrive: follow-up at age 8. *Pediatrics.* 2006;120:59–69

247. Sturm L, Drotar D. Maternal perceptions of the etiology of nonorganic failure to thrive. *Fam Syst Med.* 1991;9:53–59

248. Black M, Feigelman S, Cureton P. Evaluation and treatment of children with failure to thrive: an interdisciplinary perspective. *J Clin Outcomes Manage.* 1999;6:60–73

249. Black MM, Teti L. Promoting mealtime communication between adolescent mothers and their infants through videotape. *Pediatrics.* 1997;99:432–437

250. McDonough SC. Interaction guidance: understanding and treating early infant-caregiver relationship disturbances. In: Zeanah CH, ed. *Handbook of Infant Mental Health.* New York, NY: The Guilford Press; 1993:414–426

251. McDonough SC. Promoting positive early parent-infant relationships through interaction guidance. *Child Adolesc Psychiatric Clin North Am.* 1995;4:661–672

252. Koniak-Griffin D, Verzememnieks I, Cahill D. Using videotape instruction and feedback to improve adolescents' mothering behaviors. *J Adolesc Health.* 1992;13:570–575

253. Wolke D, Skuse D. The management of infant feeding problems. In: Cooper P, Stein A, eds. *Feeding Problems and Eating Disorders in Children and Adolescents.* Chur, Switzerland: Harwood Academic Publishers; 1992:27–59

254. Block RW, Krebs NF. Failure to thrive as a manifestation of child neglect. *Pediatrics.* 2005;116:1234–1237

255. Mackner LM, Starr RH, Black MM. The cumulative effect of neglect and failure to thrive on cognitive functioning. *Child Abuse Negl.* 1997;21:691–700

256. Kerr M, Black M, Krishnakumar A. Failure-to-thrive, maltreatment and the behavior and development of 6-year-old children from low-income, urban families: a cumulative risk model. *Child Abuse Negl.* 2000;24:587–598

257. Skuse DH. Failure to thrive and the risk of child abuse: a prospective study. *J Med Screen.* 1995;2:145–149

258. Goldson E, Cadol RV, Fitch MU. Nonaccidental trauma and failure to thrive. *Am J Dis Child.* 1976;130:490–492

259. Koel BS. Failure to thrive and fatal injury as a continuum. *Am J Dis Child.* 1969;118:565–567

260. Kreiger I. Food restriction as a form of child abuse in ten cases of psychological deprivation dwarfism. *Clin Pediatr.* 1974;13:127–133

261. Wyatt DT, Simms MD, Horwitz SM. Widespread growth retardation and variable growth recovery in foster children in the first year after initial placement. *Arch Pediatr Adolesc Med.* 1997;151:814–816

262. Fitch MJ. Cognitive development of abused and failure to thrive children. *J Pediatr Pscyhol.* 1976;1:32–37

263. Karniski W, VanBuren L, Cupoli JM. A treatment program for failure to thrive: a cost/effectiveness analysis. *Child Abuse Negl.* 1986;10:471–478

Munchausen Syndrome by Proxy

Donna Andrea Rosenberg

Department of Pediatrics, University of Colorado Medical Center

Munchausen syndrome by proxy (MSBP) is an unusual form of abuse involving the persistent fabrication of illness in a child by an adult. It was first described in 1977 by Meadow,[1] an English pediatrician. The name is derived from Munchausen syndrome, the condition of self-inflicted illness in adults. In the decades since its initial description, and compared with other forms of child abuse, MSBP has proven to be a form of child maltreatment fraught with rather different diagnostic and legal problems. The perpetrator of MSBP, usually the child's mother, often evades the early detection of her noxious ministrations because the symptoms and signs she reports seem plausible and because she appears attentive and concerned. The perpetrator's history often sounds cogent to the physician, bespeaking a serious illness. Although doctors are educated to evaluate critically the reliability of a historian, pediatricians do not expect that a history is an elaborate lie. Once the diagnosis has been considered, definitive inclusion or exclusion may be technically problematic. In consequence, ensuring civil court–ordered protection of a victim and any siblings also may prove difficult. Evaluation of the family, information from which is intended to shape therapy and which is useful only when the perpetrator is forthcoming, is often stymied by the mother's refusal to participate or her indignant denial of her malfeasance, however compelling the evidence.[2] Awareness of MSBP also varies significantly among mental health professionals,[3] and the mother may be very persuasive, even to experienced evaluators.[4] Criminal court proceedings undertaken against the perpetrator are still relatively rare,[5] even in homicidal MSBP. Medical professionals continue to struggle with this form of child abuse, which now goes by various names including pediatric condition falsification[6] or fabricated or induced illness.[7]

Definition

In MSBP, illness in a child is persistently and secretly simulated (lied about or faked) and/or produced by a parent or someone who is in loco parentis, and the child repeatedly is presented for medical assessment and care. This often results in multiple medical procedures, both diagnostic and therapeutic. The definition specifically excludes physical abuse only, sexual abuse only, and non-organic failure to thrive that is solely the result of nutritional/emotional deprivation.

Simulated illness means that lies are told by the mother about the child's symptoms. For example, the mother may repeatedly report that her child has episodes of stiffening, shaking, or decreased level of consciousness, when in fact these never occurred, or she may tell the pediatrician that the child has hematuria, and bring in a urine sample that she has contaminated with her own menstrual blood. Produced illness means that the mother secretly interferes with the child's body (eg, by surreptitious suffocation or by the administration of unprescribed and unnecessary medicines or substances) to produce symptoms or signs in the child, the fact or the extent of which are not proffered on history.

Demographics

Hundreds of cases of MSBP have been reported worldwide, although it is likely that most cases of MSBP go unreported in the literature. Most of the literature concerning this form of maltreatment originates in the United Kingdom and the United States. Cases of MSBP also have been reported from Canada; Australia; New Zealand; Western, Central, and Eastern Europe; Scandinavia; the Middle East; South America; the Indian subcontinent; Central America; Africa; Sri Lanka; Japan; and Singapore.[8] Clearly, MSBP is not a culture-specific disorder, nor is it confined to either a

socialized or privatized medical system. It also seems that the perpetration of MSBP is not as uncommon as originally thought, although getting a purchase on actual incidence is difficult. One study in the United Kingdom estimated the combined annual incidence of MSBP, non-accidental poisoning, and non-accidental suffocation as at least 2.8 per 100,000 in children younger than 1 year.[9] Extrapolation of this data to the United States suggests somewhere between 200 new cases of serious MSBP per year[10] to at least 600 new cases per year of suffocation or intentional poisoning.[6] A New Zealand study reported an incidence rate of 2 per 100,000 in children younger than 16 years.[11]

In most cases of MSBP, the perpetrator is the biological mother,[12] although fathers,[13,14] adoptive mothers,[15] other relatives,[16,17] babysitters,[18] and nurses[19] occasionally are implicated.

Boys and girls are victimized almost equally, and no special trend is noted as to birth order.[20] Curiously, however, although several children in a family may be victimized sequentially, it is unusual for more than one child to be victimized within any given period,[21] except during relatively brief transition periods. Typically, if the original victim survives, that child's medical troubles melt away when another child comes along and develops unusual and inexplicable troubles.

Most victims of MSBP are infants and toddlers.[9,12,20] Presumably, the younger children are more commonly affected because they lack the verbal skills necessary to disclose their abuse and are relatively helpless physically. They are therefore easier to manipulate and assault. Although victimization of the children commonly begins in infancy or toddlerhood, there is usually a delay in making the correct diagnosis. In 2 series, the average time from onset of symptoms and signs to diagnosis was 15 to 22 months,[12,20] but it might be as long as 20 years[20] or never.[22] A rare report describes cessation of MSBP not because of medical diagnosis, but because the school-aged victim threatened to disclose her mother's long-standing, painful, and disfiguring abuse.[23] Older child victims of MSBP, whose abuse may have begun years earlier, may adopt the false symptoms and signs as their own.[24] These children are less likely than young children to have illness produced, and more likely to have falsified reports of symptoms and medical history.[25] Some evidence suggests that these children may go on to develop Munchausen syndrome themselves[26] or some type of personality disorder.[27,28]

In one series, 25% of MSBP cases involved simulation only, 25% involved production only, and 50% involved both simulation and production of illness.[20] Another larger series showed that 57% of illness was produced.[12] In 50% to 95% of cases, depending on the meta-analytic series, the perpetrator continued victimizing the child in the hospital,[12,20] often in the most egregious ways,[29] and even in closely monitored settings, such as the pediatric intensive care unit.[30]

Short-term morbidity for the children, by definition, is 100%, much of it related to the diagnostic and therapeutic procedures ordered by the doctor. Long-term morbidity, defined as pain and/or illness that causes permanent disfigurement or impairment, is harder to assess statistically. About 8% of the surviving victims of MSBP have some kind of long-term morbidity as a result of complications of the attack or, rarely, complications from medical procedures.[12,20,31] This figure is probably an underestimate, however, and does not include long-term psychological morbidity, which may be considerable.[32]

Although it is currently impossible, for methodological reasons, to assess the mortality rate from MSBP, it is important to state that some children die because of an ultimate fatal attack. Perhaps the perpetrator accidentally goes too far, having meant to make the child ill but not to kill the child. Perhaps it is a final act of unbridled hostility toward the child. Whatever the intent, children are at some risk of death. Series death rates vary, from 6% to 33%.[12,20,31] In the largest series to date, apnea was the most commonly repeated symptom that preceded death.[12] Almost all victims were infants and toddlers, and the causes of death notably featured suffocation and poisoning. Other causes of death have been described,[20] and still others, as yet undescribed, are possible. Children as old as 8 years have been killed in the context of MSBP.[12] Furthermore, siblings of victims of MSBP tend to die in alarming numbers, often with the misdiagnosis of sudden infant death syndrome (SIDS), and there is every reason to believe that they died in a homicidal manner.[12,31,33–36] Child fatality review teams are now common throughout the country and, with their ability for multidisciplinary review, are occasionally discovering cases of MSBP that had previously but incorrectly been designated as accidental, natural, or undetermined manner of death.

A few cases of adult victims of adult perpetrators of MSBP have been reported.[37–40] The methods of assault included repeated injection of gasoline or turpentine under the skin, injection of insulin, and poisoning with benzodiazepines.

Clinical and Laboratory Findings

Symptoms, signs, and laboratory findings in MSBP cover an enormous spectrum, but the most common serious presentation seems to be apnea. Seizures, feeding problems, bleeding, central nervous system depression, diarrhea, vomiting, fever (with or without sepsis or other localized infection), rash, allergy, and behavioral problems also are reported quite commonly.[12,20] At no time, however, should any list be considered inclusive as we continually expand our understanding of the breadth of presentations of this syndrome. Table 16.1 lists some of the presentations of MSBP.

Nissen fundoplications are unnecessarily performed with distressing frequency in victims of MSBP, as are operations for the installation of a central venous catheter. Both procedures result in direct-line access to the child and therefore the possibility of further intraluminal assaults on the child with feces, saliva, contaminated water, drugs, salt, air, and many other substances.[41] Some child victims of MSBP are developmentally delayed as a result of the damage done by the inflicted illness or as a result of chronic hospitalization, enforced invalidism, or lack of stimulation. Malnutrition may be the result of the chronically inflicted illness; surreptitious withholding of food; prolonged emetic, laxative, or other drug assault; or other causes. Munchausen syndrome by proxy also may present in the context of a bona fide chronic disease, when the caretaking parent has intentionally and surreptitiously withheld treatment to significantly exacerbate the child's illness.[42,43]

The perpetration of MSBP may terminate with the homicide of the child. Probably the most common cause of death in homicidal MSBP is suffocation, but there are many causes of death, among which are poisoning with various drugs, inflicted bacterial or fungal sepsis, hypoglycemia, and salt or potassium poisoning. Too frequently, suffocation and other homicidal deaths are signed out incorrectly as to cause and manner. Either the significantly positive clinical history is undiscovered or ignored; a scene investigation is delayed or inadequate; or the autopsy, if performed, has not included all necessary dissections or tests.

A significantly positive clinical history of a deceased child would feature one or

TABLE 16.1

Some Clinical Presentations of Munchausen Syndrome by Proxy[a]

System	Symptom, Sign, or Laboratory Finding
Head, eyes, ears, nose, throat, mouth	Bleeding from ears, nose, throat Conjunctivitis External otitis Hearing/speech impairment Nasal excoriation Nystagmus Otorrhea Parotitis/orbital cellulitis Tooth loss
Respiratory	Apnea and/or acute life-threatening event Asthma Bleeding from upper respiratory tract Choking/dyspnea Cyanosis (and other color changes including pallor) Cystic fibrosis Hemoptysis Respiratory arrest Respiratory infection Sleep apnea
Cardiovascular	Bradycardia Cardiomyopathy Cardiopulmonary arrest Hypertension Rhythm abnormalities (including bradycardia, tachycardia, ventricular tachycardia, and others) Shock
Gastrointestinal	Abdominal pain Anorexia Bleeding from nasogastric tube/ileostomy Celiac disease Chronic intestinal pseudo-obstruction Crohn disease Diarrhea Esophageal burns Esophageal perforation Feculent vomiting Feeding problems Gastrointestinal ulceration Hematemesis Hematochezia or melena Hemorrhagic colitis Malabsorption syndromes Polyphagia Pseudomelanosis coli Retrograde intussusception Vomiting (cyclic or otherwise)

TABLE 16.1

Some Clinical Presentations of Munchausen Syndrome by Proxy,[a] *continued*

System	Symptom, Sign, or Laboratory Finding
Genitourinary	Bacteriuria Hematuria Menorrhagia Nocturia Polydipsia Polyuria and/or impaired urinary concentrating ability Proteinuria Pyuria Renal failure Urination from umbilical micropenis Urethral stones Urine gravel
Neurologic, musculoskeletal, developmental, psychiatric	Arthralgia Arthritis Ataxia Behavioral/personality (including anxiety, autism spectrum disorders, panic reactions, rage, disorientation, and others) Cerebral palsy Developmental delay (failure to attain and/or loss of milestones) Headache Hyperactivity Irritability Learning/attention disability Lethargy Morning stiffness Psychotic symptoms Sleep disturbances: prolonged sleep/other Seizures Syncope Tourette syndrome Unconsciousness Weakness
Skin	Abscesses Burns Eczema Excoriation Rash
Infectious, immune, allergic	Allergies (to food, drugs, others) Bacteremia (unimicrobial and/or polymicrobial) Fevers Immunodeficiency Osteomyelitis Septic arthritis Sinopulmonary disease Soft tissue/skin infection Urinary tract infection

TABLE 16.1

Some Clinical Presentations of Munchausen Syndrome by Proxy,[a] *continued*

System	Symptom, Sign, or Laboratory Finding
Abnormalities of growth Hematologic	Failure to gain weight or weight loss Anemia Bleeding diathesis Bleeding from specific sites (see system) Easy bruising Leukopenia
Metabolic, endocrine, fluid and electrolyte	Acidosis Alkalosis Biochemical chaos Creatine kinase and aldolase increase Cystinosis Dehydration Diabetes Glycosuria Hyperglycemia Hyperkalemia Hypernatremia Hypochloremia Hypoglycemia Hypokalemia Hyponatremia MELAS (mitochondrial encephalopathy lactic acidosis and stroke-like syndrome)
Other	Abuse (sexual, physical, other) Diaphoresis Fatigue Foreign-body ingestions Hypothermia Pain Peripheral edema Poisonings Premature birth

[a]Including items reportedly observed by mother or actually observed by medical staff.

more items listed in Box 16.1. If any of these factors figure in the clinical history, MSBP should be included in the differential diagnosis, along with possible genetic, metabolic, other natural, toxicological, or environmental causes of death. These factors are not diagnostic criteria for MSBP. They are historical flags that should spur further investigation, and in particular an exhaustive autopsy.

The usefulness of the autopsy as an investigative tool for determining cause and manner of death is obviously enhanced when it is done in the most thorough manner. Specifically, evidence of poisoning should be diligently searched for, with the necessary toxicological studies done from vitreous, blood, urine, gastric contents, tissues, or other sources. A "routine toxicology study" may be inadequate and, in any case, includes somewhat different studies, depending on the laboratory.[44] Specific requests may be necessary to have certain tests done. For example, though ipecac is no longer recommended as a household staple, intentional ipecac poisoning still occurs. It is useful to know that its alkaloids persist in urine for weeks, whereas they are detectable in blood for only a few hours.[45] Consulting

BOX 16.1
Review of Clinical History in a Dead Child: Circumstances Suggestive of Munchausen Syndrome by Proxy

A history of repeated medical visits for unusual, poorly defined, unpredictable, or unresponsive illness, especially apnea and seizures, which had never been confirmed to be witnessed at their starting moment by anyone other than the mother; *and* a full medical evaluation of the child that revealed no organic abnormality that could *fully* account for the child's reported illness, *or* a partial medical evaluation of the child that excluded major causes for the child's reported illness, or any medical evaluation that came to a conclusion about the child's diagnosis but whose accuracy, on review, is seriously questioned

OR

Ill sibling of decedent, especially if child was or is ill with chronic, poorly defined medical problems

OR

Dead sibling of decedent, or dead unrelated child in the same home as decedent, especially if any of the following is found:

a. Other child's death was signed out as sudden infant death syndrome;
b. Death followed a poorly defined or chronic illness;
c. Cause of death was allegedly an illness that overwhelmingly is nonfatal in childhood;
d. Cause of death was related to poisoning/intoxication;
e. Cause of death was the result of an unusual accident;
f. Death followed a presumed illness that was either unsubstantiated or excluded at autopsy; *or*
g. Explanation for the death was inadequate

OR

Mother with chronic, poorly defined medical problems

with the laboratory director as to best method to detect suspected agents or drugs often is useful. Identifying a substance may be more specifically delineated with gas chromatography/mass spectrophotometry. The laboratory should be asked to preserve the samples securely, with proper chain of evidence documented, because they may be needed later for repeated studies or other studies not originally considered. If both serum sodium and urine sodium are elevated and the child is not dehydrated, salt poisoning should be suspected. The premortem blood sodium or the postmortem vitreous sodium may be useful. Postmortem vitreous urea nitrogen is a reliable study and may be useful as a reflection of hydration status. It is interpreted in the context of other renal function studies, in the same way as is blood urea nitrogen. As with all young children suspected of having been maltreated, a skeletal survey should be done to look for fractures. Classic physical abuse injuries have been reported in victims of MSBP.[12] Microbiology studies may be central to determining whether the child was the victim of inflicted microbial assault. When postmortem microbiology blood samples are positive, care must be taken to discriminate between those that reflect infection in the child and those that are the result of postmortem blood contamination with bowel, skin, or other organisms. The condition and contents of any lines into the child (central venous catheter, gastrostomy, endotracheal tube, shunt, pacemaker, etc) should be examined closely, and it may be prudent to preserve them. As in a clinical situation, there should be careful attention paid to chain of evidence for laboratory specimens and biomedical appliances.

Homicidal suffocation deaths[36,46] deserve further comment because they are still too commonly misdiagnosed as SIDS. It is reemphasized here that if any significant history precedes death, then SIDS, by definition, is excluded. The current definition of SIDS is the unexpected death of an infant younger than 1 year that remains unexplained after a complete review of the clinical history, death scene investigation, and autopsy. For reasons having more to do with a combination of good intentions and/or politicking than with scientific durability, it is still common practice to use the term SIDS as a cause of death on a death certificate, with manner of death as natural. Sudden death in a child who had repeated apnea or acute life-threatening events before death, especially episodes that featured attacks beginning only in the mother's presence, and when the mother called someone to see the baby, the child was hypoxic (ie, cyanotic, gray, gasping, and limp) are cause for concern.[36,47] The physical findings of suffocation more commonly seen in adult victims (head and neck petechiae and/ or bruising, defensive marks, etc) are almost always absent in young children.[48] Intra-alveolar hemosiderin found at autopsy may be a marker of past smothering,[49] but this is neither definitive nor specific.[50]

Perpetrators

What are the characteristics of the perpetrator of MSBP, and why does she do this? First, it is important to state that no psychological test can include or exclude perpetration of MSBP. Second, there is no classic profile for a perpetrator, meaning that possessing certain characteristics does not entirely implicate a suspect, and lacking certain characteristics does not entirely exclude a suspect.

The perpetrator of MSBP is usually the mother. She sometimes has had nursing, medical, or paramedical training, perhaps never completed. She may be married, single, or divorced, but if married, the relationship with her husband, although perhaps seemingly satisfactory, is often shallow, with the husband at arm's length from the child's illnesses. One occasionally sees a husband who vehemently endorses his wife's history of the child, even when it is proven definitively to have been untrue. Although she was originally described as generally affable with medical and nursing staff, broader experience shows that she may have a hostile, difficult, and demanding personality. Some mothers, in their roles as champions of their ill children, have had good success at enlisting the admiration of their communities; making useful, powerful, or lucrative contacts; or obtaining benefits consequent on the child's illness, including wish-fulfillment trips.[51] Features of Munchausen syndrome[20,52] and a history of problems related to her reproductive system (including spontaneous abortions during motor vehicle crashes), unsubstantiated by her medical records, are not uncommon in these mothers, but they may lack a documented psychiatric history, or it may be unavailable for review.

Mothers have been variably diagnosed psychiatrically as normal, depressed, borderline, hysterical, narcissistic, or with various other personality disorders.[12,53] Munchausen syndrome by proxy in the context of postpartum depression also has been reported.[54] It is not to be understood from this that the mother has some kind of disease that renders her incapable of discerning right from wrong, that makes her compulsively perform acts outside her consciousness, or that makes her either the unwilling or unwitting captive of an irresistible impulse. Only rarely is the mother deemed to be psychotic or delusional.[12,20] Some reports cite a history of significant childhood maltreatment in these mothers,[55] including physical and sexual abuse,[32] with the generational legacy of abuse in some way "medicalized," from the mother's exposure to the medical field, either as a patient or a close party to a sick person. One fascinating single case study proposes that the perpetration of MSBP is related to transgenerational transmission of an attachment disorder; the perpetrator, having been insecurely attached as a child then demonstrates abnormalities of caregiving and care-eliciting when she herself becomes a mother.[56] When the behavior of mothers who suffocated their infants was recorded on covert video surveillance, 3 groups emerged: normal, hostile, and paucity of interaction.[57] These are psychodynamic interpretations. Other authors emphasize observable maternal behavior, with the perpetrator first needing to "discharge dysphoric affects" (ie, anger, anxiety, and others); next, having a breakdown in internal inhibitions; and finally, neutralization of external inhibition, all resulting in the "habit strength" of the assaultive behavior.[58] The primary motivation, according to another, is the "use of a sick child as a vehicle to maintain and regulate a relationship with doctors and other medical personnel and later with other people seen as powerful,"[51] with motivation going beyond needing to be in the limelight; it is, rather, "a dare, a challenge, engaged in compulsively about who is going to be able to outsmart whom."[51] My clinical impression is that the personality styles, backgrounds, and motivations to perpetrate MSBP (when inferable) are quite diverse, though I would agree that "(T)he difficulty that besets the endeavor to understand Munchausen by Proxy is how to judge the veracity of a person who repeatedly dissimulates."[51]

The mother may become suicidal when her duplicity is uncovered or when she becomes aware of professional suspicions. Psychiatric interventions should be offered and available. Why MSBP is overwhelmingly a female-perpetrated form of child abuse is not clear, although female patterns of learned behavior and expression of hostility have been proposed. It certainly stands in contrast to almost every other form of child abuse and neglect (except sexual abuse), in which male and female perpetrators figure in approximately equal numbers.

No evidence whatsoever suggests that the perpetrator of MSBP is unaware of her actions. On the contrary, the planning and organization often involved, the minute attention to secrecy, the fact that the assaults are committed without witnesses, and the carefully woven fabric of lies presented to the doctor all suggest great awareness. The perpetration of MSBP is volitional. It is also violent. The fact that the violence is encased in duplicity only hides, but does not diminish, its aggression.

Most mothers do not have a criminal history, but occasionally one does. They may break into their own homes to stage thefts, or set fires, sometimes collecting insurance settlements. They also may be dangerous to others in their midst, with the homicide of relatives or children in their charge, for example, having occasionally been proven or highly suspected. Fabricating factitious illness in pets also has been reported.[59,60]

Perpetrators also may be dangerous to medical professionals. They have been known to undertake criminal behavior such as stalking, breaking and entering, theft, fraud, destruction of property, and death threats. It is no longer uncommon for the perpetrator of MSBP to make false allegations of malpractice by the doctor to professional or licensing bodies, or to sue the doctor and/or hospital on one or several of a number of pretexts: defamation of character, malicious reporting, malpractice, wrongful detention of the child, or wrongful death.

Diagnostic Strategies

Failure to diagnose MSBP means that a fundamentally healthy child and his siblings could be irreversibly damaged or killed. Conversely, the failure to exclude MSBP may mean that necessary treatment is withheld from an ill child, a family is not offered prognostic information or genetic counseling, or the child is separated from his family. The single largest impediment to making a diagnosis of MSBP is the failure to include it in the differential diagnosis. Once the diagnosis is entertained and a diagnostic strategy designed, the diagnosis is usually included or excluded relatively quickly.

Once MSBP is considered, the difficulties in pursuing the diagnosis generally revolve around the dilemma of not wishing to expose the child to any more potential risk and yet needing reasonably definitive proof. This clinical judgment call is best made with the assistance of the director of medical services, the head nurse, the primary care nurse, the hospital child protection team and, if necessary, the hospital lawyer. It is at this point that social services and their representative lawyer should be notified of a possible child abuse case. The diagnostic strategy (or strategies) must maximize diagnostic capability while minimizing risk to the child and must obviously take into account access to, and condition of, the child.

When MSBP is suspected, confirmation or elimination of the diagnosis may be undertaken through one or several of a number of strategies: the search for evidence of illness fabrication, the search for evidence of an explanation other than MSBP, the separation of the child from the suspected perpetrator, and records review.

The first diagnostic strategy, the search for evidence of illness fabrication, includes such tests as toxicology studies if poisoning is suspected; blood group typing, subtyping, or DNA typing if contamination with exogenous blood is suspected; or hidden video monitoring if surreptitious suffocation is suspected. The medical literature contains some fascinating accounts in which evidence of commission has been thus captured: ipecac poisoning is uncovered by finding a postmortem blood sample positive for the alkaloids in ipecac[61] or by toxicologic studies in a living child[62]; factitious bleeding is exposed by minor blood group typing of erythrocytes in urine,[63] injecting radiolabeled erythrocytes as comparisons to the child's "bleeding sites,"[64] DNA typing of the bloody towel presented by the parent compared with that of the child's buccal cells,[65] and comparing the hemoglobin F concentration of an infant's blood to that of the blood stains on the child's bedclothes[66]; factitious diabetes mellitus is confirmed by using ascorbic acid as a marker for the child's own urine[67]; factitious hyperinsulinemic hypoglycemia is discovered by finding simultaneous low C-peptide and high insulin levels in a first critical blood sample of a hypoglycemic child[68,69]; and factitious intractable apnea is uncovered by covertly videotaping mothers suffocating their children.[29,70–72]

To a great extent, one must choose, or even design, the test depending on the fabrication that is suspected. The search for evidence of illness fabrication must be very carefully planned and executed. Depending on the situation, this involves proper chain of evidence, preservation of laboratory specimens, continuous monitoring and recording of video units with plans to intervene immediately and decisively if assault is seen, and precise coordination with law enforcement and/or social services. The advantage of this diagnostic strategy is that, if positive evidence is uncovered and is reliable, it is more likely to be accepted as definitive, medically and legally. The disadvantage is that the child is potentially exposed to at least one more assault. If the test is negative, then it is often not possible to distinguish between absence of assault, failure to capture the assault, or a false-negative test.

One diagnostic strategy in the search for evidence of illness fabrication is covert videomonitoring. It is a highly useful, if somewhat controversial, strategy. A video camera with its lens hidden in, for example, what seems to be a sprinkler head or smoke alarm, may be installed and linked to a monitoring and recording unit in a nearby room. Tertiary care hospitals should seriously consider the diagnostic benefits of such a system, especially when undertaking remodeling. Obviously, this type of system must be in place before the child's admission. If the hospital room has a private bathroom, it is wise to close it off to avoid the possibility of an assault to the child outside the range of the video.

Useful clinical data may be accrued with videotaping.[29,70–73] One investigator who videotaped mothers smothering their children noted,

> Smothering has been labeled "gentle" battering. We reject this. The video and physiological recordings showed that both children struggled violently until they lost consciousness. Considerable force was used to obstruct their airways, and this force was needed for at least 70 seconds before electroencephalographic changes, probably associated with loss of consciousness, occurred. Interestingly, in both cases a soft garment was used to smother the children and no marks were seen on the lips or around the nose.[29]

The authors further delineated features of the multichannel recordings, "a combination of which may in future prove to be pathognomonic of this type (smothering) of apnea…." The features included the sudden onset of large body movements during a relatively regular breathing pattern (from struggling induced by airway obstruction); a series of large breaths at about 1 minute after the onset of the episode, with a characteristically prolonged expiratory phase, at a relatively slow rate (a response to severe arterial hypoxia); a severe degree of sinus tachycardia; and last, at about 1 minute after the onset of the episode, large slow waves and a subsequent isoelectric baseline on the electroencephalogram typical of hypoxia.[29]

If videotaping is planned, the multidisciplinary team may want to consult with the hospital attorney. Continuous observation of the videotape by real-time monitoring is essential, and it is wise to notify hospital security and the local police department, because their participation often is needed.

The subject of diagnostic, covert videomonitoring in the hospital has engendered some animated debate, with authors addressing the legal, ethical, and logistic aspects of videotaping.[72,74–82] Some are concerned with the rights of privacy of parents in the hospital or suggest that a warrant for covert videomonitoring be obtained beforehand.[78] Other authors point out that the parental rights to privacy are abrogated when that parent is the agent of the child's possible destruction. In this pediatrician's opinion, the videotape may be considered the equivalent of other tests undertaken in the usual diagnostic process that do not individually require consent; the general medical consent form signed on behalf of the child at the time of admission to the hospital covers most procedures. Furthermore, child abuse statutes in every state permit the taking of pictures without parental consent if child abuse is suspected. In one covert videomonitoring study of 41 patients, the authors note that "specific permission to monitor was included in the admission form for consent to treat given to families on admission to the hospital. Contained within this form is the statement, 'Closed circuit monitoring of patient care may be used for educational or clinical purposes.' In addition, a sign at the entrance to the hospital informs visitors that this facility is monitored and recorded by hidden cameras."[72] The authors also note that in 4 of 41 cases, MSBP was definitely

excluded, a very useful diagnostic milestone that informs further investigation.

The second diagnostic strategy, the search for an explanation other than MSBP, has often been extensive by the time that MSBP is suspected, but it has not necessarily been exhaustive. There are certain situations in which an exhaustive search for an explanation other than MSBP is the best diagnostic strategy: when there exists neither the opportunity nor the diagnostic test that could capture evidence of commission or when the search for evidence of illness fabrication would expose the child to grave risk. The contending diagnoses on the differential should be those that are subject to definitive inclusion or exclusion. For example, if a child is repeatedly presented to the hospital with apnea that begins only in the presence of the mother, the disorders that might be causing the child's apnea (however unlikely, for example, a cerebral space-occupying lesion or gastroesophageal reflux) can be searched for, and can therefore be definitively included or excluded. Positive test results must be carefully scrutinized to ensure that they are positive neither as a result of maternal contamination/intervention, nor as a result of being "overcalled" (ie, the range of normal for the test is not reliably delineated, or minimally positive findings are said to account for substantial symptomatology). Certain gastrointestinal tests seem to be especially vulnerable to this problem, in particular gastrointestinal motility studies[83] and esophageal pH probe studies. Normal gastrointestinal motility excludes the diagnosis of chronic intestinal pseudo-obstruction.[84,85] The advantage of this diagnostic strategy is that the gathering of diagnostic evidence does not involve exposing the child to the possibility of another assault. The disadvantage is that it can be time consuming and expensive, and there may be risks to the patient of various diagnostic procedures or prolonged hospitalization.

The third diagnostic strategy, the separation of the child from the parent, may be a very useful diagnostic strategy. In certain circumstances, it carries the most diagnostic weight and is the least malignant. It is important to have a baseline against which to compare the child's subsequent course during separation, whether that separation occurs in a hospital or in a foster home. The baseline is the well-documented history of the child's symptoms and signs as provided by the mother. Therefore, it is important that the only major change that is made in the child's care during the separation is the presence of the caretaker. It is sometimes the case that the fabrication of illness causes irreversible medical problems, or that the fabrication of illness is piled onto an already existing illness. Only reversible conditions of the child can be expected to improve, and these only to the degree and at a rate that is consonant with the condition itself. The advantage of this diagnostic strategy is that it can be definitive without exposing the child to further risk. The disadvantage is that, if it turns out that it is not MSBP, then an ill child has been separated unnecessarily and perhaps harmfully from his or her mother, and correct diagnosis has been delayed. One way to minimize the possible disadvantages is to have supervised visits with the mother. The supervision must be constant and scrupulous, with no foods, medications, or candy permitted.

The fourth diagnostic strategy is records review. This diagnostic strategy involves the reformulation of a differential diagnosis—one that is comprehensive without being promiscuous—and the critical reevaluation of this differential. This strategy, which one would suppose to have been implicit in the medical care already provided, follows from the observation that the pivotal facts, although present in the medical record, are frequently obscured by the sheer volume of information accumulated. In other words, the crucial data are there, but are buried. Furthermore, the importance of a comprehensive survey of the child's medical presentation may have been repeatedly overshadowed by the immediacy of the crises. Curiously, the more chronic and intractable the child's problem, the less likely it may be that it is given a fresh, comprehensive look. Finally, a sort of colonial system of medical care sometimes evolves, with fragments of the child's condition being parceled off to subspecialists, whose purview extends only to the edge of their organ systems of interest. They accept without question the "fact" of abnormalities in another system. Overview is neglected. The totality of the presentation is lost.

Records review may be the preferred diagnostic strategy, because it is low risk and often definitive. Records review may be the only diagnostic strategy available when, for example, the child is alive but unavailable for some reason, when the symptoms and signs of fabrication are long gone, when the child has received medical care at multiple institutions, or when the child is dead.

For most pediatric patients, a thorough records review is straightforward: We read, we remember. Records are relatively brief and come from a small number of medical facilities. That a substantially different approach to records review is in order when MSBP is suspected is a consequence of 3 typical features: the record is mammoth, the legal implications are broad, and the stakes are high. Records often run to thousands of pages, sometimes from dozens of medical facilities. The doctor may be called to testify in civil and/or criminal proceedings, where the medical facts— perhaps hundreds of thousands of them—may be minutely tracked and challenged, as may the process by which the diagnosis was distilled from the facts. A computerized system for data entry, storage, organization, and retrieval is often indispensable, and any of a number of commercially available database-management systems can be adapted for this purpose. Records pages should be numbered immediately, so that data can be noted with their corresponding page numbers and later retrieved.

Because the medical and nursing records often are complicated, it is best if someone (or several people) experienced in both inpatient and outpatient pediatrics reviews the records. There are advantages and disadvantages to working with original medical records. The advantages are that poor quality or missed duplication of records is not an issue, and that vital information on oversized pages is accessible. The disadvantages are considerable: pages cannot be numbered; accessibility, space, and the simultaneous availability of the record and the necessary computer equipment are generally problematic. In reality, it is commonly impossible to review original records because of geographic or logistic problems. In these usual circumstances, care must be taken to ensure, as far as possible, that photocopied records, or records scanned onto a CD-ROM, are complete. In the process of the records review, it is often helpful to compile a cumulative dated list of such things as prescribed medications, operations, consultations, hospitalizations, diagnoses explored, diagnostic tests performed and their results, interventions attempted, and school days missed.

The diagnostic strategies used to detect MSBP in its most common presentations are outlined in Table 16.2. Obviously, these diagnostic strategies will not fit every type of suspected event, and one must tailor the diagnostic strategy to the type of perpetration suspected. This effort may involve contacting colleagues in related fields for information or to seek help. Commonly, one must combine various diagnostic strategies. An excellent example of evaluating seizures by Barber and Davis[86] appears in Box 16.2 and the comprehensive approach can be adapted to many presentations.

TABLE 16.2
Some Methods of Fabrication and Corresponding Diagnostic Strategies in Munchausen Syndrome by Proxy[a]

Presentation	Method of Simulation and/or Production	Method of Diagnosis
Apnea	Manual suffocation	■ Videomonitoring ■ Implantable ECG recorder ■ Diagnosis by exclusion ■ Patient with pinch marks on nose ■ Mother caught
	Poisoning Tricyclic antidepressants Hydrocarbon	■ Toxicology (gastric/blood) ■ Toxicology of IV fluid
Seizures	Lying	■ Diagnosis by exclusion

	Poisoning
	
	  Phenothiazines
	
	  Hydrocarbons
	  Salt
	  Sulfonylurea
	  Tricyclic antidepressants
		■ Toxicology/assay of blood, urine, IV fluid, milk
		■ Serum and urine sodium concentrations

	Suffocation/carotid sinus pressure	■ Witnessed ■ Forensic photos of pressure points
Diarrhea	Phenolphthalein/other laxative poisoning	■ Stool/diaper positive
	Salt poisoning	■ Assay of formula/gastric contents
Vomiting	Emetic poisoning	■ Assay for drug
	Injection of air into gastrostomy tube Lying	■ Videomonitoring ■ Hospital observation

TABLE 16.2

Some Methods of Fabrication and Corresponding Diagnostic Strategies in Munchausen Syndrome by Proxy,ᵃ *continued*

Presentation	Method of Simulation and/or Production	Method of Diagnosis
CNS depression	Drugs	■ Assays of blood, gastric contents, urine, IV fluid, hair; analysis of insulin type; videomonitoring
	Diphenoxylate and atropine (Lomotil) Insulin Chloral hydrate Clonidine Barbiturates/narcotics Benzodiazepines Aspirin Diphenhydramine Tricyclic antidepressants Acetaminophen Hydrocarbons Chlordiazepoxide Phenytoin Phenobarbital Carbamazepine	
	Suffocation	■ See "Apnea" and "Seizures"
Bleeding	Rodenticide (warfarin) poisoning	■ Toxicology
	Phenolphthalein poisoning	■ Diapers positive
	Exogenous blood applied	■ Blood group antigen profiling; DNA typing ■ ⁵¹Cr labeling of erythrocytes
	Exsanguination of child	■ Single-blind study ■ Mother caught in the act
	Addition of other substances (paint, cocoa, dyes)	■ Testing; washing
Rash	Drug poisoning	■ Assay
	Scratching	■ Diagnosis of exclusion
	Caustics applied/painting skin	■ Assay/wash off

TABLE 16.2
Some Methods of Fabrication and Corresponding Diagnostic Strategies in Munchausen Syndrome by Proxy,[a] *continued*

Presentation	Method of Simulation and/or Production	Method of Diagnosis

Fever	Contamination with infected material
	■ Materials
	    Saliva
	    Feces
	    Dirt
	    Contaminated water
	    Coffee grounds
	    Vaginal secretions
	    Others
	■ Target tissues
	    Blood
	    Skin
	    Bones
	    Bladder
	    Others
		■ Caught in the act
		■ Improper taping of line discovered
		■ Type of organism growing from infected sites
		■ Trial separation
		■ Epidemiology (relative-risk assessment)
		■ Diagnosis by exclusion

	Falsifying temperature Falsifying chart	■ Careful charting, rechecking (especially urine for core body temperature) ■ Careful charting, rechecking ■ Duplication (ghost record) of temperature chart in nursing station

Abbreviations: ECG, electrocardiographic; IV, intravenous; CNS, central nervous system.
[a]Adapted with permission from Rosenberg DA. Web of deceit: a literature review of Munchausen syndrome by proxy. *Child Abuse Negl.* 1987;11:547–563.

Differential Diagnosis

Most pediatric patients who present persistently for medical care are not victims of MSBP. Waring[87] discusses the 2 questions that are asked with any pediatric patient: What is the matter with the patient? Why is this child being brought for care at this moment? The answer to the first question is taught in medical schools and during residency training, whereas the ability to answer both questions, in Yudkin's words, is "the beginning of real medicine."[87,88]

Most children have a primary organic illness that accounts for the totality of their presentation, but there are other possibilities that may account for the persistence. Box 16.3 gives the differential diagnosis of persistent presentation.

Genuine illness and MSBP may coexist. The discovery of a real illness in a child who is persistently brought for medical care does not exclude MSBP; the question then becomes, Does this illness reasonably explain the severity, extent, and

BOX 16.2
Practical Guidelines: How to Avoid Making a False Diagnosis of Epilepsy[a]

- The starting point is a meticulous history supplemented by carefully chosen diagnostic tests.

- Consider first the differential diagnosis of paroxysmal events (gastroesophageal reflux, gratification phenomena, breath-holding attacks, cardiac arrhythmia, syncope, metabolic disturbances, reflex anoxic seizures, and pseudoseizures).

- Look for clinical epilepsy syndromes with typical supporting electroencephalogram (EEG) findings.

- Ask the caregiver to video "episodes." Most families have the means to do this and some hospitals may be able to loan equipment.

- Do not start treatment until sure. As a minimum, seek independent corroboration of a parent's history or supportive EEG findings. It is rarely necessary to start anticonvulsant medication immediately, and it is good practice to have EEG information beforehand.

- Be especially wary of making the diagnosis if the EEG is normal. Seek confirmation from purported witnesses early on in the course of investigations, preferably an independent third party.

- Beware of the caregiver who uses the threat of harm coming to the child to influence clinical decision-making.

- Consider hospital admission if the reported episodes are frequent. Cessation of episodes during periods of observation is suspicious.

- Actively seek to verify details given by the caregiver regarding seizures or other aspects of history.

- Question discrepancies—children with severe, polymorphic epilepsy do not generally have normal neurodevelopment.

- Take and analyze blood and urine from any child presenting for the first time with a seizure—they may have been poisoned. Ensure that the urine is screened for relevant substances, not just drugs of abuse. Store serum so future quantitative analysis is possible.

- In the sick child glucose and electrolytes will usually be checked. An electrocardiogram should also be routine—it may provide a clue to poisoning with tricyclics.

- If poisoning is suspected, collect other body fluids (eg, vomitus or fluid from gastric lavage).

- Look for subtle signs of smothering (eg, petechial bruising to the face or nasal bleeding).

- Arrange appropriate supportive investigations including prolactin levels, raised glucose and white blood count (following prolonged generalized seizures), prolonged EEG or video-EEG records, pH studies, or tilt table tests.

[a]Adapted with permission from Barber M, Davis P. Fits, faints, or fatal fantasy? Fabricated seizures and child abuse. *Arch Dis Child.* 2002;86:230–233.

BOX 16.3
Differential Diagnosis of Persistent Presentation

Organic illness

Anxious parent

Developmentally delayed parent

Vulnerable child syndrome

Psychogenic illness

Munchausen syndrome by proxy

Munchausen syndrome

type of the child's symptoms and signs? Occasionally, the distinction between MSBP and pathologic doctor shopping, or magnification of a child's real but minimal illness for the parent's own psychological or fiscal gain, may not be clear. For those cases that seem to fall at the edges of the definition of MSBP, it is worth remembering that the name applied to the child's circumstances is not so material as a careful assessment of the threatened harm to the child.

Diagnostic Criteria

When MSBP is suspected, the strength of the known facts may extend from weak to definitive. Thus there may be different degrees of diagnostic conviction, not only from case to case but also within a case, depending on the stage of the assessment. Here, therefore, diagnostic criteria for a definitive diagnosis and a possible diagnosis of MSBP are provided. Because the gathering of evidence in a case may, ultimately, diminish the likelihood or altogether exclude MSBP, diagnostic criteria for the uncertain diagnosis and the definitely excluded diagnosis also are provided.[89]

Diagnostic criteria serve to discriminate efficiently between one particular diagnosis and all others. Collectively, the diagnostic criteria for a disorder are the smallest set of findings that must be present to make a diagnosis.

Each diagnostic criterion must be present to make a diagnosis. Each criterion must be pivotal, meaning that its presence is required for, and its absence excludes, the diagnosis. Each finding must be credibly observable by human senses. Other competent observers, using the same method, would observe the finding the same way. Thus the observation would be replicable.

To summarize, each criterion is necessary, and collectively the criteria are sufficient for diagnosis.

Definitive Diagnosis

The definitive diagnosis of MSBP is the clear diagnosis. One can make a definitive diagnosis in 1 of 2 ways: by inclusion or by exclusion.

A diagnosis by inclusion is one supported by incontrovertible evidence of commission. For example, if a mother smothers the child she had previously and repeatedly presented for apnea, and if her act were captured with covert videotaping in the hospital, then the definitive diagnosis of MSBP would be one by inclusion. Box 16.4 lists the criteria for the definitive diagnosis by inclusion of MSBP.

A diagnosis by exclusion is one in which all other possible explanations for the child's condition have been considered and excluded. A diagnosis by exclusion

BOX 16.4
Munchausen Syndrome by Proxy: Criteria for a Definitive Diagnosis by Inclusion[a]

1. Child has been repeatedly presented for medical care.
   AND

2. Test/event is positive for tampering with child, or with child's medical situation.
   AND

3. Positivity of test/event is not credibly the result of test error or misinterpretation, nor of miscommunication or specimen mishandling.
   AND

4. No explanation for the positive test/event other than illness falsification is medically possible.
   AND

5. No findings credibly exclude illness falsification.

[a]Reprinted with permission from Rosenberg DA. Munchausen syndrome by proxy: medical diagnostic criteria. *Child Abuse Negl.* 2003;27:421–430.

is the only diagnosis left standing after an exhaustive investigation. For example, if a child presents with recurrent apnea that begins exclusively in one person's presence and results in observable clinical compromise, if the child is conclusively shown to not otherwise exhibit apnea, and if all possible medical conditions that could account for the apnea are properly investigated and definitively excluded, then the definitive diagnosis of MSBP would be one by exclusion. Box 16.5 lists the criteria for the definitive diagnosis by exclusion of MSBP.

Possible Diagnosis

A possible diagnosis of MSBP is one among several likely diagnoses. Box 16.6 lists the criteria for the possible diagnosis of MSBP. Medical professionals are legally mandated to report child abuse to the local authority when they have a reasonable suspicion of it. *Reasonable suspicion* is not a term of art

in medicine, but roughly translates into the set of diagnostic criteria here noted as possible diagnosis.

Inconclusive Determination: Can't Know

It is obvious that, rather than increasing the weight of medical evidence in support of a diagnosis of MSBP, accumulating data may instead diminish its likelihood. Medical criteria for inconclusive findings—that is, for MSBP being indeterminate—are therefore articulated here. *Can't know* means that, although the collection of data is complete, the data are insufficient to determine the diagnosis. One can confidently neither establish nor eliminate MSBP as the diagnosis. Can't know differs from possible diagnosis because implicit in a can't know determination is the assertion that all relevant and available strategies for diagnosis have been exhausted. This is in contrast to a possible diagnosis, in which there is an

BOX 16.5
Munchausen Syndrome by Proxy: Criteria for a Definitive Diagnosis by Exclusion[a]

1. Child has been repeatedly presented for medical care.
   AND

2. All diagnoses other than illness falsification have been credibly eliminated, so that
   a. If the child is alive, the competing diagnoses are those that took into account the child's major medical findings and that account for the entirety of the child's presentation. (A major medical finding is one that is objectively observed, sufficiently specific as to help formulate the range of diagnoses, and verifiable in the record.)
   OR
   b. If the child is alive, separation of the child from the alleged perpetrator results in resolution of the child's reversible medical problems, in accordance with their degree and speed of reversibility. No variable other than the separation can logically and fully account for the child's improvement.
   OR
   c. If the child is dead, autopsy examination does not reveal a cause of death that is credibly of accidental, natural, or suicidal manner.
   AND

3. No findings credibly exclude illness falsification.

[a]Reprinted with permission from Rosenberg DA. Munchausen syndrome by proxy: medical diagnostic criteria. *Child Abuse Negl.* 2003;27:421–430.

BOX 16.6
Munchausen Syndrome by Proxy: Criteria for Possible Diagnosis[a]

1. Child has been repeatedly presented for medical care.
   AND

2. a. Test/event is presumptively positive for tampering with child, or with child's medical situation. No other explanation is readily apparent. No findings seem to exclude illness falsification.
   OR
   b. Child has a condition that cannot be fully explained medically, despite a respectable initial evaluation at least. Cogent hypothesis suggests a faked medical condition. No findings seem to exclude illness falsification.

[a]Reprinted with permission from Rosenberg DA. Munchausen syndrome by proxy: medical diagnostic criteria. *Child Abuse Negl.* 2003;27:421–430.

expectation of further diagnostic strategy. Box 16.7 lists the criteria for an inconclusive (can't know) determination.

Definitely Not

Definitely not MSBP means that the diagnosis can be absolutely eliminated because a wholly credible alternative explanation is at hand. To allow degrees of certainty within this diagnostic option, the physician might want to use some kind of qualifier, for example, *probably not* MSBP. Probably not MSBP is about the same as saying that, in all likelihood, an alternative explanation is at hand. The fact that diagnostic criteria for the exclusion of MSBP are included means that, as with other pediatric disorders, it is inevitable that there will be more suspected than actual cases. Recognizing this means also recognizing the need for the swiftest and most decisive diagnostic test, but one whose risk

to the child does not seem to be excessive. Extreme care must be taken not to overdiagnose MSBP, or to marry oneself to the diagnosis in the absence of sufficient evidence simply because one has considered it. Cases of misdiagnosed MSBP[90] are a real tragedy for the family and child. Box 16.8 lists the criteria for excluding the diagnosis of MSBP.

Intervention

It would be folly to give a list of directives to take in all cases in which MSBP is suspected. The reader, however, may find the following considerations useful:

1. Optimally, the child can be protected and the definitive data either to include or exclude the diagnosis can be simultaneously collected. Realistically, this is often not the case. Professionals find themselves poised between weighing the eventual use-

---

BOX 16.7
Munchausen Syndrome by Proxy: Criteria for Inconclusive Determination[a]

1. Child has been repeatedly presented for medical care.
   AND

2. The relevant and available information has been reviewed and/or the child appropriately evaluated.
   AND

3. One is left with a differential diagnosis, rather than a single diagnosis.
   AND

4. It is not possible to conclusively confirm one diagnosis.
   AND

5. It is not possible to exclude all but one diagnosis conclusively on the differential diagnosis.
   AND

6. It is not possible to conclusively exclude all but one diagnosis on the differential diagnosis.

[a]Reprinted with permission from Rosenberg DA. Munchausen syndrome by proxy: medical diagnostic criteria. *Child Abuse Negl.* 2003;27:421–430.

BOX 16.8
Munchausen Syndrome by Proxy: Criteria for Excluding the Diagnosis[a]

1. Child has been repeatedly presented for medical care.
   AND

2. What had seemed to be possible falsification of illness has been wholly and credibly accounted for in some other way.

[a]Reprinted with permission from Rosenberg DA. Munchausen syndrome by proxy: medical diagnostic criteria. *Child Abuse Negl.* 2003;27:421–430.

fulness of these data against the possibility of a mishap occurring to the child during the data collection process. When further diagnostic procedures place the child in a situation of untenable risk, the protection of the child is always the paramount consideration. Because child protection is a civil matter, the legal burden of proof is preponderance of the evidence. Thus absolute diagnostic proof is not necessary, and in its absence, epidemiological evidence pertaining to the case may be sufficiently compelling (see later discussion).

2. Involve a multidisciplinary team early on. It is suggested that the county department of social services be contacted before any discussion with the family so that the medical concerns are understood and the county is involved in the plan development, including the possibility of being prepared with a restraining order. Contacts, meeting, and planning must sometimes be done on an emergency basis, so that the child is not exposed to potential harm.

   Some individuals who are not customarily members of a hospital child protection team might be included. The social worker from the county to which the case has been reported is a pivotal person. Much will depend on the social worker's communication with the medical staff and understanding of the case. Given the volume and complexity of the data to digest and the generally high rate of staff turnover among county social workers, it is preferable for the social workers to work in pairs. Any way to circumvent the widespread and inefficient practice of having an "intake worker" start the case and then an "ongoing worker" continue it should be pursued. The supervisor of the social workers and the county attorney should similarly be included in the multidisciplinary team from the start.

   Two psychiatrists and/or psychologists should be engaged to participate. Optimally, one is assigned to the family and the other to the medical and nursing staff. The family needs not only extended evaluation but also support. After confrontation of the family with the suspected diagnosis, the mother, who is generally the alleged perpetrator, is at increased risk for suicide.[20,91] The child also needs to be at least developmentally and, if of sufficient age, psychologically evaluated. Interactional assessments by an experienced developmental psychologist may be useful.

Assigning a psychiatrist for the medical and nursing staff is not superfluous. Multidisciplinary teams break down over these cases. It is axiomatic that cases of MSBP cause polarization of opinions and emotions among the hospital staff, who have often worked with the family for years. The sense of betrayal experienced by some staff members can be enormous and painful. One nurse commented, "On an intellectual level, the diagnosis was sensible, but on an emotional level, the suspicion was almost impossible to accept."[92] Others simply cannot fathom that this situation is possible; unfortunate and unnecessary rifts may occur among the staff. Anticipating the need for a mental health professional to help all staff with their feelings is good primary prevention.

Police and other law enforcement personnel also should be involved early, especially if videotaping in the hospital is anticipated. Should an episode of intentional infliction of harm come to light during the videotaping, the police generally prefer to have prior knowledge of the case and may want to be prepared with an arrest warrant. A decision must be undertaken between the hospital and law enforcement as to which entity will undertake videomonitoring.

The primary care nurse and the head nurse should be included in the multidisciplinary child protection team. The primary care nurse is often the person who has spent the most time with the child and the family over an extended period and multiple hospitalizations. He or she often has valuable information about a case that may not be known to the others on the team. This individual certainly must be included in any plans that involve diagnostic procedures for MSBP. The primary care nurse often becomes responsible for important items such as documentation and chain of evidence of specimens.

Finally, if available, it is often advisable to have a good clinical epidemiologist participating with the multidisciplinary team from the beginning, because data of commission (eg, a videotape showing the mother suffocating the baby; a definitive blood test showing exogenous insulin in the child's body) often are unobtainable. The diagnostic alternative to these data is the calculation of the relative risk to the child of being in maternal care. For example, if the child has an unspecified illness characterized by vomiting, failure to thrive, and multiple hospitalizations, an epidemiologist can review the child's records and calculate the relative risk to the child of losing weight at home compared with that of losing weight in the hospital. In the absence of data of commission, relative-risk data may be the most compelling evidence to present to the court. It is helpful if the data can be interpreted to the court in lay language by the epidemiologist or by the attending clinician.

The multidisciplinary child protection team is under no obligation to include the mother's attorney (if she has engaged one) or any other professionals who may divulge either the diagnostic strategies planned or the content of the proceedings to the family.

3. Because medical records in cases of suspected MSBP often are voluminous, efficient review must be organized prospectively. Otherwise, the result of the records review is a mass of detail from which no trends can be elicited and therefore no conclusions drawn. Therefore, in beginning the review of the records, one shortly recognizes certain patterns and then formalizes these preliminary observations into questions one asks of the data: In a child with a chief complaint of intractable vomiting, did the child have any documented episodes of vomiting while in the presence of a doctor or nurse? In a child with repeated episodes of apnea, how many episodes, if any, actually began in the presence of someone other than the mother? In a child with recurrent fevers in the hospital, who actually took and charted the temperatures when the child was febrile? Some of these data may not be discernible from written medical records.

4. All medical records of all siblings must be reviewed, including autopsy reports and death certificates. It often requires some vigor to obtain these records, but they are vital. Neither police summaries nor social work records are sufficient.

5. Review the parents' medical, educational, and work history, as far as possible from documents, especially if the parent claims various illnesses or some medical education.

6. Several methods may be used, singly or in combination, to gain access to records. Sometimes it is possible to have signed parental consent to obtain the records. Otherwise, the lawyers on the multidisciplinary team may advise canvassing the area with subpoenas or requesting court-ordered discovery of records.

7. Presentation of the review of records to the multidisciplinary team should include a brief chronological review, followed by a review of discrepancies, if any. How does the mother's history compare with the observed clinical findings in the child? How do the laboratory test results compare with the given histories (eg, are drug levels continually subtherapeutic or toxic with a history of absolute compliance)? It is impossible to list all of the possible questions, but the data will tell the reviewer which questions are important. In reviewing a case of suspected MSBP, it is essential to consider and explore all possible organic explanations.

8. When presenting a case of MSBP to the civil or juvenile court, some strategies of presentation may assist the trier of fact in coming to a conclusion.

Despite the many hours spent in reviewing records and making an extensive chronological compilation of the child's medical history, presentation of the information to the court in long, narrative form often only confuses, rather than elucidates, the material. A short summary is often better. Questions may then be asked to clarify or expand on particular events.

Graphs and charts, clearly readable and with a single issue to illuminate, often better illustrate a complex issue than a long, verbal narrative. For example, a growth chart may show that the child consistently gains weight in the hospital but loses weight at home. A histogram may show the number of apnea episodes that originated in the presence of the mother compared with the number that originated in the presence of the nursing staff or grandmother.

Cases typically involve conflicting medical opinions, and the parents usually have medical experts testify in their behalf. These experts may be one's colleagues. A clear grasp of the medical and epidemiological evidence and a professional, non-adversarial attitude is always best.

The perpetrator only rarely admits to MSBP but, curiously, she will more often agree to voluntary services as long as the court is not involved and a dependency petition is not filed. No success with this approach has been reported. Experience has shown that court-ordered intervention is necessary if there is any hope of successful protection of the child.

9. It is prudent to recommend out-of-home placement for the child.[20,32] This measure ensures protection of the child and a diagnostic period of separation to see how the child's health fares. The fact that a mother has hitherto only simulated but not produced illness is no guarantee that she will not do something more nefarious to the child in the future. Simulators may become producers of illness. Confrontation of the parent with the news of the suspected diagnosis does not, in and of itself, ensure safety for the child.[20,32,93]

The reader is cautioned in particular about the dangers of placing the child with a family member or friend. This is always a difficult situation because, for the child, the easiest transition may be to an aunt or grandmother, but the perpetrator may have access to the child, despite that relative's or friend's promises to the contrary. This places the child at potential dire risk.

10. If the child is to remain in the hospital for a time, all visits with all family members must be supervised by a medically experienced person to ensure that no one is tampering with the child's medical care. Sometimes the best course of action is to ask the court for a short (ie, 10-day to 2-week) period of hospitalization with only supervised parental visits as a diagnostic trial to determine if the child's symptoms floridly persist. If they do not, concern about MSBP is

heightened. If they do, ask the court to vacate the order and turn attention to a fresh look for an organic diagnosis. This approach is useful only if the child's symptoms and signs, if induced, would reasonably be expected to abate rather quickly in the absence of ongoing assault.

11. It is prudent to recommend out-of-home placement of siblings, because they may become the next victims if they remain in the home. At least, all siblings must have court-ordered medical evaluations and review of records.

12. Once the child is in foster care, his or her health status must be monitored and documented closely by the same physicians. Although often it is optimal to have the original doctor or set of doctors involved in the child's ongoing care, this arrangement sometimes is not practical for reasons of geography or temperament.

13. When is it safe to send the child home? If the diagnosis is indeed MSBP, it seems sensible that the same guidelines that apply to other forms of maltreatment apply in MSBP cases (ie, the perpetrator must acknowledge that she committed these acts, she must have some insight into the reasons for it, and she must provide reasonable assurance that not only insight but also sufficient change has occurred to ensure the safety of the child). Very little information is available on family reunification after maternal psychiatric intervention. In one

study, family reunification was thought to be feasible in certain cases, but the authors cautioned that long-term follow-up is necessary to monitor the safety of the child and assess whether the perpetrator's mental health has deteriorated.[93] The mother's therapist will discuss with the court those issues that concern the safety of the child. If the mother and the psychiatrist insist that all the information is privileged, the court has no way to determine that the children will be safe at home, and other permanent arrangements must be made for them.

14. Even if the children are removed permanently and parental rights are terminated, subsequent children born to the mother are at high risk of being victims of MSBP. Sometimes no formal method is available by which to keep track of the mother's pregnancies and peregrinations, but every effort must be made to protect future children.

Legal Considerations

Because a diagnosis of MSBP can lead to various legal proceedings in which the physician's testimony is requested, it is necessary to keep a few guideposts in view.

In a courtroom or out, you are not required to translate your degree of diagnostic conviction into a legal equivalent. Terms such as *probable cause, reasonable suspicion, preponderance of the evidence, clear and convincing evidence,* and *evidence beyond a reasonable doubt* have a specific meaning in the law. If asked if the evidence conforms to any of these burdens, or if you have a reasonable degree of medical certainty about the diagnosis (a popular question), use the medical language that is meaningful to you and distill it to lay terms that best embody your meaning. You are cautioned against using legal terminology unless definitions have been precisely rendered for you and are in the court record.

Be alert to attempted manipulation by lawyers. The disputatious lawyer is no more a threat, in this regard, than the pleasingly respectful lawyer. Do not let yourself be badgered. Equally, do not let yourself be flattered or lulled into a small, but medically unjustifiable, resizing of your opinion, or into being persuaded that you are a standard-bearer for a good and righteous cause. Remind the lawyer that you are in court only to provide as balanced, thorough, and comprehensible an interpretation of the medical data as is possible. Remember: All practicing attorneys have jobs that are different from those of all doctors.

A diagnosis of MSBP may have been based, at least in part, on the information you have reviewed in records. You may be asked if your opinion would change given different or additional information. In reality, there are few instances in which you can be absolutely sure that you have reviewed all existing records. If you are asked if you might change your diagnosis, or your degree of conviction about it, should you be given new information, often the most accurate answer is that it is possible but, absent the information and the time to

think it over, you have no way of gauging the likelihood of that possibility.

It is the job of the trier of fact (ie, the judge or jury), not yours, to determine if your conclusion and the reasons for it contribute to a finding that the burden of proof has been met.

Doctors and MSBP

The pathogenic role of a health care system that over-investigates and prescribes testing and therapy unnecessarily has been rightly identified as contributing to MSBP.[94] But this is perhaps too abstract. After all, what is a system other than people? Doctors are some of those people. And doctors are driven by many things: They see many children with persistent illness, most of which is identifiably organic, some of which follows an expected course, but some of which is peculiar or does not conform tidily to textbook descriptions. They don't expect a false history. Young doctors are worried by the cautionary tales of missed diagnoses that they have absorbed throughout training; seasoned doctors are haunted by their own experiences of having missed a timely diagnosis of serious illness, for this is almost universal in a long and busy primary care practice. Most want to be thorough and helpful. The hierarchy in the medical world places subspecialty opinion above that of the generalist. Indeed, a curious and paradoxical weakness of famous children's hospitals is the greater likelihood of attributing exotic, but wrong, organic diagnosis when the real problem is MSBP. There is relief at having a consultant label with an organic diagnosis in a hitherto inexplicable case, even when the label is doubtful. A well-founded fear of litigation pervades the practice of medicine. What used to be known as *defensive medicine* has now become almost mainstream medicine. There is little time for pondering.

Then there are the personal, rarely discussed vulnerabilities of doctors, some of them enhanced by the unhappy rigors of medical training: difficulty saying, "I don't know" or a certain pride that "Only I can manage this case"[95] or marrying oneself to an obscure or pet diagnosis, even when the accumulating evidence argues against it.

These realities, combined with the diversity of perpetrators of MSBP, has led to the sensible suggestion that the prevention of MSBP "might not be from understanding perpetrators better, but from better understanding of doctors and the health system."[96] But how to do this? It is almost impossible to escape the culture of investigation and subspecialty referral. Besides which, such a culture sometimes helps a patient. Therefore, because the most useful warning sign for MSBP is symptoms, signs, and tests that are incongruent, perhaps the most practical answer is that MSBP should routinely be on the differential diagnosis for *persistence with incongruence,* just as pneumonia is routinely on the differential diagnosis for dyspnea. Every physician knows that most possible diagnoses on a differential will be wrong, hopes that one will be right, and realizes that, as the old saying goes, "If you never think of it, you'll never see it." Importantly and by corollary, you will never exclude it. Warning

signs are not diagnoses, just features that could mean one of several possibilities. But it is possible that if a child's presentation doesn't make sense, it is because it doesn't make sense for a reason.

Conclusion

A child who is a victim of MSBP is at high risk of harm. The fact that the perpetrator abruptly desists from the assault does not ensure that the situation is even minimally adequate for the child. The impetus to attack the child repeatedly, the ability to objectify the child in the first place and use the child as a tool, generally reflect a lack of empathy so profound as to likely hobble the overall capacity for mothering. Regrettably, cases involving MSBP may first be identified by a multidisciplinary child fatality review board, but even though it is too late to help the child who died, other children in the family may be protected as a result. The dangerousness of perpetrators of MSBP should never be underestimated.

References

1. Meadow R. Munchausen syndrome by proxy: the hinterland of child abuse. *Lancet.* 1977;2:343–345
2. Feldman MD. Denial in Munchausen syndrome by proxy: the consulting psychiatrist's dilemma. *Int J Psychiatry Med.* 1994;24:121–128
3. Ostfeld BM, Feldman MD. Factitious disorder by proxy: awareness among mental health practitioners. *Gen Hosp Psychiatry.* 1996;18:113–116
4. Szajnberg NM, Moilanen I, Kanerva A, et al. Munchausen-by-proxy syndrome: countertransference as a diagnostic tool. *Bull Menninger Clin.* 1996;60:229–237

5. Freckelton I. Munchausen syndrome by proxy and criminal prosecutions for child abuse. *J Law Med.* 2005;12:261–266

6. Ayoub CC, Schreier HA, Keller C. Munchausen by proxy: presentations in special education. *Child Maltreat.* 2002;7:149–159

7. Royal College of Pediatrics and Child Health. *Fabricated or Induced Illness by Carers—Report of the Working Party.* London, UK: Royal College of Pediatrics and Child Health; 2002

8. Feldman MD, Brown RM. Munchausen by proxy in an international context. *Child Abuse Negl.* 2002;26:509–524

9. McClure RJ, Davis PM, Meadow SR, et al. Epidemiology of Munchausen syndrome by proxy, non-accidental poisoning, and non-accidental suffocation. *Arch Dis Child.* 1996;75:57–61

10. Schreier HA. Error in Munchausen by proxy defined. *Pediatrics.* 2004;113:1851–1852

11. Denny SJ, Grant CC, Pinnock R. Epidemiology of Munchausen syndrome by proxy in New Zealand. *J Paediatr Child Health.* 2001;37:240–243

12. Sheridan MS. The deceit continues: an updated literature review of Munchausen syndrome by proxy. *Child Abuse Negl.* 2003;27:431–451

13. Makar AF, Squier PJ. Munchausen syndrome by proxy: father as perpetrator. *Pediatrics.* 1990;85:370–373

14. Meadow R. Munchausen syndrome by proxy abuse perpetrated by men. *Arch Dis Child.* 1998;78:210–216

15. Wright M. *A Mother's Trial.* New York, NY: Bantam Books; 1984

16. Atoynatan TH, O'Reilly E, Loin L. Munchausen syndrome by proxy. *Child Psychiatry Hum Dev.* 1988;19:3–13

17. Lasher LJ, Feldman MD. Celiac disease as a manifestation of Munchausen by proxy. *South Med J.* 2004;97:67–69

18. Richardson GF. Munchausen syndrome by proxy. *Am Fam Physician.* 1987;36:119–123

19. Carrell S. Texas nurse found guilty of killing child. *Am Med News.* 1984:1–27

20. Rosenberg D. Web of deceit: a literature review of Munchausen syndrome by proxy. *Child Abuse Negl.* 1987;11:547–563

21. Alexander R, Smith W, Stevenson R. Serial Munchausen syndrome by proxy. *Pediatrics.* 1990;86:581–585

22. Meadow R. Mothering to death. *Arch Dis Child.* 1999;80:359–362

23. Bryk M, Siegel PT. My mother caused my illness: the story of a survivor of Munchausen by proxy syndrome. *Pediatrics.* 1997;100:1–7

24. Janofsky JS. Munchausen syndrome in a mother and daughter: an unusual presentation of folie á deux. *J Nerv Ment Dis.* 1986;174:368–370

25. Awadallah N, Vaughan A, Franco K, Munir F, Sharaby N, Goldfarb J. Munchausen by proxy: a case, chart series, and literature review of older victims. *Child Abuse Negl.* 2005;29:931–941

26. Conway SP, Pond MN. Munchausen syndrome by proxy abuse: a foundation for adult Munchausen. *Aust N Z J Psychiatry.* 1995;29:504–507

27. Raymond CA. Munchausen's may occur in younger persons. *JAMA.* 1987;257:3332

28. Roth D. How "mild" is mild Munchausen syndrome by proxy? *Isr J Psychiatry Rel Sci.* 1990;27:160–167

29. Southall DP, Plunkett BM, Banks MW, et al. Covert video recordings of life-threatening child abuse: lessons for child protection. *Pediatrics.* 1997;100:735–760

30. Kamerling LB, Black XA, Fiser RT. Munchausen syndrome by proxy in the pediatric intensive care unit: an unusual mechanism. *Pediatr Crit Care Med.* 2002;3:305–307

31. Meadow R. Suffocation, recurrent apnea, and sudden infant death. *J Pediatr.* 1990;117:351–357

32. McGuire TL, Feldman KW. Psychologic morbidity of children subjected to Munchausen syndrome by proxy. *Pediatrics.* 1989;83:289–292

33. Beal SM, Blundell HK. Recurrence incidence of sudden infant death syndrome. *Arch Dis Child.* 1988;63:924–930

34. Bools CN, Neale BA, Meadow SR. Co-morbidity associated with fabricated illness (Munchausen syndrome by proxy). *Arch Dis Child.* 1992;67:77–79

35. Meadow R. Recurrent cot death and suffocation [letter]. *Arch Dis Child.* 1989;64:179–180

36. Truman TL, Ayoub CC. Considering suffocatory abuse and Munchausen by proxy in the evaluation of children experiencing apparent life-threatening events and sudden infant death syndrome. *Child Maltreat.* 2002;7:138–148

37. Ben-Chetrit E, Melmed RN. Recurrent hypoglycaemia in multiple myeloma: a case of Munchausen syndrome by proxy in an elderly patient. *J Intern Med.* 1998;244:175–178

38. Sigal M, Altmark D, Gelkopf M. Munchausen syndrome by adult proxy revisited. *Isr J Psychiatry Rel Sci.* 1991;1:33–36

39. Sigal MD, Altmark D, Carmel I. Munchausen syndrome by adult proxy: a perpetrator abusing two adults. *J Nerv Ment Dis.* 1986;174:696–698

40. Chodorowski Z, Anand JS, Porzezinska B, Markiewicz A. Consciousness disturbances: a case report of Munchausen by proxy syndrome in an elderly patient. *Przegl Lek.* 2003;60:307–308

41. Feldman KW, Hickman RO. The central venous catheter as a source of medical chaos in Munchausen syndrome by proxy. *J Pediatr Surg.* 1998;33:623–627

42. Masterson J, Dunworth R, Williams N. Extreme illness exaggeration in pediatric patients: a variant of Munchausen's by proxy? *Am J Orthopsychiatry.* 1988;58:188–195

43. Meadow R. Neurological and developmental variants of Munchausen syndrome by proxy. *Dev Med Child Neurol.* 1991;33:270–272

44. Osterhoudt KC. A toddler with recurrent episodes of unresponsiveness. *Pediatr Emerg Care.* 2004;20:195–197

45. Yamashita M, Yamashita M, Azuma J. Urinary excretion of ipecac alkaloids in human volunteers. *Vet Hum Toxicol.* 2002;44:257–259

46. Meadow R. Unnatural sudden infant death. *Arch Dis Child.* 1999;80:7–14

47. Rosen CL, Frost JD, Glaze DG. Child abuse and recurrent infant apnea. *J Pediatr.* 1986;109:1065–1067

48. DiMaio VJ, DiMaio D. *Forensic Pathology.* Boca Raton, FL: CRC Press; 2001

49. Milroy CM. Munchausen syndrome by proxy and intra-alveolar haemosiderin. *Int J Legal Med.* 1999;112:309–312

50. Forbes A, Acland P. What is the significance of haemosiderin in the lungs of deceased infants? *Med Sci Law.* 2004;44:348–352

51. Schreier H. On the importance of motivation in Munchausen by proxy: the case of Kathy Bush. *Child Abuse Negl.* 2002;26:537–549

52. Meadow R. Different interpretations of Munchausen syndrome by proxy. *Child Abuse Negl.* 2002;26:501–508

53. Bools C, Neale B, Meadow R. Munchausen syndrome by proxy: a study of psychopathology. *Child Abuse Negl.* 1994;18:773–788

54. Gojer J, Berman T. Postpartum depression and factitious disorder: a new presentation. *Int J Psychiatry Med.* 2000;30:287–293

55. Lesnik-Oberstein M. Munchausen syndrome by proxy [letter]. *Child Abuse Negl.* 1986;10:133

56. Adsheaad G, Bluglass K. A vicious circle: transgenerational attachment representations in a case of factitious illness by proxy. *Attach Hum Dev.* 2001;3:77–95

57. Adshead G, Brooke D, Samuels M, Jenner S, Southall D. Maternal behaviors associated with smothering: a preliminary descriptive study. *Child Abuse Negl.* 2000;24:1175–1183

58. Rand DC, Feldman MD. An explanatory model for Munchausen by proxy abuse. *Int J Psychiatry Med.* 2001;31:113–126

59. Tucker HS, Finlay F, Guiton S. Munchausen syndrome involving pets by proxies. *Arch Dis Child.* 2002;87:263

60. Munro HM, Thrusfield MV. 'Battered pets': Munchausen syndrome by proxy (factitious illness by proxy). *J Small Anim Pract.* 2001;42:385–389

61. Schneider DJ, Perez A, Knilamus TE, Daniels SR, Bove KE, Bonnell H. Clinical and pathological aspects of cardiomyopathy from ipecac administration in Munchausen's syndrome by proxy. *Pediatrics.* 1996;97:902–906

62. Feldman KW, Christopher DM, Opheim KB. Munchausen syndrome-bulimia by proxy: ipecac as a toxin in child abuse. *Child Abuse Negl.* 1989;13:257–261

63. Outwater KM, Lipnick RN, Luban NLC, et al. Factitious hematuria: diagnosis by minor blood group typing. *J Pediatr.* 1981;98:95–97

64. Kurlandsky L, Lukoff JY, Zinkham WH, et al. Munchausen syndrome by proxy: definition of factitious bleeding in an infant by 51Cr labeling of erythrocytes. *Pediatrics.* 1979;63:228–231

65. Wenk RE. Molecular evidence of Munchausen syndrome by proxy. *Arch Pathol Lab Med.* 2003;127:e36–e37

66. Bolz WE, Brouwer HG, Schoenmakers CH. Measurement of HbF concentration for diagnosing a case of Munchausen by proxy syndrome. *J Pediatr.* 2006;148:145–146

67. Nading JH, Duval-Arnould B. Factitious diabetes mellitus confirmed by ascorbic acid. *Arch Dis Child.* 1984;59:166–167

68. Edidin DV, Farrell EE, Gould VE. Factitious hyperinsulinemic hypoglycemia in infancy: diagnostic pitfalls. *Clin Pediatr.* 2000;39:117–119

69. Giurgea I, Ulinski T, Touati G, et al. Factitious hyperinsulinism leading to pancreatectomy: severe forms of Munchausen syndrome by proxy. *Pediatrics.* 2005;116:e145–e148

70. Rosen CL, Frost JD Jr, Bricker T, Tarnow JD, Gillette PC, Dunlavy S. Two siblings with cardiorespiratory arrest: Munchausen syndrome by proxy or child abuse? *Pediatrics.* 1983;71:715–720

71. Southall DP, Stebben VA, Rees SV, Lang MH, Warner JO, Shinebourne FA. Apnoeic episodes induced by smothering: two cases identified by covert video surveillance. *Br Med J (Clin Res Ed).* 1987;294:1637–1641

72. Hall DE, Eubanks L, Meyyazhagan LS, Kenney RD, Johnson SC. Evaluation of covert video surveillance in the diagnosis of Munchausen syndrome by proxy: lessons from 41 cases. *Pediatrics.* 2000;105:1305–1312

73. Epstein MA, Markowitz RL, Gallo DM, Holmes JW, Gryboski JD. Munchausen syndrome by proxy: considerations in diagnosis and confirmation by video surveillance. *Pediatrics.* 1987;80:220–224

74. Evans D. The investigation of life-threatening child abuse and Munchausen syndrome by proxy. *J Med Ethics.* 1995;21:9–13

75. Johnson P, Morley C. Spying on mothers. *Lancet.* 1994;344:132–133

76. Feldman MD. Spying on mothers [letter]. *Lancet.* 1994;344:132

77. Samuels MP, Southall D. Covert surveillance in Munchausen's syndrome by proxy: welfare of the child must come first [letter]. *BMJ.* 1994;308:1101–1102

78. Connelly R. Ethical issues in the use of covert video surveillance in the diagnosis of Munchausen syndrome by proxy: the Atlanta study—an ethical challenge for medicine. *HEC Forum.* 2003;15:21–41

79. Howe EG. Criteria for deceit. *J Clin Ethics.* 2004;15:100–110

80. Leuthner SR. Covert video surveillance in pediatric care: the fiduciary relationship with a child. *J Clin Ethics.* 2004;15:173–175

81. Vaught W. Parents, lies, and videotape: covert video surveillance in pediatric care. *J Clin Ethics.* 2004;15:161–172

82. Flannery MT. First, do no harm: the use of covert videosurveillance to detect Munchausen syndrome by proxy—an unethical means of "preventing" child abuse. *Univ Mich J Law Reform.* 1998;32:105–194

83. Baron HI, Beck DC, Vargas JH, et al. Overinterpretation of gastroduodenal motility studies: two cases involving Munchausen syndrome by proxy. *J Pediatr.* 1995;126:397–400

84. Cucchiara S, Borrelli O, Salvia G, et al. A normal gastrointestinal motility excludes chronic intestinal pseudoobstruction in children. *Dig Dis Sci.* 2000;45:258–264

85. Hyman PE, Bursch B, Beck D, DiLorenzo C, Zeltzer LK. Discriminating pediatric condition falsification from chronic intestinal pseudo-obstruction in toddlers. *Child Maltreat.* 2002;7:132–137

86. Barber MA, Davis PM. Fits, faints, or fatal fantasy? Fabricated seizures and child abuse. *Arch Dis Child.* 2002;86:230–233

87. Waring WW. The persistent parent. *Am J Dis Child.* 1992;146:753–755

88. Yudkin S. Six children with coughs. *Lancet.* 1961;2:561–563

89. Rosenberg DA. Munchausen syndrome by proxy: medical diagnostic criteria. *Child Abuse Negl.* 2003;27:421–430

90. Rand DC, Feldman MD. Misdiagnosis of Munchausen syndrome by proxy: a literature review and four new cases. *Harv Rev Psychiatry.* 1999;7:94–101

91. Vennemann B, Perdekamp MG, Weinmann W, Faller-Marquardt M, Pollak S, Brandis M. A case of Munchausen syndrome by proxy with subsequent suicide of the mother. *Forensic Sci Int.* 2006;158:195–199

92. Blix S, Brack G. The effects of a suspected case of Munchausen's syndrome by proxy on a pediatric nursing staff. *Gen Hosp Psychiatry.* 1988;10:402–409

93. Berg B, Jones DP. Outcome of psychiatric intervention in factitious illness by proxy (Munchausen's syndrome by proxy). *Arch Dis Child.* 1999;81:465–472

94. von Hahn L, Harper G, McDaniel SH, Siegel DM, Feldman MD, Libow JA. A case of factitious disorder by proxy: the role of the health-care system, diagnostic dilemmas, and family dynamics. *Harv Rev Psychiatry.* 2001;9:124–135

95. Jureidini JN, Shafer AT, Donald TG. "Munchausen syndrome by proxy": not only pathological parenting but also problematic doctoring? *Med J Aust.* 2003;178:130–132

96. Eminson M, Jureidini J. Concerns about research and prevention strategies in Munchausen syndrome by proxy (MSBP) abuse. *Child Abuse Negl.* 2003;27:413–420

Chapter 17

Child Abuse by Poisoning

Frederick M. Henretig

Section of Clinical Toxicology
The Childen's Hospital of Philadelphia
The Poison Control Center

Robert T. Paschall

Child Protection Program
Washington University in St Louis School of Medicine

Marcella M. Donaruma-Kwoh

Section of Emergency Medicine
Baylor College of Medicine

Introduction

The image of Snow White, lying motionless in her glass coffin after a bite of her evil stepmother's poisoned apple is probably the first high-profile representation of child abuse by poisoning (CAP) in popular culture. Intentional poisoning as a form of child abuse was first reported in the medical literature by Dr C Henry Kempe in 1962, in his landmark article "Battered-Child Syndrome."[1] Kempe et al used the term *battered-child syndrome* to apply to child maltreatment of all forms. Similarly, in the seminal article "Munchausen Syndrome by Proxy. The Hinterland of Child Abuse," 2 of the 3 children reported by Meadow[2] had been repetitively poisoned with table salt and died from "extreme hypernatremia." The first case series of CAP was published in 1976 by Rogers and colleagues,[3] and included several children whose cases would now be classified as Munchausen syndrome by proxy (MSBP). Much of the experience with malicious poisoning in children overlaps considerably with that of MSBP.[4] A particularly compelling anecdote in the annals of both CAP and MSBP was a letter to the editor published in *Lancet* in 1978 asking readers for help in diagnosing a puzzling case of recurrent coma in a 2-year-old boy.[5] The child became unresponsive and hypotonic on more than 6 occasions while hospitalized, and extensive neurologic, metabolic, infectious, and toxicological evaluations were unremarkable. Within a month, the author wrote back to the *Lancet* with the fascinating denouncement of the story, and subsequently provided a detailed case report 2 years after in which he also thanked the many readers who had offered suggestions.[6] It had been finally discovered on repeated toxicological testing that the child was suffering from repetitive barbiturate poisoning. The medications were found in the mother's hospital room locker. By the time the diagnosis was established, the child had experienced 9 episodes of coma and 2 respiratory arrests requiring endotracheal intubation.

By the mid-1980s fewer than 100 intentional pediatric poisoning cases were reported in the medical literature, a likely underrepresentation of the true incidence.[7-10] Even though a foundation of pediatric diagnostics involves the art of thorough history taking via caregiver report, in the context of CAP the patient's guardian often is the primary informant as well as the perpetrator, and the true history is obfuscated.

This dilemma requires pediatricians to maintain a heightened level of suspicion regarding causality for all injuries to children, including those due to toxic substances. The following comment by Shnaps et al in 1981 is still relevant today: "We suggest that the dictum 'an injury other than a road accident in a child under two years of age should be suspected as battered child syndrome,' be applied to the cases in which impairment of the child's consciousness is found as well, and in each case efforts be directed to exclude the possibility of chemical abuse."[7,11] While this statement is a dramatic one, it is an effective filter through which one may construct an inclusive differential diagnosis in a child with altered mental status, frequently the cardinal sign of toxic ingestion. Other differential diagnoses in cases of intentional poisoning include sepsis, meningitis, epilepsy, head trauma, apnea, apparent life-threatening events, sudden infant death syndrome, metabolic derangements, bleeding diatheses, and gastroenteritis.[10,12,13]

This chapter focuses on the intentional administration of inappropriate medications or exogenous poisons as a form of child abuse. It reviews the epidemiology and most common clinical presentations, highlights the clinical and laboratory approach to diagnosis, and offers ways to manage what Shnaps et al[7] referred to as the "chemically abused child."

Definitions and Patterns of CAP

For this discussion, CAP refers primarily to the intentional administration of a medication or toxic substance by a parent or caretaker to a child (<19 years) for sinister purposes, as well as unintentional poisoning due to blatant lack of supervision or endangerment (neglect of environmental safety). In addition, there are several other scenarios of childhood intoxication that may raise the concern of maltreatment for health care providers and child protection agencies. It should be recognized that poisoning may occur by inhalation or aspiration, injection, and skin or mucous membrane contact, as well as via ingestion. Nevertheless, the latter is by far the most common route of exposure in CAP, as well as for unintentional poisonings in young children and intentional self-poisonings in adolescents.

On occasion, the inappropriate use of a medication may result in unintended toxicity, such as when a drug is given outside its usual therapeutic parameters with intent on the part of a caregiver to address perceived or actual signs or symptoms in a child. An example would be the intended therapeutic use in a child of a medication prescribed for another child or adult. A more concerning scenario might be when a medication is administered to take advantage of its side effects rather than its typical medicinal effects (eg, giving a substantive dose of diphenhydramine to induce sleep to make a child less likely to require the vigilant attention of caretakers). These acts may occur without intent to harm the child, but determining so requires careful consideration in each case.

Another dangerous situation may arise when parents administer unconventional medical therapy, including home remedies, herbal preparations, or large doses of vitamins in a manner not broadly recognized by the medical community as having medical efficacy and possibly being toxic as a result of chemical makeup or dosage, or by cumulative effect over time. Again, such a practice may represent well-intentioned motivation on the parent's part, but in extreme circumstances might constitute abuse. An example is in the case of recurrent poisoning in a child or sibling after the parents were given information regarding the danger of improperly stored pharmaceutical and non-pharmaceutical toxins.

Endangering the welfare of a child means the caregiver allows or supports circumstances and situations in which the child's health and general well-being are compromised. Child abuse by poisoning may occur in an environment that by its nature exposes the child to the risk of toxic exposure, such as a methamphetamine-manufacturing laboratory in the home. Using illicit drugs in the presence of a child or imprudently storing antifreeze and other hazardous materials in a readily accessible site also comprise an unsafe environment. Possibly even more dangerous is storing toxic materials in a container that looks innocuous or even enticing to a child such as a soft drink bottle or juice container. In such situations, there is no intent on the part of the caretaker to expose the child to the toxic substance, but its accessibility constitutes an unsafe, endangering, at-risk environment. Perhaps the most extreme example of a dangerous environment was recently encountered by one of the authors when a 6-year-old child presented with severe opiate toxicity requiring intensive care soon after returning to the United States from a trip to Haiti. During his hospitalization he rectally passed numerous remnants of oxycodone tablets, and later described being asked to swallow "pills in a white covering" before his departure.[14] His family had not sought to harm him, and had brought him to medical attention when he became unresponsive. But their desire to use him as a drug "mule" exposed him to life-threatening risk. Similar cases have been reported with adolescent patients.[15]

Tables 17.1 and 17.2 list several cases of CAP from various prescribed, household, and illicit substances.

Patient condition falsification (PCF) is a term first proposed by the Munchausen by Proxy Task Force of the American Professional Society on the Abuse of Children (APSAC) in a 1998 edition of the *APSAC Advisor.*[16] In 2002 the APSAC Task Force on Munchausen Syndrome by Proxy Definitions Working Group further clarified PCF and described its place in the more encompassing scenario referred to as MSBP.[17] The term *PCF* is used to focus on harm or risk of harm to the child and less on the motivation of the offending parent.

For purposes of this chapter, the 2 components of MSBP are (1) pathological health care–seeking behavior characterized by a parent, usually the mother, intentionally and repetitively falsifying the child's health history to cause the child to seem ill by health care providers and (2) resultant harm to the child. This form of health care–seeking behavior is characterized by the parent intentionally and repeatedly fabricating, exaggerating, or inducing an illness (possibly all 3) in a child. Consequently, the child is subjected to multiple medical interventions not recognized as unwarranted until the situation is viewed in retrospect through the filter of an awareness of a falsified medical history. One of the methods by which the child's condition may be falsified is by intentional poisoning, carrying with it significant morbidity and mortality. The primary motivation for some parent offenders is presumed to be for internal psychological gain by assuming

the sick role by proxy. External gain such as goods, services, or money may motivate or help sustain pathological health care–seeking behavior. Poisoning as a method for causing illness may occur in the child's home environment or in the hospital, despite the watchful eyes of medical staff. Some authors have dropped "syndrome" from MSBP, as will be done in the remainder of this chapter. This is partly to avoid court "battles" over the issue of how many features are required to cause a child to fit the syndrome and whether parent-child-health care interactions exhibit sufficient requisite features. For this reason we use the term *child abuse by condition falsification* and employ the term *Munchausen by proxy (MBP)* to describe the context of the parent-child dynamic within which the child is abused. A more detailed discussion of MBP and PCF is provided in Chapter 16.

The most extreme form of CAP is the premeditated homicide of a child by poisoning. This is not synonymous with PCF/MBP. In the period leading up to homicide by poisoning there is no repetitive pattern of pathological health care–seeking behavior on the part of the parent as there is in MBP. However, there may be a medical history of unrecognized failed attempts to murder the child.

Finally, even the common occurrence of exploratory ingestions of medications or toxic substances by young children may represent an abusive context. Such poisonings have been traditionally termed *accidental,* but most pediatric toxicologists today prefer to use the

TABLE 17.1
Child Abuse by Poisoning

Agent	Age	Gender	Clinical Features	Abuser	Admit	In Hospital	Other Types of Abuse	Survival	Comments
Barbiturate	4 d	M	None	Mother	–	+	–	Survival	MSBP
Barbiturate	2 y	M	↓LOC, coma	Mother	–	–	–	Death	Died 3 d after hospital discharge
Barbiturate	2 y	M	LOC, cardiac arrest, foot pain	Mother	–	+	–	Survival	Mom Munchausen
Barbiturate	14 y	F	↓LOC, ataxia, diplopia, nystagmus	Father	a	–	–	Survival	Father poisoned 2 other siblings at puberty
Barbiturate	20 mo	M	↓LOC, ataxia, seizures	Mother	o	–	–	Survival	Pill fragments found by lavage
Barbiturate	4 y	M	Ataxia	Mother	–	+	+	Survival	Arthralgia, hematuria, fever, phenothiazines, phentermine, methaqualone
Phenytoin	4 y	M	"Seizures," weight loss, extreme lethargy	Mother	a	+	–	Survival	No seizures once off medication in foster care
Phenytoin	8 y	M	Vomiting, ataxia, ↓LOC, nystagmus	Stepfather	–	–	–	Survival	Stepfather taking antiepileptics

Abbreviations: Admit, admission of guilt by perpetrator; in hospital, poisoning continued in hospital; M, male; MSBP, Munchausen syndrome by proxy; LOC, level of consciousness; F, female; a, admitted guilt; o, observed guilt; U, unknown; ALTE, apparent life-threatening event; PxAb, physical abuse; SIDS, sudden infant death syndrome; c, convicted; FTT, failure to thrive; V and D, vomiting and diarrhea; FB, foreign body; CPK, creatine phosphokinase; NaCl, sodium chloride; KCl, potassium chloride.

(continued on page 554)

TABLE 17.1
Child Abuse by Poisoning, continued

Agent	Age	Gender	Clinical Features	Abuser	Admit	In Hospital	Other Types of Abuse	Survival	Comments
Codeine	2 mo	M	↓LOC, apnea, miosis	Mother	–	+	–	Survival	
Benzodiazepine	12 d	M	Apnea, cyanosis, ↓LOC, jittery	Mother	–	–	–	Survival	
Benzodiazepine, codeine, phenobarbital	27 d	M	Apnea, cyanosis, hypotonia	U	–	–	–	Survival poisoned home	4 episodes ALTE, again after return
Meperidine, phenothiazine	24 d	F	Apnea, cyanosis	Father	a	–	–	Survival	Father sedated child to help mother rest
Meperidine, promethazine hydrochloride	33 d	M	Apnea, cyanosis, hypertonia	Mother	a	–	–	Survival	Mother "sedated" child
Phenothiazines	24 mo	F	↓LOC, ataxia	Stepfather	–	–	–	Survival	Prior aspirin poisoning
Amitriptyline	2 mo	F	Unresponsive	Mother	a	–	–	Death	16-year-old mother, pills found in endotracheal tube at autopsy
Amitriptyline	10 mo	F	Recurrent loss of consciousness	Mother	o	+	–	Survival	Sibling died of PxAb

Abbreviations: Admit, admission of guilt by perpetrator; in hospital, poisoning continued in hospital; M, male; MSBP, Munchausen syndrome by proxy; LOC, level of consciousness; F, female; a, admitted guilt; o, observed guilt; U, unknown; ALTE, apparent life-threatening event; PxAb, physical abuse; SIDS, sudden infant death syndrome; c, convicted; FTT, failure to thrive; V and D, vomiting and diarrhea; FB, foreign body; CPK, creatine phosphokinase; NaCl, sodium chloride; KCl, potassium chloride.

TABLE 17.1
Child Abuse by Poisoning, continued

Agent	Age	Gender	Clinical Features	Abuser	Admit	In Hospital	Other Types of Abuse	Survival	Comments
Imipramine	4 y	M	Drowsy, ataxia	Mother	−	+	−	Survival	Mother tried homicide/suicide previously with drugs
Tricyclic	5 mo	F	Seizures, respiratory arrest	Mother	−	−	−	Survival	
Acetaminophen	20 d	M	Lethargy, icterus	Mother	−	−	−	Death	Survived initial poisoning but died of "SIDS" at 26 wk; no autopsy
Glibenclamide	11 y	F	Seizures, unconscious, hypoglycemia	Mother	−	+	−	Survival	Many medical procedures, including subtotal pancreatectomy; cured by foster placement
Insulin, phenothiazines, laxative	17 mo	F	↓LOC, hypoglycemia	Mother	a	−	−	Survival	MSBP; siblings also probably victims
Insulin	2.5 mo	M	Seizures, hypoglycemia	Mother	−	−	−	Impaired	Sibling died of diet pill overdose
Arsenic	9 y	M	Vomiting, abdominal pain	Mother	c	−	−	Death	MSBP; mother attempted suicide twice
Arsenic	8 y	M	Vomiting, abdominal pain	Mother	c	−	−	Death	MSBP; mother attempted suicide twice

(continued on page 556)

Abbreviations: Admit, admission of guilt by perpetrator; in hospital, poisoning continued in hospital; M, male; MSBP, Munchausen syndrome by proxy; LOC, level of consciousness; F, female; a, admitted guilt; o, observed guilt; U, unknown; ALTE, apparent life-threatening event; PxAb, physical abuse; SIDS, sudden infant death syndrome; c, convicted; FTT, failure to thrive; V and D, vomiting and diarrhea; FB, foreign body; CPK, creatine phosphokinase; NaCl, sodium chloride; KCl, potassium chloride.

TABLE 17.1
Child Abuse by Poisoning, continued

Agent	Age	Gender	Clinical Features	Abuser	Admit	In Hospital	Other Types of Abuse	Survival	Comments
Arsenic	U	F	Nausea, coldness	Mother	–	–	–	Survival	Sibling also similar abuse
Ipecac	1.5 mo	F	Hypotonia, poor sucking reflex, weak cry, dehydration	Mother	a	+	–	Survival	MSBP, mother added ipecac to expressed breast milk in hospital
Ipecac	4 y	F	V and D, dehydration, heart failure	Mother	a	+	–	Death	
Ipecac, ephedrine	9 mo	F	Recurrent V and D, hypotonia, FTT	Mother	–	+	–	Survival	Diagnosed at eleventh hospitalization, bulimic mother
Ipecac	12 mo	U	V and D, FTT	Mother	–	+	–	Survival	
Ipecac	1 mo	F	V and D, FTT	Mother	+	+	–	Survival	3 older siblings laxative poisoning
Ipecac	5 y	M	V and D, cardiac dysfunction	Mother	–	+	–	Death	Cardiac dysfunction; on catheter

Abbreviations: Admit, admission of guilt by perpetrator; in hospital, poisoning continued in hospital; M, male; MSBP, Munchausen syndrome by proxy; LOC, level of consciousness; F, female; a, admitted guilt; o, observed guilt; U, unknown; ALTE, apparent life-threatening event; PxAb, physical abuse; c, convicted; FTT, failure to thrive; V and D, vomiting and diarrhea; FB, foreign body; CPK, creatine phosphokinase; NaCl, sodium chloride; KCl, potassium chloride.

TABLE 17.1
Child Abuse by Poisoning, *continued*

Agent	Age	Gender	Clinical Features	Abuser	Admit	In Hospital	Other Types of Abuse	Survival	Comments
Detergent	3 y	U	V and D burning in throat and anus	Parents	–	–	+	Survival	PxAb
Black pepper	5 mo	M	Death by pepper aspiration	Mother	a	–	–	Death	Punishment for putting fingers in mouth
Black pepper	2 y	F	Death by pepper aspiration	Godfather	a	–	–	Death	Punishment for eating pepper
Black pepper	2.5 y	F	Death by pepper aspiration	Mother	a	–	+	Death	Punishment for taking sibling's bottle, PxAb
Black pepper	2.5 y	M	Death by pepper aspiration	Mother, boyfriend	c	–	+	Death	Punishment for unknown offense, PxAb
Black pepper	3.5 y	F	Death by pepper aspiration	Mother	a	–	+	Death	Punishment for taking sibling's bottle, PxAb

Abbreviations: Admit, admission of guilt by perpetrator; in hospital, poisoning continued in hospital; M, male; MSBP, Munchausen syndrome by proxy; LOC, level of consciousness; F, female; a, admitted guilt; o, observed guilt; U, unknown; ALTE, apparent life-threatening event; PxAb, physical abuse; c, convicted; FTT, failure to thrive; V and D, vomiting and diarrhea; FB, foreign body; CPK, creatine phosphokinase; NaCl, sodium chloride; KCl, potassium chloride.

(continued on page 558)

TABLE 17.1
Child Abuse by Poisoning, *continued*

Agent	Age	Gender	Clinical Features	Abuser	Admit	In Hospital	Other Types of Abuse	Survival	Comments
Black pepper	4 y	M	Death by pepper aspiration	Self	–	–	–	Death	Pica
Black pepper	5 y	M	Death by pepper aspiration	Foster mother	a	–	–	Death	Punishment for lying
Black pepper	10 y	M	Death by pepper aspiration	Adult friend	a	–	+	Death	Punishment for not eating breakfast, PxAb: forced to eat Worcestershire and Tabasco sauce by "big brother"
Metallic foreign bodies	6 mo	F	Esophageal symptoms	U	–	–	–	Survival	Thumbtack, screw, and carpet tack among multiple foreign bodies in stomach
Chloral hydrate	3 y	F	Coma	Mother	–	U	+	Survival	Prior sodium caustic ingestion
Lasix	5 y	M	V and D, Barter's?	Mother	–	+	–	Survival	
Castor oil	18 mo	M	Diarrhea	Mother	–	+	–	Survival	Mother Munchausen, phenobarbital

Abbreviations: Admit, admission of guilt by perpetrator; in hospital, poisoning continued in hospital; M, male; MSBP, Munchausen syndrome by proxy; LOC, level of consciousness; F, female; a, admitted guilt; o, observed guilt; U, unknown; ALTE, apparent life-threatening event; PxAb, physical abuse; SIDS, sudden infant death syndrome; c, convicted; FTT, failure to thrive; V and D, vomiting and diarrhea; FB, foreign body; CPK, creatine phosphokinase; NaCl, sodium chloride; KCl, potassium chloride.

TABLE 17.1
Child Abuse by Poisoning, *continued*

Agent	Age	Gender	Clinical Features	Abuser	Admit	In Hospital	Other Types of Abuse	Survival	Comments
Phenolphthalein	17 mo	M	Diarrhea	Mother	+	+	–	Survival	2 siblings hospitalized diazepam
Phenolphthalein	26 mo	M	Fever, V and D, rash, ataxia	Mother	–	+	–	Death	Death unexplained
Muriatic acid	21 mo	F	Stridor, respiratory distress	Babysitter	+	–	+	Survival	Prior forced FB ingestion
Muriatic acid	3 y	F	Croup	Babysitter	–	–	–	Survival	
Warfarin	7 y	F	Hemorrhage	Mother	–	+	+	Survival	Multiple unexplained symptoms, folic deficiency
Bisacodyl	11 y	M	Diarrhea, hypernatremia	Mother	+	+	–	Survival	
Cold medicine	6 mo	U	Coma, FTT	Mother	–	+	–	Survival	
Cooking oil	10 y	U	Vomiting, pneumonia	Mother	–	+	–	Survival	
Phenobarbital		F	Seizures, FTT	Mother	–	–	–	Survival	Sugar/corn syrup overdose
Caustics		F	Skin burns	Mother	–	–	–	Survival	

Abbreviations: Admit, admission of guilt by perpetrator; in hospital, poisoning continued in hospital; M, male; MSBP, Munchausen syndrome by proxy; LOC, level of consciousness; F, female; a, admitted guilt; o, observed guilt; U, unknown; ALTE, apparent life-threatening event; PxAb, physical abuse; SIDS, sudden infant death syndrome; c, convicted; FTT, failure to thrive; V and D, vomiting and diarrhea; FB, foreign body; CPK, creatine phosphokinase; NaCl, sodium chloride; KCl, potassium chloride.

(continued on page 560)

TABLE 17.1
Child Abuse by Poisoning, *continued*

Agent	Age	Gender	Clinical Features	Abuser	Admit	In Hospital	Other Types of Abuse	Survival	Comments
Paracetamol	3 mo	M	Hepatic failure	Father	–	–	+	U	Also warfarin and caffeine
Chlorpromazine	18 mo	F	Prolonged sleep	Mother	–	+	–	Survival	History of seizures
Phenothiazine	5 y	M	Stupor, fever	Mother	–	+	+	Survival	Blood gravel in urine, vomiting
Sugar	22 mo	F	Diabetic seizure	Mother	–	+	–	Survival	MSBP
Imipramine	7 y	M	Unconscious	Mother	+	+	–	Survival	
Ethylene glycol	6 mo	F	Lethargy, acidosis	Babysitter	–	–	–	Survival	
Ipecac	4 y	M	V and D	Mother	–	+	–	Survival	
Ipecac	8 mo	M	Recurrent V and D, hypotonia	Mother	a	+	–	Survival	Diagnosed at fourth hospitalization
Ipecac	10 mo	F	Recurrent V and D	Mother	o	+	–	Survival	Diagnosed after multiple hospitalizations; mother had bottles of ipecac in purse

Abbreviations: Admit, admission of guilt by perpetrator; in hospital, poisoning continued in hospital; M, male; MSBP, Munchausen syndrome by proxy; LOC, level of consciousness; F, female; a, admitted guilt; o, observed guilt; U, unknown; ALTE, apparent life-threatening event; PxAb, physical abuse; SIDS, sudden infant death syndrome; c, convicted; FTT, failure to thrive; V and D, vomiting and diarrhea; FB, foreign body; CPK, creatine phosphokinase; NaCl, sodium chloride; KCl, potassium chloride.

TABLE 17.1
Child Abuse by Poisoning, *continued*

Agent	Age	Gender	Clinical Features	Abuser	Admit	In Hospital	Other Types of Abuse	Survival	Comments
Ipecac	21 mo	M	Recurrent V and D, dehydration	Mother	–	+	–	Survival	Diagnosed after multiple hospitalizations
Ipecac	16 mo	M	Recurrent V and D, muscle weakness, ↑CPK, FTT	Mother	–	–	–	Survival	Diagnosed after 3 hospitalizations
Laxatives	U	U	U	Mother	–	–	–	Survival	3 siblings of child poisoned with ipecac
Laxatives	6 y	U	Seizures, apnea, vomiting, abdominal pain	Mother	–	+	–	Survival	
Epsom salts	4 mo	F	Diarrhea, dehydration, weight loss, poor	Mother	a	+	–	Survival	
Mineral oil	10 mo	M	U	Mother	a	+	–	Survival	MSBP, sibling died of "SIDS" after mother placed him in freezer until he suffocated

Abbreviations: Admit, admission of guilt by perpetrator; in hospital, poisoning continued in hospital; M, male; MSBP, Munchausen syndrome by proxy; LOC, level of consciousness; F, female; a, admitted guilt; o, observed guilt; U, unknown; ALTE, apparent life-threatening event; PxAb, physical abuse; SIDS, sudden infant death syndrome; c, convicted; FTT, failure to thrive; V and D, vomiting and diarrhea; FB, foreign body; CPK, creatine phosphokinase; NaCl, sodium chloride; KCl, potassium chloride.

(continued on page 562)

TABLE 17.1
Child Abuse by Poisoning, *continued*

Agent	Age	Gender	Clinical Features	Abuser	Admit	In Hospital	Other Types of Abuse	Survival	Comments
Toluene	13 mo	M	↓LOC, seizures, hydrocarbon odor to breath	Parents	o	–	–	Survival	Parents inhaling toluene and drinking alcohol
Isopropyl alcohol	2 y	M	Coma, hypothermia (33°C), shock	Father	–	–	+	Survival	Contusion, scald burns, ingestion of 100 mL isopropyl alcohol
Isopropyl alcohol	4 y	F	Found dead	Mother, boyfriend	a	–	+	Death	Alcohol applied to immersion burns; left alone in room for 27 h
Ethylene glycol	8 mo	F	Intoxicated, vomiting, lethargy, acidotic	Parents	–	–	–	Survival	
Caustic	11 y	F	Progressive upper gastrointestinal ulceration, esophageal stricture, recurrent sepsis	Mother?	c	+	–	Survival	MSBP, many procedures and hospitalizations, near death from induced sepsis; cured by foster placement

Abbreviations: Admit, admission of guilt by perpetrator; in hospital, poisoning continued in hospital; M, male; MSBP, Munchausen syndrome by proxy; LOC, level of consciousness; F, female; a, admitted guilt; o, observed guilt; U, unknown; ALTE, apparent life-threatening event; PxAb, physical abuse; SIDS, sudden infant death syndrome; c, convicted; FTT, failure to thrive; V and D, vomiting and diarrhea; FB, foreign body; CPK, creatine phosphokinase; NaCl, sodium chloride; KCl, potassium chloride.

TABLE 17.1

Child Abuse by Poisoning, *continued*

Agent	Age	Gender	Clinical Features	Abuser	Admit	In Hospital	Other Types of Abuse	Survival	Comments
Air freshener	28 d	M	Recurrent apnea, cyanosis, choking	Mother	o	+	–	Survival	Air freshener added to infant's bottle
Caffeine	5 wk	M	Agitated/ irritable	Father	+	–	+	Death	Died of inflicted head injury
Caffeine	14 mo	F	V and D, dehydration, ↓LOC	Mother, boyfriend	–	–	+	Death	Lacerated spleen, rib fractures, caffeine diet pills; abused by mother and sold by mother's boyfriend
Salt (NaCl and KCl)	6 y	M	Abdominal pain, collapse	Stepfather	a	–	–	Death	Salt substitute added to food as punishment for child using too much salt
Salt	3 y	F	Somnolence, dehydration, FTT, hyper-natremia	Mother?	–	–	–	Survival	Trichotillomania, water deprivation
Salt	1 y	M	Vomiting, FTT, lethargy, cardiac arrest, hypernatremia	Mother	c	–	–	Death	

Abbreviations: Admit, admission of guilt by perpetrator; in hospital, poisoning continued in hospital; M, male; MSBP, Munchausen syndrome by proxy; LOC, level of consciousness; F, female; a, admitted guilt; o, observed guilt; U, unknown; ALTE, apparent life-threatening event; PxAb, physical abuse; SIDS, sudden infant death syndrome; c, convicted; FTT, failure to thrive; V and D, vomiting and diarrhea; FB, foreign body; CPK, creatine phosphokinase; NaCl, sodium chloride; KCl, potassium chloride.

(continued on page 564)

TABLE 17.1
Child Abuse by Poisoning, *continued*

Agent	Age	Gender	Clinical Features	Abuser	Admit	In hospital	Other Types of Abuse	Survival	Comments
Salt	5 mo	F	Hypernatremia	Father	–	–	–	Death	
Salt	5 y	F	Seizures, hypernatremia	Mother	–	–	+	Survival	FTT, bizarre eating
Water	8 y	F	Unconscious, hypothermia, hyponatremia	Foster parents	a	–	–	Survival	Water drinking chosen as humane punishment after "much counseling"
Water	4 y	F	Collapse, status epilepticus, hyponatremia, FTT	Mother	a	–	+	Survival	PxAb, gained 5.5 lb in 7 d in hospital
Peppers	33 mo	M	Coma after beating	Mother, boyfriend	a	–	+	Death	20 small peppers found in esophagus; subdural and retroperitoneal bleeds at autopsy
Jalapeno peppers	7 y	U	V and D, burning in throat and anus	Parents	–	–	+	Survival	PxAb
Tabasco sauce	5 y	U	V and D, burning in throat and anus	Parents	–	–	+	Survival	PxAb

Abbreviations: Admit, admission of guilt by perpetrator; in hospital, poisoning continued in hospital; M, male; MSBP, Munchausen syndrome by proxy; LOC, level of consciousness; F, female; a, admitted guilt; o, observed guilt; U, unknown; ALTE, apparent life-threatening event; PxAb, physical abuse; SIDS, sudden infant death syndrome; c, convicted; FTT, failure to thrive; V and D, vomiting and dia rhea; FB, foreign body; CPK, creatine phosphokinase; NaCl, sodium chloride; KCl, potassium chloride.

TABLE 17.2

Child Abuse by Poisoning: Substance Abuse

Agent	Age	Gender	Clinical Features	Abuser	Survival	Comments
Cocaine	Not born	F	Death	Mother	Death	Fetal demise due to maternal cocaine use
Cocaine	3 mo	F	Seizures	U	Survival	Heavy crack smoking in home
Cocaine	9 mo	M	Drowsiness	Uncles	Survival	Uncles smoked crack in apartment
Cocaine	2 y	M	Seizures, lethargy	Babysitter	Survival	Babysitter smoked crack
Cocaine	3 y	M	Nausea, too wobbly to stand	Adult male	Survival	Adult male smoked crack all night
Cocaine	11 d	M	Seizures, apnea	Mother	Survival	Topical cocaine powder used on nipples to relieve pain
Cocaine	2 wk	F	LOC, ataxia, seizures	Mother	Survival	Breastfeeding by cocaine-using mother
Cocaine	8 wk	F	Found dead	Parents	Death	Parents didn't ask cause of death, arrested in another city for sale and use of cocaine
Cocaine	10 wk	F	Found dead, babysitter	Parents?	Death	Parents used and sold cocaine
Cocaine	4 mo	F	Seizure	Mother?	Survival	Mother may have used cocaine to sedate child
Cocaine	9 mo	F	Seizures, in stasis for 90 min	Babysitter	Survival	Drugs accessible at home of babysitter; cocaine found in gastric lavage
Cocaine	14 mo	M	Seizures	U	Survival	Use of cocaine in the home the night before
Cocaine	3 y	F	Seizures	U	Survival	Claimed child found cocaine on street and ate it
Cocaine	6 wk	M	LOC, hypothermia 31°C, diarrhea, dehydration FTT	U	Survival	Mother admitted infant frequently exposed to crack cocaine smoke

Abbreviations: F, female; U, unknown; M, male; LOC, loss of consciousness; FTT, failure to thrive; V and D, vomiting and diarrhea; LSD, lysergic acid diethylamide; PCP, phencyclidine; THC, tetrahydrocannabinol; PxAb, physical abuse.

(continued on page 566)

TABLE 17.2
Child Abuse by Poisoning: Substance Abuse, continued

Agent	Age	Gender	Clinical Features	Abuser	Survival	Comments
Cocaine	3 mo	F	V and D, seizures, cerebral infarcts, sagittal vein, thrombosis, dehydration	Parents?	Death	Parents smoked cocaine daily; said they would not "waste" cocaine on the baby
Cocaine	12 mo	M	Epistaxis, *Haemophilus influenzae* sepsis, pericardial effusion	Mother?	Survival	Mother entered drug treatment, denied all but passive exposure to infant
Cocaine	14 mo	M	Fever, ear pain, seizures	Aunt?	Survival	Aunt smoked crack while caring for infant, denied feeding him cocaine
Cocaine	20 mo	F	Drooling, vomiting, lethargy, esophagitis, epiglottitis	Mother?	Impaired	Ingested lye used in crack preparation; esophageal stricture; required hyperalimentation and gastrostomy
Cocaine	4 y	F	Anal fissure, anal laxity	Parents	Survival	Parents accused each other of hiding rock cocaine in the child's rectum
Cocaine	4 y	F	↓LOC, vomiting, bloody diarrhea, cardiovascular collapse	U	Survival	Rock cocaine lying on kitchen table at house where cocaine was used
Cocaine	9 mo	F	Seizures, apnea, hyper-thermia, hypertension	U	Survival	Infant found playing in remnants of party where cocaine was used
Cocaine	Birth	F	Intrauterine death	Mother	Death	Intrauterine cocaine toxicity
Cocaine	6 wk	M	Found dead	Stepbrother	Death	Homicide from cocaine-laced formula
Opiate	5 d	M	Death	U	Death	Accidental "overdose" with opiates

Abbreviations: F, female; U, unknown; M, male; LOC, loss of consciousness; FTT, failure to thrive; V and D, vomiting and diarrhea; LSD, lysergic acid diethylamide; PCP, phencyclidine; THC, tetrahydrocannabinol; PxAb, physical abuse.

TABLE 17.2
Child Abuse by Poisoning: Substance Abuse, *continued*

Agent	Age	Gender	Clinical Features	Abuser	Survival	Comments
Heroin	10 mo	M	Found dead	Mother	Death	Multiple injections of heroin by mother's boyfriend to stop baby crying
Methadone	5 d	M	Apnea, cyanosis, ↓LOC, hypotonia	Mother	Survival	Mother admitted giving her own methadone to treat the baby's withdrawal
LSD	22 mo	M	Crying, agitation, hallucinations	U	Survival	Mother admitted child may have ingested LSD left in house by friend
PCP	2 mo	F	7 children with symptoms	U	Survival	Deliberate poisoning of formula vs passive
PCP	10 mo	F	LOC, lethargy, coma	U	U	Passive inhalation at a party
PCP	13 mo	F	Hypotonia, ataxia	U	Survival	Passive inhalation at a party
PCP	14 mo	F	Blank stare, miosis, nystagmus	U	Survival	Passive inhalation at a party
PCP	18 mo	F	Seizure, opisthotonos, disconjugate gaze	U	Survival	Passive inhalation at a party
PCP	11 d	M	6 children with lethargy	U	Survival	Passive inhalation vs deliberate intoxication

Abbreviations: F, female; U, unknown; M, male; LOC, loss of consciousness; FTT, failure to thrive; V and D vomiting and diarrhea; LSD, lysergic acid diethylamide; PCP, phencyclidine; THC, tetrahydrocannabinol; PxAb, physical abuse.

(continued on page 568)

TABLE 17.2

Child Abuse by Poisoning: Substance Abuse, *continued*

Agent	Age	Gender	Clinical Features	Abuser	Survival	Comments
PCP	8 mo	F	Nystagmus, ataxia	U	Survival	Passive inhalation vs deliberate intoxication
PCP	13 mo	F	Irritability, coma, hypertonic, miosis	U	Survival	Passive inhalation vs deliberate intoxication
PCP	13 mo	M		U	Survival	Passive inhalation vs deliberate intoxication
PCP	18 mo	F		U	Survival	Passive inhalation vs deliberate intoxication
PCP	5 y	F		U	Survival	Passive inhalation vs deliberate intoxication
THC	U	U	3 children in coma	—	Survival	Apparently accidental ingestion of 1 g of hashish by 3 children
THC	1–2 y	F/M	5 children with symptoms; stupor, sluggish pupils, one patient required atropine and a ventilator for respiratory depression	—	Survival	Apparently accidental ingestion

Abbreviations: F, female; U, unknown; M, male; LOC, loss of consciousness; FTT, failure to thrive; V and D, vomiting and diarrhea; LSD, lysergic acid diethylamide; PCP, phencyclidine; THC, tetrahydrocannabinol; PxAb, physical abuse.

TABLE 17.2

Child Abuse by Poisoning: Substance Abuse, *continued*

Agent	Age	Gender	Clinical Features	Abuser	Survival	Comments
THC			Stupor, sluggish pupils, one patient required atropine and a ventilator for respiratory depression	—	Survival	Apparently accidental ingestion
THC	U	U	25 children, aged 5 mo to 10 y, with symptoms including sleepiness, giggling, ataxia, hyperactivity, crying	Babysitter	Survival	9 girls admitted intoxicating a total of 25 children with marijuana while babysitting from 1 to 15 times for each child
THC	2 y	F	Ataxia, hand tremor	Babysitter	Survival	Neighbor gave marijuana-laced cookies to babysitter
THC	3 y	F	Ataxia, voracious appetite. ↓LOC, labile affect, tremor. conjunctival hyperemia	Babysitter	Survival	Neighbor gave marijuana-laced cookies to babysitter
THC	4 y	M	Ataxia, voracious appetite, ↓LOC, labile affect, tremor, conjunctival hyperemia	Babysitter	Survival	Neighbor gave marijuana-laced cookies to babysitter
Alcohol			15 intoxicated toddlers	—	Survival	"Morning after" ingestion of alcohol left out after party the night before
Alcohol			4 intoxicated toddlers	—	Survival	Intoxicated while attending family celebration
Alcohol			2 intoxicated toddlers	Parent/ babysitter	Survival	Given alcohol by parent or babysitter
Alcohol			5 boys, aged 7 to 14 y	Friends	Survival	Forced to drink under duress
Alcohol			4 boys, aged 7 to 14 y	Adult men	Survival	Forced to drink as part of sexual abuse

Abbreviations: F, female; U, unknown; M, male; LOC, loss of consciousness; FTT, failure to thrive; V and D, vomiting and diarrhea; LSD, lysergic acid diethylamide; PCP, phencyclidine; THC, tetrahydrocannabinol; PxAb, physical abuse.

(*continued on page 568*)

TABLE 17.2

Child Abuse by Poisoning: Substance Abuse, *continued*

Agent	Age	Gender	Clinical Features	Abuser	Survival	Comments
Alcohol	5 y	M	Found dead	Mother, boyfriend	Death	Child died of ingestion of cologne (70% ethanol); and salicylates; mother and boyfriend pled guilty
Alcohol	4 y	M	Vomiting and drowsiness	Dad's friend	Survival	Prior poisoning with propoxyphene (Darvon)
Alcohol	6 y	F	Coma, shock, hypothermia (34°C)	Father	Survival	Father forced child to drink a cup of brandy; peritoneal dialysis required; PxAb
Alcohol	1 y	M	Found moribund	Mother's boyfriend	Death	Mother's boyfriend fed baby rum and Coke to quiet him; PxAb

Abbreviations: F, female; U, unknown; M, male; LOC, loss of consciousness; FTT, failure to thrive; V and D, vomiting and diarrhea; LSD, lysergic acid diethylamide; PCP, phencyclidine; THC, tetrahydrocannabinol; PxAb, physical abuse.

term *unintentional.* This is not a perfect descriptor either, because the young child probably did indeed intend to ingest the substance in question, though likely not with intent to inflict self-harm. A spectrum exists between the isolated occurrence of such ingestions and negligent child care. Even when caregivers take reasonable precautions and demonstrate an appropriate level of watchfulness, children often manage to access potentially dangerous substances in their environment. In some situations, unintentional self-poisoning by young children may be construed as abusive when the caregiver has not provided sufficient child supervision (eg, blatant neglect and/or endangering). The key is to identify when the guardian has failed to provide reasonable measures of oversight of the child.

The motivation for poisoning in any of these contexts seems quite variable. As noted, the life at home of some families may be so disorganized or complicated by mental health issues such that caregivers are unable to provide any modicum of supervision. For others, social and/or occupational association with the drug culture may place children at risk by exposing them to drugs and their chemical precursors as well as introducing them to criminal activities. Some cases may represent an impulsive action carried out under duress, such as using a large dose of alcohol or sedative medication to quiet a colicky baby.[18] Other motives might include bizarre or excessively punitive child-rearing practices (eg, force-feeding black or hot pepper as punishment, or force-feeding salt and/or water restriction to "treat" enuresis).

Some families might be entertained by getting their child "high" by sharing recreational illicit drugs. As noted before, the presumed motive of the parent in MBP cases is internal gain, specifically that of assuming the sick role by proxy for self-serving purposes manifested in the form of being "recognized" as a devoted and loving or well-informed parent by a spouse, family, friends, and medical staff. Lastly, the motivation in the intentional murder of a child may be internally driven by a mental health disorder, or externally motivated to collect life insurance, bring a wrongful death civil suit, or eliminate the child as an encumbrance to the parent's personal agenda.

Epidemiology of Childhood Poisoning and CAP

Poisoning is one of the most common medical emergencies in young children and accounts for a considerable proportion of emergency department (ED) visits in adolescents. Estimates of annual poisoning occurrence in children range into the millions. Among children ages 5 years or younger, most poisonings are due to exploratory behavior or willful child abuse. The American Association of Poison Control Centers (AAPCC) Toxic Exposure Surveillance System (TESS) records all voluntary telephone contacts to poison control centers in the United States and publishes annual summary statistics. In 2005 the total number of human exposure cases reported for all ages was 2.4 million, including 1,261 fatalities.[19] Of this total, 1.2 million (50.9%) were children younger than 6 years, 151,748 (6.3%)

were children aged 6 to 12 years, and 171,392 (7.1%) were adolescents aged 12 to 19 years. Among all children younger than 20 years, most cases involved children 1 year (25%) or 2 years (26%) old (Table 17.3). Fatality was rare in young children, with 24 deaths reported in children younger than 6 years (1.9% of the total 1,261 deaths) and 12 deaths in children aged 6 to 12 years (1% of total), but increased considerably in adolescents 13 to 19 years old (77 deaths, 6.1% of total).

The peak in unintentional ingestions by toddlers 1 to 2 years old is not surprising, given that at their developmental stage they have greater mobility but little impulse control. This is compounded by the fact that their primary impulse is to explore the world with their mouths,[20–21] putting them at increased risk for poisoning.

More than 90% of poison exposures occurred in the home in 2005,[19] and the most common exposures among children were ingestions of household products including cosmetics and personal care products, cleaning substances, analgesics, foreign bodies, and plants (Figure 17.1).[19]

When comparing outcomes of poisoning, the morbidity and mortality for the typical exploratory ingestions in young children is generally low compared with that of adolescents and adults. This probably reflects the more common availability of less toxic nonprescription medications and household products to young children, smaller relative toxic doses ingested due to interruption of the ingestion by parental intervention, and the usual rapid discovery by parents and subsequent emergent access to medical treatment when the child is immediately

TABLE 17.3
Age Distribution of Human Exposure Cases[a]

Age, y	Total Number of Reports	Percentage of Total Children (age <20 y)
<1	129,096	8%
1	392,270	25%
2	402,142	26%
3	174,427	11%
4	82,907	5%
5	48,274	3%
6–12	151,748	10%
13–19	171,392	11%
Exact age unknown	11,396	0.7%

[a]Adapted from Lai MW, Klein-Schwartz W, Rodgers GC, et al. 2005 annual report of the American Association of Poison Control Centers' national poisoning and exposure database. *Clin Toxicol (Phila)*. 2006;44:803–932

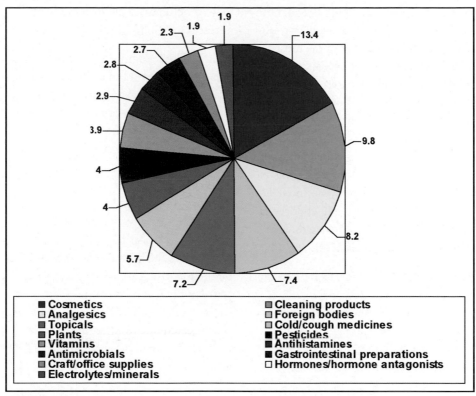

FIGURE 17.1
Percentage of top 15 substances seen in accidental pediatric ingestions.
Adapted from Lai MW, Klein-Schwartz W, Rodgers GC, et al. 2005 Annual Report of the
American Association of Poison Control Centers national poisoning and exposure database.
Clin Toxicol (Phila). 2006;44:803–932.

caught "in the act" or soon thereafter. In contrast, older children, adolescents, and adults who become poisoned by suicidal intent or recreational substance abuse often ingest large quantities of very toxic substances, and may be ill for some time before discovery and subsequent medical interventions. In this context, it is critical to note that, not surprisingly, when children are deliberately poisoned, the outcome is much more likely to be highly morbid or fatal than with unintentional ingestions.[8,9,20,23] Reported life-threatening clinical effects include deep coma, status epilepticus, respiratory compromise requiring intubation, cardiac arrhythmias, oral and esophageal corrosive injury, severe coagulopathy, and extreme metabolic aberrations. The AAPCC data are divided into 4 categories based on the reason a poisoning occurs: unintentional (eg, therapeutic errors, drug misuse, bites/stings, environmental exposures, occupational exposures, food poisoning, etc), intentional (eg, suspected suicide, drug misuse, drug abuse, etc), other (eg, withdrawal, contamination/tampering, and malicious), and adverse reaction (eg, to drugs, food, or other exposure). The malicious category "is used to capture patients who are victims of another person's intent to harm them."[19] Thus that category probably encompasses many of the most sinister cases of CAP, but probably does not reflect those likely due to severe neglect, recreational misuse, or unorthodox health practices. Nevertheless, in the 5-year period from 2000 through 2004, 2,528 cases of malicious poisoning were reported to AAPCC, thus averaging more than 500 cases per year. In 2005, of the 36 deaths reported in children younger than 13 years, 5 were due to malicious intent (Table 17.4).

Two routes of malicious, fatal pediatric poisoning are reflected in Table 17-4. However, this is certainly not a complete list of potential routes of such exposure, which might include poisoning via nasogastric or gastrostomy tube,

skin or ocular contact, or parenteral access (eg, insulin injection).

It should be recognized that the TESS system has several limitations as a tool for poisoning surveillance. It relies entirely on voluntary reporting by laypersons and health professionals. Additionally, most professional callers to poison control centers are seeking medical toxicology consultative advice, and thus do not always call if a patient has either a well-recognized and easily managed intoxication or if the patient has been in the hospital for some time before the discovery of a toxicological cause of illness and has since recovered. In the context of CAP, a further concern is that when a family member is the reporter, the data provided are necessarily subjective and likely biased, because

TABLE 17.4
Poisoning Deaths in Children Due to Malicious Intent, 2005[a]

Age	Substance	Route of Exposure	Comment
8 y	Carbon monoxide	Inhalation	Family of 4 (mother, father, 2 eight-year-olds) found dead in bedroom. Father had sealed family in room and started a charcoal fire while they slept.
8 y	Carbon monoxide	Inhalation	Sibling of above patient.
6.57 y	Carbon monoxide	Inhalation	Carboxyhemoglobin 56%
2 mo	Methadone	Ingestion	Found in cardiac arrest by police. History of neonatal cocaine and heroin withdrawal. Methadone was found by medical examiner on toxicology testing.
15 mo	Methadone	Ingestion	Methadone ingested from sippy cup. Found apneic 2 hrs later, pronounced dead in emergency department. Mother had methadone prescription.

[a]Adapted from Lai MW, Klein-Schwartz W, Rodgers GC, et al. 2005 annual report of the American Association of Poison Control Centers' national poisoning and exposure database. *Clin Toxicol (Phila)*. 2006;44:803–932

malicious intent is unlikely to be disclosed and, therefore, CAP is most likely underrepresented. Finally, medical examiners' offices do not routinely report their findings of deaths by poisoning to their regional poison control centers.

Clinical Evaluation of Potential CAP

Overview

Poisoned children most often present to medical attention with anxious caregivers who can provide a reliable and accurate history regarding the time of ingestion, substance ingested, and a reasonable estimate of total dose. This is especially true for witnessed exploratory ingestions by toddlers "caught in the act" or who are found with evidence of recent ingestion in their environment. Even adolescents who have attempted suicide or have used illicit recreational drugs will often accurately confess their actions when they become ill and are brought emergently to a hospital. However, sometimes children are exposed to a poison without being observed, subsequently become ill, and then may present as diagnostic dilemmas, having alterations in sensorium, multiorgan system dysfunction, and peculiar electrolyte or acid-base disturbances. This is probably even more the case with CAP patients, in whom the history from caregivers is not only unreliable but often deliberately misleading.

Meadow[20] outlined 4 main patterns of clinical presentation typical of CAP

1. The child is brought to medical care with a history offered by parent or caretaker as that of typical exploratory ingestion.

2. The child presents with an illness of unknown etiology, generally of acute onset (especially in the first episode of CAP).
3. The child exhibits a recurrent history of strange, unexplained clinical findings, often without a previous definitive medical diagnosis (this category is essentially MBP).
4. The child arrives at the ED moribund or dead on arrival, at times without any historical explanation.

In the cases characterized by categories 2 and 3, certain clinical features should alert the practitioner to potential CAP.[3,24,25] These include notable findings in the child's medical history, physical examination, and parental medical and social histories. Table 17.5 highlights these findings, and further discussion is provided in the following sections.

History

As is true of all forms of suspected child abuse, the differential diagnosis of poisoning must include true unintentional exposure, breech of supervision, endangerment, and deliberate poisoning with malicious intent.

There are crucial questions that must be included in the medical history when a poisoning is suspected. The most common chief complaint in a poisoned child is altered mental status. The timeline of symptoms is critical; information about the presence of a prodrome (fussiness, fever, sleeplessness) may offer insight into how a stressed caretaker attempted to "treat" the child, or can offer clues about specific substances. For example,

TABLE 17.5
Common Clinical Features Suggesting Child Abuse by Poisoning

Evaluation	Features
Medical history	<ul><li>Abrupt onset of illness, especially involving altered mental status and/or gastrointestinal (GI) symptoms (or other relevant syndromes—see Table 17.6)</li><li>Recurrent episodes of altered mental status, GI symptoms, particularly while in hospital with parent visiting</li><li>Inadequate or obviously fabricated history of toxic exposure, especially in children <10–12 months, or between 5 and 10 years old</li><li>Any symptom complex that is baffling to an experienced clinician</li></ul>
Physical examination	<ul><li>Characteristic vital sign changes — Tachycardia, hypertension, hyperthermia; bradycardia, hypotension, hypothermia; tachypnea, hyperpnea; bradypnea (see also Tables 17.6 and 17.7)</li><li>Abrupt onset of neurologic signs — Obtundation, coma; agitation, delirium, seizures</li><li>Evidence of caustic injury — Lip burns or edema, oropharyngeal ulcers</li><li>Abnormal pupillary finding</li><li>Autonomic dysfunction noted in vital signs, skin, mucous membranes, GI tract (see also Tables 17.6 and 17.7)</li><li>Dehydration</li><li>Findings suspicious for physical abuse</li><li>Any complex of signs baffling to an experienced clinician</li></ul>
Family history	<ul><li>Medications used by family members, for which the toxicity profile matches the child's clinical syndrome</li><li>Parent/caretaker recreational substance abuse or psychiatric illness</li><li>Recent psychosocial stress, or parental emotional response inappropriate for child's condition</li><li>Suspicious illness or death of a sibling</li></ul>
Social history	<ul><li>Medical or nursing background of parent/caretaker</li><li>Parent/caretaker access (occupational or recreational) to drugs or exotic chemicals with toxicity profiles that match the child's clinical syndrome</li></ul>

fever may be observed in anticholinergic drug toxicity such as cases of diphenhydramine and amitriptyline poisoning; both of these agents have been implicated in fatal CAP.[10,26]

In addition, the timeline of the child's decompensation can give an indication of the caregiver's oversight and involvement in the child's care. Timing of symptoms should not be used exclusively to estimate the amount of substance to which a child has been exposed because too many confounding factors exist for reliable interpretation.

A description of the child's home environment is important to gain insight into the environmental safety of the household, as well as identify likely toxic exposures affecting the patient. Often a substance comes to a child's attention because it was recently used or moved to a more accessible location in the home.[27] The clinician should inquire about prescription medications used by members of the patient's household, and where they are stored. Adult patients may request non–child-resistant caps on their prescription medicine containers; thus assuming all house guests' or elderly relatives' medicines are child-proof may be erroneous.[28] Vitamins are an often-overlooked ingestible substance in the home, particularly those containing high, potentially toxic concentrations of iron, and should be specifically asked about, especially if the mother is pregnant or recently postpartum. Parents may be providing the child with toxic megadoses of vitamins on the advice of alternative medicine practitioners, the media, or trusted friends.

Family hobbies and occupations should be detailed because they may be a source of a number of unusual toxins, such as toxic metals around the home workshop or artist's studio, or various hydrocarbons and solvents where painting occurs. Houseplants and the home garden, with native and cultured garden plants or mushrooms, also may be a source of toxic ingestion.[29-31] Parents who work in medical settings will have varying degrees of pharmacologic knowledge. Caretaker familiarity with both enteral and parenteral drug administration combined with easy and relatively unmonitored access to prescription medications, intravenous electrolyte solutions, and supplies to administer them may lead the caretaker to attempt to "treat" or purposefully harm a child.

A home inspection performed by law enforcement or child protective services may be indicated to determine what role the environment played in a child's toxic exposure. When deliberate poisoning is suspected, an inspection of the child's home as well as all environments where the child resides is mandatory, either with permission of the caregiver/homeowner or, if necessary, by court order.

A developmental history should be taken from the caregiver. At 7 to 9 months of age, a developmentally normal child will begin to crawl and may feed himself a piece of cat litter, a pill dropped on the floor, or part of a houseplant using a crude hand grasp. Cruising usually occurs by around 9 months of age, when the infant learns to pull up and then move around the perimeter of a supporting object. A sophisticated pincer grasp follows by 10 to 12 months, and one could reasonably expect a child to transfer a cigarette butt or rock of crack cocaine or other substance effectively from hand to mouth. An infant typically will walk at around age 12 months. Comparing a child's developmental history with typical developmental milestones helps determine the likelihood that a given poisoning was potentially an act of abuse. Unintentional or accidental self-ingestions are rare in infants younger than 10 to 12 months, in keeping with their developmental limitations of coordinating a pincer grasp, hand-mouth coordination, and ambulatory capability sufficient to elude a caretaker's notice.[10,26,32] Thus it would be unlikely for a houseplant, pill, centipede or a carpet tack to be accidentally ingested by a 6-month-old child unless it was given to him or her by an older child.[10,33,34] As demonstrated in Table 17.3, accidental ingestions are most common in toddlers and, developmentally, can be expected in children through the preschool years. Medications are the most common poisons ingested by children 2 to 3 years old, while household products are more often consumed by children in the 1- to 2-year-old age group.[35] By the age of 10, ingestions intended as suicide attempts and deliberate ingestions for amusement/intoxication increase. Typically, when young children are victims of unintentional (accidental) ingestion, there is less than a 2-hour lag between the time of the ingestion and the time to seeking medical advice.[36]

A topic that may not be routinely discussed during an acute encounter in the hospital setting is the method of discipline used to teach the child appropriate behavior. However, as noted previously, extremely punitive interventions may be encountered in CAP. Forced salt ingestion and forced water ingestion are among the most common methods used in abusive poisonings with an intent to discipline the child. The parent's history may reveal that the child was having a particularly bad day behaviorwise, which might prompt the physician to discover poisoning used as punishment. In this context, sodium abnormality on laboratory evaluation should prompt a second interview to seek a history of exogenous administration of salt or dilution of a patient's serum sodium level by forced excess water administration.[19,37]

Even more concerning in the patient history is the lack of any reasonable explanation for the child's current condition. The most prominent warning signs in the history include incomplete, unexplained, or discrepant accounts of the onset of an apparent illness. The child's developmental level must be taken into account to determine the plausibility of the history as well. Frequently, a third party is blamed for the event, either a sibling or visitor in the home. At times, third-party involvement will need to be verified by an investigative evaluation at the scene of the ingestion. Additionally, the history of similar sudden "illness" in a sibling, or a sibling death, should alarm the physician to include deliberate poisoning in the differential diagnosis, and the specter of MBP and its victim-focused component, PCF, should be raised. Recurrent unexplained episodes of symptoms with a negative medical workup are equally suspicious. Repeated poisonings raise concerns about the safety of the environment, the supervision provided by the caretaker, and the possibility of deliberate poisoning. In a 1989 study, 41% of poisoned children between the ages of 3 and 5 years had repeated ingestions. In the age group of patients who were younger than 5 years, 18% had 2 prior ingestions, and 4.4% had 3 prior ingestions. Children who deviate considerably in the number of ingestions (eg, >2) and age at time of repeat ingestion (<1 year or >5 years) should certainly raise the suspicion of CAP.[10,38] Involvement of child protective services is warranted to determine if neglect or abuse is occurring, engage the family with supportive services to identify and correct the unsafe household conditions, or remove the child from a perpetually harmful environment.

Physical Examination

General

The scope of toxin-induced physical findings is very broad but, in general, common patterns of abnormalities involve the vital signs, central nervous system (CNS), and autonomic nervous system function; eye findings; oropharynx and gastrointestinal (GI) tract injury; and characteristic skin changes.[39] In addition, characteristic breath or body fluid odors may sometimes provide helpful clues. Probably the most common consequential finding presenting in a poisoned child is altered mental status. This may manifest as decreased level of consciousness,

ranging along a continuum from drowsiness through obtundation to coma, or increased excitability, ranging from tremor and increased muscle tone through myoclonic jerks to overt seizures. Major categories of abnormal clinical findings are highlighted in Box 17.1. These clinical features represent organ systems most likely affected in toxic syndromes and, when taken together, often form a constellation of findings referred to as toxidromes (Table 17.6). Such toxidromes may be so characteristic as to provide management guidance even before precise historical or laboratory confirmation of a specific poisoning is available.

Evidence of Physical Abuse

There is a well-established association between abuse by poisoning and physical abuse.[10,26] The socioeconomic risk factors for exposing children to poisonous agents, whether deliberate or accidental, are similar risk factors for physical abuse. Often, each act is perpetrated by an isolated caregiver with a poor educational background, poor coping mechanisms in stressful situations, and poor impulse control. The diagnosis of poisoning in a child under circumstances that are either abusive or neglectful mandates an evaluation for physical abuse as is appropriate for the child's age and background. A visual inspection of the poisoned child's total body surface area for signs of inflicted injury, as well as assessing general health, growth, development, hygiene, and nutrition is mandatory.

BOX 17.1

Clinical Manifestations of Poisoning and Suspected Poisons[a]

Vital Signs

Pulse

Bradycardia
Digoxin, narcotics, organophosphates, plants (lily of the valley, foxglove, oleander), clonidine, beta-blockers, calcium channel blockers

Tachycardia
Alcohol, amphetamines/sympathomimetics, atropinics, tricyclic antidepressants, theophylline, salicylates, phencyclidine, cocaine

Respirations

Slow, depressed
Alcohol, barbiturates (late), narcotics, clonidine, sedative hypnotics

Tachypnea
Amphetamines, barbiturates (early), methanol, salicylates, carbon monoxide

Blood pressure

Hypotension
Cellular asphyxiants (methemoglobinemia, cyanide, carbon monoxide), phenothiazines, tricyclic antidepressants, barbiturates, iron, theophylline, clonidine, narcotics, beta-blockers, calcium channel blockers

Hypertension
Amphetamines/sympathomimetics (especially phenylpropanolamine in over-the-counter [OTC] cold remedies, diet pills), tricyclic antidepressants, phencyclidine, monoamine oxidase inhibitors (MAOIs), antihistamines, atropinics, clonidine, cocaine

Temperature

Hypothermia
Ethanol, barbiturates, sedative hypnotics, narcotics, phenothiazines, antidepressants, clonidine, carbamazepine

Hyperpyrexia
Atropinics, quinine, salicylates, amphetamines, phenothiazines, tricyclics, MAOIs, theophylline, cocaine

BOX 17.1

Clinical Manifestations of Poisoning and Suspected Poisons,[a] *continued*

Neuromuscular

Coma
Narcotic depressants, sedative hypnotics, anticholinergics (antihistamines, antidepressants, phenothiazines, atropinics, OTC sleep preparations), alcohol, anticonvulsants, carbon monoxide, salicylates, organophosphate insecticides, clonidine, γ-hydroxybutyrate

Delirium/psychosis
Alcohol, phenothiazines, drugs of abuse (phencyclidine, lysergic acid diethylamide [LSD], peyote, mescaline, marijuana, cocaine, heroin, methaqualone), sympathomimetics and anticholinergics (including prescription and OTC cold remedies), steroids, heavy metals, dextromethorphan

Convulsions
Alcohol, amphetamines, cocaine, phenothiazines, antidepressants, antihistamines, camphor, boric acid, lead, organophosphates, isoniazid, salicylates, plants (water hemlock), lindane, lidocaine, phencyclidine, carbamazepine

Ataxia
Alcohol, barbiturates, carbon monoxide, anticonvulsants, heavy metals, organic solvents, sedative hypnotics, hydrocarbons

Paralysis
Botulism, heavy metals, plants (poison hemlock), ticks, paralytic shellfish poisoning

---

Eyes

Pupils
Miosis
Narcotics, organophosphates, plants (mushrooms of the muscarinic type), ethanol, barbiturates, phenothiazines, phencyclidine, clonidine

Mydriasis
Amphetamines, atropinics, barbiturates (if comatose), botulism, cocaine, methanol, glutethimide, LSD, marijuana, phencyclidine, antihistamines, antidepressants

Nystagmus
Diphenylhydantoin, sedative hypnotics, carbamazepine, glutethimide, phencyclidine (both vertical and horizontal), barbiturates, ethanol, MAOIs, ketamine, phencyclidine, dextromethorphan

BOX 17.1

Clinical Manifestations of Poisoning and Suspected Poisons,[a] *continued*

Skin
Jaundice Carbon tetrachloride, acetaminophen, naphthalene, phenothiazines, plants (mushrooms, fava beans), heavy metals (iron, phosphorus, arsenic) *Cyanosis* (unresponsive to oxygen, as a result of methemoglobinemia) Aniline dyes, nitrites, benzocaine, phenacetin, nitrobenzene, phenazopyridine, dapsone *Pinkness to redness* Atropinics and antihistamines, alcohol, carbon monoxide, cyanide, boric acid
Odors
Acetone: acetone, isopropyl alcohol, phenol and salicylates Alcohol: ethanol (alcoholic beverages) Bitter almond: cyanide Garlic: heavy metal (arsenic, phosphorus, and thallium), organophosphates Oil of wintergreen: methylsalicylates Hydrocarbons: hydrocarbons (eg, gasoline, turpentine)

[a]Modified from Mofenson HC, Greensher J. The unknown poison. *Pediatrics* 1974;54:336.

TABLE 17.6
Toxidromes[a]

	Sympathomimetics (amphetamines, cocaine)	Anticholinergics (antihistamines, others)	Organophosphates (insecticides, nerve gases)	Opiates/ Clonidine	Barbiturates/ Sedative-Hypnotics	Salicylates	Theophylline
Mental status/ CNS	Agitation, delirium, psychosis, convulsions	Delirium, psychosis, coma, convulsions	Confusion, fascicula-tions, coma	Euphoria, somnolence, coma	Somnolence, coma	Lethargy, convulsions	Agitation, tremor, convulsions
Heart rate	Increased	Increased	Decreased (or increased)	Decreased			Increased
Blood pressure	Increased	Increased		Decreased	Decreased		Decreased
Temperature	Increased	Increased		Decreased	Decreased	Increased	
Respirations			Increased	Decreased	Decreased	Increased	Increased
Pupils	Large, reactive	Large, sluggish	Small	Pinpoint			
Bowel sounds	Present	Diminished	Hyperactive				
Skin	Diaphoresis	Flushed, dry	Diaphoresis				
Miscellaneous			SLUDGE[b]			Vomiting	Vomiting

Abbreviation: CNS, central nervous system.

[a]Reprinted from Osterhoudt K, Ewald MB, Shannon M, Henretig FM. Toxicologic emergencies. In: Fleisher GR, Ludwig S, Henretig FM, eds. *Textbook of Pediatric Emergency Medicine.* 5th ed. Philadelphia. PA: Lippincott, Williams & Wilkins; 2006:951–1007.

[b]SLUDGE is a mnemonic representing salivation, lacrimation, urination, defecatior, gastric cramping, and emesis.

Vital Signs

Patient assessment begins, as for all pediatric emergencies, with a rapid survey of the airway, breathing, and circulatory status (or "ABCs"). It also is critical to measure core temperature in poisoned children, even though this vital sign is sometimes forgotten in the reliance on the traditional ABC mnemonic. Alterations in respiratory rate may reflect CNS depression with bradypnea or, alternatively, hyperventilation may occur in the setting of metabolic acidosis, primary increased ventilatory drive, or direct toxin-induced pulmonary injury, such as chemical pneumonitis from hydrocarbon aspiration.

Heart rate and blood pressure are also commonly affected. Tachycardia, usually with hypertension, may accompany overdose from stimulants. Bradycardia and hypotension typically occur with beta-blocker, calcium channel blocker, or clonidine intoxication, and may also be observed in organophosphate exposure due to inhibition of acetylcholinesterase and resultant increased vagal tone.[40] Cardiac glycoside toxicity, including that due to digoxin and related plant-based alkaloids, also may result in bradycardia and lowered arrhythmia threshold. In contrast to the more common finding of tachycardia with hypotension (eg, in the context of hypovolemia or sepsis), toxin-induced hypotension often is accompanied by bradycardia (see Table 17.6).

As stated earlier, core temperature determination is critical. Life-threatening extreme hyperthermia may complicate poisonings by a number of toxins, including anticholinergic agents (eg, diphenhydramine, Jimsonweed), stimulants (eg, amphetamine or cocaine), and salicylate, as well as by neuroleptic malignant syndrome and serotonin syndrome. Hypothermia is a characteristic of poisoning from opiates, ethanol, clonidine, and several sedative-hypnotic or anticonvulsive agents with generalized CNS depressant effects.

Central Nervous System

Central nervous system depression, from drowsiness to coma, is one of the most common presenting findings in poisoned children. The CNS effects of toxic exposure may represent a direct effect of the ingested drug or toxin, including prescription medications and illicit recreational drugs, such as marijuana[41] or ethanol. Diminished responsiveness may also be secondary to metabolic effects induced by the ingested poison, reduced oxygen delivery due to carbon monoxide (CO) inhalation or methemoglobin formation, or impaired oxygen use at the cellular level as occurs in cyanide toxicity.

Central nervous system excitation also may occur, ranging from agitation, delirium, and increased muscle tone and hyperreflexia to overt generalized seizures, which commonly complicates diagnosing recreational and prescription drug overdoses. As for CNS depression, seizures may result from direct toxic effects on the brain or inadequate cerebral perfusion and loss of substrate delivery. Other movement disorders may occur and provide clues to the toxin, such as extrapyramidal findings in antipsychotic or metoclopramide overdose. Neuroleptic malignant syndrome is a rare and severe adverse drug reaction that presents with altered mental status, muscle rigidity, and hyperthermia in response to the antidopaminergic effects of both typical antipsychotic medications and several of the newer atypicals. Serotonin syndrome presents with similar findings and occurs when a drug or drug combination results in excessive CNS serotoninergic activity. This is seen most commonly when a patient is exposed to both a monoamine oxidase inhibitor class of antidepressant and any number of additional serotonergic agents, including dextromethorphan, meperidine, or the selective serotonin reuptake inhibitor antidepressants.

Eyes

The pupillary response to light should be noted. Miosis is a hallmark of opiate intoxication, and may also be seen with ethanol, barbiturate, clonidine, phencyclidine, phenothiazine, and organophosphate toxicity. Mydriasis reflects the systemic effects of amphetamines, antihistamines, atropinics, cocaine, lysergic acid diethylamide (LSD), marijuana, or methanol. Dilated pupils with sluggish pupillary response is characteristic of anticholinergic toxicity, although this finding might also be observed in patients with advanced cerebral edema as a late complication of a number of toxicological causes and hypoxic-ischemic encephalopathy. In cases of CNS dysfunction without a history of ingestion, the medical evaluation is often initially focused on intracranial injury

from mechanical forces. However, the prudent medical provider should consider obtaining body fluid specimens for toxicology screening panels and case-specific toxicological analysis concomitantly with neuroimaging. Nystagmus may be found as an ocular manifestation following phencyclidine ingestion.

Oropharynx and Gastrointestinal Tract

Certain household and industrial chemicals and common condiments may manifest corrosive effects on the mouth, pharynx, and more distal GI tract. Such findings might include visible burns and/or edema of the lips, oropharyngeal ulcers, and severe vomiting and/or diarrhea, in some cases bloody. Iron supplements in overdose will typically cause recurrent vomiting and profuse, often hemorrhagic, diarrhea. Other agents have profound local or autonomic nervous system oral and GI effects with either increased bowel motility or, conversely, inhibited peristalsis. Likewise, copious oral secretions are characteristic of organophosphate poisoning, while dry, tacky mucous membranes are observed with anticholinergic toxicity.

Skin

Caustic agents will cause skin irritation that may progress to burns given their agent-specific corrosive effect and contact time. Burns and/or soot around the nose and mouth in a smoke-exposed child should increase the level of suspicion for CO intoxication due to a house fire. In toxic plant exposures, nonspecific skin reactions (erythema, urticaria) may also occur in areas of contact with plant sap or fruit pulp. Jaundice is a hallmark of hepatotoxicity. Cyanosis is seen with hypoxia from drug-induced CNS depression or oxidant agent-induced methemoglobinemia. Hot, red, dry skin is a hallmark of anticholinergic toxicity, while cool, clammy skin is typical of sympathomimetic poisoning, and these differences in skin findings, along with the previously noted GI findings, may be helpful in distinguishing these toxidromes in patients with agitated delirium, tachycardia, hypertension, dilated pupils, and elevated temperature.

Odors

Characteristic odors that might be noted on a poisoned patient's breath, clothing, or body fluids are detailed in Table 17.6. Some of the more commonly appreciated odors in pediatric intoxications include the fruity odor of acetone or isopropyl (rubbing) alcohol, the "alcohol on breath" smell in ethanol exposure (usually due to beer, wine, or hard liquor components rather than ethanol per se), and the recognizable hydrocarbon odor of gasoline, mineral spirits, or lighter fluids.

Specific Toxic Syndromes in CAP

Not surprisingly, the range of clinical presentations that represent the scope of potential CAP cases is vast. Any single drug or chemical agent might be used to deliberately poison a child. Nevertheless, certain patterns of intoxication have been described often, especially in cases of repetitive poisoning that may constitute the PCF component of MBP. This section will attempt to categorize

the more clinically important and common patterns, which tend to particularly involve abnormalities of the CNS, GI tract, coagulation system, and metabolic state (see Table 17.7).[7,8,10,26]

Central Nervous System

Variable degrees of altered mental status, ranging from lethargy to deep coma, have characterized the cases involving psychotropic medications, anticonvulsants, alcohol, and recreational substances of abuse.[4,7,8,10,26] Additional findings include confusion, ataxia, myoclonus, seizures, and pupillary changes. In some children, improvement and subsequent "relapse" into coma, often occurring in the hospital, are particularly characteristic. Typical neurologic investigations are often initially unrevealing, although in several cases the electroencephalogram demonstrates fast-wave activity that is ultimately a clue to drug intoxication. When toxicological laboratory screens are ordered, they are often initially reported as negative (Box 17.2). In some cases, further and more specific toxicological analyses in light of clinical suspicions are eventually diagnostic.

Most psychoactive medication intoxications follow a predictable pattern of absorption, distribution, and elimination. The subsequent clinical course parallels this, with rapid development of maximum alteration in sensorium followed by steady improvement. When patients improve in the hospital, only to "relapse" while still hospitalized, intentional poisoning by a visiting parent must be suspected.

TABLE 17.7
Major Patterns of Clinical Presentation in Child Abuse by Poisoning

System	Specific Findings	Drugs/Toxins
Central nervous system	Obtundation, coma	Barbiturates, benzodiazepines, anticonvulsants; alcohols, other sedative-hypnotics; opioids; antidepressants, other psychotropics; marijuana, phencyclidine
	Agitation, irritability	Caffeine, phencyclidine
	Seizures	Cocaine, tricyclic antidepressants, salt, water, laxatives, insulin, oral hypoglycemics
Gastrointestinal	Vomiting	Ipecac, detergent, arsenic, hot peppers, alcohol, acetaminophen, salt
	Diarrhea	Ipecac, laxatives, hot peppers
	Caustic effects	Caustics, iron, hot peppers
Heme	Bleeding diathesis	Warfarin
Metabolic	Hypernatremia	Salt, water restriction
	Hyponatremia	Water
	Hyperglycemia	Sugar
	Hypoglycemia	Insulin, oral hypoglycemics, salicylate
	Metabolic acidosis	Toxic alcohols, iron

BOX 17.2
Important Drugs and Toxins Not Detected by Most Drug Screens[a]

Coma Causing	Hypotension Causing
Bromide	Beta-blockers[b]
Carbon monoxide	Calcium channel blockers[b]
Chloral hydrate	Clonidine[b]
Clonidine	Colchicine
Cyanide	Cyanide
γ hydroxybutyrate	Digitalis[b]
Organophosphates	Iron
Tetrahydrozoline (in over-the-counter eye drops)	

[a]Modified with permission from Wiley JF II. Difficult diagnoses in toxicology: poisons not detected by the comprehensive drug screen. *Pediatr Clin North Am.* 1991;38:725–737.

[b]Hypotension often is seen with bradycardia.

Gastrointestinal Tract

Severe vomiting and diarrhea have been common manifestations of CAP.[7,8,10,26,42] In particular, chronic vomiting and diarrhea that remain undiagnosed after multiple investigations and hospitalizations have been the hallmark of the MBP subset of cases of CAP. The predominant toxins reported have been syrup of ipecac and nonprescription laxatives.[43–46] In many of these cases the perpetrator-mother has had a history of anorexia/bulimia.

Patients poisoned with ipecac typically present with recurrent vomiting, which is not bilious or bloody, and intermittent diarrhea. Musculoskeletal weakness and cardiac toxicity also may complicate the course, and some patients develop potentially fatal congestive heart failure. The myopathy of ipecac is believed to result from a direct toxic effect of the alkaloid emetine on muscle fibers.[42] The skeletal muscle injury results in a predominantly proximal muscle weakness. Serum creatine phosphokinase and aldolase often are elevated. Emetine-induced cardiomyopathy is manifested by tachycardia, congestive failure, and electrocardiograph abnormalities including flattened or inverted T waves, prolonged P-R interval, and dysrhythmias. Echocardiography may reveal decreased left ventricular function and dilated chambers.

Not surprisingly, diarrhea is the primary presenting finding in children poisoned with laxatives. Again, chronic diarrhea may represent the MBP subset of CAP. In this context, children are typically subjected to extensive diagnostic investigations, including contrast radiography and endoscopy, which are unrevealing. Laxative abuse also has been reported using Epsom salts.[47]

More unusual causes of GI toxicity in CAP have been reported as well. Intentional acetaminophen abuse results in hepatotoxicity.[48,49] Injuries to the GI tract have resulted from detergents, metallic foreign bodies, and hot peppers.[8,33,50]

Metabolic Aberrations

Metabolic aberrations include altered electrolyte and/or glucose homeostasis such as hypernatremia and hyponatremia, hyperglycemia and hypoglycemia, and metabolic acidosis. Implicated drugs and toxins include table salt,[51–53] water restriction or water loading,[54,55] and diuretics[3,56]; sugar,[57] oral hypoglycemics,[58] and insulin administered parenterally[59,60]; and salicylates[61] or toxic alcohols.[60,62] Hypoglycemia caused by exogenous insulin administration may be detected by laboratory analysis demonstrating elevated insulin but low C-peptide levels.[24]

Hemorrhagic Diathesis

A number of patients have been reported with chronic anticoagulant poisoning and have presented to medical attention with a hemorrhagic diathesis.[63,64] Warfarin has been the predominant agent, and patients have manifested prolonged prothrombin and partial thromboplastin times. In some cases, the perpetrators had been treated for thrombophlebitis or similar illness and so had access to the medication.

Miscellaneous

Children have suffered ocular injury after caustic agents were repeatedly administered to their eyes.[65] Hydrocarbons have been injected intravenously, resulting in a characteristic breath odor, coma, apnea, and pneumonitis.[66] Other exotic poisonings have included ingestions of vitamin A,[67] pine oil,[68] arsenic, air freshener, and caffeine.[48,69–71]

Laboratory Evaluation

General Considerations

The laboratory evaluation of children with suspected CAP is crucial to diagnosing and initiating specific medical therapy. It is important to anticipate the need for toxicological testing early in the clinical evaluation, particularly when confronted with a child who manifests a characteristic clinical picture or poses a diagnostic dilemma. When collecting blood and urine, it is prudent to obtain extra samples when possible. In rare circumstances, laboratory evaluation of vomitus or fecal material also might be helpful. In cases of suspected CAP, careful chain of evidence precautions should be taken when obtaining, handling, and transporting specimens for analysis.

The appropriate accumulation and interpretation of laboratory information in a possible poisoning victim can be an intimidating task. The hospital chemistry laboratory director may be a good resource for advice. In addition, regional poison control centers offer immediate toxicology consultation advice by telephone (800/222-1222), often with a more in-depth evaluation available on a timely basis. In many academic medical centers, toxicologists and laboratory medicine specialists are on staff and can be of assistance in focusing the clinician's efforts in identifying a toxin in various body fluids.

In the event a child is brought to the hospital in extremis caused by an encephalopathy of obscure origin, liver failure, hemorrhagic diathesis, severe dehydration as a result of vomiting or diarrhea, and/or extreme serum chemistry or acid-base disturbances, it is critical to save blood and urine samples for later definitive toxicological testing. If the child is dead on arrival, or an initially moribund child subsequently dies, the responsible clinician must discuss with the medical examiner the possibility of occult poisoning to ensure appropriate tissue samples undergo toxicological analysis.

Specific Laboratory Tests

Blood Glucose Level

Hypoglycemia is one of the most easily detectable and treatable side effects of toxic ingestion. Exogenous insulin administration and the ingestion of sulfonylureas, ethanol, or beta-blockers all may cause abnormally elevated serum glucose levels.

Arterial Blood Gas

Arterial blood gas (ABG) analysis can be useful in evaluating the nature of significant acid-base disturbances, a common manifestation of significant poisoning. It may also indicate subtle respiratory depression before hypoventilation caused by CNS depression abruptly deteriorates and hypoxia and cyanosis ensue. The blood gas laboratory also typically performs spectrophotometric determinations on heparinized blood for abnormal hemoglobin species, such as methemoglobin and carboxyhemoglobin, which might result from toxic exposures. Such tests may be provided routinely with all ABG orders, though in some hospitals they may require a special request.

Methemoglobinemia sufficient to produce cyanosis may manifest normal or, more typically, slightly low oxygen saturation on pulse oximetry and a normal arterial partial pressure of oxygen and calculated oxygen saturation as measured by ABG. Sulfonamides, quinines, benzocaine, naphthalene (found in moth balls), nitrates, and nitrites are among the more common causes of methemoglobinemia. In CO toxicity, the pulse oximetry and ABG findings also are misleading (although CO does not produce cyanosis).

Electrolytes

Sodium imbalance may be reflective of exogenous administration of salt, water restriction, or excessive forced water intake. Typically a child will excrete excess salt in the urine but may not do so efficiently if simultaneously deprived of water. In such circumstances, the high serum sodium concentration will be reflected by an equally high sodium concentration in the urine, and the fractional excretion of sodium (FE_{Na}) will be greater than 2% (see formula). Conversely, in a child who has hypernatremia in the context of dehydration, the FE_{Na} would be less than 1% if the child has intact renal tubular function acting to preserve intravascular volume.[20,37] Salt poisoning must be distinguished from a renal concentration defect; a history of polyuria or polydipsia would be present in a central or nephrogenic cause of free water loss, such as in diabetes insipidus.

Fractional excretion of sodium (FE_{Na})

$$FE_{Na} = \frac{Urine\ Na \times Plasma_{creatinine}}{Plasma_{Na} \times Urine_{creatinine}} \times 100$$

Bicarbonate

The well-known mnemonic MUDPILES (methanol, uremia, diabetic ketoacidosis, paraldehyde, phenformin, isoniazid, iron, lactic acidosis, ethanol, ethylene glycol, and salicylates) is a useful first step in guiding the differential diagnosis of agents in poisoning cases complicated by elevated anion gap metabolic acidosis. The presence of a high anion gap metabolic acidosis in a putative case of poisoning may suggest CAP, along with corroborative clinical and laboratory findings. For example, a case report of deliberate poisoning of an infant by the administration of ground iron tablets noted that an unresolved metabolic acidosis was a red flag during a prolonged hospitalization and helped lead to an eventual diagnosis of CAP.[72]

Additional agents leading to an anion gap acidosis include CO, cyanide, caffeine, albuterol, toluene, and theophylline. If ethylene glycol is an agent of concern, the fluorescein in ethylene glycol–based antifreeze may be present in urine or gastric contents and cause them to glow when viewed with a Wood (ultraviolet) light. This effect depends on the length of time since ingestion, however, and its absence should not be used to rule out ethylene glycol consumption in cases where clinical suspicion exists. Inborn errors of metabolism, for example methylmalonic acidemia, in a symptomatic infant with an increased anion gap metabolic acidosis and hypoglycemia may mimic an ingestion.

Serum Osmolality

The osmotic properties of a liquid are a reflection of the ionic concentration of its dissolved substances per unit of solvent. For serum, osmolality is expressed in units per kilogram and typically is measured directly in the hospital chemistry laboratory. Serum osmolarity is expressed in units per liter of solvent and typically is calculated using the measured osmolar concentrations of normally present electrolytes such as sodium, blood urea nitrogen (BUN), and glucose. A serum osmolal gap may be detected by subtracting the calculated osmolarity from the actual measured osmolality (for the sake of this calculation, in common practice the values for osmolality and osmolarity are used interchangeably). The following formula is a reasonable estimate for calculated osmolarity.

This value is then subtracted from the measured serum osmolality, with caution taken to insist that the measurement be done by freezing point depression because volatiles, like alcohols, will be lost if the assay is done by vapor pressure method.

Osmolal gap = measured osmolality – calculated osmolarity (normal range 0–10)

A significantly increased osmolal gap usually reflects the presence of ethanol or non-ethanol toxic alcohols.

Blood Urea Nitrogen/Creatinine

These values may be used as an indicator of renal compromise following poisoning.

Focused Assessment Tools

Carboxyhemoglobin (HbCO)

Clinical symptoms of CO poisoning may not correlate with the HbCO level in the blood. In acute poisonings, when the patient's blood is tested soon after removal from exposure, symptoms typically begin at levels of 10% and most often accompany complaints of headache, vomiting, or syncope. As exposure increases, pediatric patients may become obtunded or deeply comatose. Postexposure neurologic sequelae are common in heavily exposed patients. There are 2 areas of limitations in this testing: chronic smokers (more likely in the adolescent population) may

---

Serum Osmolarity

Osmolarity (mOsm/L) = 2 x [Na mEq/L] + $\dfrac{[\text{Glucose mEq/L}]}{18}$ + $\dfrac{[\text{BUN mg/dL}]}{2.8}$

routinely have an HbCO level hovering around 10%, and fetal hemoglobin may also be read as an elevation of HbCO.[73] The direct myocardial toxicity of CO, compounded by the CO-induced systemic metabolic acidosis and diminished oxygen delivery, may cause myocardial ischemic injury even in children, who may manifest elevated serum markers such as creatine kinase-MB or troponin levels; however, consequential myocardial ischemia is rare in previously normal children.

Emetine Level

When surreptitious use of ipecac to induce emesis is suspected, a serum or urine emetine assay can be helpful if drawn early enough. Optimal collection time is within 3 hours of ingestion; the high volume of distribution yields almost no recovery of emetine after approximately 3 hours.[74] Chronic ingestion of ipecac has been reported to cause skeletal muscle weakness and cardiomyopathy.[75,76]

High-pressure liquid chromatography tandem mass spectrometry (LC/MS/MS) is currently believed to be the most reliable technique for detecting the emetine component of ipecac. Specimens submitted for emetine analysis must be collected and sent to the toxicology laboratory in an expedited manner; it is suggested that the laboratory be consulted for specific details on adequate volume, any required special collection/handling instructions, and the proper use of standard chain of custody procedures.

C-Peptide and Insulin Level

Factitious hypoglycemia orchestrated by exogenous administration of insulin may be detected by concomitant testing of serum insulin and serum C-peptide levels. C-peptide is a subunit of insulin cleaved from insulin in its conversion from proinsulin in pancreatic islet cells. If the insulin level is high but C-peptide is low, one may deduce that the insulin detected was not synthesized by the patient's pancreas but came from an external source, either by self-injection or injection by another person. These measurements are only interpretable under the circumstances of a blood sample drawn at the time of the hypoglycemic episode. C-peptide levels obtained after intravenous glucose therapy has been initiated and glucose homeostasis restored may be clouded by the increased insulin-production activity of the patient's own intact pancreas in response to one or more glucose boluses and, therefore, would not have diagnostic utility.

Oral Hypoglycemic Panel

Serum assays are available for measuring the presence of all drugs in the sulfonylurea class, as well as some meglitinides. The availability of these measures will vary across laboratory facilities; however, reference laboratories for "send out" analysis are available.

Toxicology Screens for Drugs of Abuse

Most hospitals use immunoassay testing in rapid screening for commonly abused illicit drugs and intentionally overdosed psychoactive medications. Such screens typically are limited to detecting barbiturates, benzodiazepines, and tricyclic antidepressants in blood, and amphetamines, barbiturates, benzodiazepines, cocaine metabolites, cannabinoids, and opiates in urine. Some hospitals also may include phencyclidine in their rapid urine drug screens (UDS). Drugs such as LSD, ketamine, and the so-called date rape drugs γ-hydroxybutyrate (GHB) and flunitrazepam (Rohypnol) are abused but are not consistently included in routine urine assays and, therefore, must be specifically ordered. Separate quantitative blood testing is usually done for alcohol, acetaminophen, and salicylates. Pediatricians should be familiar with what is included in their hospital's toxicology panels.

Important in some drug classes is that a common metabolite is detectable, rather than the parent drug. In the case of the benzodiazepines (BZPs), the metabolite is oxazepam; neither lorazepam (Ativan) nor alprazolam (Xanax), among other recent generation BZPs, yield oxazepam with their metabolism, so a false-negative would be the outcome of a UDS of those drugs. Similar caveats exist for amphetamines; 3,4-methylenedioxy-N-methylamphetamine ("Ecstasy") and paramethoxyamphetamine (street name "Death") may be missed. The same is true for synthetic opioids, such as oxycodone, hydrocodone, methadone, and fentanyl, as well as synthetic "designer drugs" like fentanyl/sufentanil, none of which are usually assayed for in a "routine" UDS.[73,77] None of these substances, as well as a number of other commonly encountered drugs such as clonidine

and a variety of toxins causing significant alteration of mental status and/or cardiovascular function, are detected on routine drug screens. Some of the more important of these compounds are highlighted in Box 17.2.

Many hospitals also offer a more comprehensive qualitative toxicology panel (Box 17.3). In such comprehensive drug panels, typically a substantially larger volume of urine is required for an adequate analysis. As with the limited screen, the breadth of such testing may vary, and the sensitivity for detection varies across substances and testing methods. Blood specimens may also be necessary for quantitative measurements. It is helpful to confer with a toxicologist and/or the laboratory medical staff regarding the patient's clinical presentation and likely drugs of interest before sending the body fluid sample.

Focused Quantitative Drug Assays

Several medications, particularly psychotropics, anticonvulsants, lithium, theophylline, caffeine, digoxin, lidocaine, and aspirin, manifest serum levels that may be routinely followed for therapeutic management. In addition, toxic alcohols methanol and ethylene glycol can be measured in blood but must be specifically requested. In many cases of deliberate poisoning or intentional misuse of a pharmacologic agent, the mere presence of the medication in the child's blood may be sufficient for the diagnosis of abuse, regardless of the absolute blood level. In situations where a medication had initially been prescribed appropriately, but the child's caretaker is suspected of intentionally overdosing the child, a quantitative blood drug level is essential. When obtaining blood samples for quantitative levels in suspected intentional poisoning cases, it always is prudent to obtain an extra aliquot consisting of blood at least twice the amount required by the laboratory for analysis. The same is true for a UDS. Saved urine and blood must be stored at the temperature required as instructed by the reference laboratory and kept in a secure location. The clinician ordering specific serum drug levels in suspected CAP should understand the turnaround time for the assay; order analysis "stat"; expedite the collection and, if it is a "send out," expedite transport of the sample by same-day or overnight mail to the reference laboratory; and maintain a proactive system for following up on reports. In the case of a suspected deliberate poisoning, discharging the child to an uncontrolled, unprotected environment before drug assay reports have been received can result in a disastrous outcome.

BOX 17.3
Representative "Comprehensive" Urine Drug Panel[a]

Acetaminophen	Glutethimide
Acetone	Isopropranolol
Amobarbital	Methanol
Butabarbital	Nordiazepam
Butalbital	Pentobarbital
Carbamazepine	Phenobarbital
Chlordiazepoxide	Phenytoin
Diazepam	Quinidine
Ethanol	Salicylates
Ethchlorvynol	Secobarbital

[a]These urine toxicology screens are qualitative tests that report detection of the presence of a given drug. Many factors can influence the detection of a substance of concern in a particular specimen: dose, half-life, cross-reactive agents, and time of sample acquisition. *This list varies among laboratories.*

Fecal Analysis

Chronic diarrhea may be caused by repetitive, covert administration of laxatives and enemas. In such cases, fecal sample measurements of both osmolality and electrolytes may prove useful. The estimated osmolality of intestinal contents is 290 mOsm/kg, reaching plasma osmolality in a normal patient as the gut contents move past the jejunum, after which the rate of intestinal salt absorption decreases. If poorly absorbable substances are ingested, such as cathartic agents that work by generating an increased osmotic gradient, fecal salt concentrations will be decreased due to the osmotic space that is occupied by the ingested agent.

Fecal Osmolality Gap = Measured fecal osmolality – Calculated fecal osmolality; Calculated fecal osmolality = 2 [fecal Na] (in mEq/L) + 2 [fecal K] (in mEq/L)

Sodium and potassium are the primary ions found in fecal water. Once they are subtracted from the stool osmolality as noted in the formula above, the difference is equal to the fecal osmotic gap. A low gap (<50 mOsm/kg) implies that the stool electrolytes (sodium, potassium, bicarbonate, and chloride) are the major contributors to the fecal osmolality. If the osmotic gap is elevated (>100 mOsm/kg), one may conclude that a poorly absorbable, unmeasured substance is responsible for the increased gap.[78] In cases of intentional laxative administration, the unmeasured ion is typically magnesium; Epsom salts, milk of magnesia, and magnesium citrate are commonly used laxatives containing magnesium.

Electrocardiogram

Characteristic dysrhythmias are caused by a variety of medications and toxins, including tricyclic antidepressants and several other psychotropic medications; digoxin, beta-blockers, and calcium channel blockers; cocaine; and the amphetamines. Tricyclic antidepressants and many antipsychotics may cause sinus tachycardia, but QRS and Q-T interval prolongation are harbingers of potential serious ventricular dysrhythmias. Digoxin may cause a wide variety of arrhythmias due to increased automaticity and decreased conduction; atrial tachycardias (narrow QRS) or junctional tachycardias with atrioventricular (AV) block are the classic findings. Toxic levels of clonidine may cause sinoatrial or atrioventricular bradycardia. Beta-blockers and calcium channel blockers typically demonstrate a sinus bradycardia and AV block of varying degrees. Of these 2 antihypertensive medications, beta-blockers may be associated with hypoglycemia, while calcium channel blockers are more typically associated with hyperglycemia, although severe intoxications may be hard to distinguish. Exposure to a toxic dose or chronic ingestion of ipecac (the metabolite of which is emetine) may show T-wave inversion in all electrocardiogram leads and prolongation of the Q-T interval.

Radiology

Radiographic imaging may detect iron (ferrous sulfate) and enteric-coated tablets in a child's GI tract. Radiopaque foreign bodies the child ingests, aspirates, or is forced to consume may be visualized in the GI or respiratory tract. However, a negative x-ray alone cannot rule out ingestion or aspiration of non-radiopaque substances. A skeletal survey might be considered in a nonverbal or preverbal poisoned child as an effective screening tool for other forms of abusive injury when coupled with a thorough history and physical examination.[79] However, a skeletal survey does not take the place of a comprehensive physical examination of the entire body surface area of the patient in search of external signs of inflicted injuries. All children 2 years old and younger suspected of being a victim of abuse of any type warrant a skeletal survey. As mentioned earlier, signs of CNS dysfunction necessitate a simultaneous evaluation for multiple etiologies including poisoning, trauma, and infection.

Management and Outcome

Overall, intentionally injured children have been found to have more severe injuries, longer intensive care unit and hospital stays, and a greater number of specialty consultations than their inpatient counterparts with unintentional injury. In addition, their injuries are more likely to be fatal.[80] Pediatric poisoning victims also follow this pattern. Furthermore, long-term sequelae, not only physical but emotional, and the child's future safety must be considered once the medical crisis has resolved.

The scant literature that addresses the outcome for pediatric poisoning victims dwells mainly on those children who were victims of poisoning in the more complicated context of MBP, and details the inner confusion of these children as well as the frequent occurrence of social dysfunction and behavior disorders.[81,82]

British and Irish researchers attempted to follow long-term outcomes in pediatric survivors of deliberate poisoning. Twenty-five percent of the study group continued to demonstrate morbidity in the form of behavior problems, physical problems, or disabilities. Children who demonstrated direct harm were less likely to have returned to their homes, and younger children in particular were more likely to be protected by removal from the home environment. Of the children who were allowed to return home, none experienced re-abuse for the duration of the study; however, in 40% of those families, the siblings of the poisoned child were likely to have suffered abuse, some fatal.[83] The authors recommend caution in returning children to their homes, along with ongoing vigilant medical surveillance.[83]

Conclusion

The timely recognition and treatment of CAP requires a high level of suspicion; "that which is not sought is not found." Clinical acumen in this context will be enhanced by a thorough knowledge of nondeliberate childhood poisoning patterns and recognition of those clinical features suggestive of CAP. The toxicological mechanisms of commonly encountered poisonous substances should be understood. Then the prepared clinician, with a thorough history and physical examination, can thoughtfully guide the laboratory and environmental evaluation of the pediatric patient who presents with the typical patterns of CAP.

References

1. Kempe CH, Silverman FN, Steele BF, Droegemueller W, Silver HK. The battered-child syndrome. *JAMA.* 1962;181:17–24

2. Meadow R. Munchausen syndrome by proxy. The hinterland of child abuse. *Lancet.* 1977;2:343–345

3. Rogers D, Tripp J, Bentovin A, et al. Non-accidental poisoning: an extended syndrome of abuse. *Br Med J.* 1976;1:793–796

4. Henretig F. The deliberately poisoned child. In: Levin A, Sheridan MS, eds. *Munchausen's Syndrome by Proxy: Issues in Diagnosis and Treatment.* New York, NY: Lexington Books; 1995

5. Lorber J. Unexplained episodes of coma in a two-year-old. *Lancet.* 1978;2:472–473

6. Lorber J, Reckless JP, Watson JB. Nonaccidental poisoning: the elusive diagnosis. *Arch Dis Child.* 1980;55:643–647

7. Shnaps Y, Frand M, Rotem Y, Tirosh M. The chemically abused child. *Pediatrics.* 1981;68:119–121

8. Dine MS, McGovern ME. Intentional poisoning of children—an overlooked category of child abuse: report of seven cases and review of the literature. *Pediatrics.* 1982;70:32–35

9. Tenenbein M. Pediatric toxicology: current controversies and recent advances. *Curr Probl Pediatr.* 1986;16:185–233

10. Bays J, Feldman KW. Child abuse by poisoning. In: Reece RM, Ludwig S, eds. *Child Abuse: Medical Diagnosis and Treatment.* Philadelphia, PA: Lippincott Williams & Wilkins; 2001:405–441

11. Berry DJ, Grove J. Emergency toxicological screening for drugs commonly taken in overdose. *J Chromatogr.* 1973;80:205–220

12. Rosenberg DA. Web of deceit: a literature review of Munchausen syndrome by proxy. *Child Abuse Negl.* 1987;11:547–563

13. Welch MJ, Correa GA. PCP intoxication in young children and infants. *Clin Pediatr (Phila).* 1980;19:510–514

14. Beno S, Calello D, Baluffi A, Henretig FM. Pediatric body packing: drug smuggling reaches a new low. *Pediatr Emerg Care.* 2005;21:744–746

15. Traub S, Hoffman RS, Neelson LS. Pediatric "body packing." *Arch Pediatr Adolesc Med.* 2004;57:174–177

16. Ayoub CC, Alexander R. Definitional issues in Munchausen by proxy. *APSAC Advisor.* 1998;11:7–10

17. Ayoub CC, Alexander R, Beck D, et al. Position paper: definitional issues in Munchausen by proxy. *Child Maltreat.* 2002;7:105–111

18. Fischler RS. Poisoning: a syndrome of child abuse. *Am Fam Physician.* 1983;28:103–108

19. Lai MW, Klein-Schwartz W, Rodgers GC, et al. 2005 annual report of the American Association of Poison Control Centers' national poisoning and exposure database. *Clin Toxicol (Phila).* 2006;44:803–932

20. Meadow R. ABC of child abuse. Poisoning. *BMJ.* 1989;298:1445–1446

21. Eddleston M. Patterns and problems of deliberate self-poisoning in the developing world. *QJM.* 2000;93:715–731

22. Shannon M. Ingestion of toxic substances by children. *N Engl J Med.* 2000;342:186–191

23. Litovitz TL, Klein-Schwartz W, White S, et al. 2000 annual report of the American Association of Poison Control Centers Toxic Exposure Surveillance System. *Am J Emerg Med.* 2001;19:337–395

24. Bauman WA, Yalow RS. Child abuse: parenteral insulin administration. *J Pediatr.* 1981;99:588–591

25. Meadow R. Munchausen syndrome by proxy. *Arch Dis Child.* 1982;57:92–98

26. Paschall RT. The chemically abused child. In: Giardino AP, ed. *Child Maltreatment.* Vol. 1. 2nd ed. St Louis, MO: GW Medical Publishing; 2005

27. Garrettson LK, Bush JP, Gates RS, French AL. Physical change, time of day, and child characteristics as factors in poison injury. *Vet Hum Toxicol.* 1990;32:139–141

28. Riordan M, Rylance G, Berry K. Poisoning in children 3: common medicines. *Arch Dis Child.* 2002;87:400–402

29. Russell AB, Hardin JW, Grand L, Fraser A. *Poisonous Plants of North Carolina.* Russell AB, ed. Raleigh, NC: North Carolina State University; 1997

30. Riordan M, Rylance G, Berry K. Poisoning in children 4: household products, plants, and mushrooms. *Arch Dis Child.* 2002;87:403–406

31. USDA, NRCS. 2007. The PLANTS Database. http://plants.usda.gov. Accessed September 2007

32. McGuigan ME. Poisoning potpourri. *Pediatr Rev.* 2001;22:295–302

33. Friedman EM. Caustic ingestions and foreign body aspirations: an overlooked form of child abuse. *Ann Otol Rhinol Laryngol.* 1987;96:709–712

34. Barnett PL. Centipede ingestion by a six-month-old infant: toxic side effects. *Pediatr Emerg Care.* 1991;7:229–230

35. Wiseman HM, Guest K, Murray VS, Volans GN. Accidental poisoning in childhood: a multicentre survey. 2. The role of packaging in accidents involving medications. *Hum Toxicol.* 1987;6:303–314

36. Yamamoto LG, Wiebe RA, Matthews WJ Jr. Toxic exposures and ingestions in Honolulu: I. A prospective pediatric ED cohort; II. A prospective poison center cohort. *Pediatr Emerg Care.* 1991;7:141–148

37. Coulthard MG, Haycock GB. Distinguishing between salt poisoning and hypernatraemic dehydration in children. *BMJ.* 2003;326:157–160

38. Litovitz TL, Flagler SL, Manoguerra AS, Veltri JC, Wright L. Recurrent poisonings among paediatric poisoning victims. *Med Toxicol Adverse Drug Exp.* 1989;4:381–386

39. Osterhoudt K, Ewald MB, Shannon M, Henretig FM. Toxicologic emergencies. In: Fleisher GR, Ludwig S, Henretig FM, eds. *Textbook of Pediatric Emergency Medicine*. 5th ed. Philadelphia. PA: Lippincott, Williams & Wilkins; 2006:951–1007

40. Yilmaz HL, Yildizdas, DR. Amitraz poisoning, an emerging problem: epidemiology, clinical features, management, and preventive strategies. *Arch Dis Child*. 2003;88:130–134

41. Bonkowsky JL, Sarco D, Pomeroy SL. Ataxia and shaking in a 2-year-old girl: acute marijuana intoxication presenting as seizure. *Pediatr Emerg Care*. 2005;21:527–528

42. Goebel J, Gremse DA, Artman M. Cardiomyopathy from ipecac administration in Munchausen syndrome by proxy. *Pediatrics*. 1993;92:601–603

43. Lacey SR, Cooper C, Runyan DK, Azizkhan RG. Munchausen syndrome by proxy: patterns of presentation to pediatric surgeons. *J Pediatr Surg*. 1993;28:827–832

44. Sutphen JL, Saulsbury FT. Intentional ipecac poisoning: Munchausen syndrome by proxy. *Pediatrics*. 1988;82:453–456

45. Weinberg D, Lande A, Hilton N, Kerns DL. Intoxication from accidental marijuana ingestion. *Pediatrics*. 1983;71:848–850

46. McClung HJ, Murray R, Braden NJ, Fyda J, Myers RP, Gutches L. Intentional ipecac poisoning in children. *Am J Dis Child*. 1988;142:637–639

47. Fenton AC, Wailoo MP, Tanner MS. Severe failure to thrive and diarrhoea caused by laxative abuse. *Arch Dis Child*. 1988;63:978–979

48. Hickson GB, Altemeier WA, Martin ED, Campbell PW. Parental administration of chemical agents: a cause of apparent life-threatening events. *Pediatrics*. 1989;83:772–776

49. Meadow R. Munchausen syndrome by proxy abuse perpetrated by men. *Arch Dis Child*. 1998;78:210–216

50. Tominack RL, Spyker DA. Capsicum and capsaicin—a review: case report of the use of hot peppers in child abuse. *J Toxicol Clin Toxicol*. 1987;25:591–601

51. Adelson L. Homicidal poisoning. A dying modality of lethal violence? *Am J Forensic Med Pathol*. 1987;8:245–251

52. Desprez PH, Vandourn G, Burquin C, et al. Privation d'eau: une forme inhabituelle de maltraitance. *Arch Francaises Pediatr*. 1990;47:287–289

53. Dockery WK. Fatal intentional salt poisoning associated with a radiopaque mass. *Pediatrics*. 1992;89:964–965

54. Tilelli JA, Ophoven JP. Hyponatremic seizures as a presenting symptom of child abuse. *Forensic Sci Int*. 1986;30:213–217

55. Keating JP, Schears GJ, Dodge PR. Oral water intoxication in infants. An American epidemic. *Am J Dis Child*. 1991;145:985–990

56. Chan DA, Salcedo JR, Atkins DM, Ruley EJ. Munchausen syndrome by proxy: a review and case study. *J Pediatr Psychol*. 1986;11:71–80

57. Verity CM, Winckworth C, Burman D, Stevens D, White RJ. Polle syndrome: children of Munchausen. *Br Med J*. 1979;2:422–423

58. Cohle SD, Trestrail JD, Graham MA, Oxley DW, Walp B, Jachimczyk J. Fatal pepper aspiration. *Am J Dis Child*. 1988;142:633–636

59. Mehl AL, Coble L, Johnson S. Munchausen syndrome by proxy: a family affair. *Child Abuse Negl*. 1990;14:577–585

60. Zitelli BJ, Seltman MF, Shannon RM. Munchausen's syndrome by proxy and its professional participants. *Am J Dis Child*. 1987;141:1099–1102

61. Pickering D, Ellis H. Neonatal hypoglycaemia due to salicylate poisoning. *Proc R Soc Med*. 1968;61:1256

62. Woolf AD, Wynshaw-Boris A, Rinaldo P, Levy HL. Intentional infantile ethylene glycol poisoning presenting as an inherited metabolic disorder. *J Pediatr*. 1992;120:421–424

63. Hvizdala EV, Gellady AM. Intentional poisoning of two siblings by prescription drugs. An unusual form of child abuse. *Clin Pediatr (Phila).* 1978;17:480–482

64. White ST, Voter K, Perry J. Surreptitious warfarin ingestion. *Child Abuse Negl.* 1985;9:349–352

65. Taylor D, Bentovim A. Recurrent nonaccidentally inflicted chemical eye injuries to siblings. *J Pediatr Ophthalmol.* 1976;13:238–242

66. Saulsbury FT, Chobanian MC, Wilson WG. Child abuse: parenteral hydrocarbon administration. *Pediatrics.* 1984;73:719–722

67. Shaywitz BA, Siegel NJ, Pearson HA. Megavitamins for minimal brain dysfunction: a potentially dangerous therapy. *JAMA.* 1977;238:1749

68. Hill RM, Barer J, Hill LL, Butler CM, Harvey DJ, Horning MG. An investiga-tion of recurrent pine oil poisoning in an infant by the use of gas chromatographic-mass spectrometric methods. *J Pediatr.* 1975;87:115–118

69. Alexander R, Smith W, Stevenson R. Serial Munchausen syndrome by proxy. *Pediatrics.* 1990;86:581–585

70. Morrow PL. Caffeine toxicity: a case of child abuse by drug ingestion. *J Forensic Sci.* 1987;32:1801–1805

71. Rivenes SM, Bakerman PR, Miller MB. Intentional caffeine poisoning in an infant. *Pediatrics.* 1997;99:736–738

72. Black J, Zenel J. Child abuse by intentional iron poisoning presenting as shock and persistent acidosis. *Pediatrics.* 2003;111:197–199

73. Hoffman RJ, Nelson L. Rational use of toxicology testing in children. *Curr Opin Pediatr.* 2001;13:183–188

74. Scharman EJ, Hutzler JM, Rosencrance JG, Tracy TS. Single dose pharmacokinet-ics of syrup of ipecac. *Ther Drug Monit.* 2000;22:566–573

75. Schneider D, Perez A, Knilamus TE, Daniels SR, Bove KE, Bonnell H. Clinical and pathological aspects of cardiomyopa-thy from ipecac administration in Munchausen's syndrome by proxy. *Pediatrics.* 1996;97:902–906

76. Rashid N. Medically unexplained myopathy due to ipecac abuse. *Psychosomatics.* 2006;47:167–169

77. Maxwell JC. Party drugs: properties, prevalence, patterns, and problems. *Subst Use Misuse.* 2005;40:1203–1240

78. Schiller LR. Chronic diarrhea. In: McNally PR, ed. *GI/Liver Secrets.* 2nd ed. Philadelphia, PA: Hanley and Belfus; 2002

79. American Academy of Pediatrics Section on Radiology. Diagnostic imaging of child abuse. *Pediatrics.* 2000;105:1345–1348

80. Wright MS, Litaker D. Childhood victims of violence: hospital utilization by children with intentional injuries. *Arch Pediatr and Adolesc Med.* 1996;150:415–420

81. Mcguire T, Feldman KW. Psychologic morbidity of children subjected to Munchausen syndrome by proxy. *Pediatrics.* 1989;83:289–292

82. Bools C, Neale BA, Meadow SR. Follow up of victims of fabricated illness (Munchausen syndrome by proxy). *Arch Dis Child.* 1993;69:625–630

83. Davis P, McClure RJ, Rolfe K, et al. Procedures, placement, and risks of further abuse after Munchausen syn-drome by proxy, non-accidental poison-ing, and non-accidental suffocation. *Arch Dis Child.* 1998;78:217–221

Chapter 18

Immersion Injury in Child Abuse and Neglect

Kenneth W. Feldman

University of Washington School of Medicine
Child Protection Team, Children's Hospital and Regional Medical Center

Drowning is the second leading cause of death from unintentional injury in children 1 to 14 years of age and is the fifth leading cause of death in children younger than 1 year,[1] causing 17.1% and 7.5% of deaths, respectively. Overall childhood drowning mortality rates are 1.75 per 100,000, but rates for 0- to 4-year-old children are highest at 3.4 per 100,000. Ninety-eight percent of drowning deaths were classified as unintentional, 1.6% homicidal, and 2.1% undetermined. Seventy-seven percent of the drownings classified as homicides occur in the 0- to 4-year-old group (0.08 homicidal drowning deaths per 100,000). Despite these statistics, drowning has received little attention in the child abuse literature.

Early case series of abused children lack reference to drowning as a result of child abuse or neglect.[2-6] However, Adelson's[7] 1961 description of 46 child homicides included 10 cases of abuse and 3 of neglect. Five children in the entire series died of drowning, including 4 who were immersed in a bathtub. It is unclear how many of the drownings fit the child abuse pattern. Subsequent studies of child homicide[8-11] and series of childhood drownings[12,13] have begun to reveal instances of inflicted immersion injury. Abuse and neglect should be considered in a variety of drownings. Events felt to be unintentional immersions may be found to have historical or physical evidence of intentional injury. With intentional drowning, physical injuries are likely to be subtle, while the history may be vague, inconsistent, or behaviorally and developmentally implausible. Abuse also should be considered when children present to care with a specious history of submersion injury, but have physical findings suggestive of other types of inflicted injury. The opposite situation is encountered when children are brought to care in extremis without a history of drowning, but with clinical or pathologic evidence of immersion. Although neonatacide has been relatively neglected in the child abuse literature, drowning is often the mode of death in these events. Judgments also must be made whether child supervision leading to unintentional submersion is beneath community standards, meeting definitions of child neglect.

Epidemiology of Childhood Drowning

Drowning rates vary widely based on climate, culture, and environmental hazards. Pearn and Nixon[14] observed freshwater immersion and drowning death rates, respectively, of 10.43 and 5.17 per 100,000 in children younger than 16 years in a total population study of Brisbane, Australia, from 1971 to 1975. The immersion rate for toddlers reached 50.01 per 100,000, and 45% of those children died. Sixty percent of the drownings were in pools, whereas 23% involved other bodies of water and 17% involved bathtubs. Hawaii had a lower immersion rate of 3.1 per 100,000 children from 1973 to 1977, but the ready access to saltwater recreation led to 41% of the incidents occurring in saltwater.[15] In King County Washington, the annual incidence and mortality rates over a 10-year period were 5.5 and 2.6 per 100,000 children.[13] Rates were highest at 12.8 in preschoolers, with 43% of immersion victims younger than 5 years. The region has many bodies of cold natural water (50% of immersions) and a moderate presence of public and private, unguarded pools (33% of immersions). Twelve percent of drownings occurred in the family bathtub. However, in contrast to the incidence throughout childhood, 24% of immersions of children younger than 5 years occurred in the bath. In spite of abundant saltwater, few (2%) instances of saltwater immersion were noted, likely because Washington State's saltwater is

cold enough to discourage swimming. In the British Isles, immersion (1.5/100,000) and immersion death rates (0.7/100,000) were lower, but a greater percentage of victims were younger than 5 years (68%).[16] In a study of drowning and near drowning in the United States, garden pools (19%) were found to pose a hazard nearly equal to that of natural bodies of water (20%), but still less than pools intended for swimming (27%). Bathtub immersion deaths accounted for 14% of all immersions, and 68% of the victims were younger than 5 years of age. In California, Arizona, and Florida, drowning was reported as the leading cause of unintentional injury death in children younger than 5 years.[17] Florida has among the highest drowning rates in the world (93/100,000 children <12 years).[18] Although private swimming pools were the single leading site of immersion in Florida, the canals, ponds, and lakes built to drain low and marshy land were the sites of 41% of immersions. Swimming pool drowning in preschoolers follows an inverse socioeconomic status incidence pattern than most childhood injuries. Because access to private pools is greater in higher income families, their rate of drowning is also increased.[14,17] Bathtub drownings comprised 9% of the fatal immersions in the United States during 1995.[19] However, 55% to 64% of infant drownings occurred in the bathtub.[19,20] Seventy-eight percent of all infant drownings occurred in the home.[19] Sixteen percent of those infants drowned in buckets. Eighty-four percent of drownings in children aged 1 to 4 years were in artificial pools or bodies of freshwater.

Intentional Submersions

In 1977 Pearn and Nixon were the first to report intentional drowning as a pattern of child abuse.[12,21–23] Three bathtub submersion cases were described. Abuse was recognized in 2 drownings: one attributed to maternal confession and one to a previous abuse report from neighbors. In one case the child sustained a subsequent compound skull fracture while also in the father's care. They note that the usual unintentional bathtub immersion involves a child between age 9 and 15 months, accompanied only by another young child in the bath or unaccompanied. Lower socioeconomic status families with several children were most often involved in such submersions. Pearn and Nixon[14] hypothesized that bathtub submersions in older children were more often inflicted. Subsequent authors have noted a high frequency of epilepsy as a cause of submersions in older children.[13,24,25] Kemp et al[26] also suggest that bathtub drownings of children outside the ages of 8 to 24 months are more concerning for abuse. Neither Pearn and Nixon nor Kemp et al emphasized that immersion injuries of infants younger than 8 to 9 months are more likely to be inflicted. Few reports of accidental or inflicted bathtub submersions of younger infants can be found. However, it seems intuitive that parents are unlikely to leave unsupervised infants who are unable to sit unassisted in the tub. In recent years, the use of bathtub seats may have provided parents with a false sense of security for their very young infants in bathtubs. The caretaker's overestimation of an older infant's ability to sit safely and of preschool peers to supervise a child is what leads to unintentional submersion. Jensen[27] found all but 1 of the 33 injuries due to submersions of all causes in infants younger than 1 year to have occurred between 6 and 11 months. Further, all but one of the fatal bathtub submersions occurred in children younger than 2 years who were bathing with another child aged 10 months to 7 years, without direct adult supervision. The final victim was 47 months old, but had a known seizure disorder and was bathing unsupervised with his twin sibling. Fifty-nine percent of the nonfatal bathtub submersion victims were both younger than 2 years and bathing with another child, but not directly supervised by an adult. In Lavelle et al's[28] review, the youngest child to sustain a bathtub injury due to abuse or severe neglect was 4 months old. Twenty-eight percent of immersions occurred while the victim was bathing with a child who was younger than 4 years. Seventy-five percent of the victims were younger than 2 years. One drowning victim among 12 child homicides reported by Hodge and Ludwig[10] was 3 months old. They did not specify whether that child drowned in the bathtub, but another child died of a beating that preceded his being placed in the bathtub. Quan et al's[13] 3 abuse or neglect submersions involved children younger than 5 years who were in the bathtub. Gillenwater et al[29] found 8% of childhood drownings to have resulted from abuse. Five of the reported 16 inflicted immersions involved infants and the remainder children younger than 4 years. However, the specific ages were not noted. Review of Gillenwater et al's original data for inflicted bathtub immersions indicates that one victim was a newborn, 2 were 4 months old, and one each were 2½, 3, and 3¼ years old. Only 3 of all 9 victims of inflicted bathtub drownings were in the typical 8- to 24-month age range of unintentional bathtub victims. They observed the victim to often be the youngest child of a large sibship. The 75% mortality for inflicted immersions was twice (38%) that of unintentional immersions, possibly due to lack of or nonstandard resuscitation.[29] As opposed to Nixon and Pearn,[21] the socioeconomic status of their families of children with inflicted immersions did not differ from that of unintentional submersion victims.[29] Fatal and nonfatal hospitalized bathtub immersion rates in California for 1996 through 1998 were 13 per 100,000 for infants 6 to 12 months of age.[20] Yet, 4 per 100,000 infants younger than 6 months, an age range when few infants can sit unassisted, also sustained bathtub immersions. In children aged 1 to 1¼ years and 1¼ to 1½ years, there were 4 and 5 per 100,000 immersions, respectively. Bathtub immersions were rare in children older than 1½ years. In all, 180 bathtub immersions were reported.

Case: A 3-year-old, who was being cared for by his 15-year-old sibling soiled his clothes. The sibling ran a bath, undressed the child, and put him in the bathtub. On returning from a phone call, the child's mother found him submerged in 3 inches of water. Medics could not revive him.

Feces were found in the bathtub, on the toilet, and on the floor. The bathtub water was very cold. Legal investigation revealed that the child had been suffocated prior to immersion.

In a recently published office study, 1 of 11 ten-month-old infants and 36 of 121 ten- to 18-month-old infants were observed to climb into a 14-inch (35.5 cm) high bathtub unassisted.[30] About half entered feetfirst and half headfirst. Thus reports that older infants or toddlers climbed into drawn bathtubs of water and drowned should be considered to be potentially developmentally plausible. Judgment about abuse in these cases should depend on additional evidence and the child's specific developmental history.

Kemp et al[26] described 2 infants younger than 2 months who slipped from their parent's arms during a bath and were briefly immersed without injury. This outcome for unintentional submersion is reassuring when compared with the cumulative 52% mortality for inflicted immersions (Table 18.1). Five of 187 drowning cases in Cuyahoga County, OH, in children and adolescents older than 10 years were judged homicidal.[31] Two of the victims had negative results for alcohol and drugs of abuse, while older accidental and suicidal drowning victims commonly had positive tests for alcohol or illicit drugs. The county's homicidal child deaths occurred in infants, 2 of whom drowned in the bathtub and 1 in a toilet.

Inflicted bathtub immersions can be difficult to recognize due to the lack of associated injuries.[7,21] Diagnosis most

TABLE 18.1
Bathtub Submersion Case Series and Child Abuse

Author	Study Years	Bathtub Immersions	Due to Abuse	Fatalities
		(N)	(N)	(N)
Pearn and Nixon (22)	1973–1977	7	1	0
Quan et al (13)	1974–1983	16	3	–
Devos et al (47)	1934–1983	12	1	1
(9 due to carbon monoxide poison)				
Kemp et al (26)	1988–1989	44	10	6
Lavelle et al (28)	1982–1992	21	6	–
Schmidt and Madea (66)	1980–1993	12	2	2
Gillenwater et al (29)	1983–1991	34	9	3
(56% of 16 inflicted submersions were in the bathtub)				
Total		146	32 (22%)	12 (52%)[a]

[a]Denominator only includes studies reporting number of fatalities associated with abuse.

often depends on discrepancies in the history, caretaker confessions, or concerns expressed by others. Bowel or toilet training accidents may trigger the event.[12] Only one of Kemp et al's[26] 10 cases had associated injuries of abuse at the time of the immersion. A second child subsequently sustained inflicted trauma. Lavelle et al[28] believed 6 bathtub immersion victims to have been abused. However, they did not state how often individual children had associated injuries. Two children had inflicted bruise patterns, 2 had fractures, and 1 had retinal bleeding. However, in the combined group of children diagnosed with either abuse or severe neglect, physical findings of abuse and/or severe neglect were found in 38% of the children, and one-quarter had prior child protective services (CPS) involvement. One of their case descriptions also included abusive physical findings. Gillenwater et al[29]

found physical evidence consistent with or suspicious for abuse in 14 of 16 inflicted immersion victims. Although they did not specify in the original article, review of the data showed 8 of the 9 bathtub immersion victims had physical evidence of abuse, as did both summaries of bathtub cases in the report. Ten of the 16 inflicted immersions of all types had histories inconsistent with the event; 4 a previous history of abuse; 3 an admission or eyewitness report; and 1 a positive radiologic finding of abuse.

Case: A mother's stories varied as to whether her 14-month-old had been alone or with a 2- year-old sibling in a bathtub or whether both had last been seen outside the bathtub. She found the infant submerged in the bathtub and sought aid from a neighbor. At the hospital, resuscitation was unsuccessful. Bilateral retinal hemorrhages, a left frontal ecchymosis with accompanying subgaleal bleeding, and 2 areas of occipital ecchymoses were present. Forearm, upper thigh, and buttock bruises were noted. Both palms had healing linear burn scars attributed to touching an oven. A healing clavicle fracture, without accompanying history, was found on skeletal radiography.[29]

The 3 inflicted bathtub immersion victims described by Greist and Zumwalt[32] had additional physical evidence of abuse, including bruising and scars. Perrot and Nawojczyk[33] found 8 of 170 victims of apparent sudden infant death syndrome to have died of unnatural death. One death occurred when a 4-month-old child's mother "blacked out" after placing the baby supine on a towel in a bathtub containing 2 to 3 inches of water. When the mother revived, she found the infant prone and apneic with its nose submerged. At autopsy a parietal hematoma and free intraperitoneal air were attributed to attempts to remove the child from the bathtub and revive her. In spite of these injuries, the authors declared the death as due to accidental immersion.

Brewster et al[8] found that 7% of the homicides of United States Air Force–dependent children between 1 day and 1 year old occurred by drowning. One of 12 child homicides seen at a Philadelphia emergency department during the early 1980s was due to drowning.[10] One additional child was brought with a history of drowning, but died of inflicted head injury, unaccompanied by evidence of drowning. In a death review study of 384 children from birth to 5 years old in Missouri from 1983 to 1986, the authors concluded retrospectively that 121 had definitely been abused, 25 probably abused, and 109 possibly maltreated.[9] Fewer than half of the definitely abused children had been previously recognized or recorded as inflicted injury victims in formal databases. Five of the probable and 16 of the possible maltreatment deaths (total 21/134, 16%) were due to drowning. The rate of drowning in the definitely abused group of children was not specified.

Other bodies of water than the bathtub have been involved in inflicted immersions. Adelson[7] observed one homicidal drowning to have been in a brook. One of Greist and Zumwalt's[32] homicidal drownings occurred in a natural hot spring. Another live-born newborn was delivered and drowned in a toilet. The final non-bathtub victim was held prone with her mouth open and was asphyxiated by water poured into her mouth. Five of the inflicted submersions reported by Gillenwater et al[29] occurred in natural bodies of water, one in a swimming pool and one in a toilet. This case was judged probably inflicted due to being developmentally unlikely.

> **Case:** The mother surmised that her 8-month-old child had climbed out of her infant walker and tipped headfirst into the toilet. The infant was found wedged, head down, in the toilet and was apneic; the toilet seat was down. She survived 3 days after rescue. Autopsy was negative for trauma except for a knee contusion and tongue tip abrasion.[29]

Resnick[34] reported in his literature review of filicide that the mode of death in 13% was drowning (17/131). However, only a small proportion (<12%) of the filicide victims followed the classic pattern of child abuse. Much more common were "altruistic" killings (49%), with 38% of them accompanied by suicide of the perpetrator. In the murder suicides, the perpetrator, overidentifying the child with himself or herself, wished to save the child from a similar adulthood fate. The other "altruistic" killings fit a pattern of euthanasia. Twenty-four percent of the killings resulted from acute perpetrator psychosis. Eleven killings were intended to dispose of an unwanted child and 2 were intended to punish or seek revenge on a spouse. This contrasts with the higher frequency of "unwanted child" and lower incidence of "altruistic" and "psychotic" killings in neonatacide. See next column.

Toddlers have been recognized to fall headfirst into and sustain drowning events in 3- to 5-gallon pails.[27,35–38] The top-heavy toddler is waist high to the rim of these buckets. Curiosity leads them to look and fall in headfirst. The buckets are stable when filled with water, so that the wedged child is unable to escape. The children reported in individual case series range from 9 to 16 months old. None of the authors note inflicted instances of pail drownings. In a larger series, using reports to the Consumer Product Safety Commission (CPSC), pail drowning victims range from 7 to 15 months old.[36] In order to fall into the pail, the child needs to at least be a cruiser. Pails are typically 25 to 28 cm (9.8–11 in.) high, a height well within the range of cruising infants. Although the 7-month-olds from the

Mann et al[36] study may have been early cruisers, the data abstract format of the CPSC reports would have been unlikely to have details about child development. Certainly the child's individual developmental ability should be reviewed to decide whether the unintentional injury scenario is plausible. Toddlers can sustain similar unintentional immersions in toilets.

Neonatacide

Neonatacide has extensive historical roots. Lacking other means of birth control, societies either sanctioned or ignored parental killing of newborns. The victim might be simply unintended and unwanted, impaired by malformation or of reduced viability, or at times simply the wrong sex.[39] In the late 19th century, Pinkham[40] reported that 28% (29/104) of homicidal deaths of all ages in Massachusetts resulted from infanticide. He cited one "notorious case" of a neonate thrown from the dock in Lynn. He also described in detail the medicolegal evaluation of an infant found dead in a privy. Resnick[41] reviewed the case literature of neonatacide in an attempt to understand its psychiatric underpinnings. Drowning, suffocation, strangulation, head trauma, exposure, and stabbing were the common methods of death for the 37 reported infants. He noted that drowning most often occurred in the toilet. The baby was killed by its mother in 34 of the instances, by the father in 2, and by both parents in 1. Motivations were divided between murder of an unwanted infant (33), psychotic acts (5), and altruistic (1) and accidental (1) motivations. Altruistic murders were intended to relieve suffering, and accidental murders in this study and his 1969 study[34] of older children contained many motivations, including classic "battered child syndrome." The unwanted infant cases often included young, unmarried primiparas who either denied pregnancy or naively anticipated a stillbirth. There was a lack of preparation for the birth and the murder. Many of the mothers were afraid to reveal the pregnancy to their mother and/or family. Included among these were instances of incest. A second group of mothers were older, egotistic, and promiscuous women who disposed of their encumbering infant with premeditation. Some were married women who bore newborns by men other than their husband. Common among both motivations was a lack of empathy for the neonate and failure to view the baby as a person. Finkelhor[42] also comments on the predominance of young mothers with unintended pregnancies and no prenatal care in the killing of unwanted newborns. Drowning was a prototypic mode. Greist and Zumwalt[32] reported a premature infant delivered into a toilet by a 17-year-old, unwed mother. Walther and Faust's[43] forensic study of 89 stillborns and liveborns revealed during postmortem examination that 20 deaths were violent. Two additional children also had postmortem evidence of prenatal death. Histology and scene investigation led to a determination of violent causes of death in 11 of the remaining 67 cases not diagnosed at autopsy. Five of the children died from birth into a toilet, pail, or another water container. After investigation, the cause of death remained unclear due to the advanced state of decomposition of 49 infants who had been left in water or otherwise concealed for prolonged periods. A violent cause of death was found in 33 of the 40 cases for which a pathologic determination could be made.

In neonatacide, as in drowning in general, local customs and the local environment contribute to patterns of injury. In the Hokkaido district of Japan, 57% (24/42) of neonatacide were by drowning.[44] This most often occurred in a cistern under a toilet. In all, 29 bodies were discovered in a toilet and 2 in a bath. Some neonates had been killed by other means than drowning before disposal.

Pathology of Drowning

One of the difficulties assessing drowning as a cause of death is the lack of consistent and specific pathologic findings. As Knight[45] so aptly indicated: "Many corpses are recovered from water, but not all have drowned." Death from natural disease may precede or occur after entering the water. Natural disease may also decrease endurance, contributing to a drowning death. Other injuries in the water can cause death. Other effects of immersion, such as vagal-induced bradycardia in the intoxicated victim with cold-water exposure, may cause death. Review of 58 childhood drowning deaths by Smith et al[46] found no inflicted events, but 6 who died of natural causes. In 4 cases, epileptic events lead to the immersion. One child died of a ruptured intracranial aneurysm and one of a coronary anomaly. Devos et al[47] reported carbon monoxide (CO) poisoning to be a frequent cause of unintentional bathtub immersion deaths in Belgium. Exposure to CO likely would remain unrecognized without careful scene investigation and a high level of suspicion because children in the United States are less likely to have CO exposure.

The final common pathway in drowning is asphyxia, although cold stress and electrolyte abnormalities often contribute.[45] Freshwater drowning may induce washout of pulmonary surfactant, with alveolar overdistension. Betz et al[48] observed that alveolar macrophages also are washed out in the pulmonary edema fluid, but that the number of residual macrophages is not different between drowning victims and other fatalities. Frothy, often bloody, pulmonary edema fluid is commonly observed. It is not until macrophages per area of alveolar lining are quantitated morphometrically that differences are noted between drowning and other causes of death. This reflects the macrophage washout plus "emphysema aqueosum" (the alveolar overdistension of the drowning victim). Such morphometric analysis is not suitable for routine case evaluation. Attempts to diagnose drowning by differences in electrolytes and chemistries on the right and left side of the circulation have also yielded inconsistent and unreliable results.[45] Certainly aspirated or swallowed water is absorbed into the circulation and in freshwater drowning, hyponatremia may occur. This finding has been observed in infant swimming/drownproofing programs.[49]

> **Case:** A breastfed infant was admitted to the hospital at 3 weeks of age, then later at 6 weeks of age with

altered consciousness, seizures, and hyponatremia (114 mEq/L and 133 mEq/L). During the first hospitalization a computed tomography scan of the brain, renal and endocrine studies, and human milk electrolytes were normal. Further history revealed that the family had been supplementing the baby's diet with tap water by bottle and the hyponatremia was attributed to that. Concerns about the father's rough play with and yelling at the baby led to CPS referral for parenting skills. Both parents had childhood histories of abuse and rejection.

On the second hospitalization respiratory distress led to finding a right upper lobe infiltrate as well as multifocal pulmonary atelectasis on the chest film. The infant was again hospitalized after an apneic event a week later. Pneumogram demonstrated moderate gastroesophageal reflux and she was discharged on therapy for reflux.

Three weeks later she presented in irreversible shock with abdominal bruising, rib fractures, and a lacerated liver. In retrospect, she had been in her father's presence at the onset of all 4 events. Her father subsequently admitted immersing her in water when she was fussy. The hyponatremia likely resulted from aspiration of water, as did the pulmonary infiltrates of the second hospitalization.

Lung weights in drowning are inconsistently increased and fluid may exude from the cut surface of the lung.[45]

"Dry lung" drowning may result from laryngospasm or from reflex bradycardia. Intrapulmonary hemorrhage may be noted.[45]

Attempts have been made to document drowning by noting the presence of foreign materials in the lung and body. Diatoms are present in most freshwater and saltwater bodies. They commonly enter the lungs along with aspiration of water, then pass into the circulation. Unfortunately the potential for specimen contamination is great and their presence in the lungs may be a postmortem artifact of water entry.[45] Diatoms are less likely to enter the circulation and other body tissues postmortem. Because there are a great number of diatom species with differing morphology, they may have a role in matching immersion victims with a specific body of water, through identifying species homology.[50] Similarly other foreign materials (silt, weeds, sand, bath salts [which may contain fluorescein],[51] toilet paper,[37] and cesspool contents)[44] have been described as links between a victim and a specific body of water. Middle-ear hemorrhage has been proposed as an indication of drowning,[52] but it seems too nonspecific.[45] In neonatacide, the first pathologic consideration is not whether the infant died by drowning, but whether the child was born alive.

Those conducting pathologic and scene evaluation should also assess whether caretakers have given a false history of unintentional drowning to obscure findings of other inflicted injury.

Case: Medics were called to the home of a 26-month-old foster child who had been found apneic in the bathtub after being left alone for an indeterminate time. However, they observed her to be lying on the floor beside the bathtub. She was dry and was wearing a dry diaper. Fresh hair dryer grid imprint burns were observed on her face and granulating scald burns were seen at the angles of her mouth. Multiple bruises were observed about her face and body. Hair was avulsed from her scalp and petechiae noted at the empty follicles. Right-sided retinal hemorrhage was present. She was resuscitated, but died a day later. At autopsy, an occipital scalp contusion, an acute subdural hemorrhage, and massive brain swelling were observed. The left humerus had a well-healed shaft fracture and deformity suggestive of a healed proximal metaphyseal injury. No evidence of drowning was seen at autopsy. Her foster mother subsequently pleaded guilty to charges of physical assault.

Neglect in Drowning

Most neglect fatalities result from common childhood unintentional injuries.[53] Drowning represents a classic injury scenario in which caretakers must balance the child's needs for education about safety and independence of activity with the need for supervision. The younger child lacks the cognitive ability to learn how to avoid hazards, whereas the older child can incorporate safety learning. The older child needs to begin independent exploration of the world. If there is misunderstanding by the caretaker of the child's ability on this scale of protection versus independence or an imbalance between the caretaker's actions and the child's needs, problems result. At the younger end of the scale, the caretaker fails to protect the child from hazards he or she is unable to understand or avoid. At the older end of the scale, the child's learning and independence are stunted and a symbiotic relationship of the parent, with the overprotected child, may develop. One of the commonest causes of fatal, unintended injury is drowning. Lapses in supervision expose children to hazards beyond their mastery. Within these supervision lapses are those that are common or fit the community standard for most caretakers. Alternatively, individual events may represent pervasive patterns of lack of supervision or significantly fail to meet community standards of supervision. The former might result in unintentional or "accidental" child injury or death, while death or injury in the latter case would be termed *injury due to child neglect*. Child neglect accounts for a similar number of child deaths as does child abuse.[42,54] Among child deaths from neglect, drowning is frequent. At least 26% (9/34 cases) of fatal neglect reported by Margolin[55] was the result of drowning. Six resulted from bathtub drownings and 2 from bucket drownings. Lavelle et al[28] felt 67% of 21 bathtub immersions constituted either simple or severe neglect. Feldman et al[56] observed that clinicians had sufficient concern to refer 25% of 12 bathtub immersions to CPS. Three of 4 reported neglect fatalities from Oregon during 1985 and 1986 resulted from drowning.[53] Three of 18 pediatric

neglect deaths over 25 years in South Carolina resulted from drowning.[57] Included were drownings in a container of bleach, a pool, and a lake. Victim ages ranged from 9 months to 3 years.

As stated previously in this chapter, the peak ages for unintentional bathtub immersions are 8 to 24 months old.[22,26] Byard et al[58] reported that all 17 deaths in cobathing infants were 8 to 22 months old. They had been left in the bathtub with 19- to 48-month-old siblings. Santer and Stocking,[59] surveying medically indigent families in Chicago, found that 89% of children between ages 35 and 59 months and 6% of those younger than 3 years sometimes bathe without supervision. In 2003, 31% of parents of children younger than 5 years reported sometimes leaving children alone in the bath.[60] This suggests that the supervisory milieu in which unintentional drowning occurs affects many infants and toddlers. Bathtub drowning incidents, whether ruled neglect or not, follow a similar pattern of occurring in families with other children in the family[23,56] when the younger child is left to bathe with preschool-aged siblings. All of Lavelle et al's[28] bathtub submersion victims had been left unattended by an adult and 28% had a peer under age 4 years in the bathtub with them. Infants also sustain bathtub drownings when left unsupervised in bath seats. From 1989 to 2004, 5 of 36 bathtub drownings of infants in the United Kingdom had been left in bath seats.[61] The seats seem to provide caretakers with a false sense of safety. Margolin[55] found that older children were victims of fatal neglect more often than fatal abuse (2.8 vs 1.8 years old), and fatalities from either form of maltreatment were infrequent in children older than 3 years. Fatal neglect occurred in larger families (mean 4.9 vs 3.5 family members) having more children (mean 3.3 vs 1.8 children). A single parent (44% vs 31%) frequently headed families of both fatal neglect and fatal abuse victims. Lavelle et al[28] also found 43% of bathtub drowning victims to be from a single-parent home. These incidents are commonest in lower socioeconomic status families[22,56] with significant psychosocial problems.[22,28] Besharov[62] observed that neglect is 4 times as likely to involve low-income families on public assistance and single parent families (45% of reports). The household routine may be upset, whereas with inflicted bathtub immersions, a frustrating event such as a toileting accident or a child crying, may trigger the abusive event.[21]

Health care professionals who were provided scenarios of childhood submersions were only slightly more likely than not to consider neglectful a "welfare mother who left a 1- and 4-year-old alone in the bathtub" and a "father who left a 16-month-old alone in the bathtub in order to answer the phone."[56] Further they were slightly more likely not to report the incident to CPS. Clinicians were even less likely to consider a "3-year-old child who wandered off at a picnic and drowned in a lake" to have been neglected. However, parental impairment seemed most likely to result in a neglect diagnosis. A "2-year-old who drowned in the family pool while under

the care of his intoxicated father" elicited clinicians' strongest opinion of neglect. These judgments, that most drownings are not neglect, contrast with the opinion of Reece and Gorlin,[63] who felt that lack of infant bath supervision constitutes "passive abuse." They felt that cases of drowning in which the victim is younger than 1 year should be considered and managed as "nonaccidental" injury. Margolin[55] also equated any fatal childhood injury in the absence of direct caretaker supervision with neglect. All of the neglect deaths he reported, except 4 involving failure to follow medical advice and 2 from failure to seek medical care expeditiously, resulted from injuries. Although others have also observed neglect deaths from malnutrition, exposure to the elements, and failure to provide needed medical care, this raises the problem of screening for risk of unintentional injury fatality due to neglect. He suggested that 61% of the families would have been identified by 3 items on Polansky's Childhood Level of Living Scale.[64] However, the items that were suggested, such as "mother sometimes leaves child in the care of an insufficiently older sibling," seem to lack precision and would likely encompass most families.

Besharov[62] felt that CPS involvement was not warranted in injury due to neglect, unless the pattern of neglect was pervasive. Alter[65] also described neglect as a sustained pattern of inadequate parenting that must be judged in light of community standards. She suggested that when making decisions to involve CPS, the danger to the child should be quantified by documenting the degree of injury, age of the child, and frequency with which the child was exposed to hazard. Further qualitative judgments about parental behavior, including its willfulness, other attributes and effectiveness of the parent-child interaction, level of parental social deviance, and willingness to change, should be included in decision-making. Feldman et al[56] suggested that clinicians consider the utility of reporting borderline cases of neglect. Reports and requests for home evaluation to public health nursing, rather than initially to CPS, might in some cases allow better information gathering and preventive intervention. In any case, the focus should be less on establishing blame for past neglect than on identifying behavior that creates future risk to the child or family. Evaluators should seek solutions to these risks.

Conclusion

As in any other type of childhood injury, the clinician should consider whether the injury scenario is behaviorally and developmentally plausible. The child should be examined for other indications of maltreatment. The strengths, weaknesses, and coping style of the family should be considered. If those procedures are followed, child abuse or neglect may be recognized as the cause of a childhood immersion event. This knowledge is required for the clinician to appropriately intervene to protect the victim and siblings.

References

1. National Safety Council. *Accident Facts-1998 Edition.* Itasca, IL: National Safety Council; 1998

2. Gregg GS, Elmer E. Infant injuries: accident or abuse? *Pediatrics.* 1969;44:434–439

3. Holter JC, Friedman SB. Child abuse: early case finding in the emergency department. *Pediatrics.* 1968;42:128–138

4. Kempe CH, Silverman FN, Steele BF, et al. The battered-child syndrome. *JAMA.* 1962;181:17–24

5. O'Neill JA Jr, Meacham WF, Griffin PP, et al. Patterns of injury in the battered child syndrome. *J Trauma.* 1973;13:332–339

6. Smith SM, Hanson R. 134 battered children: a medical & psychological study. *British Med J.* 1974;3:666–670

7. Adelson L. Slaughter of innocents: study of forty six homicides in which the victims were children. *N Engl J Med.* 1961;264:1345–1349

8. Brewester DR, Nelson JP, Hymel KP, et al. Victim, perpetrator, family, and incident characteristics of 32 infant maltreatment deaths in the United States Air Force. *Child Abuse Negl.* 1998;22:91–101

9. Ewigman B, Kivilahan C, Land G. The Missouri child fatality study: underreporting of maltreatment fatalities among children younger than five years of age, 1983 through 1986. *Pediatrics.* 1993;91:330–337

10. Hodge D, Ludwig S. Child homicide: emergency department recognition. *Pediatr Emerg Care.* 1985;1:3–6

11. Muscat JE. Characteristics of child homicide in Ohio, 1974–84. *Am J Public Health.* 1988;78:822–824

12. Pearn J, Nixon J. Attempted drowning as a form of non-accidental injury. *Aust Paediatr J.* 1977;13:110–113

13. Quan L, Gore EJ, Wentz K, et al. Ten-year study of pediatric drownings and near-drownings in King County, Washington: lessons in injury prevention. *Pediatrics.* 1989;83:1035–1040

14. Pearn J, Nixon J. Freshwater drowning and near-drowning accidents involving children. *Med J Aust.* 1976;2:942–946

15. Pearn JH, Wong RYK, Brown J III, et al. Drowning and near drowning involving children: five-year total population study from the city and county of Honolulu. *Am J Public Health.* 1979;69:450–454

16. Kemp A, Sibert JR. Drowning and near drowning in children in the United Kingdom: lessons for prevention. *BMJ.* 1992;304:1143–1146

17. Wintermute GJ. Childhood drowning and near-drowning in the United States. *Am J Dis Child.* 1990;144:663–669

18. Rowe MI, Arango A, Allington G. Profile of pediatric drowning victims in a water-oriented society. *J Trauma.* 1977;17:587–591

19. Brenner RA, Trumble AC, Smith GS, Kessler EP, Overpeck MD. Where children drown, United States 1995. *Pediatrics.* 2001;108:85–89

20. Agran PF, Anderson C, Winn D, Trent R, Walton-Haynes L, Thayer S. Rates of pediatric injuries by 3-month intervals for children 0 to 3 years of age. *Pediatrics.* 2003;111:e683–e692

21. Nixon J, Pearn J. Non-accidental immersion in bathwater: another aspect of child abuse. *Br Med J.* 1977;1:271–272

22. Pearn J, Nixon J. Bathtub immersion accidents involving children. *Med J Aust.* 1977;1:211–213

23. Pearn JH, Brown J, Wong R, Bart R. Bathtub drownings: report of seven cases. *Pediatrics.* 1979;64:68–70

24. Diekema DS, Quan L, Holt VL. Epilepsy as a risk factor for submersion injury. *Pediatrics.* 1993;91:612–616

25. Saxena A, Ang LC. Epilepsy and bathtub drowning: important neuropathological observations. *Am J Forensic Med Pathol.* 1993;14:125–129

26. Kemp AM, Mott AM, Sibert JR. Accidents and child abuse in bathtub submersions. *Arch Dis Child.* 1994;70:435–438

27. Jensen LR, Williams SD, Thurman DJ, et al. Submersion injuries in children younger than 5 years in urban Utah. *West J Med.* 1992;157:641–644

28. Lavelle JM, Shaw KN, Seidl T, et al. Ten-year review of pediatric bathtub near-drownings: evaluation for child abuse and neglect. *Am J Emerg Med.* 1995;25:344–348

29. Gillenwater JM, Quan L, Feldman KW. Inflicted submersion in childhood. *Arch Pediatr Adolesc Med.* 1996;150:298–303

30. Allaisio D, Fisher H. Immersion scald burns and the ability of young children to climb into a bathtub. *Pediatrics.* 2005;115:1419–1421

31. Gorniak JM, Jenkins AJ, Felo JA, Balraj E. Drug prevalence in drowning deaths in Cuyahoga County, Ohio: a ten-year retrospective study. *Am J Forensic Med Pathol.* 2005;26:240–243

32. Griest KJ, Zumwalt RE. Child abuse by drowning. Pediatrics. 1989;83:41–46

33. Perrot LJ, Nawojczyk S. Nonnatural death masquerading as SIDS (sudden infant death syndrome). *Am J Forensic Med Pathol.* 1988;9:105–111

34. Resnick PJ. Child murder by parents: a psychiatric review of filicide. *Am J Psychiatry.* 1969;126:73–82

35. Jumblic MI, Chamblis M. Accidental toddler drowning in 5-gallon buckets. *JAMA.* 1990;263:1952–1953

36. Mann NC, Weller SC, Rauchschwalbe R. Bucket-related drownings in the United States, 1984–1990. *Pediatrics.* 1992;89:1068–1071

37. Scott PH, Eigen H. Immersion accidents involving pails of water in the home. *J Pediatr.* 1980;96:282–284

38. Walker S, Middelkamp N. Pail immersion accidents. *Clin Pediatr.* 1981;20:341–343

39. McGowan J. Little girls dying: an ancient and thriving practice. *Commonwealth.* 1991;118:481–482

40. Pinkham JG. Some remarks upon infanticide, with report of a case of infanticide by drowning. *Boston Med Surg J.* 1883;109:411–413

41. Resnick PJ. Murder of the newborn: a psychiatric review of neonatacide. *Am J Psychiatry.* 1970;126:58–64

42. Finkelhor D. The homicides of children and youth: a developmental perspective. In: Kantor GK, Jasinski J, eds. *Out of Darkness: Contemporary Perspectives on Family Violence.* Thousand Oaks, CA: Sage Publications; 1997

43. Walther G, Faust G. Kausalitatsprobleme beim Nachweis der Totung des Neugeborenen [Problems in the diagnosis of homicide in newborns]. *Z Rechtsmed.* 1970;67:109–118

44. Shionono H, Maya A, Tabata N, et al. Medicolegal aspects of infanticide in Hokkaido District, Japan. *Am J Forensic Med Pathol.* 1986;7:104–106

45. Knight B. Immersion deaths. In: Knight B, ed. *Forensic Pathology.* New York, NY: Oxford University Press; 1991:360–373

46. Smith NM, Byard RW, Bourne AJ. Death during immersion in water in childhood. *Am J Forensic Med Pathol.* 1991;12:219–221

47. Devos C, Timperman J, Piette M. Deaths in the bath. *Med Sci Law.* 1985;25:189–200

48. Betz P, Nerlich A, Penning R, et al. Alveolar macrophages and the diagnosis of drowning. *Forensic Sci Int.* 1993;62:217–224

49. Kropp RM, Schwartz JF. Water intoxication from swimming. *J Pediatr.* 1982;101:947–948

50. Pollanen M. Diatoms and homicide. *Forensic Sci Int.* 1998;91:29–34

51. Mukaida M, Kimura H, Takada Y. Detection of bath salts in the lungs of a baby drowned in a bathtub. *Forensic Sci Int.* 1998;93:5–11

52. Liu C, Babin RW. A histological comparison of the temporal bone in strangulation and drowning. *J Otolaryngol.* 1984;13:44–46

53. Oregon Department of Human Services. *Fatal Child Abuse and Neglect in Oregon, 1985 and 1986.* Salem, OR: Oregon Children's Services Division; 1988

54. Anderson R, Ambrosino R, Valentine D, et al. Child deaths attributed to abuse and neglect: an empirical study. *Child Youth Serv Rev.* 1983;5:75–89

55. Margolin L. Fatal child neglect. *Child Welfare.* 1990;69:309–319

56. Feldman KW, Monestersky C, Feldman GK. When is childhood drowning neglect? *Child Abuse Negl.* 1993;17:329–336

57. Knight LD, Collins KA. A 25-year retrospective review of deaths due to pediatric neglect. *Am J Forensic Med Pathol.* 2005;26:221–228

58. Byard RW, de Kening C, Blackbourne B, Nadeau JM, Krous HF. Shared bathing and drowning in infants and young children. *J Paediatr Child Health.* 2001;37:542–544

59. Santer LJ, Stocking CNB. Safety practices and living conditions of low-income urban families. *Pediatrics.* 1991;88:1112–1118

60. Simon HK, Tamura T, Colton K. Reported level of supervision of young children while in the bathtub. *Ambul Pediatr.* 2003;3:106–108

61. Sibert J, John N, Jenkins D, et al. Drowning of babies in bath seats: do they provide false reassurance? *Child Care Health Dev.* 2005;31:255–259

62. Besharov DJ. *Recognizing Child Abuse: A Guide for the Concerned.* New York, NY: The Free Press/MacMillan; 1990:99–107, 108–113

63. Reece RM, Grodin MA. Recognition of nonaccidental injury. *Pediatr Clin North Am.* 1985;32:41–57

64. Polansky N, Chalmers MA, Buttenweiser E, et al. Assessing adequacy of child caring: an urban scale. *Child Welfare.* 1978;57:439–449

65. Alter CF. Decision-making factors in cases of child neglect. *Child Welfare.* 1985;64:99–111

Chapter 19

Unusual Manifestations of Child Abuse

Rebecca R. S. Socolar

Departments of Pediatrics and Social Medicine, University of North Carolina School of Medicine at Chapel Hill
University of North Carolina Hospitals

Desmond K. Runyan

Department of Social Medicine, The University of North Carolina at Chapel Hill

How might manifestations of child abuse be considered unusual? Is it the behavior or parental act that is unusual or is it the manifestation of harm? In this chapter, we will consider both of these issues—behaviors that are unusual and results that are uncommon. Unusual might mean infrequent manifestations of abuse or bizarre variations of common manifestations. Our judgment about what is rare is usually determined by clinical experience rather than by epidemiological data.

Rare or unusual forms of child maltreatment have a history of becoming more widely recognized and losing the appellation "rare." Child maltreatment itself was once thought to be quite rare. Gill[1] noted the existence of just 6,000 officially reported cases of child abuse in the United States in 1967. Sexual abuse was considered rare; in 1955, the total number of incest cases in the United States was estimated to be 500, and in 1969, the estimated number was 5,000.[2]

Annual maltreatment incidence estimates now border on 47 per 1,000 children per year by parent self-report, and the total number of cases identified by professionals is 5.7 per 1,000 children per year.[3] In the United States, there are about 1 million substantiated cases per year.

In the 1940s, 1950s, and 1960s, fractures were recognized as a principal manifestation of child abuse[4,5] and the battered child syndrome was described.[6] At that time, these were new and unusual findings, and were reported as such in the literature. Early case reports of some unusual types of maltreatment from the 1960s and 1970s were later recognized to represent more common patterns. For example, in 1975, Kempe[7] specified a number of clinical signs of child abuse as uncommon manifestations of the battered child syndrome, including human bites, handprint bruising, intramural hematoma of the bowel, and whiplash–shaken infant syndrome. Today these would not be considered uncommon manifestations of physical abuse. A review of the literature in the subsequent decades reveals that reports of findings that were originally viewed as unusual or bizarre have come to be incorporated into standard knowledge about maltreatment and they are now covered in some detail in other chapters of this volume. Munchausen syndrome by proxy (MSBP), for example, was once considered an unusual manifestation of abuse; it has now become the topic of a separate chapter in this volume, although epidemiological estimates of the frequency still characterize this problem as one of relatively low frequency.

The purpose of a catalog of unusual manifestations is not to titillate the reader but to help extend the differential diagnostic possibilities for the clinician and to help ensure that maltreatment is included among the diagnostic possibilities when an unusual clinical presentation is noted. In this chapter we begin with a discussion of the role of culture in determining what is unusual, and then we address perpetrated behaviors of abuse and summarize a variety of reported forms of maltreatment organized by organ system to assist the clinician in the recognition of unusual physical manifestations of maltreatment. In addition to the type of abuse and the involved organ system, other aspects of abuse might make it unusual. For example, in some cases, the implement used for the abuse is what is unusual, such as an air weapon, needles, a microwave, or a candle; in other cases, a characteristic of the perpetrator or victim is the unusual feature, such as male

perpetrators of MSBP, perpetrators with mental illness, or twin victims of the shaken baby syndrome. To avoid duplication, we have categorized perpetrators, victims, and behavior by type of abuse and organ system that was affected.

Behaviors and Culture

Determining what is rare or unusual is filtered through the lens of culture. What is rare in one culture may be more common and carry quite a different connotation in another. A specific behavior or form of abuse may seem to be uncommon not because the experience is uncommon within a culture or ethnic group of people but because that group is a small segment in the larger society. Alternatively, a behavior may be normative in the larger society but be very uncommon and unacceptable within a minority cultural group. For example, in the 2004 report, "Epidemiologic Features of Physical and Sexual Maltreatment in the Carolinas," only 6% of US parents reported slapping a child on the face, head, or ears, whereas 45% reported spanking a child in the last year.[8] Similar data from India indicate that 57% of parents use slapping their child on the face or head as discipline. The same percentage (57%) report using spanking as discipline.[9] When the International Society for the Prevention of Child Abuse and Neglect convened more than 50 professionals in 30 countries to design an instrument to assess the frequency of child abuse, they included items such as "twisting his or her ear"; "hit him/her on the head with knuckles"; "threaten to invoke ghosts, evil spirits, or harmful people"; "put chili pepper, hot pepper, or spicy food in mouth"; "pinching him or her"; and "forcing the child to stand or kneel in a painful area such as hot sand or with an added burden." These types of items had been left out of the US-developed parent-child conflict tactics scale as possible means of discipline because of the anticipated rarity of these behaviors.[10]

One study, from one rural area in one developing country, reported that 12 per 1,000 parents had used inflicting a burn as punishment; in a similar survey in the United States, only 2 per 1,000 parents admitted burning a child as discipline in an anonymous telephone survey.[8,11] Putting hot pepper in the mouth or on the tongue was included recently in a survey of parents in North and South Carolina, and the rate of endorsement for use in the past year was 3 per 1,000 parents. Conflict tactics scale data from another developing country suggested some of the same manifestations of maltreatment were seen there.[12] Interestingly, cases of the use of pepper as punishment have been reported as unusual manifestations of maltreatment in the United States.[13,14] In developing countries, there were reports of a relatively high frequency of forcing the children to stand in one place with an added burden or in hot sand. In one of the countries, nearly 2% of the children had been tied up off the ground by a parent (Table 19.1).

These international data help to put the US experience in context. It is likely that forms of maltreatment that are common in other countries occur in the United States, although perhaps at lower rates.

TABLE 19.1
Unusual Forms of Maltreatment Used by Parents in Population Surveys (Self-Report)

	Behavior Rates United States[a] (Last Year)	Rate for Developing Country[b] (Last 6 mo)	Rate for Developing Country[c] (Last 6 mo)
Slapped face	61/1,000	578/1,000	210/1,000
Burned or scalded	2/1,000	12/1,000	5.9/1,000
Threatened with knife or gun	0/1,000	12/1,000	0/1,000
Choked	Not asked	16/1,000	7.4/1,000
Beat up	3/1,000	Not asked	27/1,000
Kicked	3/1,000	104/1,000	56/1,000
Hot pepper in mouth	3/1,000	26/1,000	7.7/1,000

[a]Theodore A, Chang JJ, Runyan DK, Hunter WM, Bangdiwala SI, Agans R. The epidemiology of the physical and sexual maltreatment of children in the Carolinas. *Pediatrics*. 2005;3:e331–e337.
[b]Hunter WM, Jain D, Sadowski LS, Sanhueza AI. Risk factors for severe child discipline practices in rural India. *J Pediatr Psychol.* 2000;25:435–447.
[c]Runyan DK, Wattam C, Ikeda R, Hassan F, Ramiro L. Child abuse and neglect by parents and other caretakers. In: Krug E, Dahlberg L, Mercy J, Zwi A, Lozano R, eds. *World Report on Violence and Health*. Geneva, Switzerland: World Health Organization; 2002.

It is difficult to know the extent to which the rates reported here represent true differences in behavior in different countries, as opposed to different willingness to report behaviors. It seems likely that societal norms affect actual behavior as well as willingness to report about behaviors.

Physical Abuse

Skin

Microwave Burns

The cases of 2 children, 5 weeks old and 14 months old, with full-thickness burns as a result of being placed in microwave ovens have been reported.[15] The 5-week-old infant had burns over 11% of her body surface, was hospitalized for 33 days, and survived after 4 surgeries including amputations, escharotomies, and skin grafts (Figure 19.1). Biopsies showed characteristic microwave burn patterns (see Chapter 1), with sparing of the subcutaneous fat level between burned dermis/epidermis and muscle. The 14-month-old toddler had second- and third-degree burns of the midback, which required skin grafting, but these lesions would not have been recognized

as the result of microwave burns had the babysitter not confessed. The child recovered fully with no evidence of any long-term physical or psychological sequelae at approximately age 10 years.

Grease Burns

Recently a case of inflicted burns using hot cooking oil to heat a metal spatula for burning the child was reported.[16] A review of 215 hospitalized cases of burns caused by hot grease/oil[17] revealed only one case of child abuse, although 4% to 8% of all pediatric burns are reported to be caused by hot grease or oil.[18] This suggests that abuse by burning a child with grease is unusual. Hot water is reported to be the thermal medium that burns 82% of child abuse burn victims,[19] whereas flame and hot solids are the medium of burn in 8% to 10% of child abuse burns.

Subcutaneous Emphysema

A 2-month-old girl presented with extensive swelling of her head and neck as well as subcutaneous emphysema over her scalp, neck, and chest, with crepitus.[20] Further studies revealed a hypopharyngeal perforation that caused

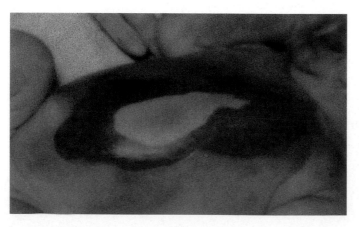

FIGURE 19.1
Ventral burns. There are full-thickness burns to left abdomen and thorax and partial-thickness burns to left anterior thigh. Extensive circumferential burns of right foot and left hand are not seen. This infant presumably was placed on her back in a micro-wave oven.

pneumomediastinum and subcutaneous emphysema. In addition, she had multiple rib fractures. There now have been several reported cases of subcutaneous emphysema associated with perforations of the hypopharynx or esophagus of abused children (see Chapter 4).

Tattooing and Scarring

Cases of children who were given tattoos or scars have been reported, including a 7-year-old boy whose arm was forcibly tattooed with his name, 2 children with other signs of abuse who had been tattooed on their hands, and a 9-year-old girl who had a cross cut in her forehead when her mother heard voices that told her to cut crosses in her forehead and her daughter's forehead.[21]

Gastrointestinal/Thoracic

Hypopharynx and Esophagus

More than 22 cases of traumatic perforation of the hypopharynx have been reported since 1984[22] (see Chapter 4). Although this seems to be a relatively rare manifestation of abuse, it has now been reported multiple times. Examples include infants[23,24] who were diagnosed when laryngoscopy revealed hemorrhagic lesions of the posterior pharyngeal wall, and radiography revealed interstitial emphysema. Toddlers have been reported as well and, as with infants,[25] frequently have other substantial injuries in addition to the pharyngeal/esophageal perforation.[26–28] Often these inflicted perforations result in associated infections.[29,30]

One case of esophageal foreign bodies associated with a child fatality has been described.[31] In this case, coins were repeatedly inserted into the esophagus of a 5-month-old infant. The child was seen initially at 4 months with numerous coins in the esophagus, and a history given that a piggy bank had spilled into the crib and the child ingested the coins. The child was hospitalized, and 7 coins were retrieved by esophagoscopy. One month later, the child was brought dead on arrival to the same emergency department (ED) with multiple fractures of extremities and 3 coins in the esophagus. The mechanism of death was not clear.

Small Bowel

When intestinal intramural hematomas secondary to child abuse were first described,[32] they were thought to be unusual. By now, intramural duodenal hematomas and perforations have been described numerous times, and in a recent study represented 2.8% of the injuries from all child abuse admissions.[33] Jejunal hematomas are recognized as less common than duodenal, but still not rare. Hematomas and perforations of the small bowel, particularly of the young child, should raise the suspicion of abusive injury. Strictures of the duodenum and jejunum have been described as an unusual complication of hematomas and perforations secondary to child abuse in a 15-month-old.[34]

Pancreas

After pseudocysts of the pancreas secondary to child abuse were first described,[35] it was not long before it was recognized that pseudocysts of the pancreas were due to child abuse more commonly than the literature had previously indicated.[36] More than 25 years after pseudocysts of the pancreas were first described in cases of abuse, they are still considered relatively rare.

Chylothorax and Chylous Ascites

An 11-month-old with respiratory distress had chest radiography that showed complete opacification of the right lung field. Thoracentesis revealed odorless, sterile, creamy fluid. There were multiple fractures of ribs, spine, and long bone, as well as a probable inflicted burn.[37] There are now several reports of chylothorax as a manifestation of child abuse.[38]

Chylous ascites is an extremely rare complication of abdominal trauma in children. Some of the first cases of posttraumatic chylous ascites in children were first reported in the 1960s, and recognized as a manifestation of child abuse in the 1970s.[39] Since that time, there have been several reports of chylous ascites secondary to child abuse.[40,41] The diagnosis is made by the milky appearance of fluid obtained from paracentesis, a sterile culture, the presence of fat globules on Sudan stain, and an alkaline pH. It is estimated that child abuse accounts for approximately 10% of all cases of chylous ascites in children.[42] The leakage caused by trauma has consistently been found at the root of the mesentery of the small bowel rather than at the thoracic duct or cisterna chyli.

Cardiac Lacerations and Commotio Cordis

Six cases of fatal abusive cardiac lacerations in children from age 9 weeks to 2.5 years were reported.[43] All were the result of severe blunt-force trauma, and all had evidence of other significant trauma. In 5 cases, the right atrium was lacerated; the left ventricle was lacerated in the remaining case. The authors pointed out that this type of injury is the result of motor vehicle accidents or very violent assault, and not minor trauma.

Commotio cordis is an impact injury that disrupts the electrical activity of the heart without cardiac contusion or laceration. There have been a few reported cases of such child abuse injuries in which young children were punched in the chest with the immediate onset of symptoms and collapse.[44]

Head/Neurologic

Shaken Baby/Shaken Impact Syndrome

This is not an uncommon form of maltreatment, but the incidence is fortunately low at about 30 per 100,000 live births in the first year of life and a tenth of that rate in the second year of life.[45] Some unusual variations of the syndrome have been reported. A case of a 6-week-old infant with a traumatic aneurysm as a complication of shaking with impact has been described.[46] Initially the infant presented with a large left subdural hemorrhage, interhemispheric hemorrhage, and cerebral edema. The infant improved for 20 days and then developed seizures again. A repeated computed tomography (CT) scan showed parafalcine subarachnoid blood and fresh intraventricular hemorrhage. Ultimately, a saccular traumatic aneurysm was removed. A reviewer of this article made the point that the phenomenon of traumatic aneurysm is different from re-bleeding in an old subdural hemorrhage.[47] In the case of traumatic aneurysm, the location of the bleeding is different, and the subdural hemorrhage had resolved before the second clinical deterioration occurred.

Intracranial Foreign Body

A 2-month-old baby presented with a 4-mm circular laceration on his forehead with a history that the baby pulled a coffee table over onto his head.[48] Radiographs showed an intracranial airgun pellet. The father then changed his story and reported that his air pistol had gone off accidentally. The mother, who was interviewed separately, said that the father held the pistol several inches from the baby's head and said "shut up or I'll shoot you," and then fired the weapon. The skeletal survey was negative, and the infant recovered well after surgical removal of the pellet.

Spinal Cord Injury

Spinal cord injury without spinal fracture and without head injury is a rare presentation of child abuse, and may escape detection unless other signs of abuse are detected. A recent report of cervical spine injuries found that all cases of injury due to child abuse had spinal cord injury without radiographic abnormality but also had severe associated injuries.[49] Isolated spinal cord injury is usually due to hyperflexion/hyperextension injuries. Cervical

magnetic resonance imaging (MRI) examination can provide specific information about the trauma, but is not routinely recommended to evaluate the shaken baby/shaken impact syndrome.[50,51] The case of a 15-month-old girl with unexplained quadriplegia has been reported.[52] At presentation there were fresh and old suggestive bruises, an old facial burn, and an old clavicular fracture, in addition to flaccid quadriplegia with an MRI that showed fusiform swelling of the midcervical spinal cord with hematomyelia. The child survived, but quadriplegia persisted with an MRI after 2 months that showed atrophy of the spinal cord where it had previously been swollen (Figure 19.2). It should be noted that spinal cord injury without radiographic abnormality is limited to infants, because at this age, the spinal column can be deformed to the point of spinal cord injury without fracture of vertebrae or rupture of ligaments. In addition, thorough postmortem examination demonstrates upper cervical cord lesions in a substantial fraction of infants who die of their head injuries, but these injuries are seldom recognized before death.

Eye

Two cases of inflicted keratoconjunctivitis with additional signs of child abuse have been reported in infants.[53] It is unclear whether the mode of injury was traumatic or chemical, but in each case the lower half of the cornea and conjunctiva were affected. The authors speculate that this may be due to protection of the upper cornea by Bell reflex.

Ear

The tin-ear syndrome is defined by the clinical triad of isolated ear bruising, hemorrhagic retinopathy, and a small ipsilateral subdural hematoma with severe cerebral swelling. This injury is thought to be caused by blunt injury to the ear that results in significant rotational acceleration of the head, and represents an unusual manifestation of child abuse (see Chapter 2). Four cases of this injury have been reported, all children were aged 2 to 3 years and all had a fatal outcome.[54]

Nose

Two reports involving 4 children ranging in age from 6 months to 8 years indicated that mothers became obsessed with nasal hygiene to the point of significant injury to the nasal tip, columella, and distal septum[55] (Figure 19.3). There is a report of successful surgical correction in 2 of the children, although one child showed signs of failure of nasal growth.[56] In each case, other causes such as congenital aplasias, congenital syphilis, and leishmaniasis were ruled out.

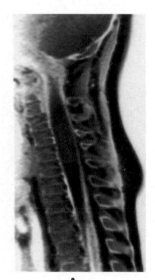
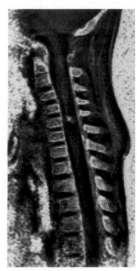

A   B

FIGURE 19.2
A. A sagittal T1-weighted image of the cervical spine demonstrated fusiform swelling of the midcervical spinal cord (black arrowheads). **B.** A sagittal T2-weighted image of the cervical spine exhibited several globular (white arrowhead) and linear low-signal lesions within the substance of the spinal cord that were interpreted as hematomyelia.

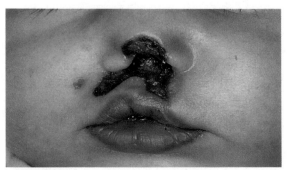

FIGURE 19.3
Nasal destruction in a 6-month-old infant.

Teeth

Dental injuries that occur as the result of blunt trauma to the face are frequent manifestations of abuse (see Chapter 5). There has been a case report of 3 children in a family of 6 (ages 13 and younger) who were each found to have multiple missing permanent incisors.[57] Eventually it was discovered that their parents were extracting teeth as punishment. Although the loss of a single tooth could have been the result of accidental trauma, the loss of multiple teeth at the ages of the children seen in this family did not have a plausible medical explanation.

Skeletal

Sternum

Injuries of the sternum are rare in young children. Abusive sternal injuries are thought to be the result of direct blows or compression of the chest[50] (see Chapter 3). In the absence of a history of massive force applied to the thorax by accidental means, child abuse is thought to be likely.

Pelvis

Fractures of the pelvis are seldom reported in abused children (see Chapter 3). If there is no history of a motor vehicle crash or other severe trauma, then intentional trauma should be considered the etiology for these injuries because the force required to produce such an injury is tremendous. The cases that have been described have always entailed multiple fractures and severe trauma.[58] The case of a 4-year-old girl who was brought to the hospital in full cardiopulmonary arrest was described.[59] Multiple injuries including skin bruising, abrasions, and scars were noted all over the body, as well as laceration of the external genitalia, hymen, and vagina. Radiographs showed multiple humeral fractures and a questionable area over the left acetabulum/pubic ramus. At autopsy this area was confirmed as a fracture of the superior pubic ramus and anterior acetabular margin. Pelvic fractures are rare in abused children, but pelvic fractures are associated with signs of sexual abuse as well as physical abuse. Radiography of the pelvis may be helpful in selected cases of sexual abuse that involved signs of significant blunt-force trauma to the soft tissues overlying the pelvis.[60]

Spine

Spinal injury is an uncommon manifestation of child abuse and, when seen, it occurs in young children. The average age in reports of these injuries is 22 months, with half of them younger than 1 year.[61] Cervical spine injuries occur in 1% to 2% of abusive head injury and should be considered in any infant who has a severe shaking injury; however, despite the tremendous acceleration and deceleration forces on the head in the prevalent non-accidental shaking injuries, cervical spine injuries are unusual.[62] There have been several reports of thoracolumbar fracture with listhesis, most commonly at L1-L2.[63] Spinal fracture and spinal cord injury may occur simultaneously in abuse cases, although this is rare.[62] Another report described twin infant girls with hyperflexion-extension injuries of the lower cervical spine that resulted in cervical spine fracture-dislocation and cord compression.[64]

Reports of hangman's fracture (C2 fracture) are rare and must be differentiated from congenital spondylolysis, but have now been described for abused children aged 5 months,[65] 6 months,[66] and 23 months.[67] A hangman's fracture results from forced hyperextension of the neck and has occurred in conjunction with shaken baby syndrome.

Hands and Feet

Fractures of the hands and feet are unusual compared with other fractures in abused children, but when found, particularly in infants, are highly suggestive of abuse. A recent review of abused children younger than 2 years found that these fractures were often subtle radiographic findings that require high-detail imaging systems. Buckle fractures of the phalanges likely resulted from forced hyperextension[68] (see Chapter 3).

Systemic: Inhalants, Ingestions, Withholding Nourishment

Cocaine

A number of reports of cocaine intoxication emerged in the 1980s.[69–71] Although it is unclear which of these cases was due to breastfeeding, intentional administration, accidental ingestion, or passive inhalation of crack vapors, any of these represents abuse or supervisory neglect (see Chapter 17). There has been a case report of the homicide of a 10-month-old due to crack cocaine ingestion.[72] Cocaine intoxication may not be an unusual form of abuse/neglect. Of all children younger than 5 years seen in one urban ED, 2.5% had cocaine metabolites in their urine.[73] Thus in this setting, this form of abuse/neglect could not be considered unusual. Clinical presentations of cocaine intoxication that were reported included tachycardia, hypertension, and a range of neurologic symptoms from drowsiness, tremulousness, and unsteady gait to seizures.

Pepper

Fatal pepper aspiration has been reported several times in the literature.[13,14] Abusive and accidental incidents have been reported. In cases of abuse, the pepper was given as punishment to children ranging in age from 4 months to 10 years. About half of the children had evidence of previous abuse, and about half of families initially gave incorrect histories. Mechanical obstruction and mucosal edema were the 2 mechanisms of death. In a survey of parent discipline practices for mothers of children younger than 18 years in 2 states, the use of hot pepper in the mouth as discipline was reported at a rate of 3 per 1,000 children.[8] About 2 in 10,000 calls to poison centers are related to black pepper ingestions.[14]

Withholding Water and Water Intoxication

Hypernatremic dehydration from water deprivation has been reported as a form of abuse in children ranging from 2 to 8 years old, often in children who are enuretic, either as a form of managing the enuresis or to punish the child for wetting.[74] The degree of hypernatremia in each case was extreme (with serum sodium concentrations ranging from 183–201 mEq/L) and required hospitalization. On the other end of the hydration spectrum are accounts of water intoxication produced, for example, by forcing a garden hose into a 4-year-old boy's mouth and making him swallow large quantities of water. The boy developed hyponatremia (serum saline concentration was 117 mEq/L) accompanied by coma and convulsions, but he survived.[75] Other reports of fatal forced water intoxication have been associated with other physical abuse,[76] and one case of compulsive water drinking leading to severe hyponatremia and brain edema as a psychological reaction to abuse has been reported.[77] In one case series the most common kind of abusive poisoning was excessive salt ingestion with water restriction and the second most common was water intoxication.[78]

Other Unusual Poisoning

Poisoning may be one of the more common mechanisms for perpetration of MSBP (see also Chapter 17); however, the incidence of MSBP by any mechanism is unknown and is thought to be uncommon. Various substances have been used to poison or infect children who are victims of MSBP, including prescription and nonprescription drugs.[79,80] In addition, a case of choral hydrate poisoning causing coma in a 3-year-old girl on 4 separate occasions, in the context of MSBP, has been described.[81] Ipecac poisoning of 3 children younger than 2 years, resulting in symptoms including chronic vomiting and diarrhea as well as other gastrointestinal, neurologic, and cardiovascular symptoms has been described. In each case the perpetrator was the biological mother,[82] and each was thought to represent MSBP.

Another early case of MSBP involved the intentional poisoning of 2 siblings by prescription drugs.[83]

Other substances besides pepper and water withholding or intoxication have been used as punishment or to abuse a child. A case of fatal child abuse has been reported in which a 6-year-old was forced by the live-in babysitter to consume large doses of sodium bicarbonate to make the child vomit as punishment. Included in the ingestion were vinegar, dishwashing liquid, and red pepper. Multiple electrolyte abnormalities ensued, and the child was removed from the ventilator after 6 days of flatline electroencephalogram.[84] Intentional iron poisoning of a 7-week-old has also been reported.[85]

Other Trauma

Needles

Insertion of needles into various body parts as a form of abuse has been described. An 11-year-old boy from India presented to the hospital with an acute abdomen presumed to be secondary to appendicitis. Radiographs of the abdomen revealed 7 needles in the abdomen and 1 in the right lower chest. He reported that this stepmother disliked him and had inserted a sewing needle in his abdomen once a week, and threatened to kill him if he complained.[86] A report of 3 children with abusive needle injuries included a 4-week-old infant who died of pneumonia and was found to have 3 sewing needles embedded in the occipital lobe. The sibling of this infant had 4 needles in the soft tissues of the head, neck, and forearm. A third baby had 4 needles removed from the abdomen.[87] A 13-month-old boy had fragments of nails or tacks in both feet and sewing needles in the perineum and gluteal soft tissues.[88]

Pencils

A 4-year-old boy had a deep penetrating wound of the right hand inflicted with a pencil. Although initially the parents said the wound was accidental, questioning of the child revealed that it was inflicted by the mother because the boy had failed to complete his homework properly.[89]

Other Systemic Manifestations of Trauma Due to Child Abuse

Myositis with elevation of creatinine phosphokinase levels is a known manifestation of muscle trauma. It is unclear how common this manifestation of abuse may be. A case was reported of a 2-year-old boy with myositis secondary to the battered child syndrome; it was not recognized as abuse until there had been multiple ED visits, fractured bones, and intracranial bleeding.[90] Hemoglobinuria has been reported in 2 children (20 and 32 months old) after severe beatings. One went on to develop transient oliguria, and the other transient renal failure.[91]

Genitourinary

Penis

Inflicted incisions of the penis have been reported in a 6-month-old and a 3-year-old. In each case the inconsistent or conflicting histories provided did not adequately explain the injury. In one case, the incision was clean but involved all skin layers, and in the other, there was a gaping wound at the base of the shaft[92] (Figure 19.4).

Penile strangulations have been reported in cases of parents who have become frustrated with nocturnal enuresis. Patients have presented with penile edema, ulceration, or urethral fistula. Three cases of penile strangulation have been reported from Turkey in children aged 4 to 7 years; one was due to ligation with thread, the other 2 to ligation with hair.[93] When the penis is ligated, the urethra may be completely or partially transected. The degree of damage is variable and is correlated with the duration of strangulations.

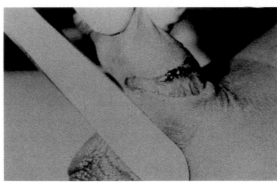

FIGURE 19.4
Incision at base of penis.

Unusual Perpetrators

Munchausen Syndrome by Proxy

The incidence rate for MSBP (see also Chapter 16) and the prevalence of various methods used for inducing MSBP are unknown. Although confirmed cases of MSBP remain rare, it seems likely that many cases of MSBP go unreported, and so it is uncertain how unusual the diagnosis or its various manifestations might be. We do know that the perpetrator of MSBP is almost always the mother.[94] Meadow,[95] in the largest series reported of fathers as perpetrators, described 15 men, 12 of whom were acting out the need to assume a sick role by proxy or were engaged in attention-seeking behavior.

Mental Illness Related

Folie á deux is an uncommon disorder in which the dominant person imposes his or her delusions on a younger/more submissive person. Several cases have been reported of fatal or near-fatal child abuse at the hands of parents with folie á deux. In each case, there had not been a previous diagnosis of psychopathology in either parent. When the abuse occurred, it was based on shared religious delusions, with subsequent diagnoses of psychotic disorder in at least one parent.[96] Several of the cases reported involved "beating the faith" into a child or ridding a child of Satan by beating or killing the child.

Neglect

Neglect has been associated primarily with poverty and parental problems with emotional health and substance abuse (see Chapter 14). Neglect secondary to religious beliefs and practices is an uncommon but pernicious form of child maltreatment.

In a case of fatal child neglect of an adolescent with ulcerative colitis, a 15.5-year-old girl had intermittent abdominal cramps and watery diarrheal stools 6 months before her death.[97] Her devout Christian Scientist parents allowed her to be evaluated by a gastroenterologist 4 months before her death because of the urging of other family members. The parents refused the recommended therapy and instead instituted a liquid health-food diet and sought the care of a chiropractic/health food clinic. Eventually she presented to the hospital obtunded and with severe anemia, electrolyte abnormalities, malnutrition, and fatal gram-negative sepsis.

A review of the cases of 172 children who died between 1975 and 1995 in the United States whose parents withheld medical care because of religious beliefs revealed that most of the fatalities were from conditions for which survival rates with medical care would have exceeded 90%[98] (Table 19.2). The denominations represented most commonly for the fatalities reviewed were Faith Assembly; First Church of Christ, Scientist (Christian Scientist); Church of the First Born; Faith Tabernacle; and End Time Ministries. The incidence of nonfatal medical neglect due to religious beliefs and practices is unknown, but it is likely to be higher than 172 cases over 20 years.

TABLE 19.2

Child Fatalities Associated With Religion-Motivated Medical Neglect

Diagnoses	N	Ages (y, Unless Specified)[a]	Expected Outcome
General or miscellaneous			
Cachexia, gastric aspiration	1	9	Excellent
Dehydration	6	4 mo, 5 mo, 1, 5, 8, 12	Excellent
Diabetes, type 1	12	3, 7, 10 (2), 11, 12 (2), 13 (2), 15 (2), 16	Excellent
Epilepsy, withheld medications	1	17	Excellent
Burns, 50% total burn surface area	1	1	Good
Hydrocephaly, myelomeningocele	1	2 mo	Excellent
Foreign-body aspiration	1	2	Good
Renal failure	3	15 (3)	Excellent
Trauma, motor vehicle accident	1	2	No benefit
Infections			
Diphtheria	3	3, 4, 9	Excellent
Laryngotracheobronchitis	1	18 mo	Excellent
Measles (with complications)	7	1, 5, 9 (2), 13, 14, 16	Excellent
Meningitis, *Haemophilus influenzae*	9	4 mo, 1 (7), 4	Excellent
Meningitis, *Streptococcus pneumoniae*	4	2 mo, 5 mo, 1, 7	Excellent
Meningitis, bacterial, nonspecified	1	1	Excellent
Meningitis, posttraumatic	1	15	Excellent
Pericarditis, *S pneumoniae*	1	1	Excellent
Pertussis	1	1 mo	Excellent
Pneumonia (varying etiologies)	22	Range 1 mo–2 y	Excellent
Pneumonia/myocarditis	1	1	Good
Rocky Mountain spotted fever	1	4	Excellent
Toxic shock syndrome, staphylococcus	1	17	Excellent
Abdominal surgical disorders			
Intussusception	3	8 mo, 9 mo, 14	Excellent
Appendicitis, ruptured	7	Range 5–14	Excellent
Small bowel obstruction	1	6	Excellent
Strangulated hernia	1	6	Excellent
Volvulus	2	9 days, 26 mo	Excellent
Congenital heart lesions			
Common atrioventricular canal	1	7 mo	Good
Double-outlet right ventricle	1	12	No benefit
Ventricular septal defect, pneumonia	2	9 mo, 10 mo	Excellent
Tumors			
Ewing sarcoma	1	13	Good
Leukemia, acute lymphocytic	3	4, 5, 7	Good
Leukemia, nonspecified	1	2	Fair
Lymphoma, Burkitt	1	13	Good
Lymphoma, non-Hodgkin	1	3	Good
Neuroblastoma	1	1	Fair
Osteogenic sarcoma	3	6, 12, 14	Fair
Posterior fossa, nonspecified	1	2	Fair
Rhabdomyosarcoma	2	4, 5	Fair
Wilms tumor	1	2	Good
Total		113	

[a]Numbers in parentheses indicate number of cases.

Sexual Abuse

Foreign Bodies and Objects

The prevalence of the use of objects to perpetrate sexual abuse is undetermined. A case was reported of a 20-month-old girl who was sexually assaulted by a male babysitter with a candle. The parents took the child for an evaluation after she moaned and cried all night. Surgeons removed a 12×2-cm wax candle from her peritoneal cavity. Other injuries included a tear in the perineum and posterior fourchette, ruptured levator ani muscle, and perforation of the posterior vaginal fornix.[99]

Sometimes it is hard to determine whether injuries of the genitalia are accidental or inflicted. Sharp penetrating injuries to the hymen have been seen secondary to abuse and accidents. Four cases of girls who had genital injuries caused by sharp objects including 3 accidental injuries from a nail, sharp projections from the edge of a swimming pool, and a toy vacuum cleaner, and one abusive injury from a sharp wooden object have been reported.[100]

Vaginal foreign bodies are rare in prepubertal girls, with an incidence of about 0.017% in a general clinic, and 1.4% to 4% in the presence of a vaginal discharge. A review of cases of girls presenting to a general pediatric clinic with vaginal foreign bodies including paper, hair, cotton, and a plastic cap indicated that sexual abuse was suspected or confirmed in 11 of 12 cases.[101] It is unclear whether vaginal foreign bodies are related to sexual abuse in any given case, but it is an uncommon manifestation of sexual abuse.

Rectovaginal Trauma

Severe trauma, including perforation of the vagina, is unusual in sexually victimized children. The case of a 4-year-old with a rectovaginal fistula has been reported. The child had been abused by penile penetration of her mouth, vagina, and anus, and digital penetration of her vagina and anus 2 months earlier. A large defect of the posterior rim of the hymen and thickened perineal tissue was present on physical examination. In the knee-chest position, yellow mucoid material was visualized throughout the vagina and anus, and a fistula required a diverting colostomy and a vaginal flap to repair the defect.[102] Perforation of the vagina was certainly present at the time of the abuse.

Genital Care Practices

Rarely children are subjected to bizarre, invasive, and/or abusive genital care practices, including painful washing, frequent and ritualistic inspections, application of creams/medicines, and enlistment of medical intervention for supposed genital or urinary problems. A record review of 790 children seen in a clinic specializing in abuse evaluation found 17 cases with abnormalities due to unusual genital care practices; all were girls.[103] The behaviors involved in genital care practices fell into 3 categories: a ritualistic excessive parental focus on the child's genitals, parents giving a long history of genital problems in their children that may have been the result of parental fabrication or inducements of disorders, and overt sexual abuse in which the father used cream on the daughter's genitalia as an excuse for the genital touching. Explanations given by parents for their behavior included that they had been washed this way or thought these hygiene practices were necessary to stop odor, or that at some point an event such as a diaper rash or other medical problem occurred that legitimized their behavior in their own minds. Another report of aberrant genital care practices in 3 children was reported more recently.[104]

Conclusion

The litany of inhumanity to children in this chapter is sobering and painful. Fortunately, most of the cases reported here are uncommon. Despite high workloads, most clinicians and child protection social workers will see few of these manifestations of abuse or neglect in their careers. Case reports are published because of the variation from normal and the information they can shed on the diagnostic process or prognosis. Caution should be taken against generalizing case reports as characteristic of the underlying phenomena. Although a compilation of case reports may serve some purpose, it cannot be used as epidemiological data. As child abuse has become better recognized, the state of our knowledge may have matured to the point that what is currently considered unusual may actually be so. However, in the decades to come, it may be that we again recognize that some of what we currently consider to be unusual is not so.

References

1. Gill D. Violence against children: physical abuse in the United States. Cambridge, UK: Harvard University Press; 1970
2. Greenberg N. The epidemiology of childhood sexual abuse. *Pediatr Ann.* 1979;8:16–28
3. Theodore A, Runyan D. A medical research agenda for child maltreatment: negotiating the next steps. *Pediatrics.* 1999;104:168–177
4. Caffey J. Multiple fractures in the long bones of infants suffering from chronic sudural hematoma. *AJR Am J Roentgenol.* 1946;56:163–173
5. Silverman FN. The roentgen manifestations of unrecognized skeletal trauma in infants. *Am J Roentgenol Radium Ther Nucl Med.* 1953;69:413–427
6. Kempe CH, Silverman FN, Stelle BF, et al. The battered child syndrome. *JAMA.* 1962;181:105–112
7. Kempe CH. Uncommon manifestations of the battered child syndrome. *Am J Dis Child.* 1975;129:1265
8. Theodore A, Chang JJ, Runyan DK, Hunter WM, Bangdiwala SI, Agans R. The epidemiology of the physical and sexual maltreatment of children in the Carolinas. *Pediatrics.* 2005:e331–e337
9. Jain D. India safe. Presented at: International Conference on Child Abuse Research; June 29, 1997; Durham, NH
10. Straus M, Hamby S, Finkelhor D, et al. Identification of child abuse with the Parent Child Tactics Scale (PCCTS): development and preliminary psychometric data from a national sample of American parents. *Child Abuse Negl.* 1998;22:249–270
11. Hunter WM, Jain D, Sadowski LS, Sanhueza AI. Risk factors for severe child discipline practices in rural India. *J Pediatr Psychol.* 2000;25:435–447
12. Hassan F, Refaat A, El-Sayed H, El-Defrawi MH. Disciplinary practices and child maltreatment among Egyptian families in an urban area in Ismailia City. *Egypt J Psychiatry.* 1999;22:172–189

13. Adelson L. Homicide by pepper. *J Forensic Sci.* 1964;9:391–395

14. Cohle SD, Trestrail JD, Graham MA, et al. Fatal pepper aspiration. *Am J Dis Child.* 1988;142:633–636

15. Alexander RC, Surrell JA, Cohle SD. Microwave oven burns to children: an unusual manifestation of child abuse. *Pediatrics.* 1987;79:255–260

16. Mukadam S, Gilles E. Unusual inflicted hot oil burns in a 7-year-old. *Burns.* 2003;29:83–86

17. Murphy JT, Purdue GF, Hunt JL. Pediatric grease burn injury. *Arch Surg.* 1995;130:478–482

18. Parish RA, Novack AH, Heimbach DM, et al. Pediatric patients in a regional burn center. *Pediatr Emerg Care.* 1986;2:165–167

19. Purdue GF, Hunt JL, Prescott PR. Child abuse by burning: an index of suspicion. *J Trauma.* 1988;28:221–224

20. Bansal BC, Abramo TJ. Subcutaneous emphysema as an uncommon presentation of child abuse. *Am J Emerg Med.* 1997;15:573–575

21. Johnson CF. Symbolic scarring and tattooing: unusual manifestations of child abuse. *Clin Pediatr.* 1994;33:46–49

22. Reece RM. Editor's note. *Q Child Abuse Med Update.* 1999;6:5

23. Ramnarayan P, Qayyum A, Tolley N, Nadel S. Subcutaneous emphysema of the neck in infancy: under-recognized presentation of child abuse. *J Laryngol Otol.* 2004;118:468–470

24. McDowell HP, Fielding DW. Traumatic perforation of the hypopharynx: an unusual form of abuse. *Arch Dis Child.* 1984;59:888–889

25. Tavill MA, Trimmer W, Austin MB. Pediatric esophageal perforation secondary to abusive blunt thoracic trauma. *Int J Pediatr Otorhinolaryngol.* 1996;35:263–269

26. Morzaria S, Walton JM, MacMillan A. Inflicted esophageal perforation. *J Pediatr Surg.* 1998;33:871–873

27. Reece RM. Unusual manifestations of child abuse. *Pediatr Clin North Am.* 1990;37:905–921

28. Reece RM, Arnold JE, Splain J. Pharyngeal perforation as a manifestation of child abuse: report of three cases. *Child Maltreat.* 1996;1:364–367

29. Ablin DS, Reinhart MA. Esophageal perforation with mediastinal abscess in child abuse. *Pediatr Radiol.* 1990;20:524–525

30. Golova N. An infant with fever and drooling: infection or trauma? *Pediatr Emerg Care.* 1998;13:331–333

31. Nolte KB. Esophageal foreign bodies as child abuse: potential fatal mechanisms. *Am J Forensic Med Pathol.* 1993;14:323–326

32. Eisentein EM, Delta BG, Clifford JH. Jejunal hematoma: an unusual manifestation of the battered-child syndrome. *Clin Pediatr.* 1965;4:436–440

33. Gaines BA, Shultz BS, Morrison K, Ford HR. Duodenal injuries in children: beware of child abuse. *J Pediatr Surg.* 2004;39:600–602

34. Shah P, Applegate KE, Buonomo C. Stricture of the duodenum and jejunum in an abused child. *Pediatr Radiol.* 1997;27:281–283

35. Bongiovi JJ, Logosso RD. Pancreatic pseudocyst occurring in the battered child syndrome. *J Paediatr Surg.* 1969;4:220–226

36. Pena DJ, Medovy H. Child abuse and traumatic pseudocyst of the pancreas. *J Pediatr.* 1973;83:1026–1028

37. Guleserian K, Gilchrist B, Luks F, et al. Child abuse as a cause of traumatic chylothorax. *J Pediatr Surg.* 1996;31:1696–1697

38. Geismar SL, Tilelli JA, Campbell JB, Chiaro JJ. Chylothorax as a manifestation of child abuse. *Pediatr Emerg Care.* 1997;13:386–389

39. Boysen BE. Chylous ascites: manifestation of the battered child syndrome. *Am J Dis Child.* 1975;129:1338–1339

40. Hilfer CL, Holgersen LO. Massive chylous ascites and transected pancreas secondary to child abuse: successful non-surgical management. *Pediatr Radiol.* 1995;25:117–119

41. Olazagasti JC, Fitzgerald JF, White SJ, Chong SK. Chylous ascites: a sign of unsuspected child abuse. *Pediatrics.* 1994;94:737–739

42. Benhaim P, Strear C, Knudson M, et al. Posttraumatic chylous ascites in a child: recognition and management of an unusual condition. *J Trauma Injury Infect Crit Care.* 1995;39:1175–1177

43. Cohle SD, Hawley DA, Berg EE, et al. Homicidal cardiac laceration in children. *J Forensic Sci.* 1995;40:212–218

44. Denton JS, Kalelkar MB. Homicidal commotio cordis in two children. *J Forensic Sci.* 2000;45:734–735

45. Keenan HT, Runyan DK, Marshall SW, Nocera MA, Merten DF, Sinal SH. A population-based study of inflicted traumatic brain injury in young children. *JAMA.* 2003;290:621–626

46. Lam CH, Montes J, Farmer JP, et al. Traumatic aneurysm from shaken baby syndrome: case report. *Neurosurgery.* 1996;39:1252–1255

47. Hymel KP. Reviewer's note. *Q Child Abuse Med Update.* 1999;6:6

48. Campbell-Hewson GL, D'Amore A, Busuttil A. Non-accidental injury inflicted on a child with an air weapon. *Med Sci Law.* 1998;38:173–176

49. Brown RL, Brunn MA, Garcia VF. Cervical spine injuries in children: a review of 103 patients treated consecutively at a Level 1 pediatric trauma center. *J Pediatr Surg.* 2001;36:1107–1114

50. Kleinman PK, cd. *Diagnostic Imaging of Child Abuse.* 2nd ed. St Louis, MO: Williams & Wilkins; 1998

51. Ghatan S, Ellenbogen RG. Pediatric spine and spinal cord injury after inflicted trauma. *Neurosurg Clin North Am.* 2002;13:227–233

52. Piatt J, Steinberg M. Isolated spinal cord injury as presentation of child abuse. *Pediatrics.* 1995;96:780–782

53. Ong T, Hodgkins P, Marsh C, Taylor D. Blinding keratoconjunctivitis and child abuse. *Am J Ophthalmol.* 2005;139:190–191

54. Hanigan WC, Peterson RA, Njus G. Tin ear syndrome: rotational acceleration in pediatric head injuries. *Pediatrics.* 1987;80:618–622

55. Fischer H, Allasio D. Nasal destruction due to child abuse. *Clin Pediatr.* 1996;35:165–166

56. Orton CI. Loss of columella and septum from an unusual form of child abuse. *Plast Reconstr Surg.* 1975;56:345–346

57. Carrotte PV. An unusual case of child abuse. *Br Dent J.* 1990;168:444–445

58. Starling SP, Heller RM, Jenny C. Pelvic fractures in infants as a sign of physical abuse. *Child Abuse Negl.* 2002;26:475–480

59. Prendergast NC, deRoux SJ, Adsay NV. Non-accidental pediatric pelvic fracture: a case report. *Pediatr Radiol.* 1998;28:344–346

60. Kleinman P. Editor's note. *Q Child Abuse Med Update.* 1999;6:7

61. Diamond P, Hansen C, Christofersen M. Child abuse presenting as a thoracolumbar spinal fracture dislocation: a case report. *Pediatr Emerg Care.* 1994;10:83–86

62. Smith W. Editor's note. *Q Child Abuse Med Update.* 1998;5:5

63. Levin TL, Berdon W, Cassell I, Biltman NM. Thoracolumbar fracture with listhesis—an uncommon manifestation of child abuse. *Pediatr Radiol.* 2003;33:305–310

64. Rooks VJ, Sisiler C, Burton B. Cervical spine injury in child abuse: report of two cases. *Pediatr Radiol.* 1998;28:193–195

65. Van Rijn RR, Kool DR, de Witt H, Majoie CB. An abused five-month-old girl: hangman's fracture or congenital arch defect? *J Emerg Med.* 2005;29:61–65

66. Kleinman PK, Shelton YA. Hangman's fracture in an abused infant: imaging features. *Pediatr Radiol.* 1997;27:776–777

67. Ranjith RK, Mullett JH, Burke TE. Hangman's fracture caused by suspected child abuse. A case report. *J Pediatr Orthop B.* 2002;11:329–332

68. Nimkin K, Spevak MR, Kleinman PK. Fractures of the hands and feet in child abuse: imaging and pathologic features. *Radiology.* 1997;203:233–236

69. Bateman DA, Heagarty MC. Passive freebase cocaine ("crack") inhalation by infants and toddlers. *Am J Dis Child.* 1989;143:25–27

70. Ernst AA. Unexpected cocaine intoxication presenting as seizures in children. *Ann Emerg Med.* 1989;18:774–777

71. Rivkin M, Gilmore HE. Generalized seizures in an infant due to environmentally acquired cocaine. *Pediatrics.* 1989;84:1100–1102

72. Havlik D, Nolte KB. Fatal "crack" cocaine ingestion in an infant. *Am J Forensic Med Pathol.* 2000;21:245–248

73. Kharasch S, Vinci R, Glotzer D, et al. Unsuspected cocaine exposure in young children. *Am J Dis Child.* 1991;145:204–206

74. Pickel S, Anderson C, Holliday MA. Thirsting and hypernatremic dehydration: a form of child abuse. *Pediatrics.* 1970;45:54–59

75. Mortimer JG. Acute water intoxication as another manifestation of child abuse. *Arch Dis Child.* 1980;55:401–403

76. Arieff AI, Kronlund BA. Fatal child abuse by forced water intoxication. *Pediatrics.* 1999;103:1292–1295

77. Lin CY, Tsau YK. Child abuse: acute water intoxication in a hyperactive child. *Acta Paediatr Taiwan.* 2005;46:39–41

78. Dine MS, McGovern ME. Intentional poisoning of children—an overlooked category of child abuse: report of seven cases and review of the literature. *Pediatrics.* 1982;70:32–35

79. Feldman KW, Christopher DM, Opheim KB. Munchausen syndrome/bulimia by proxy: ipecac as a toxin in child abuse. *Child Abuse Negl.* 1989;13:257–261

80. Valentine JL, Schexnayder S, Jones JG, et al. Clinical and toxicological findings in two young siblings and autopsy findings in one sibling with multiple hospital admission resulting in death. *Am J Forensic Med Pathol.* 1997;18:276–281

81. Lansky LL. An unusual case of childhood chloral hydrate poisoning. *Am J Dis Child.* 1974;127:275–276

82. McClung HJ, Murray R, Braden NJ, et al. Intentional ipecac poisoning in children. *Am J Dis Child.* 1988;142:637–639

83. Hvizdala EV, Gellady AM. Intentional poisoning of two siblings by prescription drugs. *Clin Pediatr.* 1978;17:480–482

84. Huntington RW, Weisberg HF. Unusual form of child abuse [letter]. *Forensic Sci Int.* 1977;22:5–6

85. Black J, Zenel JA. Child abuse by intentional iron poisoning presenting as shock and persistent acidosis. *Pediatrics.* 2003;111:197–199

86. Swadia ND, Thakore AB, Patel BR, et al. Unusual form of child abuse presenting as an acute abdomen. *Br Surg.* 1981;68:668

87. Fearne C, Kelly J, Habel J, et al. Needle injuries as a cause of non-accidental injury [letter]. *Arch Dis Child.* 1997;77:187

88. Lukefahr JL, Angel CA, Hendrick EP, Torn SW. Child abuse by percutaneous insertion of sewing needles. *Clin Pediatr.* 2001;40:461–463

89. Lee ACW, So KT, Wong HL, et al. Penetrating pencil injury: an unusual case of child abuse. *Child Abuse Negl.* 1998;22:749–752

90. Ben-Youssef I., Schmidt TL. Battered child syndrome simulating myositis. *Pediatr Orthoped.* 1983;3:392–395

91. Rimer RL, Roy S. Child abuse and hemoglobinuria. *JAMA.* 1977;238:2034–2035

92. Lukschu M, Bays J. Inflicted incision of the penis. *Child Abuse Negl.* 1996;20:979–981

93. Gultekin EY, Ozdamar AS, Gokalp A, et al. Penile strangulation injuries. *Pediatr Surg Int.* 1996;11:279–280

94. Rosenberg DA. Web of deceit: a literature review of Munchausen syndrome by proxy. *Child Abuse Negl.* 1987;11:547–563

95. Meadow R. Munchausen syndrome by proxy abuse perpetrated by men. *Arch Dis Child.* 1998;78:210–216

96. Kraya NAF, Patrick C. Folie á deux in a forensic setting. *Aust N Z Psychiatry.* 1997;31:883–888

97. Jackson DL, Korbin J, Younger S, et al. Fatal outcome in untreated adolescent ulcerative colitis: an unusual case of child neglect. *Crit Care Med.* 1983;11:832–833

98. Asser SM, Swan R. Child fatalities from religion-motivated medical neglect. *Pediatrics.* 1998;101:625–629

99. Gromb S, Lazarini HJ. An unusual case of sexual assault on an infant: an intraperitoneal candle in a 20-month-old girl. *Forensic Sci Int.* 1998;94:15–18

100. Hostetler B, Muram D, Jones CE. Sharp penetrating injuries to the hymen. *Adolesc Pediatr Gynecol.* 1994;7:94–96

101. Herman-Giddens MD. Vaginal foreign bodies and child sexual abuse. *Arch Pediatr Adolesc Med.* 1994;148:195–200

102. Kellog ND, Para JM. A rectovaginal fistula in a sexually assaulted child. *Clin Pediatr.* 1996;35:369–371

103. Herman-Giddens ME, Berson NL. Harmful genital care practices in children. *JAMA.* 1989;261:577–579

104. Hornor G, Ryan-Wegner NA. Aberrant genital practices: an unrecognized form of child sexual abuse. *J Pediatr Health Care.* 1999;13:12–17

Pathology of Fatal Abuse

Thomas Andrew

Dartmouth Medical College
State of New Hampshire Medical Examiner's Office

Jordan Greenbaum

Child Protection Center
Children's Healthcare of Atlanta

Introduction

This chapter presents an overview of fatal child abuse injuries to serve as a reference for all disciplines to help improve our system of child death investigation. In presenting the forensic pathologist's perspective we hope to make clear the impact of apparent scientific conflicts on the ultimate certifier of death of a fatally abused child. In that role, the forensic pathologist must consider what can be stated in reports and court proceedings given the sometimes confusing legal phrases such as "preponderance of the evidence," "to a reasonable degree of medical certainty," and "beyond reasonable doubt."

The importance of thorough investigation of *all* sudden, unexpected deaths in children who were *both* previously healthy and ill but stable cannot be overstated. Such deaths are nearly universally reportable to the medico-legal authority (medical examiner or coroner). Once proper jurisdiction is established, a complete investigation of the death, including autopsy of the deceased, must be carried out before the cause and manner of death can be certified with any degree of medical, scientific, and/or legal certainty. *Cause of death* is the disease state, injury, or combination of the two that initiates an ultimately lethal train of events and without which death would not have occurred. Whatever is listed as the underlying or proximate cause of death must be etiologically specific. In the case of fatal trauma this is usually self-evident. Contributory but non-causative factors may be listed in a separate area on the certificate if they serve to clarify the proximate cause. *Mechanism of death* refers to the physiological derangement—physical, biochemical, or functional—that triggers death, for example, exsanguination, electrolyte perturbation, or ventricular arrhythmia. With the notable exception of asphyxia, mechanism of death rarely appears on death certificates unless it serves in some way to explain the proximate cause of death. *Manner of death* is an opinion of the certifier as to how the death came about and typically there are 5 choices: natural, accident, suicide, homicide, or undetermined.

The Death Investigation

Presented with a fatally battered child, the task of the forensic pathologist is less diagnostic and more documentary in character. The autopsy is at times relegated to an ancillary role while the investigation of the scene of and circumstances surrounding an infant's or child's death becomes paramount. The death investigation is to the forensic pathologist what the history is to the clinician. As in clinical settings, the history taken from an adult who may also be the abuser must be put into proper perspective. Without the collaboration of all parties—emergency medical personnel, law enforcement, clinical child abuse specialists, radiologists, child protection workers, forensic pathologists, and prosecutors—such investigations are doomed to confusion and perhaps failure.

The development and promulgation of various standardized protocols for the investigation and autopsy of child deaths have enhanced the quality of child death investigation. The forensic pathologist relying solely on postmortem morphological or laboratory observations to properly assign manner and occasionally even cause of death will err at an unacceptably high rate. Lacking a multidisciplinary approach, the forensic pathologist may never even see all of the

evidence. Thus a homicidal asphyxia could be certified as sudden infant death syndrome (SIDS) or an accidental head injury could be ruled a homicide. The following is a case in point:

> **Case:** Paramedics responded to a call for an unresponsive infant at 10:30 am. On arrival they encountered an apneic, pulseless, mottled, cold, stiff 2-month-old male. No resuscitation efforts were initiated, but the body was transported by ambulance to the emergency department (ED), where he was pronounced dead at 10:45 am. History elicited from the infant's mother in the ED was that he had a respiratory illness the previous week. He was fussy at 4:00 am. An attempt at bottle-feeding was met with vomiting and the infant was placed prone in his crib. His mother found him unresponsive at approximately 10:00 am. A diagnosis of SIDS was rendered in the ED.

Interview of the mother by police and the medical examiner's death investigator yielded much the same information with the notable additions of a description of bright red fluid from the nostrils confirmed by inspection of the bedding. The mother confirms finding the infant cold and stiff at 10:00 am. She called her own mother, then called 911 at 10:30 am. The mother lived alone with the infant and described him as colicky.

A detailed examination of the apartment with the mother's consent later that morning revealed a notebook in plain view on the kitchen table with references to Charles Manson and Son of Sam and a handwritten note in large block letters stating, "KILL THE BOY." In the course of a long interrogation by police the mother admitted to holding the infant tightly against her chest until he stopped moving.

Gross autopsy, microscopic examination, skeletal survey, and ancillary laboratory studies were negative, save for bloody fluid from the nose and an odd abrasion over the vertex. The cause of death was certified as asphyxia due to smothering and the manner of death as homicide, based on the investigative data. Predictably, at trial the mother recanted her statement to police and defense council vigorously suggested the cause of death was SIDS. The mother was convicted of second-degree murder.

Requirements for Qualified Personnel

The need for qualified personnel begins at the scene of death if a child dies outside a hospital. Investigators working for coroners and medical examiners should have specific training in the approach to infant and child death investigation. Certification of investigators by the American Board of Medicolegal Death Investigators is optimal. The breadth of information to be obtained regarding the child's prenatal, birth, and postnatal medical history; environmental risk factors; family history; and sensitive re-creation of the circumstances of the death or discovery with the parent or caretaker requires more from an

investigator than the ability to fill out a checklist of standard questions.

Whether an area is served by a coroner or medical examiner, the examination of an infant or child who dies suddenly, unexpectedly, or violently is best performed by an experienced forensic pathologist, preferably one certified by the American Board of Pathology. If the death investigation is the history, the autopsy is the physical examination. The hospital pathologist, performing a very small number of autopsies annually and serving occasionally as a coroner's pathologist, lacks the necessary experience to recognize and interpret trauma and postmortem artifacts. A Canadian group has advocated for all sudden unexpected infant deaths to be autopsied "in centers with expertise in pediatric pathology,"[1] but this is unlikely to occur in the United States. Consultation with other specialists as the need arises is the mark of a diligent and thorough forensic examination. For example, trying to interpret healed and partially healed injuries without the input of the clinical child abuse pediatrician who followed the patient from admission to death is needlessly difficult. A pediatric radiologist should read the postmortem skeletal series and assist the forensic pathologist in his or her understanding of any antemortem radiologic studies. A neuropathologist with expertise in the developing brain is an invaluable resource. While such specialists do not exist in great numbers, establishing working relationships with available experts greatly enhances the pathologist's work.

Review of Records

The forensic pathologist rarely has the entire record prior to autopsy, but all available records should be reviewed before examining the body. The initial summary by the medical examiner investigator may provide important information regarding the scene, the basic background history regarding the child's past medical conditions, and the events leading to death. It is critical for the pathologist to obtain and review records from primary sources. These records should be obtained by whatever means are available to the coroner or medical examiner. It should be noted that medical examiners and coroners are specifically exempt from Health Insurance Portability and Accountability Act of 1996 restrictions if their request for records is in the normal course of their duties.[2] Hospital administrators and risk managers are often unaware of this exemption. A complete record review will include emergency run sheets, police reports, child protective services reports, and past medical records including birth records. A birth certificate may yield important information, such as both parents' names in some cases, other names for the mother of the child, and prior addresses. These data may lead to information, perhaps of forensic significance, such as previous police or social services interactions in the current or other jurisdictions.

Paramedics and emergency medical technicians should not be overlooked as a source of information. A personal interview by the death investigator or the forensic pathologist is recommended. Their impressions regarding the environment where the child was found, interactions with those at the scene, and specific details about the ease or difficulty with which lines and airways were or were not established can prevent the forensic pathologist from making interpretive errors that can damage credibility in legal proceedings. Notation of the presence of unusual items at the scene, including a plastic bag near the child, drug paraphernalia, or open medication containers, should be made. A recorded body temperature on transport, particularly low body temperatures, is extremely valuable to the forensic pathologist. This objective information may be important in time of death estimations or suggest specific issues such as sepsis, head injury, or even cold-water immersion.

Critical information is also contained in ED records and medical records from the hospital stay if the child was admitted. An infant who has multiple minor oral and facial abrasions or contusions observed prior to resuscitative efforts may have been smothered. Traces of blood in the nasopharynx and/or oropharynx may be another important but undocumented observation.

The first priority in the hospital setting is preservation of life, but detailed description and photodocumentation of all injuries should be done as soon as possible after stabilization. These images may be of critical importance if sufficient time has elapsed prior to death for healing or partial healing to occur. Timed and dated images can aid the forensic pathologist in interpreting findings at autopsy. Prior medical records and birth records are important to review to rule out organic contributors to death, including complications related to prematurity or preexisting disease. The child's primary medical provider may be able to give important information regarding prior concerns of abuse or neglect involving the deceased child or a sibling.

Law enforcement reports and witness statements should be reviewed by the forensic pathologist. These documents may add data that the forensic pathologist may not have otherwise considered. Detailed statements from caregivers regarding the physical state of the child in the hours and days to death are important in determining whether the child showed evidence of illness or injury. And as with all physical abuse investigations, a description by the caretaker who witnessed any trauma should be compared with the autopsy findings to look for inconsistencies in mechanism, forces, and timing of injury, or in the known developmental capabilities of the child.

Family History

Thorough questioning during the death investigation, and ideally to autopsy, will provide a verbal report regarding the child's and family's medical and social history that may be compared with the written record. Investigators or the pathologist should attempt to obtain detailed family history, including signs and symptoms of bleeding disorders, bone disorders or frequent fractures, metabolic diseases, sudden infant death, seizures, and other disorders that may help explain autopsy findings.

Significant illness and especially deaths of other siblings should be sensitively but methodically probed. For example, previous SIDS deaths raise the legitimate concern for serial infant suffocation[3] or, less likely, a rare metabolic disorder. Carpenter et al[4] reexamined this question and came to the conclusion that "repeat sudden infant deaths are most probably natural." Most forensic pathologists would likely share the cautious concern expressed by Bacon and DiMaio[5] in response to this recent study. Should a previous death have occurred involving very similar circumstances or the same caretaker, the index of suspicion may rise substantially. A previous infant death in the same family in another jurisdiction, perhaps under a different last name, will likely be missed by death investigators unless explicitly described by the caretakers.

Family members can also provide information regarding the child's history of signs and symptoms of bleeding, neurologic disease, developmental delays, and other conditions. While autopsy provides information about existing pathology in the child's body it is limited in its ability to test for many disorders diagnosable in the living child. Laboratory testing is necessarily limited and functional studies impossible, making the child's medical history and the family history more important.

Scene and Circumstance Investigation

The importance of thorough scene investigation was demonstrated by Bass et al[6] in 1986. Despite the flaws in the paper identified by experienced forensic and pediatric pathologists,[7,8] the paper revealed the wealth of potential information missed when the scene of death is not directly viewed by the death investigator. Twenty-six consecutive infant deaths certified by the New York City Office of Chief Medical Examiner as SIDS were independently investigated by the Bass group. A significant percentage of those yielded information suggesting the possibility of other, more specific causes of death. While the study raised ethical questions, no one today would deny the critical importance of the scene investigation.

> **Case:** A 6-week-old female went to stay overnight for the first time with her biological father. She had previously slept in a crib in her mother's home. The infant was found unresponsive on a mattress on the floor of the father's apartment. An unusual livor pattern under the chin matched the edge of a control knob of a stereo unit on the floor between the mattress and the wall. The father subsequently admitted to finding the infant wedged between the mattress and the stereo with her neck hyperextended and the stereo knob under her chin.

The scene should be investigated as soon as possible after death is reported. The environment, already altered by the discovery of the child and efforts to render aid prior to transport, is inevitably further altered either inadvertently or with the specific intent to obscure the circumstances of death. If necessary, dolls can be effectively used by a skillful investigator to assist the caretakers in re-creating the events in question,

including the precise location of certain events, as well as the location and position of the child as discovered.

In the case of infants in particular, in the absence of trauma, a well-performed and documented scene investigation is likely to be far more important in reaching a conclusion as to cause and manner of death than the autopsy alone. (See Chapter 21.)

No environmental observation can be considered insignificant until autopsy findings render it so. Guntheroth and Spiers[9] have outlined the role of thermal stress as an environmental risk factor. Moon et al[10,11] have pointed out the significance of a simple change in environment from home to child care. Their retrospective study of 1,916 SIDS cases over 10 years revealed 20.4% of deaths occurred in child care versus a 7% rate predicted by time spent by infants in out-of-home child care. Sixty percent of these were in noncommercial settings. Infants in child care were more likely to be placed or found prone, particularly when the usual sleep position was side or supine. Such a change for the supine-sleeping infant placed prone for the first time seems to dramatically heighten the risk of SIDS. A similar study by deJonge et al[12] in the Netherlands corroborated these findings.

Environmental cleanliness, safety hazards, pets, quantity and quality of food, the presence of drugs and/or unusual quantities of alcohol, and other factors may or may not prove important to the examining pathologist. The degree of danger of environmental hazard depends on the child's developmental capacity. Therefore the investigator should understand the basics of motor and cognitive development of infants and children.

Case: A 9-month-old female was heard "screaming hysterically" at 10:00 am. She quieted but was not physically checked until 5:30 pm, at which time she was found with her head wedged between the "frame" and "headboard" of an inflatable toddler bed placed on top of a mattress. When extricated she was noted to have a plume of pulmonary edema foam exuding from the mouth. A crib was available in the house, but she was perceived to have "slept better" in the toddler bed.

Case: A 6-month-old infant was found unresponsive and when first responders arrived they were presented with the infant prone in a crib. Death was evident and no resuscitation was attempted. The investigator questioned the caretakers based on observations of the pattern of livor on the infant's back, a rectangular pressure mark on his back, and a clearly faulty crib with a broken side rail. Caretakers subsequently admitted to having found the infant had slipped between the railing and mattress. Crying was not evident in that the infant's chest movement was severely restricted.

Observation and photographs of the scene help to recognize an implement used as a weapon inflicting patterned blunt impact or burn injuries on the body. The injuries may vary in age, but a consistent pattern suggests a specific object. Short falls of various types are common historical features in abuse cases. Photographs with orienting tape measures of the furniture or other surfaces from which the child might have fallen along with any obstacles they might have contacted during the fall are helpful. When there are cases of scald burns, the dimensions of any tub or sink implicated in the event should be documented. The height of the faucets, degree of strength or dexterity needed to operate them, the maximum hot-water temperature, and the time required to reach maximum temperature should be recorded. Similar principles apply to stoves and other hot surfaces, or objects claimed to be responsible for burns on a child.

Reconstruction of fatal events through an interview requires sensitivity. The medical death investigator is not an arm of law enforcement so this should be a medically oriented interview that is neutral and non-accusatory. For example, determining that an infant died while awake should alert the pathologist to the higher likelihood of significant cardiac pathology as the true cause of death.[13] When possible, all adults and verbal children in the company of the deceased in the hours preceding and at the time of death should be individually interviewed. Significant issues involving historical consistency and plausibility may emerge even in this initial stage of inquiry. Reenactment of events in alleged falls, scald burns, and other injuries may be consistent with observed injuries or be questionable based on pattern and distribution of injuries and/or developmental capability of the child.

Perhaps the reddest of historical red flags is the "shifting scenario" phenomenon. History "A" at the initial interview that becomes history "B" when autopsy findings are revealed that strongly correlated with abuse. Equally worrisome is the claimed total lack of knowledge as to how a child sustained a significant, common injury in cases ultimately proven to be abuse.

Injury Time Window

Establishing the probable time range for a child's injuries often is the responsibility of the forensic pathologist or clinical child abuse specialist. Doing so requires coordinating investigative, physical and, in fatal cases, autopsy findings. The initial window is established based on information about when the child was last known to be awake and alert. If there was a survival interval between injury and death, with treatment in the ED or hospital, these records should be reviewed. Gross and microscopic observations at autopsy may further help to narrow the time frame of injury based on the relatively predictable physiological sequence of events in tissue inflammation and repair. Subdural hematoma is a classic example in which good gross and microscopic documentation can fix the time of injury with a reasonable degree of scientific certainty.[14] Of note, these data are based on adult data, and may or may not reflect the resolution of subdural hematoma in infants and children.

There are limitations of investigative data and, to a lesser extent, medical and pathological evidence. A false history that reasonably accounts for the pattern and distribution of injuries in a child of appropriate development and fits the time frame in which the injury is believed to have occurred may go undetected unless refuted by an independent witness or confession. Anecdotal experience and a "hunch" or "bad feeling" about a given case should not be substituted for good evidence.

The Autopsy

Translated from its Greek roots *autos* (self) and *opsis* (sight), the autopsy is literally to "see for one's self." There is no substitute for the postmortem examination. Most autopsies in the United States are being done under the auspices of coroners' and medical examiners' offices. A hospital-based generalist is likely to be unfamiliar with the specialized requirements and interpretive issues posed by the forensic autopsy, especially that of a child. A forensic pathologist with pediatric autopsy experience is the individual best suited to perform this examination.

Given its critical role in the investigative process, a well-conducted and well-documented autopsy has the potential to move the inquiry forward or change its direction. Properly synthesizing information from the death scene and circumstances, record review, and the autopsy itself, the forensic pathologist may be able to opine whether death was due or contributed to by injury or neglect. The details on injury patterns can allow more critical assessment of the proffered history. The injuries can be placed in context with the timeline of the fatal incident developed by investigation, particularly if there was a delay in seeking treatment that cannot otherwise be explained. The autopsy may reveal remote or occult injury in addition to the injuries causing death, evidence of intoxicants or poisons, or the existence of metabolic disorders.

The importance of thorough documentation of the autopsy cannot be overemphasized. The forensic pathologist must communicate the results of the autopsy to a wide variety of individuals, such as other pathologists, clinicians, law enforcement personnel, attorneys, child protective workers, and the family itself. Photographic documentation should be extensive and organized with images captured in such a way as to clarify the narrative protocol. In addition to the "as is" images, injuries should be cleansed of surrounding blood and other distracters and photographed with and without a scale.

Identification

Without proper identification of the deceased, no homicide investigation can proceed. In most child abuse autopsies identification is not an issue, but in some cases of abandoned newborns and other neonaticides or fragmented, decomposed, mummified, or skeletonized remains, the forensic pathologist must rely on tools and consultation beyond the simple visual identification. Footprints of infants may be a starting point if there are antemortem prints on file at the hospital of birth. In older children, radiologic or dental identification may be possible provided there are adequate antemortem records for

comparison. Serologic markers and DNA analysis also can be used. In the absence of an antemortem DNA sample (perhaps from a hairbrush or toothbrush), this technology can be used to establish the relationship of the deceased child to a putative parent.

Time of Death Determination

Few issues are shrouded in more myth and lore than determining approximate time of death. Standard textbooks of forensic pathology[15-18] are sources of such information. The issue is significant in that an opinion as to time of death may implicate a specific caretaker when more than one is suspected, or may be used to refute a caretaker's story if discrepant. In adults, the anticipated sequence of early postmortem changes of rigor mortis, livor mortis, algor mortis, and ocular changes may be altered by a variety of environmental and antemortem physiological factors, rendering time of death an opinion subject to challenge. These same factors can more profoundly affect the body of a small child, and interpretive adjustments need to be made in rendering such opinions.

Rigor mortis is the postmortem stiffening of muscle. It is a passive phenomenon representing the spontaneous breakdown of adenosine triphosphate to adenosine diphosphate and resultant locking of actin/myosin filaments. It proceeds in all muscles at the same rate, but the process is completed in smallest muscles first. This gives the impression of a "march" down the body from the jaw and neck, where stiffness is detectable minutes after death, to the lower extremities. Once rigor is complete, the body remains stiff until decomposition begins to affect actin and myosin so that muscle returns to a flaccid state. This sequence can be slowed by hypothermia, cold environmental temperatures, and low total body muscle mass such as that seen in infants, children, debilitated persons, and the elderly. It may be accelerated by vigorous muscular activity (exercise, struggle, seizure), uremia, acidosis, electrocution, hyperpyrexia, and high environmental temperatures.

Livor mortis is the term for purple to purplish red discoloration of the body's dependent region due to postmortem settling of noncirculating blood. Livor remains fluid for several hours postmortem and then becomes fixed. This information is used in conjunction with the observed degree of rigor mortis to determine if rigor is on its upslope or downslope. *Algor mortis,* or the anticipated equilibration of body temperature with its surrounding environment, may be the least predictable of all the postmortem changes. This is particularly true in infants. Various formulae, nomograms, and algorithms for postmortem heat loss have been offered, but none is widely used routinely. Confounding variables include amount of body fat and clothing (insulation), active air currents, and body temperature at the moment of death (high or low). While a rectal temperature, whether recorded in the ED or at the death scene by an investigator, may be critical for other purposes, its utility in time of death estimates is limited.

Postmortem ocular changes consist of gradual corneal clouding to the point of virtual opacification by roughly 72 hours after death. This too can be altered by environment and must be considered in the context of all other observed postmortem changes. More objective, but still fraught with variable degrees of error, is the use of postmortem potassium concentrations in vitreous fluid.[19,20] In theory, 2 samples are drawn hours apart and the results plotted on a graph, whereupon an equation yields an approximate postmortem interval. This type of analysis is not widely used because of analytical difficulties posed by vitreous fluid and a lack of standards for the results. It should also be remembered that the most valuable observations of time of death–related changes are at the scene of death, not in the autopsy suite hours or even a day after initial discovery of the body.

Gastric content has been touted as another tool to assess time of death based on the assumption that gastric emptying time across the spectrum of ages is generally less than 2 hours. This, however, must be put in context by an accurate history of what and how much was eaten by the deceased; gastric emptying time is greatly influenced by the type and quantity of food as well as the baseline health of the individual. Ultimately, the forensic pathologist's time of death estimate is going to be framed by the window of when the child was last known to be alive and when he or she was found dead. In some cases, despite the diligent synthesis of all data collected, the window may not be able to be narrowed further.

In the case of long-dead remains, such as abandoned newborns and discarded bodies, the extent of decomposition is evaluated in the context of the environmental conditions. In the case of observable maggot, fly, or beetle activity, a forensic entomologist should be consulted to fix an approximate postmortem interval by analyzing the life stages of the insects. Occasionally the expertise of a qualified botanist can also help determine time of death. Skeletal remains require consultation with an experienced forensic anthropologist who cannot only provide accurate estimates of age and stature, but a systematic analysis of taphonomic changes to the skeleton that can be used to estimate a postmortem interval.[21]

Ultimately the forensic pathologist must not place too much emphasis on any single criterion. Time of death *estimates* require correlation of investigative and demonstrative evidence. Rigid adherence to set schemes and formulae lend a false sense of security and introduce the potential of a large degree of error.

Photography

Photographic images do not replace the narrative investigative report or autopsy protocol, but they should substantially augment and enhance these. Photographic documentation begins at the actual death scene. Typically a wide shot of the entire environment is followed by images of successively narrow focus ultimately depicting the body and any visible injuries. In the autopsy suite the first series of images are taken of the body as it is received. The body is then undressed and photographed again.

A third series of images is taken after the body is cleansed of blood, dirt, and other debris. Lastly, detailed photographs of individual injuries or groups of injures are taken with and without an orienting scale. A color guide may be a useful adjunct if bruises of varying color are depicted. A macro lens allowing one-to-one, close-range imaging is ideal.

Every effort should be made to keep distracting items out of photos, particularly detailed photos of the injuries. While digital technology allows for editing of images such as cropping extraneous background distractions, a well-constructed original is preferred for evidence. Much has been made of the ease of manipulation of digital images, but edits are internally tracked and a log can be generated. Ultimately the onus is on the expert witness, who must testify under oath that the images presented into evidence are a true and accurate representation of the findings as viewed at the time of autopsy.

At present, 35-mm and/or high-resolution digital imaging is the current standard for autopsy photography and should be routinely used in the clinical setting. Polaroid photographs do not offer the resolution and color balance of 35-mm images and make interpretation very difficult. A wide variety of specialized photographic techniques are available to the forensic pathologist to enhance the visualization of certain types of injuries, such as bite marks and older bruises. Ultraviolet (250–400 nm) light is absorbed by hemoglobin and melanin that migrate to the periphery of wounds. Infrared (700–960 nm) light is capable of penetrating below the skin surface and is absorbed by the blood.[22]

Radiologic Documentation

Clinicians have long known the markedly increased diagnostic sensitivity afforded by tightly collimated views of various anatomical regions as separate images—the skeletal survey. Except for fiscal restrictions, most coroners and medical examiners would welcome the option of obtaining separate views of the skull, chest, abdomen, and extremities. The standard survey as outlined by the American College of Radiology in conjunction with the National Association of Medical Examiners[23] is ideal, but the views delineated previously will serve reasonably well. Such images can guide the forensic pathologist in sampling specific metaphyseal injuries or spinal or digital fractures that would otherwise escape detection. Computed tomography (CT) and magnetic resonance imaging are used nearly exclusively in the clinical realm, particularly in the area of craniocerebral trauma, but the clinical images are useful adjuncts to the forensic pathologist, who consults with the pediatric neuroradiologic imaging specialist.

Clinical correlation is essential. Preautopsy images can guide sampling, but there are frequently instances of fractures discovered at autopsy that were not detected radiologically. These include acute, non-displaced rib and skull fractures and/or discrepancies in the interpretation of antemortem neuroradiologic images and gross autopsy findings, particularly in the area of sub-dural versus subarachnoid hemorrhages. Review of antemortem films becomes more important when there has been a significant survival interval, with changing radiologic findings, partial healing, and/or surgical treatment of injuries. Nowhere is this more important than in infants or children with head injuries.

Discovering the occasional radiodense foreign body in the airway, alimentary tract, or elsewhere represents time and resources well spent in obtaining a preautopsy skeletal survey. Such a finding and its recovery at autopsy may mean the difference between diagnosing an etiologically specific cause of death, such as asphyxia due to aspiration of a button battery, and certifying the death as undetermined.

Recovery of Evidence

It is rare that an investigator finds an unaltered child death scene. Even if not purposefully altered by an abuser, the scene is typically contaminated by the actions of the individual discovering the body or by resuscitative efforts at the scene. Paradoxically, the truly undisturbed scene on arrival of first responders may serve to raise concerns about the circumstances of the death given the regularity with which there is some effort on the part of those encountering the body to initiate resuscitation. Most fatal abuse takes place where the child normally resides or spends significant time. The other occupants of these spaces, child and adult, are inevitably among the "persons of interest" in such cases. Daily contact between the deceased and these other individuals all but negates Locard's principle of linking victim and perpetrator by documenting the transfer of trace evidence.

Transport to an ED and further resuscitative efforts introduce further contamination of evidence because lines and tubes are placed, clothing may be cut away, body surfaces washed, and diapers and clothing may be discarded. Nevertheless, seeking detailed information about the original appearance of the child, and recovery of all personal effects, falls to the professionals investigating the death. A direct interview with first responders and ED personnel may fill critical information gaps that may otherwise hover over a given case as "reasonable doubt."

Once in the custody of the forensic pathologist, clothing should be inspected for fabric defects, biological stains (vomit, feces, urine, blood, semen) and, in selected cases, trace evidence. Trace evidence should be labeled promptly after collection and proper identification and chain of custody need to be maintained at all times. Formula containers or other food items brought to the autopsy suite are inspected and, if appropriate, may be submitted for chemical and/or toxicological analysis. Should contamination within the original container of a commercial product such as formula or infant food be discovered, notification of appropriate local, state, and/or federal agencies, as well as the manufacturer of the product, should be made as soon as possible.

Documentation of Injuries

Injuries Related to Cardiopulmonary Resuscitation

Many children who succumb to injuries related to maltreatment have undergone some form of resuscitation. Questions arise during the investigation or during trial regarding the contribution of cardiopulmonary resuscitation (CPR) to the trauma documented at autopsy. Price et al[24] compared cases of fatal inflicted abdominal injury (n=33) with cases of death due to natural causes (n=324) in children up to 10 years old. Of the children dying of abdominal trauma, 73% received CPR. There was no difference in the nature or severity of injuries documented at autopsy when these cases were compared with homicide victims who had received no CPR. Even more compelling is the finding that only 4 of 324 children who died of natural causes sustained any injury attributable to resuscitation, and 3 of 4 injuries were minor. The fourth patient developed a life-threatening complication unrelated to chest compressions, which involved puncture of the underlying lung during central line placement.

Similar findings were noted by Bush et al,[25] who found that 7% of children dying of non-traumatic causes sustained CPR-related injuries. Notably, CPR was performed by laypersons in a large proportion of cases (47%). Chest wall abrasions and contusions were by far the most common injuries sustained and were observed in 50% of the children who were injured. Only 3% of children had complications that were potentially life-threatening, according to the

Kirschner et al[26] classification system. These included a "small" pneumothorax, epicardial hematoma, and pulmonary interstitial hemorrhage and hemoperitoneum. Bilateral rib fractures involving the sternochondral junction were identified in a single case: a 3-month-old infant who died of SIDS who had received 75 minutes of CPR by lay and professional rescuers. The anterior location of these fractures is in contrast to the classic posterior location of inflicted rib injuries. Other studies have similarly indicated that CPR-related rib fractures are uncommon and, when present, tend to be anterior in location.[27-30] The rarity of rib fractures in children contrasts sharply with the high incidence seen in adults receiving CPR. In their literature review, Hoke and Chamberlain[31] found a 13% to 97% incidence of rib fractures in adults receiving conventional CPR, but an incidence of only 0% to 2% in children.

While Ryan et al[27] found a much higher incidence of CPR-related injuries than the studies cited previously (42% of children resuscitated, with 20% sustaining more than one injury), their results confirmed the rarity of serious trauma, with no children sustaining life-threatening injury. Almost 70% of the injuries were cutaneous contusions or abrasions. Bruising after death is possible, at least while the blood is still fluid. Not surprisingly, postmortem injuries are most likely to occur within the first few hours of death.[32] Determining the antemortem versus postmortem natures of injuries can be extremely difficult and, at times, impossible. Robertson and Mansfield[33] considered the various criteria commonly used to distinguish these injuries and drew several conclusions.

1. A "very large" bruise is unlikely to have been caused after death, given the lack of blood pressure under these circumstances. However, the maximum possible size of a postmortem bruise is not known, and a "small" bruise may have occurred either antemortem or postmortem.
2. Postmortem disruption of blood vessels can lead to infiltration of tissues by extravasated blood, making this an unreliable parameter for judging whether the bruise was sustained antemortem or postmortem.
3. Abrasions can and do occur postmortem.
4. Color changes in a bruise indicative of hemolysis and degradation do not occur after death.
5. An absence of vital reaction on histopathologic examination does not preclude antemortem injury.
6. Changes to the injured tissues or to the regional lymph nodes may provide more information regarding the antemortem versus postmortem nature of a contusion than does the local reaction to the extravasated blood.

Cutaneous Injuries

One of the authors (JG) performed a detailed physical examination on a battered child in the intensive care unit, documenting several cutaneous injuries and assuming all had been identified. The child was declared brain dead later that morning, and at autopsy the next day at least 3 or 4 additional contusions were noted on the scalp and back, once the head hair had been shaved and strong lamps and a magnifying glass had been used to inspect the body. Medical equipment, less than optimal room lighting, and limited patient mobility can significantly hinder the external examination of a living child.

The location, size, color, and shape of contusions and abrasions should be documented. Several studies of cutaneous injuries in abused and non-abused pediatric populations have repeatedly demonstrated that the distribution of injuries differs significantly.[34] Very few cutaneous injuries are noted on young, nonmobile, non-abused children,[35-37] which is in contrast with young children dying of inflicted trauma. Of 24 cases of fatal inflicted head injury involving infants and young children (mean age 9 months), 71% had "new" external bruises and 63% had "old" bruises.[38] Mobile non-abused children tend to incur accidental cutaneous trauma to the anterior aspect of the body, primarily over bony prominences, with the forehead, shins, and forearms absorbing the brunt of the injuries. They infrequently injure areas of the body ordinarily protected, such as the trunk, neck, soft portion of the cheeks, inner thighs, and buttocks.[35-37,39] In contrast, abused children often show injuries in these areas.

There is scant literature addressing the relative size of contusions and abrasions on abused versus non-abused children.[37,39] However, there is evidence to suggest that abused children tend to have larger cutaneous bruises than children sustaining their trauma through accidental means. Dunstan et al[40] used the maximum dimension of contusions from specific body locations to design a scoring system that successfully discriminated between abused and non-abused children. Depending on the score threshold used, specificity was as high as 99% (with sensitivity somewhat lower at 69%–77%).

Patterned injuries are those that have a shape that partially replicates the edges of the impacting object. They are common in abused children and uncommon in non-abused children. In their study of children aged 1 to 14 years, Dunstan et al[44] found pattern contusions in 57% of abused children and only 2% in those who had not been abused. Patterned injuries are significant and should be described and photographed at autopsy, with measurements not only of bruised areas but of intervening spared skin, and indications of regular spacing, curved versus straight edges, and the existence of angles. This will help in later comparisons with possible weapons retrieved by scene investigation. It is not unusual to have bruising that is detailed enough to replicate the idiosyncrasies of a belt or kitchen utensil. Photographs should include a "location" shot that includes an obvious body part to clarify where the injury lies, as well as one or more close-up shots to highlight detail. To compare injury dimensions with the suspected object used to inflict the injury, it is important to obtain photographs with the lens held parallel to the injury to minimize distortion. Photographs of injuries should include a measurement device (placed in the plane of the injury) and a color strip. When possible (facial injuries being a notable exception), external description of the injury should be followed by a vertical incision into the skin and subcutaneous tissue to document the depth of the bleeding. The scalp should be examined carefully because injuries here are common and may be subtle. Shaving parts of the scalp to better visualize contusions, abrasions, and other injuries should be considered.

In children with dark skin, extensive bruising may be difficult to discern, especially over the buttocks. The autopsy should include one or more incisions into the back, buttocks, posterior thighs, and upper arms to look for very subtle soft tissue hemorrhage. This is often performed at the end of the autopsy, when most of the blood has been drained from the body. Even children with very pale skin may have subtle bruises that are easily overlooked if lighting is inadequate or the external examination is hasty. Bruising to the posterior aspect of the body, especially the buttocks, is suspicious for inflicted injury as these areas are not usually involved in typical accidental trauma sustained by young children.[35,36,39–41] Finally, the skin should be re-examined 24 hours after the autopsy to detect subtle injuries that may have been missed initially. It is not unusual for very slight, relatively pale cutaneous contusions and abrasions to become visible after blood drainage at autopsy and extended refrigeration of the body.

While skin lacerations are relatively unusual in non-accidental trauma, it is important to accurately identify and describe them too, distinguishing them from incised wounds. Lacerations are the result of splitting of soft tissue from blunt-force trauma and typically involve soft tissues overlying bone (very commonly the scalp). Lacerations differ from incised and stab wounds—injuries related to sharp-force trauma—in that they show tissue bridging within the wound (tiny strands of preserved tissue that bridge the gap between lacerated edges) and typically have abraded edges with varying degrees of bruising. There is undermining of the injury edges, the degree and direction of which depends on the angle of the delivering force.[17,42] Descriptions of a laceration should include its location, dimensions, the degree of abrasion/contusion of the edges, and the direction and degree of undermining.

Incised and stab wounds are caused by sharp-edged objects, the former representing wounds that are longer than they are deep, and the latter involving wounds that are deeper than they are long.[46] These sharp-force injuries lack abraded edges, tissue bridging, and undermining of wound margins, making them distinguishable from lacerations (blunt-force trauma). Again, location, size, and description of edges are important. Measurement should occur with the wound in its resting state, but also when the margins are gently re-approximated so as to eliminate gaping from naturally occurring tension within the skin. One should also determine the depth of the wound (including the organs involved) and its direction (eg, a stab wound to the chest may be directed left to right, and downward.)

Samples of cutaneous injuries should be obtained for histopathologic examination. This allows estimates of injury age and, in some cases, determinations that injuries are of different ages. Histologic dating has distinct limitations, as do all other methods of injury dating, but it can provide helpful information to the pathologist and to investigators. Details of histologic changes occurring during the healing phase follow.

Bite Marks

Documentation of bite mark injuries deserves special mention because this type of cutaneous injury has the potential to aid significantly in the investigation by eliminating or implicating potential perpetrators. Bite marks are unusual but certainly not rare injuries in fatal child abuse, and may be identified anywhere on the child's body. They may be classic in their appearance— 2 areas of interrupted marks oriented toward one another—or they may be relatively distorted and difficult to accurately identify. They may be in the form of abrasions (from teeth crushing the child's skin or being drawn across the skin in parallel linear abrasions), contusions (from disruption of small blood vessels within the dermis and/ or subcutaneous tissue), or even small lacerations. One may often see combinations of these blunt injuries. There may be central bruising composed of clustered or confluent petechiae related to suction of the child's skin within the mouth of the biter and compression of the skin against the biter's palate (Figure 20.1).

The common practice of measuring the intercanine distance and assuming that a value greater than 3 cm indicates an adult jaw is unreliable and may lead to serious error. A forensic odontologist may be able to make a more reliable estimate by measuring the size of individual teeth to determine if the biter was an adult or a child. Establishing whether the biter was a human or other animal is relatively straightforward. Human bite marks form a circle or shallow oval, whereas those from household animals (those typically blamed for bites) have a narrow, deep U-shape. The teeth of an animal also are more likely to penetrate the skin than are the relatively blunt teeth of a human.

It is important that professionals evaluating a fatally injured child in the intensive care unit describe and photograph possible bite marks immediately, rather than assuming the child will be declared brain dead within a few hours and deferring examination to the medical examiner at autopsy. Frequently the decision to remove life support is

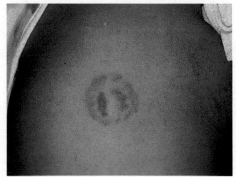

FIGURE 20.1
Child with well-demarcated bite mark. Note the individual bruises corresponding to teeth and the central bruises related to suction applied by the biter.

delayed by hours to a few days, and the bite marks are likely to become blurred and/or faded over time as the contusions spread out and begin healing. It also is important to obtain swabs of the bite marks for potential DNA recovery from saliva.

Photographs are extremely important in bite-mark documentation, and the expertise of a forensic odontologist may prove helpful. Photographs should be obtained from multiple angles, especially if the bite mark is located on a markedly curved surface such as the child's arm. This allows compensation for potential distortion related to a non-flat surface. Camera angles should be determined by attempting to obtain perpendicular views of all aspects of the curved injured surface. Lighting is critical and side lighting allows subtle indentations within the bite mark to be identified. A ruler should be positioned in the plane of the injury and should include measurements in 2 dimensions (American Board of Forensic Odontology ruler). This mitigates distortion along either the x-axis or y-axis related to slight variations in camera angle.

If the pathologist intends to consult a forensic odontologist, he or she should communicate with that person before beginning the dissection at autopsy so that arrangements can be made for impression molds to be obtained without artifactual distortion of the bite mark related to proximal incisions.

Burns

Inflicted trauma accounts for a minority of burns seen in pediatric patients,[43–46] with estimates ranging from less than 1%[47] to 28%[48] of patients seeking medical attention, which reflects differences in populations studied, criteria used for identifying abuse, and types of burns studied (all types vs tap-water scald burns). Advances in medical care have significantly improved the chances of survival.[49]

At the time of the autopsy, the pathologist should document all injuries carefully, including taking photographs of the body in the anatomical position, and with repositioning of the child the way he or she was thought to have been at the time of injury. Parts of the scalp may need to be shaved to assess the extent and borders of head burns.

If the child survived for a significant period after the injury, the autopsy may be considerably less helpful in injury documentation. Commonly resuscitation and the body's widespread inflammatory response to the burn leads to massive third spacing of fluids with severe edematous changes. Surgical debridement, with biomembrane placement or grafting, will change the appearance of the burns. Healing will have intervened, as may have secondary progression of the burn from hypotension, sepsis, and/or wound infection. Nonetheless, liberal sampling for histopathologic examination should be performed, and such analysis may aid in ascertaining the depth of injury (full vs partial thickness) and the burn age.[50] Discussion of wound age estimation by histologic methods is described later in the chapter, but one should keep in mind the many factors that may affect progression of inflammatory changes, especially in a child experiencing massive body burns, with their associated complications.

Contact Burns

The need for adequate documentation, including photographs, detailed measurements of the burned and spared areas, as well as histopathologic sampling of injuries at the time of autopsy, cannot be overemphasized. It is much easier to obtain careful measurements and photographs at the time of autopsy than it is when the child is awake and moving, or comatose but immobilized by extensive medical equipment.

Flame Burns

Fatal flame burns are typically associated with accidental house fires, and the circumstances may be related to severe caretaker neglect. Elaborate description of postmortem findings in these cases is beyond the scope of this chapter and is described in detail in various forensic textbooks.[17,32,42] However, a few points are worth mentioning. Most victims of house fires ultimately succumb to smoke inhalation rather than fatal burns.[51] The burns one sees at autopsy may well have occurred after death, and gross distinction between antemortem and postmortem burns can be very difficult. Histologic evidence of significant inflammation establishes a pre-mortem injury, but the absence of an inflammatory reaction does not rule it out because death may have occurred before the reaction. Extensively charred bodies may develop changes that can be mistaken for pre-mortem injuries. These include skull fractures from steam pressure within the skull, skin rupture from

contraction of hot skin, bony fractures of extremities from shrinking of the musculature, and epidural "heat hematomas" related to blood and marrow originating in the skull bones.

Estimating the Age of Injury With Histopathology

Estimating the timeframe of injury using histopathologic methods is potentially valuable although, as with all other methods, it has limitations and only a range of inexact time can be estimated. Several factors influence the process of inflammation and wound healing, including the age and health of the child, the type and location of the injured tissue involved, the size of the wound and its nature (laceration vs contusion), blood flow to the injured region, and the ability of the body to mount a response. The inflammatory response can continue during a child's resuscitation if perfusion continues and cells remain alive. One must also consider the ability of some inflammatory cells to function for several hours after "death" (eg, leukocytes survive for hours and can marginate after "death") and fibroblasts may survive for days.[17] Much of the research published regarding wound healing considers injuries of the skin (often incised wounds) or of the central nervous system (CNS) and is performed on animals. This must be kept in mind when extrapolating information to other types of injuries involving other organ systems. Nonetheless, there are some general guidelines to consider when the pathologist evaluates wounds and evidence of associated inflammation, and these help establish broad timeframes for the trauma.[17,32,42,52,53]

Initial 4 hours after injury: Fresh hemorrhage, fibrin deposition; margination of leukocytes within blood vessels (this can appear within minutes); and appearance of a few extravascular polymorphonuclear leukocytes, mostly in the perivascular region. Existing tissue histiocytes begin to show reactive changes.

4 to 12 hours after injury: Leukocyte infiltration, primarily polymorphonuclear (per Betz,[52] most wounds will show this after 15 hours). Macrophages are typically not evident until after approximately 12 to 15 hours. Edema of the tissues is seen. There may be swelling of vascular endothelium. Fibroblasts become reactive.

12 to 24 hours: Increasing infiltration of leukocytes (granulocytes and macrophages). Fibroblasts may show mitotic activity. A peripheral wound zone is demarcated by the inflammatory cells.

24 to 72 hours: Fibroblast infiltration may begin, especially toward the end of this period. Necrotic tissue is apparent and the ground substance may take on a bluish tinge.

3 to 6 days: Granulation tissue becomes apparent, with neovascular and fibroblast proliferation, collagen deposition, and the appearance of giant cells in areas of foreign debris. The Perls test for hemosiderin becomes positive after about 72 hours (some studies suggest a shorter interval and in many cases, the reaction may be delayed beyond 3 days). Erythrophages begin to appear.

1 week to several months: Hematoidin may be seen after approximately 8 days.

Spot-like lymphocyte infiltrations may be seen within this period. Eventually the inflammatory infiltration subsides, as does the neovascularization. Fibroblasts continue to produce collagen and gradually a scar is formed. Eventually the scar becomes relatively avascular and heavily fibrosed.

A few caveats should be kept in mind.

- A small contusion may not ever develop a significant cellular inflammatory response if tissue damage is slight.[32] This does not necessarily mean that the injury occurred immediately before the child's death or in the early postmortem period.
- Wound infection can substantially alter the timing of the inflammatory response.
- Red blood cell hemolysis may be patchy and irregular, with cells remaining intact for many days. Thus rupture of these cells is an unreliable indicator of injury age.[17]

Betz[52] studied progressive inflammatory reactions to human skin lacerations and surgical and stab/cut wounds in adults (contusions were not included) using histopathologic and histochemical evaluation. Results of this study are summarized in Table 20.1. Along with a thorough literature review, Betz goes on to make several important points that should be kept in mind when attempting to estimate the age of an injury involving any organ.

- Positive findings (eg, the presence of a given cell type or other reactive change) help estimate the minimum age of an injury. Negative findings are much less helpful because the absence of a given phenomenon may be related to methodological factors (eg, sampling error), individual variation, or any number of confounding factors that delay wound healing.

- The literature shows wide variation in some parameters of wound age estimation, and some of this variation may be due to differences in definition of a phenomenon and/or criteria for a "positive" finding (eg, a few macrophages vs a definite infiltrate). The pathologist should base age estimates on an unambiguous detection of the reactive change.

- Studying cell populations within areas of hemorrhage can be misleading because passive accumulation of cells ordinarily residing in the blood vessels (granulocytes, macrophages, and lymphocytes) can occur in postmortem injuries. Therefore attention should be paid to cell infiltrates *outside* the areas of hemorrhage.

- Betz[52] found a marked variability in the time required for macrophages to predominate over neutrophils within the inflammatory infiltrate. This variability continued until 12 days posttrauma, when all wounds had made this transition. Therefore this ratio seems to be of limited usefulness, especially in wounds that are relatively recent.

- Hematoidin pigment was seen only infrequently within wounds, limiting its use as an estimate of wound age.

- Similarly, "spot-like" lymphocyte infiltrates were not regularly seen, although their presence outside the area of hemorrhage suggested a wound age of at least 8 days.

- Using "time to completion of re-epithelialization" as an age estimate depends on the size of the skin defect and applies to "standardized epidermal defects" (including surgically treated and primarily healing wounds), so that this parameter cannot be used on abrasions of different size. In his study, Betz[52] found the minimum interval to complete re-epithelialization was 5 days; all wounds had re-epithelialized by 21 days.

TABLE 20.1

Age Estimation of Human Skin Wounds by Histologic Examination[a]

Histologic Parameter	Earliest Appearance	Time of Regular Appearance
Neutrophils	20–30 min	>15 h
Macrophages	3 h	>15 h
Macr/gran ratio[b]	20 h	>11 d
Siderophages/hemosiderin	3 d	>7 d
Hematoidin	8 d	Many never positive
Increased fibroblasts	25 h	≥6 d

[a]Adapted from Betz P. Histological and enzyme histochemical parameters for the age estimation of human skin wounds. *Int J Legal Med.* 1994;107:60–68.
[b]Ratio of macrophages to granulocytes within inflammatory infiltrate.

Estimating the age of a contusion may be more difficult than a laceration. In their analysis of commonly used methods of distinguishing antemortem versus postmortem injuries, Robertson and Mansfield[33] suggested that extravasated blood may not be a strong irritant to surrounding tissues so may not incite a strong reaction. This was supported by their finding that some cutaneous bruises several days old showed relatively little inflammatory reaction, although macrophage ingestion of erythrocytes was observable.

There is evidence to suggest that histopathologic evaluation may be more useful in estimating the age of abrasions than contusions.[53] This should be kept in mind when the pathologist is sampling injuries consisting of abraded contusions. Fortunately this type of combined injury is not at all uncommon. Table 20.2 summarizes histologic stages of healing within abraded skin.

Fractures

The evaluation of fractures at the time of autopsy involves several steps.[54] A skeletal survey should be performed, preferably using a standard protocol implemented for surveys in living children and encompassing the views recommended by Kleinman.[55] The survey should be interpreted by a pediatric radiologist whenever possible. The importance of this radiographic evaluation cannot be overemphasized. If a child with suspected abuse dies at a children's hospital, serious consideration should be given to having the child undergo a formal skeletal survey (with staff radiologist interpretation) before the body is transported to the medical examiner's office. A good skeletal survey can alert the pathologist to fractures that otherwise may be overlooked. This is especially true for long-bone fractures since standard autopsy procedure does not involve careful dissection of all long bones, and some radiographically identified fractures (confirmed by histology) may be invisible at the time of gross autopsy even when the area is exposed by dissection.[56]

At autopsy, the pathologist should evaluate the rib cage very carefully, looking for evidence of hemorrhage and/or callus formation. Hyperemia and edema may be noted if the fracture is recent.[54] Hemorrhage at the fracture site may persist for 3 to 4 weeks[54] so it is not necessarily an indication of extremely recent injury. Connective tissue callus bridging the fracture site may be seen within days. In fact, the pathologist may be able to palpate a healing rib fracture before it is identifiable on radiograph.[56] While it is tempting to use the size of the callus in one's estimation of injury timing, it is important to note that callus size does not correlate with injury age. The callus is fibrocartilaginous in its early stages, only becoming bony later in the process. Thus a callus that is easily sliced with a scalpel is indicative of a more recent injury.

Rib fractures should be described noting location and gross appearance and photographed in situ. Photographs should include a view of the entire hemithorax as well as one or more close-up views of the fracture site. The area of fracture should be resected and this specimen

TABLE 20.2
The Histology of Healing Skin Abrasions

Finding	Earliest Appearance	Clearly Visible
Stage 1: Scab* Formation		
Perivascular infiltration of neutrophils	2 h	4–6 h
Zone of neutrophils below abrasion surface		8 h
Abrasion has 3 visible layers		12 h
1: surface zone of red blood cells/fibrin or crushed epithelium		
2: infiltrating neutrophils		
3: damaged collagen)		
Zone of damaged collagen clearly demarcated from underlying healthy collagen		48 h
Stage 2: Epithelial Regeneration		
Early epithelial regeneration seen at edges of abrasion and in hair follicles (clear cells)	24 h	48 h
Layer of epithelial cells begins growing below scab[a]	30 h	3 d
Complete epithelial regenerative layer below scab	Day 4–5	
Stage 3: Subepidermal Granulation		
Granulation tissue seen below scab		5–8 d
Subepithelial repair and epithelial hyperplasia most prominent; new collagen seen		9–12 d
Stage 4: Regression		
Decrease in epidermal and dermal cellular activity		~12 d
Epithelium becomes atrophic		After 12 d

Adapted from Robertson I, Hodge PR. Histopathology of healing abrasions. *Forensic Sci.* 1972;1:17–25.
[a]A scab consists of red blood cells, fibrin, infiltrating leukocytes, damaged collagen, and necrotic epithelium.

photographed and radiographed (alternatively, repeat radiographs of the thoracic cavity after evisceration may be obtained). The pathologist should resect suspicious areas for further evaluation. Skeletal survey is much less sensitive than specimen radiography and histology in identifying fractures. In their study of 31 infants dying with inflicted skeletal injuries, Kleinman et al[57] found that specimen radiography substantially increased the yield of detected fractures (92% vs 58%), and much of this difference was due to improved recognition of rib fractures. Skeletal survey was especially poor at detecting fractures of the rib heads and the costochondral junction.

Resected bone fragments should be fixed in formalin prior to histologic examination. They may need to be decalcified to avoid distortion and artifactual disruption while cutting through calcified bone. Sections may be stained with hematoxylin-eosin; special staining for collagen may also be used.

For other types of fractures, a similar process is recommended. Skeletal survey will almost always be needed to identify fractures outside the axial skeleton because the extremities are not routinely dissected to the bone at the time of autopsy and external indications of fractures are unusual. However, incisions in the soft tissues of the upper arms and the lower extremities may reveal deep soft tissue bruising, which may indicate an underlying fracture. Again, areas of fracture should be resected, photographed, radiographed, and examined histologically.

One of the most important advantages to histopathologic evaluation of suspected bony fractures is to estimate the age of the injury. Timing of trauma is critical to a child abuse investigation, yet most of the techniques used in clinical medicine give poor estimates of injury age. For example, Prosser et al[58] performed a literature review to examine the evidence for radiologic dating of fractures in children. They concluded that the evidence base for radiologic dating practice is scant. Further, radiologic estimates of injury age are made in terms of weeks, not days. For example, periosteal reaction may be seen as early as 4 days after trauma and is present in at least 50% of cases by 2 weeks. However, this also implies that a sizable number of cases show no periosteal reaction by 2 weeks, making the range of possible injury age fairly large. In addition, there are problems generalizing study results to abused children.

Many studies lack patients in the relevant age group, and most studies involve children with casted (immobilized) fractures so do not address the influence of movement and repeated trauma on the healing process.

Histology offers another method to estimate fracture age[54,56] and is especially useful if the information gathered from this technique is used in conjunction with that obtained through other means, such as radiographic evaluation, clinical history, and gross examination at autopsy. In some cases, histopathologic estimates are more precise than radiographic ones.[56] Histopathologic dating of injuries is not without its limitations, however. As Zumwalt and Hirsch[54] point out in their literature review of fracture age estimation, the information regarding infant rib fractures is limited. Much of that information is based on animal models, human birth injuries, and extrapolation from adult data. The latter practice should be undertaken with caution because it is thought that infant fractures heal more rapidly than adult injuries since immature bone is more osteogenically active, and remodeling is faster when skeletal growth has not stopped.

Given limitations in the research on fracture repair, the healing process has been described and crude estimates of age may be made.[54,56] Immediately after the injury, there will be bleeding from torn blood vessels at and near the fracture site. Re-bleeding may occur with movement of the fractured bone. Hemorrhage, fibrin deposition, acute inflammation, and necrosis of the injured bone and marrow develop within the first few weeks. Osteolytic activity (breakdown of bone) is usually seen within 4 to 7 days. Osteoblasts may be identified within 2 to 4 days and new bone may be seen within 5 to 10 days of injury, continuing for weeks to months. The initial granulation tissue (callus) that begins to appear within 5 to 7 days of injury consists of osteoblasts, osteoclasts, fibroblasts, chondroblasts, and neovasculature. The callus will develop cartilage so that the initial bridge between fracture fragments is fibrocartilaginous; this bridge will eventually become bony (the union of the fracture). The new bone is laid down over preexisting bony trabeculae. Based on data regarding growth rate of fiber and lamellar bone, experienced osteopathologists may be able to estimate the age of a fracture in part by looking at the width of new trabeculae. Remodeling, which involves replacement of the woven bone by both lamellar bone and medullary cavity, gradually restores normal bone to the site of injury. This is a long process that begins relatively early in the repair process and continues for months to years.

Thoracic Injuries

Children with major intrathoracic inflicted injuries may present in a variety of ways. While cardiac rupture with tamponade or exsanguination may occur rapidly in some cases, in others perforation is delayed and symptoms may occur hours or days later. Myocardial contusions may gradually evolve to transmural necrosis and eventual perforation or aneurysm formation.[59] Significant cardiac injury may be accompanied by no external signs of trauma and a normal initial cardiac examination.

Because intrathoracic trauma may be unexpected at the time of autopsy, care must be taken even when opening the chest wall. A lacerated intercostal vessel may be the cause of a major hemothorax. Traumatically fractured ribs must not be confused with iatrogenically fractured ones. The dissection of the heart must include careful inspection of all chambers and examination of the junction of the vena cava with the right atrium. Traumatic interventricular septal defect is rare[59] but should be excluded. Lacerations to the pericardial sac should be identified and differentiated from iatrogenic incisions. Injuries should be sampled liberally for histologic evaluation. This may be critical in determining whether a perforation was acute and affecting normal myocardium or delayed and secondary to contusion necrosis. As described elsewhere in this chapter, limited information regarding injury timing may be obtained from examination of the degree and nature of the inflammatory infiltrate.

In rare cases of fatal inflicted cardiac injury, there may be no sign of trauma to the heart. This is seen in cases of commotio cordis (also called *cardiac concussion*). While this type of injury typically occurs in young people engaging in sports,[60] it has been described in physical abuse as well, although rarely.[61] There may or may not be evidence of cutaneous chest wall injury; Maron et al[60] found minor abrasions or contusions over the precordium in 12 of 22 pediatric commotio cordis cases. Thorough examination of the heart reveals no evidence of clinically significant disease, and no trauma to the myocardium, valves, or coronary arteries. The proposed mechanism involves induction of a lethal ventricular dysrhythmia by a sudden blow to the precordium that occurs at an electrically vulnerable time during the cardiac cycle.

Abdominal Injuries

Most significant abdominal injuries in young children are not abusive. In one study of children younger than 6 years, only 26% of those admitted with abdominal injuries were felt to have been abused. In turn, major intra-abdominal injury is a relatively uncommon form of physical abuse,[62] representing fewer than 0.5% of cases of abuse requiring hospital admission in one study.[63] However, this type of trauma carries a high mortality rate. In the latter study, 45% of the abuse victims died of their injuries. A significant number of children who succumb to inflicted abdominal trauma are never brought for medical attention, or are brought only when in extremis and beyond rescue.[24] Thus in many cases the autopsy is the only source of medical information regarding the child's fatal injury. There may have been no opportunity to obtain pre-mortem laboratory testing, physical examination, or monitoring of pre-death events. This makes the gross autopsy all the more important because it may be the only opportunity to answer key questions of the investigation. Careful and thoughtful dissection of the abdominal organs is very impor-

tant. A precise description of injury location and type, as well as evidence of inflammation and healing, is critical.

Case: A 3-year-old female collapsed on the way home from child care and was immediately rushed to the nearby hospital, but was unable to be resuscitated. She had complained of abdominal pain when greeted by her mother and had seemed weak and listless. Autopsy revealed a full-thickness laceration of the proximal small bowel in the region of the ligament of Treitz, as well as "extensive laceration of the transverse mesocolon." No further description of the mesocolonic laceration was provided and photographs added little to the description. "Brownish-red fluid was noted in the peritoneal cavity (volume unspecified)."

In determining the mechanism of death, and providing some information to investigators about the timing of the injury and likelihood of associated symptoms, vital information has been omitted. How large was the small bowel laceration? Was it a small perforation or near-complete transection? What, if any, blood vessels were lacerated within the transverse mesocolon? Careful dissection of the lacerated mesocolon may have revealed a transection of the middle colic artery, a relatively large vessel that would likely have bled profusely. On the other hand, the mesocolon could have been extensively lacerated without interruption of a major blood vessel, resulting in only limited bleeding. Approximately how much fluid was noted in the peritoneal cavity and did it appear to be predominantly blood or a mixture of bowel contents and inflammatory exudate? Was pus visible on the serosa of abdominal organs? This type of information helps determine the relative roles of exsanguination and peritonitis with sepsis in the mechanism of death and whether the time interval between injury and collapse was likely to have been short or more prolonged, and perhaps provides clues regarding the child's likely symptomatology during the period before death.

In most cases the autopsy cannot definitively answer questions about time of death and the antecedent clinical presentation. Children with similar abdominal injuries may have markedly different clinical courses. The gross and histologic evaluations provide additional information but are not a panacea for investigators.

Sometimes a child dies of inflicted trauma after a prolonged hospital admission, well after undergoing extensive resuscitation and abdominal surgery. In these cases, the potential for the autopsy to provide key information may be limited. The injured tissue may have been resected during emergency surgery; there may have been substantial interval healing and resolution; and complications of surgery (adhesions, inflammation, secondary infection) may make visualization and dissection difficult, if not impossible. In such cases, the pathologist should try to examine the specimens resected during the initial surgery, both grossly and microscopically. Gross specimens are fixed in formalin and retained by the hospital

pathology department for varying periods and are often available for review by the medical examiner. Histologic slides are retained for many years. Consultation with the pediatric pathologist who initially examined the specimen may prove invaluable since that person viewed the injured tissue prior to formalin fixation and may even have had the opportunity to view it in situ.

If the child had any antemortem medical intervention, the pathologist should review related reports and correlate the findings with those of the autopsy. Emergency medical services and ED records may provide key information regarding the child's presentation. Liver function tests and amylase and lipase levels (and trends) may suggest liver and pancreatic injury, respectively. Postmortem measurement of these enzymes is not helpful because changes occur rapidly after death.[42] Abdominal and pelvic CT scans may help direct the dissection, although significant injury may not be identifiable.[64]

In most cases, external examination of the abdominal wall will show no cutaneous bruising.[24,65] Fatal cases of abdominal trauma may be more likely to show abdominal wall bruising than nonfatal ones. Price et al[24] found such bruising in 42% of fatal cases, which is a rate far greater than the author (JG) has seen among surviving victims of inflicted abdominal trauma. The low rate of cutaneous injury with significant abdominal trauma may be related to a number of factors. The child's thin abdominal wall may be somewhat protected by clothing, and the lack of underlying bone allows the tissue to distort considerably, transmitting the force of the blunt impact to the underlying organs. In addition, the blow may be delivered over a relatively large surface area, making focal skin injury less likely. However, in some cases bruising is seen and it may be quite prominent, especially if the blood has tracked far from the site of vessel disruption. Occasionally blood may track through the inguinal canal and accumulate in the scrota or labia.[17] This should not be confused with local trauma to the genitalia. Abrasions to the abdominal wall are unusual but may occur if a rough surface such as the sole of a shoe contacts bare skin, either perpendicularly (crushing the epidermis) or tangentially (scraping it).

Inflicted abdominal injuries often involve structures in the central upper abdomen, including duodenum, pancreas, and jejunum.[17] The liver is often involved[24,66,67] and this may be related to its large size, prominent location in the right upper quadrant, and limited ability to compress in response to external trauma. Anatomy in the young child may contribute to the distribution of injuries. The costal margins are widely flared and the abdominal musculature relatively thin, allowing protuberance of the internal organs and affording little protection from external trauma. Also important is the relatively narrow anteroposterior diameter of the abdomen.[66] A blow to the abdomen, typically involving a punch or kick, causes sudden distortion of the abdominal wall and underlying abdominal structures, displacing them posteriorly. If enough force is applied, structures may be compressed against the vertebral column.

Compressive, tensile, and shear stresses associated with crushing, rapid deceleration of mobile structures, and differential movement of adjacent tissues lead to solid and hollow organ lacerations and contusions and disruption of vascular structures. The latter may reside within the mesenteric structures, elsewhere in the peritoneal cavity, on the posterior abdominal wall, or within the end organ itself.

Solid organ injuries involving the liver, spleen, and kidney are more common than hollow viscus trauma in abused children,[68,69] but small bowel and mesenteric injuries are often seen. The stomach is much less commonly injured, although such trauma is described,[70] and affected children are typically at risk because of a stomach distended by food and/or air. Forceful compression of the bowel mesentery against the vertebral column or sudden displacement and shearing stress may lead to laceration and contusion of this tissue. Large mesenteric blood vessels may be torn, leading to brisk and life-threatening bleeding. Alternatively, vessels may be injured and thrombose, leading to gradual ischemia and necrosis of bowel supplied by that vessel. Ultimately the necrotic bowel may perforate and set into motion the lethal complications of peritonitis and overwhelming sepsis. Mesenteric injury typically occurs toward the intestinal margin of the membrane.[17,64] At times the lacerations are multiple and leave a "shredded" appearance to the mesentery. Pancreatic trauma may lead to chemical peritonitis and widespread fat necrosis.

Blows to the child's abdomen and flank may cause blunt trauma to the kidneys or adrenals. Renal injury is less common than other solid organ injury[24,66,72] but may occur from direct impact to the kidney parenchyma, from traction on the hilar vessels with laceration and/or thrombosis, and from disruption of the pelvis and/or uretero-pelvic junction with leakage of urine. Young children lack the abundant peri-renal fat that offers so much protection to adults, rendering the kidneys and adrenal glands relatively vulnerable to trauma. Adrenal trauma is relatively unusual in both accidental and inflicted abdominal injury[77] and typically in-volves hemorrhage. However, lacera-tions have been documented in cases of massive trauma with polyorgan injury and may serve as a marker of an injury event involving major forces.[24,72] The most common mechanism of adrenal injury is thought to be compression,[71] and this is supported by the common finding of associated trauma to nearby organs.

Of major concern to child abuse inves-tigators is establishing the time frame of the injury. There are several factors to be considered when the pathologist attempts to provide answers to this question.

1. **Type and character of the injury**
    Vascular injury: Major blood vessels such as the inferior vena cava may sustain shear injury, leading to rapid exsanguination. Rarely they may develop pseudoaneurysms, with major symptoms and complications only developing months to years later. Contusions and lacerations of

various sizes lying deep within solid organs may tamponade relatively quickly, causing little hemodynamic instability and playing only a minor role in the child's death. On the other hand, a smaller but superficial injury that involves transection of the cap-sule may allow continued bleeding into the peritoneal cavity, leading to hypovolemic shock. Blood pressure and flow within the lacerated organ will also affect the rate of blood loss: Hemorrhage from the liver paren-chyma tends to be slow relative to the spleen, given the low pressure in the hepatic sinusoids. Nonetheless, disruption of major vessels in either organ or within the thin pediatric mesentery will yield brisk bleed-ing.[17,63] In still other cases, a super-ficial injury that does not disrupt the capsule may undergo slow continued bleeding over ensuing hours, leading to an increasingly large subcapsular hematoma. Over time, the distended capsule may rupture, leading to hematoma disruption, brisk bleed-ing, and consequent exsanguination. In the latter case, a large accumula-tion of blood within the peritoneal cavity may lead to the false conclu-sion that the child experienced rapid exsanguination immediately after the injury rather than after a significant interval. To avoid that mistake, the pathologist needs to examine the injured organ carefully and look for signs of a ruptured subcapsular hematoma.

Determining the possible role of exsanguination in death may not be simple or straightforward. Even assuming that the blood volume of a young child is approximately 75 cc/kg body weight and that loss of approximately one-third of the total blood volume leads to shock, with loss of half or more leading to death, one cannot necessarily rely on measuring the blood in the peritoneal cavity to determine whether the child exsanguinated from abdominal injury. There may be little intraperitoneal blood but massive blood loss into the retroperitoneal tissues or the mesentery. Inflammatory exudate and bowel contents may contribute to the volume of intraperitoneal fluid. Documenting laceration of a major blood vessel increases the likelihood that exsanguination played a major role, but one must also consider possible tamponade, vessel spasm and shunting, shock related to other processes, etc. Postmortem leakage of blood from lacerated vessels may also add substantial volume to the intraperitoneal blood, making this measurement hard to interpret. Regardless, massive intra-abdominal bleeding with shock seems to be the mechanism of death in many cases of fatal inflicted abdominal trauma. Of the 10 abused children who died in the Cooper et al[63] study, 90% suffered massive intra-abdominal bleeding.

Hollow organ injury: Injury to hollow viscus organs is common in cases of fatal inflicted abdominal trauma, occurring in 30% of children in one study.[24] Such trauma may involve primarily hemorrhage (typically a duodenal wall hematoma) or

partial versus full-thickness wall laceration. In one study of blunt abdominal trauma from all causes,[64] perforation was the most common injury, occurring in 65% of children, with avulsion of the intestine comprising the next most common injury, accounting for 8%. The most common sites of bowel injury are the duodenum and proximal jejunum.[55] The retroperitoneal location of the duodenum renders it especially susceptible to crush injury against the vertebral column. The relative immobility of the proximal jejunum adjacent to the ligament of Treitz increases the risk of injury in this area. In estimating the time frame of injury, it is important to determine not only the size and depth of wall disruption (partial vs full-thickness), but also the location of the injury relative to other abdominal and retroperitoneal structures. Transection of the bowel will lead to leakage of bowel contents into the peritoneal cavity and/or retroperitoneal tissues. The size of the laceration contributes to the speed of the egress. But the omentum, mesentery, and adjacent organs may also influence the process by slowing the spread of irritating fluid and effectively confining it to a limited space. The greater omentum is somewhat mobile in that the inferior and lateral margins are unattached. Thus it moves with gut peristalsis. It can adhere to injured tissue and thereby help prevent the spread of contaminating fluid throughout the peritoneal cavity.[73] This may affect the timing of the child's pain from peritonitis, delaying severe symptoms for some hours. (The visceral peritoneum lacks afferent pain fibers, but the parietal peritoneum is quite sensitive.) However, it must be remembered that young children have a less well-developed greater omentum with relatively little fat, which renders organs and the abdominal wall less well protected from trauma and contaminating bowel contents than in older children and adults.

Bowel transections may not occur at the time of injury and the pathologist must look for evidence of wall necrosis with secondary (delayed) perforation versus immediate and complete transection of previously healthy wall. The delayed perforation may be related to a thrombosed mesenteric vessel with end-organ infarction or to direct tissue damage of the bowel wall related to crush injury, with gradual evolution of necrosis and tissue sloughing. Again, this distinction has major implications for estimating the time frame of the injury and the child's likely symptoms   (eg, signs of peritonitis within a   few hours vs more nonspecific signs   and symptoms over hours to days, followed by rapid progression to   evidence of peritonitis and shock). Secondary perforation may be delayed up to 2 to 5 days after the initial trauma.

2. **Single versus multiple injuries**
   Inflicted abdominal injury may involve trauma to more than one site,[67,74] and head injury may ultimately have played the major role

in a given child's death. Thorough autopsy and dissection of all major organs will help identify significant parenchymal injuries, as well as major soft tissue hemorrhage within the retroperitoneum and extremities.

3. **Coexisting disease or previous injury**
   A child with significant chronic disease may well succumb more quickly to the effects of major abdominal trauma than would a previously healthy child. Underlying immune deficiency, anemia, coagulopathy, or respiratory or heart disease may all affect a child's clinical course, adversely affecting his or her ability to react to hemorrhage, shock, and/or infection. In addition, a child who has had prior significant abdominal trauma or abdominal surgery may have developed adhesions, which affect the freedom of the organs to move in response to sudden blunt trauma to the abdominal wall, leading to altered injury patterns. A child who has focal bowel wall weakening from subacute, healing trauma may sustain a full-thickness perforation if the same region of bowel is retraumatized, even if the forces involved in the second traumatic event are not as great as the first.

4. **History of the child passing stool**
   When a child who has died of abdominal injuries is found to have a history of stooling within the recent past, investigators may ask if this indicates the child must have been injured at some point after that time. The answer is no. Children may pass

stool even if they have already sustained significant bowel or other intra-abdominal injury. Indeed, stooling may be a terminal event in some deaths.

5. **Stomach contents**
   The presence of identifiable food fragments in a child's stomach may help to confirm parts of the caretaker history. For example, the 3-year-old described on page 662 was said to have consumed half of a toaster pastry and some orange juice approximately 1 hour before collapsing. Results of the laboratory analysis of gastric contents were consistent with this history. However, it is important to note that the presence of this food does not necessarily imply that the small bowel transection occurred after breakfast. It is possible for children to eat (although they may lack a normal appetite) after sustaining major gastrointestinal injury.

6. **Gross appearance at autopsy**
   The appearance of the injured organs and the surrounding structures can provide very crude estimates of the injury time frame. As noted previously, volume of blood accumulation in the peritoneal cavity can be misleading. The time required for a given volume of inflammatory fluid to accumulate in cases of bowel transection cannot be determined with certainty since many factors will affect the rate of accumulation. The volume of intraluminal bowel contents leaking into the abdominal cavity will influence the total volume of intraperitoneal fluid, as will the rate of third-spacing and fluid shifts. The serosal surfaces of intra-abdominal organs become dull from inflammation relatively early on in the process, within a few hours, while frank pus accumulation takes longer. Devitalized, necrotic bowel may take hours to days to perforate.

7. **Histopathologic examination**
   Much of the research published regarding wound healing considers injuries of the skin or CNS, and this must be kept in mind when extrapolating to abdominal injuries. Nonetheless, some general guidelines to help establish broad time frames for the trauma are described in the section on estimating the age of wounds.

   When sampling areas of inflamed tissue for histopathologic examination, it is important to understand that dispersion of bowel contents throughout the peritoneal cavity may be delayed. The degree of inflammation at the wound site (eg, the proximal jejunum) may be much greater than that at a distant serosal surface (distal descending colon). Tissue should be obtained from several intraperitoneal sites, and information from these sites may help determine the time course of evolving peritonitis and corresponding symptoms. In addition, the wound borders and immediately adjacent tissue should be generously sampled to estimate the age of the injury and to help determine whether the perforation occurred at the time of injury or later, when necrotic tissue finally gave way to transmural disruption.

8. **Comparison of wound site to other injuries** *(abdominal and extra-abdominal)*

    Samples of injuries from other sites of the body should be obtained and their associated inflammatory changes compared with those in the abdomen to estimate whether the child likely sustained trauma on more than one occasion. Histo pathologic examination of abdominal wall bruising may help estimate the timing of intra-abdominal trauma, especially if the contusion directly overlies injured internal organs.

    When children are in extremis after sustaining inflicted abdominal trauma they may aspirate, and histopathologic examination of the ensuing pneumonitis may also help estimate the lower limits of survival time.

Intentional Asphyxia

The autopsy findings in fatal cases depend on the type of mechanical asphyxia inflicted. In children subjected to neck compression (manual or ligature strangulation), isolated obstruction of the jugular veins, with preservation of arterial flow through the carotid vessels, may lead to showers of petechiae over the skin of the face and postauricular region, the conjunctivae, oral mucosa, the temporalis muscles, and undersurface of the scalp (Figure 20.2). The presence of petechiae is related to increased intravascular pressure, with consequent rupture of small venules.[75] Some children show intense facial congestion. It

is important to keep in mind, however, that the presence of petechiae is a nonspecific finding and may be observed in children dying of natural causes, as well as from asphyxia. In living children it may be seen in benign processes associated with an intense Valsalva maneuver.

Increased force applied to the child's neck may lead to *both* arterial and venous obstruction, with or without accompanying airway occlusion. Such a situation lacks the sudden and severe increase in venous pressure associated with isolated venous occlusion, so the child will show no prominent facial congestion or edema and no showers of petechiae. The same lack of findings would be expected in cases involving

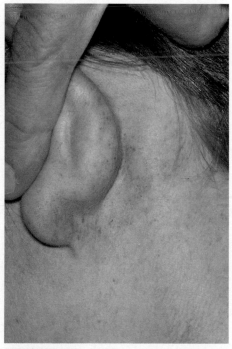

FIGURE 20.2
Postauricular petechiae in a 9-year-old boy who was victim of attempted strangulation.

reflex bradycardia and asystole, provided this occurred very early during the course of the neck compression.

In children sustaining forceful neck compression there may or may not be injuries to the neck structures.[17,75–79] Skin abrasions from the fingernails of the child or perpetrator may result from scraping or crushing of the epidermis. These injuries may be linear or curvilinear (in either direction), and the shape of the abrasion is determined by multiple factors, including the distortion of the child's skin under pressure, the shape of the fingernail, and the orientation of the adult's hands.[75] Bruises from the perpetrator's fingerpads may be seen. While clusters of small bruises on one side of the neck and a single bruise on the other side *may* reflect the fingers and thumb of the adult, the pathologist should be very careful with such an interpretation, since in some cases fingers may leave no visible marks (especially over the firm surface of the posterior neck) and/or a finger may be repositioned during the struggle, yielding more than one bruise. Further, the size of the fingerpad bruises does not necessarily reflect the size of the adult's fingertips, as seeping blood may expand the size of a contusion well beyond the area of direct trauma.

In some cases of homicidal neck compression, there may be evidence of internal injury, typically involving small areas of hemorrhage within the strap muscles of the neck or beneath the thyroid capsule. The cartilaginous nature of the hyoid, cricoid, and thyroid cartilage precludes fracture of these structures in children, in contrast to the not infre-

quent fractures of these heavily calcified structures in older adults.[17,80] Although infrequent, the carotid arteries may show evidence of direct trauma, including dissection or perivascular hemorrhage.[81,82] Sometimes the pathologist will observe submucosal hemorrhage of the epiglottis or base of the tongue, the latter occurring when the tongue is pushed up against the soft palate.

In some cases, examination of internal organs will show intrathoracic petechiae; congested, edematous, and atelectatic lungs; aspiration of gastric contents (this reflects a common and very nonspecific agonal event); and cerebral edema. However, such findings are not invariable. If there is a sufficient period of survival, cerebral edema may be extreme, and the global softening and necrosis indicative of "respirator brain" may be prominent. Some children may have developed cystic infarcts with widespread encephalomalacia, indicative of severe global hypoxia-anoxia.[83]

The autopsy may be completely negative in a case of intentional smothering, making the diagnosis extremely difficult, if not impossible. More than half of the infants in Meadow's[84] study of covert homicides showed no bruises, petechiae, or oronasal blood at the time of autopsy. In his study of 18 fatal suffocation victims, DiMaio[85] documented only one young child with petechial hemorrhages (2 hemorrhages in the eyes). When findings are present, they are typically subtle and may include minor facial, oral, or nasal abrasions and contusions, or a few subconjunctival hemorrhages. Injuries are related to pressure from the perpetrator's hand or other occlusive object. Older victims tend to show more prominent and numerous cutaneous injuries than are typically seen in young infants.[86] As discussed previously, very small and seemingly minor orofacial injuries may be falsely attributed to iatrogenic causes in those cases involving attempted resuscitation, making interview of medical providers critical in correctly interpreting autopsy findings. Studies of complications related to CPR potentially shed some light on this issue. In their study of pediatric injuries from CPR, Price and colleagues[24] found no facial injuries and only one oral injury among 324 children dying of natural causes. The oral trauma consisted of a frenulum laceration related to intubation. Bush et al[25] documented no orofacial injuries among 211 children younger than 12 years. In contrast, Ryan et al[27] found 9 lip injuries among 153 resuscitated children and 31 contusions/abrasions to the scalp or face. Nine cases of minor nasal mucosal trauma resulted in epistaxis and 9 other minor injuries of the "airway" were observed. Unfortunately, the authors did not indicate the total number of children sustaining these orofacial injuries, nor did they provide the maximum number of injuries sustained by any one child. Nonetheless, results of these studies suggest that minor orofacial trauma is certainly a possible complication of CPR, a conclusion most clinicians are likely to feel is supported by their own experience. Additional research is needed to document the average number of orofacial injuries attributable to CPR among children dying of non-traumatic causes.

Evidence suggests oronasal bleeding may be more common in cases of asphyxia than in SIDS. In their study of sudden infant death, Krous et al[87] found that only 3% of those who died of SIDS had evidence of frank oronasal blood that could not be attributed to CPR. This number rose to 14% in victims of known accidental suffocation.

Studies of pulmonary pathology in sudden infant death have addressed the possibility that differences in the amount of pulmonary hemorrhage and/or hemosiderin may help distinguish asphyxial deaths from SIDS.[88–92] Results of some studies suggest that asphyxia may be associated with increased pulmonary hemorrhage, and multiple asphyxial events over time may be associated with increased hemosiderin-laden macrophages within the lungs. However, other data fail to support this theory[93] and, at this point, the relationship, if any, remains to be clarified. Other factors potentially confound the relationship, and these must be considered and excluded.[94] It is important to note, however, that pulmonary hemorrhage, old or new, is relatively nonspecific and insensitive because many entities are associated with these findings (including small amounts of pulmonary hemorrhage in SIDS cases), and many cases of asphyxia lack substantial hemorrhage.

Sexual Assault/Abuse

While it is very unusual to die because of acute sexual assault,[95] a maltreated child may die from other causes after having been sexually abused/assaulted, acutely or in the past. If there is any possibility of acute sexual abuse/assault in a child victim, the pathologist should consider testing for trace evidence by obtaining a sexual assault evidence kit. The pathologist should collaborate with the local crime laboratory to ensure proper protocol is followed when collecting specimens. Swabs should be collected from oral, vaginal, cervical (in pubertal and postpubertal patients), and anal regions. Appropriate hair samples should be collected and fingernails examined for blood or tissue (one may cut the nails and submit these or swab the fingertips). The body should be examined carefully for trace evidence such as foreign pubic hairs or dried secretions. Any grossly visible trace evidence should be photographed before being collected (eg, a pubic hair on a prepubertal girl's labia). Scanning the body with a Wood light may help detect semen, although the specificity and sensitivity of this technique is limited.[96,97] Attention should be focused especially on breasts and genital regions, as well as neck and face. Semen may be identified in the child's hair. Urine and blood may be sent to test for date rape drugs.

A careful skin examination should be followed by a thorough oral examination, looking for evidence of trauma (eg, petechiae on the palate in cases of penile-oral contact). Anogenital examination should be performed using labial separation and traction; a cotton swab may be helpful in visualizing the entire hymen in adolescent females. The examination may be challenging in some cases, especially in large children with fully developed rigor mortis. A good light source is mandatory, and a source

of magnification extremely helpful. Photographs should be obtained that document the findings, even if normal. One should remember that postmortem relaxation may cause artifactual "gaping" of orifices, which may be falsely interpreted as evidence of prior penetration. It is not at all unusual for the anal opening to appear dilated (similar to the appearance when a child is under anesthesia) and the vulvar tissues to "gape." Artifacts related to refrigeration and congealing subcutaneous fat, as well as to postmortem lividity, can also lead to false interpretations of trauma and abnormality.

A good external examination must be supplemented with a careful internal examination, looking for evidence of trauma, pelvic inflammatory disease, pregnancy, and/or coexisting organic disease. This includes careful examination of the rectum and anal canal, vagina, cervix, and uterus with associated reproductive organs. The pathologist should look for evidence of foreign body insertion and/or of perforation into the peritoneal cavity. In many cases it is advisable to remove the relevant organs en bloc to allow a very careful dissection, photography, fixation in formalin, and ample tissue sampling for histology. Removing the reproductive organs (typically with the bladder and urethra), rectum, perineum, and vulvar tissues in the female, and the rectum, anus, and perianal tissues in the male, is a radical procedure. However, one can repair the resulting deformity by suturing the surrounding soft tissues together to close the pelvic wall defect and this allows for proper embalming procedures. In cases of penetrating trauma, the pathologist should look carefully for evidence of trauma in the soft tissues of the pelvic floor, hemorrhage or healing trauma to the pouch of Douglas or elsewhere in the peritoneal cavity, and evidence of fistula formation (recto-vaginal or cysto-vaginal). Any trauma should be liberally photographed and sampled for histopathologic examination. Contusions and lacerations to the anal canal or rectum should be described carefully in terms of location from external anal sphincter, size of traumatic lesion, and gross appearance. Histologic sampling will allow some estimation of the age of the injury based on the nature and degree of inflammatory infiltrate, as well as presence and degree of fibrosis.

Hypothermia

Fatal acute hypothermia may be related to inadequate supervision (as when a young child leaves the home and wanders outside in the cold for a prolonged period) or physical abuse. The prevalence of inflicted hypothermia involving cold-water baths/showers or forced exposure to cold ambient temperature is unknown. The literature on this topic is scarce but suggests that it is an uncommon cause of fatal abuse,[98] and this is supported by data from general studies of pediatric homicide.[99-101] Indications of hypothermia as the cause of death in a child may be evident in the history of premorbid events and clinical findings. The core body temperature measured at the scene or in the ED may indicate severe hypothermia <80.6°F–82.4°F). Sometimes, however,

thermometers in the ED do not register below a certain level (85°F) so an exact core body temperature may not be available. It is worth a telephone call to the ED to assess whether the recorded temperature was a true reading or simply a reflection of the lowest recordable temperature. While medical personnel may have found an unresponsive, floppy, comatose child, there may be a recent history of signs/symptoms indicative of mild, moderate, or severe hypothermia. Caretakers may report that the child appeared lethargic, confused, dysarthric, and/or ataxic. There may have been initial rapid breathing, followed by hypoventilation and, ultimately, apnea. Shivering may have been prominent during the phase of mild hypothermia, only to disappear over time as the child's temperature dropped. (There is a fairly wide range of temperatures below which shivering ceases, with values quoted between 75.2°F–95°F.)[102]

> **Case:** A 6-year-old boy was found by paramedics asystolic and apneic, with wet hair and cold, pale skin. The father said the child had been taking a bath in lukewarm water with his brother and had showed no evidence of illness or injury. He had collapsed shortly after the bath and was unable to be resuscitated by his father or medical personnel. Rectal temperature in the ED was 85°F (lowest recordable temperature on thermometer). Investigation ultimately revealed, through a disclosure by the older sibling, that the decedent had been forced to sit in a cold bath as punishment (duration unknown),

then had been made to get out of the bathtub and do push-ups while naked. He collapsed during the exercise. While struggling to get out of the bath, the child had slurred his words, lost his balance, and appeared disoriented.

In deaths from hypothermia, there may be few to no pathologic changes at autopsy, which makes history and investigation that much more critical. On the other hand, some cases show multiple external and internal findings to suggest the diagnosis. This is especially true in cases of death from exposure to cold ambient temperatures. One may see patches of pink skin discoloration over large joints and along extensor surfaces, purportedly due to pooling of oxygenated blood in capillaries of cold, hypometabolic tissues.[17] Elsewhere, the extremities may be pale and/or cyanotic. Excoriations of the fingers, ears, or nose may be seen.[42] There may be cold, firm, pale areas of frostbite (which may appear red and swollen if the child survived long enough to undergo rewarming).[103] Internal examination may reveal varying numbers of Wischnewsky spots: small brownish-black, slightly raised dots scattered over the gastric mucosa, which are neither erosions nor ulcers but are accumulations of hemoglobin, perhaps related to antemortem hemorrhage and red blood cell breakdown.[104] There may be evidence of acute pancreatitis, with fat necrosis and/or hemorrhage. There may be sludging of red blood cells related to cold agglutinins and accompanying microinfarcts of various organs. Pulmonary edema and hemor-

rhage may be seen. Children who have survived for a period may show evidence of acute respiratory distress syndrome and/or disseminated intravascular coagulation. There may be superimposed infection related to the child's immunocompromised state.

Fatal Neglect

Neglect constitutes the leading cause of child maltreatment deaths in the United States, accounting for 36% of the 1,500 cases of confirmed fatal child maltreatment in 2003.[105] Young children are at especially high risk. In 2003, 79% of child maltreatment deaths involved children younger than 4 years; 44% were younger than 1 year.[105] In a study of pediatric deaths due to neglect, 16 cases were identified over a 25-year period. The largest group (5/16, 31%) comprised children succumbing to chronic processes related to malnutrition with or without dehydration, while the remaining cases were related to acute events: 4 drowning/aspiration, 2 toxic ingestions, 2 hyperthermia/hypothermia, 1 electrocution, 1 dehydration plus blunt-force trauma to buttocks and thighs, and 1 delay in seeking medical attention for a ruptured appendix.[106]

Because of the variety of manifestations of fatal child neglect, the forensic pathologist must always consider the possibility that this form of maltreatment has played a central or contributing role in a child's death. Information obtained outside the autopsy suite may be critical in making this decision. The scene investigation may yield evidence of severe environmental neglect that placed the child at risk for health or safety complications (one or more of which may have contributed to death). Investigation may reveal evidence of a failure to adequately supervise the child, leading to a fatal injury. Review of medical records may reveal signs of medical neglect, which may be corroborated by autopsy findings of untreated (or inadequately treated) organic disease. Finally, the autopsy may reveal evidence of physical neglect, of which the most extreme form is fatal starvation.

It is clear, then, that evaluation for child neglect requires collaboration between the child's primary care physician and other medical providers, the medical examiner investigators (who obtain photographs of the home and interview the caretakers and medical providers), child protective services workers (who may have information regarding prior referrals for abuse or neglect in the family), and the pathologist. The meetings of the child fatality review team often provide the forum for important information exchange that can aid the neglect investigation.

Failure to Thrive and Starvation

In their 25-year retrospective review of child deaths attributable to neglect, Knight and Collins[110] documented malnutrition with or without dehydration as the most common cause of death. The manner of death in all but one of these cases was ruled a homicide. The average age of the victims was 2.4 months (range, 1.5–4 months). While fatal cases of starvation are more likely to involve very young children,[107] older children may be at risk as well, especially if they are disabled or otherwise dependent on others.

At the time of the autopsy, the pathologist may lack full medical records; these should be obtained and reviewed as soon as possible. The child's body should be weighed and measured, with weight, height, and head circumference plotted on appropriate growth charts.[108] Special growth charts may be required for premature infants, or for children with chronic conditions (eg, cerebral palsy). When available, these measurements should be compared with previous growth records. If the child showed evidence of failure to thrive, it will be important to review medical records for prior diagnostic evaluations and, to the extent possible, combine this information with that obtained at autopsy to rule out organic disease. The differential diagnosis for organic failure to thrive is vast.[109] Children experiencing failure to thrive typically show significant changes in the weight for age parameter before decreasing their linear growth velocity; the head circumference is the last parameter to show the effects of decreasing growth.[108] The pathologist should look for evidence of wasting (low weight for height), stunting (low height for age), and decreased velocity of head growth.

On external examination, the pathologist should look for evidence of physical neglect. Is the clothing insufficient for the environmental conditions? Is it excessively dirty, ill-fitting, or damaged? The child's state of hygiene should be assessed. Is the skin inordinately dirty? (Look for evidence of long-standing poor hygiene, such as dirt beneath most nails, dirt in generally protected areas [behind the ears, on the trunk and neck, etc]; dirt within skin creases; and "ground-in" dirt that is difficult to remove.) Is there evidence of untreated skin conditions such as severe eczema, scabies, or irritation dermatitis? While relatively severe diaper dermatitis can develop rapidly, especially when the child has a history of diarrhea, a lack of such history; the presence of heavily soiled diapers; and widespread, very severe dermatitis (often with evidence of long-standing irritation such as hypopigmentation) would lead one to suspect inadequate care and attention to hygiene. Infants who regurgitate on themselves and are left alone may show severe excoriation of the skin on the neck from irritation related to the pooled acidic gastric contents.

The skin should also be assessed for untreated cutaneous injuries and/or secondary wound infections. The state of the hair should be assessed as well. Very dirty, matted hair with trapped food or other filth; severe head lice; or untreated, advanced scalp conditions suggest physical neglect. Pressure sores on the scalp or elsewhere suggest prolonged placement in one position, as do occipital alopecia and bony deformities such as marked plagiocephaly. The condition of the teeth and gums should be assessed. Bottle caries is common in neglected children, and older children may show numerous caries from chronic lack of care. It is important to mention, however, that accessibility to dental care should be considered when interpreting the significance of poor dental hygiene.

Generally full medical records are only available to the pathologist after the autopsy. However, review of these records can be extremely helpful, yielding information regarding prior organic disease, the results of workups for failure to thrive, prior concerns on the part of medical personnel for abuse or neglect, or caretaker noncompliance with regular primary care and immunizations. There may be clear evidence of noncompliance with treatment recommendations for chronic disease, often with documented complications (eg, multiple admissions to the pediatric intensive care unit for asthma exacerbations or ketoacidosis), or documentation of suspicious injuries noted by prior medical providers. Direct phone conversations with medical providers can be fruitful because the pathologist may ask specific questions and elicit information not previously considered by medical personnel, or information that had been considered but not documented in written records.

In cases of failure to thrive, premorbid workup is supplemented with postmortem examination and investigation. Careful gross dissection and histologic examination of organs may identify congenital anomalies or chronic disease. The pathologist should seek the expertise of pediatric pathologists as necessary, as well as other specialists, such as neuropathologists, gastroenterologists, geneticists, or endocrinologists. Correlation of autopsy findings with clinical information obtained by medical providers and by death investigators, who may conduct lengthy, detailed interviews of caretakers regarding family history, birth history, the child's medical history, feeding regimens and eating patterns, possible concerns on the part of caretakers for the child's poor weight gain, and signs/symptoms of illness prior to death, is essential. The investigator may seek corroboration of caretaker information by conducting interviews of multiple caretakers, child care providers, relatives, public health nurses, and other medical providers. A more detailed discussion of failure to thrive is contained in Chapter 15.

Starvation

Long-standing food deprivation may result in death. Fatal starvation occurs most often in infants, young children, and debilitated children, who are dependent on others for food supply. The features of starvation may vary, with children showing characteristics of *edematous* protein/energy malnutrition (PEM) (kwashiorkor) or *non-edematous* PEM (marasmus). Protein and energy intake are similar in the 2 types of PEM, but when a chronically malnourished child encounters extra stress acutely, he may develop leaky cell membranes, efflux of cellular ions, and consequent increased interstitial fluid volume and edema (kwashiorkor). Thus intercurrent illness in a malnourished child may lead to features of edematous PEM.[110]

Autopsy in a child who died of starvation typically reveals multiple external, internal, gross, and microscopic findings (Box 20.1). The classic emaciated appearance of marasmus, with prominence of large joints, facial bones, and ribs, is secondary to profound loss of subcutaneous adipose

tissue and muscle atrophy. The routine thoracoabdominal "Y" incision may reveal layers of abdominal musculature and fatty tissue only 2- to 3-mm thick. Sunken eyes are related to the absence

BOX 20.1
Gross, Radiographic, and Microscopic Findings in Fatal Starvation

Gross
General emaciation
Prominent joints, facial bones, and ribs
Generalized loss of subcutaneous fat
Muscle atrophy
Temporal wasting
Loss of orbital fat (sunken eyes)
Loss of Bichat's fat pad (sunken cheeks)
Redundant skin (especially on thighs, buttocks)
Skin hyperpigmentation or hypopigmentation
Loose, dull, coarse scalp hair
Scalp hair reddish brown, blond, or gray
Edema of limbs, face
Edema of internal organs
Abdominal distention
Empty stomach/small bowel
Small and hard versus mucoid stools
Duodenal stress ulcers
Bowel wall thinning
Decreased organ weights

Radiographic
Delayed bone age
Osteopenia
Nutritional rickets

Microscopic
Fatty infiltration of liver
Atrophic lymph nodes/thymus
Atrophy of brown fat
Decreased size and mass of skeletal muscle fibers
Cardiac myofibrillar degeneration
Atrophy of small bowel mucosa
Decreased white pulp in spleen
Stress involution of adrenals
Hyperkeratosis; epidermal atrophy of skin

of orbital fat and, possibly, concomitant dehydration. Hollow cheeks are secondary to loss of Bichat's fat pad in the buccal region (this effect may occur relatively late in the course of malnutrition). There may be prominent temporal wasting and dry, flaky, thin skin. Loss of buttock fat leaves pelvic bones and the perianal region prominent. There may be decubitus ulcers from prolonged immobilization, especially over bony prominences such as the spine. Redundant skin folds may be seen on the proximal limbs and over the buttocks. In edematous PEM, dermatitis may lead to hyperpigmentation of the skin, although in contrast to pellagra, this does not occur in skin exposed to sunlight. There may also be areas of hypopigmentation. Scalp hair may be loose, dull, thin, and coarse and may turn a streaky reddish brown, blond, or gray from hypopigmentation. Edema may be present peripherally in the limbs and in the face but is also notable in the internal organs.[101] Abdominal distention is related to weakened abdominal muscles, intestinal distention (from intestinal hypomotility and gas production), and enlarged liver rather than to ascites.

Internally, the starved child may have an empty stomach and small bowel, with small, dry lumps of stool distally, indicative of chronic constipation. However, in some children with non-edematous PEM there is starvation diarrhea with mucousy stools. One may see a gastric bezoar[107] related to the child's consumption of hair, threads, or other bits of material. Small fragments of these materials may be seen in the substance of the stool as well. Duodenal stress ulcers may

be present and the wall thickness of the gastrointestinal tract may be reduced. Organs are often decreased in weight. It is important to compare organ weights to recent standards because use of older tables may be deceptive.[111] A skeletal survey may reveal evidence of delayed bone age,[107] osteopenia, or nutritional rickets. It may also show acute or healing fractures suspicious for concomitant physical abuse. Kellogg and Lukefahr[107] found histories or physical findings consistent with recent physical abuse in 6 of 12 starved children, and this tendency for coexisting abuse should be kept in mind when performing the autopsy because it may guide the pathologist to obtain skeletal surveys in children outside the typical age group.

Microscopically, one may find fatty infiltration of the liver with corresponding hepatomegaly; atrophic lymph nodes and thymus; atrophy of brown fat; and muscular, as well as cardiac, degenerative changes. Cardiac myofibrillar fragmentation may be prominent. Skeletal muscle fibers are decreased in size and mass.[112] There is a decrease in the total mass and protein content of the pancreas and the intestinal mucosa, with flattened villi and atrophic mucosa. There may be bone marrow hypoplasia involving red cell and leukocyte production. The spleen may show poorly developed white pulp.[106] There may be stress involution of the adrenal glands. The skin may show basal layer atrophy in the epidermis and hyperkeratosis, as well as collagen loss.[110]

It is important for the pathologist to carefully document all of the signs of starvation with detailed written descriptions and appropriate photographs. The degree of malnutrition should be estimated using an accepted classification system such as the Waterlow classification[113] or the Gomez criteria.[114] Adequate documentation is critical for a number of reasons, not the least of which is to address the legal issue of whether the caretaker would have been aware of the child's severe condition. Full body and close-up photographs provide stark evidence of the severity of fatal malnutrition and the lack of subtlety in its presentation.

Often there is autopsy evidence of coexisting dehydration,[106,107] most reliably documented by raised vitreous sodium and blood urea nitrogen values.[115] Physical stigmata of dehydration may be present in the form of dry organs, dry mucous membranes (although care must be taken to consider the effect of postmortem desiccation), sunken eyes, and tacky subcutaneous fat.[116] Estimation of dehydration using skin turgor is problematic in deceased children because refrigeration can cause subcutaneous fat to congeal and affect apparent turgor.

In cases of malnutrition, it is important for the pathologist to look for signs of coexisting vitamin and mineral deficiencies. For example, follicular hyperkeratosis may reflect vitamin A or C deficiency, as may corkscrew hairs.

Dermatitis may be the result of zinc, niacin, or riboflavin deficiency, or reflect lack of essential fatty acids. Bleeding and/or receding gums may signal a lack of vitamins A, C, K, or folate.

The mechanism of death from starvation is incompletely understood and likely involves a number of factors. Starvation leads to bone marrow suppression with a decrease in production of white blood cells and alterations in cell-mediated immunity. A decrease in complement and neutrophil dysfunction lead to a reduced ability to kill bacteria. The child is at increased risk for opportunistic infections, which can become quite severe in the absence of the body's ability to mount an adequate inflammatory response. Some children die of pneumonia. The markedly reduced mass and impairment of metabolism involving the respiratory muscles affects the child's ability to breathe and adequately inflate the lungs. Victims of starvation have a decrease in vital capacity and tidal volume. This, combined with their impaired immunity, makes pneumonia a very high risk. Generalized muscle atrophy and weakness may impair a child's ability to swallow and protect the airway from aspiration and subsequent pneumonia.

Dehydration contributes to death by decreasing the already depleted intravascular volume and adding to the existing electrolyte abnormalities. Starvation leads to loss of cardiac muscle mass and myofibrillar fragmentation. Patients can develop very low cardiac output and low blood pressure, resulting in inadequate blood flow to the vital organs. It can also lead to abnormal, potentially lethal, cardiac rhythms.[110]

While the pathologist must be ready to testify to the severity and manifestations of fatal starvation, he or she may also be asked about the degree of suffering the child may have experienced during the process. This, of course, is a difficult question, but one must consider not only the chronicity of the starvation process but also the child's ability to experience hunger, to be aware of his surroundings (to know whether he is alone or whether others are available but unresponsive to his needs), to be able to signal his distress, and the phy-sical dis-comfort of the manifestations of mal-nutrition and avitaminoses. Decubitus ulcers may be extremely painful until the process becomes severe enough to destroy afferent nerve fibers in the area; photophobia and dermatitis may be uncomfortable, as may angular stomati-tis or paresthesias. Severe nutritional neglect may also be accompanied by profound emotional neglect, and chil-dren may be left for long periods alone, and even confined in small   areas such as closets.

> **Case:** A 15-year-old male with cere-bral palsy was found dead by his family one morning. He weighed 23 pounds at death, equivalent to the weight of an average 2 ½-year-old child with cerebral palsy. He had last seen a physician and had last attended school approximately 2 years prior to death. He had had "no recent medical problems." According to family members, the child spent much of his time on a blanket in the middle of the family room, through which there was constant traffic of mother and multiple siblings. Dirt and feces stained the carpet beneath the child. Clothing, toys, refuse, and debris, including food matter, sur-rounded the space where he lay.

While the child was immobile and incapable of feeding himself, he had clearly been aware of his surround-ings and when healthy had been able to communicate with others at a basic level. He was starving, yet there was "edible" food on the floor inches away, which he could no doubt see. He was unable to change his own diaper and at death was found with feces covering his buttocks and embedded within large, necrotic skin ulcers. Investigators eventually learned that as the child gradually became more and more emaciated and weak, the family argued more about who was going to care for him. The child, who had reasonable receptive language skills, likely heard this and understood it.

This case illustrates several historical characteristics that are common in cases of fatal and nonfatal starvation. In their evaluation of 12 such cases, Kellogg and Lukefahr[107] found that most caretakers minimized the extreme nature of the child's physical condition. The victim typically lived with other children who were not malnourished, and most vic-tims had not attended school or been seen by medical providers for an extended period. It was common for families to have one parent absent or uninvolved with child care (7 of 12 cases).

In some cases, it is possible to estimate the duration of a child's starvation, and this may be helpful in aiding laypersons to understand the degree of depriva-tion.[117,118] Meade and Brissie[118] calculated this in a 6-week-old infant, taking into account computed caloric deficit (expected weight minus actual weight, with adjustment for dehydration, then conversion of this weight deficit into caloric deficit) and dividing this by the average daily caloric requirement. This gave a very approximate estimate of the number of days of nutritional deprivation. Nagao et al[117] estimated the caloric deficit of a slightly older child (3 years). This entailed consideration of daily physical activity as it affected the caloric requirement, and the authors pointed out the difficulty in calculating caloric deficits in mobile young children (as opposed to very young infants). Multiple assumptions may be made in the calculation of the estimates, but these tend to underestimate the duration of starvation rather than overestimate it. For example, a child may not have been continually deprived of food, but given scant food sporadically. This would prolong the starvation process by intermittently providing external sources of energy. Similarly, Meade and Brissie assumed that the body's "self-digestion" was 100% efficient. Were this not the case (and it probably isn't), the lack of perfect efficiency would lead to even greater caloric deficits (and greater interval of deprivation).

Inadequate Supervision

Unintentional injury is the leading cause of death in children 1 to 4 years old, and many "accidental" deaths are related to poor caretaker supervision. Drowning, fire/burns, and suffocation are all events that frequently involve inadequate supervision of small children and all are included in the top 10 causes of unintentional injury deaths (Table 20.3).[119]

TABLE 20.3
Leading Causes of Fatal Unintentional Injuries, Children 1–4 Years Old, 2002

Cause of Death	No. of Deaths	% of Deaths
1. Motor vehicle traffic	533	32.5
2. Drowning	454	27.7
3. Fire/burn	226	13.8
4. Suffocation	139	8.5
5. Pedestrian, other	83	5.1
6. Fall	37	2.3
7. Poisoning	31	1.9
8. Natural/environment	29	1.8
9. Struck by or against	26	1.6
10. Other	83	5.0
Total:	**1,641 deaths**	

Adapted from National Center for Injury Prevention and Control, Centers for Disease Control and Prevention. WISQARS database. http://www.cdc.gov/ncipc/maps/default.htm.

The issue of caretaker culpability in "accidental" pediatric deaths is a complex one[62] and beyond the scope of this chapter. Clearly in the very young, non-ambulatory child, intense supervision is required. But for older children, most adults agree that some degree of independence is necessary. The crucial question is whether the caretaker ensured the child was in a safe environment and whether basic protective measures were in place to adequately respond to a crisis. If not, one should ask whether the adult realized these conditions were not met and what, if anything, the caretaker could have done about it. These questions lead to many others regarding issues of inherent caretaker ability, community standards, and societal responsibility. The difficulty in finding adequate answers makes these cases among the most challenging for members of the pediatric fatality review team.

Medical providers play an important role in this analysis by providing epidemiological and clinical data regarding modifiable and non-modifiable risk factors for injury and death, as well as input regarding the physiology and developmental skills of a child that render him particularly susceptible to injury.

Hyperthermia

Childhood death from environmental hyperthermia is unusual but not rare, and case reports typically describe infants and young children found in enclosed vehicles[120–124] or in bed.[125] When evaluating the potential role of child neglect, investigators frequently ask medical examiners questions about the duration the child may have been left alone in the hot environment, and the ambient and body temperatures associated with death. Several published studies show unequivocally that temperatures in enclosed parked vehicles may rapidly reach levels incompatible with life.[121,123,126] The vehicle acts like a greenhouse, absorbing and trapping long wavelength radiant energy.[121] Experiments with various cars parked in sun or shade on warm or hot days (temperatures ranging from 83°F–100.4°F) demonstrate internal car temperatures as high as 172°F.[121,123,126] King et al[123] demonstrated that at least 75% of the rise in temperature within cars of various sizes and colors occurred within 5 minutes of closing the doors. Factors influencing maximum internal car temperatures include car size,[126] external car color,[123] degree of ventilation afforded through windows,[121,123,126] and position of the vehicle in the direct sun versus shade.[121,126] The most dangerous situation seems to be a small, dark-colored car with closed windows parked in direct sun. Importantly, windows "cracked" a few inches provide inadequate ventilation to protect children inside. Significant temperature reduction is only accomplished when windows are left at least half open.[123,126] With this data indicating that dangerously elevated temperatures may be reached within a few minutes, it is tragic but not surprising to learn of a toddler dying of hyperthermia after being left unattended for only 1 hour.[121] While healthy children are vulnerable to hyperthermia in unattended vehicles, those with risk factors such as pre-existing fever, recent poor fluid intake, or chronic disease are particularly susceptible.

The body dissipates heat by evaporation, convection, and conduction; in hot environments evaporation plays a major role.[121] However, infants and young children may be compromised in their ability to regulate body temperature with evaporation because of excessive clothing/bedding (especially if the material is resistant to moisture) and cushioned seats that surround much of the body and decrease the surface area available for evaporation of sweat.[122] Environments with relatively high local humidity decrease evaporation efficiency further. Children who are restrained in car seats may also be at a disadvantage because their position below the level of the cracked window limits heat loss through convection (transfer of heat by movement of air). Further, if the thin layer of air surrounding the skin is not circulated (because of overlying clothing or bedding and a lack of general airflow from the car windows or in the bedroom), then it may eventually become saturated with water from evaporation and further evaporation is precluded.[127] Finally, conduction may actually increase body heat if a child's body is pressed up against a hotter object, such as a seat buckle or hot vinyl upholstery.

The risk of heat stroke significantly increases when core temperatures rise above 104°F, and at 109°F there is major disruption of hepatic and cerebral function.[32] Hyperpyrexia causes thermal damage to many vital organs. Findings at autopsy vary, in part depending on survival time,[118,123] degree of hyper-thermia,[32] and time since death, the latter determining the extent of post-mortem decompositional changes. There are no findings that are "diagnostic" of heat stroke, and changes one sees at autopsy may be very nonspecific.[127] When evaluating an infant or young child who has been exposed to environmental hyperthermia, one may find evidence of profuse sweating (soaked clothing and wrapping), vomiting, and/or dehydration. Investigators may report that the child's skin felt very hot at the time the child was discovered. The body temperature may be significantly elevated, especially if the child has not been subjected to cooling efforts. Temperatures as high as 108°F have been recorded in victims,[121,124,128] and Krous et al[125] reported a case in which body temperature was 106°F when measured 3 hours after death. There may be cutaneous and/or conjunctival petechiae, purpura, skin slippage, and/or cutaneous burns. Internal examination may demonstrate intrathoracic petechiae; pulmonary edema, congestion, or hemorrhage; cerebral edema; adrenal hemorrhage; and/or evidence of disseminated intravascular coagulation in the form of widespread hemorrhages. Microscopically, there may be fibrin thrombi within small vessels, hepatic necrosis, acute tubular necrosis of the kidneys, and myocardial degeneration.[120,124,125,127] Hepatic necrosis and disseminated intravascular coagulation are typically seen in victims who survive at least 6 hours after exposure.[122]

When considering the possibility of heat stroke as a cause of death, history and scene investigation become vitally important, since autopsy findings may be nonspecific. The National Association of Medical Examiners (NAME) recommends that the diagnosis of a heat-related death be "based on a history of exposure to high ambient temperature and a reasonable exclusion of other causes of hyperthermia."[124] If core body temperature measured at the time of collapse is at least 105°F, the cause of death should be certified as heat stroke (given the above diagnostic requirements). Lower body temperatures may also be accepted if there is a history of attempts to cool the body, or if there is a history of mental status changes and elevated liver and muscle enzymes.

In cases of children found in parked vehicles, it is important for investigators to measure (or estimate) ambient and vehicular temperatures, determine humidity, and describe whether the car was parked in the sun or shade (this may change over time if the child was left for a prolonged period); whether any windows were open and to what degree; and the color, model, and size of the car. The type of the child's clothing should be described, as should the position of the child when left by the caretaker and when found (a doll should be placed and photographed as a demonstration). Photographs of the vehicle's location and the inside of the vehicle should be obtained. Witnesses may be able to help determine how long the child was alone in the car and when the child may have collapsed.

In the case of an infant who may have sustained heatstroke while in bed, the ambient temperature should be measured or estimated and the bedding should be described (type, amount, position in relation to baby), photographed, and retained. Investigators should determine if there were other persons and/or items in the bed with the child. The source of excessive heat should be determined (bedding, central heating, space heater, etc). If the source is a room heater, then diagrams should be constructed to document the child's position in relation to the heat source and to sources of ventilation. The infant's clothing should be described and retained. Toxicological studies can help rule out the influence of medications on body temperature and regulation. Caretakers should be questioned about signs and symptoms of prior illness.

Evaluating the Role of Neglect in Pediatric Deaths

In many cases of child deaths related to unintentional injuries, the role of neglect is clear. The child who dies after being left unattended in a hot car for 3 hours while his father conducts drug sales inside is clearly the victim of neglect. But in many other cases, the role of neglect is much less obvious, and the decision is heavily influenced by societal standards and personal judgment. This decision is not the sole purview of the medical examiner. In fact, in many cases considered neglectful by authorities, the medical examiner has ruled the manner of death an accident rather than a homicide.[106] Evaluating the contribution of neglect has obvious consequences for the caretaker and surviving siblings. The parent may lose custody of other children and/or undergo criminal prosecution for negligence. In assessing these cases a number of factors need to be considered.

Case: A 12-month-old infant was found submerged in the bathtub, cyanotic and apneic after being left alone there with his 2-year-old sister while the mother left the home "briefly" to speak with an electrician outside. The mother reported she had only been gone for "about 5 minutes" when she heard the older sibling yelling. She came back to the bathroom and found the submerged infant. The child was ultimately resuscitated but suffered extensive anoxic brain injury and remained in a persistent vegetative state. He eventually succumbed to pneumonia approximately 6 months after the event.

Investigators and district attorneys were divided in their opinion of whether this mother should be prosecuted for neglect and whether the 2-year-old should be allowed to remain in her care. Ultimately, the 2-year-old was taken into custody and the mother charged with neglect. She pled guilty but served no time in prison.

In analyzing this case and others like it, investigators need to consider a number of factors.

The immediate circumstances and history provided by the caretaker
- Does the history make sense? Does it change over time? Are there indications that the history being pro-

vided is inaccurate? (For example, interview of the electrician indicated the time the mother was outside was in the range of 15 minutes, rather than the 5 minutes she stated.)
- Does scene investigation support the history?
- Is there evidence that an acute, stressful environmental event occurred immediately before the injury, which may have distracted the caretaker from appropriately supervising the child?
- Are there signs of other types of neglect noted at the scene, such as a filthy, unsafe home; evidence from neighbors of chronic poor supervision of young children; drug paraphernalia in the home to suggest caretaker intoxication in the presence of children?
- Is there evidence that the caretaker is suffering from mental health issues that compromise his or her ability to supervise a child or that he or she has cognitive limitations?
- Is there evidence of caretaker intoxication at the time of the incident or of chronic intoxication?

Background investigation
- Have there been prior child protective service referrals for neglect or other maltreatment?
- Has this child or others living in the home been seen by medical providers for "accidental" injuries in the past which, in retrospect, suggest an element of poor supervision?
- Have there been prior concerns on the part of medical providers that this child has suffered from medical neglect in the past? Educational neglect?

Community and societal issues

- Are there laws addressing the circumstances surrounding the child's death (drug possession and sales, unregistered guns, swimming pool security ordinances, etc)?
- Is the potentially neglectful behavior something commonly practiced by others in the caretaker's community and viewed as acceptable?
- Is it common knowledge that the caretaker's behavior would likely place a child's health at substantial risk?
- Was the caretaker's behavior under his or her control and the product of a conscious decision? Were there other options that would not have placed the child at risk?
- Had the caretaker been warned about this behavior in the past or had prior experience with such events?

To adequately answer these questions, there should be thorough case investigation and good collaboration between agencies. Communication among the various disciplines must be stressed so that a decision can be made based on all available information. The child fatality review team is an excellent forum for sharing information and making a decision regarding the role of neglect in a child's death.

Routine Histopathologic Evaluation at Autopsy

In addition to generously sampling injuries as described in the preceding sections, the pathologist also routinely samples all major organs for histopathologic examination. It is important to rule out organic disease as a contributor to death, and many pathologic processes are not identifiable on gross inspection. The presence of disease occasionally helps in the determination of time of injury, as in the case of a severely head-injured infant who is left alone for hours and who develops terminal aspiration pneumonia. Secondary changes emanating from the primary trauma may affect a multitude of organs and contribute to a general understanding of the patient's clinical course and demise. Special stains are occasionally ordered, including stains for hemosiderin, infectious organisms, or specific pathophysiological changes (eg, ß-amyloid precursor protein as an indicator of axonal damage).

It is not uncommon to find evidence of concomitant disease in a fatally abused child. The issue to consider, therefore, is whether the disease contributed to death. For example, mild tracheitis is quite common and of no clinical significance in the death of a severely beaten child. Evidence of congenital bone disease will have significant implications for interpretation of a child's multiple healing fractures, although may not have any impact on determination of the cause of death. Presence of disease must be considered along with all elements of the autopsy and investigation in ultimately determining cause of death.

Laboratory Studies

Postmortem Chemistry

Blood chemistries begin to change nearly immediately in the postmortem period, but the vitreous fluid is a matrix in which certain analytes remain relatively stable and a mirror of blood chemistries for 18 to 24 hours after death, barring any unusually accelerated decomposition. Sodium, urea nitrogen, and creatinine can provide scientifically supportable evidence of dehydration in selected cases. The relationship to blood chemistries is not one-to-one, and each laboratory analyzing vitreous chemistries should establish its own normal range for use in interpreting reported results. Vitreous potassium will increase rapidly postmortem as it does in the serum but does have some limited utility in calculating an approximate postmortem interval as outlined previously in this chapter. Postmortem evaluation of antemortem potassium abnormalities is not possible. Hyperkalemia cannot be diagnosed and hypokalemia is unlikely to be detected. Analysis of vitreous glucose is useful only in cases of hyperglycemia, particularly if done in tandem with analysis for acetone. Vitreous glucose rapidly diminishes to undetectable levels postmortem, thus negating this technique for investigating the possibility of hypoglycemia as a consequence of inborn errors of metabolism or inappropriate administration of insulin.

The latter continues to be a vexing situation for forensic pathologists because increasingly few commercial laboratories will stand behind their analysis of postmortem serum levels of insulin and C-peptide. These 2 protein moieties are, in theory, stable for up to 24 hours postmortem. Analytic difficulties, however, seem to make these measurements subject to challenge. One of the authors of

this chapter (TA) has had moderate success with obtaining reliable postmortem analysis in serum of other stable, large molecules (thyroid hormones, hemoglobin electrophoresis, lipid profiles, gamma globulin), but has been unable to obtain results for others of diagnostic significance, such as protein S and protein C.

Proper interpretation of vitreous electrolyte concentrations involves consideration of more than simply the reported value. Sample procurement is technique-sensitive. Excessive negative pressure applied to the sampling syringe can draw bits of retinal tissue into the sample, skewing results. Any degree of decomposition may call the results to question. All things considered, a normal vitreous electrolyte panel may well be of more diagnostic significance than abnormal results without clinical correlation. Nevertheless, vitreous electrolytes coupled with autopsy findings of dehydration (sunken eyes and/or fontanels, tacky serosal surfaces, dry bladder, empty bowel) in the complete absence of the appropriate clinical history requires closer scrutiny of the proffered history (Table 20.4).

Hypernatremia or hyponatremia may reflect processes other than disease. Forced ingestion of salt, salted water, or copious amounts of plain water are well-documented forms of child abuse, usually in infants or toddlers. A review of 12 cases of abusive salt poisoning by Meadow[128] saw most cases in children younger than 6 months and in 10 of 12 the abuse was carried out by the mother. Antemortem serum sodium has been

TABLE 20.4
Vitreous Electrolyte Patterns

Classification	Sodium/Chlorine (mEq/L)	Potassium	Vitreous Urea Nitrogen (mg/dL)
Normal	130–155/105–135	<15	<40
Dehydration	>155/>135	—	40–100
Low salt	<130/<105	<15	—
Uremic	Variable	Variable	Marked elevation
Decomposition	<130/<105	>20	—

reported as high as 190 to 205 mEq/L in such cases. This information may be used to calculate the excess salt load by the child, which can be graphically demonstrated to a jury, thus refuting the exceedingly unlikely explanation that the child spontaneously or accidentally ingested the salt on his or her own.

Dilutional hyponatremia due to water intoxication has been reported in infants fed diluted formula for a long period,[129] and fatalities have occurred in children forced to drink large quantities of water as a form of punishment.[130] The latter paper does not report postmortem vitreous sodium concentrations, but all 3 presented with seizures, encephalopathy, and profound hyponatremia (plasma sodium 112 ± 2 mmol/L). At autopsy, all 3 had cerebral edema as a prominent finding.

Toxicology

Toxicological screening for a wide range of drugs of abuse and therapeutic drugs is a very common, albeit not uniform, procedure in most forensic autopsies. Despite its relatively low yield in infant and child deaths, these cases should not represent an exception to this practice.

Case: An 8-year-old male with attention-deficit/hyperactivity disorder ran out into the street into the path of an oncoming car. The child was pronounced dead at the scene of blunt impact injuries of the head. Postmortem toxicological testing revealed the presence of cocaine and benzoylecgonine in the blood. The source of cocaine was never discovered, but a referral was made to child protective services, which investigated the issue of safety of the remaining children in the household.

Whatever the age of the child, the presence of excessive or unprescribed therapeutic agents and/or illicit drugs in postmortem blood warrants careful thought. Toxicological results, like any laboratory data, must be interpreted in light of the totality of case information. This may include reviewing other cases examined in the autopsy suite the same day. Fatal intoxication may be the result of intentional poisoning or access to the drug by the child in an environment of neglect. Agents may not be those typically thought of as agents of abuse. In 2003 Black and Zenel[131] published a case of intentional iron poisoning presenting as shock and acidosis.

Postmortem drug levels do not necessarily mirror blood levels at death given the vagaries of postmortem toxicology. The first interpretive consideration is the sample source. An antemortem specimen on presentation to a health care facility is ideal. The best postmortem specimens are those from the periphery, usually drawn from the femoral region. Absent a good peripheral sample, central blood from the heart, vena cava, or aorta may be submitted, but results from this sample may be more difficult to interpret owing to postmortem redistribution (Table 20.5). Alternative toxicology samples include vitreous fluid, liver, bile, brain, kidney, muscle, and other tissues. Hair may be used to evaluate chronic toxic exposures such as lead. Most scalp hair grows approximately 1 cm per month. Sampling can be done of hair segments from proximal to distal in order to establish a pattern of exposure.

Postmortem redistribution is a particular problem involving basic lipophilic drugs with large distribution volumes. Routes of redistribution typically follow these patterns:

Stomach/gastrointestinal → liver, lungs, and heart
Liver → lungs, heart
Lungs → heart, aorta
Myocardium → heart chambers

Thus one can easily see the distinct advantage of submitting a peripheral specimen for analysis. In addition to redistribution there are other controversial issues in the interpretation of postmortem toxicology. Calculation of total dose based on postmortem levels is fraught with error. In toxicity, a given drug is not likely to be at equilibrium and the amount of unabsorbed drug may be large. Furthermore, most drugs have nonlinear kinetics, there may be genetic variations in how a given drug is metabolized, drugs will accumulate with repeated usage, and elimination will underestimate the amount of drug originally consumed. Proposed formulae claiming to provide a "back calculation" to dose taken have shown to have errors of +150% to -75%.

It is recommended that the forensic pathologist collect and have analyzed blood from more than one site, avoid interpreting toxicological results without consideration of case history and autopsy findings, and avoid interpreting postmortem blood levels from clinically derived tables of "normal" ranges. Postmortem concentrations in clear-cut drug fatalities may completely overlap concentrations wherein the drug is an incidental finding. There are no normals in postmortem toxicology.

Metabolic and Genetic Disorders

Now some 20 years after the first reports of fatty acid disorders and medium-chain acyl-coenzyme A dehydrogenase

TABLE 20.5
Impact of Sampling Site

Site	Amitriptyline (ng/mL)	Doxepin (ng/mL)
Femoral	3.4	3.8
Subclavian	7.3	6.4
Left heart	6.6	5.9
Right heart	4.6	5.0

(MCAD) deficiency, in particular, presenting as sudden unexplained infant death,[132,133] the availability of economical screening for a wide variety of inborn errors of metabolism using tandem mass spectrometry technology has made such screening relatively routine. Actual diagnostic yield of these screens tends to be low; however, a definitive diagnosis, particularly in the context of more than one sudden, unexpected infant death in a household, is enormously significant. These disorders are inherited, usually in an autosomal-recessive fashion, and can be managed if diagnosed properly. Proposed mechanisms for sudden death in infancy include rapid onset of hypoglycemia with intercurrent stress and toxicity of elevated free fatty acids and/or their metabolic intermediates.

Despite assertions that MCAD deficiency alone may be responsible for up to 5% of sudden unexplained infant deaths, one author's (TA) 15-year experience with routine postmortem metabolic screening has yielded but 2 diagnoses, both of type I glutaric aciduria. In neither case were there the elements of subdural hemorrhage (SDH) or retinal hemorrhage (RH), but given the known association between SDH/RH and this disorder,[134] a correct diagnosis will surely prevent the incorrect allegation of abuse.[135,136] Other amino acidemias can be screened for, as well as a wide range of other metabolic disturbances, making this an effective screening tool despite its low yield. It is important for the forensic pathologist to note that diagnoses have been made even in the absence of gross or microscopic evidence of fatty change of the liver. All that is required is several drops of whole blood dried on filter paper. Bile is another testable matrix and can be collected in the same manner. More extensive testing may require frozen liver, cardiac, or skeletal muscle.

More recently testing has become commercially available for detection of the most common genetic mutations associated with inherited forms of long QT syndrome (LQTS). Mutations have been identified in genes that encode ion channels with resultant inactivation of sodium channels.[137,138] Ion/current flow derangements prolong the cardiac muscle action potential and lead to early-after depolarizations and ultimately a prolongation of the QT segment that can degenerate into torsade de pointes then ventricular fibrillation. While prohibitively expensive to do in every infant autopsy for most resource-strapped medicolegal jurisdictions at present, such testing may eventually be added to the routine armamentarium of the forensic pathologist faced with an otherwise unexplained infant death. Identification of a sentinel case could have significant impact on the family, and all first-degree relatives should be screened.[139]

In selected cases genetic screening for inheritable thrombophilias may yield information of importance to families. Factor V Leiden and prothrombin G20210A mutations can be detected postmortem[140] and should be considered in cases of venous thrombosis absent any clearly defined risk factor such as recent trauma, prolonged immobilization, or morbid obesity.

Microbiology

Postmortem microbiological testing is rarely the diagnostic linchpin of the autopsy. Excellent samples of cerebrospinal fluid for culture are easily obtained postmortem, but with increasing postmortem interval, blood cultures become increasingly difficult to interpret given the likelihood of contamination by enteric flora. At autopsy, a sterilely collected spleen specimen for culture has higher diagnostic yield. In any case, microbiological data, like all other postmortem laboratory data, must be considered in the context of the whole case. A blood culture with *Escherichia coli* in the total absence of any demonstrable locus for sepsis does not confirm a diagnosis of sepsis.

Culturing the genital tract and oral cavity for sexually transmitted agents can be done and is best obtained very soon after death. Clinicians are cautioned that such procedures should never occur without the knowledge and consent of the coroner or medical examiner. Ideally the forensic pathologist or his or her designee will be present for the procurement of such specimens if this is done somewhere other than the autopsy facility.

More success has been achieved using serology, antigen testing, DNA or RNA probes, and other indirect microbiological techniques. The testing procedures are quite specific and are less subject to problems of postmortem contamination than are cultures.

Limitations of the Autopsy

Despite the tremendous value of the autopsy, it is no greater than the value of its weakest element, whether that be the scene investigation, the gross examination, histologic examination, or ancillary laboratory studies. The findings cannot be accurately interpreted without correlation of all elements, any one of which may be compromised, perhaps by circumstances beyond control of the forensic pathologist charged with assigning cause and manner of death. Unrealistic expectations of what the forensic pathologist can present as scientifically sound conclusions can be a disadvantage to the pathologist unprepared to address these issues.

Special Problems in Child Autopsies

The concepts of cause and manner of death have been previously discussed. There are in every forensic pathology practice, however, cases in which determination of one or both poses particular difficulty. Consider the situation in which abuse is strongly suspected or is obvious but the precise cause of death remains undetermined after autopsy. In contrast is the case in which the immediate cause of death is evident but its relationship to clear-cut abuse is uncertain. There are also cases in which a clearly abusive injury is the cause of death but intense dispute arises over the timing of the fatal injury. Occasionally an antemortem diagnosis of abuse is made but is refuted by findings at autopsy. The forensic pathologist must be willing and able to assist in the resolution of such cases when resolution is possible. There will be, despite the best efforts of all concerned, a small subset of cases in which cause and manner of death must be most accurately classified as undetermined.

Precision in the use of language for cause and manner of death, as well as examination reports and opinion statements, is of paramount concern to the forensic pathologist and to the clinician as well. The former, in particular, must have a clear understanding of *medicolegal* causation. For example, if it is more likely than not a given child would have died on a specific day at a specific time because he or she had suffered the inflicted injury documented at autopsy, the manner of death is homicide. The rules of evidence in the courtroom are often bewildering to the medical witness. Despite the relatively privileged position of the expert witness, it behooves the conscientious expert to understand the basics of what can be stated "to a reasonable degree of medical and/or scientific certainty" in legal proceedings. These concepts are discussed in detail in Chapter 24.

Perinatal Deaths

The central issue in perinatal deaths presenting to the forensic pathologist is the question of stillbirth versus live birth. Fetal loss in most jurisdictions is reportable to the coroner or medical examiner when that loss comes beyond a certain gestational age (typically 20 weeks) and/or fetal weight and if that loss could be attributable to some nonnatural cause such as substance abuse, accidental injury, or assault. Direct trauma to the pregnant abdomen can cause premature rupture of membranes, induce premature labor, or cause catastrophic placental abruption or uterine rupture. Direct fetal trauma is uncommon without penetrating trauma of the maternal abdomen, although it can occur.[141] In a 3-year retrospective descriptive study, Weiss et al[142] reported traumatic fetal death at a rate of 3.7 per 100,000 live births, with vehicular crashes responsible for 82%, firearms 6%, and falls 3%. Younger mothers (15–19 years old) were at significantly higher risk of traumatic fetal loss, with a rate of 9.3 per 100,000 live births.

> **Case:** A 34-week gestation fetus was stillborn after no fetal heart tones were detectable 2 days prior to delivery. The mother presented to the ED after having been in a minor vehicular collision with a low-speed impact sustained to the rear left side of the mother's vehicle. Maternal vital signs were stable on arrival, and there was no evidence of hemorrhage or other signs of abruption. The ED physician stated he "thought he may have heard fetal heart tones," but this was negated by ultrasound and intrauterine fetal demise was diagnosed. Labor was induced with Pitocin with delivery of the stillbirth.
>
> Based on the appearance of the macerated, stillborn fetus, the delivering obstetrician opined that death occurred prior to the vehicular crash. Parental consent for autopsy was obtained, but hospital pathologists refused to perform the examination because of the parents' insistence that the vehicular crash caused the

death, and the case was referred to the medical examiner. Based on autopsy findings and their comparison to features described by Genest et al[143–145] (Table 20.6), the medical examiner estimated death to have occurred 3 to 5 days prior to delivery, thus eliminating the crash as an etiology for the fetal loss. A perinatal consultant retained by the medical examiner opined death occurred 2 to 3 days prior to delivery, and the case went on to litigation.

The possibility of neonaticide raises the medicolegal stakes in the case by a substantial margin. Birth is invariably unattended by any medical personnel and occurs in concealment after a variably successful attempt to conceal the pregnancy itself. Delivery into a toilet presents the additional problem of the difficult diagnosis of death of a live-born infant by drowning. Even without this confounding variable the basic questions of viability and death due to natural or nonnatural causes remain extant. If nonnatural, it must be further determined whether the death was due solely to abandonment or inflicted injury to the live-born infant. The stereotypical case involves a naïve or cognitively impaired primiparous teen who denies, conceals, or is truly unaware of her pregnancy; receives no prenatal care; then acts impulsively on the delivery of the infant. There are, however, substantial mental health issues in these cases.[146,147]

Case: A 17-year-old girl, 5 feet 2 inches, 97 pounds at baseline, concealed her pregnancy from teachers, classmates, her boyfriend, and her boyfriend's family, with whom she was residing. One day after sexual intercourse with the boyfriend, a term female was delivered in the bathroom overnight and the infant was wrapped in towels and sheets then placed under the mother's bed. The family dog pulled the now-dead infant out from under the bed and was discovered with the remains, which were then placed in a laundry basket prior to the paternal grandmother's call to 911. Autopsy confirmed the presence of postmortem anthropophagy by the dog as well as live birth.

The burden of proof of live birth rests on the pathologist. The mother will nearly always state she believed the infant was stillborn, and this is the presumed starting point with objective, documented proof of live birth required to refute the proffered history. The medicolegal significance in this lies in the fact that the fetal death certificate does not provide for a manner of death determination. Autopsy should include examination of the placenta and umbilical cord, and the investigation is seriously compromised without such an examination. The placenta can provide objective gestational age data and yield case-defining information such as chorioamnionitis, meconium-related changes, atherosis of arterioles related to preeclampsia, fetal thrombotic vasculopathy, circumvallate placenta with chronic marginal separation, fetomaternal hemorrhage, villitis, congenital syphilis, or other TORCH (toxoplasmosis, other agents, rubella, cytomega-

TABLE 20.6
Assessment of Fetal Maceration[a]

Intrauterine Duration of Retention	Gross Fetal Examination	Fetal Organ Histology	Placental Histology
4 hours		Kidney: loss of tubular nuclear basophilia	
6 hours	Desquamation of patches >1 cm; brown or red discoloration of umbilical stump		Intravascular karyorrhexis
12 hours	Desquamation on face, back, or abdomen		
18 hours	Desquamation of 25% of body OR 2 or more body regions		
24 hours	Brown or tan skin discoloration on abdomen Moderate desquamation	Liver: loss of hepatocyte nuclear basophilia Inner half of myocardium: loss of nuclear basophilia	
36 hours	Any cranial compression		
48 hours	Desquamation of >50% of body	Outer half of myocardium: loss of nuclear basophilia	Multifocal stem vessel luminal abnormalities
72 hours	Desquamation of >75% of body		
96 hours	Overlapping cranial sutures (4–5 days)	Loss of nuclear basophilia in bronchial epithelial cells and liver cells	
1 week	Widely open mouth	Gastrointestinal tract: Maximal loss of nuclear basophilia Adrenal glands: maximal loss of nuclear basophilia Trachea: chondrocyte loss of nuclear basophilia	

[a]From Genest DR, Williams MA, Greene MF. Estimating the time of death in stillborn fetuses: I. Histologic evaluation of fetal organs: an autopsy study of 150 stillborns. *Obstet Gynecol.* 1992;80:575–584; Genest DR. Estimating the time of death in stillborn fetuses: II. Histologic evaluation of the placenta: a study of 71 stillborns. *Obstet Gynecol.* 1992;80:585–592; Genest DR, Singer DB. Estimating the time of death in stillborn fetuses: III. External fetal examination: a study of 86 stillborns. *Obstet Gynecol.* 1992;80:593–600.

lovirus, herpes simplex) syndrome infections and amnion nodosum reflecting oligohydramnios.

A thorough assessment of gestational age and fetal maturity should be made using the appropriate, standardized physical measurements (crown-heel, crown-rump, occipitofrontal circumference, chest and abdomen circumference, foot length) and observations.[148] Observed trauma is documented and evaluated for the possibility of being related to the birthing process or post-natal trauma. Cephalohematoma, for example, would not be a particularly suspicious finding, but skull fracture and/or intracranial injury is not typically seen in unattended, out-of-hospital births in which no forceps or vacuum extraction device has been used. Facial and/or conjunctival petechiae cannot be presumed to be related to homicidal compression of the neck or chest because these may also be seen as a result of pressure exerted during passage through the birth canal. By the same token, their presence is a reliable sign of live birth. Organ weights should be recorded and compared to weights seen on standard, population-based organ weight tables.[149]

Pre-autopsy radiographs of a non-decomposed infant without any history of attempted resuscitation showing an air bubble in the stomach strongly suggests live birth. Further signs of live birth are sought during the internal examination. Again, presuming an un-documented attempt at resuscitation, a whole lung or portion of lung may be placed in water or formalin with a por-tion of liver of comparable size. If the lung floats and the liver sinks, aeration of the lungs and, therefore, live birth may be inferred. If both sink, the lungs are not likely aerated, but live birth cannot be categorically ruled out. If both float the suggestion is that de-composition will prohibit a definitive opinion as to whether the infant was stillborn (Figure 20.3). Histologically, the lungs of the live-born infant should have relatively uniform expansion, but this alone is not a reliable indicator. Note maceration as opposed to decom-position is diagnostic of intrauterine fetal death. Clearly, the presence of milk (formula) or colostrum in the stomach proves live birth. Some have used the presence of a polymorphonuclear in-flammatory cell infiltrate at the dis-rupted end of the umbilical cord and/or periumbilical skin as evidence supporting live birth.

Even if live birth is more likely than not, extreme prematurity; lethal malformations or birth injuries; sepsis; and birth asphyxia due to placental abnormalities, cord catastrophes, or aspiration of meconium may bring about death even under optimal birth conditions. A manner of death determi-nation of homicide requires that the live-born infant would not have died but for abandonment, exposure, inflicted trauma, intoxication, or poisoning. In that neonaticide often involves conceal-ment, it is important for the forensic pathologist to retain samples for DNA should a putative mother be identified in the course of the investigation. The Autopsy Committee of the College of American Pathologists has promulgated practice guidelines for the perinatal and

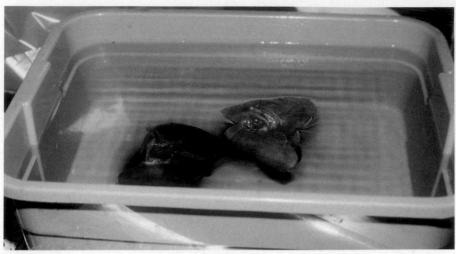

FIGURE 20.3
Float test as evidence of live birth. Aerated lungs float, whereas liver sinks.

pediatric autopsy that can prove useful.[150]

Fatal Abuse Without "Fatal" Injury

These cases demonstrate the axiom that the forensic pathologist solely dependent on anatomical findings to rule on cause and manner of death is doomed to repeated failure. Abuse and neglect can kill without a demonstrably fatal anatomical lesion. Failure to seek or obtain treatment for what might otherwise be a nonfatal condition, particularly in a chronically ill or abused child with compromised physiological reserves, may prove fatal. The child may present to the pathologist with a significant underlying medical condition or multiple injuries in various stages of healing that fit the profile of inflicted injury and a lethal bronchopneumonia. The underlying condition may have seemed stable, and no single injury ended this child's life, but the constellation of findings may still provide suffi-

cient evidence to certify the manner of death as homicide by neglect or abuse.

The capacity for repeated or prolonged abuse to compromise a child's immune system has support in the literature. Similarly, an acutely or chronically ill child who is subsequently abused is less likely to successfully cope with the additional physiological stress of the abuse. Evaluation of any given case ultimately comes down to the "But for..." question of causation. If the injuries aggravated an underlying disease or further impaired the child's health to any extent contributing to death, the manner of death is most accurately classified as homicide.

Rarely an infant or child will present to the forensic pathologist with extensive, acute, inflicted soft tissue trauma, but autopsy reveals no internal visceral injury sufficient to bring about death. Typically the injuries are distributed posteriorly (back, buttocks, and legs). Incision into these areas reveals confluent subcutaneous and intramuscular hemorrhage (Figure 20.4). The *mechanism* of death in these cases is not demonstrable by autopsy, but several mechanisms can be reasonably posited. So-called stress cardiomyopathy refers to widely scattered microscopic foci of individual myocyte necrosis (Figure 20.5), believed to be caused by high circulating levels of catecholamines in response to the severe stress of repetitive or prolonged trauma.[151] It should be noted that these foci are patchy and their absence does not necessarily negate the diagnosis. High levels of myoglobin, tissue lipases, and/or other tissue damage-related enzymes dumped into the systemic circulation may provoke catastrophic cardiovascular collapse. Given the volume of blood that can accumulate in these tissue spaces, simple exsanguination may be yet another mechanism of death. Finally, special stains for fat on fresh frozen or formalin-fixed frozen tissue may reveal the presence of lethal amounts of fat embolization to lungs or brain.

An otherwise well cared for child who dies of a treatable medical or surgical condition poses special difficulties. Some conditions, such as fulminating sepsis, meningitis, or pneumonia, may catch even the vigilant parent off guard, but in some cases parental impairment, mental illness, ignorance, or neglectful indifference may be responsible for a delay in seeking treatment. Alternatively, there are those who eschew medical intervention for religious reasons. In these cases the forensic pathologist may likely rule the manner of death natural and allow the legal system to take its course in determining if there is criminal culpability on the part of caretakers.

"Negative" Autopsy

This may be considered the terminus of the spectrum of fatal abuse without demonstrable fatal injury. The prototypical example would be the "gentle homicide" of asphyxiating an infant.

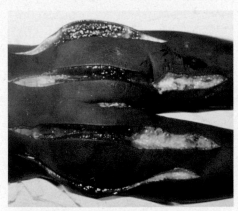

FIGURE 20.4
Subcutaneous hemorrhage demonstrated at autopsy.

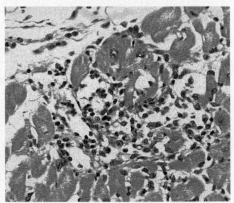

FIGURE 20.5
Histology of stress cardiomyopathy.

Poisoning may also present in this fashion. So too, however, will SIDS, metabolic disorders, and certain types of accidental asphyxia. Within the peak SIDS age range of 2 to 4 months, 80% to 82% of sudden, unexplained infant deaths will be certified as SIDS.[152] The overall percentage is declining at present, due mainly to better scene investigation, the documentation of unsafe sleep environments and, to a lesser extent, more detailed ancillary testing such as toxicological and metabolic screening. This has brought about a "diagnostic shift" of some concern to those who study SIDS.[153-155]

The definition of SIDS since 1989 has been "the sudden death of an infant under one year of age which remains unexplained after performance of a complete postmortem investigation, including an autopsy, an examination of the scene of death and a review of the case history." In 2004 a multispecialty team met in San Diego to revisit the definition of SIDS.[156] While a slight modification was added to the definition (sudden, unexpected death of an infant younger than 1 year, *with onset of the fatal episode apparently occurring during sleep,* that remains unexplained after a thorough investigation, including performance of a complete autopsy and review of the circumstances of death and the clinical history), the more practical information to emerge from the San Diego group was a stratified classification of sudden unexplained infant deaths that more closely reflects current case profiles.

- *Category IA SIDS:* classic features and complete documentation
- *Category IB SIDS:* classic features but incomplete documentation
- *Category II SIDS:* meets category I criteria with specific exceptions
- *Unclassified Sudden Infant Death:* does not meet category I or II criteria, alternative diagnoses of natural or unnatural conditions are equivocal, including cases in which autopsy is not performed

It remains to be seen if this newly proposed diagnostic stratification of the SIDS diagnosis will be assigned a specific coding scheme, but this would provide improved diagnostic and epidemiological clarity.[157] Low birth weight, prematurity, maternal smoking and/or other substance abuse, poverty, single motherhood, maternal age younger than 20 years, short intergestational intervals, and lack of prenatal care continue to be risk factors.[158]

Autopsy findings, when present at all, are non-diagnostic. Observed lesions that are insufficient to cause death include thymic, pleural, and epicardial petechiae (Figures 20.6 and 20.7); pulmonary engorgement and patchy intra-alveolar hemorrhage, seen in two-thirds of SIDS cases and more than 5% of non-SIDS cases; minimal to moderate aspiration with foamy macrophages and granulomata, seen in 15% of SIDS and 10% of non-SIDS cases; and small, focal, perivascular CNS hemorrhages, an agonal phenomenon seen in 17% of SIDS and 16% of non-SIDS cases.

Thymic involution is indicative of chronic stress and is not a specific marker for SIDS. Other nonspecific findings include subendocardial hemorrhage, minimal acute bronchopneumonia, extramedullary hematopoiesis, nonspecific portal inflammation, slight hepatic steatosis, old germinal matrix hemorrhage, and red blood cell sickling in hepatic sinusoids. Matturri et al[159] have advocated routine, in-depth histological evaluation of the brain stem nuclei and cardiac conduction system in all such cases, and while this is acknowledged as valuable, it is not likely to become standard practice in the United States.

The medical examiner or coroner best serves families by having a coherent follow-up strategy for sudden, unexplained infant death. He or she should contact the family immediately after autopsy to report whatever has (or has not) been observed and where the case will go from that point. Referral to appropriate bereavement/informational services should be made. Contact should be formally made again when the case is ultimately finalized to explain results and answer any questions that remain.

As has been previously noted, fatal suffocation (obstruction of the mouth and nose) of an infant, whether accidental or homicidal, has no morphological correlate at autopsy. Petechiae of the face, conjunctivae, or visceral serosal surfaces have not proven to be of discriminatory diagnostic value in separating one type of death from another. A conclusion of asphyxia is better supported by the constellation of conjunctival petechiae, acute pulmonary

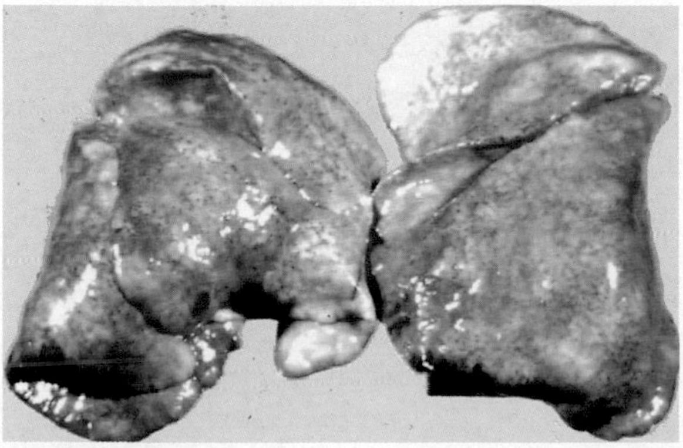

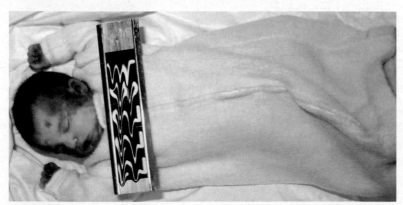

FIGURE 20.6
Thymic petechiae.

FIGURE 20.7
Pleural petechiae.

emphysema, and patchy atelectasis in the absence of CPR (the latter a rarity) and, in older children capable of a fight, facial or mucosal injuries.

> **Case:** A 3-week-old infant was dead in her crib and 2 older siblings were dead in their beds in another room. One child had a prominent plume of edema fluid at the mouth while the other showed curvilinear facial abrasions and small mucosal tears of the buccal mucosa corresponding to her teeth. Their mother was also dead in her bed. All had been strangled and/or suffocated by the father of the children who wanted a new life with his paramour.

The presence of cerebral edema will cast doubt on a diagnosis of SIDS. As opposed to what is believed to be rapid death due to some functional chemical or electrical mechanism, cerebral edema suggests either trauma or, in the absence of other markers of trauma, a prolonged interval between physiological insult and death as may be seen in asphyxia or metabolic, toxic, or encephalopathic disorders. Its presence indicates the need for specific inquiry into possible etiologies as opposed to simply passing the finding off to SIDS.

A history of recurrent apnea and/or an apparent life-threatening event (ALTE) lacking a diagnosis after a competent medical workup is another situation with an increased index of suspicion. A recent study has shown no link between such episodes and eventual SIDS.[160] DiFiore et al[161] studied 119 preterm infants using respiratory inductance plethysmography, heart rate and oxygen saturation monitoring, and esophageal pH. They found that there was no temporal relationship between acid-based gastroesophageal reflux (GER) and apnea, nor did GER prolong apnea in preterm infants. An ALTE unrelated to diagnosable cardiac, respiratory, or gastrointestinal conditions has a reasonable likelihood of representing factitious apnea and/or repetitive, induced, sublethal asphyxia. The tragedy of the serial murders such as those reported by Stanton and Simpson[162] and documented in detail in Firstman and Talan's *The Death of Innocents*[163] represents an extreme example of this phenomenon. Faced with repetitive *unexplained* infant deaths within a family today most forensic pathologists would certify the second death as cause and manner un-determined and the third as an asphyxial homicide. Recently published papers have suggested ways in which SIDS can be distinguished from non-accidental causes of sudden, unexplained infant death.[164-166] The American Academy of Pediatrics Committee on Child Abuse and Neglect, with input from NAME,[157,167,168] has recommended the following:

- Accurate history taking at the time of death made available to the medical examiner or coroner
- Prompt death scene investigation
- Appropriate use of available medical specialists by the medical examiner or coroner
- Complete autopsy, including skeletal survey, toxicological and metabolic screening within 24 hours of death
- Thorough review of medical history and records

- A supportive approach to parents during the death review process
- Consideration of intentional asphyxiation in cases with problematic ALTE histories
- Use of accepted diagnostic categories on death certificates
- Prompt informing sessions with parents
- Review of all cases by the local child fatality review team

The foregoing discussion has been heavily weighted toward infants, but the occasional deceased toddler or older child may also present the forensic pathologist with a "negative autopsy." As in the infant, this more often reflects a natural cause of death such as an inheritable dysrhythmia (eg, LQTS, seizure disorders or, more rarely, fulminant sepsis). Sudden death in epilepsy is well described,[169] though clinicians are often incredulous of the diagnosis as a cause of death. Blood levels of prescribed anticonvulsants may be absent, sub-therapeutic, or therapeutic in such cases. These diagnoses may depend entirely on investigative and/or record review data. Nonnatural causes of death with no findings may include commotio cordis (ventricular fibrillation triggered by a blow to the chest during repolarization of cardiac muscle),[170] hypothermia or hyperthermia, asphyxia, electrocution, and undetected poisoning. The child with commotio cordis may or may not have a suggestive contusion, and the episode is usually witnessed because they tend to occur in the context of athletic events such as baseball or hockey games. Hypothermia and hyperthermia have

subtle and variably present autopsy findings such as Wischnewski spots in the former[171] and serosal petechiae in the latter. It is decidedly more difficult to asphyxiate the older child capable of resistance than the infant, and their struggle may be reflected by findings previously noted and depicted. Low-voltage electrocution leaves burns at contact points in a minority of cases. Once again, thorough investigation remains the key to diagnosis in these cases as well as cases of subtle abusive trauma because objective findings may not be readily apparent. The Zumwalt and Hirsch[172] article from 1980 on the latter issue is as cogent today as it was the day of publication.

Determination of Manner of Death

Determination of manner of death falls to the medical examiner or coroner if it is anything other than natural. A significant number of natural deaths also come, by statute, under the jurisdiction of the medicolegal authority in a given municipality, county, or state. Table 20.7 is a simplified scheme of how to correlate investigative and autopsy findings to most accurately assign manner.

Even in high-quality death investigation systems, some 2% to 3% of cases (with sudden, unexplained infant death as a unique category) may be certified as of undetermined cause and/or manner. Neglect cases can pose especially difficult in this regard. All professionals involved in the death investigation, including the forensic pathologist, must

TABLE 20.7
Sudden Deaths in Infants and Children: Determination of Manner of Death

Autopsy	Investigation	Manner
Natural disease No injury	a. Negative b. Inconclusive (FTT, impaired parent, neglect) c. Positive (neglect, MSBP)	a. Natural b. Undetermined or natural c. Homicide
Negative autopsy No disease, no injury	a. Negative b. Inconclusive (history of abuse, neglect, prior SIDS/ SUID) c. Positive (≥SIDS/SUID, physical evidence, confession)	a. Natural b. Undetermined c. Homicide
Fatal injury	a. Negative (documented circumstance consistent with accident) b. Inconclusive (timing, multiple suspects) c. Positive (consistent with injuries)	a. Accident b. Undetermined c. Homicide
Nonfatal injury Aggravating disease process	a. Confirmed accidental injury, medical complication b. Injury due to abuse c. Inconclusive d. Injury due to abuse, no anatomical cause of death	a. Accident b. Homicide c. Undetermined d. Homicide or undetermined

Abbreviations: FTT, failure to thrive; MSBP, Munchausen syndrome by proxy; SIDS, sudden infant death syndrome; SUID, sudden, unexplained infant death.

always remain cognizant of the significant social and economic difficulties faced by so many families and strive for a sense of impartiality and compassion. By the same token, every child has the right to be shielded from harm and to receive the physical and emotional care necessary to permit normal growth and development.

References

1. Cote A, Russo P, Michaud J. Sudden unexpected death in infancy: what are the causes? *J Pediatr.* 1999;135:437–443

2. United States Department of Health and Human Services. OCR Summary of the HIPAA Privacy Rule. April 11, 2003. http://www.hhs.gov/ocr/hipaa/privacy.html. Accessed May 31, 2007

3. DiMaio VJM, Bernstein CG. A case of infanticide. *J Forensic Sci.* 1974;19:744–754

4. Carpenter RG, Coombs RC, Daman-Willems C, McKenzie A, Huber J, Emery JL. Repeat sudden unexpected and unexplained infant deaths: natural or unnatural? *Lancet.* 2005;365:29–35

5. Bacon C, DiMaio VJ. Repeat sudden unexpected infant deaths [letter]. *Lancet.* 2005;365:1137–1138

6. Bass M, Kravath RE, Glass I. Death-scene investigation in sudden infant death. *N Engl J Med.* 1986;320:507–511

7. Gross EM, Leffers B. Investigation of SIDS [letter]. *N Engl J Med.* 1986;315:1675

8. Valdes-Dapena MA, Mandell F, Merritt TA. Investigation of SIDS [letter]. *N Engl J Med.* 1986;316:1675

9. Guntheroth WG, Spiers PS. Thermal stress in sudden infant death: is there an ambiguity with the rebreathing hypothesis? *Pediatrics.* 2001;107:693–698

10. Moon RY, Patel KM, Shaefer SJM. Sudden infant death syndrome in child care settings. *Pediatrics*. 2000;106:295–300

11. Moon RY, Sprague BM, Patel KM. Stable prevalence but changing risk factors for sudden infant death syndrome in child care settings in 2001. *Pediatrics*. 2005;116:972–977

12. deJonge GA, Lanting CI, Brand R, Ruys JH, Semmekrot BA, van Wouwe JP. Sudden infant death syndrome in child care settings in the Netherlands. *Arch Dis Child*. 2004;89:427–430

13. Dancea A, Cote A, Roblicek C, Bernard C, Oligny LL. Cardiac pathology in sudden unexpected infant death. *J Pediatr*. 2002;141:336–342

14. Hirsch CS. Craniocerebral trauma. In: *Handbook of Forensic Pathology* Northfield, IL: College of American Pathologists; 1990

15. Perper JA. Time of death and changes after death. In: Spitz WU, ed. *Spitz and Fisher's Medicolegal Investigation of Death: Guidelines for the Application of Pathology to Crime Investigation*. 3rd ed. Springfield, IL: Charles C. Thomas; 1993

16. DiMaio VJM, DiMaio D. *Forensic Pathology*. 2nd ed. Boca Raton, FL: CRC Press Inc; 2001

17. Saukko P, Knight B. *Knight's Forensic Pathology*. 3rd ed. New York, NY: Oxford University Press; 2004

18. Dolinak D, Matshes E, Lew E. *Forensic Pathology—Principles and Practice*. Boston, MA: Elsevier Academic Press; 2005

19. Coe JI. Chemical considerations. In: Spitz WU, ed. *Spitz and Fisher's Medicolegal Investigation of Death: Guidelines for the Application of Pathology to Crime Investigation*. 3rd ed. Springfield, IL: Charles C. Thomas; 1993

20. Coe JI. Vitreous potassium as a measure of the postmortem interval: an historical review and critical evaluation. *Forensic Sci Int*. 1989;42:201–213

21. Sorg MH, Haglund WD, eds. *Advances in Forensic Taphonomy*. Boca Raton, FL: CRC Press; 2005

22. Wright PD. Photography in bite-mark and patterned injury documentation—Part I. *J Forensic Sci*. 1998;43:877–880

23. Society for Pediatric Radiology, National Association of Medical Examiners. Post-mortem radiography in the evaluation of unexpected death in children less than 2 years of age whose death is suspicious for fatal abuse. *Pediatr Radiol*. 2004;34:675–677

24. Price EA, Rush LR, Perper JA, Bell MD. Cardiopulmonary resuscitation-related injuries and homicidal blunt abdominal trauma in children. *Am J Forensic Med Pathol*. 2000;21:307–310

25. Bush CM, Jones JS, Cohle SD, Johnson H. Pediatric injuries from cardiopulmonary resuscitation. *Ann Emerg Med*. 1996;28:40–44

26. Krischer JP, Fine EG, Davis JH, Nagel EL. Complications of cardiac resuscitation. *Chest*. 1987;92:287–291

27. Ryan MP, Young SJ, Wells DL. Do resuscitation attempts in children who die cause injury? *Emerg Med J*. 2003;20:10–12

28. Betz P, Liebhardt E. Rib fractures in children—resuscitation or child abuse? *Int J Legal Med*. 1994;106:215–218

29. Spevak MR, Kleinman PK, Belanger PL, Primack C, Richmond JM. Cardiopulmonary resuscitation and rib fractures in infants. A postmortem radiologic-pathologic study. *JAMA*. 1994;272:617–618

30. Feldman KW, Brewer DK. Child abuse, cardiopulmonary resuscitation, and rib fractures. *Pediatrics*. 1984;73:339–342

31. Hoke RS, Chamberlain D. Skeletal chest injuries secondary to cardiopulmonary resuscitation. *Resuscitation*. 2004;63:327–338

32. Gordon I, Shapiro HA, Berson SD. *Forensic Medicine: A Guide to Principles*. 3rd ed. New York, NY: Churchill Livingstone; 1988:37

33. Robertson I, Mansfield RA. Ante-mortem and post-mortem bruises of the skin: their differentiation. *J Forensic Med*. 1957;4:2–10

34. Maguire S, Mann MK, Sibert J, Kemp A. Are there patterns of bruising in childhood which are diagnostic or suggestive of abuse? A systematic review. *Arch Dis Child.* 2005;90:182–186

35. Sugar NF, Taylor JA, Feldman KW. Bruises in infants and toddlers: those who don't cruise rarely bruise. Puget Sound Pediatric Research Network. *Arch Pediatr Adolesc Med.* 1999;153:399–403

36. Carpenter RF. The prevalence and distribution of bruising in babies. *Arch Dis Child.* 1999;80:363–366

37. Mortimer PE, Freeman M. Are facial bruises in babies ever accidental? *Arch Dis Child.* 1983;58:75–76

38. Atwal GS, Rutty GN, Carter N, Green MA. Bruising in non-accidental head injured children; a retrospective study of the prevalence, distribution and pathological associations in 24 cases. *Forensic Sci Int.* 1998;96:215–230

39. Labbe J, Caouette G. Recent skin injuries in normal children. *Pediatrics.* 2001;108:271–276

40. Dunstan FD, Guildea ZE, Kontos K, Kemp AM, Sibert JR. A scoring system for bruise patterns: a tool for identifying abuse. *Arch Dis Child.* 2002;86:330–333

41. Pascoe JM, Hildebrandt HM, Tarrier A, Murphy M. Patterns of skin injury in nonaccidental and accidental injury. *Pediatrics.* 1979;64:245–247

42. Spitz WU, ed. *Spitz and Fisher's Medicolegal Investigation of Death: Guidelines for the Application of Pathology to Crime Investigation.* 3rd ed. Springfield, IL: Charles C. Thomas; 1993: 217–235, 252, 413–443, 660–661, 664

43. Hight DW, Bakalar HR, Lloyd JR. Inflicted burns in children. Recognition and treatment. *JAMA.* 1979;242:517–520

44. Hummel RP III, Greenhalgh DG, Barthel PP, et al. Outcome and socioeconomic aspects of suspected child abuse scald burns. *J Burn Care Rehabil.* 1993;14:121–126

45. Rosenberg NM, Marino D. Frequency of suspected abuse/neglect in burn patients. *Pediatr Emerg Care.* 1989;5:219–221

46. Andronicus M, Oates RK, Peat J, Spalding S, Martin H. Non-accidental burns in children. *Burns.* 1998;24:552–558

47. Hobson MI, Evans J, Stewart IP. An audit of non-accidental injury in burned children. *Burns.* 1994;20:442–445

48. Feldman KW, Schaller RT, Feldman JA, McMillon M. Tap water scald burns in children. *Pediatrics.* 1978;62:1–7

49. Sheridan RL, Remensnyder JP, Schnitzer JJ, Schulz JT, Ryan CM, Tompkins RG. Current expectations for survival in pediatric burns. *Arch Pediatr Adolesc Med.* 2000;154:245–249

50. Baur PS, Parks DH, Larson DL. The healing of burn wounds. *Clin Plast Surg.* 1977;4:389–407

51. Squires T, Busuttil A. Child fatalities in Scottish house fires 1980–1990: a case of child neglect? *Child Abuse Negl.* 1995;19:865–873

52. Betz P. Histological and enzyme histochemical parameters for the age estimation of human skin wounds. *Int J Legal Med.* 1994;107:60–68

53. Robertson I, Hodge PR. Histopathology of healing abrasions. *Forensic Sci.* 1972;1:17–25

54. Zumwalt RE, Hirsch CS. Subtle fatal child abuse. *Hum Pathol.* 1980;11:167–174

55. Kleinman PK, ed. *Diagnostic Imaging of Child Abuse.* 2nd ed. St Louis, MO: Mosby; 1998: 252, 422

56. Klotzbach H, Delling G, Richter E, Sperhake JP, Puschel K. Post-mortem diagnosis and age estimation of infants' fractures. *Int J Legal Med.* 2003;117:82–89

57. Kleinman PK, Marks SC Jr, Richmond JM, Blackbourne BD. Inflicted skeletal injury: a postmortem radiologic-histopathologic study in 31 infants. *AJR Am J Roentgenol.* 1995;165:647–650

58. Prosser I, Maguire S, Harrison SK, Mann M, Sibert JR, Kemp AM. How old is this fracture? Radiologic dating of fractures in children: a systematic review. *AJR Am J Roentgenol.* 2005;184:1282–1286

59. Karpas A, Yen K, Sell LL, Frommelt PC. Severe blunt cardiac injury in an infant: a case of child abuse. *J Trauma.* 2002;52:759–764

60. Maron BJ, Poliac LC, Kaplan JA, Mueller FO. Blunt impact to the chest leading to sudden death from cardiac arrest during sports activities. *N Engl J Med.* 1995;333:337–342

61. Baker AM, Craig BR, Lonergan GJ. Homicidal commotio cordis: the final blow in a battered infant. *Child Abuse Negl.* 2003;27:125–130

62. Gaines BA, Shultz BS, Morrison K, Ford HR. Duodenal injuries in children: beware of child abuse. *J Pediatr Surg.* 2004;39:600–602

63. Cooper A, Floyd T, Barlow B, et al. Major blunt abdominal trauma due to child abuse. *J Trauma.* 1988;28:1483–1487

64. Canty TG, Canty TG Jr, Brown C. Injuries of the gastrointestinal tract from blunt trauma in children: a 12-year experience at a designated pediatric trauma center. *J Trauma.* 1999;46:234–240

65. Bensard DD, Beaver BL, Besner GE, Cooney DR. Small bowel injury in children after blunt abdominal trauma: is diagnostic delay important? *J Trauma.* 1996;41:476–483

66. Philippart AI. Blunt abdominal trauma in childhood. *Surg Clin North Am.* 1977;57:151–163

67. Ng CS, Hall CM, Shaw DG. The range of visceral manifestations of non-accidental injury. *Arch Dis Child.* 1997;77:167–174

68. Sivit CJ, Taylor GA, Eichelberger MR. Visceral injury in battered children: a changing perspective. *Radiology.* 1989;173:659–661

69. Wood J, Rubin DM, Nance ML, Christian CW. Distinguishing inflicted versus accidental abdominal injuries in young children. *J Trauma.* 2005;59:1203–1208

70. Case ME, Nanduri R. Laceration of the stomach by blunt trauma in a child: a case of child abuse. *J Forensic Sci.* 1983;28:496–501

71. Iuchtman M, Breitgand A. Traumatic adrenal hemorrhage in children: an indicator of visceral injury. *Pediatr Surg Int.* 2000;16:586–588

72. deRoux SJ, Prendergast NC. Adrenal lacerations in child abuse: a marker of severe trauma. *Pediatr Surg Int.* 2000;16:121–123

73. Snell RS. *Clinical Anatomy for Medical Students.* 2nd ed. Boston, MA: Little, Brown & Company; 1981

74. Cameron CM, Lazoritz S, Calhoun AD. Blunt abdominal injury: simultaneously occurring liver and pancreatic injury in child abuse. *Pediatr Emerg Care.* 1997;13:334–336

75. Ely SF, Hirsch CS. Asphyxial deaths and petechiae: a review. *J Forensic Sci.* 2000;45:1274–1277

76. Camps FE, Hunt AC. Pressure on the neck. *J Forensic Med.* 1959;6:116–135

77. Harm T, Rajs J. Types of injuries and interrelated conditions of victims and assailants in attempted and homicidal strangulation. *Forensic Sci Int.* 1981;18:101–123

78. Luke JL, Reay DT, Eisele JW, Bonnell HJ. Correlation of circumstances with pathological findings in asphyxial deaths by hanging: a prospective study of 61 cases from Seattle, WA. *J Forensic Sci.* 1985;30:1140–1147

79. Taff ML, Boglioli LR. Strangulation. A conceptual approach for courtroom presentation. *Am J Forensic Med Pathol.* 1989;10:216–220

80. Feldman KW, Simms RJ. Strangulation in childhood: epidemiology and clinical course. *Pediatrics.* 1980;65:1079–1085

81. Malek AM, Higashida RT, Halbach VV, et al. Patient presentation, angiographic features, and treatment of strangulation-induced bilateral dissection of the cervical internal carotid artery. Report of three cases. *J Neurosurg.* 2000;92:481–487

82. Clarot F, Vaz E, Papin F, Proust B. Fatal and non-fatal bilateral delayed carotid artery dissection after manual strangulation. *Forensic Sci Int.* 2005;149:143–150

83. Simpson RK Jr, Goodman JC, Rouah E, Caraway N, Baskin DS. Late neuropathological consequences of strangulation. *Resuscitation.* 1987;15:171–185

84. Meadow R. Unnatural sudden infant death. *Arch Dis Child.* 1999;80:7–14

85. DiMaio VJ. Homicidal asphyxia. *Am J Forensic Med Pathol.* 2000;21:1–4

86. Banaschak S, Schmidt P, Madea B. Smothering of children older than 1 year of age-diagnostic significance of morphological findings. *Forensic Sci Int.* 2003;134:163–168

87. Krous HF, Nadeau JM, Byard RW, Blackbourne BD. Oronasal blood in sudden infant death. *Am J Forensic Med Pathol.* 2001;22:346–351

88. Berry PJ. Intra-alveolar haemorrhage in sudden infant death syndrome: a cause for concern [comment]? *J Clin Pathol.* 1999;52:553–554

89. Yukawa N, Carter N, Rutty G, Green MA. Intra-alveolar haemorrhage in sudden infant death syndrome: a cause for concern? *J Clin Pathol.* 1999;52:581–587

90. Hanzlick R, Delaney K. Pulmonary hemosiderin in deceased infants: baseline data for further study of infant mortality. *Am J Forensic Med Pathol.* 2000;21:319–322

91. Schluckebier DA, Cool CD, Henry TE, Martin A, Wahe JW. Pulmonary siderophages and unexpected infant death. *Am J Forensic Med Pathol.* 2002;23:360–363

92. Stiffman MN, Schnitzer PG, Adam P, Kruse RL, Ewigman BG. Household composition and risk of fatal child maltreatment. *Pediatrics.* 2002;109:615–621

93. Jackson CM, Gilliland MG. Frequency of pulmonary hemosiderosis in Eastern North Carolina. *Am J Forensic Med Pathol.* 2000;21:36–38

94. Forbes A, Acland P. What is the significance of haemosiderin in the lungs of deceased infants? *Med Sci Law.* 2004;44:348–352

95. Orr CJ, Clark MA, Hawley DA, Pless JE, Tate LR, Fardal PM. Fatal anorectal injuries: a series of four cases. *J Forensic Sci.* 1995;40:219–221

96. Gabby T, Winkleby MA, Boyce WT, Fisher DL, Lancaster A, Sensabaugh GF. Sexual abuse of children. The detection of semen on skin. *Am J Dis Child.* 1992;146:700–703

97. Santucci KA, Nelson DG, McQuillen KK, Duffy SJ, Linakis JG. Wood's lamp utility in the identification of semen. *Pediatrics.* 1999;104:1342–1344

98. Bouska I. Causes of death in fatal cases of child abuse 1964–1988. *Cas Lek Cesk.* 1995;134:344–346

99. de Silva S, Oates RK. Child homicide—the extreme of child abuse. *Med J Aust.* 1993;158:300–301

100. Brewster AL, Nelson JP, Hymel KP, et al. Victim, perpetrator, family, and incident characteristics of 32 infant maltreatment deaths in the United States Air Force. *Child Abuse Negl.* 1998;22:91–101

101. Lucas DR, Wezner KC, Milner JS, et al. Victim, perpetrator, family, and incident characteristics of infant and child homicide in the United States Air Force. *Child Abuse Negl.* 2002;26:167–186

102. Mallet ML. Pathophysiology of accidental hypothermia. *QJM.* 2002;95:775–785

103. Behrman RE, Kliegman RM, Jenson HB, eds. *Nelson Textbook of Pediatrics.* 17th ed. Philadelphia, PA: Saunders; 2004:133–134, 170–173, 338

104. Tsokos M, Rothschild M, Madea B, Rie M, Sperhake J. Histological and immunohistochemical study of Wischnewsky spots in fatal hypothermia. *Am J Forensic Med Pathol.* 2006;27:70–74

105. US Government Printing Office. Child maltreatment 2003. www.acf.hhs.gov/programs/cb/pubs/cm03/index.htm. Accessed April 29, 2005

106. Knight LD, Collins KA. A 25-year retrospective review of deaths due to pediatric neglect. *Am J Forensic Med Pathol.* 2005;26:221–228

107. Kellogg ND, Lukefahr JL. Criminally prosecuted cases of child starvation. *Pediatrics.* 2005;116:1309–1316

108. Centers for Disease Control and Prevention. Clinical growth charts. http://www.cdc.gov/nchs/about/major/nhanes/growthcharts/clinical_charts.htm

109. Frank DA, Silva M, Needlman R. Failure to thrive: mystery, myth and method. *Contemp Pediatr.* 1993;10:114–133

110. Feldman M, Friedman LS, Sleisenger MH, eds. *Sleisenger & Fordtran's Gastrointestinal and Liver Disease: Pathophysiology/Diagnosis/Management.* 7th ed. Philadelphia, PA: Saunders; 2002: 272–275

111. Thompson WS, Cohle SD. Fifteen-year retrospective study of infant organ weights and revision of standard weight tables. *J Forensic Sci.* 2004;49:575–585

112. Shetty PS. Adaptation to low energy intakes: the responses and limits to low intakes in infants, children and adults. *Eur J Clin Nutr.* 1999;53(suppl 1):S14–S33

113. Waterlow JC. Classification and definition of protein-calorie malnutrition. *Br Med J.* 1972;3:566–569

114. Gomez F, Galvan RR, Frank S, et al. Mortality in second and third degree malnutrition. *J Tropical Peds.* 1956;2.77–83

115. Coe JI. Postmortem chemistries on human vitreous humor. *Am J Clin Pathol.* 1969;51:741–750

116. Gilbert-Barness E, Debich-Spicer DE. *Handbook of Pediatric Autopsy Pathology.* Totowa, NJ; Humana Press; 2005

117. Nagao M, Maeno Y, Koyama H, et al. Estimation of caloric deficit in a fatal case of starvation resulting from child neglect. *J Forensic Sci.* 2004;49:1073–1076

118. Meade JL, Brissie RM. Infanticide by starvation: calculation of caloric deficit to determine degree of deprivation. *J Forensic Sci.* 1985;30:1263–1268

119. National Center for Injury Prevention and Control, Centers for Disease Control and Prevention. WISQARS database. http://www.cdc.gov/ncipc/maps/default.htm. Accessed May 31, 2007

120. Hiss J, Kahana T, Kugel C, Epstein Y. Fatal classic and exertional heat stroke—report of four cases. *Med Sci Law.* 1994;34:339–343

121. Roberts KB, Roberts EC. The automobile and heat stress. *Pediatrics.* 1976;58:101–104

122. Gibbs LI, Lawrence DW, Kohn MA. Heat exposure in an enclosed automobile. *J La State Med Soc.* 1995;147:545–546

123. King K, Negus K, Vance JC. Heat stress in motor vehicles: a problem in infancy. *Pediatrics.* 1981;68:579–582

124. Donoghue ER, Graham MA, Jentzen JM, Lifschultz BD, Luke JL, Mirchandani HG. Criteria for the diagnosis of heat-related deaths: National Association of Medical Examiners. Position paper. National Association of Medical Examiners Ad Hoc Committee on the Definition of Heat-Related Fatalities. *Am J Forensic Med Pathol.* 1997;18:11–14

125. Krous HF, Nadeau JM, Fukumoto RI, Blackbourne BD, Byard RW. Environmental hyperthermic infant and early childhood death: circumstances, pathologic changes, and manner of death. *Am J Forensic Med Pathol.* 2001;22:374–382

126. Surpure JS. Heat-related illness and the automobile. *Ann Emerg Med.* 1982;11:263–265

127. DiMaio DJ, DiMaio VJM. *Forensic Pathology.* Boca Raton, FL: CRC Press; 1993

128. Meadow R. Non-accidental salt poisoning. *Arch Dis Child.* 1993;68:448–452

129. Keating JP, Shears GJ, Dodge PR. Oral water intoxication in infants: an American epidemic. *Am J Dis Child.* 1991;145:985–990

130. Arieff AI, Kronlund BA. Fatal child abuse by forced water intoxication. *Pediatrics.* 1999;103:1292–1295

131. Black J, Zenel JA. Child abuse by intentional iron poisoning presenting as shock and persistent acidosis. *Pediatrics.* 2003;111:197–199

132. Roe CR, Millington DS, Maltby DA, et al. Recognition of medium-chain acyl-CoA dehydrogenase deficiency in asymptomatic siblings of children dying of sudden infant death or Reye-like syndrome. *J Pediatr.* 1986;108:13–18

133. Arens R, Gozal D, Jain K, et al. Prevalence of medium-chain acyl-coenzyme A dehydrogenase deficiency in the sudden infant death syndrome. *J Pediatr.* 1993;123:415–418

134. Kohler M, Hoffmann GF. Subdural hematoma in a child with glutaric aciduria type I. *Pediatr Radiol.* 1998;28:582

135. Hartley LM, Khwaja OS, Verity CM. Glutaric aciduria type I and nonaccidental head injury. *Pediatrics.* 2001;107:174–175

136. Gago LC, Wegner RK, Capone A, Williams GA. Intraretinal hemorrhages and chronic subdural effusions: glutaric aciduria type 1 can be mistaken for shaken baby syndrome. *Retina.* 2003;23:724–726

137. Ackerman MJ. The long QT syndrome: ion channel diseases of the heart. *Mayo Clinic Proc.* 1998;73:250–269

138. Schwartz PJ, Priori SG, Duhaime R, et al. A molecular link between the sudden infant death syndrome and the long-QT syndrome. *N Engl J Med.* 2000;343:262–267

139. Miller MD, Porter CJ, Ackerman MJ. Diagnostic accuracy of screening electrocardiograms in long QT syndrome I. *Pediatrics.* 2001;108:8–12

140. Andrew TA, Fairweather RB. Prothrombin G20210A mutation and sudden death. *Am J Forensic Med Pathol.* 2003;24:377–380

141. Alley JR, Yahagi Y, Moncure MM, Strickler JC. A case of in utero fetal brain trauma after motor vehicle collision. *J Trauma.* 2003;55:782–785

142. Weiss HB, Songer TJ, Fabio A. Fetal deaths related to maternal injury. *JAMA.* 2001;286:1863–1868

143. Genest DR, Williams MA, Greene MF. Estimating the time of death in stillborn fetuses: I. Histologic evaluation of fetal organs: an autopsy study of 150 stillborns. *Obstet Gynecol.* 1992;80:575–584

144. Genest DR. Estimating the time of death in stillborn fetuses: II. Histologic evaluation of the placenta: a study of 71 stillborns. *Obstet Gynecol.* 1992;80:585–592

145. Genest DR, Singer DB. Estimating the time of death in stillborn fetuses: III. External fetal examination: a study of 86 stillborns. *Obstet Gynecol.* 1992;80:593–600

146. Spinelli MG. A systematic investigation of 16 cases of neonaticides. *Am J Psychiatry.* 2001;158:811–813

147. Spinelli MG. Maternal infanticide associated with mental illness: prevention and the promise of saved lives. *Am J Psychiatry.* 2004;161:1548–1557

148. Ballard JL, Noval KK, Driver M. A simplified score for assessment of fetal maturation of newly born infants. *J Pediatr.* 1979;95:769–774

149. Schulz DM, Giordano DA, Schulz DH. Weights of organs of fetuses and infants. *Arch Pathol.* 1962;74:244–250

150. Bove KE, CAP Autopsy Committee. Practice guidelines for autopsy pathology: the perinatal and pediatric autopsy. *Arch Pathol Lab Med.* 1997;121:368–376

151. Cebelin MS, Hirsch CS. Human stress cardiomyopathy: myocardial lesions in victims of homicidal assaults without internal injuries. *Hum Pathol.* 1980;11:123–132

152. Hunt CE. Sudden infant death syndrome and other causes of infant mortality: diagnosis, mechanisms, and risk for recurrence in siblings. *Am J Respir Crit Care Med.* 2001;164:346–357

153. Malloy MH, MacDroman M. Changes in the classification of sudden, unexpected infant deaths: United States, 1992–2001. *Pediatrics.* 2005;115:1247–1253

154. Mitchell E, Krous HF, DonaldT, Byard RW. Changing trends in the diagnosis of sudden infant death. *Am J Forensic Med Pathol.* 2000;21:311–314

155. Beckwith JB. Defining the sudden infant death syndrome. *Arch Pediatr Adolesc Med.* 2003;157:286–290

156. Krous HF, Beckwith B, Byard RW, et al. Sudden infant death syndrome and unclassified sudden infant deaths: a definitional and diagnostic approach. *Pediatrics.* 2004;114:234–238

157. American Academy of Pediatrics Task Force on Sudden Infant Death Syndrome. The changing concept of sudden infant death syndrome: diagnostic coding shifts, controversies regarding the sleeping environment, and new variables to consider in reducing risk. *Pediatrics.* 2005;116:1245–1255

158. Paris CA, Remler R, Daling JR. Risk factors for sudden infant death syndrome: changes associated with sleep position recommendations. *J Pediatr.* 2001;139:771–777

159. Matturri L, Ottaviani G, Bendetti G, Agosta E, Lavessi AM. Unexpected perinatal death and sudden infant death syndrome: anatomopathologic and legal aspects. *Am J Forensic Med Pathol.* 2005;26:155–160

160. Kiechl-Kohlendorfer U, Hof D, Peglow UP, Traweger-Ravanelli B, Kiechl S. Epidemiology of apparent life threatening events. *Arch Dis Child.* 2005;90:297–300

161. DiFiore JM, Arko M, Whitehouse M, Kimball A, Martin RJ. Apnea is not prolonged by acid gastroesophageal reflux in preterm infants. *Pediatrics.* 2005;116:1059–1063

162. Stanton J, Simpson A. Murder misdiagnosed as SIDS: a perpetrator's perspective. *Arch Dis Child.* 2001;85:454–459

163. Firstman R, Talan J. *The Death of Innocents.* New York, NY: Bantam Books; 1997

164. Meadow R. Unnatural sudden infant death. *Arch Dis Child.* 1999;80:7–14

165. Levene S, Bacon CJ. Sudden unexpected death and covert homicide in infancy. *Arch Dis Child.* 2004;89:443–447

166. Craft AW, Hall DMB. Munchausen syndrome by proxy and sudden infant death. *BMJ.* 2004;328:1309–1312

167. American Academy of Pediatrics Committee on Child Abuse and Neglect. Distinguishing sudden infant death syndrome from child abuse fatalities. *Pediatrics.* 2001;107:437–441

168. American Academy of Pediatrics Committee on Child Abuse and Neglect. Addendum: distinguishing sudden infant death syndrome from child abuse fatalities. *Pediatrics.* 2001;108:812

169. Tomson T, Walczak T, Sillanpaa M, Sander JW. Sudden unexpected death in epilepsy: a review of incidence and risk factors. *Epilepsia.* 2005;46(suppl 11):54–61

170. Vincent GM, McPeak H. Commotio cordis: a deadly consequence of chest trauma. *Physician Sports Med.* 2000;28:30–39

171. Turk EE, Sperhake JP, Pueschel K, Tsokos M. An approach to the evaluation of fatal hypothermia. *Forensic Sci Med Pathol.* 2005;1:31–35

172. Zumwalt RE, Hirsch CS. Subtle, fatal child abuse. *Human Pathol.* 1980;11:167–174

Chapter 21

Sudden Infant Death Syndrome and Fatal Child Abuse

Henry F. Krous

Department of Pathology, Children's Hospital-San Diego
Department of Pathology, University of California at San Diego

Roger W. Byard

Department of Pathology, University of Adelaide

Introduction

Distinguishing sudden infant death syndrome (SIDS) from death due to inflicted injury continues to challenge professionals.[1] The pediatrician, family physician, or pathologist must know which course to follow in relating to the family. If child abuse is suspected, the physician must fulfill mandated legal obligations to report the case to the appropriate authorities. If the reason for death is SIDS, sympathy and support are required. Complicating this decision is the potential polarization between those who believe that a sympathetic approach to parents losing their infant is the highest priority, and those whose training and experience have convinced them that fatal child abuse is distressingly common, especially because SIDS cases can generally not be distinguished from "soft suffocation" in the absence of a confession by the perpetrator. However, a non-accusatory approach to caregivers is optimal given that it ensures that all parties are treated fairly. Medical exam-

iners and coroners have the added medicolegal responsibility to determine the cause and manner of death. Our knowledge in this area is incomplete, and ambiguity exists in some cases. The purpose of this chapter is to present the scientific evidence about SIDS and fatal child abuse to help reduce ambiguity and enhance the likelihood that a correct determination can be made.

A case of sudden and unexpected infant death was first described in the Bible (I Kings 3:19,22). For centuries, it was accepted as a natural phenomenon, defying explanation. In the mid-20th century, spurred by parents suffering the loss of infants to this poorly explained condition, the scientific community entered a period of fruitful research as to why these infants were dying suddenly and unexpectedly. At the same time, the medical community, which had previously repressed the abhorrent concept of caretakers harming their children, was being informed by new literature describing this phenomenon.

In 1946 Caffey[2] published his seminal article on multiple fractures and subdural hematomas, and in 1953 Silverman[3] postulated that such injuries were the result of unrecognized trauma. In 1961 Adelson[4] added to the factual information about fatal child abuse. In 1962 Kempe et al[5] coined the phrase *battered child syndrome* and further raised the consciousness of the medical community about the unpleasant truth that infants and children were being physically abused and killed. The stage was being set for a controversy about death in infancy, its causes, and the possibility of a caretaker's culpability for those deaths.

High-profile cases of serial child homicides focused attention on fatal child abuse as a reason for some sudden, unexpected deaths in infants, especially because some had initial diagnoses of SIDS. In upstate New York, Waneta Hoyt was charged with suffocating 5 of her children, all of whom had their deaths initially attributed to SIDS. Two of these children were among 5 cases included in the 1972 report of Steinschneider[6] who postulated that SIDS was the result of prolonged apnea, using these 2 deaths from SIDS as examples of this disorder. This article, heralded as a breakthrough despite the small numbers and questionable interpretation of data, elevated prolonged apnea to the top of the list of hypotheses for SIDS. This in turn spurred the development of research about apnea and subsequently the proliferation of the concept of testing for apnea and home-monitoring programs. In their book, *The Death of Innocents,* Firstman and Talan[7] skillfully analyzed this case, the implications it had for the SIDS research community, and the impact that it had on pediatrics professionals and many of their patient families. The media accounts of the Hoyt case raised public awareness about the possibility of infant murders being mistaken for SIDS or other medical illness. For those parents who had lost babies to SIDS, and for many health care providers, the suggestion that even some SIDS deaths were actually child murders was painful and unacceptable. They feared that by raising the old specter of infanticide, the 25-year effort of parents and professionals to provide compassion for families losing their babies to SIDS would evaporate. It became apparent that an objective and integrated approach to the ascertainment of sudden, unexpected infant deaths must occur.

Sudden Infant Death Syndrome

Definition

Defining SIDS continues to present a dilemma because pathognomonic postmortem findings have yet to be identified. Sudden infant death syndrome therefore remains a diagnosis of exclusion despite dramatic developments in our understanding of its epidemiology and pathology occurring during the last decade.

The definition of SIDS has evolved during the last 37 years. Initially defined in 1969 as "the sudden death of any infant or young child, which is unexpected by history, and in which a thorough postmortem examination fails to demonstrate an adequate cause for death."[8] Twenty years later, the definition was changed by an expert panel convened by the National Institute of Child Health and Human Development (NICHD) to "the sudden death of an infant under one year of age which remains unexplained after a thorough case investigation, including performance of a complete autopsy, examination of the death scene, and review of the clinical history."[9] In the intervening years, literally thousands of publications enhancing our knowledge (and sometimes unfortunately having the opposite effect) appeared in the medical literature. With this increase in knowledge, it became increasingly evident that a general definition should exist for purposes of death certification and vital statistics, and another for research.[10-15] With this in mind, another expert panel composed primarily of pathologists experienced in pediatric forensic pathology, death certification, and SIDS research proposed the following general definition in 2004: "the sudden and unexpected death of an infant under 1 year of age, with onset of the fatal episode apparently occurring during sleep, that remains unexplained after a thorough investigation including performance of a complete autopsy, and review of the circumstances of death and the clinical history."[16] The general definition was then stratified to provide specific criteria for different categories to enhance research and to provide a diagnostic framework to make SIDS a more inclusive diagnosis. This is especially important given the increased proportion of SIDS cases that have atypical clinical presentations, potentially unsafe sleeping environments, and/or more "severe" pathologic findings at postmortem examination.[17,18] The subcategories of SIDS are delineated elsewhere, as well as another category, unclassified sudden infant death, which was created for cases whose death did not meet "the criteria for Category l or II SIDS, but where alternative diagnoses of natural or unnatural conditions are equivocal. This includes cases where autopsies have not been performed."[16]

Incidence and Risk-Reduction Campaigns

The National Center for Health Statistics reported that there were 5,476 SIDS cases in the United States in 1988, representing an overall rate of 1.4 deaths per 1,000 live births, making it the second leading cause of death in infancy (including the neonatal period) among white infants, accounting for 14.5% of all deaths and representing a rate of 1.[24] per 1,000 live births. In contrast, for black infants, SIDS was the leading cause of death, accounting for 12.8% of all deaths and representing a rate of 2.26 per 1,000 live births.

A multitude of epidemiological studies have identified factors that increase the risk of SIDS. As a result, public awareness initiatives such as the Reduce the Risk campaigns in New Zealand, Australia, and Western Europe[19-22] and the Back to Sleep campaign in the United States were undertaken to eliminate exposure of infants to these risk factors by modifying infant care practices. They included recommendations for supine placement of infants to sleep, use of a firm sleep surface, avoidance of excessive wrapping or bundling of infants while sleeping, and avoidance of prenatal and postnatal exposure to cigarette smoke. Implementation of these campaigns was followed by dramatic declines in the overall incidence of SIDS. Rates declined by 50% or more in Western Europe, New Zealand, Australia, and the United States.[23] By 1995 the number of cases declined to approximately 3,000 deaths in the United States, yielding a rate of approximately 0.5 deaths per 1,000 live births.[24] Nevertheless, SIDS remains a significant cause of postneonatal infant death, in part because these public health initiatives have not equally reached all segments of the population, for example certain minority communities.[25] Willinger et al[26] have reported that significant predictors of prone placement in the United States included maternal black race, maternal age between 20 and 29 years, residence in the mid-Atlantic or southern states, maternal parity, and infant age younger than 8 weeks. In this study, it was encouraging that the prevalence of infants placed in the prone sleep position declined by 66% between 1992 and 1996, and at the same time, SIDS rates declined by approximately 38%. In California, there were 3,508 SIDS cases from 1990 to 1995; SIDS rates per 1,000 live births declined from 2.69 to 2.15 for black infants and from 1.04 to 0.61 for all others.[27]

Clinical Presentation

Sudden infant death syndrome occurs most frequently in infants between 2 and 4 months of age.[28] Fewer than 5% of cases occur during the first month of life, the rate peaks during the second to the fourth months, and decreases progressively such that 90% of SIDS deaths occur by the age of 6 months.[28] In most studies, SIDS occurs more often in male infants (60%).[23,28] Deaths have occurred more frequently during the fall and winter months in both the northern and southern hemispheres, suggesting that temperature alone is not a causative factor. Since implementation of the Back to Sleep campaign *(vide supra)*, SIDS cases are more evenly distributed throughout each of the seasons.[29,30] The typical presentation of SIDS is the discovery of a lifeless young infant who had been fed and then put down to sleep. The infant may have had a minor upper respiratory infection or gastro-esophageal symptoms, but not of such a serious nature to have suggested that sudden death was imminent. In general, upper respiratory infections occur at rates similar to those of controls,[31] but gastrointestinal symptoms are slightly more common.[32] No outcry is heard, and the infant is often in the position in which he or she had been placed at bedtime. Emergency personnel are contacted, and often initiate cardio-pulmonary resuscitation (CPR) in the home and continue these measures until reaching the hospital, where the infant is pronounced dead. When discovered, some show clenching of the fists, occasionally with clutched blanket fibers. Pink, frothy, and/or mucoid oronasal secretions are often reported in cases of SIDS, but the description of "blood" is very uncommon.[33] Lividity and rigor mortis are not uncommon.

Risk Factors

Despite rare studies to the contrary,[34] there are innumerable reports from New Zealand, Australia, Western Europe, Hong Kong, and the United States that being placed prone to sleep significantly increases an infant's risk for SIDS.[35–42] Sudden infant death syndrome rates have declined as fewer infants have been placed prone.[26] Certain segments of the US population have not adopted the supine sleep position for infants, consequently the incidence of SIDS has not declined in these groups at the same rate as that of the general population.[26]

Cigarette smoking has emerged as an even more important risk factor for SIDS as the supine sleep position has replaced the prone position.[43–45] Maternal smoking before and/or during gestation and after delivery all increase the risk of SIDS.[46–58] Paternal smoking also increases the risk of SIDS, but this association may be a reflection of a higher rate of passive smoke exposure by a coexisting smoking mother.[45] At postmortem examination, pericardial levels of cotinine, a nicotine metabolite, are higher in SIDS cases than in controls.[52]

Bed sharing (occasionally equated with co-sleeping, which may merely signify sleeping in the same room, as opposed to sharing the same sleep surface) as a potential risk factor for SIDS continues to generate controversy between breastfeeding advocates who believe that bed sharing promotes maternal-infant bonding and epidemiologists and forensic pathologists whose concerns center on risk factors that increase the risk for SIDS. To date, dozens of articles devoted to this issue have appeared in the medical literature. Mosko and colleagues[59–61] have provided arguments, based principally on evolutionary and laboratory analysis of mother-infant pairs, favoring the hypothesis that the comparatively sensory-rich environment of bed sharing might be protective against SIDS in some contexts. After studying mother-infant pairs, these investigators concluded that bed sharing promoted infant arousals[60] and reduced stage 3 to 4 sleep; in addition, the mother's responsiveness to infant arousals during bed sharing may contribute to the protective effects of bed sharing. From an epidemiological viewpoint, however, investigators in the New Zealand Cot Death Study found that bed sharing significantly increased the risk of SIDS among infants of mothers who smoked.[62–64] To date, while rare studies show no increase in SIDS risk associated with bed sharing,[65] essentially none of the remainder have shown a protective effect.[18,23,63,64,66–69] There are 2 recent studies showing an increased risk of SIDS even when the infant was bed sharing with nonsmoking parents.[17,70] Therefore, the American Academy of Pediatrics (AAP), which strongly supports breastfeeding, has recommended that infants are safest when sleeping alone.[71] Challenges presented by breastfeeding advocates[72–75] to the recommendation that infants sleep separate from the mother have been soundly refuted.[76]

An increasing body of literature suggests that pacifier use can reduce the risk of SIDS.[77] A meta-analysis of 7 published case-control studies calculated summary odds ratios (SORs) for "usual" and "last sleep" pacifier use and SIDS risk.[78] The

SORs for pacifier use with "usual" and during "last sleep" were 0.71 (95% confidence interval [CI], 0.59–0.85) and 0.39 (95% CI, 0.31–0.50), respectively with multi- variate odds ratios.

Ethnicity affects SIDS rates. Black,[79] Alaska natives,[80] and most, but not all, Native American infants have higher SIDS rates than do white and Asian infants.[27,81,82] However, in some studies, the excess mortality among black infants disappears when adjusted for maternal education and income.[83] Sudden infant death syndrome rates in Native Americans residing in the northern United States are higher than those in the southwestern part of the country, possibly as a result of the high prevalence of smoking among the former. Other studies suggest the higher prevalence of other SIDS risk factors accounts for the higher SIDS rates in Native Americans compared with whites.[84] It is now apparent that alcohol abuse may contribute to higher SIDS rates among Native Americans.[85,86] Others concluded from their studies on the effect of various factors on the rate of SIDS within certain populations that SIDS rates and socioeconomic status are inversely related, but socioeconomic status may act as a confounder, effect modifier, or intermediate variable.[87] Recent reports indicate decreases in SIDS rates among Native Americans and Alaska natives.[88,89]

Infants of illegal substance-abusing mothers (ISAM) are also at higher risk of SIDS compared with control subjects.[90–97] In a study from Los Angeles County, CA, the SIDS rate was 8.87 cases per 1,000 ISAM, compared with 1.22 cases per 1,000 infants for non-ISAM in the general population, a highly significant statistical difference.[93] The significantly greater incidence of SIDS in male infants, with a higher rate in winter months, and among black infants and non-Hispanic white infants in the non-ISAM population was not observed in the ISAM group. Conversely, symptomatic apnea was reported significantly more frequently before SIDS for the ISAM group than for the non-ISAM group. In another study from New York City, the SIDS rate in drug-exposed infants was 5.8 per 1,000 infants, compared with 1.4 per 1,000 who were not drug-exposed.[98] The risk ratios for SIDS were 3.6 with methadone, 2.3 with heroin, 3.2 with methadone and heroin combined, 1.6 with cocaine, and 1.1 with cocaine and methadone combined or heroin exposure.[98] However, in a study from Detroit, MI, 44% of 2,964 infants screened by meconium sampling had positive results for cocaine, opiates, or cannabinoids, and studies of mortality rates during the first 2 years of life showed no difference between the drug-positive and drug-negative groups. Similarly, the incidence of SIDS was no different between the 2 groups.

Many studies have shown that the risk of SIDS is not increased after diphtheria, tetanus, and pertussis immunization; indeed, it is purported that the association is coincidental rather than causal.[99–105] However, a Vaccine Adverse Events Reporting System study in 2004 identified a statistical increase in SIDS within 3 days following whole-cell pertussis vaccines, but not acellular vaccines, among those residing in the United States from 1997 to 1999; this is an interesting observation given there are approximately 3,000 proteins, including known neurotoxins (endotoxin, pertussis toxin, and adenylate cyclase) in the cellular vaccine, as opposed to only 2 to 5 proteins in the acellular vaccine.[106]

Descriptions of infants being overdressed, overwrapped, hot, and sweaty when discovered dead have prompted the suggestion that overheating and hyperthermia may be important risk factors in SIDS.[107-111] One suggested mechanism is that of a febrile seizure. Elevated ambient temperatures have been associated with apnea in premature babies,[96] suggesting that apnea might occur in older infants with increased body temperatures. Hyperthermia as a factor contributing to SIDS deaths requires more carefully crafted studies to determine the relative importance of this factor. One such study,[112] using a case-control method, examined 41 SIDS victims by measuring thermal conditions at the death scene and at the scene of last sleep for control infants. A questionnaire was also administered to all the parents. The results showed that SIDS victims had greater thermal insulation for their given room temperature than did the matched controls ($P = .009$). There are also experimental studies showing the adverse effect of hyperthermia on respiratory function. Decerebrated, vagotomized, neonatal piglets aged 3 to 15 days show substantially prolonged inhibition of the laryngeal chemoreflex after infusions of distilled water when the body

temperature was elevated approximately 2.5°C, suggesting that elevated body temperature may contribute to the pathogenesis of SIDS by increasing the inhibitory effects of the laryngeal chemoreflex.[113] Others have shown that 21-day-old mice exposed to hyperthermia (40.5°C–43.5°C) and hypoxia have an increasingly frequent failure to arouse during the first and after multiple hypoxic exposures.[114] Gasping duration and frequency increased with body temperature elevation. Observations from these studies suggest that thermal stress may be important in SIDS as a result of its adverse effect on arousal, gasping, and laryngeal chemoreflex.

In many studies, twins and triplets are at greater risk of SIDS than singletons,[115-118] although this has been contested.[119] Studies showing a higher twin risk for SIDS have generally attributed this to lower birth weights of twins, compared with singletons. Sudden unexpected death in both twins has been the subject of numerous articles.[120-124] Beal[120] reported that 6 of 625 surviving twins (1%) had subsequently died of SIDS. In a large study in 1999, Malloy and Freeman[119] studied twin pairs over a 5-year period in the United States to determine whether there was an increased risk of SIDS in this population. There were 767 matched twin pregnancies in which one or both twins died of SIDS. Compared with twin pregnancies in which no SIDS deaths occurred, the victims of SIDS both had lower mean birth weights and younger gestational ages and were likely to be black, with mothers having a lower than 12th-grade education.[64] In the 767 SIDS twin deaths, there were only 7 sets in which both twins died, and in only one of these sets were the deaths on the same day. The authors concluded that, independent of birth weight, twins do not seem to be at greater risk for SIDS compared with singletons.[119]

The simultaneous deaths of twins allegedly due to SIDS have been reported.[125,126] Based on published series, Beal[120] estimated that 12 (2%) of 637 twin infant pairs died simultaneously of SIDS. A review of simultaneous twin deaths cited in the world literature from 1900 to 1998 identified 41 pairs, but also found that the deaths of only 12 (29.2%) pairs of twins fulfilled 3 criteria that included evaluation of the location of death, the circumstances of death, and the SIDS definition.[127] Given the statistical improbability of such an event, it is far more likely that their deaths were the result of an environmental factor. For example, Ramos et al[128] reported 45-day-old twins dying within hours of one another and after death scene investigation and postmortem examination, concluded that the combination of sublethal blood levels of carbon monoxide, overwrapping of the infants with bedclothes, and mechanical upper airway obstruction caused their deaths. Others have also suggested the possibility of not only accidents, but also of inflicted injuries causing such simultaneous deaths.[129]

Recurrence of SIDS within a family is an important counseling issue for future pregnancies, given that many parents of infants who die of SIDS may wish to have subsequent children. The possibility of genetically transmitted inborn

errors of metabolism or other conditions must be considered, and questions of a forensic nature should also be raised. In a 14-year study of subsequent siblings of SIDS victims in Norway[130] and in a Washington state study over 16 years,[131] the SIDS risk in siblings was almost 4 times that of the SIDS risk among the general population. A comparison of SIDS occurrences between siblings of SIDS victims and infants from maternal age—and birth rank—matched control families; however, it revealed no statistically significant difference in SIDS rates or in total infant mortality rates in families with a history of SIDS, compared with families in which there had been no SIDS deaths. Thus the notion was challenged that having an infant die of SIDS increases the likelihood of having another who dies of SIDS. With the exclusion from the SIDS statistics of some of the deaths now thought to be due to inborn errors of metabolism, the chances for recurrent SIDS in families seem even less likely. It should be noted that these studies were reported before implementation of initiatives promoting supine sleep position and avoidance of smoke exposure. There is a growing impression among pediatric and forensic pathologists that an increasingly higher proportion of SIDS cases have more complex risk factor interactions than was found before the implementation of the Back to Sleep campaign.[18] In a setting of socioeconomic deprivation, unsafe sleep environments, along with persistence of the prone sleeping position and continued exposure to tobacco smoke, the recurrence risk may be increased. Newer studies focusing on the emerging profile characterizing many of the current cases of SIDS are needed to address this issue.

Pathology

The postmortem findings in SIDS have been extensively described.[4,132-135] Minor abnormalities that should not be considered lethal are common. For example, respiratory system inflammatory infiltrates are frequently identified, but not more often than among controls.[31] Similarly, the results of postmortem microbiological cultures are not significantly different between SIDS and control cases.

Although autopsies often reveal minor pathologic changes, the etiology and mechanisms of death in SIDS are not understood. Nevertheless, an autopsy, especially when supplemented by review of the clinical history and circumstances of death, is still considered essential in determining the cause and manner of sudden and unexpected death in infancy.[136,137] A study by Kumar et al[138] reviewed the autopsy findings in 107 cases of postneonatal patients who had died during a 10-year period at a large suburban medical center. Sixty of these patients were younger than 1 year. In 34%, a new diagnosis was made at autopsy, whereas complete concordance was seen in 66%. This is a convincing argument supporting the value of well-conducted pediatric autopsies.

Sturner[139] described the need for careful examination and thorough photography of the external aspects of the body and coverings, including the orifices, as well as patterns of lividity and external drains and markings before the body is washed or altered; extensive histologic study of the upper respiratory tract and lungs; and consultation with clinical colleagues and a detailed review of the potential significance of findings before a diagnosis is rendered.

A standardized protocol, which has been endorsed by the Society for Pediatric Pathology (SPP), the National Association of Medical Examiners (NAME), and the SIDS Global Strategy Task Force, has been developed for pathologists performing postmortem examinations on infants who die suddenly and unexpectedly.[140] This protocol prompts recording of positive and negative observations required to reach a diagnosis in cases of sudden and unexpected infant death by using a checklist. It also encourages narrative descriptions of abnormalities, supplemented by microscopic, microbiological, and toxicological analyses, as well as the use of radiographic and photographic imaging.

A pathognomonic marker for SIDS has not been found, and it seems unlikely that such a marker will ever be found given the likelihood that SIDS consists of more than one entity and has more than one cause.

The bodies of SIDS victims appear well nourished and well developed, but their weights are typically below the 50th percentile expected for age.[28] It has been suggested that their growth rates are slow,[141] but this notion has been challenged in a study comparing each of 78 SIDS cases with 2 controls matched for postnatal age, season, neighborhood, and date of parental interview.[142]

No differences were observed between SIDS victims and controls with respect to the growth rates between their births and last live weights and between their last 2 live weights. Stratification of these infants by gender, gestational age, maternal smoking during pregnancy, breastfeeding versus bottle-feeding, or age at death did not change the results. Similarly, no difference in bone growth plates has been detected between SIDS infants and controls.[143] The significance of reduced levels of docosahexaenoic acid, a substance involved in neural maturation, in the brains of bottle-fed infants compared with breastfed infants remains uncertain.[144]

Fibers from bedclothes may be found in the often-clenched hands of infants who die of SIDS.[28] Signs of resuscitation and postmortem changes must be distinguished from non-accidental trauma. Reddish-blue mottling of the skin indicative of postmortem lividity may occur in dependent portions of the body. The blood in the heart is liquid and often oozes from venipuncture sites. The bladder and rectum are empty. A variety of reported subtle, but nonlethal, anomalies are neither diagnostic nor specific.[145]

Oronasal secretions are observed frequently in SIDS, but oronasal blood is uncommonly reported. In the San Diego SIDS/Sudden Unexplained Death in Childhood (SUDC) Research Project database, some type of oronasal secretion was described in 155 (38%) of 406 cases of sudden infant death.[33] Oronasal blood was described in only 28 (7%) of 406 cases of sudden infant death and could not be attributed to CPR in 14 cases, including 10 (3%) of 300 SIDS

cases, 2 (14%) of 14 accidental suffocation cases, and 2 (15%) of 13 undetermined cases. Importantly, 8 of the 10 children in the SIDS cases were bed sharing and 5 were with both parents; in 2 cases, the infant was between them. One of the infants was from a family with 3 child protective services (CPS) referrals. This analysis found that oronasal blood not attributable to CPR was rare in SIDS when an infant had been sleeping supine, alone, and in a safe environment.

Intrathoracic petechiae are the most common abnormality seen macroscopically and are identified in more than 80% of SIDS cases.[146,147] Despite opinions to the contrary,[148] facial and conjunctival petechiae are exceedingly rare in SIDS cases, and their presence should provoke a search for another cause of death. Experimental evidence and observations in human postmortem examinations suggest that petechiae limited to the thorax can result from attempting to breathe against an obstructed upper airway in the moments preceding death.[132,147,149–151] Alternatively, it also has been suggested that bronchiolar obstruction could cause the same finding.[152] Poets et al[153] identified intrathoracic petechiae in monitored infants who were gasping deeply before dying of SIDS.

The relationship between intrathoracic petechiae and a facedown position has been studied. In the San Diego SIDS/SUDC Research Project database, 36.7% of infants were found with their faces straight down.[154] Those infants were similar with respect to age, gender, and gestational age to infants found with the face in any other position, and intrathoracic petechiae were identified in more than 92% of both groups. The severity of intrathoracic petechiae, whether measured by the number of involved intrathoracic organs or by the extent of thymic involvement, was also similar between the 2 groups. These data argue against external oronasal obstruction as a mechanism of death in SIDS victims found facedown, but they do not exclude pharyngeal or laryngeal obstruction, rebreathing, or hyperthermia.

The lungs in SIDS victims are congested and variably edematous, but not consolidated. Pneumonia evidenced by pulmonary consolidation is not seen with the naked eye. Microscopic interstitial lymphocytic infiltration of the lungs is common, but is mild and not to be considered lethal.[31]

Occasionally there are mild interstitial lymphocytic infiltrates within the epicardium and/or myocardium,[155,156] but a diagnosis of myocarditis is precluded by the absence of myocardial necrosis as defined by the Dallas criteria.[157-160] However, recent immunochemical studies of the myocardium in cases of sudden infant death with little or no evidence of myocardial necrosis and inflammation by routine light microscopy have shown evidence of early stages of inflammation with viral proteins and early myocardial injury.[161-163] Future studies should help to clarify the significance of earlier findings.

Although it has been proposed that laryngeal basement membrane thickening is a marker for SIDS,[164-166] Krous et al[167] were unable to confirm this finding

when a large number of cases from the Chicago Infant Mortality Study were analyzed.

Pathophysiology

There is general consensus that SIDS is a catastrophic consequence involving the simultaneous intersection of 3 elements: a critical period of development, an exogenous stressor, and an underlying vulnerability. This is known as the triple-risk model.[168-170] These 3 facets incorporate widely recognized epidemiological, physiological, and postmortem findings in SIDS.

It has been proposed that infants may die of SIDS as a result of a deficiency in the medullary serotonergic network, and this has been the subject of recent comprehensive reviews.[171,172] During the first half of infancy, rapid changes occur in respiratory and cardiovascular physiology in association with rapid brain growth and development. This renders the at-risk infant vulnerable to exogenous risk factors such as prone sleep position, which can cause fatal hypercarbia, hypoxia, and/or acidosis. Abundant literature has long emphasized the prevalence of respiratory abnormalities in SIDS, be they physiological, infectious, or developmental.[132,151,173-186] The concept that an internal stressor precipitates sudden death was derived in part from epidemiological studies indicating that minor respiratory or gastrointestinal illnesses occur around the time of death in some SIDS victims, as well as observations of symptoms suggestive of more severe illness in the 2 days before death.[187,188] Endogenous stressors associated with SIDS, such as fever and infection, tend to cause an increased rate of carbon dioxide production, alter the demand for cardiac output and/or thermoregulation, and/or decrease arousal. The prone sleeping position is associated with a facedown sleeping position in some infants,[24] and the facedown position is associated with rebreathing of exhaled gases and an increase in end-tidal carbon dioxide in normal infants, particularly those sleeping on soft bedding where pockets of exhaled gas form and trap carbon dioxide.[32]

The possibility of upper airway obstruction has been postulated by several investigators.[28,58,111,147,189] Partial or complete upper airway obstruction may be caused by posterior repositioning of the mandible with pharyngeal occlusion or by compressing the nose directly.[190,191] As many as 25% to 50% of SIDS victims are found in the facedown position, approximately three quarters of whom are found prone, and one quarter found with their faces covered by bedcovers.[20,192,193]

Other authors have suggested high negative intrathoracic pressure as the cause of the prominent intrathoracic petechiae, and have proposed that airway obstruction causes negative pressure.[28,132,147,150,189] Pharyngeal obstruction, because of backward displacement of the tongue, pharyngeal collapse during sleep, or neck flexion leading to obstruction, have all been suggested as capable of producing upper airway obstruction.[182,190,194–196] In another study,[197] obstructive sleep apnea was identified in 19 (95%) of 20 infants from families who had histories of

SIDS, apparent life-threatening events (ALTEs), or obstructive sleep apnea. In contrast, obstructive sleep apnea was present in only 31 (30%) of 105 infants whose family histories were negative for the same variables.

Confirming observations made a decade earlier, Folgering et al[198] and Filiano and Kinney[199] developed their hypothesis of deficiency of the medullary serotonergic system after performing a series of elegant studies beginning initially with the demonstration of arcuate nucleus abnormalities that were evident during routine light microscopy of the brain stem of SIDS victims. In subsequent studies, deficient receptor binding for serotonin and other neurotransmitters was identified in rhombic lip-derived neurons that are critical for the regulation of respiration, upper airway reflexes, chemosensing, cardiovascular function, thermoregulation, motor activity, pain, and arousal.[86,200–207]

Subsequently, genetic studies of the promoter region of the serotonin transporter gene revealed variable tandem repeat sequence polymorphisms in the protein (5-HTT) gene that were associated with an increased risk of SIDS in Japan[208] and in black infants in the United States.[209] In Japan, long and extra-long alleles were more frequently found in SIDS victims than in age-matched controls.[208] In black infants, significant positive associations were found between SIDS and the long/long and long allele genotype distribution.[208] At the same time, a significant negative correlation between SIDS and the short/short genotype was also observed.[209,210] This polymorphism differentially regulates 5-HTT expression, with the long allele (the SIDS-associated allele) being a more effective promoter than the short allele.

Circumstances of Death and Scene Investigation

The NICHD definition of SIDS required that investigation of the death scene should not reveal any explanation for the sudden death of an infant.[9] The 2004 San Diego definition expanded the requirement for a death scene examination into an investigation of the circumstances of death that includes not only the actual scene of death but other environments in which the infant may have been before death.[16] In uncomplicated cases of SIDS, investigation of the circumstances of death and the scene where the infant was found lifeless do not reveal causes or contributing factors to death. However, along with the decline in SIDS cases has been a reduction in the number of uncomplicated cases.[18] As a result, a higher proportion of cases is complicated by a complex social milieu, lower socioeconomic status, chaotic living conditions, and less than pristine postmortem findings.[18] The sleep site may not have been completely safe because of an unstable bed, soft sleep surfaces, or the presence of pillows and/or overstuffed toys. The infant may have been in an uncontrolled bed sharing situation with adults. Consequently, in many cases the diagnosis of SIDS has become more difficult and contentious.

The scene investigation is critical to the forensic pathologist's interpretation of postmortem findings, and to facilitate this the Centers for Disease Control and Prevention has produced and published *Guidelines for the Scene Investigation of Sudden Unexpected Infant Death,* which have been endorsed by NAME, SPP, and the SIDS Global Strategy Task Force. This has recently been revised and updated.[211, 212]

Hanzlick[213] has listed the impediments to high-quality death investigations. These include regional variations in death investigation requirements, lack of peer review, lack of specified standards, credentialing inconsistencies, variations in coroner and/or medical examiner systems, inadequate funding, manpower shortages, lack of government interest, legal influences on medical decisions, and operation of medical examiner/coroner offices outside health care delivery systems. He proposed forming a national office of death investigation affairs to facilitate improvements.

Other Causes of Sudden Infant Death

In 1982 prolongation of the QT interval was proposed as a cause of SIDS.[214] In a prospective study of 4,205 infants, prolongation of the corrected QT (QTc) interval was identified in 3 cases that were initially diagnosed as SIDS. Subsequently, it was suggested that unbalanced maturation of sympathetic neural pathways could produce ventricular tachyarrhythmias in electrically unstable hearts and cause death.[215] A prospective study of 34,442 newborn infants at 1-year follow-up revealed 34 deaths (24 of which were diagnosed as SIDS) with longer QTc than that in the survivors and in infants who had died of other causes.[214] However, this study received intense criticism.[216–220] Subsequently, a prospective study identified SCN5A mutations in 2 of 93 SIDS victims: a 6-week-old white male with an A997S missense mutation in exon 17 and a 1-month-old white male with an R1826H mutation in exon 28.[221] Based on these data it was concluded that approximately 2% of SIDS cases have an identifiable SCN5A channel defect that may lead to a fatal arrhythmia.

Defects in fatty acid metabolism account for a small percentage of sudden infant deaths that have been diagnosed as SIDS,[222,223] although others have found markers for medium-chain acyl-CoA dehydrogenase (MCAD) deficiency to be no more common in SIDS than in control cases.[224] Mild hepatic steatosis is common in SIDS, but severe lipid accumulation in the liver, renal tubular epithelium, and muscle tissues increases the likelihood that a defect in fatty acid metabolism is present. Medium-chain acyl-CoA dehydrogenase deficiency, with autosomal-recessive inheritance, is the most common, and usually presents with recurrent episodes of hypoglycemia and lethargy mimicking Reye syndrome, or with features clinically indistinguishable from SIDS.[225] Mortality in MCAD deficiency is 60% in the first 2 years of life, but when recognized, the disease can be managed effectively. A single mutation, A985G, in the MCAD gene accounts for more than 90% of the cases among whites; DNA testing can identify most patients with and carriers of MCAD deficiency.[223,226,227] If death occurs during the first week of life,

when SIDS is rare, and microscopic lipid is found in the tissues, then the G583A mutation variant of MCAD deficiency should be considered.[226] Blood from the affected individual, or tissue or blood from both parents, can be used to identify carriers.[228,229] There are also defects in short-chain acyl-CoA dehydrogenase, long-chain acyl-CoA dehydrogenase, and very-long-chain acyl-CoA dehydrogenase that can also cause sudden unexpected infant death. Postmortem or newborn blood specimens taken at delivery can be used to make the diagnosis after death.[228,229]

As previously noted, hyperthermia has been associated with infant and early childhood death, and careful scene investigation is again critical in establishing this diagnosis. Krous et al[230] reported 10 cases of children ranging in age from 53 days to 9 years. When the authors' cases were grouped with others reported in the literature, distinct subgroups emerged. Children who died of hyperthermia in vehicles were older, were exposed more quickly to higher temperatures, and often had more severe skin damage. Those who died in bed were primarily infants exposed to lower environmental temperatures. The presence of intrathoracic petechiae, which were present in nearly all the cases, suggested terminal gasping in failed attempts at autoresuscitation before death.

Myocarditis is an important but uncommon cause of sudden infant death.[231,232] Twenty-four cases of isolated myocarditis were found among 3,196 pediatric autopsies at the Children's Hospital of Winnipeg, Canada, over a 40-year period, and 21 of these were infants.[233] Myocarditis is usually caused by coxsackievirus B, but other viruses have been identified.[234–237] Microscopic examination of the heart reveals lymphocytic infiltration of degenerating, necrotic, and edematous myocardium. Myocardial apoptosis seems to be an important mechanism of myocardial destruction.[238] Death is usually caused by an arrhythmia, although in some cases there is chronic heart failure. There is also a very unusual case of a 26-day-old boy who died of eosinophilic endomyocarditis without extracardiac disease, the etiology of which remained unexplained after review of the medical and family histories and circumstances of death; extensive light and immunofluorescence microscopy; and microbiological, metabolic, and toxicological testing.[239]

Accidents are another cause of sudden infant death; their accurate recognition often rests on not only the autopsy, but also on careful scene examination and reconstruction. Accidental causes of death that have been recognized include hangings, wedgings, and foreign body aspiration.[1,192,240–250] Byard et al[246] reported 30 cases of unexpected death from asphyxia caused by unsafe sleeping conditions, including hanging from loose dental retainers, clothing, or curtain cords; positional asphyxia; and suffocation from plastic bed covers. Infant deaths while breastfeeding have also been described and are presumably caused by oronasal obstruction.[248,251,252]

A variety of benign and malignant neoplasms have been associated with sudden infant and childhood death. In the study of 68 such cases reported by Krous et al,[253] most (84%) involved the heart and brain. Another recent publication has described sudden infant and childhood deaths occurring over a 20-year period as a result of undiagnosed neoplasms.[254] In this latter study, acute lymphoblastic leukemia and lymphoblastic lymphoma accounted for 4 of the 8 identified cases; 2 other deaths were caused by medulloblastoma complicated by intraventricular hemorrhage and intraperitoneal rupture of bilateral Wilms tumor. Review of the literature reveals that leukemia, lymphoma, and Wilms tumor are the most common tumors associated with sudden unexpected death in infants and children.[1,255–258]

A host of other infectious, neoplastic, traumatic, and toxicological disorders and congenital anomalies associated with sudden death in infancy have been comprehensively reviewed elsewhere.[1]

Differentiating Between SIDS and Child Abuse

Although the etiology of cases labeled as SIDS is heterogeneous, most are likely to be of a natural origin. While there is no doubt that some cases are homicides,[259–263] the actual percentage of undiagnosed infanticides (especially those caused by soft suffocation) within the SIDS group is unknown, and will probably remain so for the foreseeable future. Estimates vary widely. After studying the problem of infant deaths in Sheffield, England, for more than 25 years, Emery[264] concluded, "filicide is the probable mechanism of death in approximately 1 in 10 of the unexplained unexpected deaths." Others estimate that less than 3% of SIDS deaths are undiagnosed infanticides. During an 18-year interval in California, rates of infanticide did not change at the same time that SIDS rates declined dramatically.[265] As a result, the proportion of infant deaths caused by inflicted injuries increased. Correct ascertainment is confounded by those who propound that the first sudden infant death in a family is SIDS, the second undetermined, and the third homicide.[259] The intensely negative emotional response to such a statement derives from its inherent injustice—each case must be thoroughly judged on its own merits. It must be remembered that genetic disorders, such as those associated with fatal arrhythmias,[221] or abnormalities of metabolism,[228] may cause several sudden infant deaths in families and may remain undiagnosed even after adequate postmortem evaluations. Inadequate death scene investigations and reconstructions may also result in failure to recognize accidental deaths. As death review teams become more common and more information is made available, these issues will be clarified. It is also our belief that a compassionate and non-accusatory approach to families can yield information that is vital in ascertaining the correct cause and manner of death, even when the death may have resulted from inflicted injury.

There have been numerous attempts to identify a postmortem marker that could reliably distinguish "soft" suffocation from SIDS. Oronasal blood is one such candidate that was observed in 60% of previous ALTEs experienced by 4 children and in 3 other unrelated infants who were being cared for by the same person. Attempted suffocation of these infants was videotaped.[266] Oronasal blood may also be a postmortem sign of accidental suffocation, but it has been reported in SIDS victims found supine in a safe sleep enviroment.[33]

The presence of intra-alveolar siderophages has also been proposed as evidence of past attempts at inflicted suffocation. The earlier suggestion[267] that pulmonary interstitial hemosiderin may represent a histologic marker of previous "near-miss" SIDS events, which are now known as ALTEs, was not confirmed by Byard et al.[268] Based on the presence of intra-alveolar siderophages in 2 pairs of siblings who had been repeatedly hospitalized for evaluation of ALTEs before their sudden deaths at home, Becroft and Lockett[269] proposed they may have been victims of imposed suffocation. Dorandeu et al[270] reported that intra-alveolar siderophages were significantly more abundant in the lungs of murdered infants and children between 1 and 48 months of age who had been chronically abused, compared with control infants who died of either natural or accidental causes. The potential role of undetected chest trauma is not clear in these cases. Hanzlick and Delaney[271] identified 6 cases of sudden infant death from causes other than SIDS (one being asphyxia) in which the total iron levels were at least twice the mean of the entire group, and also proposed that high intra-alveolar siderophage counts suggest a cause of death other than SIDS. Conversely, Jackson and Gilliland[272] reported 110 SIDS cases and identified intra-alveolar siderophages in 7, but none in infants who had died of asphyxia or abusive injuries. However, imprecise reporting of results and a complex system of quantifying intra-alveolar siderophages make it difficult to draw comparisons or conclusions. Schluckebier et al[273] concluded that intra-alveolar siderophages may be present in cases of repeated asphyxia or hypoxia, but not in cases of SIDS, after comparing 43 cases of infants whose deaths were attributed to SIDS, asphyxia, trauma (accidental or inflicted), or undetermined causes, or whose deaths were preceded by probable hypoxia. After review of the literature, Forbes and Acland[274] concluded that previous episodes of asphyxiation are not proven by the presence of intra-alveolar siderophages. In a San Diego SIDS/SUDC Research Project report of 91 SIDS cases and 29 cases of death due to suffocation (27 accidents and 2 homicides), neither the means of the log-transformed intra-alveolar siderophage counts nor the medians of the raw intra-alveolar siderophage counts were significantly different between the SIDS and control suffocation groups, although the range was wider in the SIDS group than in the suffocation control group.[275] Only 6% of each group had a history of prior ALTEs. Approximately three-fourths of the families from both groups had no prior referral to CPS. The investigators concluded that intra-alveolar siderophage counts cannot be used as an independent variable to ascertain past attempts at suffocation and that the number of intra-alveolar siderophages varies widely in cases of sudden infant death caused by SIDS and accidental or inflicted suffocation.

Pulmonary intra-alveolar hemorrhage has also received attention as a marker that might distinguish SIDS from suffocation. But the literature is contradictory due to inconsistent inclusion criteria, absence of control cases, and lack of uniform assessment. In the National Institute of Child Health and Human Development Co-operative Epidemiological Study, pulmonary intra-alveolar hemorrhage was observed in 66% of more than 700 SIDS cases, but comparisons with infants who died from other causes were not made.[276] Yukawa et al[277] suggested that pulmonary intra-alveolar hemorrhage of at least moderate severity may be a postmortem marker of overlaying or smothering and that SIDS may be an inappropriate diagnosis. However, infants without a clinical history that suggested either accidental or inflicted suffocation revealed similar severe pulmonary intra-alveolar hemorrhage as did cases with those histories. Using a grading system similar to that devised by Yukawa et al[277] in their assessment of 115 SIDS cases, Becroft et al[278] suggested that pulmonary intra-alveolar hemorrhage might be more frequent in infant deaths caused by accidental or inflicted suffocation than in SIDS, even though their study included no control cases and lacked standardized histologic sections of the lungs. They also grouped their cases by those with and without pulmonary intra-alveolar hemorrhage rather than by the severity of the hemorrhage. After assessing 4 microscopic sections taken from the anterior and posterior portions of both upper lobes from 60 infants who had died from a variety of causes, Hanzlick[279] found that pulmonary intra-alveolar hemorrhage was common and was possibly enhanced by attempts at CPR and longer postmortem intervals. Given that the infants whose deaths were caused by SIDS, trauma, congenital anomalies, infections, overlaying, drowning, metabolic disorders, and undetermined causes were analyzed in a single group, specific conclusions cannot be drawn. The grading scale for hemorrhage ranging from 0 to 24 was also complex. Potter et al[280] found more severe pulmonary intra-alveolar hemorrhage in 151 infants who died of SIDS than in 15 infants who died of accidental or inflicted suffocation. Their data are published only in abstract form; however, data from the San Diego SIDS/SUDC Research Project was retrospectively analyzed using a semiquantitative measure for pulmonary intra-alveolar hemorrhage in 419 cases of SIDS, 37 cases of accidental suffocation, and 3 cases of inflicted suffocation.[281] Pulmonary intra-alveolar hemorrhage was graded as absent (0), mild (1), moderate and focal (2), moderate and multifocal (3), and severe and diffuse (4). Grade 3 or 4 hemorrhage occurred in 35% of deaths attributed to suffocation, but in only 11% of the SIDS cases. Victims of SIDS with pulmonary intra-alveolar hemorrhage of this severity were more likely to have been bed sharing, with more than one other co-sleeper, than those with grades 0 or 1 hemorrhage. Thus it seems clear that neither the presence nor the severity of pulmonary intra-alveolar hemorrhage can be used in isolation to differentiate SIDS from suffocation, whether accidental or inflicted.

Child Abuse Fatalities

Infanticide has been reported more often in poorer countries, as opposed to the murder of children 1 to 4 years old, which seems to be uniformly distributed across all nations.[282] Approximately 2,000 children die annually in the United States from maltreatment.[283] In the United States, 10,370 deaths from injuries occurred over a 9-year period at a rate of 29.7 per 100,000 live births.[284] In the US state of Georgia, the child abuse fatality rate in poor, rural, white families was 3.3 per 100,000 children compared with 2.4 per 100,000 children in poor, urban, black families. Important risk factors were young age (relative risk [RR] 6:1), parental teenage childbearing (RR 4:1), and low socioeconomic status.[285] When the entire United States is considered, different sociological theories may be required to account for the regional variation in the rates of infanticide.[286] Declining SIDS rates and recent recommendations to differentiate SIDS and child abuse have generated speculation that some cases of infanti-cide were misdiagnosed as SIDS. During an 18-year interval encompassing the years before and after the Back to Sleep campaign in California, the ratio of in-fanticide to SIDS increased from 4.3 in 1981 to 10.2 in 1998.[265] However, the increase in the ratio of infanticide to SIDS deaths was due to a decrease in SIDS deaths, and not to an absolute increase in infanticides.

Review of specific reports provides insights into the murder of children. In 1961 Adelson[4] reported details of 46 child homicides in Cuyahoga County, OH, from 1944 to 1960. Ten of the children were younger than 1 year. Of those, 5 drowned and 3 died of starvation. The causes of death of the other 2 are unknown. Adelson concluded that "Failure to perform autopsies on infants found dead (or said to have been found dead) because they are 'crib deaths' . . . will inevitably result in the missing of many cases of this type of homicide." In a follow-up article in 1991, Adelson[287] reported 194 child homicides in Cuyahoga County between 1976 and 1980: 16 occurred in infants between the ages of 1 month and 1 year, and 7 occurred between the ages of 1 and 6 months. All were fatally and obviously battered, and no cases were likely to have been confused with SIDS.

Emery and Taylor[288] described a 24-year period in Sheffield, England (1960–1984), during which post-perinatal deaths (birth–2 years) were investigated by gathering information about the death scene, obstetric and pediatric care, and autopsy findings, and by conducting home visits. Accidental suffocation was thought to be the cause of death in 10% of these cases, and the possibility of active intervention on the part of one or both parents was raised in another 10%, a rate consistently double that of overt child abuse in this age group. Specific data on infants between the ages of 1 month and 1 year were not reported.

Asch[289] hypothesized that many cases of sudden infant death were "infanticides, perpetrated by the mother as a specific manifestation of a postpartum depression." Although data do not bear out the numbers proposed by Asch, there are convincing descriptions wherein postpartum depression and other psychiatric disturbances, particularly in mothers who had histories of maltreatment themselves, have led to infanticide.[121,290-294]

In 1985 Christoffel et al[295] examined 43 unexpected deaths in children brought to the Children's Memorial Hospital in Chicago, IL, from 1980 to 1981. Nine of those deaths were the result of child abuse, and in 3 cases the correct diagnosis was established only by postmortem examination. The 2 factors having the highest predictive value for child abuse, according to the authors, were "dead on arrival" (DOA) and the subjects being younger than 1 year. An interesting observation, however, was that this study included 6 SIDS infants who arrived DOA and who were in the appropriate age group (1–7 months), and yet when subjected to postmortem examination, the results in every instance were consistent with SIDS. In the same journal issue, Kirschner and Stein[296] described 10 cases in which the diagnosis of child abuse was made on the basis of incomplete or erroneous medical observation and interpretations (eg, lividity, postmortem anal sphincter dilation, and mongolian blue spots being confused with traumatic lesions). Five of these cases were subsequently diagnosed as SIDS. Both of these articles underscore the need for appropriate evaluation of pre-mortem and post-mortem variables for all unwitnessed fatalities.

In a report from the Arkansas Children's Hospital covering the period between October 1983 and May 1987, 8 of 170 cases referred to hospital with a diagnosis of SIDS were selected for review because of concern that the diagnosis of SIDS was erroneous. The diagnosis in all 8 was changed after postmortem and death scene investigation.[297] Perrot suggested an even greater number of cases would have their initial diagnosis changed had all 170 cases been subjected to such review (LJ Perrot, personal communication).

Emery et al[298] reviewed the autopsy findings of 60 infant deaths registered as SIDS victims between 1974 and 1985 in Madison, WI.[298] The authors claimed that 10 of those infants had medical diagnoses suggestive of abuse sufficient to explain their deaths. This high rate (17%) has not been seen in other such analyses and calls into question the criteria for making the diagnoses.

Suffocation and Munchausen Syndrome by Proxy

The term Munchausen syndrome by proxy (MSBP) was introduced by Meadow[299] in 1977. It is a form of parent-induced illness that has been recognized as causing bizarre symptoms and signs that have puzzled clinicians and pathologists.[299] Because parent-induced apnea may be a manifestation of lethal MSBP, it is now in the differential diagnosis when ALTEs are being evaluated.

In 1979 Berger[300] reported 2 cases of child abuse simulating near-miss SIDS. The first case involved a 5-month-old girl who had a history of apnea and cyanotic spells and was extensively evaluated in the hospital for 5 weeks. During unwitnessed bathing of the infant by the mother, the mother ran out of the bathroom calling for help, and the infant was found cyanotic and limp,

with bleeding gums and fresh pinch marks on her nose. The second case was a 6-week-old girl with apnea and cyanosis, also hospitalized for several weeks, who had "spells" only when her mother visited. On one of those visits, the mother was discovered holding her hand over the infant's nose and mouth. Rosen et al[301] reported 2 siblings with recurrent cardiorespiratory arrest who, when removed from the care of the mother, stopped having the episodes. In 1986 Rosen et al[302] described 6 infants referred for evaluation of recurrent infant apnea requiring multiple resuscitation efforts. In 2 cases, the mothers were proven conclusively, by means of video surveillance, to be the perpetrators of the apneic episodes. In a third, the mother had an overt psychiatric disorder. For these 3 infants, the apneic episodes stopped when they were placed with other caretakers. The 3 other infants died within 1 month of leaving the hospital. Southall et al[303] reported 2 cases of apneic episodes induced by smothering and detected by covert video surveillance. Griffith and Slovik[304] reported 2 infants who were referred to a center for sleep disorders because of apnea and near-miss SIDS, both of whom were found to be victims of MSBP.

Meadow[305] reviewed and reported 27 cases of young children suffocated by their mothers. Twenty-four of the children had histories of previous episodes of apnea, cyanosis, or seizure, and 11 had experienced 10 or more episodes, either invented or caused by their mothers. Eighteen of the children were alive, and 9 were dead. In the families of these

27 cases, there were 15 older living siblings and 18 who had died suddenly and unexpectedly, 13 of whom had histories of recurrent apnea, cyanosis, or seizures, and most had been certified as SIDS. Meadow drew the distinction between the features seen in this group of suffocated infants and in infants dying of SIDS (Table 21.1). In an article in 1999 Meadow[306] reported details of 81 children from 50 families in which 42 deaths had been attributed to SIDS and 29 to other causes. Family and criminal courts had determined that all 81 of these children had been killed by their parents.

In 1991 Burchfield and Rawlings[307] described 10 hospitalized neonates from a variety of referring hospitals who had ALTEs or who had died of unexplained causes in the hospital. Five of the patients died, and autopsies performed on 4 of the 5 yielded no adequate explanations for the deaths. Evaluation of the survivors also failed to reveal a cause for the ALTEs. Four of the survivors had severe neurologic impairment. These cases are puzzling in that they occurred in a hospital environment, presumably while under nursing supervision.

Southall et al[266] reported their experience with 39 children referred for evaluation. While in the hospital, the children, ranging in age from 2 months to 44 months, were studied by means of covert video surveillance. Thirty-six had been referred for ALTEs, one for suspected seizure disorder, one for failure to thrive, and one for suspected strangulation. The number of ALTEs reported by the parents ranged from 2 to more than 50 (median = 7). Forty-six children constituted a control group and were being investigated for ALTEs due to proven medical conditions. Covert video surveillance was accomplished by placing a video camera in each corner of the patients' rooms and a microphone in the ceiling. The infants and children underwent continuous monitoring of transcutaneous oxygen saturation with pulse oximetry and monitoring of breathing movements and electrocardiography. The median time of surveillance was 29 hours. In 30 cases, covert video surveillance revealed attempts at intentional suffocation of the infant. Frank oronasal hemorrhage was reported in 11 of 38 patients with ALTEs, but in none of the 46 control children, as has been observed in other

TABLE 21.1
Features Present in Suffocated Infants and in SIDS Victims[a]

Features	Suffocation (%)	SIDS (%)
Previous apnea	90	<10
Previous unexplained disorder	44	<5
>6 months old	55	<15
Dead sibling	48	2

Abbreviation: SIDS, sudden infant death syndrome.
[a]Used with permission from Meadow R. Suffocation, recurrent apnea, and sudden infant death. *J Pediatr.* 1990;117:351–354.

studies evaluating attempted suffocation.[269,300,305,306,308] Twelve of the 41 siblings of the children undergoing covert video surveillance had died suddenly and unexpectedly, with 11 being classified as SIDS. After video surveillance, 4 parents admitted to suffocating 8 children, and one child died of deliberate poisoning. In the 52 siblings of the 46 children in the control group, 2 had died: one of a hypoplastic left heart at the age of 5 days, and the other of SIDS. Studies such as these underscore the need for comprehensive medical and scene investigation due to the non-specificity of postmortem findings.

Substance Abuse and Its Relation to Child Fatalities

The relationship between child abuse and substance abuse is well established. Wallace[309] found that 34.3% of 70 mothers who used crack cocaine had Bureau of Child Welfare involvement as a result of the mother's drug use, and the neglect or abuse that followed.[309] Wallace concluded that most (53%) crack-cocaine smoking mothers had become dysfunctional as parents and no longer cared about their children. She further stated, "Crack-related deterioration in mothers' ability to care for their children reveals a shocking decline in psychosocial functioning compared with a pre-crack level of functioning." Famularo et al[310] showed a strong association between substance abuse and child maltreatment. During the period of study, 67% of the abused or neglected children seen in a juvenile court system in Massachusetts lived with substance-abusing parents. The rates of fatal child abuse directly attributable to substance

abuse are unknown, but it is logical to assume that a fatal outcome is an inevitable consequence in a proportion of these reported instances of maltreatment.

Twins and Child Abuse

In 1982 Groothuis et al,[311] in a retrospective study of twins in Nashville, TN, reported an increased incidence of child abuse in families with twins. Forty-eight families with twins were compared with control singleton births (matched for hospital of delivery, birth date, maternal age, race, and socioeconomic status). Three control families (2.4%) and 9 families with twins (18.7%) had been reported for maltreatment. One child died, and 8 children from 6 families were removed from their homes. When analyzing the variables in the families studied, the authors concluded that twin status had the greatest impact on the risk of subsequent child abuse, suggesting that the stress of rearing twins, added to other burdens of child rearing in already marginally functioning families, was a significant determinant for subsequent abuse. A nationwide study from Japan revealed that 10% of child abuse victims were products of multiple births and in only a few cases were both twins abused.[312] The likelihood that both twins would be abused increased when there were serious parental or family problems; in contrast, abuse limited to one twin was linked to the child's medical problems or to non-home care. There is also a report of a family in which both twins were repeatedly admitted to the hospital for apparent hemoptysis following which the mother was proven to have simulated the episodes, and to have evidence of MSBP herself.[313]

Radiographic Studies

The use of radiography as an ancillary study in postmortem examinations is routine in most jurisdictions. Kleinman and colleagues[314] noted that "The babygram is an inadequate examination to assess for skeletal injuries, particularly when they are inflicted. The babygram should be strenuously condemned, as it not only may fail to identify critical forensic data, but the apparent absence of fractures may give unjustified reassurance that no trauma has occurred." Belanger[315] described the elements of the skeletal survey. The skeletal survey consists of 19 images collimated to each anatomical body region, with frontal views of the appendicular skeleton and frontal and lateral views of the axial skeleton (Box 21.1).

In 1984 Kleinman et al[316] subjected 12 cases of unexplained infant deaths to complete radiographic skeletal surveys by pediatric radiologists using high-resolution film–screen cassettes or direct-exposure techniques to yield maximal osseous detail. Autopsies were performed, supplemented with resection and high-detail radiography, and histologic study of all non-cranial sites of suspected osseous injury or sites of high risk of injury (distal femoral, proximal and distal tibial, and proximal humeral metaphyses). Eight of the infants were found to have evidence of inflicted injury. Four of the abused infants had an initial history of apnea or ALTEs. A history of having been shaken

---

BOX 21.1
Required Views of the Skeletal Survey in Cases of Unexpected Infant Death[a,b]

Anteroposterior skull
Lateral skull
Lateral cervical spine
Anteroposterior thorax
Lateral thorax
Anteroposterior pelvis
Lateral lumbar spine
Anteroposterior humeri
Anteroposterior forearms
Oblique hands
Anteroposterior femora
Anteroposterior tibias
Anteroposterior feet

[a]Used with permission from Kleinman PK. *Diagnostic Imaging in Child Abuse*. St Louis, MO: Mosby; 1998.
[b]All positive sites should be viewed in at least 2 projections.

was noted in 3 cases. The cause of death in 6 of the 8 cases was head trauma. In 3 of those infants, multiple rib fractures were found at autopsy, and in the other 3 only postmortem evidence of head injury was found. In total, 34 bony injuries were found, including 13 metaphyseal injuries. Eleven of the 13 metaphyseal injuries were evident on skeletal survey, 12 on specimen radiography, and all on histologic analysis. Fifteen posterior rib fractures were identified at autopsy, 8 of which were not visible on skeletal survey because of their acuteness. Three skull fractures and one thoracic spine fracture were found. Fractures of the clavicle, vertebrae, and long-bone diaphyses were indistinguishable from fractures resulting from accidental injury. Kleinman et al[314] later studied 165 fractures in 31 fatally abused infants whose average age was 3 months. Fifty-one percent of the fractures were in the rib cage and 44% in the long bones (of which 89% were classic metaphyseal lesions). In their report of 108 dead infants, Williamson and Perrot[317] determined that when parenchymal lung disease was present, bone abnormalities at the autopsy were often not identified in the postmortem radiographs. Multiple fractures were seen in all of the child abuse cases, with no radiographic findings in the SIDS cases.

Perpetrators of Fatal Child Abuse: Is There a Profile?

In 37 of the 46 homicides reported by Adelson,[4] children were killed either by their parents, close relatives, or by persons who stood in loco parentis. Eight were slain by unrelated persons, and one assailant was never identified. Frankly psychotic assailants were identified in 17 cases, 4 were classified as "borderline psychotic," and suicidal intent with the desire to "take the children" with them accounted for 3 cases. Nine children were killed by fathers during violent outbursts, 4 girls and 1 boy were killed during sexual assault, 3 infants died of starvation, and 1 child died of burns inflicted by a father throwing flammable liquid onto the bed in which the mother and child were sleeping. One child died of repeated beatings.

In a 1973 English study of 29 children killed by their fathers, Scott[318] found the following characteristics. First, nearly two thirds of the fathers were not married to their partners, and more than one half were not the biological father of the child. Second, in one quarter of this group the work and child-caring roles were reversed, with the father being the primary caretaker. Finally, the fathers had unrealistic expectations of the children and failed to understand that the behaviors of the victims were typical for infants and children, and viewed the infant as having adult motivations. Three fourths of the cases had unmistakable warnings of the subsequent outcome. In 27% of the cases, the fathers had records of violent crimes. Personality disorders, broadly characterized as "immature" or "aggressive," were seen in 75% of fathers. Most of the fathers had themselves experienced parental violence or hostility.

Korbin[291] examined the childhood histories of 9 women imprisoned for inflicting fatal child abuse and found that all had a history of childhood abuse, and that "abuse in one's childhood is an enduring potentiating factor." Five of the women had experienced spousal abuse and had a "dearth of support or compensatory factors." They also were seen as unable to seek and obtain effective assistance. Korbin[290] described the mothers' faulty perceptions of their children as being rejecting and having developmental abnormalities. The author found that the mothers had provided warning signals to professionals and their personal networks before the abusive incidents.

These and other retrospective studies have been criticized because of methodological flaws. Later studies drawing a connection between child victimization and subsequent abusive parental behaviors have also suffered from poor study designs.[48] Conversely, evidence suggesting that childhood victimization does not lead to abusive parenting behavior has been provided by Miller and Challas.[319] In their longitudinal study over a 25-year period, they found that 45% of persons abused as children were rated as not being at risk of abusing their children. However, Egelund et al[320] found that 70% of 47 mothers who had themselves been abused as children were currently mistreating their children. Kaufman and Zigler[321] concluded from review of the literature that the link between being maltreated and becoming abusive was "far from inevitable"[321] and Widom[322,323] supported this contention. Hunter and Kilstrom[324] reported 40 families in which this pattern was broken and identified factors relating to "a broad network of resources, a degree

of self-differentiation, an attitude of realistic optimism, and the ability to marshall extra resources to meet crisis situations."

Schloesser et al[325] studied 104 abuse-related fatalities occurring in Kansas from 1975 to 1980 and then from 1983 to 1989. Among their findings were these indicators: very young age of the parents at the first pregnancy, high rate of single parenthood, significantly lower educational achievement of victims' mothers, inadequate prenatal care, complications during pregnancy, and low birth weight among the victims.

Starling et al[326] studied 151 victims of head injury and found that males were more often perpetrators of that form of abuse. Fathers accounted for 37%, the mother's male partner 21%, female babysitters 17%, and mothers 13%. There was no determination of the identity of the perpetrator in some of the cases.

Lee[313] found that children were 8 times more likely to die of abuse if they were not in households with 2 biological parents (adjusted odds ratio [AOR], 8.8; 95% CI, 3.6–21.5). The risk of abusive death was also increased for children residing with stepparents, foster parents, or adoptive parents (AOR, 4.7; 95% CI, 1.6–12.0). In another population-based, case-control study of 149 children younger than 5 years, Schnitzer and Ewigman[327] found that children residing in households with unrelated adults were nearly 50 times more likely to die of abusive injuries compared with children residing with 2 biological parents (AOR, 47.6; 95% CI, 10.4–218).[327]

In this study, most known perpetrators were male (71.2%), and most were the child's father (34.9%) or the male partner of the child's mother (24.2%). In households with unrelated adults, most perpetrators (83.9%) were an unrelated adult household member, and in only 2 cases (6.5%) were the perpetrators the biological parent of the child.

Although studies of perpetrators have provided useful information for the analysis of unexpected infant death, the construction of standard profiles may predispose to misdiagnosis. The importance of risk factors derives from their incorporation into the larger landscape of infant death review.

Death Certification

Death certification typically requires determining both the cause and manner of death: the cause being the physiological and/or anatomical abnormalities leading to death, and the manner being the medicolegal category of natural or unnatural, such as accident, homicide, suicide, or undetermined. In the last few years, there has been a trend toward attributing sudden, unexpected infant death that is unexplained by medical history review, scene investigation, and postmortem examination as "undetermined" with respect to both cause and manner.[328,329] This is unfortunate because the use of the term SIDS acknowledges that the exact cause of death is uncertain, while recognizing that most of these deaths are natural. Labeling these cases "undetermined" may raise concerns similar to those of the Scottish finding of "'unproven'" (ie, it may be perceived that the parents have some-

how escaped detection and prosecution for murder). As has been discussed already, autopsy findings are often nonspecific, and even prior referral to child protection service agencies does not discriminate with any level of certainty between homicide and SIDS.[330,331]

Correct ascertainment of the cause and manner of death is critically important for allocating adequate public resources to improve the health of infants and children. A recent study from Colorado compared data collected by a multidisciplinary child fatality review team with vital records for all children aged from birth to 16 years during a 9-year interval and found that only half of the death certificates for children who died of maltreatment were completed correctly.[332] Violent deaths were more likely to be identified than nonviolent deaths, and maltreatment by an unrelated perpetrator was 8.71 times (95% CI: 3.52–21.55) more likely to be recognized than maltreatment by a parent.

Child Fatality Review Teams

The first interagency child fatality review team in the United States was formed in 1978 in Los Angeles County under the direction of Michael Durfee (The Interagency Council on Child Abuse and Neglect). By 1999 child fatality review teams existed in 49 states. In California, nearly 100% of the population now lives in communities served by child fatality review teams. The composition of these teams varies, but usually consists of representatives from the medical examiner/coroner's office and the district attorney's office; a representative from CPS; and a pediatrician familiar with pediatric diseases, child abuse, and childhood injury. Including a pediatric pathologist, as well as personnel from the police/sheriff's office and public health nursing, can significantly enhance the expertise of the teams. This approach has been described in 4 manuals prepared by the Child Maltreatment Fatalities Project of the American Bar Association Cen-ter on Children and the Law and the AAP, supported by the Robert Wood Johnson Foundation.[333–336]

Review of cases of childhood death has been shown to have a variety of applications. In a report from the US state of Georgia, team members reviewed 255 cases of 1,889 childhood deaths. In 87% of cases, the child fatality review team concurred with causes of death as stated on death certificates.[337] In 21 cases the review team disagreed with the death certificate and 5 of the cases were re-classified as child abuse based on the team's recommendations. Certain public health initiatives, such as stronger child passenger restraint laws and installation of a traffic signal at dangerous intersections, were other positive results of this child fatality review team's activities.

In another report on the activities of a child fatality review team, Herman-Giddens et al[338] reviewed all child homicides in North Carolina from 1985 to 1994. Two hundred and twenty of the total were homicides involving child abuse, but the *International Classification of Diseases, Ninth Revision, Clinical Modification (ICD-9-CM)* code E967 (homicide and injury purposely inflicted by other persons/child battering and other maltreatment) was assigned

to only 68 of the 220 cases. This reporting underascertainment of almost 60% indicated that significant problems exist in accurately recording the cause and manner of death in children.

Conclusions

This chapter has reviewed relevant literature and provides an overview of SIDS, infanticide, and child fatalities, as well as addressed issues important to other causes of sudden infant death, investigation of the circumstances of death, postmortem examination, death certification, and child death review teams. It concludes with guidelines for differentiating SIDS from infanticide.

The literature provides some parameters for making the distinction between SIDS and fatal child abuse that may be grouped into 3 categories: highly consistent with SIDS, less likely to be SIDS, and suggestive or diagnostic of abuse.

To reach the best decision in these sometimes ambiguous and complex cases, we recommend the following steps:

1. Use endorsed standardized death scene protocols to obtain details of the medical history from emergency responders, medical personnel, and medical records, with death scene investigation by knowledgeable individuals, including careful and supportive interviews of the infant's household members.
2. Use endorsed standardized postmortem examination and data collection protocols.

3. Conduct comprehensive postmortem examinations within 24 hours of death, including toxicology, metabolic screening, microbiological studies, vitreous electrolyte, urea and creatinine analysis, and full skeletal surveys. Resuscitation paraphernalia should be examined by a medical examiner/pathologist before it is removed.

4. Use infant death review teams organized locally to review the data collected.

5. Use accepted diagnostic categories on death certificates as promptly as possible, including *ICD-9-CM* E codes, after case review has occurred.

6. Maintain a supportive approach to parents during the death review process.

7. Allocate adequate funds to support the critical process of ascertaining the cause and manner of death and, secondarily, encourage the protection of all infants and children.

8. Stimulate and support more research into the etiology of both SIDS and child abuse.

References

1. Byard RW. *Sudden Death in Infancy, Childhood and Adolescence.* 2nd ed. Cambridge, UK: Cambridge University Press; 2004

2. Caffey J. Multiple fractures in the long bones of infants suffering from chronic subdural hematoma. *AJR Am J Roentgenol.* 1946;56:163–173

3. Silverman F. The roentgen manifestations of unrecognized skeletal trauma in infants. *Am J Roentgenol Rad Ther.* 1953;69:413–426

4. Adelson L. Slaughter of the innocents. A study of forty-six homicides in which the victims were children. *N Engl J Med.* 1961;264:1345–1349

5. Kempe CH, Silverman FN, Steele BF, Droegemueller W, Silver HK. The battered-child syndrome. *JAMA.* 1962;181:17–24

6. Steinschneider A. Prolonged apnea and the sudden infant death syndrome: clinical and laboratory observations. *Pediatrics.* 1972;50:646–654

7. Firstman R, Talan J. SIDS and infanticide. In: Byard RW, Krous HF, eds. *Sudden Infant Death Syndrome: Problems, Progress & Possibilities.* London, UK: Arnold; 2001:291–300

8. Beckwith JB. Discussion of terminology and definition of the sudden infant death syndrome. In: Bergman AB, Beckwith JB, Ray CG, eds. *Proceedings of the Second International Conference on the Causes of Sudden Death in Infants.* Seattle, WA: University of Washington Press; 1970:14–22

9. Willinger M, James LS, Catz C. Defining the sudden infant death syndrome (SIDS): deliberations of an expert panel convened by the National Institute of Child Health and Human Development. *Pediatr Pathol.* 1991;11:677–684

10. Beckwith JB. Defining the sudden infant death syndrome. *Arch Pediatr Adolesc Med.* 2003;157:286–290

11. Krous HF. Reflections on redefining SIDS. *Arch Pediatr Adolesc Med.* 2003;157:291–292

12. Berry PJ. Pathological findings in SIDS. *J Clin Pathol.* 1992;45(11 suppl):11–16

13. Guntheroth WG, Spiers PS, Naeye RL. Redefinition of the sudden infant death syndrome: the disadvantages. *Pediatr Pathol.* 1994;14:127–132

14. Taylor EM, Emery JL. Categories of preventable unexpected infant deaths. *Arch Dis Child.* 1990;65:535–539

15. Rognum TO. Sudden infant death syndrome: need for simple definition but detailed diagnostic criteria. *Arch Pediatr Adolesc Med.* 2003;157:293

16. Krous HF, Beckwith JB, Byard RW, et al. Sudden infant death syndrome and unclassified sudden infant deaths: a definitional and diagnostic approach. *Pediatrics.* 2004;114:234–238

17. Carpenter RG, Irgens LM, Blair PS, et al. Sudden unexplained infant death in 20 regions in Europe: case control study. *Lancet.* 2004;363:185–191

18. Blair PS, Sidebotham P, Berry PJ, Evans M, Fleming PJ. Major epidemiological changes in sudden infant death syndrome: a 20-year population-based study in the UK. *Lancet.* 2006;367:314–319

19. Dwyer T, Ponsonby AL. Sudden infant death syndrome: after the "Back to Sleep" campaign. *BMJ.* 1996;313:180–181

20. Dwyer T, Ponsonby AL. The decline of SIDS: a success story for epidemiology. *Epidemiology.* 1996;7:323–325

21. Fleming PJ, Blair PS, Bacon C, et al. Environment of infants during sleep and risk of the sudden infant death syndrome: results of 1993–5 case-control study for confidential inquiry into stillbirths and deaths in infancy. Confidential Enquiry into Stillbirths and Deaths Regional Coordinators and Researchers. *BMJ.* 1996;313:191–195

22. Mitchell EA, Brunt JM, Everard C. Reduction in mortality from sudden infant death syndrome in New Zealand: 1986–92. *Arch Dis Child.* 1994;70:291–294

23. Hauck FR. Changing epidemiology. In: Byard RW, Krous HF, eds. *Sudden Infant Death Syndrome: Problems, Progress & Possibilities.* London, UK: Arnold; 2001:31–57

24. Anderson RN, Kochanek KD, Murphy SL. Report of final mortality statistics, 1995. *Mon Vital Stat Rep.* 1997;45(suppl 2):66–69

25. Sudden infant death syndrome—United States, 1983–1994. *MMWR Morb Mortal Wkly Rep.* 1996;45:859–863

26. Willinger M, Hoffman HJ, Wu KT, et al. Factors associated with the transition to nonprone sleep positions of infants in the United States: the National Infant Sleep Position Study. *JAMA.* 1998;280:329–335

27. Adams EJ, Chavez GF, Steen D, Shah R, Iyasu S, Krous HF. Changes in the epidemiologic profile of sudden infant death syndrome as rates decline among California infants: 1990–1995. *Pediatrics.* 1998;102:1445–1451

28. Beckwith JB. The sudden infant death syndrome. *Curr Probl Pediatr.* 1973;3:1–36

29. Arnestad M, Andersen M, Vege A, Rognum TO. Changes in the epidemiological pattern of sudden infant death syndrome in southeast Norway, 1984–1998: implications for future prevention and research. *Arch Dis Child.* 2001;85:108–115

30. Beal SM. Sudden infant death syndrome: is the winter preponderance due to some infants having the head covered? *J Paediatr Child Health.* 2000;36:612

31. Krous HF, Nadeau JM, Silva PD, Blackbourne BD. A comparison of respiratory symptoms and inflammation in sudden infant death syndrome and in accidental or inflicted infant death. *Am J Forensic Med Pathol.* 2003;24:1–8

32. Hoffman HJ, Damus K, Hillman L, Krongrad E. Risk factors for SIDS. Results of the National Institute of Child Health and Human Development SIDS Cooperative Epidemiological Study. *Ann N Y Acad Sci.* 1988;533:13–30

33. Krous HF, Nadeau JM, Byard RW, Blackbourne BD. Oronasal blood in sudden infant death. *Am J Forensic Med Pathol.* 2001;22:346–351

34. Klonoff-Cohen HS, Edelstein SL. A case-control study of routine and death scene sleep position and sudden infant death syndrome in Southern California. *JAMA.* 1995;273:790–794

35. Mitchell EA, Scragg R, Stewart AW, et al. Results from the first year of the New Zealand cot death study. *N Z Med J.* 1991;104:71–76

36. Mitchell EA, Aley P, Eastwood J. The national cot death prevention program in New Zealand. *Aust J Public Health.* 1992;16:158–161

37. Mitchell EA, Ford RP, Taylor BJ, et al. Further evidence supporting a causal relationship between prone sleeping position and SIDS. *J Paediatr Child Health.* 1992;28 (suppl 1):S9–S12

38. Taylor JA, Krieger JW, Reay DT, Davis RL, Harruff R, Cheney LK. Prone sleep position and the sudden infant death syndrome in King County, Washington: a case-control study. *J Pediatr.* 1996;128:626–630

39. Tirosh E, Becker T, Mansour Y, Cohen A, Jaffe M. Sleep position, bedding and heating practices in high- and low-risk ethnic groups for unexpected death in infancy (UDI). *Eur J Epidemiol.* 2000;16:281–286

40. Mehanni M, Cullen A, Kiberd B, McDonnell M, O'Regan M, Matthews T. The current epidemiology of SIDS in Ireland. *Ir Med J.* 2000;93:264–268

41. Paris CA, Remler R, Daling JR. Risk factors for sudden infant death syndrome: changes associated with sleep position recommendations. *J Pediatr.* 2001;139:771–777

42. Nelson T, To KF, Wong YY, et al. Hong Kong case-control study of sudden unexpected infant death. *N Z Med J.* 2005;118:U1788

43. Blair PS, Fleming PJ, Bensley D, et al. Smoking and the sudden infant death syndrome: results from 1993–5 case-control study for confidential inquiry into stillbirths and deaths in infancy. Confidential Enquiry into Stillbirths and Deaths Regional Coordinators and Researchers. *BMJ.* 1996;313:195–198

44. MacDorman MF, Cnattingius S, Hoffman HJ, Kramer MS, Haglund B. Sudden infant death syndrome and smoking in the United States and Sweden. *Am J Epidemiol.* 1997;146:249–257

45. Schoendorf KC, Kiely JL. Relationship of sudden infant death syndrome to maternal smoking during and after pregnancy. *Pediatrics.* 1992;90:905–908

46. Alm B, Milerad J, Wennergren G, et al. A case-control study of smoking and sudden infant death syndrome in the Scandinavian countries, 1992 to 1995. The Nordic Epidemiological SIDS Study. *Arch Dis Child.* 1998;78:329–334

47. Bulterys MG, Greenland S, Kraus JF. Chronic fetal hypoxia and sudden infant death syndrome: interaction between maternal smoking and low hematocrit during pregnancy. *Pediatrics.* 1990;86:535–540

48. Cooke RW. Smoking, intra-uterine growth retardation and sudden infant death syndrome. *Int J Epidemiol.* 1998;27:238–241

49. Haglund B, Cnattingius S. Cigarette smoking as a risk factor for sudden infant death syndrome: a population-based study. *Am J Public Health.* 1990;80:29–32

50. Klonoff-Cohen HS, Edelstein SL, Lefkowitz ES, et al. The effect of passive smoking and tobacco exposure through breast milk on sudden infant death syndrome. *JAMA.* 1995;273:795–798

51. Little RE, Peterson DR. Sudden infant death syndrome epidemiology: a review and update. *Epidemiol Rev.* 1990;12:241–246

52. Milerad J, Rajs J, Gidlund E. Nicotine and cotinine levels in pericardial fluid in victims of SIDS. *Acta Puediatr.* 1994;83:59–62

53. Milerad J, Sundell H. Nicotine exposure and the risk of SIDS. *Acta Paediatr Suppl.* 1993;82(suppl 389):70–72

54. Mitchell EA, Ford RP, Stewart AW, et al. Smoking and the sudden infant death syndrome. *Pediatrics.* 1993;91:893–896

55. Naeye RL. Hypoxemia and the sudden infant death syndrome. *Science.* 1974;186:837–838

56. Ponsonby AL, Couper D, Dwyer T. Features of infant exposure to tobacco smoke in a cohort study in Tasmania. *J Epidemiol Community Health.* 1996;50:40–46

57. Shiono PH, Klebanoff MA, Rhoads GG. Smoking and drinking during pregnancy. Their effects on preterm birth. *JAMA*. 1986;255:82–84

58. Tonkin S, Beach D. The vulnerability of the infant upper airway. In: Harper R, Hoffman H, eds. *Sudden Infant Death Syndrome. Risk Factors and Basic Mechanisms*. New York, NY: PMA Publishing; 1988:417

59. Mosko S, McKenna J, Dickel M, Hunt L. Parent-infant cosleeping: the appropriate context for the study of infant sleep and implications for sudden infant death syndrome (SIDS) research. *J Behav Med*. 1993;16:589–610

60. Mosko S, Richard C, McKenna J. Infant arousals during mother-infant bed sharing: implications for infant sleep and sudden infant death syndrome research. *Pediatrics*. 1997;100:841–849

61. Mosko S, Richard C, McKenna J, Drummond S, Mukai D. Maternal proximity and infant CO2 environment during bedsharing and possible implications for SIDS research. *Am J Phys Anthropol*. 1997;103:315–328

62. Scragg R, Mitchell EA, Taylor BJ, et al. Bed sharing, smoking, and alcohol in the sudden infant death syndrome. New Zealand Cot Death Study Group. *BMJ*. 1993;307:1312–1318

63. Mitchell EA, Tuohy PG, Brunt JM, et al. Risk factors for sudden infant death syndrome following the prevention campaign in New Zealand: a prospective study. *Pediatrics*. 1997;100:835–840

64. Scragg RK, Mitchell EA. Side sleeping position and bed sharing in the sudden infant death syndrome. *Ann Med*. 1998;30:345–349

65. Blair PS, Platt MW, Smith IJ, Fleming PJ. Sudden infant death syndrome and sleeping position in pre-term and low birth weight infants: an opportunity for targeted intervention. *Arch Dis Child*. 2006;91:101–106

66. Beal SM, Byard RW. Accidental death or sudden infant death syndrome? *J Paediatr Child Health*. 1995;31:269–271

67. Gessner BD, Ives GC, Perham-Hester KA. Association between sudden infant death syndrome and prone sleep position, bed sharing, and sleeping outside an infant crib in Alaska. *Pediatrics*. 2001;108:923–927

68. Hauck FR, Herman SM, Donovan M, et al. Sleep environment and the risk of sudden infant death syndrome in an urban population: the Chicago Infant Mortality Study. *Pediatrics*. 2003;111:1207–1214

69. Stray-Pedersen A, Arnestad M, Vege A, Sveum L, Rognum TO. Bed sharing and sudden infant death [in Norwegian]. *Tidsskr Nor Laegeforen*. 2005;125:2919–2921

70. Tappin D, Ecob R, Brooke H. Bedsharing, roomsharing, and sudden infant death syndrome in Scotland: a case-control study. *J Pediatr*. 2005;147:32–37

71. The changing concept of sudden infant death syndrome: diagnostic coding shifts, controversies regarding the sleeping environment, and new variables to consider in reducing risk. *Pediatrics*. 2005;116:1245–1255

72. Gessner BD, Porter TJ. Bed sharing with unimpaired parents is not an important risk for sudden infant death syndrome. *Pediatrics*. 2006;117:990–991; author reply 994–996

73. Eidelman AI, Gartner LM. Bed sharing with unimpaired parents is not an important risk for sudden infant death syndrome: to the editor. *Pediatrics*. 2006;117:991–992; author reply 994–996

74. Bartick M. Bed sharing with unimpaired parents is not an important risk for sudden infant death syndrome: to the editor. *Pediatrics*. 2006;117:992–993; author reply 994–996

75. Pelayo R, Owens J, Mindell J, Sheldon S. Bed sharing with unimpaired parents is not an important risk for sudden infant death syndrome: to the editor. *Pediatrics*. 2006;117:993–994; author reply 994–996

76. Kattwinkel J, Hauck FR, Moon RY, Malloy MH, Willinger M. In reply. *Pediatrics*. 2006;117:994–996

77. Li DK, Willinger M, Petitti DB, Odouli R, Liu L, Hoffman HJ. Use of a dummy (pacifier) during sleep and risk of sudden infant death syndrome (SIDS): population based case-control study. *BMJ.* 2006;332:18–22

78. Hauck FR, Omojokun OO, Siadaty MS. Do pacifiers reduce the risk of sudden infant death syndrome? A meta-analysis. *Pediatrics.* 2005;116:e716–e723

79. Black L, David RJ, Brouillette RT, Hunt CE. Effects of birth weight and ethnicity on incidence of sudden infant death syndrome. *J Pediatr.* 1986;108:209–214

80. Adams MM. The descriptive epidemiology of sudden infant deaths among natives and whites in Alaska. *Am J Epidemiol.* 1985;122:637–643

81. Grether JK, Schulman J. Sudden infant death syndrome and birth weight. *J Pediatr.* 1989;114:561–567

82. Grether JK, Schulman J, Croen LA. Sudden infant death syndrome among Asians in California. *J Pediatr.* 1990;116:525–528

83. Kraus JF, Greenland S, Bulterys M. Risk factors for sudden infant death syndrome in the US Collaborative Perinatal Project. *Int J Epidemiol.* 1989;18:113–120

84. Irwin KL, Mannino S, Daling J. Sudden infant death syndrome in Washington State: why are Native American infants at greater risk than white infants? *J Pediatr.* 1992;121:242–247

85. Iyasu S, Randall LL, Welty TK, et al. Risk factors for sudden infant death syndrome among northern plains Indians. *JAMA.* 2002;288:2717–2723

86. Kinney HC, Randall LL, Sleeper LA, et al. Serotonergic brainstem abnormalities in Northern Plains Indians with the sudden infant death syndrome. *J Neuropathol Exp Neurol.* 2003;62:1178–1191

87. Kraus JF, Bultreys M. The epidemiology of sudden infant death syndrome. In: Kiely M, ed. *Reproductive and Perinatal Epidemiology.* Boca Raton, FL: CRC Press; 1991

88. Decrease in infant mortality and sudden infant death syndrome among Northwest American Indians and Alaskan Natives— Pacific Northwest, 1985–1996. *MMWR Morb Mortal Wkly Rep.* 1999;48:181–184

89. Muhuri PK, MacDorman MF, Ezzati-Rice TM. Racial differences in leading causes of infant death in the United States. *Paediatr Perinat Epidemiol.* 2004;18:51–60

90. Bauchner H, Zuckerman B, McClain M, Frank D, Fried LE, Kayne H. Risk of sudden infant death syndrome among infants with in utero exposure to cocaine. *J Pediatr.* 1988;113:831–834

91. Bauchner H, Zuckerman B. Cocaine, sudden infant death syndrome, and home monitoring [editorial]. *J Pediatr.* 1990;117:904–906

92. Ward SL, Schuetz S, Kirshna V, et al. Abnormal sleeping ventilatory pattern in infants of substance-abusing mothers. *Am J Dis Child.* 1986;140:1015–1020

93. Ward SL, Bautista D, Chan L, et al. Sudden infant death syndrome in infants of substance-abusing mothers. *J Pediatr.* 1990;117:876–881

94. Chasnoff IJ, Burns WJ, Schnoll SH, Burns KA. Cocaine use in pregnancy. *N Engl J Med.* 1985;313:666–669

95. Durand DJ, Espinoza AM, Nickerson BG. Association between prenatal cocaine exposure and sudden infant death syndrome. *J Pediatr.* 1990;117:909–911

96. Peterson DR. SIDS in infants of drug-dependent mothers [letter]. *J Pediatr.* 1980;96:784–785

97. Thomas D. Infants of drug-addicted mothers. *Aust Paediatr J.* 1988;24:167–168

98. Kandall SR, Gaines J, Habel L, Davidson G, Jessop D. Relationship of maternal substance abuse to subsequent sudden infant death syndrome in offspring. *J Pediatr.* 1993;123:120–126

99. Bouvier-Colle MH, Flahaut A, Messiah A, Jougla E, Hatton F. Sudden infant death and immunization: an extensive epidemiological approach to the problem in France—winter 1986. *Int J Epidemiol.* 1989;18:121–126

100. Hoffman HJ, Hunter JC, Damus K, et al. Diphtheria-tetanus-pertussis immunization and sudden infant death: results of the National Institute of Child Health and Human Development Cooperative Epidemiological Study of Sudden Infant Death Syndrome risk factors. *Pediatrics.* 1987;79:598–611

101. Mitchell EA, Stewart AW, Clements M. Immunisation and the sudden infant death syndrome. New Zealand Cot Death Study Group. *Arch Dis Child.* 1995;73:498–501

102. Silvers LE, Ellenberg SS, Wise RP, Varricchio FE, Mootrey GT, Salive ME. The epidemiology of fatalities reported to the vaccine adverse event reporting system 1990–1997. *Pharmacoepidemiol Drug Saf.* 2001;10:279–285

103. Jonville-Bera AP, Autret-Leca E, Barbeillon F, Paris-Llado J. Sudden unexpected death in infants under 3 months of age and vaccination status—a case-control study. *Br J Clin Pharmacol.* 2001;51:271–276

104. Beal SM. SIDS and immunization [letter]. *Med J Aust.* 1990;153.117

105. Byard RW, Mackenzie J, Beal SM. Vaccination and SIDS: information from the South Australian SIDS Database [letter]. *Med J Aust.* 1995;163:443–444

106. Geier DA, Geier MR. An evaluation of serious neurological disorders following immunization: a comparison of whole-cell pertussis and acellular pertussis vaccines. *Brain Dev.* 2004;26:296–300

107. Sudden-infant-death syndrome. *N Engl J Med.* 1982;307:891–893

108. Bass M, Kravath RE, Glass L. Death-scene investigation in sudden infant death. *N Engl J Med.* 1986;315:100–105

109. Stanton AN. Sudden infant death. Overheating and cot death. *Lancet.* 1984;2:1199–1201

110. Stanton AN, Oakley JR. Pattern of illnesses before cot deaths. *Arch Dis Child.* 1983;58:878–881

111. Stark AR, Thach BT. Mechanisms of airway obstruction leading to apnea in newborn infants. *J Pediatr.* 1976;89:982–985

112. Ponsonby AL, Dwyer T, Gibbons LE, Cochrane JA, Jones ME, McCall MJ. Thermal environment and sudden infant death syndrome: case-control study. *BMJ.* 1992;304:277–282

113. Curran AK, Xia L, Leiter JC, Bartlett D Jr. Elevated body temperature enhances the laryngeal chemoreflex in decerebrate piglets. *J Appl Physiol.* 2005;98:780–786

114. Kahraman L, Thach BT. Inhibitory effects of hyperthermia on mechanisms involved in autoresuscitation from hypoxic apnea in mice: a model for thermal stress causing SIDS. *J Appl Physiol.* 2004;97:669–674

115. Standfast SJ, Jereb S, Janerich DT. The epidemiology of sudden infant death in upstate New York: II: birth characteristics. *Am J Public Health.* 1980;70:1061–1067

116. Daltveit AK, Vollset SE, Otterblad-Olausson P, Irgens LM. Infant mortality in Norway and Sweden 1975–88: a cause-specific analysis of an increasing difference. *Paediatr Perinat Epidemiol.* 1997;11:214–227

117. Rintahaka PJ, Hirvonen J. The epidemiology of sudden infant death syndrome in Finland in 1969–1980. *Forensic Sci Int.* 1986;30:219–233

118. Getahun D, Demissie K, Lu SE, Rhoads GG. Sudden infant death syndrome among twin births: United States, 1995–1998. *J Perinatol.* 2004;24:544–551

119. Malloy MH, Freeman DH Jr. Sudden infant death syndrome among twins. *Arch Pediatr Adolesc Med.* 1999;153:736–740

120. Beal S. Sudden infant death syndrome in twins. *Pediatrics.* 1989;84:1038–1044

121. Kraus JF, Borhani NO. Post-neonatal sudden unexplained death in California: a cohort study. *Am J Epidemiol.* 1972;95:497–510

122. Smialek JE. Simultaneous sudden infant death syndrome in twins. *Pediatrics.* 1986;77:816–821

123. Spiers PS. Estimated rates of concordancy for the sudden infant death syndrome in twins. *Am J Epidemiol.* 1974;100:1–7

124. Valdes-Dapena MA. Sudden infant death syndrome: a review of the medical literature (1974–1979). *Pediatrics*. 1980;66:597–614

125. Ladham S, Koehler SA, Shakir A, Wecht CH. Simultaneous sudden infant death syndrome: a case report. *Am J Forensic Med Pathol*. 2001;22:33–37

126. Balci Y, Tok M, Kocaturk BK, Yenilmez C, Yirulmaz C. Simultaneous sudden infant death syndrome. *J Forensic Leg Med*. 2007;14:87–91

127. Koehler SA, Ladham S, Shakir A, Wecht CH. Simultaneous sudden infant death syndrome: a proposed definition and worldwide review of cases. *Am J Forensic Med Pathol*. 2001;22:23–32

128. Ramos V, Hernandez AF, Villanueva E. Simultaneous death of twins. An environmental hazard or SIDS? *Am J Forensic Med Pathol*. 1997;18:75–78

129. Bass M. The fallacy of the simultaneous sudden infant death syndrome in twins. *Am J Forensic Med Pathol*. 1989;10:200–205

130. Irgens LM, Skjaerven R, Peterson DR. Prospective assessment of recurrence risk in sudden infant death syndrome siblings. *J Pediatr*. 1984;104:349–351

131. Peterson DR, Sabotta EE, Daling JR. Infant mortality among subsequent siblings of infants who died of sudden infant death syndrome. *J Pediatr*. 1986;108:911–914

132. Beckwith JB. Observations on the pathologic anatomy of SIDS. In: Bergman AB, Beckwith JB, Ray CG, eds. *Proceedings of the Second International Conference on the Causes of Sudden Death in Infants*. Seattle, WA: University of Washington Press; 1970:83–107

133. Valdes-Dapena M. The pathologist and the sudden infant death syndrome. *Am J Pathol*. 1982;106:118–131

134. Valdes-Dapena M, Huff D. *Perinatal Autopsy Manual*. Washington, DC: Armed Forces Institute of Pathology; 1983

135. Krous HF. The pathology of sudden infant death syndrome: an overview. In: Culbertson JL, Krous HF, Bendell RD, eds. *Sudden Infant Death Syndrome. Medical Aspects and Psychological Management*. Baltimore, MD: The Johns Hopkins University Press; 1988:18–47

136. Byard RW, Carmichael E, Beal S. How useful is postmortem examination in sudden infant death syndrome? *Pediatr Pathol*. 1994;14:817–822

137. Mitchell E, Krous HF, Donald T, Byard RW. An analysis of the usefulness of specific stages in the pathologic investigation of sudden infant death. *Am J Forensic Med Pathol*. 2000;21:395–400

138. Kumar P, Taxy J, Angst DB, Mangurten HH. Autopsies in children: are they still useful? *Arch Pediatr Adolesc Med*. 1998;152:558–563

139. Sturner WQ. Common errors in forensic pediatric pathology. *Am J Forensic Med Pathol*. 1998;19:317–320

140. Krous H. Instruction and Reference Manual for the International Standardized Autopsy Protocol for Sudden Unexpected Infant Death. *J SIDS Infant Mortal*. 1996;1:203–246

141. Kelmanson IA. Differences in somatic and organ growth rates in infants who died of sudden infant death syndrome. *J Perinat Med*. 1992;20:183–188

142. Brooks JG, Gilbert RE, Flemming PJ, Berry PJ, Golding J. Postnatal growth preceding sudden infant death syndrome. *Pediatrics*. 1994;94:456–461

143. Byard RW, Byers S, Moore A, Leppard P, Fazzalari NL. Morphometric assessment of bone and growth plate in sudden infant death syndrome. *J SIDS Infant Mortal*. 1997;2:151–160

144. Byard RW, Makrides M, Need M, Neumann MA, Gibson RA. Sudden infant death syndrome: effect of breast and formula feeding on frontal cortex and brainstem lipid levels. *J Paediatr Child Health*. 1995;31:14–16

145. Vawter GF, Kozakewich PHW. Aspects of morphologic variation amongst SIDS victims. In: Tildon JT, RoederRL, Steinschneider A, eds. *Sudden Infant Death Syndrome.* New York, NY: Academic Press; 1983:163–170

146. Beckwith JB. The sudden infant death syndrome: a new theory. *Pediatrics.* 1975;55:583–584

147. Krous HF. The microscopic distribution of intrathoracic petechiae in sudden infant death syndrome. *Arch Pathol Lab Med.* 1984;108:77–79

148. Kleemann WJ, Wiechern V, Schuck M, Troger HD. Intrathoracic and subconjunctival petechiae in sudden infant death syndrome (SIDS). *Forensic Sci Int.* 1995;72:49–54

149. Beckwith JB. Intrathoracic petechial hemorrhages: a clue to the mechanism of death in sudden infant death syndrome? *Ann N Y Acad Sci.* 1988;533:37–47

150. Krous HF, Jordan J. A necropsy study of distribution of petechiae in non-sudden infant death syndrome. *Arch Pathol Lab Med.* 1984;108:75 76

151. Farber JP, Catron AC, Krous HF. Pulmonary petechiae: ventilatory-circulatory interactions. *Pediatr Res.* 1983;17:230–233

152. Martinez FD. Sudden infant death syndrome and small airway occlusion: facts and a hypothesis. *Pediatrics.* 1991;87:190–198

153. Poets CF, Meny RG, Chobanian MR, Bonofiglo RE. Gasping and other cardiorespiratory patterns during sudden infant deaths. *Pediatr Res.* 1999;45:350–354

154. Krous HF, Nadeau JM, Silva PD, Blackbourne BD. Intrathoracic petechiae in sudden infant death syndrome: relationship to face position when found. *Pediatr Dev Pathol.* 2001;4:160–166

155. Anderson WR, Edland JF, Schenk EA. Conduction system changes in the sudden infant death syndrome. *Am J Pathol.* 1970;59:35A

156. Anderson RH, Bouton CT, Smith A. Sudden death in infancy: a study of cardiac specialized tissue. *Br Med J.* 1974;2:135–139

157. Aretz HT. Diagnosis of myocarditis by endomyocardial biopsy. *Med Clin North Am.* 1986;70:1215–1226

158. Aretz HT. Myocarditis: the Dallas criteria. *Hum Pathol.* 1987;18:619–624

159. Billingham ME, Mason JW. The role of endomyocardial biopsy in the management of acute rejection in cardiac allograft recipients. In: Fenoglio JJ, ed. *Endomyocardial Biopsy: Techniques and Applications.* Boca Raton, FL: CRC Press; 1982:57–64

160. Billingham ME. Acute myocarditis: a diagnostic dilemma. *Br Heart J.* 1987;58:6–8

161. Dettmeyer R, Schlamann M, Madea B. Immunohistochemical techniques improve the diagnosis of myocarditis in cases of suspected sudden infant death syndrome (SIDS). *Forensic Sci Int.* 1999;105:83–94

162. Dettmeyer R, Kandolf R, Schmidt P, Schlamann M, Madea B. Lympho-monocytic enteroviral myocarditis: traditional, immunohistological and molecularpathological methods for diagnosis in a case of suspected sudden infant death syndrome (SIDS). *Forensic Sci Int.* 2001;119:141–144

163. Dettmeyer R, Baasner A, Schlamann M, et al. Role of virus-induced myocardial affections in sudden infant death syndrome: a prospective postmortem study. *Pediatr Res.* 2004;55:947–952

164. Shatz A, Hiss J, Arensburg B. Basement-membrane thickening of the vocal cords in sudden infant death syndrome. *Laryngoscope.* 1991;101:484–486

165. Shatz A, Hiss J, Arensburg B. Myocarditis misdiagnosed as sudden infant death syndrome (SIDS). *Med Sci Law.* 1997;37:16–18

166. Shatz A, Hiss Y, Hammel I, Arensburg B, Variend S. Age-related basement membrane thickening of the vocal cords in sudden infant death syndrome (SIDS). *Laryngoscope.* 1994;104:865–868

167. Krous HF, Hauck FR, Herman SM, et al. Laryngeal basement membrane thickening is not a reliable postmortem marker for SIDS: results from the Chicago Infant Mortality Study. *Am J Forensic Med Pathol.* 1999;20:221–227

168. Caddell JL. A triple-risk model for the sudden infant death syndrome (SIDS) and the apparent life-threatening episode (ALTE): the stressed magnesium deficient weanling rat. *Magnes Res.* 2001;14:227–238

169. Guntheroth WG, Spiers PS. The triple risk hypotheses in sudden infant death syndrome. *Pediatrics.* 2002;110:e64

170. Filiano JJ, Kinney HC. A perspective on neuropathologic findings in victims of the sudden infant death syndrome: the triple-risk model. *Biol Neonate.* 1994;65:194–197

171. Kinney HC, Filiano JJ, White WF. Medullary serotonergic network deficiency in the sudden infant death syndrome: review of a 15-year study of a single dataset. *J Neuropathol Exp Neurol.* 2001;60:228–247

172. Kinney HC. Abnormalities of the brainstem serotonergic system in the sudden infant death syndrome: a review. *Pediatr Dev Pathol.* 2005;8:507–524

173. Guilleminault C, Ariagno R, Korobkin R, et al. Mixed and obstructive sleep apnea and near miss for sudden infant death syndrome: 2. Comparison of near miss and normal control infants by age. *Pediatrics.* 1979;64:882–891

174. Guilleminault C, Ariagno RL, Forno LS, Nagel L, Baldwin R, Owen M. Obstructive sleep apnea and near miss for SIDS: I. Report of an infant with sudden death. *Pediatrics.* 1979;63:837–843

175. Guilleminault C, Souquet M, Ariagno RL, Korobkin R, Simmons FB. Five cases of near-miss sudden infant death syndrome and development of obstructive sleep apnea syndrome. *Pediatrics.* 1984;73:71–78

176. Kahn A, Blum D, Waterschoot P, Engelman E, Smets P. Effects of obstructive sleep apneas on transcutaneous oxygen pressure in control infants, siblings of sudden infant death syndrome victims, and near miss infants: comparison with the effects of central sleep apneas. *Pediatrics.* 1982;70:852–857

177. Kahn A, Blum D, Rebuffat E, et al. Polysomnographic studies of infants who subsequently died of sudden infant death syndrome. *Pediatrics.* 1988;82:721–727

178. Schechtman VL, Harper RM, Kluge KA, Wilson AJ, Hoffman HJ, Southall DP. Cardiac and respiratory patterns in normal infants and victims of the sudden infant death syndrome. *Sleep.* 1988;11:413–424

179. Schechtman VL, Harper RM, Kluge KA, Wilson AJ, Southall DP. Correlations between cardiorespiratory measures in normal infants and victims of sudden infant death syndrome. *Sleep.* 1990;13:304–317

180. Schechtman VL, Harper RM, Wilson AJ, Southall DP. Sleep apnea in infants who succumb to the sudden infant death syndrome. *Pediatrics.* 1991;87:841–846

181. Schechtman VL, Lee MY, Wilson AJ, Harper RM. Dynamics of respiratory patterning in normal infants and infants who subsequently died of the sudden infant death syndrome. *Pediatr Res.* 1996;40:571–577

182. Tonkin SL, Davis SL, Gunn TR. Upper airway radiographs in infants with upper airway insufficiency. *Arch Dis Child.* 1994;70:523–529

183. Gillan JE, Curran C, O'Reilly E, Cahalane SF, Unwin AR. Abnormal patterns of pulmonary neuroendocrine cells in victims of sudden infant death syndrome. *Pediatrics.* 1989;84:828–834

184. Cutz E, Perrin DG, Hackman R, Czegledy-Nagy EN. Maternal smoking and pulmonary neuroendocrine cells in sudden infant death syndrome. *Pediatrics.* 1996;98:668–672

185. Cutz E, Ma TK, Perrin DG, Moore AM, Becker LE. Peripheral chemoreceptors in congenital central hypoventilation syndrome. *Am J Respir Crit Care Med.* 1997;155:358–363

186. Cutz E, Jackson A. Airway inflammation and peripheral chemoreceptors. In: Byard RW, Krous HF, eds. *Sudden Infant Death Syndrome: Problems, Progress & Possibilities.* London, UK: Arnold; 2001:156–181

187. Kleemann WJ, Hiller AS, Troger HD. Infections of the upper respiratory tract in cases of sudden infant death. *Int J Legal Med.* 1995;108:85–89

188. Krous HF. Sudden infant death syndrome: pathology and pathophysiology. *Pathol Annu.* 1984;19:1–14

189. Krous HF. Pathological considerations of sudden infant death syndrome. *Pediatrician.* 1988;15:231–239

190. Tonkin S. Sudden infant death syndrome: hypothesis of causation. *Pediatrics.* 1975;55:650–661

191. Tonkin SL, Gunn TR, Bennet L, Vogel SA, Gunn AJ. A review of the anatomy of the upper airway in early infancy and its possible relevance to SIDS. *Early Hum Dev.* 2002;66:107–121

192. Kemp JS, Unger B, Wilkins D, et al. Unsafe sleep practices and an analysis of bedsharing among infants dying suddenly and unexpectedly: results of a four-year, population-based, death-scene investigation study of sudden infant death syndrome and related deaths. *Pediatrics.* 2000;106:e41

193. Kemp JS, Thach BT. Rebreathing of exhaled air. In: Byard RW, Krous HF, eds. *Sudden Infant Death Syndrome: Problems, Progress & Possibilities.* London, UK: Arnold; 2001

194. Thach BT, Davies AM, Koenig JS. Pathophysiology of sudden upper airway obstruction in sleeping infants and its relevance for SIDS. *Ann N Y Acad Sci.* 1988;533:314–328

195. Tonkin SL, Partridge J, Beach D, Whiteney S. The pharyngeal effect of partial nasal obstruction. *Pediatrics.* 1979;63:261–271

196. Tonkin SL, Stewart JH, Withey S. Obstruction of the upper airway as a mechanism of sudden infant death: evidence for a restricted nasal airway contributing to pharyngeal obstruction. *Sleep.* 1980;3:375–382

197. McNamara F, Sullivan CE. Obstructive sleep apnea in infants: relation to family history of sudden infant death syndrome, apparent life-threatening events, and obstructive sleep apnea. *J Pediatr.* 2000;136:318–323

198. Folgering H, Kuyper F, Kille JF. Primary alveolar hypoventilation (Ondine's curse syndrome) in an infant without external arcuate nucleus. Case report. *Bull Eur Physiopathol Respir.* 1979;15:659–665

199. Filiano JJ, Kinney HC. Arcuate nucleus hypoplasia in the sudden infant death syndrome. *J Neuropathol Exp Neurol.* 1992;51:394–403

200. Kinney HC, Filiano JJ, Sleeper LA, Mandell F, Valdes-Dapena M, White WF. Decreased muscarinic receptor binding in the arcuate nucleus in sudden infant death syndrome. *Science.* 1995;269:1446–1450

201. Kinney HC, Filiano JJ, Assmann SF, et al. Tritiated-naloxone binding to brainstem opioid receptors in the sudden infant death syndrome. *J Auton Nerv Syst.* 1998;69:156–163

202. Panigrahy A, Filiano JJ, Sleeper LA, et al. Decreased kainate receptor binding in the arcuate nucleus of the sudden infant death syndrome. *J Neuropathol Exp Neurol.* 1997;56:1253–1261

203. Nachmanoff DB, Panigrahy A, Filiano JJ, et al. Brainstem 3H-nicotine receptor binding in the sudden infant death syndrome. *J Neuropathol Exp Neurol.* 1998;57:1018–1025

204. Panigrahy A, Filiano J, Sleeper LA, et al. Decreased serotonergic receptor binding in rhombic lip-derived regions of the medulla oblongata in the sudden infant death syndrome. *J Neuropathol Exp Neurol.* 2000;59:377–384

205. Mansouri J, Panigrahy A, Filiano JJ, Sleeper LA, St John WM, Kinney HC. Alpha2 receptor binding in the medulla oblongata in the sudden infant death syndrome. *J Neuropathol Exp Neurol.* 2001;60:141–146

206. Panigrahy A, Filiano J, Sleeper LA, et al. Decreased serotonergic receptor binding in rhombic lip-derived regions of the medulla oblongata in the sudden infant death syndrome. *J Neuropathol Exp Neurol.* 2000;59:377–384

207. Kinney HC, Myers MM, Belliveau RA, et al. Subtle autonomic and respiratory dysfunction in sudden infant death syndrome associated with serotonergic brainstem abnormalities: a case report. *J Neuropathol Exp Neurol.* 2005;64:689–694

208. Narita N, Narita M, Takashima S, Nakayama M, Nagai T, Okado N. Serotonin transporter gene variation is a risk factor for sudden infant death syndrome in the Japanese population. *Pediatrics.* 2001;107:690–692

209. Weese-Mayer DE, Berry-Kravis EM, Maher BS, Silvestri JM, Curran ME, Marazita ML. Sudden infant death syndrome: association with a promoter polymorphism of the serotonin transporter gene. *Am J Med Genet.* 2003;117A:268–274

210. Weese-Mayer DE, Zhou L, Berry-Kravis EM, Maher BS, Silvestri JM, Marazita ML. Association of the serotonin transporter gene with sudden infant death syndrome: a haplotype analysis. *Am J Med Genet.* 2003;122A:238–245

211. Iyasu S, Hanzlick R, Rowley D, Willinger M. Proceedings of "Workshop on Guidelines for Scene Investigation of Sudden Unexplained Infant Deaths"—July 12–13, 1993. *J Forensic Sci.* 1994;39:1126–1136

212. Iyasu S, Rowley D, Hanzlick R. Guidelines for death scene investigation of sudden, unexplained infant deaths: recommendations of the Interagency Panel on Sudden Infant Death Syndrome. *MMWR Morb Mortal Wkly Rep.* 1996;45:1–6

213. Hanzlick R. On the need for more expertise in death investigation (and a National Office of Death Investigation Affairs?). *Arch Pathol Lab Med.* 1996;120:329–332

214. Schwartz PJ, Montemerlo M, Facchini M, et al. The QT interval throughout the first 6 months of life: a prospective study. *Circulation.* 1982;66:496–501

215. Schwartz PJ. The quest for the mechanisms of the sudden infant death syndrome: doubts and progress. *Circulation.* 1987;75:677–683

216. Hodgman JE, Siassi B. Prolonged QTc as a risk factor for SIDS. *Pediatrics.* 1999;103:814–815

217. Hoffman JI, Lister G. The implications of a relationship between prolonged QT interval and the sudden infant death syndrome. *Pediatrics.* 1999;103:815–817

218. Martin RJ, Miller MJ, Redline S. Screening for SIDS: a neonatal perspective. *Pediatrics.* 1999;103:812–813

219. Southall DP. Examine data in Schwartz article with extreme care. *Pediatrics.* 1999;103:819–820

220. Tonkin SL, Clarkson PM. A view from New Zealand: comments on the prolonged QT theory of SIDS causation. *Pediatrics.* 1999;103:818–819

221. Ackerman MJ, Siu BL, Sturner WQ, et al. Postmortem molecular analysis of SCN5A defects in sudden infant death syndrome. *JAMA.* 2001;286:2264–2269

222. Bennett MJ, Powell S. Metabolic disease and sudden, unexpected death in infancy. *Hum Pathol.* 1994;25:742–746

223. Levinson G, Coulam CB, Spence WC, Sherins RJ, Schulman JD. Recent advances in reproductive genetic technologies. *Biotechnology.* 1995;13:968–973

224. Arens R, Gozal D, Jain K, et al. Prevalence of medium-chain acyl-coenzyme A dehydrogenase deficiency in the sudden infant death syndrome. *J Pediatr.* 1993;122:715–718

225. Harpey JP, Charpentier C, Paturneau-Jouas M. Sudden infant death syndrome and inherited disorders of fatty acid beta-oxidation. *Biol Neonate.* 1990;58 (suppl 1):70–80

226. Brackett JC, Sims HF, Steiner RD, et al. A novel mutation in medium chain acyl-CoA dehydrogenase causes sudden neonatal death. *J Clin Invest.* 1994;94:1477–1483

227. Nagao M. Frequency of 985A-to-G mutation in medium-chain acyl-CoA dehydrogenase gene among patients with sudden infant death syndrome, Reye syndrome, severe motor and intellectual disabilities and healthy newborns in Japan. *Acta Paediatr Jpn.* 1996;38:304–307

228. Chace DH, DiPerna JC, Mitchell BL, Sgroi B, Hofman LF, Naylor EW. Electrospray tandem mass spectrometry for analysis of acylcarnitines in dried postmortem blood specimens collected at autopsy from infants with unexplained cause of death. *Clin Chem.* 2001;47:1166–1182

229. Bennett MJ, Rinaldo P. The metabolic autopsy comes of age. *Clin Chem.* 2001;47:1145–1146

230. Krous HF, Nadeau JM, Fukumoto RI, Blackbourne BD, Byard RW. Environmental hyperthermic infant and early childhood death: circumstances, pathologic changes, and manner of death. *Am J Forensic Med Pathol.* 2001;22:374–382

231. Smith NM, Bourne AJ, Clapton WK, Byard RW. The spectrum of presentation at autopsy of myocarditis in infancy and childhood. *Pathology.* 1992;24:129–131

232. Rasten-Almqvist P, Eksborg S, Rajs J. Myocarditis and sudden infant death syndrome. *APMIS.* 2002;110:469–480

233. deSa DJ. Isolated myocarditis as a cause of sudden death in the first year of life. *Forensic Sci Int.* 1986;30:113–117

234. Shimizu C, Rambaud C, Cheron G, et al. Molecular identification of viruses in sudden infant death associated with myocarditis and pericarditis. *Pediatr Infect Dis J.* 1995;14:584–588

235. Sun CC, Smith T. Sudden infant death with congenital cytomegalic inclusion disease. *Am J Forensic Med Pathol.* 1984;5:65–67

236. Lozinski GM, Davis GG, Krous HF, Billman GF, Shimizu H, Burns JC. Adenovirus myocarditis: retrospective diagnosis by gene amplification from formalin-fixed, paraffin-embedded tissues. *Hum Pathol.* 1994;25:831–834

237. Dettmeyer RB, Padosch SA, Madea B. Lethal enterovirus-induced myocarditis and pancreatitis in a 4-month-old boy. *Forensic Sci Int.* 2006;156:51–54

238. Kyto V, Saraste A, Saukko P, et al. Apoptotic cardiomyocyte death in fatal myocarditis. *Am J Cardiol.* 2004;94:746–750

239. Krous HF, Haas E, Chadwick AE, Wagner GN. Sudden death in a neonate with idiopathic eosinophilic endomyocarditis. *Pediatr Dev Pathol.* 2005;8:587–592

240. Byard RW, Moore L, Bourne AJ. Sudden and unexpected death—a late effect of occult intraesophageal foreign body. *Pediatr Pathol.* 1990;10:837–841

241. Byard RW, Bourne AJ, Beal SM. Mesh-sided cots—yet another potentially dangerous infant sleeping environment. *Forensic Sci Int.* 1996;83:105–109

242. Byard RW, Beal SM. V-shaped pillows and unsafe infant sleeping. *J Paediatr Child Health.* 1997;33:171–173

243. Moore L, Bourne AJ, Beal S, Collett M, Byard RW. Unexpected infant death in association with suspended rocking cradles. *Am J Forensic Med Pathol.* 1995;16:177–180

244. Moore L, Byard RW. Pathological findings in hanging and wedging deaths in infants and young children. *Am J Forensic Med Pathol.* 1993;14:296–302

245. Moore L, Bourne AJ, Beal S, Byard RW, Collett M. An association between suspended rocking cradles and infant death? *Med J Aust.* 1993;159:215–216

246. Byard RW, Beal S, Bourne AJ. Potentially dangerous sleeping environments and accidental asphyxia in infancy and early childhood. *Arch Dis Child.* 1994;71:497–500

247. Smialek JE, Smialek PZ, Spitz WU. Accidental bed deaths in infants due to unsafe sleeping situations. *Clin Pediatr (Phila).* 1977;16:1031–1036

248. Byard RW. Is breast feeding in bed always a safe practice? *J Paediatr Child Health.* 1998;34:418–419

249. Collins KA. Death by overlaying and wedging: a 15-year retrospective study. *Am J Forensic Med Pathol.* 2001;22:155–159

250. Byard RW, Beal S, Blackbourne B, Nadeau JM, Krous HF. Specific dangers associated with infants sleeping on sofas. *J Paediatr Child Health.* 2001;37:476–478

251. Byard RW, Gallard V, Johnson A, Barbour J, Bonython-Wright B, Bonython-Wright D. Safe feeding practices for infants and young children. *J Paediatr Child Health.* 1996;32:327–329

252. Krous HF, Chadwick AE, Stanley C. Delayed infant death following catastrophic deterioration and breast-feeding. *J Paediatr Child Health.* 2005;41:215–217

253. Krous HF, Chadwick AE, Isaacs H Jr. Tumors associated with sudden infant and childhood death. *Pediatr Dev Pathol.* 2005;8:20–25

254. Somers GR, Smith CR, Perrin DG, Wilson GJ, Taylor GP. Sudden unexpected death in infancy and childhood due to undiagnosed neoplasia: an autopsy study. *Am J Forensic Med Pathol.* 2006;27:64–69

255. Yamashita M, Chin I, Horigome H, Umesato Y, Tsuchida M. Sudden fatal cardiac arrest in a child with an unrecognized anterior mediastinal mass. *Resuscitation.* 1990;19:175–177

256. Levin H, Bursztein S, Heifetz M. Cardiac arrest in a child with an anterior mediastinal mass. *Anesth Analg.* 1985;64:1129–1130

257. Whybourne A, Zillman MA, Miliauskas J, Byard RW. Sudden and unexpected infant death due to occult lymphoblastic leukaemia. *J Clin Forensic Med.* 2001;8:160–162

258. Zakowski MF, Edwards RH, McDonough ET. Wilms' tumor presenting as sudden death due to tumor embolism. *Arch Pathol Lab Med.* 1990;114:605–608

259. Di Maio DJ, Di Maio VJM. *Forensic Pathology.* New York, NY: Elsevier; 1989

260. Dimaio VJ. SIDS or murder? *Pediatrics.* 1988;81:747–748

261. Cashell AW. Homicide as a cause of the sudden infant death syndrome. *Am J Forensic Med Pathol.* 1987;8:256–258

262. Bohnert M, Grosse Perdekamp M, Pollak S. Three subsequent infanticides covered up as SIDS. *Int J Legal Med.* 2005;119:31–34

263. Bajanowski T, Vennemann M, Bohnert M, Rauch E, Brinkmann B, Mitchell EA. Unnatural causes of sudden unexpected deaths initially thought to be sudden infant death syndrome. *Int J Legal Med.* 2005;119:213–216

264. Emery JL. Infanticide, filicide, and cot death. *Arch Dis Child.* 1985;60:505–507

265. Krous HF, Nadeau JM, Silva PD, Byard RW. Infanticide: is its incidence among postneonatal infant deaths increasing?: an 18-year population-based analysis in California. *Am J Forensic Med Pathol.* 2002;23:127–131

266. Southall DP, Plunkett MC, Banks MW, Falkov AF, Samuels MP. Covert video recordings of life-threatening child abuse: lessons for child protection. *Pediatrics.* 1997;100:735–760

267. Stewart S, Fawcett J, Jacobson W. Interstitial haemosiderin in the lungs of sudden infant death syndrome: a histological hallmark of 'near-miss' episodes? *J Pathol.* 1985;145:53–58

268. Byard RW, Stewart WA, Telfer S, Beal SM. Assessment of pulmonary and intrathymic hemosiderin deposition in sudden infant death syndrome. *Pediatr Pathol Lab Med.* 1997;17:275–282

269. Becroft DM, Lockett BK. Intra-alveolar pulmonary siderophages in sudden infant death: a marker for previous imposed suffocation. *Pathology.* 1997;29:60–63

270. Dorandeu A, Perie G, Jouan H, Leroy B, Gray F, Durigon M. Histological demonstration of haemosiderin deposits in lungs and liver from victims of chronic physical child abuse. *Int J Legal Med.* 1999;112:280–286

271. Hanzlick R, Delaney K. Pulmonary hemosiderin in deceased infants: baseline data for further study of infant mortality. *Am J Forensic Med Pathol.* 2000;21:319–322

272. Jackson CM, Gilliland MG. Frequency of pulmonary hemosiderosis in Eastern North Carolina. *Am J Forensic Med Pathol.* 2000;21:36–38

273. Schluckebier DA, Cool CD, Henry TE, Martin A, Wahe JW. Pulmonary siderophages and unexpected infant death. *Am J Forensic Med Pathol.* 2002;23:360–363

274. Forbes A, Acland P. What is the significance of haemosiderin in the lungs of deceased infants? *Med Sci Law.* 2004;44:348–352

275. Krous HF, Wixom C, Chadwick AE, Haas EA, Silva PD, Stanley C. Primary intra-alveolar siderophages in SIDS and suffocation: A San Diego SIDS/SUDC Research Project. *Pediatr Dev Pathol.* 2006;9:103–114

276. Valdes-Dapena M, McFeeley PA, Hoffmanh HJ, et al. *"Classic" or Typical Histologic Findings in SIDS.* Washington, DC: Armed Forces Institute of Pathology; 1993

277. Yukawa N, Carter N, Rutty G, Green MA. Intra-alveolar haemorrhage in sudden infant death syndrome: a cause for concern?. *J Clin Pathol.* 1999;52:581–587

278. Becroft DM, Thompson JM, Mitchell EA. Nasal and intrapulmonary haemorrhage in sudden infant death syndrome. *Arch Dis Child.* 2001;85:116–120

279. Hanzlick R. Pulmonary hemorrhage in deceased infants: baseline data for further study of infant mortality. *Am J Forensic Med Pathol.* 2001;22:188–192

280. Potter S, Berry PJ, Fleming P. Pulmonary haemorrhage in sudden unexpected death in infancy. *Pediatr Dev Pathol.* 1999;2:394–395

281. Krous HF, Chadwick AE, Haas EA, Stanley C. Pulmonary intra-alveolar hemorrhage in SIDS and suffocation. *J Clin Forensic Leg Med.* 2007;14:461–470

282. Moniruzzaman S, Andersson R. Age- and sex-specific analysis of homicide mortality as a function of economic development: a cross-national comparison. *Scand J Public Health.* 2005;33:464–471

283. Stiffman MN, Schnitzer PG, Adam P, Kruse RL, Ewigman BG. Household composition and risk of fatal child maltreatment. *Pediatrics.* 2002;109:615–621

284. Brenner RA, Overpeck MD, Trumble AC, DerSimonian R, Berendes H. Deaths attributable to injuries in infants, United States, 1983–1991. *Pediatrics.* 1999;103:968–974

285. Jason J, Andereck ND. Fatal child abuse in Georgia: the epidemiology of severe physical child abuse. *Child Abuse Negl.* 1983;7:1–9

286. Lester D. Regional variation in homicide rates of infants and children. *Inj Prev.* 1996;2:121–123

287. Adelson L. Pedicide revisited. The slaughter continues. *Am J Forensic Med Pathol.* 1991;12:16–26

288. Emery JL, Taylor EM. Investigation of SIDS [Letter]. *N Engl J Med.* 1986;315:1676

289. Asch SS. Crib deaths: their possible relationship to post-partum depression and infanticide. *J Mt Sinai Hosp N Y.* 1968;35:214–220

290. Korbin JE. Incarcerated mothers' perceptions and interpretations of their fatally maltreated children. *Child Abuse Negl.* 1987;11:397–407

291. Korbin JE. Childhood histories of women imprisoned for fatal child maltreatment. *Child Abuse Negl.* 1986;10:331–338

292. Steele BF. Parental abuse of infants and small children. In: Anthony AJ, Benedek T, eds. *Parenthood: Its Psychology and Psychopathology.* Boston, MA: Little, Brown; 1970

293. Steele BF. Psychodynamic factors in child abuse. In: Helfer ME, Kempe RS, Krugman RD, eds. *The Battered Child.* 5th ed. Chicago, IL: University of Chicago Press; 1997

294. Steele BF, Pollock C. A psychiatric study of parents who abuse infants and small children. In: Hefner RE, Kempe CH, eds. *The Battered Child.* Chicago, IL: University of Chicago Press; 1968

295. Christoffel KK, Zieserl EJ, Chiaramonte J. Should child abuse and neglect be considered when a child dies unexpectedly? *Am J Dis Child.* 1985;139:876–880

296. Kirschner RH, Stein RJ. The mistaken diagnosis of child abuse. A form of medical abuse? *Am J Dis Child.* 1985;139:873–875

297. Perrot LJ, Nawojczyk S. Nonnatural death masquerading as SIDS (sudden infant death syndrome). *Am J Forensic Med Pathol.* 1988;9:105–111

298. Emery JL, Chandra S, Gilbert-Barness EF. Findings in child deaths registered as sudden infant death syndrome (SIDS) in Madison, Wisconsin. *Pediatr Pathol.* 1988;8:171–178

299. Meadow R. Munchausen syndrome by proxy. The hinterland of child abuse. *Lancet.* 1977;2:343–345

300. Berger D. Child abuse simulating "near-miss" sudden infant death syndrome. *J Pediatr.* 1979;95:554–556

301. Rosen CL, Frost JD Jr, Bricker T, Tarnow JD, Gillette PC, Dunlavy S. Two siblings with recurrent cardiorespiratory arrest: Munchausen syndrome by proxy or child abuse? *Pediatrics.* 1983;71:715–720

302. Rosen CL, Frost JD Jr, Glaze DG. Child abuse and recurrent infant apnea. *J Pediatr.* 1986;109:1065–1067

303. Southall DP, Stebbens VA, Rees SV, Lang MH, Warner JO, Shinebourne EA. Apnoeic episodes induced by smothering: two cases identified by covert video surveillance. *Br Med J (Clin Res Ed).* 1987;294:1637–1641

304. Griffith JL, Slovik LS. Munchausen syndrome by proxy and sleep disorders medicine. *Sleep.* 1989;12:178–183

305. Meadow R. Suffocation, recurrent apnea, and sudden infant death. *J Pediatr.* 1990;117:351–357

306. Meadow R. Unnatural sudden infant death. *Arch Dis Child.* 1999;80:7–14

307. Burchfield DJ, Rawlings DJ. Sudden deaths and apparent life-threatening events in hospitalized neonates presumed to be healthy. *Am J Dis Child.* 1991;145:1319–1322

308. Makar AF, Squier PJ. Munchausen syndrome by proxy: father as a perpetrator. *Pediatrics.* 1990;85:370–373

309. Wallace BC. *Crack Cocaine: A Practical Treatment Approach for the Chemically Dependent.* New York, NY: Brunner/ Magel; 1991

310. Famularo R, Stone K, Barnum R, Wharton R. Alcoholism and severe child maltreatment. *Am J Orthopsychiatry.* 1986;56:481–485

311. Groothuis JR, Altemeier WA, Robarge JP, et al. Increased child abuse in families with twins. *Pediatrics.* 1982;70:769–773

312. Tanimura M, Matsui I, Kobayashi N. Child abuse of one of a pair of twins in Japan. *Lancet.* 1990;336:1298–1299

313. Lee DA. Munchausen syndrome by proxy in twins. *Arch Dis Child.* 1979;54:646–647

314. Kleinman PK, Marks SC Jr, Richmond JM, Blackbourne BD. Inflicted skeletal injury: a postmortem radiologic-histopathologic study in 31 infants. *AJR Am J Roentgenol.* 1995;165:647–650

315. Belanger PL. Quality assurance and skeletal survey standards. In: Kleinman PK, ed. *Diagnostic Imaging in Child Abuse.* St Louis, MO: Mosby; 1998

316. Kleinman PK, Blackbourne BD, Marks SC, Karellas A, Belanger PL. Radiologic contributions to the investigation and prosecution of cases of fatal infant abuse. *N Engl J Med.* 1989;320:507–511

317. Williamson SL, Perrot LL. The significance of postmortem radiographs in infants. *J Forensic Sci.* 1990;35:365–367

318. Scott PD. Parents who kill their children. *Med Sci Law.* 1973;13:120–126

319. Miller D, Challas G. Abused children as adult parents: a twenty-five year longitudinal study. Paper presented at: National Conference for Family Violence Researchers, University of New Hampshire; July 21–24, 1981; Durham, NC

320. Egelund B, Jacobvitz D, Papatola K. Intergenerational continuity of abuse. In: Gelles R, Lancaster J, eds. *Child Abuse and Neglect: Biosocial Dimensions.* New York, NY: Aldine Press; 1987

321. Kaufman J, Zigler E. The intergenerational transmission of child abuse. In: Cicchetti D, Carlson V, eds. *Child Maltreatment Theory and Research on the Causes and Consequences of Child Abuse and Neglect.* New York, NY: Cambridge University Press; 1989

322. Widom CS. Does violence beget violence? A critical examination of the literature. *Psychol Bull.* 1989;106:3–28

323. Widom CS. The cycle of violence. *Science.* 1989;244:160–166

324. Hunter RS, Kilstrom N. Breaking the cycle in abusive families. *Am J Psychiatry.* 1979;136:1320–1322

325. Schloesser P, Pierpont J, Poertner J. Active surveillance of child abuse fatalities. *Child Abuse Negl.* 1992;16:3–10

326. Starling SP, Holden JR, Jenny C. Abusive head trauma: the relationship of perpetrators to their victims. *Pediatrics.* 1995;95:259–262

327. Schnitzer PG, Ewigman BG. Child deaths resulting from inflicted injuries: household risk factors and perpetrator characteristics. *Pediatrics.* 2005;116:e687–e693

328. Malloy MH. Trends in postneonatal aspiration deaths and reclassification of sudden infant death syndrome: impact of the "Back to Sleep" program. *Pediatrics.* 2002;109:661–665

329. Malloy MH, MacDorman M. Changes in the classification of sudden unexpected infant deaths: United States, 1992–2001. *Pediatrics.* 2005;115:1247–1253

330. O'Halloran RL, Ferratta F, Harris M, Ilbeigi P, Rom CD. Child abuse reports in families with sudden infant death syndrome. *Am J Forensic Med Pathol.* 1998;19:57–62

331. Krous HF, Haas EA, Manning JM, et al. Child Protective Services referrals in cases of sudden infant death: a 10-year population-based analysis in San Diego County, California. *Child Maltreat.* 2006;11:247–256

332. Crume TL, DiGuiseppi C, Byers T, Sirotnak AP, Garrett CJ. Underascertainment of child maltreatment fatalities by death certificates, 1990–1998. *Pediatrics.* 2002;110:e18

333. Anderson TL, Wells SJ. *Data Collection for Child Fatalities: Existing Efforts and Proposal Guidelines.* Chicago, IL: American Bar Association; 1992

334. Granik LA, Durfee M, Wells SJ. *Child Death Review Teams: A Manual for Design and Implementation.* Chicago, IL: American Bar Association; 1992

335. Kaplan SR. *Child Fatality Legislation in the United States.* Chicago, IL: American Bar Association; 1992

336. Kaplan SR, Granik LA. *Child Fatality Investigative Procedures Manual.* Chicago, IL: American Bar Association; 1992

337. Luallen JJ, Rochat RW, Smith SM, O'Neil J, Rogers MY, Bolen JC. Child fatality review in Georgia: a young system demonstrates its potential for identifying preventable childhood deaths. *South Med J.* 1998;91:414–419

338. Herman-Giddens ME, Brown G, Verbiest S, et al. Underascertainment of child abuse mortality in the United States. *JAMA.* 1999;282:463–467

Photodocumentation and Other Technologies

Lawrence R. Ricci

The Spurwink Child Abuse Program
Department of Pediatrics, University of Vermont College of Medicine

Robert A. Shapiro

Cincinnati Children's Hospital Medical Center
University of Cincinnati School of Medicine

Introduction

Technological tools such as cameras and computers offer health care professionals various ways to document physical examination findings, illustrate findings for legal purposes, collaborate and consult with colleagues, and network for educational and quality assurance purposes. This chapter will be broken up into 2 sections, the first, authored by Lawrence Ricci, will discuss photodocumentation including traditional 35-mm film, digital still, and digital video photography. The second, authored by Robert Shapiro, will discuss computer-based technologies such as e-mail and videoconferencing. It is important to remember that even though some of the equipment discussed in this chapter may be outdated by the time of publication, the principles will continue to hold. It is equally important to remember that equipment always remains subservient to the needs of abused children and their families and

is only of use if it enhances the ability of the professional to address those needs.

Photodocumentation

Lawrence R. Ricci

Since the first edition of this book in 1994, a revolution of sorts has occurred in technologies available for child abuse evaluation, including the emergence and wide acceptance of digital still and video imaging. However, the guiding principles are the same since the first days of daguerreotype and silver halide photography: good equipment, adequate lighting, and planned composition.

Photographic documentation of visual findings is an important component of any child abuse evaluation. High-quality photographs of physical findings may be valuable in influencing courts to adjudicate that child abuse has taken place.[1] Photographs may be used for consultation, peer review, and teaching of concepts such as cutaneous injury patterns, hymen anatomy, and trauma.

Although some institutions have access to professional photographic staff, many do not.[2] It is incumbent on the medical care providers who evaluate abused children to ensure adequate photographic documentation of visible lesions, either by taking the photographs themselves or by arranging for someone to take them. Even when photographs are taken by professional photographers, law enforcement officials, or child protective services workers, the medical provider still is responsible for seeing that all areas of importance are documented adequately. Indeed, many states require reporting medical professionals to make reasonable efforts "to take or cause to be taken" color photographs of any areas of visible trauma.[2]

Medical care providers who care for abused children should be familiar with the basic principles and techniques of clinical photography. These principles include good equipment, adequate lighting, and planned composition. The key equipment concerns are camera, lens, and lighting. A quality lens, adequate flash, and proper technique are of far greater importance than brand or features of a camera.[3] No particular system is best. Decisions should be based on the needs of the photographer and the cost of the system. The ideal system not only produces consistent, reliable results, but also is comfortable and easy to use.

Cameras

Camera systems for photographing the physically abused child range from expensive and sophisticated 35-mm (and now digital single-lens reflex [SLR]) close-up systems[4-8] to less expensive and simpler instant or self-developing cameras.[9] Systems recommended for photographing a victim of sexual abuse range from expensive colposcopic cameras[6-8] to 35-mm close-up systems[4,5] and, most recently, simple video cameras. Although it has been said that 35-mm photography is the standard for patient documentation,[10] digital still and video cameras are increasingly supplanting silver halide–based still cameras in photodocumentation.

Instant-processing cameras have the advantage of simple operation and low cost. Their disadvantages include poor resolution and poor color rendition.[2] This deficiency is particularly problematic when photographing faint bruises or small lesions. Because of their limited close-up capability, instant-processing cameras generally are unsuitable for photographing of the genitorectal area. Additionally, they require expensive film that is difficult to reproduce and store. The only argument for using an instant-processing camera is that the print develops just after the photograph is taken, thus guaranteeing at least some form of documentation. One compromise, particularly when immediate documentation is needed, is to take instant and 35-mm or high-quality digital photographs.[11] One model of instant processing camera specifically designed for medical and dental photography is the Polaroid Macro 5 SLR-1200.

It allows 1× to 3× magnification, has dual flashes for even lighting, and has a dual-light range finder for focusing. The quality of imaging and magnification is quite impressive; however, reproduction and storage of the images remains a problem.

Fixed-focus lens point-and-shoot or compact 35-mm cameras are inexpensive and easy to use yet, much like instant-processing cameras, they offer limited close-up capability and expandability. Typically, the viewfinder does not view the same image as the lens. This feature, coupled with fixed-focus that can focus no closer than 6 to 7 ft, often creates blurred images when the photographer attempts to magnify the image by moving in closer than the close-focusing limit of the lens. These cameras often have fixed aperture and shutter speed, limiting their range in varying photographic situations. Compact cameras, much like instant-processing cameras, have little to recommend them in the clinical setting.[11]

Serious medical photography requires a camera that offers control over aperture, focusing, and shutter speed. Also, the camera should be able to accept a variety of lenses and other attachments. The 35-mm format offers an unrivaled choice of cameras, lenses, and accessories and, hence, excellent resolution and close-up capability. The most widely used 35-mm camera is the 35-mm SLR. Newer consumer-priced digital SLR cameras, particularly those at the 8 megapixel and above range and with a sensor that approaches 35-mm film size, are quite comparable.

A reflex camera is one in which the viewing system uses a mirror to reflect the image directly from the lens onto the viewing screen. The mirror flips out of the way to expose the film when the shutter is released. A 35-mm SLR uses 35-mm film and a single lens for both viewing and recording the image while a digital SLR uses a digital sensor instead of film and a single lens. The photographer then sees the same image as the lens and the film, important when using close-up or zoom lenses.

The most versatile system for the relatively skilled photographer combines an SLR camera body with a series of lenses (eg, 50 mm, 105 mm, 35- to 105-mm zoom, macro lens) and both hot shoe and ring flash.[5] The accessories are used in various combinations depending on the particular clinical circumstances. Attached to an SLR camera, a macro lens allows photographs showing fine anatomical detail to be taken (Figure 22.1).

Prepackaged 35-mm camera systems that allow true macro reproduction (1×) include the Canon EOS EF 100 mm f/2.8 macro autofocus with ML-3 macro ring lite (camera body separate) or the Yashica/Contax Dental Eye II. Comparable digital SLR systems exist.

These systems offer totally integrated (dedicated) flash that self-adjusts during shooting. Their versatility and expandability make them unequaled (Figure 22.2). They compare favorably with and are significantly less expensive than colposcopic cameras for photographing the sexually abused child. Unfortunately, their technical requirements may be prohibitive for the occasional user.

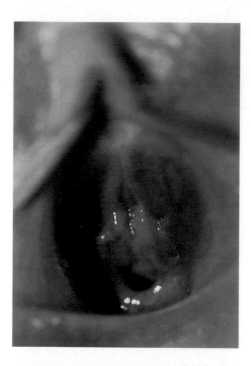

FIGURE 22.1
A 5-year-old girl photographed during a sexual abuse examination using the camera in Figure 22.2. Magnification is 1× (1:1). Lighting and resolution are excellent. The chief complaint was vaginal bleeding reportedly after a self-inflicted fingernail scratch while bathing. A vertical linear abrasion located to the left of the urethra is consistent with the history. Note how depth of field is limited both in front of and behind the lesion. Also note the vertical format or orientation of the image to best show neighboring anatomy.

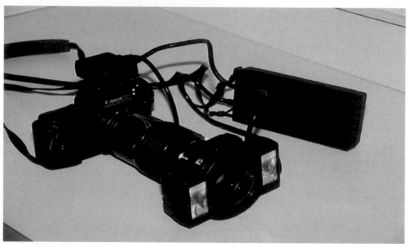

FIGURE 22.2
Example of a true macro (1:1) 35-mm camera system, a Canon T50 camera body with databack and motor drive, Kiron 105-mm 1× (1:1) manual-focus macro lens, and Canon ML-1 ring flash. This kind of system with magnification range of 0.1× (1:10) to 1× (1:1) is unrivaled in versatility and photographic quality.

Lenses

Lens quality more than anything else determines picture quality. Lenses come in 3 basic types: normal focal length, wide angle, and long or telephoto. The labeling of a particular focal length is dictated by the format (negative or transparency image size) of the camera. A normal lens is one in which the focal length approximately equals the diagonal measurement of the camera film format (the diagonal of 24 by 36 mm). For a 35-mm camera (35 mm refers to the total film width including sprockets), a normal focal length would be 50 to 55 mm. A wide-angle lens would then be 28 to 35 mm, whereas a long lens would be 80 mm or greater. See the discussion of digital still cameras for differences from 35-mm cameras.

The ideal lens for medical photography should have good optics, medium telephoto focal length to minimize distortion (85–105 mm), and macro or close-up capability up to 1×. (The image on the negative or transparency is magnified to life size.)

Magnification is the ratio of image size on the negative or transparency to actual object size (image size/object size). It can be expressed as a ratio (1:2), a fraction (1/2), a decimal (0.5×), or a percentage (50%). Close-up is 0.1× to 0.5×, extreme close-up is 0.5× to 1×, and true macro is 1× to 35×. For example, photographing an 8-year-old child by using a 35-mm format would produce the following images at different magnifications: 0.05×, full body; 0.1×, half body; 0.2×, face, hand; 0.5×, ear, lips, eye, genitorectal area; 1×, fingernail, introitus; 2×, hymen.

The maximal magnification of a lens can be checked by focusing the camera on a metric ruler at the closest focusing distance of the lens.[11] With a 35-mm SLR, the viewfinder screen and film are both 36 mm wide. Thus if the screen or the film "sees" 36 mm of ruler horizontally (at the closest working distance of the lens), the magnification is 1×. If the screen sees 72 mm, the magnification is 0.5× (m = 36 mm/number of millimeters "seen" horizontally on the viewfinder screen).

A 90- to 110-mm lens is recommended for close-up work, particularly involving the face, when using a 35-mm camera.[12] Long lenses compress or flatten perspective. This flattening is advantageous in face shots because features such as the nose are less distorted. For torso or full-length photography, a 50- or 55-mm lens is adequate.[13] In general, a medium telephoto lens, such as a 105-mm lens, is best for everything from 0.2× to 1× (head and neck down to fingernails), whereas a 55-mm lens should be used for full- and half-body lengths only (0.05×–0.1×).[2,13]

In close-up work, an additional advantage of longer focal length is greater working distance. A typical 50-mm lens at 0.1× has a close working distance of 25 cm. A 100-mm lens doubles this working distance. Children may be less fearful if the camera is farther away (ie, subject-to-lens distance is increased). In addition, flash illumination becomes more uniform as the distance increases.[4]

Zoom lenses offer variable focal length, which allows one lens to be used for both close-up and distant work. By changing the focal length to bring the subject closer, they allow the photographer to remain stationary while changing the magnification. Some zoom lenses provide macro capability up to 0.25×.

Macrophotography

For close work greater than 0.5×, a macro lens offers the best solution.[5] Although the term is often used to describe any close-focusing lens, a true macro lens is capable of providing 1× or greater magnification. Lenses sold as "zoom with macro focusing" are not true macro lenses and often magnify only up to 0.25×. True macro lenses have their barrels embossed with magnification, especially from 0.5× to 1×. Examples of true macro lenses include

the Canon 100 mm f/2.8 1:1 macro autofocus and the Nikon 105 mm f/2.8 1:1 micro autofocus. As used here, the "f" rating signifies the widest aperture or lens diaphragm opening. An f-number (or f-stop) is a numeric representation of the diameter of the diaphragm opening or aperture of the lens. A sequence of f-numbers on the lens dial calibrates the aperture in regular steps or stops. The f-numbers generally follow a standard sequence such that the interval between one stop and the next represents a halving or doubling in image brightness. As the numbers become higher, the aperture is reduced.

A relatively inexpensive alternative to a macro lens is a set of close-up or supplementary lenses placed over the normal lens to magnify the image.[11] These auxiliary lenses may provide

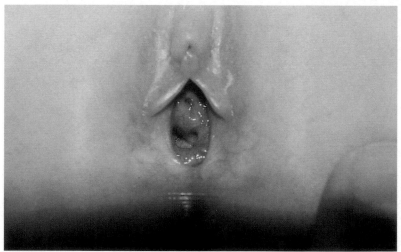

FIGURE 22.3
A 4-year-old girl photographed with the camera in Figure 22.2 during a sexual abuse examination. Magnification of 0.5× (1:2) is achieved by adding a supplementary close-up lens (+6 diopter). Although the hymen is visualized adequately at least for major trauma, resolution is fair and the image is a bit overexposed. Shadow at bottom is from the top-mounted flash blocked by the lens.

reasonable magnification up to 0.5×
(Figure 22.3); however, using close-up
lens attachments to achieve magnification greater than 0.5× significantly
reduces image quality. Beyond 0.5×,
a macro lens offers the best option.
Bellows and extension tubes, although
cumbersome and difficult to use, are
another option. Colposcopic camera
attachments use the extension-tube
principle to achieve 1× or greater
magnification.

A problem particular to close-up work
is narrow depth of field.[11] Depth of field
is the zone of sharpness extending in
front of and behind the center of focus.
It is determined by aperture, lens focal
length, and subject-to-lens distance.
The larger the aperture (the smaller the
f-number), the narrower the depth of
field. In the close-up range, depth of

field can be quite narrow (a typical 105-
mm macro lens at 1× magnification and
f-22 has a maximal depth of field of 6
mm). This limitation can be a significant
problem when photographing cavities,
such as the rectum, that may have a
greater depth than the depth of field
of the lens (Figure 22.4). This problem
may necessitate a series of photographs,
each focused at different points near and
far, none of which captures the entire
area. When depth of field is a problem,
it is important not only to focus carefully but also to try to position the subject and/or the camera so that all of the
important parts to be photographed fall
in a plane parallel to the film. A powerful flash can improve depth of field by
allowing a smaller aperture.

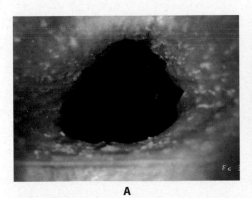
A

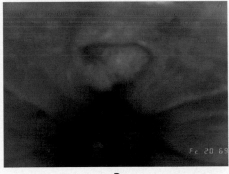
B

FIGURE 22.4
Examples of anal-rectal photography. **A.** A 15-year-old girl in the prone knee-chest position
with gentle buttock traction is photographed with the camera in Figure 22.2. Magnification
is 1× (1:1). Entire dilated anal-rectal area with adequate angle of view and adequate depth of
field are shown. **B.** A subacute fissure is evident at 12 o'clock position in a 4-year-old boy using
the camera in Figure 22.5. Photographic magnification is 2× (2:1), whereas viewing magnification through the binoculars is 16 power. The lesion is well delineated, but depth of field
is limited as is the angle of view. Variable magnification, particularly from 4 to 16 power,
is a useful option in colposcope photography.

Colpophotography

The colposcope is a binocular viewing device (often with varying magnification) with an attached light source. It was originally developed for the study of cervical pathology and was first used to study sexual assault–related genital injuries in 1982 by Teixeira.[6] Subsequently, Woodling and Heger[7] and then others applied the colposcope to the study of genital and rectal anatomy in children. Colposcopy enhances the ability to examine genitalia in a noninvasive manner with excellent magnification and lighting. Perhaps most importantly, it allows for close-up photographic documentation of findings. This high-quality documentation has supported the development of a common anatomical language, peer consultation, and research. A camera can be added by an extension tube for photographic documentation (Figure 22.5). Typically, a standard 35-mm or digital SLR camera body is used. Many examiners now attach a video camera for teaching and documentation.[14]

A drawback to colposcopic photography, basically macrophotography through an extension tube rather than a macro lens, is limited depth of field (≤4 mm) compared with better macro lenses (6–8 mm) and, at magnifications greater than 1×, limited viewing angle (Figure 22.4). The singular advantage of the colposcope, however, is that the same instrument provides illuminated and magnified viewing along with photographic capability so that examination and documentation can occur simultaneously.

Colposcopes can differ significantly from one manufacturer to another in quality, accessories, and cost. Ease of use, quality of optics and light source, magnification, and photographic capabilities are important features. The most useful magnification range is between 4 and 16 power. Four power, which refers to the magnification in the eyepiece, is equal to 0.5× or 1:2 reproduction on the 35-mm slide or negative. Eight power equals 1× or 1:1, whereas 16 power creates an image on the slide that is 2 times life size, 2× or 2:1. Features to consider for photographing through a colposcope include a beam splitter rather than a mirror, a high-quality ring flash with rapid recycle time (<5 seconds is good; <2 seconds is ideal), and databack for the camera. A remote shutter release, either

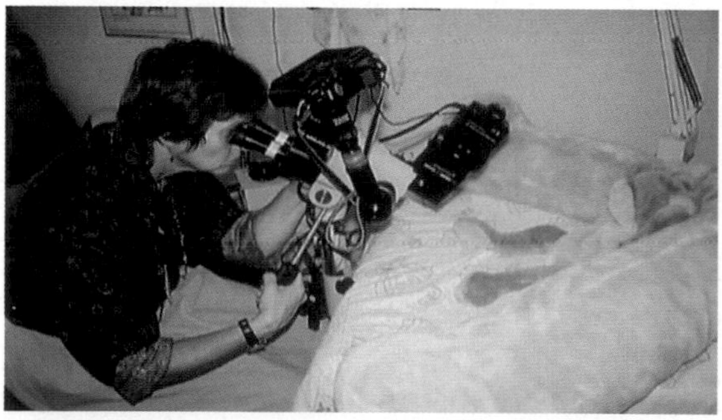

FIGURE 22.5
Example of a colposcope with T-mounted camera allowing 2× (2:1) photographic magnification and simultaneous 16-power viewing, a Frigitronics colposcope with Canon T90 camera body (databack, motor drive, and remote shutter release), and Vivitar hot shoe–mounted flash. This system only allows viewing at 16 power and photography at 2× (2:1), although quality of photographic image is excellent. Quantum Turbo battery attached to the flash allows 2-second recycle time.

hand or foot controlled, allows both of the examiner's hands to be free for picture taking by an assistant or even the child.

Photographing genitorectal findings may be difficult through the colposcope because of rapid changes in genitorectal shape, excessive magnification (narrow angle of view), and narrow depth of field (Figure 22.4).[15] A good lighting source for the camera is critical. The colposcope must provide adequate resolution, exposure, and depth of field (Figures 22.6 and 22.7). Any system chosen must be tested thoroughly by the examiner before clinical use. It is vital that the viewing lens be cleaned regularly. Colposcopically obtained still and video images are usually out of focus because the examiner assumed that if the image through the binocular lens is in focus, then the camera image will be in focus. This is incorrect. The examiner should

first focus the camera—the still camera through the eyepiece of the camera, the video camera on the monitor—then focus the colposcope using only the focusing rings on the eyepieces rather than moving the scope itself so that both the camera and the eyepieces have the same focus point. Because of movement of the focusing rings on the eyepiece, this refocusing should be done daily. Bypassing the eyepieces and viewing the image directly on a monitor avoids this problem and, if the monitor is of adequate size and quality, can offer excellent viewing capability.

A less expensive and quite adequate alternative to colposcopic photography is the use of a 35-mm camera equipped with macrofocusing lens and ring flash (Figures 22.2 and 22.5).[11] Even less expensive, although with limited magnification and resolution, is a fixed lens camera with supplementary close-up lenses (Figure 22.8).

Recently, video alternatives to colposcopes have been introduced.[16] In general, these alternatives incorporate a close-up video camera attached to a stand, with the image projected onto a monitor and saved on videotape or digital media. These systems are less expensive than colposcopes, provide the same quality of video documentation, and allow viewing of the findings on a monitor rather than through the eyepiece of the colposcope. An even simpler solution to

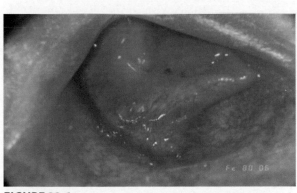

FIGURE 22.6
A 2-year-old girl photographed with the colposcope in Figure 22.5 during a sexual abuse examination. Magnification is 2× (2:1). Lighting and resolution are excellent. Three punctate submucosal hemorrhages are located on the vaginal surface of the hymen at 5 o'clock position consistent with penetrating trauma. These subtle findings would not have been documented as well using less magnification. Note the databack identification code in the lower right-hand corner.

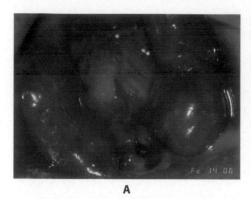
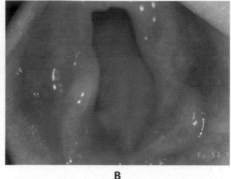

A   B

FIGURE 22.7
A 2-year-old girl with extensive penetrating trauma to the hymen and vagina at 6 o'clock position photographed using the colposcope in Figure 22.5. **A.** Three days after the trauma. **B.** Months later. Magnification is 2× (2:1). Detail and lighting are excellent, although had trauma been more extensive, such a narrow angle view would have been inadequate. Figure 22.7 was useful legally in demonstrating that the injury required significant penetration. Note the databack identification code in the lower right-hand corner.

video documentation is to use a commercial video camera mounted on a dolly tripod (Figure 22.9). These cameras allow close-up viewing and recording at a very reasonable price.

Lighting

No single aspect affects the quality and usefulness of a medicolegal photograph more directly than lighting. Proper lighting can show texture, color, depth, and contour. Improper lighting can hide detail in shadow, wash out bruises, and even misrepresent evidence.[2,13,17]

Short of 3-source studio lighting, electronic flash offers the best light for indoor color medical photography.[10,17] The 2 basic types of electronic flash units are a traditional point source flash mounted to the side or top of the camera and a ring flash encircling the camera lens (Figures 22.2 and 22.8, respectively).

A ring flash provides the best overall lighting in the form of shadowless, uniform illumination.[11] It is particularly useful when photographing cavities and recesses such as the mouth, vagina, and rectum. Shadowing for detail, important in black-and-white photography, is less important when using color film, which uses varying colors and hues to separate detail. Controlled shadowing, however, may still be effectively used to demonstrate texture in bites and abrasions.

With modern through-the-lens (TTL) metering systems, flash use has become simple.[11] Dedicated flashes are designed to work best with a particular camera. Connection of the flash to the shutter for synchronization may be through a coaxial cable or direct through a shoe fitting on the camera (hot shoe). Many electronic flash guns have automatic exposure control. Light from the flash

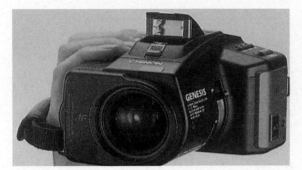

FIGURE 22.8
An early example of a simple
yet versatile point-and-shoot
35-mm camera with a single
non-interchangeable 35- to
80-mm lens, small built-in flash,
autofocus, and limited macro
capability to 0.25× (1:4). Addition
of accessory close-up lenses can
increase magnification
to 0.5× (1:2).

is reflected from the subject back to a sensing cell. When sufficient light has been reflected, the cell cuts off the current, and the light is switched off. The light-producing power of a flash is measured by its guide number (guide number = the distance in feet × f-stop). A higher guide number represents a more powerful flash. A more powerful flash allows a smaller aperture and, hence, greater depth of field.

Limitations of an electronic flash include reflections, particularly from mucous membranes and dark skin; loss of 3- dimensional quality of textured areas, such as abrasions; washout of subtle colors by overexposure; and inadequate lighting, especially if a hot shoe–mounted flash is blocked by a long lens (Figure 22.8).[2,13] Reflections and loss of texture can be minimized by taking photographs from differing perspectives or angles. The lens-shadowing problem can be obviated by using a ring flash. Bracketing of the shot that is shooting at 3 different apertures, very easy to do with modern digital SLR cameras, can prevent overexposure or underexposure. When using electronic flash, it is important to remove or neutralize other point light sources prone to create exposure imbalance, such as shadow-producing operative lights or partially illuminating sunlight.

Flash-recycle time, the time it takes the flash capacitor to recharge and be ready to fire again, is especially important when photographing children.[11] The difference between 2 to 5 seconds and 10 to 15 seconds may be the difference between a good photograph and none at all with a child who is unwilling to sit still for the several seconds it takes a slow flash to recycle. As batteries discharge, recycle time lengthens; thus fresh batteries should always be used. Spare batteries should be readily available. Lithium ion or rechargeable nickel metal hydride batteries, although more expensive, shorten recycle time and last significantly longer.

Film

Prior to the emergence of high-resolution digital cameras, 35-mm color slide film, sometimes called color transparency or color reversal film, was considered the standard for medical photography.[10,17] Color film offers a distinct advantage over black-and-white in that color film uses the various hues of the subject to separate details more effectively.[2]

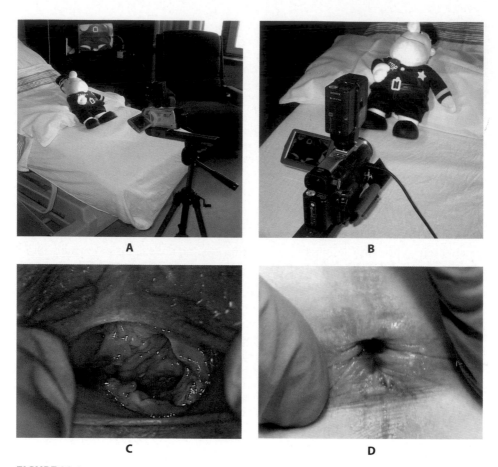

FIGURE 22.9
A. Sony digital video camera set up for sexual abuse examination. Camera is on tripod, which should have a leveling device and either built in or attached wheels. **B.** A wheeled monopod could also be used. Camera also has a hotshoe mounted auxiliary video light, which is essential for correct lighting. Autofocus can be used, as can variable zoom. Stills captured from the video using proprietary video editing software. **C.** Genital injuries in a 14-year–old, including hymenal laceration and perihymenal bruising at 9 o'clock along with an avulsive laceration from 3 o'clock extending to 6 o'clock. **D.** A 6-month-old child who had been digitally penetrated, showing a laceration external to the anal verge at 6 o'clock.

Color also portrays the findings more realistically. Care should be taken, however, to not assume that the color on the print is a totally accurate representation of the color of the finding, given the vagaries of processing and printing. Just as color assignment and bruise age interpretation are problematic in the living subject, even more care should be used when interpreting an image for color and injury age. Color slides are relatively inexpensive, quickly developed, and easy to file, and they can be converted into satisfactory color prints if necessary.[10,17] Although color negative or print film offers greater exposure and contrast latitude and, hence, is more forgiving of exposure mistakes, color slide film provides a first-generation image that can be projected. Color negative film necessitates a second-generation conversion into a print, sometimes resulting in color-balance distortion. Conversion of color negatives to slides or color slides to prints can result in loss of sharpness and color balance.

Duplicating slides or prints may alter color and resolution.[2] Magnification should be accomplished in the original photograph by varying camera distance and/or lens focal length, and not in the print- or slide-making process (Figures 22.10 and 22.11; see also Figures 22.1, 22.6, and 22.7). As a rule, only one patient should be photographed on each roll of film. Even if a roll has only a few exposures, it should be developed rather than kept in the camera, thus avoiding accidental exposure of the film or confusion of subjects.

Film speed is the sensitivity of the film emulsion to light, as measured by its International Standards Organization (ISO) rating. A film rated at 400 ISO is twice as light sensitive or "fast" as one rated at 200 ISO. Slower film (lower ISO rating) offers finer grain, which in turn means greater sharpness and definition. Slower film, however, requires more light and/or a larger aperture. A larger aperture results in narrower depth of field. Film should be fast enough to provide an aperture of f-11 or f-16. Medium-speed (100–200 ISO) daylight film allows a smaller aperture for greater depth of field yet minimal grain.[17] Digital cameras allow varying ISO settings,

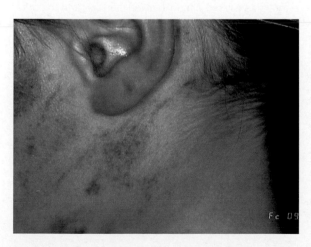

FIGURE 22.10
A 3-year-old boy with classic hand imprint pattern injury to the face photographed with the camera in Figure 22.2. Magnification is 0.25× (1:4). This magnification clearly reveals not only the thin linear markings characteristic of a handprint, but also the bruising extending behind the ear. This photograph alone demonstrates that the injury could not have occurred from a fall, as alleged. Note the databack identification code in the lower right-hand corner.

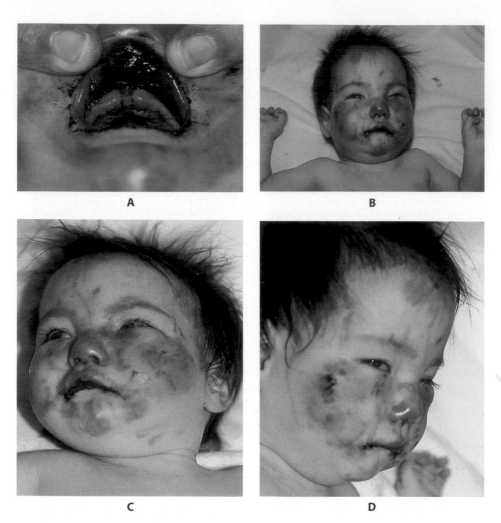

FIGURE 22.11
A 1-year-old girl with extensive injury to the face and upper lip photographed with the camera in Figure 22.2. **A.** Magnification is 0.5× (1:2). This view at this magnification dramatically illustrates the force required to produce such an injury and was instrumental in convincing the court judge that an adult caretaker, not a 3-year-old sibling, had inflicted this and the other facial trauma. **B–D.** Varying perspective facial views at 0.25× (1:4) magnification. **C.** Best shows the left scleral hemorrhage, whereas D best shows the dramatic edema of the left periorbital region.

in effect changing the sensitivity of the sensor. As with film, however, higher ISO settings create more "grain" or, in digital parlance, "noise."

A flash should always be used when shooting indoors with daylight film.[11] Daylight film is color balanced to give accurate color rendition in average daylight. The color temperature of daylight is 5,000°K. Normal indoor lighting has a color temperature of 3,000°K and will create significant color distortion if daylight film is used without a flash. Electronic flash is standardized to the same color temperature as average daylight.[18] The same concepts hold true for digital cameras.

Film may be refrigerated or frozen to prolong its effective shelf life. Film that is refrigerated, however, requires 3 hours at room temperature to reach a usable temperature; 24 hours is needed if the film is frozen.[18]

Differences in image processing may be noted between film laboratories, as well as at the same laboratory, with development of successive roles of film if quality control of the development process is not maintained.[17] Using Kodak processing laboratories ensures quality control and standardization.[19]

After the film is developed, each image should be reviewed for both technique and content. No photographs, even poor ones, should be discarded. This action could be misconstrued as destruction of evidence.[10,20]

A storage/filing system should be established in a cool, dry, and low-light loca-

tion. Each slide should be stored in a clear plastic sheet to minimize handling of the slide and to allow viewing and easy storage. Stored slides last many years with proper use, care, and storage.[18] A slide used for lectures or left out in the light, however, will fade after only a few years.[21]

In contrast to color slides, self-processing Polaroid film is expensive, difficult to reproduce, and difficult to store. Thirty-five millimeter and Polaroid film can be mechanically damaged and can deteriorate, especially if exposed to light. Videotape can be affected by magnets, and the iron oxide matrix making up the tape has been known to deteriorate over time. Computer floppy disks seem to have a fairly long shelf life if not exposed to a magnetic field. Compact discs (CDs) store data using optical laser technology (as opposed to magnetic floppy disks or chemical film). Images can be stored on CD using a read-write CD drive and can then be read by any other CD drive. Caution should be exercised, however, when saving to rewritable CDs because many older CD drives may not be able to read them. Compact discs will not deteriorate but can be mechanically damaged.

Whatever storage media is used, whether 35-mm prints or slides, Polaroid film, videotape, or CDs, images should be stored and released according to specific institutional policies. Guidelines such as those developed by the American Professional Society on the Abuse of Children[22] for photographing the abused child should be consulted.

Photographic Composition

Composition is the proper arrangement of the elements in a photograph. The compositional goal of medical photography is accurate documentation of the patient's condition. Artistic composition is less important than consistency of technique and reproducibility of results.

Medical photography must show injuries as realistically as possible and should not be used to enhance or exaggerate trauma. It is useful to photograph burns, dirty abrasions, and even unkempt children before and after cleaning. Lesions should be rephotographed as they change over time.[2] Just as varying perspective can add a 3-dimensional quality, photographs of the same child over time can add a fourth dimension (Figure 22.7).

Perspective or viewpoint refers to the relation between objects at different distances from the camera as well as the angle from which the objects are viewed. Proper perspective is important in accurately depicting a scene. Perspective can be altered by subject-to-lens distance, lens focal length, magnification, point of view, and size of the final photograph.[20]

The following compositional principles should be kept in mind when photographing abused children (Table 22.1):

1. At least one, if not several, pictures should contain an anatomical landmark (Figures 22.12 and 22.13). The inclusion of an elbow or knee allows the viewer to identify the location of a wound. Anatomical or background material unnecessary to the photograph, however, should be left out. By adhering to this principle, the main subject will occupy a larger part of the picture and will be easier to study, and unneeded and possibly confusing visual information will be omitted.[3,17,23]

TABLE 22.1
Photography Shooting Tips

Before	Establish a protocol or checklist for operation. Decide in advance who will use the camera. Always test a camera before using a new system.
During	Compose the picture the way you usually look at the area. Keep the photographer and subject at the same level. Arrange the subject so that the surface of interest is parallel to the film plane. Take several shots from different angles and distances. Take one photograph with landmarks and one of the lesions alone as close as possible. Magnify in the original, not in a blow up. Bracket shots if correct exposure is uncertain. Take a photograph of patient's name. Take a photograph of the face to identify the patient.
After	Review pictures. Label prints, slides, or digital files and store appropriately.

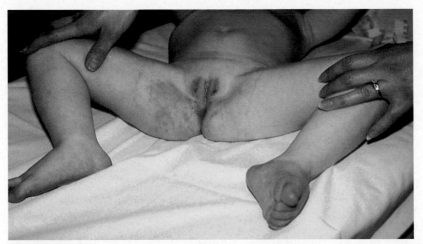

FIGURE 22.12
A 2-year-old girl with extensive bruising of the labia and perianal region photographed with
the camera in Figure 22.9 at the 55-mm setting on the zoom (equivalent to a standard 55-mm
lens). Magnification is 0.1× (1:10). View demonstrates extent of trauma in relation to surrounding anatomy but is limited in detail. Close-up views would help, particularly in assessing
trauma to the vagina and rectum. Nevertheless, this view, showing the bruising into the rectal
area, was particularly useful in convincing the trial judge that sexual assault had occurred.

2. At least 2 photographs should be taken of each finding, one including identifying landmarks and one close-up with the lesion filling the frame. Magnification should be obtained in the original and not achieved in a blow-up (Figures 22.1, 22.6, 22.7, 22.9C and D, 22.10, and 22.11). The finding of interest should occupy as much of the frame as the camera allows.

3. The subject should be arranged so that the surface of interest is parallel to the film surface or plane. Likewise, the camera and the subject should be at the same level.[3,17,23] An exception to this rule applies to colposcopic photography, in which the upward-tilting genitalia of a child requires that the camera be tilted down from above.[14]

4. Varying perspective—taking a number of exposures from different angles and distances—is useful, particularly because electronic flash may produce unpredictable reflections.[17,19] Likewise, because the skin is a curved surface, some lesions may require several photographs to reveal the pathologic findings fully (Figures 22.11 and 22.14). Areas of trauma that have texture or are swollen (contusions, lacerations, abrasions, and blisters) may lose their 3-dimensional quality when light strikes them directly. Offsetting the camera-to-subject axis by 15 degrees allows the light source to glance off the lesion and create contour shadowing.

5. The picture should be composed in the way the examiner would normally look at the anatomical area.

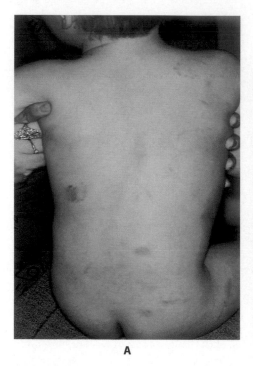
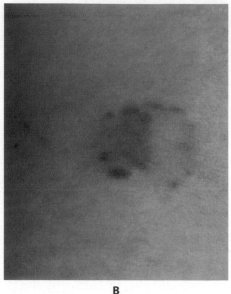

A   B

FIGURE 22.13
A 3-year-old boy with bites on his back photographed with the camera in Figure 22.2.
Magnifications are 0.1× (1:10) **(A)** and 0.5× (1:2) **(B)**. **A.** Full back view demonstrates 2 bites
(right shoulder and left flank) in relation to neighboring anatomy. **B.** Close-up view of the
flank bite demonstrates detail of teeth imprint. Size of teeth and arch suggest the bite came
from another child as alleged. A measuring tape in the viewing field would have been
helpful even though precise measurements were documented in the record.

The horizontal format is standard.
When necessary, however, such as
for full-body images, the vertical
format is used (Figure 22.1).

6. The size of lesions may be documented on the photograph by positioning a measuring device, such as
an adhesive metric scale, directly
above or below the injury.[2,20] Size
along with color may be distorted
in the photograph. A standardized
color bar, although awkward to use,
may be placed in the photographic
plane for comparison with the color
of the lesion. This step ensures that if
color is distorted in the developing
process, adequate comparisons can
still be made. If color is a significant
concern, however, as when trying
to age a bruise, it is more useful to
document the color carefully in writing than to rely on the photograph.

7. It is desirable, but not always possible, to have a standard set of views
for each area photographed.[13] The
4 cardinal anatomical positions—
anteroposterior, posteroanterior,

A

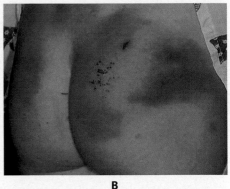

B

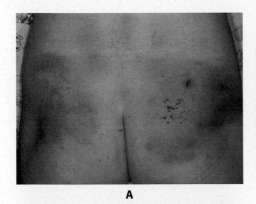

C

FIGURE 22.14
A 5-year-old girl hit with a paddle and photographed with the camera in Figure 22.2. Magnification is 0.2× (1:5). **A–C.** Three views were required to illustrate the extent of the buttock pattern injury. Multiple views showing a curving multi-planar injury are useful in illustrating how such an injury could not have resulted from an accidental fall.

and right and left lateral—should be kept in mind when photographing children. Young children may not cooperate with such positioning plans, however, again reinforcing the usefulness of multiple views from varying perspectives (Figure 22.14).

8. Forensic bite-mark photography is a specialized branch of medical photography and is best performed by or interpreted by a forensic dentist or pathologist. The basic objective of photographing bites is the accurate recording of all aspects of the mark. Size, shape, color, depth of indentations, and 3-dimensional contours must be preserved. No one medium is suitable for all these functions. Photographs, both black-and-white and color, can record the first 3 features, whereas dental impressions show the last 2 features. Ultimately, the photographs may be enlarged to life size and compared with a representation of the suspect's teeth.[19] The same principles described throughout this chapter apply to photographing bite marks. Multiple views from multiple perspectives are particularly important in delineating texture and shape. Parallel views best depict shape and size, whereas obliquely directed views and lighting highlight texture. Some views should show neighboring anatomy; others should magnify the bite as much as the camera and lens will allow (Figure 22.13).

9. Keeping a record or log of photographic data (date, time, location, case number, camera, lens, aperture, shutter speed, film, light source, subject distance, and macro lens magnification) helps reconstruct cases, particularly for courtroom verification; aids in learning and teaching; and encourages consistent technique if the child requires more photographs later. Digital cameras record much of this information as metadata inside the digital image file.

10. Background is important.[10,13,23] The background wall should be non-reflective, ideally a matte-finish neutral gray, green, or blue. Glossy background surfaces can produce a glare. A cluttered room makes a poor background for medical photographs. Materials unnecessary for the photograph should be deleted. A back drop may be useful.

11. Before photographing children, it is important to establish both a protocol and a checklist for operation. Who will take the photographs and how the film will be handled after picture taking should be identified. The photographer should always test shoot several images when using a new camera setup.

Common Photographic Errors

Despite the advent of simple and sophisticated electronic cameras, camera-operation errors continue to occur.

1. The subject is blurred. This problem is usually caused by improper focusing, often because the photographer was trying to get closer than the minimal focusing distance of the lens in an attempt to magnify the image. This problem is particularly common with viewfinder fixed-focus compact cameras. Sometimes movement of subject or camera will cause blurring. Shutter speeds less than 1/90 of a second for normal lens and less than 1/125 of a second for tele photo lens should not be used. If the camera is on autofocus, a problem will occur if the subject of interest is outside the center focusing ring. For example, if the subject is in the foreground and off to the side, the camera may focus on a centered background object, throwing the foreground out of focus. Another problem with autofocus is when it is ignored or over ridden. This can happen if the autofocus has not been given enough time to set, if the camera is too close, or if the natural lighting is so low that the autofocus can't find the subject.

2. The negative is clear or the transparency is black. Most likely the film was never exposed because it did not advance in the camera. The most common cause of this problem is failure to load the film properly (the film sprocket holes never caught properly in the film-transport sprockets). It is important to load film correctly and to ensure that the film is being transported through the camera by checking that the rewind knob turns as the film is advanced. Because of this problem, some centers recommend shooting a backup set of instant prints with a Polaroid camera. Newer, nearly foolproof electronic

cameras either fail to shoot at all or show on the data screen that the film is not advancing.

3. The film is overexposed or underexposed. Incorrect exposure continues to be a problem in photography despite advances in automatic exposure control. Exposure depends on the brightness of the image, the camera aperture, the length of time the photographic material is exposed (shutter speed), and film speed. The usual cause of incorrect exposure is incorrect setting of the aperture, film speed, shutter speed, or flash. Camera and flash settings should be checked carefully. An exposure technique some professionals use to avoid overexposure or underexposure is bracketing. If the final combination of film and flash indicates an aperture of f-16, 3 frames are exposed: one at a setting of f-16, one overexposed at f-11, and the third underexposed at f-22. One of the 3 should be perfectly exposed.[17,19] Newer, high-end digital still cameras have the option of automatic bracketing.

4. The print or slide has distorted color, often yellow or green. This error occurs most commonly because color daylight film is used indoors without a flash or because the photographer did not wait for the flash to recharge before shooting the next picture. Always use a flash indoors, even if the room is bright. This is equally true for digital cameras, which assume daylight color temperature.

Photographing Children

When photographing children, it is important to explain to the child what is going to happen in language the child will understand.[11] Allowing the child to try out the camera and flash often aids in gaining trust. Most cameras, particularly those mounted on a colposcope, can be provided with a remote switch that the child may control. Children should be allowed to assume a position of comfort. It is better to have a cooperative child, somewhat out of optimal photographic position yet not moving, than an uncooperative, moving child. The photographer can compensate for incorrect anatomical position with multiple views. If the child will not move, the photographer should.

It is often useful to involve a trusted support person in the photographic session. Infants and toddlers may be photographed more easily if they are held in the lap of a guardian or assistant. Apart from being a comfort to the child in unfamiliar surroundings, such a person provides an extra pair of hands.[24]

Film-advancing motor drives are almost mandatory when photographing children with traditional 35-mm SLR cameras, as is a fast recycling flash. Because an unexpected flash may be alarming, children should be allowed to preview and even try out the flash.

The photographer must at all times be cognizant of the potential traumatic effect of photographs on the abused child, with regard to both the photographic process itself and the use of these photographs in court. Some children may refuse photographic documentation, despite the photographer's best efforts. This refusal should, as much as possible, be respected. Similarly, the adverse effects of photographing children, particularly sexually abused children, should not be underestimated. These issues should be addressed openly and sympathetically before and after the evaluation. In terms of anxiety, Siegel and colleagues[16] reported no significant difference in comparing an intraoral camera or a colposcope to visual inspection. Using a 6-point scale for anxiety (0–5) rated by the child using happy to sad faces, camera mean anxiety was 2, colposcope was 2.16, and visualization was 2.16.

Video

Obtaining a photograph that adequately represents the findings of an abused child can be challenging, given both the inherent plasticity of some of these structures and general motion by the child.[14] This problem has led many to use video photographic techniques for both documentation and teaching.[14]

Video cameras combined with high-resolution printers make examination and documentation easier and more precise for both sexual and physical abuse. Modern video technology uses optical sensing semiconductor devices (charged coupled device) to transfer light to digital electronic information, which is then stored on videotape. Traditional analog VHS or super-VHS (S-VHS) cameras record an analog signal, whereas newer digital video cameras record a digital signal on the tape. Video cameras are easy to use and satisfactory for many

uses. The image produced can be reviewed immediately, eliminating the wait for film development. Video offers a 3-dimensional quality to documentation, can capture the movement of the subject itself, and can offer a near infinite number of perspectives.[25]

The original consumer format for videotape was VHS. The subsequent 8-mm format allowed use of a smaller audio-cassette-sized tape and, hence, a smaller camera. Eight millimeter is comparable in quality to standard VHS and is easier to store. Hi-8 and S-VHS video cameras offer a significant improvement in image quality or resolution over 8 mm and VHS. Digital video cameras are better still (VHS and 8-mm video record 200 lines of resolution; S-VHS and Hi-8 can record 400 lines; digital video, 500 plus lines).[25] The newer high definition (HD) digital video cameras further boost the resolution of the video image and allow even higher resolution still capture. For example, current HD cameras allow 720 lines or, depending on the format, up to 1,080 lines of horizontal resolution. Although lines of resolution, a video construct, is not directly translatable to pixels, one can see that increasing the number of lines of horizontal resolution by as much as 100% over standard digital video should not only increase the resolution of the video but should significantly increase the resolution of a still later grabbed from the video.

One of the drawbacks of video documentation is the inability to produce 35-mm quality still photographs. Some examiners record both video and 35-mm or digital still images. Video can be converted to digital stills for printing by using a video capture card or transferred directly to a usable still using a video printer. The use of a video camera either colposcopically mounted or standalone to document findings combined with a video printer for immediate still-image production is a versatile combination. Many modern digital video cameras include still capture capability up to 3 megapixels. Because the video camera lens is different from a still camera lens, these still images do not match the quality of stills from a dedicated still camera with the same pixel count. Even so, these stills are often quite satisfactory. Additionally, as the resolution of video cameras has increased, grabbed stills from video using standard video editing software now have fairly good resolution in the order of 0.5 to 1 megapixel.

Digital Still Imaging

The same principals as applied to traditional film cameras apply to digital cameras. Digital cameras offer the distinct advantage of an image that can be immediately viewed via an LCD screen on the camera and the ability to shoot many pictures in rapid succession without having to change film canisters. For example, a 1-gigabyte storage card in a camera that shoots 8 megapixel images at full resolution can store 300 or more images. A significant problem of early digital still cameras was the delay in capturing the image after the shutter release is pressed. Newer cameras have reduced these delays to an insignificant time.

Newer 5+ megapixel digital still cameras challenge traditional 35-mm still cameras in image quality. Such megapixel cameras can produce an 8- by 10-inch photograph that rivals 35 mm. Estimates of the resolution of 35-mm film have varied from 10 to 20 (or even 30) megapixels depending on the grain and speed of the film being used. A digital camera's pixel count is its horizontal resolution multiplied by its vertical resolution. For example, an image 2,048 pixels across and 1,536 pixels high is 3 megapixels, while an image 2,560 by 1,920 pixels is 5 megapixels. The important point is that as digital still cameras approach 10 megapixels, they effectively match the resolution of 35-mm film. For most technical work where an 8- by 10–inch print is being made without cropping, 3 to 5 megapixels is quite adequate (Figures 22.15 and 22.16). Of course if the image is cropped significantly and blown up, even a 35-mm print can show significant grain or in the case of a digital image, pixilation.

Digital still cameras typically save the image in JPEG format. When setting the camera up for operation, it is important to set the resolution at the highest setting and the compression at the lowest. Given the price of modern memory cards, there is really no reason to record at anything but the highest resolution and lowest compression. RAW formatting, as opposed to JPEG, is available on some cameras. A RAW image contains all of the details captured by the image sensor, unaffected by the camera's settings for white balance and exposure compensation among other things. Such files are generally quite large but offer the skilled photographer the option of varying these settings when editing the

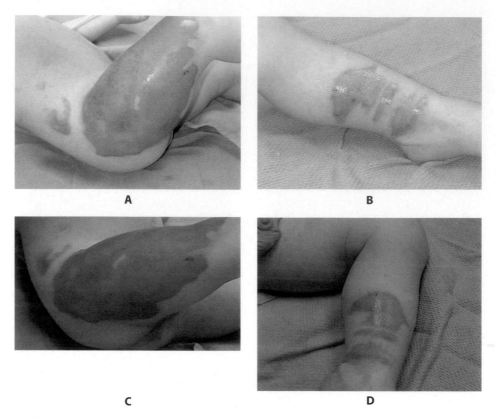

FIGURE 22.15
A, B. Digital still images using a Nikon Coolpix 9500 with attached flash of the hot-liquid spill burns sustained by a 6-month-old child. **C, D.** The same child photographed with a Sony digital video camera. These images are frames grabbed from the video. Ambient fluorescent lighting was used.

image rather than when taking the picture.

When purchasing a digital still camera it is important to recognize that the sensor size is typically smaller than 35-mm film. Thirty-five millimeter film captures a 36 by 24 rectangle, while all except the most advanced digital camera sensors capture a significantly smaller image. This affects how one interprets lens specifications. For example, using the Canon EOS Digital Rebel XT and a

50-mm lens is not the same as using a 50-mm lens on a 35-mm film camera. The focal length of the Digital Rebel 50-mm lens must be multiplied by 1.6. This creates an effective focal length of 80 mm.

Digital image storage is quite easy because such images are easily stored on a hard drive or network drive (eg, in a folder identifying the patient's name). As the resolution of images increases, however, the size of a file can create

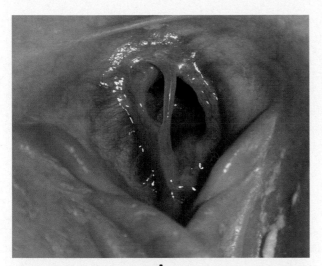

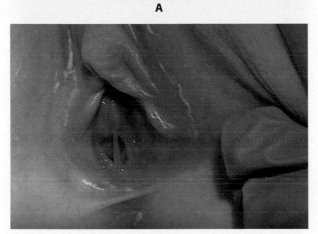

FIGURE 22.16
A. Digital still image using a Nikon Coolpix 9500 with attached flash of a hymenal examination of a 14-year-old girl, showing hymenal band. **B.** The same child photographed with a Sony digital video camera. The frame was grabbed from the video. Ambient fluorescent lighting was used.

storage space problems. An 8-megapixel camera can create a 4-megabyte JPEG and an 8-megabyte camera RAW image while digital video can create huge video files that can quickly overwhelm even the largest storage drives. Whatever system is used, it must have adequate backup capability. Of course images can be stored in the patient's chart using CDs for stills and DVDs for video.

As digital imaging becomes more and more the norm, monitoring of quality

and accuracy become quite important. Of particular importance is the accuracy of the monitor in representing the color as provided by the digital image. One way to ensure accurate color rendition is to use calibration software and hardware such as the ColorVision Spyder[2] Color Calibration System, which uses a colorimeter to measure and adjust the color balance of the monitor to ensure accurate color rendition. With regard to printing, most modern ink jet printers can provide excellent representations of the digital image, provided of course the image is printed at the highest quality using photo quality paper and appropriate print settings for the paper being used. Printing on plain paper at standard quality is often inadequate for assessing injuries. Photocopier black-and-white images are virtually worthless.

Digitized images—whether digitized primarily by using a digital still or digital video camera or secondarily by scanning a slide, negative, or print or by capturing a frame from a video—can be transmitted via the Internet or direct computer-to-computer connection to colleagues for discussion. Telemedicine communication techniques have emerged as a powerful tool in child abuse consultation and education.[25] Combining digital images with medical consultation listservs such as SIGCA-MD allows practitioners worldwide to share findings and solicit opinions from colleagues. Benefits are obvious, but the potential dangers are less so. Poor-quality images could elicit incorrect interpretation particularly around subtle anogenital findings and around color interpretation. Because opinions are unscreened and, in some cases, the credentials of the provider offering an opinion are unknown, such opinions should be used cautiously and never interpreted as either a formal second opinion or a consensus opinion.

Alternative Imaging and Visualization Tools

Ultraviolet (UV) photography has an established role in clinical forensic med-icine and is beginning to see limited use in child abuse assessments.[26] Reflected UV photographs can reveal long-healed bite marks, belt imprints, and wound remnants. A drawback of UV 35-mm photography is that the image cannot be seen until after development. A hand-held, image-intensifier UV viewer has been developed by Hamamatsu that allows direct and immediate viewing and recording of UV images from skin.[27] Vogeley and colleagues[28] report the use of Wood lamp illumination and digital photography in the documentation of bruises. They used direct UV illumina-tion as an alternative to reflective UV. They reported on 3 patients whose bruises were only visible using the Wood lamp. They used a Sony Digital Mavica camera in low ambient light with illumination from the Wood lamp held 10 cm from the skin. Images were contrast enhanced 10% to 40% using Photoshop.

Visualization and illumination aids are often used for examination of the ano-genital area of children. The most ex-pensive, of course, is the colposcope. However, significantly less expensive, adequate alternatives are available. Probably the least expensive is the use of a pair of optical loupes attached to eye glasses plus a halogen head lamp. A more expensive alternative is the use of dedicated binocular magnifying glasses with attached headlamp.

Legal Issues

In child abuse litigation, photographs of the injured child may be impor-tant in proving non-accidental injury.

For photographs to be used as court evidence, they must be properly verified and relevant to the issue.[29]

Verification requires that the photographer or medical provider testify that the pictures accurately portray the findings.[2] A medical provider who examined the child, even though not the photographer, may verify that they accurately represent the findings. The photographer/medical provider should be able to state how the photograph was taken. Practitioners should not, however, portray themselves as photography experts. Such a portrayal might lead to questions on obscure optical and film concepts and potentially discredit the medical witness.

From a medicolegal perspective, photographs of abused children should convey a fair and accurate representation of the scene. Pictures that are inadmissible because of technical error (out of focus, distorted, unidentifiable, too dark, etc) must be avoided.[30] Seeking a second opinion from a photograph requires that the image reasonably reflect the original findings. To help verify that the photographs are actually of a particular child, 2 pictures can be taken: one of the child's name and one of the child's face. Likewise, an identifying sign may be placed in front of the patient for each picture. The inclusion of such signs or labels in the photograph, however, is time consuming and distracting.[3] An alternative for identification is the use of a camera databack. Many 35-mm and digital cameras have databack capability that imprint the time, date, and an identifying code on each frame (Figures 22.4, 22.6, 22.7, 22.10).

Relevance is a judicial decision.[31] Photographs may have evidentiary value yet be deemed prejudicial to the defendant. Whether the probative value outweighs the prejudicial danger remains a decision for the trial judge. Photographs are generally considered admissible, however, if they shed light on the issue, enable a witness to describe better the objects portrayed, permit the jury to understand the testimony better, or corroborate testimony. Courts generally permit medical providers to explain and illustrate their testimony with a photograph. Some states require that reasonable efforts be made by the reporting hospital or medical provider "to take or cause to be taken" color photographs of any areas of visible trauma on the child.[2] Many provide for immunity from civil or criminal prosecution for the person arranging for or taking photographs if done in good faith.

Many child abuse laws state that permission is not needed for the taking of photographs as a part of a child abuse evaluation. Going through the process of obtaining consent, however, can establish an alliance with the family. A variety of consent forms are available, including a model form drafted by the American Medical Association.[3,4,17]

Each institution should have a policy for the handling and the release of photographs.[2] Outside laboratory processing may be acceptable because sending film out is the normal business procedure for the institution.[20]

Although concerns have been expressed that digital images will not be accepted in court, there is no case law excluding digitally obtained images. An often-stated concern about digital photographs is that such photographs are easily manipulated. Of course, changing 35-mm slides and negatives by color or contrast or brightness manipulation has always been possible. The new concern over digital image alteration seems to be based both on the ease with which such changes can be made and on the possibility of drastic, substantive change, such as selectively enhancing one element of the image over another. Original images for courtroom use should of course never be altered. If a copy is altered to improve viewing, such as by enlargement or by brightening, such changes should be clearly noted. Ultimately, however, photographs are useful only as demonstration aids for the examiner to explain the findings. As such, they should be as fair and accurate a representation of the findings as possible. Capturing and recording a digital image on a memory card is really no different from capturing and recording a chemical image on silver-based film.[25]

Because of the fear of image alteration, some manufacturers have provided security software that guarantees an unaltered image. However, most if not all of these programs are expensive and cumbersome to use. In some cases the image is actually degraded in storage. Courts do not require that images be certified unedited but that they simply accurately represent what they purport to represent. Digital still files in addition have what is known as metadata imbedded in them, which can identify if and when an image has been altered. Metadata information includes the time the

photo was taken (from the clock in the camera), whether the photo was altered and resaved, and a wealth of technical information such as camera, lens, shutter speed, aperture, and flash setting. Many photoediting programs such as Photoshop allow easy access to this metadata.

Digital images have been used in the courtroom since at least 1991 and are now almost exclusively being used as the preferred photodocumentation modality. The combination of peer acceptance, court acceptance, widespread usage, and the lack of successful court challenge have demonstrated that digital imaging is here to stay.

Online Technologies and Tools

Robert A. Shapiro

Computers and Internet Connectivity

Few clinicians will require very high-end computer gear. Most computers have adequate memory and speed to access the Internet, display graphics and video, and allow live-interactive online sessions. The price of these computers is well within reach. In 2006 a complete computer system, including a 17-inch monitor and color printer, sold for less than $1,000, often close to $500 if purchased on sale. Less-expensive computers are slower and will become obsolete before more expensive computers. When purchasing a new computer system, a reasonable guideline to follow is not to buy the cheapest machine offered, but don't spend too much more. Even laptops are within this price range. If a computer is too old to run a current operating system and cannot quickly view Web pages, graphic files, or video, it is probably time to replace it with a newer machine. The choice of computer brand or operating system is an individual one. Checking the Web for reports of reliability can help make an informed decision. A computer assembled by a local shop might be as reliable as one sold by a national retailer. Do invest in a good monitor. An LCD monitor can be purchased for little more than a CRT monitor and requires less power (green), offers great resolution, and occupies little space on a desktop. Don't purchase anything smaller than a 17-inch LCD, and consider a 19-inch display.

A more expensive and powerful computer is desirable for work that requires more computer processing power. Examples of this include extensive video editing or work with large or RAW graphic files.

Any computer might require repair and will almost certainly need some maintenance. Over time, spyware, viruses, rogue programs, and assorted junk work to slow a computer down and may cause programs to stop working. No computer should be run without protection against attacks from the Internet. Antivirus software is a must, and virus definitions must be kept up to date. Use the software's automatic update feature to keep your software current. Defense against spyware is often included in antivirus software. If it is not, a program to monitor this threat, and a firewall, is recommended. Retail antivirus and anti-spyware programs are sold by Microsoft, Symantec, McAfee,

and many others. They typically must be purchased and renewed each year. There are some programs that are available at no cost for individual use. Currently, antivirus programs from AVG and Avast can be used free of charge at home, and free versions of spyware protection and firewall software also can be found. Search the Internet for current offerings.

Fast and reliable connectivity to the Internet is another essential component. In order to connect you must have a physical connection to the Internet and an Internet service provider (ISP) that will deliver content to you. Connecting to the Internet requires a modem or modem-like device that sends the digital signal to and from your computer. The oldest connection technology is dial-up. Avoid this if possible; dial-up is very slow and ties up your phone line while you are online. Other connection methods are referred to as broadband, and include DSL, cable, satellite, and power lines (the power outlets in your wall). All of these methods are more similar to each other than they are different, and choosing one typically is a matter of availability and price. Depending on which provider you select as your local Internet company (DSL, cable, satellite, etc), you may or may not be offered a choice of ISP. If you are a user of America Online (AOL), for example, AOL is already your ISP and there is no need to pay another ISP monthly fee. In this case, look for a broadband provider that allows you to separate the costs of your Internet connection and your ISP. America Online can also be your broadband connection company, which may reduce monthly fees.

Online Tools for Consultation and Collaboration

See Table 22.2 for a summary of the features of the Internet communication tools detailed in the following paragraphs.

E-mail

E-mail is the simplest and most available online tool to share images and collaborate or consult with distant colleagues. E-mail is best when used as a communication tool between a reasonably finite group of individuals. An e-mail distribution list can contain a very large number of e-mail addresses, and managing the list becomes tedious.

When sending information that requires confidentiality per Health Insurance Portability and Accountability Act guidelines, special handling is required. Using a corporate e-mail system, which provides a method to send secure messaging, may require special procedures before mail is sent securely. If no such built-in confidentiality mechanism is available, messages sent through e-mail

TABLE 22.2
Attributes of Internet Communication Tools

	Size of Group	Privacy	Type of Information That Can Can Be Shared or Exchanged	Cost
E-mail	1:1 or distribution list	Not ensured without encryption.	Any electronic document; text, images, video; limitation on file size	Nothing or very low
Discussion list	Many	Can be limited to those with a username and password.	Typically limited to text and images	Often nothing or very low
Bulletin board	Many	Can be limited to those with a username and password.	Typically limited to text and images	Often nothing or very low
Internet meeting	1:1 or many	Not ensured without encryption.	Any electronic document; text, images, video	Low to moderate: charged per minute per user; encryption may cost extra
Video-conference	1:1 or many	ISDN is private; IP can be encrypted.	Voice and video, documents imaged with a document camera	Inexpensive to very expensive depending on technology used and need for bridging

Abbreviations: ISDN, integrated services digital network; IP, Internet protocol.

should be treated as if they may be intercepted. Removing patient identifiers before sending the e-mail will help protect patient confidentiality. If information containing patient identifiers must be sent through unsecured e-mail, sending an encrypted e-mail will protect the patient's confidentiality. This can be done using readily available software and then sending the encrypted message as an attachment to an e-mail message. Microsoft now includes a built-in feature to compress and password-protect files as part of the Windows operating system. More robust and flexible software can be used such as WinZip, WinRar, and PKZip. A popular program for the Macintosh platform is made by SmithMicro software. The password needed to open the compressed file can be sent in a separate e-mail message or mailed. Frequent correspondents may agree on a password ahead of time to facilitate the process. As with any system that adds a layer of complexity, some users will find an encrypted file inaccessible without support.

Most e-mail services enforce a limitation on message file size. This limitation will vary from service to service and exists to prevent an e-mail system server from becoming overloaded. Users will face this limitation when they attach large files to e-mail messages. Video files are almost always too big to pass through e-mail system filters. Photographs (digital images) sent as attachments will also cause the e-mail to fail if the total size of the attachments exceeds the allowed limit. The only way to know how many attachments you can reliably send to another user is to know the limi-

tation imposed by your service provider and then, not exceeding this limit, try and send the message. If the recipient's e-mail server rejects your message, send it again but with fewer attachments or with attachments that are smaller in size. You may need to send multiple messages, each containing a portion of the attachments that you need to transmit. Video and still digital images can often be saved as smaller files than the original file size. Reducing the file size in this way may allow transmission through e-mail, but may also reduce the quality of the image sent.

Discussion Lists

Subscription to a discussion list allows a large number of people to post questions or comments about a particular topic to the entire group. Posts to the list are usually sent by e-mailing the message (the post) to a specific e-mail address. These posts can then be read by all other members of the list through e-mail messages sent to them or by logging onto the list Web page and browsing or searching for postings. Subscription to a particular list may be open, so that anyone can join, or closed, which limits and controls the membership. Subscription lists may also employ a moderator who may screen posts before they are distributed or who may organize posts in some fashion that makes them more accessible to list members. If a list maintains an archive, members can search and download old messages. At the time of this writing, the child abuse community has discussion lists available by subscription.

Internet Bulletin Boards

Internet bulletin boards are similar to discussion lists in that they allow a large group of people with similar interests to post messages and read responses from others. One of the main differences between these 2 Internet communication tools is that, unlike the discussion list, posts to the bulletin board are not usually sent out by e-mail to board subscribers. Rather, subscribers select when they will choose to read posts by visiting the board's Web site. This fundamental difference creates a very different type of Internet community compared with the discussion list. Bulletin boards are typically organized by topic, and their screen layout and query tools invite the visitor to first read through prior posts to search for an answer already given to their query before posting a new question to the online community. There is typically much less interaction among bulletin board members compared with discussion list members because members must actively seek to read the discussion threads rather than receiving the messages passively in their e-mail inbox. Bulletin boards, however, are a great tool to find answers to timely questions because they are readily available and accessible to board members. At the time of this writing, there are no active medical child abuse bulletin boards known to the authors.

Internet and Videoconferencing

The terms *Internet* and *Web conferencing* refer to online meetings. Depending on the type of online interaction required, these online meetings can be held between just a few participants (or sites) up to hundreds or more participants. Obviously, a meeting can be more interactive when the numbers of participants are restricted. At the time of this writing, there are many Internet meeting companies to choose from. A quick Internet search is all that is needed to find them.

The main benefit of Internet conferencing is that participants need not travel in order to meet. Although there is a cost to conducting the Internet meeting, there is no time spent traveling, and there are no costs associated with that travel. An Internet meeting includes audio and visual presentation. The audio portion of the meeting can be conducted over the telephone using a conference manager (just like any telephone conference call), or it can be conducted using voice over Internet protocol (VOIP). VOIP phone calls compete with regular telephone service in homes and businesses. VOIP calls can be less expensive but may require equipment not available to all conference participants. The visual portion of the conference requires a computer, an Internet connection, and conferencing software. At the time of this writing, most of the conferencing software is provided online by the Internet conferencing host or company. Participants are given a Web address before the meeting starts and are asked to log in to the meeting on that site. In addition, some hosting companies require a small software download onto the participant's computer.

The visual presentation can include display of a slide show (ie, PowerPoint or equivalent) or documents such as word processor files, spreadsheets, drawings, photographs, software, and Web pages. Depending on the speed of each user's Internet connection, video may also be viewed as a group. In addition to viewing, small groups can collaborate on document editing or software development. Typically, one site is the leader or presenter of information, and the role of presenter can change from one site to another during the meeting. The meeting presenter should be familiar with the software ahead of time to minimize any online time spent learning how to conduct the meeting. Each participant's computer will display the same image at the same time. On-screen editing tools allow each participant to comment on or indicate a portion of the screen to the others. Individual conferencing software includes other features, such as written chat between participants in real time, real-time tests or quizzes, a list of participants online, and the ability to save a record of the completed conference for later playback.

Individuals or small groups who participate at each site need only a telephone with a speakerphone option and a computer. If there are more participants at a particular site than can view a computer monitor together, an LCD projector can be connected to the computer and a conference phone can be used to enhance the meeting experience.

Internet conferences often must be planned ahead. The meeting won't happen for those who unexpectedly lose their Internet connection and for some who are connecting for the first time and encounter technical problems with either their computer or with the firewall. (In corporate and health care environments, a firewall may be placed between the user's computer and the Internet by the information technology department in order to restrict and prevent intrusive Internet traffic. Some individuals may find that they cannot participate in an Internet conference without the prior support of their information technology department.)

The privacy concerns regarding the transmission of information over an Internet conference meeting is similar to those challenges faced when transmitting information over e-mail. The connection may not have a guarantee of security, and users should consider stripping patient identifiers from the material displayed. Meetings can be password protected and unlisted, making intrusion rather unlikely, but not impossible. Some meeting programs allow for an extra measure of security by providing an option to encrypt the Internet conference.

Videoconferencing technology refers to live video from one site to another. The video call can be a "point-to-point" call with only 2 sites connected to one another, or it can be a multisite call with many separate participants. The resources required, as well as the cost, may depend on whether the call is point to point and the type of technology used to transmit the video signal.

Many videoconference calls are placed over digital phone lines referred to as integrated services digital network (ISDN). Calls placed using this system, known as h.320, are as secure as a telephone call, so patient privacy should not be an issue if confidential information needs to be shared. Real-time transmission of video requires the use of 3 ISDN phone lines simultaneously. The 3 lines are combined by the videoconferencing equipment to provide a transmission rate of 384K. The video quality is almost guaranteed to be very good, but the equipment costs can be expensive and the ISDN lines may require a monthly rental cost as well as a per-call cost. As with all technology, the cost has been decreasing.

Another way to place a video call is over the Internet (Internet protocol [IP] based). Like all IP solutions, and unlike ISDN, privacy concerns must be considered. Internet protocol–based calls, known as h.323, have a bandwidth of 384K, just like ISDN calls, but because transmission is over the Internet and not rented telephone lines, the bandwidth is not guaranteed and may be inconsistent, resulting in poor video quality. Depending on the amount of Internet traffic, the video quality may be great one day and only marginal another day. The cost of making an IP-based video call is a fraction of ISDN calls. The equipment is relatively inexpensive, and the cost during the call may be nothing. Some videophones include encryption technology that allows guaranteed privacy during the call, like an ISDN call.

When multiple sites connect to a videoconference or call, complexity is added to the technology. Decisions must be made regarding who will see whom, how many sites will be visible on the screen simultaneously, if the presenting site changes, or if there is dialog; does the image switch back and forth between speakers or do you place images of both sites on the screen? The combining of multiple sites during a video call and the decision-making regarding the above questions are handled by a video bridge. Paying for this service will typically require added costs to a video call, and the bridge may impose other technical limitations on the call and therefore limit participation by those with dissimilar equipment.

Videoconferencing is not a direct substitute for meeting in person. Adding video to a meeting provides some visual contact with your other conferees, but it is not the same as sitting at a conference table with them. There can be some frustrating "out of sync" times between the audio and video call components, and depending on the quality of the rooms being used for the video call, poor lighting, wide camera angles, and distractions can limit the usefulness of a video call.

At the time of this writing, there are incompatibilities between some videoconferencing systems so that one system may not be able to connect with another. This should become less and less prevalent and the quality of the video call should improve as the technology changes and as faster options to connect become more commonplace.

Using Online Tools to Enhance Education and Patient Care

The Internet has become a great tool to find educational resources. Professionals in all fields have opportunities for interactive learning by subscribing to a relevant discussion list. These lists may be discovered through discussions with colleagues or through an Internet search. Other online learning opportunities, including continuing education credit, are offered through Internet meetings and videoconferences from colleagues and their related institutions.

Collaboration between colleagues can be enhanced by using Internet communication tools such as those discussed previously. Many of these resources can be used as an interactive meeting place, either providing real-time meeting opportunities, as with Internet meetings and videoconferencing, or by exchanging information but without the real-time interaction.

Collegial support may be sought to request a second opinion regarding case findings, discuss an unusual finding, or seek advice. For those physicians who have few or no local colleagues, e-mail, Internet meeting, and videoconferencing technologies can reduce the limitations imposed by geography. E-mail is virtually cost-free, available to practically everyone, and a great resource to communicate text and images one-to-one between colleagues. Using an Internet meeting site allows the consultant to view images and documents "alongside" the colleague, and it is interactive. Using videoconferencing technology allows for real-time interaction with a colleague or patient. When connected to a video colposcope, videoconferencing equipment can enable real-time supervision of others, allowing the distant site to view the colposcope findings and provide direction or diagnosis. The choice of technology depends on the type of information to share, the need for real-time collaboration versus delayed communications, requirements for privacy, equipment availability, and the cost to use each resource.

If providing distant consultation, there are other issues to consider than which technology to use. This type of consultation may be referred to as *telemedicine*. If the distant site is in another state and includes interaction with a patient, there are likely professional licensing requirements. And if the patient is being seen within another institution, the remote expert may need hospital credentials. There may be opportunities for financial reimbursement, requiring background investigation and procedures. The distant expert should maintain clinical records of the encounter and advice just as he or she would normally do if locally involved with a patient.

There are many reasons to pursue quality assurance activities in an individual's practice or clinical environment. By creating shareable documentation of clinical activities, many opportunities for quality assurance become available. Recorded clinical findings or methods can be shared with other colleagues using e-mail, Internet meetings, or videoconferencing, allowing comparisons and some measure of practice. In addition, Internet meetings are an inexpensive method to conduct regular peer review with distant colleagues (Table 22.3).

Conclusion

Because photographs offer the only certain method of preserving perishable visual findings, they serve several useful purposes. Photographs can be reviewed after the examination to double-check findings or perhaps even to discover previously unnoticed findings. If the magnification is precisely known, measurements can be obtained directly from the photograph. Photographic findings can be discussed among colleagues and consultants or can be compared with recent published data. The development of regional peer-review groups to enhance technical and interpretive skills is to be encouraged. Photographs taken during an initial examination can provide a standard for subsequent comparison. Likewise, if a second opinion is required, photographs may save the child from the trauma of reexamination. In court, photographs can provide a powerful and convincing statement, whereas a simple verbal description

might fail (Figures 22.7, 22.11, and 22.12). Even when not used directly in court, photographs may enhance testimony by jogging the examiner's memory of specific findings.[11]

Whether child abuse has occurred and who is responsible is a legal issue for the courts to decide. Corroborative physical evidence photographically documented can be an important adjunct to the legal process. A normal examination, particularly of the sexually abused child, does not exclude the possibility of abuse, however, because many children present without current physical evidence. The need for a sensitive medicolegal history continues to be paramount.

The guiding principles of medical photography are good equipment, adequate lighting, and planned composition. Equally important is a working knowledge of camera equipment, print development, and medicolegal implications. Medical providers who provide medicolegal examinations of abused children must have access to adequate photographic equipment and a working knowledge of photographic techniques.

TABLE 22.3
Applications Suitable to Internet Communication Tools

	Education	Collaboration	Consultation	Quality Assurance
E-mail	x	x	x	x
Web browsing	x			
Discussion list	x	x		
Bulletin board	x	x		
Internet meeting	x	x	x	x
Videoconference	x	x	x	x

The development of several Internet communication tools has made it possible for widespread collaboration, consultation, education, and quality assurance within the field of child abuse documentation. E-mail, discussion lists, bulletin boards, Internet meetings, and videoconferencing can allow text, images, and videos to be shared among professionals, depending on the mode of communication used.

References

1. Ladson S, Johnson CF, Doyt RE. Do physicians recognize sexual abuse? *Am J Dis Child.* 1987;141:411–415

2. Ford RJ, Smistek BS. Photography of the maltreated child. In: Ellerstein NS, ed. *Child Abuse and Neglect: A Medical Reference.* New York, NY: John Wiley and Sons; 1981

3. Sebben JE. Office photography from the surgical viewpoint. *J Dermatol Surg Oncol.* 1983;9:763–768

4. Cordell W, Zollman W, Karlson H. A photographic system for the emergency department. *Ann Emerg Med.* 1980;9:210–214

5. Ricci LR. Medical forensic photography of the sexually abused child. *Child Abuse Negl.* 1988;12:305–310

6. Teixeira WRG. Hymenal colposcopic examination in sexual offenses. *Am J Forensic Med Pathol.* 1981;2:209–215

7. Woodling BA, Heger A. The use of the colposcope in the diagnosis of sexual abuse in the pediatric age group. *Child Abuse Negl.* 1986;10:111–114

8. Woodling BA, Kossoris P. Sexual misuse: rape, molestation and incest. *Pediatr Clin North Am.* 1981;28:481–499

9. Baum E, Grodin MA, Alpert JJ, et al. Child sexual abuse, criminal justice, and the pediatrician. *Pediatrics.* 1987;79:437–439

10. Gilmore J, Miller W. Clinical photography utilizing office staff: methods to achieve consistency and reproducibility. *J Dermatol Surg Oncol.* 1988;14:281–286

11. Ricci LR. Photographing the physically abused child: principles and practice. *Am J Dis Child.* 1991;145:275–281

12. Morello D, Converse J, Allen D. Making uniform photographic records in plastic surgery. *Plast Reconstr Surg.* 1977;59:366–373

13. Williams AR. Positioning and lighting for patient photography. *J Biol Photogr.* 1985;53:131–143

14. McCann J. Use of the colposcope in childhood sexual abuse examinations. *Pediatr Clin North Am.* 1990;37:863–880

15. Adams JA, Phillips P, Ahmad M. The usefulness of colposcopic photographs in the evaluation of suspected child sexual abuse. *Adolesc Pediatr Gynecol.* 1990;3:75–82

16. Siegel RM, Hill TD, Henderson VA, Daniels K. Comparison of an intraoral camera with colposcopy in sexually abused children. *Clin Pediatr.* 1999;38:375–376

17. Weiss CH. Dermatologic photography of nail pathologies. *Dermatol Clin.* 1985;3:543–556

18. Freehe CL. Photography in dentistry: equipment and technique. *Dent Clin North Am.* 1983;27:3–73

19. Bernstein ML. The application of photography in forensic dentistry. *Dent Clin North Am.* 1983;27:151–170

20. Spring GE. Evidence photography: an overview. *J Biol Photogr.* 1987;55:129–132

21. Eaton GT. Proper storage of photographic images. *J Audiov Media Med.* 1985;8:94–98

22. American Professional Society on the Abuse of Children. *Photographic Documentation of Child Abuse.* Charleston, SC: American Society on the Abuse of Children; 1995

23. Whitesell J. The basics of medical photography in plastic surgery. *J Plast Reconstr Surg Nurs.* 1981;1:89–92

24. Reeves C. Pediatric photography. *J Audiov Media Med.* 1986;9:131–134

25. Finkel MA, Ricci LR. Documentation and preservation of visual evidence in child abuse. *Child Maltreat.* 1997;2:322–330

26. Barsley RE, West MH, Fair JA. Forensic photography: ultraviolet imaging of wounds on skin. *Am J Forensic Med Pathol.* 1990;11:300–308

27. Hubbard SB. Ultraviolet photography. *Photo Electronic Imaging.* 1992;35:40–42

28. Vogeley E, Pierce MC, Bertocci G. Experience with wood lamp illumination and digital photography in the documentation of bruises on human skin. *Arch Pediatr Adolesc Med.* 2002;156:265–268

29. Flower MS. Photographs in the court room "Getting it straight between you and your professional photographer." *North Ky State Law Forum.* 1974;2:184–211

30. Scott CC. *Photographic Evidence.* 2nd ed. St Paul, MN: West Publishing; 1969

31. Myers JEB, Carter LE. Proof of physical child abuse. *Mo Law Rev.* 1988;53:189–224

Further Reading

Evidence Photographers International Council, Inc. *Standards for Evidence Photography Criminal and Civil.* Honesdale, PA: Evidence Photographers International Council, Inc.; 1998

Hedgcoe J. *The New Manual of Photography.* New York, NY: DK Publishing; 2003

US Department of Justice Office of Justice Programs. *Photodocumentation in the Investigation of Child Abuse.* Washington, DC: Office of Justice Programs; 1996

Chapter 23

Neurobiology and the Long-term Effects of Early Abuse and Neglect

John Stirling

Santa Clara Valley Medical Center

Medical service to victims of child abuse and neglect does not end with detection of the abuse. Physicians and nurses must help patients and their caregivers understand the role played by early trauma in altering the child's responses to events and assist them in finding safer and more effective ways to help the victim adapt to their world. This chapter will explore the neurobiological underpinnings of behavioral adaptation and the role played by early stress in guiding these changes. The coevolution of biology and behavior will be considered with an eye toward helping victims' caregivers guide the children on the road to normal social development.

These children come to pediatric offices and emergency departments daily because their caretakers turn to primary care providers to resolve bothersome behavioral issues. The physician may be asked to prescribe treatments for school-yard violence, oppositional and defiant behavior, and academic inattention. When abuse, neglect, or other complex childhood trauma has occurred recently, the diagnosis may be easier, though treatment options always remain a challenge. When the trauma is more remote, as when the child presents with a foster or adoptive parent years after being removed from the abusive or neglectful environment, the clinician may see the behavior as unprecedented, inexplicable decisions made by an aberrant personality. The story is a familiar one to the practitioner: A child persists in behaviors that are clearly unsuitable to the environment, often in the face of clear and consistent attempts by the caregivers to teach more acceptable behaviors. Techniques that work for other children, even with other children in the same household, simply fail. At times it can seem as though victims of early abuse, neglect, or other adverse childhood experiences are left unable to learn from those experiences.

Recent advances in developmental neurobiology have helped to inform psychological theory to explain this peculiar inability. Technological advances have demonstrated that early trauma can result in alterations to the developing brain and bias the child's response to stressful events. Traumatized individuals can, in effect, develop an altered physiological response to external stimuli. When children react differently than their peers, a caregiver's conventional responses to misbehaviors will often provoke unexpected reactions. Indeed, a caregiver's standard responses to misbehavior (a louder voice, a more stern approach, escalating disciplinary measures) may prove counterproductive by inducing further stress.

Rather than viewing such alterations to the traumatized child's brain as "damage," it is probably more useful to see them as examples of *adaptation,* albeit adaptation to an unusual, idiosyncratic environment. Unfortunately, these adaptations are seldom generalizable to other, more conventional environments, and they give rise to the problem behaviors that challenge parents, teachers, and medical professionals. The child is asked to function in a different world than that to which his or her brain has adapted. This "war of the worlds" must be understood by the child's caretakers if successful adaptation is to be achieved.

Neurobiology: First Principles

In its ability to settle the earth, the human race has proven itself among the most successful of species. Humans have populated the planet from the seacoasts to the heights of the Himalayas, and from the arctic to the antarctic. To a large extent, this success reflects the amazing adaptability of the human brain. Biologists note that human offspring are far less capable at birth than the progeny of other large mammals, and that our children remain dependent on their parents far longer than do the young of other animals. The unfinished character of the newborn human brain allows for a considerable degree of "customization" in its adaptation to the environment in which it finds itself. After all, a newborn human child may find itself in the darkest jungle or among the ice floes, on a mountain or a beach. Some environments favor visual acuity, some auditory. In some, social skills will be paramount; in others, secondary. The newborn human brain has the ability to become the type of brain most needed for success in the environment in which it finds itself. This adaptation is a lifelong process. The most dramatic changes are accomplished during the first few years and involve 3 sequential processes, each step reflecting the child's environment: myelination, synaptogenesis, and apoptosis, or neuronal pruning.

Myelination

The first and most dramatic of the brain's postnatal building projects is the development of myelin. This fatty substance is contained in Schwann cells, cells that wrap around the axons and dendrites of developing neurons and in effect insulate them from neighboring cells. Effective myelination is dependent on good nutrition, requiring high-quality, long-chain fatty acids such as those found in human milk. The myelin sheath promotes efficient and rapid conduction of the nerve impulse, and the clinical appearance of myelination reflects this more efficient function. Myelin primarily appears in the newborn brain over the first 6 months and, as it does, the infant's movements become more coordinated and to some extent more purposeful, in ways that mirror the new areas of myelination.

Synaptogenesis

The term *synaptogenesis* refers to the development of axonal connections (synapses) between neurons leading to effective neural communication. Neuro-anatomists have noted that the brain in early childhood is host to a wild prolif-eration of neural connections as newly matured neurons grow and establish new contact with others, often in areas remote from their origin. This growth is not uniform across the brain, but varies by region and function. The visual cor-tex, for example, reaches its peak den-sity of neural connection after the first 3 or 4 months of life. Synaptogenesis in the speech and language centers, in the angular gyrus and Broca area, peaks later, at around 8 or 9 months, perhaps because speech and language are so dependent on perception. In turn, neurons in the prefrontal cortex, seat of our executive functions of judgment and self-regulation, reach their maxi-mal synaptic density sometime before 3 years of age.[1,2] One can speculate that these regions themselves mature under the influence of the speech and language capacities developed earlier. It is this plethora of potential connections that gives the young child's brain its remark-able ability to learn quickly and retain information well, an ability that seldom fails to amaze his or her parents.

Apoptosis

Apoptosis refers to the involution of neural cells, a process in which excess neurons appear to be "pruned." This pruning seems to follow the regional burgeoning of neural connections described previously and can be quite dramatic, with adult synapse counts throughout the brain being much lower than those seen in childhood. Scientists have hypothesized that this process of growing and pruning neuronal connec-tions is necessary to refine our percep-tions and higher cerebral functions.

Whether a new neural connection is maintained seems to depend on experi-ence. In some cases, the brain seems almost to expect a certain amount of input for normal development and will shut down the circuits if that input is not received. This is especially the case when the input would be expected for all members of the species, as with the sensory cortex. With sensory depriva-tion, as when a cataract (or an experi-menter's blindfold) obscures the vision in a newborn animal's eye, the eye may remain *anatomically* normal, but it will be *functionally* blind, having failed to develop necessary connections to the visual cortex. If the vision remains ob-scured long enough (the *critical period),* the blindness will persist, even after the obstruction is removed.[3] For visual function in kittens, the critical period is 2 to 3 months; for humans, it may be reckoned in years. While most of the rigorous work on neural development has involved sensory modalities, this pattern of proliferation and pruning is typical of most cortical tissue. It is believed that each area of the developing cortex follows this sequence in its turn, and that each has its period of relatively greater sensitivity and need for formative input to guide its growth.

However long the period of vulnerability, it is evident that experience determines which connections will persist and which will perish. Circuits not used are lost, while those used repeatedly are strengthened. Neurons that fire together, as the neurobiologists say, wire together. As opposed to the young child's brain, which is optimized for learning, the mature brain is optimized for efficient function, using those skills it has already learned.

Imaging the Brain

It has always been difficult for the human brain to study itself. Scientists and physicians have learned about the gross anatomy of the brain via gross and microscopic dissection, but this can reveal little about its function. To study the brain's abilities, researchers have relied on "accidents of nature," individuals in whom disease or trauma have resulted in focal injury, which itself could only be verified postmortem. The functional state of the brain was a mystery that spawned a great deal of informed conjecture (and the occasional "interrogation" of a living brain during surgery).

With the advent of computed tomography and magnetic resonance imaging (MRI), physicians were finally able to assess loci of injury in living patients, accurately correlating lesions with functional impairments. Subsequent advances in imaging (functional MRI,

positron emission tomography) have opened a window into the brain's metabolic function in "real time," allowing a researcher to watch which areas of the brain function in situ while the patient thinks, speaks, senses the environment, and feels emotion.

The venerable electroencephalogram, once restricted to quietly eavesdropping on the brain's electrical activity, has benefited from the new technologies of computer analysis to appreciate subtle changes in function ranging from subclinical seizures to alterations in cerebral dominance. Improved electron microscopy and new methods of chemical analysis have allowed further insight into brain function at the synaptic level.

Lifelong Learning

To say that the brain undergoes experience-dependent structural and functional modification is merely a way to say that it is doing what brains do best: learning. While there is no doubt that younger brains learn more, and faster, we continue to acquire knowledge (and brain modifications) throughout our lives.[4,5]

These changes occur on a relatively large scale and involve modifications that can be seen on scans or on microscopic counts of neurons and synapses. The brain undergoes more subtle structural modifications with learning as well. Experience can bring about changes in the number of glia, cells that act to support neural growth and function. "Experienced" neural regions also contain more blood vessels than their less-stimulated counterparts, which helps to ensure their survival.[6] Investigators using electron microscopy and chemical tagging techniques have found that experience can bring changes in sensitivity at the level of the neuronal receptor site, in effect making the neuron more or less aware of its surroundings.[7] Even the synthesis of neurotransmitters, the chemical agents so vital to the transmission of information, varies with experience. Recent research has shown increased neurotransmitter synthesis in the cerebellum when subjects receive proprioceptive input, as when a baby is held, carried, and rocked.[8,9]

Attachment: The Importance of the Other

It is clear that the child's brain follows a developmental trajectory, and that timing and experience work together to determine its arc. The importance of stimulation to brain development suggests the next major point: The brain cannot develop its capabilities in isolation. The adaptability of the human brain comes at a price: A prolonged period of development requires stable and reliable caregivers. The newborn human child needs relationships with other human beings to provide a safe environment, effective stimulation, and models of appropriate behavior. It is meaningless to discuss the early structural and functional development of the human brain without acknowledging the importance of other human beings in the process, especially when we come to consider the effects of early neglect and other forms of abuse.

A baby left alone will die. A baby given sustenance without personal interaction may live but, like the blindfolded kittens in the experiment, will grow up lacking in critically important abilities. This human experiment has been inadvertently conducted over the years, by neglectful parents or by the state, and the results are striking. Clinicians describe children that seem to lack the capacity to form a trusting attachment to other human beings.[10,11] They may be delayed in achieving their motor milestones and in developing speech.[1,12] Neuroimaging of these severely neglected children shows decreased metabolism and lack of development in the prefrontal cortex, an area vital to the brain's executive functions,[13] and in the temporal lobes, areas concerned with speech, language, and emotional communication.[14] Even children less severely affected risk developing an emotional "blind spot."

The price we pay for our adaptability is a prolonged period of relative incompetence, which means dependence on others to provide more than calories. The newborn requires that a mature human being be present for the first years for protection from and gradual introduction to his environment. When this support is missing or seriously flawed, the child's brain adjusts accordingly.

In his investigation of refugee children after the atrocities of World War II, social researcher John Bowlby[10] described a process he termed *attachment,* in which the child seeks proximity to some "preferred individual, usually perceived as older or wiser," behavior that ensures the child's safety. He explained that, in the child's interactions with a mature individual, the child develops an "internal working model" of relationships. The child comes to expect that needs will be filled (or not), and learns to behave according to the expectations taught by that relationship.[10] When the behavior of the parent is predictable and nurturing, the child perceives the world as safe and predictable and feels free to explore. Neural pathways in the developing cerebral cortex associate the parent figure's presence with feelings of security. This confidence in one's protectors is called *secure attachment.* If the caregiver is not perceived as ever-present and supportive, the child must devote more time and effort to ensuring his own security, and attachment is said to become less secure. The cortical connections develop quite differently in this case, associating the parent figure with anxiety or distress. Insecure attachment may result in a variety of behaviors—from continual attention-seeking to apparent indifference to the caregivers—but whatever its manifestation, *insecure attachment* impairs the child's freedom to learn from his world.

Bowlby's successors in attachment research carried on his work. Using the so-called Strange Situation paradigm, Ainsworth and colleagues[15] delineated several distinct and stable categories of attachment between children and caregivers. In the experimental situation, the experimenters observed a child's behaviors on separation from the parent figure, in the company of a stranger, and

on reunification with the known adult. In the most common, "stable" attachment category (56%–65%), the child was able to tolerate brief separation and be comforted by the parent on her or his return. Another group (20%–25%) was "avoidant," tolerating separation well but appearing disinterested in the parent figure on her or his return. Other children (10%–20%) were categorized as "ambivalent," showing much more distress and anxiety and taking much longer to reassure. Children whose parents were frankly abusive or mentally ill were seen to have what researchers termed *disordered attachment* styles, with behavior in the experimental setting that was dramatic and unpredictable, with components of both approach and avoidance. Fortunately, such disorganized attachment, which presents a nearly impossible challenge to the child, was seen in only 5% to 10% of the families studied.[11]

Not surprisingly, parental assessments show styles that correlate well with their children's behaviors. While securely attached children are seen to have nurturing and supportive parents, children in the avoidant group had parents who acted in a dismissive or disinterested fashion. The parents of the ambivalent subjects responded to their children in a style that was described as preoccupied and distant.

It is important in the context of abuse and neglect to remember that the parent-child relationship is a *reciprocal* one, in which each member responds to the actions of the other and influences them in turn. When a supportive parent recognizes and meets a child's needs, the infant learns patience and self-regulation.[16] Confident that needs will be met, securely attached children are less demanding and easier to parent well. Insecurely attached children aren't as easy to rear. Some are very demanding, as they continually seek to prove the parent's availability; others, having been too often dismissed, become themselves dismissive and thus often appear disobedient or disrespectful. Such behavior can provoke angry—and sometimes dangerous—responses, or deliberate neglect, from a stressed parent. A cycle of abuse or neglect can be initiated, which will serve only to reinforce the child's maladaptive behavior, rather than helping extinguish it.[17]

Children raised in violent or neglectful homes often lack the tools they would need to break this cycle. Language skills and cognitive abilities are often delayed in this population. These deficiencies may be a reflection of prenatal challenges such as malnutrition and exposure to toxins such as drugs and alcohol, or of postnatal neglect, but they deny the children the tools they need to readapt successfully.[18]

The process of attachment is also the path by which the child develops self-esteem. Through the responses of the primary caregivers, the child begins to learn about himself as well as about others. He comes to see himself as worthy of attention or not, to regard others as important or irrelevant, and behaves accordingly. The responses of others—punishing a misbehavior or merely ignoring a very quiet child—serve to confirm the child's worldview, and reinforce his behavior patterns.

Early lessons in human relationships are not easily unlearned. These behavioral variations constitute what psychologists term *attachment styles* and remain stable over long periods. It seems that the lessons learned in this early relationship are soon generalized to others. In effect, in his relationship to the primary caregiver, the child acquires a lens through which he views all future interpersonal relationships. When viewed through that lens, the responses of those around him may easily be taken to confirm the child's impression that the world is an unpredictable and arbitrary place and that other people cannot be trusted. Unless the others in the child's environment are sensitive and skillful in their responses, the maladaptive behavior will be reinforced.

This may be most apparent when a maltreated child experiences a change in his life circumstances, and he must function in a world different from that to which his young brain has adapted. A previously abused boy or girl may continue in a maladaptive behavior pattern despite several years in a consistent and supportive foster home. The child of a parent who has left an abusive relationship, or renounced drug or alcohol abuse, may continue to display challenging behaviors despite the parent's best efforts. The stability of such maladaptive behavior is no doubt due in part to the developing brain's sensitivity to new input, as the new brain develops structurally in response to environmental stresses. In many cases, it also reflects the tendency of the child's attachment style to influence his perceptions and behaviors, and thus the behaviors of his caregivers, in a "dance" of unintended reinforcement.

Neurobiology of Stress

A newborn human brain comes into the world ready to adapt, to become the kind of brain needed for survival in its new environment. Life with parents whose behavior is abusive or neglectful is stressful in the extreme and places demands on the developing brain. The child necessarily adapts—learns—to cope with the demands of this stressful environment, and the learning process involves structural modification on many levels. To understand the consequences of these adaptations, it is necessary to consider the biological concomitants of the stress response as they relate to the child's plastic central nervous system (CNS).

All animals undergo stress, and it can be very important to respond quickly, especially when the stress in question might be life-threatening. Over millions of years, mammals have developed efficient mechanisms to optimize their physiology for flight from, or combat with, an aggressor. This *fight or flight* mechanism increases blood flow to skeletal muscles, increases blood glucose to provide fuel, and raises blood pressure and heart rate. In its extreme manifestations, it may be termed the *fight, flight, or freeze* mechanism, as an excessive stress response results in a paralysis. This extreme reaction may have a selective value when the threat is so severe as to be unavoidable.[19]

On a cellular level, these temporary adaptations to stress are mediated by circulating hormones, principally by cortisol released from the adrenal cortex. When an environmental threat is registered by the hypothalamus in the brain, adrenocorticotropic hormone is secreted by the pituitary gland, stimulating the adrenals to release cortisol. This steroid hormone has direct effects on metabolism, increasing supplies of circulating glucose by antagonizing insulin and converting body protein to sugar. It is essential to a proper stress response from the vascular system and facilitates the action of glucagon, growth hormone, and other hormones. While the blood vessels in muscles are adjusting, the pupils are dilating, and the heart is racing to supply needed nutrients, the cortisol is also having an effect on the specialized cells of brain structures. Physiologists have noted increased excretion or blood concentrations of adrenal cortical hormones in many situations that involve novelty and challenge, ranging from job stress to final examinations to anticipation of surgery. Spikes of cortisol can be observed in experimental subjects undergoing stressful interviews or even watching exciting movies. It has been suggested that learning proceeds faster in the presence of the hormone.[20]

Chronic elevations of the stress hormones, however, prompt the brain to adapt, with consequences for long-term function. Childhood abuse and neglect have been shown to correlate with altered responses to cortisol in children,[2,3] adolescent[4], and adult[5-7] populations. While baseline cortisol levels in abuse victims are normal or even diminished, the victim's hypothalamic-pituitary axis often becomes hyperresponsive to stressful stimuli. These adaptations result in symptoms of emotional numbing and hyperarousal, well-recognized criteria of post-traumatic stress disorder.[8] Though adaptive to a high-threat environment, these modifications to the developing brain impair the victim's social adjustment.

At the same time as the body is adjusting to overcome the environmental threat, the brain, under the influence of cortisol, is planning to avoid future problems by ensuring that the current one is not easily forgotten. The mechanism involves 2 structures in the temporal lobe long known to be instrumental in the formation, storage, and retrieval of memories, the amygdala and the hippocampus. Neurologists have observed that damage to the hippocampus, as by stroke or trauma, can leave the individual unable to store memories, while damage to the amygdala deprives them of their emotional content. By stimulating the amygdala, a small structure in the limbic system, the stress hormone ensures that memories of the current event are specially tagged and handed off to an adjacent structure, the hippocampus. When marked and stored in this fashion, memories of traumatic events are kept in an easily retrievable form, immediately accessible for reference in event of another threat.

The brain seems to store emotional memories differently that it does more routine ones. Emotional memories are recalled as a gestalt, often complete with sensory impressions like smells and sounds. Recall of an emotional event can often be triggered by an associated sensory impression, as when a combat veteran hears a firecracker and relives a battle, or a lover smells his girl's perfume and is transported back to their last tryst. More commonplace events are recalled in a more analytic fashion, piece by piece. The difference seems to be an association with strong emotion. The emotions that initiate this labeling can be positive or negative, but in either event serve to perform a sort of triage on the associated sensory impressions: When an event is extraordinarily stressful, it is to be recalled immediately and vividly.

Why Two Brains Are Better Than One

These styles of recall are reminiscent of the different modes of information processing favored by the 2 cerebral hemispheres. Though roughly symmetrical in shape and size, the 2 halves of the cerebral cortex handle information in very different ways. The damage done by a cerebral stoke depends on the side affected. While strokes on either side can result in muscular paralysis, damage to the left temporal region often results in loss of the ability to understand or produce speech, while similar injury to the right temporal region does not. In the 1950s, patients with intractable seizure disorders underwent transection of the corpus callosum, the thick bundle of nerve fibers connecting each cortex to the other. Scientists following patients who had survived this radical procedure found themselves able to study each hemisphere individually by presenting stimuli in the opposite visual field, and measuring responses in the opposite limb. These so-called split-brain studies revealed that the right cerebral hemisphere, far from being silent, was busy processing nonlinguistic data, and was very active.[21]

The researchers found that the left cerebral hemisphere specialized not only in sending and receiving language, rather its talent for written and spoken speech reflected a predilection for a particular way of processing information, which might be described as analytic thought. Analytic (or symbolic) thought involves breaking down an event into its component parts and comparing them to other stored patterns, then recombining them into a new whole to solve a problem. Our distant ancestor, for example, might have needed to cross a river, and by combining his current mental image of the river with a previous memory of a fallen tree, he might imagine building a bridge. This recombination of symbols, of course, is similar to the mental process involved in choosing the right word to convey a given meaning, so it's not surprising that speech would come to reside in an area favoring this type of information processing, as selection favored efficient problem-solvers.

The problem with analytic thought, however, is that it is slow. When threatened by a bear, we don't have time to analyze the situation before calling up our hormonal cavalry. Split-brain findings suggest that our right hemispheres in fact provide just that type of rapid response processing. The right brain, though unable to create verbal speech, has proven adept at pattern recognition. Faces, for example, are recognized when shown to the right hemisphere, but not when projected to the left. Similarly, songs and simple rote verbal phases are retained after a left-hemisphere stroke that would wipe out other verbal capabilities. These pattern-based memories seem to be retained by the right side. This specialization of the cerebral hemispheres allows both systematic problem-solving when time permits and rapid pattern recognition when crises loom.

The right hemisphere's talents for pattern recognition are not, of course, used only in emergencies. An emerging body of research is revealing the importance of such pattern recognition during the first years of a child's development, as the baby learns to recognize its parents and assess the meaning of caregivers' facial expressions. The young child could be said to live in a world of patterns, associating stimulus and response to lay the groundwork for later development of analytic thought that characterizes so much of adult interaction. Pioneering developmentalist Jean Piaget referred to early childhood as a "preoperational" phase, in which the child has yet to learn how to break down and recombine input analytically.[22] The right brain is felt to develop first, as patterns are laid down well before the acquisition of symbolic language. Babies' behavior is characterized by strong emotions, and the brain's response to stress can help guarantee that these memories of distress and relief are tagged and stored for immediate recall. Though early memories often defy verbal expression, emotional recollections from our earliest times can return as gestalt patterns summoned by association.

These patterns of emotion, though not readily accessible to verbal analysis, are among our most vivid memories, and inform the baby's, the child's, and eventually the adult's interactions with others. They constitute the neurologic basis of the "lens" provided by early attachment, determining the child's pattern-based biochemical response to the actions of those around him. Necessarily, such patterns are not readily accessible to verbal analysis by the opposite hemisphere but, under ideal circumstances, the hemispheres can work together. The left and right brains, as mentioned, are connected by thick bands of axons in the corpus callosum and lesser commissures. These pathways permit rapid communication and allow each hemisphere to recognize the other, integrating its functions with those of its cortical partner.[23]

Stress and Memory: Ghosts From the Past

A child raised in an abusive or neglectful home naturally experiences a different set of emotional associations than one raised in a more supportive environment. The abused child might be expected to undergo strong emotion more often, and perhaps to feel relief less, or at least under different circumstances. The abused or neglected child experiences a different world, one that calls forth different responses from the developing brain. As the brain grows and adapts to its environment, generating synapses and pruning them, it will become a different brain, one that has

adapted to an environment characterized by stress. Indeed, using modern tools to image brain development, researchers have begun to delineate several important characteristics that distinguish the traumatized brain. As we learn more about the brain's development, neurobiology continues to dovetail with behavioral science and clinical observation.

That traumatic events can affect the manner in which memories are recorded and stored is well known. That previous trauma leads to troubling memories and erratic behavior has been a recurring theme in literature since the time of ancient Greece. In 1859 the French psychiatrist Briquet called attention to the association between hysterical symptoms and early trauma.[24] In 1889 his colleague Janet described what he termed *l'automatisme psychologique,*[25] postulating that trauma altered memory processing and observing that trauma memories tended to return unbidden, and at times inappropriately. In doing so, he was foreshadowing the description of what we now term *post-traumatic stress disorder (PTSD).* This term, which was widely publicized by the American Psychiatric Association in its 1980 *Diagnostic and Statistical Manual of Mental Disorders, Third Edition,* refers to a set of characteristic symptoms and responses after exposure to an extreme stressor, one that involved intense fear, helplessness, or horror. These may be summarized as (1) a tendency to persistently *reexperience* the traumatic event (through intrusive thoughts, dreams, and flashback recollections); (2) *numbing* of general responsiveness; (3) *avoidance* of stimuli that trigger this reexperience (seen as social withdrawal, restricted range of affect, and constriction of play); and (4) persistent symptoms of arousal (hypervigilance, exaggerated startle, and other physiological measures).[26] Post-traumatic stress disorder has been extensively studied in combat veterans and adult rape victims, and has been described in the aftermath of natural disasters as well as kidnappings and other examples of human brutality. In any event, the victim feels doomed to relive the traumatic events, as they are recalled by seemingly innocent stimuli from the external world.[27,28]

It seems that there may be great variation among the events that inspire this long-lived reaction pattern, but it is clear that these extreme stressors initiate a process of rapid, pattern-based recall for the traumatic events. Recall of the fearful occasion calls forth the same physiological state of arousal, complete with all the stress hormones. The victim has learned to recognize a life-threatening event and optimized the rapid retrieval of the previous state of arousal ;so as to avoid getting into the same fix again. Of course, in the case of the veteran at home, or the rape victim who fears all men, this physiological state is emphatically not adaptive.

As discussed previously, this type of gestalt memory, in which recall of an entire pattern is triggered by a sensory association, is the specialty of the right cerebral hemisphere. It is interesting in this context to note that the most effective mode of therapy for PTSD has involved an approach that works to

assert cognitive control over problem behaviors. In cognitive-behavioral therapy, patients are encouraged to construct a verbal narrative description of the maladaptive behaviors, in effect bringing them more closely under control of the usually dominant, verbal left hemisphere.[29]

Children who undergo severe or prolonged (so-called complex) trauma also develop the diagnostic features of PTSD, which is perhaps all the worse for the plasticity of the victim's young CNS. Consider that the child's brain is optimized for learning, and remember that the fight or flight response to life-threatening stimuli is initially adaptive, and it is apparent that a child growing in a threatening environment will adapt by frequent use of this memory pathway. One could hypothesize that the right-hemisphere, pattern-recognition mode might even become the abused child's default mode, that pattern storage and rapid retrieval are more the rule than the exception.

Computer analysis of electroencephalogram (EEG) patterns suggests just that. Teicher[7] studied brain wave coherence in patients who had been victims of severe abuse. The coherence of EEG signals is correlated with the structural complexity and thus the development of the underlying brain tissue. The findings suggested that these severely affected individuals had undergone a reversal of the usual pattern of left-brain dominance. Where healthy control individuals all showed greater development in their left cerebral hemispheres, abuse and neglect victims were more developed in the right, though all were right-handed. They had learned, in effect, to lead with the right brain, preferring to solve problems by gestalt pattern recognition as opposed to a more analytic, reasoned approach.

Functional and anatomical studies lend credence to this model. Prolonged exposure to high circulating levels of cortisol alter the sensitivity and even the size of the amygdala and hippocampus, and can affect its ability to grow and adapt later in life as well.[9,10,30,31] Alterations in the function of these important regions might be expected to affect the storage and retrieval of memories, especially those associated with strong emotion.

Researchers studying hemispheric function in adult abuse victims describe preferential activation of the right hemisphere in recalling emotionally disturbing memories, while control subjects used the hemispheres in a more balanced way.[32] Seeking the cause of this lack of hemispheric coordination, others have confirmed that the corpus callosum is measurably smaller in victims of abuse, especially neglect.[33] Fewer neurons in this important commissure mean less communication and less chance for the analytic/verbal and the gestalt/emotional halves of the brain to cooperate in problem solving.

This cooperation is usually a good thing, but it can be slow. In a high-threat environment, right-brain, pattern-recognition processing has traditionally been safer. For a young child, there is no more threatening environment than a home in which the adults are abusive, violent, or unavail-able. From an evolutionary standpoint, it makes good sense that a child from such a home would learn to react emotionally first, and ask questions later (if at all). From a neurodevelopmental perspective, we can see how those early reactions work to determine the structure of the young brain, and how such early adaptations might prove very difficult to reverse.

This is not to say that every child whose home is abusive or neglectful develops full-blown PTSD; most do not live out this worst-case scenario. Nonetheless, the behaviors seen in abuse victims suggest that these changes are common enough. Patients rarely present to the pediatric office wearing signs that identify them as abuse sufferers, much less ones saying, "I have PTSD." They do, however, present with chief complaints like school violence, as relatively innocent events such as a teacher's attempts at discipline or a playground scuffle trigger a disproportionate fight or flight response. Their caretakers may question whether they have attention-deficit disorder when the children seem to find it hard to concentrate on schoolwork, not realizing that an early childhood spent looking for the next threat has trained them to avoid the very type of concentration needed to succeed in school. Social withdrawal and constricted affect of PTSD can present as extreme shyness or depression, but this maladjustment is rarely seen as the consequence of early adaptation.

Positive Feedback Isn't Always Good

Less sophisticated caregivers, especially foster or adoptive parents, often see the abuse victim's exaggerated responses as a sign of willful disobedience, as part of a struggle for control or an attempt to "manipulate" them. They set out to teach the child more appropriate behaviors, using techniques they've learned in their own childhood or tested in raising their own children. These usually include the tried and tested practices of emotional confrontation, scolding, or otherwise punishing their charges while explaining the connection of the punishment to the behavior. Unfortunately, while those techniques may have proven effective enough on normal children, they can be counterproductive when they fail to take into account the particular neurobiological adaptations of the abused or neglected child: immediate pattern recognition and an exaggerated fight or flight response.

The abused child may overreact physically to the caretaker's raised voice or fierce countenance, as these often trigger emotional memories of the previous abuse. The resultant spike of adrenaline and cortisol may trigger explosive angry behavior, which in turn provokes a more dramatic response from the adult, as he or she seeks to regain control of the situation. The usual child may experience a physiological reaction, but it is relatively mild, and may be overcome by the tempering, analytic influence of the left cerebral hemisphere. In this scenario, each individual influences the other in a way that only provokes more anger in a "dance" of positive feedback. In a classic positive feedback loop, the response to a stimulus acts to perpetuate the stimulus, not to extinguish it. The tools commonly used by parents to change problem behaviors in their children can result in uncontrolled escalation when employed against the threat-adapted brain.

Moreover, this escalation, if it becomes a pattern of interaction, can continue to affect the child's neurologic development, in another, larger loop of positive feedback. By triggering the emotional memories again and again, the caretaker's actions confirm the associations, reminding the developing brain that this is, indeed, a threatening world, one that demands heightened reflexes. As neurons fire together, they "wire" together, and behavior, influenced by existing anatomy, influences new anatomy in turn. In this way the abused child travels an ever-deepening rut of behavior and maladaptive response, learning to behave in less and less appropriate ways.

Intervention

Outcome studies of the victims of abuse and neglect show a bewildering variety of pathologies, spanning multiple domains of function. Ineffective regulation of behavior and emotion, poor self-concept, and impaired learning capacity are common presentations to the pediatric office. Severe cases may show problems with anxiety, depression, social helplessness, and symptoms of bipolarity. By adulthood, many victims have developed cardiovascular or endocrine disorders from the persistent effects of the stress response.[34]

Foster parents, adoptive parents, and biological parents who now find themselves better able to care for previously abused or neglected children face daunting obstacles. They are often asked to take responsibility for the behaviors of a child whose responses to their mutual environment are dramatically different from their own, a child who treats their well-meant attempts at correcting behavior as if they were life-threatening attacks. To make matters worse, their young charge often does not trust them, nor anyone else in particular. They have often been participating involuntarily in a positive feedback loop of escalating, counterproductive behaviors. It shouldn't be surprising that their complaint on presentation to the doctor's office is often that, "Nothing I do seems to work!"

The key to meaningful intervention, whether in the professional's office or at home, lies in the recognition that children who have been subjected to complex trauma are quantifiably different from their non-abused peers, that they have spent their early years adapting to a world quite different than that in which they are now expected to perform. This adaptation has occurred on a deep neurologic level and by late childhood can be very difficult to undo. Moreover, attempting the change by using the same old tools that work for other children can be counterproductive, confirming the child's mistaken impressions and entrenching the very behaviors they want to eliminate.

Therapy must be directed toward reshaping the victim's perceptions and emotional responses. The younger the children, the more this difficult task falls to the caregivers, but it is necessary to involve all parties whatever the child's age.

The pediatric provider plays a primary role in recognizing and helping the caregivers to appreciate the critical link between the child's troublesome behavior and earlier trauma. In doing so, the pediatrician can help them understand that the child's problems are more than just simple "defiance" or willful misbehavior, and that their inability to change the behavior is neither a sign that the child is incorrigible, nor that they lack good parenting skills. The newly explored links between the abuse victim's behavior and the new brain's anatomy and physiology help remove the child's actions from the "black box" of mental illness. The mind and the body need no longer to be seen as dichotomous. When our perceptions of alcohol dependence underwent such a change in the 1950s, society moved from condemnation of alcoholism (as a character flaw) to a more practical concern with effective treatment (of alcohol dependence, a disease). When a physiological origin is understood, response can be more than a moral judgment.

The physician can help the adults appreciate that there are evidence-based interventions that can help put the child and family back on a more normal developmental path. Treatment research has shown that the amount of support received from parents and guardians is one of the most important factors for increasing the children's resilience.[35] By providing a new perspective on their dependents' misbehavior, the practitioner can guide the caregivers toward a more effective response, and begin to break the cycles of destructive feedback that have characterized their relationship with the child.

Effective interventions in severe cases, of course, will require more than simply reframing the caregiver's perceptions or even increasing empathy. As mentioned previously, trauma-specific therapy involving a cognitive-behavioral approach has demonstrated the best efficacy. Cognitive-behavioral therapy includes education about abuse and typical reactions to it, and teaches safety skills and stress management. With children who are ready and able, therapists facilitate a coherent narrative of the traumatic events and help the client regulate the emotions the narrative elicits. Telling the story of the trauma recruits the verbal/analytic left brain, and encourages cooperation with its more emotional counterpart on the right. By increasing cognitive processing, the therapist helps correct any distorted ideas the child may have developed about how and why the trauma occurred, and can defuse the explosive stress response to which the child has been conditioned. Especially with younger children, cognitive-behavioral therapists or multisystem therapists can work with caregivers to ensure therapy continues at home.[36,37]

Medications have been widely used to help manage the more troublesome physiological manifestations of the stress response, especially hyperarousal.

Abuse victims can suffer sleep disturbance, nightmares, and high anxiety long after the stressful events. Adrenergic blocking agents are often used for these symptoms of hypervigilance and arousal. Children suffering the long-term consequences of early trauma also demonstrate difficulties with concentration and mood disorders such as depression. Stimulants and serotonin reuptake inhibitors can relieve these unwelcome souvenirs of bad times. Though clinicians have found medications to be of some value in reducing these symptoms, it must be remembered that the evidence base for such pharmacologic interventions in children with symptoms of PTSD lags behind that for adults, and that management does not equate with cure. Even so, by helping victims of early maltreatment—and those around them—overcome their maladaptive physiology, medications can play a valuable role in breaking the cycle of reinforcement and let the family work on building strengths.

Conclusions

- The newborn child's brain undergoes a burst of neural development in its first years to suit it for the world in which it finds itself. This process of growth, connection, and pruning among neurons is guided by the child's perceptions of that environment, as reflected in their stimulation and use together. The bulk of this adaptation is completed by the time the child is 3 or 4 years old.
- Neural development is dependent on the presence of another, protective human, usually a parent. When such a figure is inconsistent, absent, or

abusive, offspring are denied many skills, such as emotional recognition and regulation, necessary for learning and adaptation. The child's ability to learn is severely impaired, often for life.

■ When the child's early environment is at odds with the current one, the learned responses may not be appropriate. The maladapted child is then recognized as having problem behaviors. This is especially true when the child has experienced neglectful or abusive caregivers and a high-threat environment.

■ Persistent exposure to high levels of threat, with actuation of the hypothalamic-pituitary axis, can result in habituation to high levels of cortisol and other stress hormones. The resultant changes in brain structures such as the amygdala, hippocampus, and corpus callosum are difficult or impossible to reverse, as are their behavioral concomitants.

■ A high-threat environment also encourages the child to learn to depend on rapid, emotional responses to threatening patterns, rather than a more analytic approach. These rapid responses seem to depend on actuation of the right, nonverbal hemisphere and are also facilitated by anatomical changes that, once undertaken, are difficult to reverse. They may be difficult to access or influence through verbal, left-hemisphere channels.

■ Clinicians presented with a child's stubborn behavior problems need to consider consequences of early maltreatment in the differential diagnosis.

■ When an aberrant stress response is felt to underlie the behaviors, therapeutic interventions may require a team approach, with the primary caregiver playing a central role.

■ Shifting the focus on maladaptive behaviors from psychology to physiology removes much of the social stigma and allows the family to concentrate on healing, rather than blame.

References

1. Huttenlocher PR. Synaptic density in human frontal cortex—developmental changes and effects of aging. *Brain Res.* 1979;163:195–205

2. Huttenlocher PR, Dabholkar A. Regional differences in synaptogenesis in human cerebral cortex. *J Comp Neurol.* 1997;387:167–178

3. LeVay S, Wiesel TN, Hubel DH. The development of ocular dominance columns in normal and visually deprived monkeys. *J Comp Neurol.* 1980;191:1–51

4. Eriksson PS, Perfilieva E, Bjork-Eriksson T, et al. Neurogenesis in the adult human hippocampus. *Nat Med.* 1998;4:1313–1317

5. Gould E, Tanapat P, Hastings NB, Shors TJ. Neurogenesis in adulthood: a possible role in learning. *Trends Cogn Sci.* 1999;3:186–192

6. Black J, Isaacs K, Anderson B, Alcantara A, Greenough W. Learning causes synaptogenesis, while motor activity causes angiogenesis, in cerebellar cortex of adult rats. *Proc Natl Acad Sci USA.* 1990;87:5568–5572

7. Teicher MH. Wounds that time won't heal: the neurobiology of child abuse. *Cerebrum.* 2000;2:50–67

8. Anderson CM, Teicher MH, Polcari A, Renshaw PF. Abnormal T2 relaxation time in the cerebellar vermis of adults sexually abused in childhood: potential role of the vermis in stress-enhanced risk for drug abuse. *Psychoneuroendocrinology.* 2002;27:231–244

9. De Bellis MD, Giedd JN, Boring AM, Frustaci K, Ryan ND. Developmental traumatology, part 2: brain development. *Biol Psychiatry.* 1999;45:1271–1284

10. Bowlby J. *Attachment.* Vol 1. New York, NY: Basic Books; 1982

11. James B. *Handbook for the Treatment of Attachment-Trauma Problems in Children.* New York, NY: The Free Press; 1994

12. Spitz R. Hospitalism: an inquiry into the genesis of psychiatric conditions in early childhood. *Psychoanal Study Child.* 1945;1:53–74

13. Shore A. *Affect Regulation and the Self: The Neurobiology of Emotional Development.* Hillsdale, NJ: Lawrence Erlbaum Associates; 1994

14. Chugani H. A critical period of brain development: studies of cerebral glucose utilization with PET. *Prev Med.* 1997;27:184–188

15. Ainsworth MS, Blehar MC, Waters E. Patterns of attachment: a psychological study of the strange situation. Oxford, England: Lawrence Earlbaum Associates; 1978

16. Beeghley M, Cicchetti D. Child maltreatment, attachment, and the self system: emergence of an internal state in toddlers at high social risk. In: Hertzig M, Farber E, eds. *Annual Progress in Child Psychiatry and Child Development.* Philadelphia, PA: Brunner/Mazel; 1996:127–166

17. Carlson E, Sroufe L. Contribution of attachment theory to developmental psychopathology. In: Cicchetti D, Cohen D, eds. *Theory and Methods.* Vol 1. New York, NY: J Wiley & Sons; 1995

18. Rossman B. Longer term effects of children's exposure to domestic violence. In: Graham-Bermann S, Edelson J, eds. *Domestic Violence in the Lives of Children.* Washington, DC: American Psychological Association; 2001:35–65

19. Perry BD, Azad I. Posttraumatic stress disorders in children and adolescents. *Curr Opin Pediatr.* 1999;11:310–316

20. Vander A, Sherman J, Luciano D. *Human Physiology: Mechanisms of Body Function.* New York, NY: McGraw-Hill; 1975

21. Buklina SB. The corpus callosum, interhemisphere interactions, and the function of the right hemisphere of the brain. *Neurosci Behav Physiol.* 2005;35:473–480

22. Piaget J. The stages of the intellectual development of the child. *Bull Menninger Clin.* 1962;26:120–128

23. Gazzaniga MS. Cerebral specialization and interhemispheric communication: does the corpus callosum enable the human condition? *Brain.* 2000;123:1293–1326

24. Crocq L, De Verbizier J. Le traumatisme psychologique dans l'oeuvre de Pierre Janet. *Annales Medico-psychologiques.* 1989;60:983–987

25. Janet P. *L'automatism psychologique.* Paris, France; 1889

26. American Psychiatric Association. Task Force on DSM-IV. *Diagnostic and Statistical Manual of Mental Disorders: DSM-IV-TR.* 4th ed. Washington, DC: American Psychiatric Association; 2000

27. Brett E. The classification of posttraumatic stress disorder. In: van der Kolk B, McFarlane A, Weisaeth L, eds. *Traumatic Stress: The Effects of Overwhelming Experience on Mind, Body, and Society.* New York, NY: The Guilford Press; 1996

28. Drake E, Bush S, von Gorp W. In: Eth S, ed. *PTSD in Children and Adolescents.* Washington, DC: American Psychiatric Association; 2001

29. Kolko D, Swenson C. *Assessing and Treating Physically Abused Children and Their Families.* Thousand Oaks, CA: Sage Publications; 2002

30. Mirescu C, Gould E. Stress and adult neurogenesis. *Hippocampus.* 2006;16:233–238

31. Mirescu C, Peters JD, Gould E. Early life experience alters response of adult neurogenesis to stress. *Nat Neurosci.* 2004;7:841–846

32. Schiffer F, Teicher MH, Papanicolaou AC. Evoked potential evidence for right brain activity during the recall of traumatic memories. *J Neuropsychiatry Clin Neurosci.* 1995;7:169–175

33. Teicher MH, Dumont NL, Ito Y, Vaituzis C, Giedd JN, Andersen SL. Childhood neglect is associated with reduced corpus callosum area. *Biol Psychiatry.* 2004;56:80–85

34. Cook A, Blaustein M, Spinozolla J, van der Kolk B. Complex trauma in children and adolescents. http://www.nctsnet.org/nctsn_assets/pdfs/edu_materials/ComplexTrauma_all.pdf. Accessed May 17, 2007

35. Deblinger E, Heflin A. *Treating Sexually Abused Children and Their Non-Offending Parents.* Thousand Oaks, CA: Sage Publications; 1986

36. Deblinger E, Stauffer L, Steer R. Comparative efficacies of supportive and cognitive behavioral group therapies for young children who have been sexually abused and their non-offending mothers. *Child Maltreat.* 2001;6:332–343

37. Saunders B. Closing the quality chasm in child abuse treatment: identifying and disseminating best practice. In: Saunders B, ed. *Kauffman Best Practices Project.* Kansas City, MO: Kauffman Foundation; 2004:1–48

Chapter 24

Legal Aspects of Child Abuse

John E. B. Myers

University of the Pacific
McGeorge School of Law

The medical profession plays a key role in protecting abused and neglected children. This chapter discusses the impact of law on medical practice related to child abuse and neglect. The chapter also addresses the role medical professionals play in the investigation and ensuing legal process related to child maltreatment. The chapter provides a general overview of legal principles without focusing on the law of individual states, which varies significantly. Consult a local attorney about the laws of your state.

The Medical Provider's Role in the Legal System

The medical provider's role in the legal system has expanded considerably over the last 2 decades. In addition to the medical provider's traditional roles of examining children, reporting cases of child abuse, and testifying as an expert witness, medical providers increasingly participate in the review of cases outside the traditional medical setting. Medical providers participate on multidisciplinary teams that review cases to determine whether abuse has occurred. In several states, this process is mandated by statute. Similar procedures have evolved for the review of child fatalities.

Child death review teams include medical examiners, pediatricians, public health officials, and other professionals.

The medical provider's judgment about whether a child's injury or death is the result of abuse is central to the investigative process in physical abuse and child homicide cases. Coordination between the medical provider and investigating agencies is essential to ensure that conclusions are accurate.

Medical providers recognize the value of actively participating in training efforts to improve other professionals' knowledge of medical issues. Many medical professionals serve as "medical mentors," sharing medical literature and training materials with attorneys and other professionals, conducting meetings to discuss current developments, and giving lectures and seminars.

Mental health professionals have also witnessed an expansion of their role in the legal system. Psychologists and psychiatrists are now involved with sexually violent predator cases that involve detailed assessments of sex offenders to decide whether the offenders should be civilly committed, often after their criminal sentence has been served. Mental health professionals are involved with assessments of offenders to inform judicial decisions on the placement of offenders. The assessment may include psychosexual assessments as part of the sentencing process, determination of issues involving risk management in the community, and recommending appropriate probation conditions or levels of community supervision or registration. Laws in many states mandate mental health treatment for offenders, in addition to services afforded to victims. Psychological assessments of juvenile sex offenders are used to determine rehabilitative needs and occasionally to determine whether such juveniles should be transferred to the adult criminal justice system.

As practice in this area continues to expand, medical and mental health providers can anticipate that their roles in the legal system will continue to develop.

Forensic Implications of Children's Disclosure Statements During Physical Examinations and Interviews

Many children disclose abuse to medical professionals. The diagnostic importance of children's disclosure statements is described elsewhere in this text. In addition to their diagnostic implications, children's statements during examinations and interviews have forensic value. Children's statements can be admitted in court as evidence when certain conditions are satisfied.

Children's Statements Describing Abuse Are Hearsay*

Medical professionals understand the forensic importance of medical and laboratory evidence of abuse but may be less cognizant of the forensic importance of children's words. When a child's statements are properly documented, the statements may be admissible in subsequent legal proceedings (ie, the child's words become legal evidence of abuse or neglect). Indeed, in many cases, the child's statements to professionals are the most compelling evidence of maltreatment. Suppose, for example, that while 4-year-old Beth is being examined by a physician, the child points to her genital area and says, "Daddy put his pee-pee in me down there. Then he took it out and shook it up and down and white stuff came out." Beth's words are compelling evidence of abuse. In subsequent criminal proceedings against Beth's father, the prosecutor calls the examining physician as a witness and asks the physician to repeat Beth's words and to describe her gesture. Before the doctor can speak, however, the defense attorney objects that Beth's words and gesture are hearsay. The rule in all states is that hearsay statements are inadmissible unless the statements meet the requirements of an exception to the rule against hearsay. To determine whether Beth's description of abuse is hearsay, the judge analyzes Beth's words in terms of the following definition. A child's words are hearsay when (a) the child's words were intended by the child to describe something that happened, (b) the child's words were spoken before the court proceeding at which the words are repeated by someone who heard the child speak, and (c) the child's words are offered in court to prove that what the child said actually happened.

Analysis of Beth's words reveals that they are hearsay. First, Beth intended to describe something that happened. Second, Beth made her statement before the proceeding where the prosecutor asks the physician to repeat Beth's words. Finally, the prosecutor is offering Beth's words to prove that what Beth said actually happened.

Beth's words are not the only hearsay, however. Her gesture pointing to her genital area also is hearsay. The gesture was nonverbal communication intended by Beth to describe abuse. The judge will sustain the defense attorney's hearsay objection unless the prosecutor persuades the judge that Beth's words and gesture meet the requirements of an *exception to the rule against hearsay.* In Beth's case, as in many other child abuse cases, the prosecutor's ability to convince the judge that Beth's hearsay statement meets the requirements of an exception to the hearsay rule depends as much on the documentation of the physician as on the legal acumen of the prosecutor. If the doctor knew what to document when Beth disclosed abuse, the prosecutor has a much better chance of persuading the judge to allow the doctor to repeat Beth's words and gesture.

---

*On occasion, a child's statement to a medical professional can be used in court as non-hearsay. The intricacies of non-hearsay uses of children's statements are beyond the scope of this chapter.

Exceptions to the Hearsay Rule
Although the rule against hearsay has at least 30 exceptions, only a few play a day-to-day role in child abuse and neglect litigation. Four hearsay exceptions follow. For extensive analysis of children's hearsay statements see Myers.[1]

The Excited Utterance Exception
An excited utterance is a hearsay statement that relates to or describes a startling event. The statement must be made while the child is under the emotional stress caused by the startling event. The theory behind the excited utterance exception is that statements made under significant stress are generally reliable. All states have a version of the excited utterance exception. The following factors are considered by the judge in determining whether a hearsay statement is an excited utterance:

1. **Nature of the event.** Some events are more startling than others, and judges consider the likely impact a particular event would have on a child of similar age and experience. In most cases, sexual or physical abuse is sufficiently startling to satisfy the excited utterance exception.

2. **Amount of time elapsed between the startling event and the child's statement relating to the event.** The more time that passes between a startling event and a child's statement describing the event, the less likely a judge is to conclude that the statement is an excited utterance. Although passage of time is important, elapsed time is not dispositive. Appellate courts and trial judges have approved delays ranging from a few

minutes to many hours. The professional should document as precisely as possible how much time passed between the abuse and the child's statement—minutes count.

3. **Indications the child was emotionally upset when the child spoke.** Judges consider whether the child was crying, frightened, or otherwise upset when the statement was made. If the child was injured or in pain, the judge is more likely to find an excited utterance.

4. **Child's speech pattern.** In some cases the way a child speaks, such as pressured or hurried speech, indicates excitement.

5. **Extent to which the child's statement was spontaneous.** Spontaneity is a critical factor in the excited utterance exception. The more spontaneous a statement, the more likely it meets the requirements of the exception.

6. **Questions used to elicit the child's statement.** Asking questions does not necessarily destroy the spontaneity required for the excited utterance exception. As questions become suggestive, however, spontaneity may dissipate, undermining applicability of the exception.

7. **First safe opportunity.** In many cases, abused children remain under the control of the abuser for hours or days after an abusive incident. When the child is finally released to a trusted adult the child has the first safe opportunity to disclose what happened. A child's statement at the first safe opportunity may qualify as an excited utterance even though considerable time has elapsed since

the abuse occurred. It is important to document threats communicated to the child, experiences of physical abuse or corporal punishment, and the child's expressions of fear.

8. **Rekindled excitement.** A startling event such as abuse may be followed by a period of calm during which excitement abates. If the child is subsequently exposed to a stimulus that reminds the child of the startling event, the child's excitement may be rekindled. Rekindled excitement sometimes satisfies the excited utterance exception to the rule against hearsay.

Professionals are encouraged to document the foregoing factors and any additional evidence that a child was distraught when describing maltreatment.

Medical Diagnosis or Treatment Exception

Nearly all states have a "diagnosis or treatment" exception to the hearsay rule for certain statements to professionals providing diagnostic or treatment services. The professional to whom the child speaks may be a physician, psychiatrist, psychologist, nurse, social worker, paramedic, emergency medical technician, or technician. The exception includes the child's statements describing medical history and statements describing present symptoms, pain, and other sensations. Finally, the exception includes the child's description of the cause of illness or injury.

In many cases, the child is the one who provides the information that is admissible under the diagnosis or treatment exception. Sometimes, however, an adult describes the child's history and symptoms to the professional. As long as the adult's motive is to obtain treatment for the child, the adult's statements are admissible under the exception.

The primary rationale for the diagnosis or treatment exception is that hearsay statements to professionals providing diagnostic or treatment services are reliable because the patient has an incentive to be truthful with the professional. This rationale is applicable for many older children and adolescents. Some young children, however, may not understand the need for accuracy and candor with health care providers. When a child does not understand that personal well-being may be affected by the accuracy of what is said, the rationale for the diagnosis or treatment exception evaporates, and the judge may rule that the child's hearsay statement does not satisfy the exception.

The diagnosis or treatment exception has its clearest application with children receiving traditional medical care in a hospital, clinic, or physician's office. Most children have at least some understanding of doctors and nurses, and the importance of telling the clinician "what really happened." Judges are less certain about the applicability of the diagnosis or treatment exception with psychotherapy, where the child may not understand the importance of accuracy. Yet when there is evidence that the child understood the need for accuracy with a mental health professional, judges generally conclude that the diagnosis or treatment exception extends to psychotherapy.

To increase the probability that a child's statement describing maltreatment satisfies the diagnosis or treatment exception to the rule against hearsay, professionals are encouraged to take the following steps:

1. Discuss with the child the clinical importance of providing accurate information and of being completely forthcoming. The physician might say, "Hello, I'm Doctor Jones. I'm a doctor and I'm going to give you a checkup to make sure everything is okay. While you are here today, I'll ask you some questions so I can help you. It's important for you to listen carefully to my questions. When you answer my questions, be sure to tell me everything you know. Tell me only things that really happened. Don't pretend or make things up. Your answers to questions help me to do my job as a doctor, so it is important for you to tell me only things that really happened."

2. The diagnosis or treatment exception requires that information supplied to the professional be pertinent to diagnosis or treatment. Thus it is important to document why information disclosed by a child is pertinent to diagnosis or treatment. For example, the medical provider could document in the child's record that the provider decided to conduct testing for sexually transmitted infections (STIs) and to collect forensic materials (rape kit) after listening to the child's medical history.

The medical diagnosis or treatment exception to the hearsay rule relates to both diagnosis and treatment. Treatment can consist of the medical treatment provided as part of the medical examination itself or treatment at a later time, which may include mental health treatment. However, the fact that no treatment is necessary following completion of the examination does not vitiate the exception. Since only a small percentage of cases involve positive medical findings, the principle diagnostic information obtained in the typical medical examination is the child's history. Accordingly, the medical provider should document that the medical history is pertinent to diagnosis.

3. If the child identifies the perpetrator, the professional should document why knowing the identity of the perpetrator is pertinent to diagnosis or treatment. For example, knowing the identity of the perpetrator is important in deciding whether it is safe to send the child home. The professional needs to know the perpetrator's identity if there is a possibility the child was exposed to an STI. The decision to refer a child for mental health services is influenced in some cases by the identity of the abuser, making identity pertinent to treatment.

Residual and Child Hearsay Exceptions

Most states have a hearsay exception known as a residual or catch-all exception that allows use in court of reliable hearsay statements that do not meet the requirements of one of the traditional exceptions (eg, excited utterance, medical diagnosis, or treatment). In addition to the general residual exception, most states have a special residual exception for statements by children in child abuse cases.

When a child's hearsay statement is offered under a residual or child hearsay exception, the most important question is whether the statement is reliable. Professionals who interview, examine, and treat children play an indispensable role in documenting the information judges consider to determine whether children's statements are sufficiently reliable to be admitted under residual or child hearsay exceptions. Professionals should document the following:

1. **Spontaneity.** The more spontaneous a child's statement, the more likely a judge will find it reliable.
2. **Statements elicited by questioning.** The reliability of a child's statement may be influenced by the type of questions asked. When questions are suggestive or leading, the possibility increases that the questioner influenced the child's statement. It should be noted, however, that suggestive questions are sometimes necessary to elicit information from children, particularly when the information is embarrassing. The smaller the number of suggestive and leading questions, the more likely a judge is to conclude that a child's statement is reliable.
3. **Consistent statements.** Reliability may be enhanced if the child's description of abuse is consistent over time.
4. **Child's affect and emotion when hearsay statement was made.** When a child's emotions are consistent with the child's statement, the reliability of the statement may be enhanced.

5. **Play or gestures that corroborate the child's hearsay statement.** The play or gestures of a young child may strengthen confidence in the child's statement. For example, the child's use of dolls may support the reliability of the child's statement.

6. **Developmentally unusual sexual knowledge.** A young child's developmentally unusual knowledge of sexual acts or anatomy supports the reliability of the child's statement.

7. **Idiosyncratic detail.** Presence in a child's statement of idiosyncratic details of sexual acts points to reliability. Jones wrote, "The interview can be examined for signs of unique or distinguishing detail. This may be found both within the account of the sexual encounter and/or in unrelated recollections. Examples include children who describe smells and tastes associated with rectal, vaginal, or oral sex."[2]

8. **Child's belief that disclosure might lead to punishment of the child.** Children hesitate to make statements they believe may get them in trouble. If a child believed disclosing abuse could result in punishment, confidence in the child's statement may increase.

9. **Child's or adult's motive to fabricate.** Evidence that the child or an adult had or lacked a motive to fabricate affects reliability.

10. **Medical evidence of abuse.** The child's statement may be corroborated by medical evidence.

11. **Changes in child's behavior.** When a child's behavior alters in a way that corroborates the child's description of abuse, it may be appropriate to place increased confidence in the child's statement.

None of the foregoing factors is a litmus test for reliability. Judges consider the totality of circumstances to evaluate reliability, and professionals can assist the legal system by documenting anything that indicates the child was or was not telling the truth when describing abuse.

Fresh Complaint of Sexual Assault

A child's initial disclosure of sexual abuse may be admissible in court under an ancient legal doctrine called fresh complaint of rape or sexual assault. In most states, a child's fresh complaint is not, technically speaking, hearsay. The law of fresh complaint varies considerably across the country. In most states, a child's initial disclosure of sexual abuse may be admissible as evidence of "fresh complaint" or, as it is called in some states, "outcry."

Impact of the Constitution on Hearsay

There are 2 sources of law that limit the admission of hearsay evidence in court. First is the rule against hearsay, discussed previously, which is part of the law of evidence. Hearsay exceptions (eg, excited utterance, medical diagnosis, or treatment) are also part of evidence law. Second, in addition to the law of evidence and its hearsay rule, the US Constitution places limits on hearsay. The US Constitution's Sixth Amendment, with its Confrontation Clause, dictates that certain hearsay statements are inadmissible against defendants in criminal cases. To be admissible against the defendant in a criminal trial, hearsay must satisfy both the Confrontation Clause and an exception to the rule against hearsay. In some situations, hearsay that fits an exception is inadmissible because it violates the Confrontation Clause.

Two decisions of the US Supreme Court—*Crawford v Washington*[3] and *Davis v Washington*[4]—define the impact of the Confrontation Clause on the admission of hearsay in criminal cases. Before discussing *Crawford* and *Davis,* however, it is important to mention 2 subsidiary rules. First, if the child who made a hearsay statement is able to testify in court and be cross-examined by the defense attorney about the hearsay, then the Confrontation Clause is satisfied and the child's hearsay can be admitted without affront to the Confrontation Clause. (Of course, the hearsay still has to meet the requirements of an exception to the rule against hearsay.) Second, the limits on hearsay imposed by the Confrontation Clause apply only in criminal cases. Thus in child protection proceedings in juvenile or family court—which are civil not criminal—the Confrontation Clause is inapplicable. *Crawford* and *Davis* do not apply in protective proceedings in juvenile or family court or in proceedings to terminate the parent-child relationship.

In a criminal prosecution, when the prosecutor offers hearsay against the defendant, *Crawford* and *Davis* come into play. As stated previously, if the child can testify and be cross-examined

about the hearsay, the Confrontation Clause is satisfied. However, when the child is unable to testify in court, the question under *Crawford* and *Davis* is whether the child's hearsay statement was testimonial when it was made. If the child's hearsay was testimonial, then it cannot be admitted against the defendant. On the other hand, if the child's statement was non-testimonial, then the Confrontation Clause places no limit on use of the statement against the defendant.

Under *Crawford* and *Davis,* the word *testimonial* is a term of art. A hearsay statement can be testimonial even though it bears no resemblance to testimony in court. Hearsay is testimonial when a reasonable person in the position of the speaker would appreciate that the statement could be used in later criminal proceedings. For example, a person's answers to questions during formal police interrogation at a police station are testimonial because a reasonable person in that situation understands that the police are asking questions to conduct an investigation and gather evidence for possible use in court.

Children's hearsay statements to parents, relatives, teachers, friends, foster parents, babysitters, and other non–law enforcement individuals are typically non-testimonial. Statements to child protection social workers are sometimes testimonial, sometimes not. A statement to a social worker is testimonial if the social worker's primary purpose in questioning a child is to gather evidence. Judges generally rule that children's statements during formal forensic interviews at child advocacy centers are testimonial, although the Minnesota Supreme Court held to the contrary in *State v Bobadilla*.[5]

Although many statements to police officers are testimonial, some are not. The answer depends on the circumstances in which the officer questions the child. Statements to police are most likely to be non-testimonial when the police ask questions in the context of an ongoing emergency. Thus a police officer's initial questions on arriving at the scene in response to a 911 call are typically intended to assess the situation, see whether medical help is necessary, and determine whether the victim and the officer are safe. Answers to such initial questions are typically non-testimonial. As the initial emergency abates, and the officer's questions turn from securing the scene to gathering evidence, statements become testimonial. In deciding whether statements to police officers are testimonial, judges consider the following: (a) Is there an ongoing emergency? (b) Is the child safe or in present danger? (c) Is medical assistance necessary? (d) Is the child alone or protected by others? (e) Is the child seeking help? (f) Is the child describing events that are happening as the child speaks? Or is the child describing past events? (g) How much time has elapsed since the events transpired? (h) What is the level of formality of the questioning?

Hearsay statements to physicians, nurses, and other medical providers are non-testimonial when the provider's primary motive for questioning the child is clinical.[6] The fact that the provider is aware of the forensic implications of communicating with children about maltreatment does not alter this conclusion. In *State v Moses*,[7] the Washington Court of Appeals concluded that a domestic violence victim's statements to a doctor were non-testimonial. The court wrote, "Courts that have addressed *Crawford's*[3] impact on statements admitted under the medical diagnosis or treatment exception focus on the purpose of the [victim's] encounter with the health care provider…. In cases where courts have found such statements to health care providers are testimonial, the prosecutorial purpose of the medical examination has been clear."[7] The Maryland Court of Special Appeals' decision in *Griner v State*[8] is instructive. In *Griner*, 4-year-old Chase made hearsay statements to a hospital admitting nurse. The Maryland court wrote, "Chase's statements to [nurse] Kaur were not testimonial. Kaur examined and questioned Chase as a routine preliminary procedure necessary prior to admitting him to the pediatrics ward. Kaur's questioning of Chase was not the equivalent of a police interrogation. Kaur was a nurse on the pediatrics ward performing her regular duties…. Chase was unafraid, smiling, wanted to play, and told Nurse Kaur that he was not in any pain. Under the standards enunciated in *Crawford*,[3] Chase's statements to Kaur were not testimonial.[8]" In *Commonwealth v DeOliveria*,[9] the Massachusetts Supreme Judicial Court considered a 6-year-old's hearsay statements to a pediatrician in the emergency department. Concluding that the child's statements were non-testimonial, the court wrote, "Patricia's statements cannot persuasively be said to have been made in response to police interrogation. Although police officers were present at the hospital, there is no indication in the record that they were present during the doctor's examination of Patricia, or that they had instructed the doctor on the manner in which his examination should proceed. Nothing in the record would support a determination that the doctor acted as an agent of law enforcement. Indeed, the doctor's testimony as to his role as a physician entirely independent from law enforcement, and the judge's findings in connection with his medical evaluation of Patricia, are all to the contrary. Police presence at a hospital cannot turn questioning of a patient by a physician during a medical examination into interrogation by law enforcement."[9] Finally, the Mississippi Supreme Court concluded in *Hobgood v State*[10] that a 5-year-old's statements to a therapist and a physician were nontestimonial. The court wrote, "These individuals were not working in connection with the police…. Had the police directed the victim to seek treatment from a doctor and a therapist for the purpose of discovering evidence to aid in the investigation then it might be possible for the statement to implicate the Confrontation Clause."[10] Hearsay statements to medical providers are non-testimonial when the provider's primary purpose in questioning the child is provision of medical care.

Importance of Documentation

Medical professionals are in an excellent position to document children's hearsay statements. Without careful documentation of exactly what questions are asked and exactly what children say, the professional will not likely remember months or years later when the professional is called as a witness and asked to repeat what the child said. Documentation is needed not only to preserve the child's words, but also to preserve a record of the factors indicating that the child's hearsay statements meet the requirements of an exception to the hearsay rule.

Confidential Records and Privileged Communications

Abused and neglected children interact with many professionals. Each professional who comes in contact with the child documents the interaction. Much of this information is confidential and must be protected from inappropriate disclosure. Confidentiality arises from 3 sources: (1) the broad ethical duty to protect confidential information, (2) laws that make certain records confidential, and (3) privileges that apply in legal proceedings.

Ethical Duty to Safeguard Confidential Information

The ethical principles of medicine, nursing, and other professions require professionals to safeguard confidential information revealed by patients. The principles of medical ethics of the American Medical Association require physicians to "safeguard patient confidences within the constraints of the law."[11] The Hippocratic oath states, "whatsoever I shall see or hear in the course of my profession…if it be what should not be published abroad, I will never divulge, holding such things to be holy secrets." The Code of Ethics for Nurses of the American Nurses Association states that nurses safeguard the patient's right to privacy by carefully protecting information of a confidential nature.[12]

Laws That Make Patient Records Confidential

Every state has laws that make certain records confidential. Some of the laws pertain to records compiled by government agencies such as child protective services, public hospitals, and the juvenile court. Other laws govern records created by professionals and institutions in the private sector such as physicians, psychotherapists, and private hospitals. The federal Health Insurance Portability and Accountability Act also controls the confidentiality of some of these records.

Despite legal protections, confidential records may be ordered to be produced in child abuse proceedings through a variety of means. Records may be subpoenaed by a grand jury or an attorney. A judge may order release of records. In appropriate cases the judge considering release of records conducts a private or "in camera" inspection of the records to determine their appropriateness for release.

Privileged Communications

The ethical duty to protect confidential information applies in all settings. In legal proceedings, however, certain professionals have an additional duty to protect confidential information. The law prohibits disclosure during legal proceedings of confidential communications between certain professionals and their patients. These laws are called *privileges*.

Unlike the across-the-board ethical obligation to protect confidential patient information, privileges apply only in legal proceedings. Privileges clearly apply when professionals testify in court and are asked to reveal privileged information. Privileges also apply during legal proceedings outside the courtroom. For example, in most civil cases, and in some criminal cases, attorneys take pretrial depositions of potential witnesses. During a deposition, questions may be asked that call for disclosure of privileged information. If this occurs, the professional or one of the attorneys should raise the privilege issue.

Communication between a patient and a professional is privileged when 3 requirements are fulfilled. First, the communication (oral or written) must be between a patient and a professional with whom privileged communication is possible. All states have some form of physician-patient and psychotherapist-patient privilege. Not all professionals are covered by privilege statutes, however. For example, if a patient communicates with a psychotherapist who is not covered by privilege law, no privilege applies. (A privilege may apply if the therapist not covered by a privilege is working under the supervision of a therapist who is covered by a privilege.) Of course, the fact that a privilege does not apply does nothing to undermine the therapist's ethical duty to protect confidential information.

In legal proceedings, the presence or absence of a privilege is important. In court, a professional may have to answer questions that require disclosure of information the professional is ethically bound to protect. By contrast, the professional generally does not have to answer questions that require disclosure of privileged information. Thus in legal proceedings a privilege gives protection to confidentiality that is not available under the ethical duty to protect confidential information.

The second requirement for a privilege to apply is that the patient must seek professional services. The patient must consult the professional to obtain advice or therapy. If the patient enters therapy, the privilege applies to confidential communications leading up to and during therapy. If the patient does not formally enter therapy, the privilege may nevertheless apply to confidential communications between the patient and the professional. For example, a patient may consult a physician who refers the patient to a second professional. Communication between the patient and the referring physician is privileged even though the patient does not receive treatment from the referring physician.

The third requirement of privilege law is that only communications that the patient intends to be confidential are privileged. The privilege covers confidential statements from the patient to the professional. The privilege also covers statements by the professional to the patient. Thus privilege is a 2-way street. Privilege generally does not attach to communications that the patient intends to be released to other people.

The fact that a third person is present when a patient discloses information may or may not eliminate the confidentiality required for privilege. The deciding factor usually is whether the third person is needed to assist the professional. For example, suppose a physician is conducting a physical examination and interview of a child. The presence of a nurse during the examination does not undermine the confidentiality of information revealed to the doctor. Furthermore, the presence of a child's parents need not defeat privilege. Again, the important factor is whether the third person is needed to assist the professional. A privilege is not destroyed when colleagues consult about cases.

Privileged communications remain privileged when the relationship with the patient ends. In most situations, the patient's death does not end the privilege.

The privilege belongs to the patient, not the professional. In legal parlance, the patient is the "holder" of the privilege. As the privilege holder, the patient can prevent the professional from disclosing privileged information in legal proceedings. For example, suppose a treating physician is subpoenaed to testify about a patient. While the physician is on the witness stand, an attorney asks a question that calls for privileged information. At that point, the patient's attorney should object. The patient's attorney asserts the privilege on behalf of the privilege holder—the patient. The judge then decides whether a privilege applies.

If the patient's attorney fails to object to a question calling for privileged information, or if the patient is not represented by an attorney, the professional may assert the privilege on behalf of the patient. Indeed, the professional has an ethical duty to assert the privilege if no one else does. The professional might turn to the judge and say, "Your Honor, I would rather not answer that question because answering would require disclosure of information I believe is privileged." When the judge learns that a privilege may exist, the judge decides whether the question should be answered.

Disclosure of Confidential and Privileged Information

Patient Consent

Patient consent plays the central role in release of confidential or privileged information. As Gutheil and Appelbaum observed, "With rare exceptions, identifiable data can be transmitted to third parties only with the patient's explicit consent."[13] A competent adult may consent to release of privileged information to attorneys, courts, or anyone else. The patient's consent should be informed and voluntary. The professional should explain any disadvantages of disclosing confidential information. For example, the patient may be told that release to third persons may waive privileges that would otherwise apply.

A professional who discloses confidential information without patient consent can be sued. With an eye toward such lawsuits, Gutheil and Appelbaum wrote, "It is probably wise for therapists always

to require the written consent of their patients before releasing information to third parties. Written consent is advisable for at least 2 reasons: (1) it makes clear to both parties involved that consent has, in fact, been given and (2) if the fact, nature, or timing of the consent should ever be challenged, a documentary record exists. The consent should be made a part of the patient's permanent chart."[13]

When the patient is a child, parents normally have authority to make decisions about confidential and privileged information. When a parent is accused of abusing or neglecting a child, however, it may not be appropriate for the parent to make decisions regarding the child's confidential information. In the event of a conflict between the interests of the child and a parent, a judge may appoint someone else, such as a guardian *ad litem,* to make decisions about confidential and privileged information. Unfortunately, appointment of a guardian *ad litem* cannot always be accomplished in a timely fashion. Two examples among many possible scenarios illustrate the problem.

The first involves the request for authorization to donate organs when a child sustains fatal injuries as a result of abuse. This situation occurs particularly in abusive head trauma cases. The child may be declared brain dead and remain on life support to prolong opportunities to harvest organs. In this situation, the parent may be a suspect in the investigation while at the same time asked to authorize medical procedures that may affect the evidence uncovered in a subsequent autopsy. The necessity of harvesting the organs at a particular time may not permit the time necessary to appoint a guardian *ad litem* to authorize the procedure. In some jurisdictions, laws authorizing the harvesting of organs from donors may override even the ability of the medical examiner to intercede.

The second example involves situations where a child has been removed from a parent's care as a result of allegations of abuse or neglect. Despite removal, the parent retains certain parental rights and therefore may have authority to authorize release of confidential records to themselves or their attorney. Parents may desire to obtain therapeutic records of the child or other confidential records to discredit the child as a witness or to support the parent's defense. In many instances, the child's attorney or the prosecutor are not aware that such records are being sought and are not in a position to object. Moreover, the custodian of the records may be unaware that a criminal or juvenile court proceeding is underway against the parent, suggesting the need for caution in the release of records.

Limitations of the Physician-Patient Privilege

Privileges are not absolute. In many states, for example, the physician-patient privilege applies only in civil cases and is not applicable in criminal trials. Thus in a criminal trial, confidential communications between patient and doctor that would normally be privileged may have to be revealed. In most states, the psychotherapist-patient priv-

ilege applies in civil and criminal cases, making the psychotherapist-patient privilege broader than the physician-patient privilege.

Subpoenas

A subpoena is issued by a court, typically at the request of an attorney. A subpoena is a court order and cannot be ignored. Refusal to obey a subpoena can be punished as contempt of court.

The 2 types of subpoenas are a subpoena requiring an individual to appear at a designated time and place to provide testimony, sometimes called a *subpoena ad testificandum,* and a subpoena requiring a person to produce records or documents. A subpoena for records is sometimes called a *subpoena duces tecum.*

A subpoena does not override privileges such as physician-patient and psychotherapist-patient. The subpoena for testimony requires the professional to appear, but the subpoena does not mean the professional has to disclose privileged information. A judge decides whether a privilege applies and whether a professional has to answer questions or release records.

Before responding to a subpoena, the professional should contact the patient or, in the case of a child, a responsible adult. The patient may desire to release confidential or privileged information.

It is often useful, with the patient's permission, to communicate with the attorney issuing the subpoena. In some cases, the conversation lets the attorney know the professional has nothing that can assist the attorney, and the attorney withdraws the subpoena. Even if the attorney insists on compliance with the subpoena, the conversation may clarify the limits of relevant information in the professional's possession. Care should be taken during such conversations to avoid disclosing confidential or privileged information.

If doubts exist concerning how to respond to a subpoena, consult an attorney. Legal advice should not be obtained from the attorney who issued the subpoena.

Reviewing Client Records Before or During Testimony

When a professional is asked to testify, portions of the child's record may be reviewed to refresh the professional's memory. In some cases, the professional leaves the record at the office. In other cases the record is taken to court. Generally, it is entirely appropriate to review pertinent records before testifying. Indeed, such review is often essential for accurate and detailed testimony. Professionals should be aware, however, that reviewing records before or during testimony may compromise the confidentiality of the records.

Reviewing records before testifying

While the professional is on the witness stand, the attorney for the alleged perpetrator may ask whether the professional reviewed the child's record and, if so, may request the judge to order the record produced for the attorney's inspection. In most states, the judge has authority to order the record produced. In favor of disclosure, the judge consid-

ers the attorney's right to cross-examine the professional and the extent to which the record will assist cross-examination. Against disclosure, the judge evaluates the impact on the child of disclosing confidential information. The outcome turns on which of these factors predominates.

Referring to records while testifying

When records are reviewed before testifying, the judge may or may not order the records disclosed to the attorney for the alleged perpetrator. If the professional takes the record to court and refers to it while testifying, however, the judge is very likely to order the record disclosed.

Protecting records from disclosure

Whether a professional reviews a child's record before or during testimony, a judge is more likely to require disclosure of non-privileged records than of records that are protected by the physician-patient or psychotherapist-patient privileges. Unfortunately, in most states, the law is unsettled regarding the impact of record review on privileged communications. With the law unsettled, steps can be taken to reduce the likelihood that reviewing records will jeopardize confidentiality or privilege.

It is often advisable to determine what information has already been released to the parties as part of the legal process. If the parties already have access to the entire record as part of the discovery process, then there is less reason for the professional to be concerned that their review of the record will implicate concerns of privileged or confidential records.

When reviewing a child's record before going to court, consider limiting review to portions of the record that are needed to prepare for testifying. Document the parts of the record reviewed and not reviewed. In this way, if a judge orders the record disclosed to the attorney for the alleged perpetrator, an argument can be made that disclosure should be limited to portions of the record actually used to prepare for testifying.

Recall that records containing privileged communications probably have greater protection from disclosure than non-privileged records. With this distinction in mind, professionals may wish to organize records so that privileged information is maintained separately from non-privileged information. When a record that is organized in this manner is reviewed before testifying, it is sometimes possible to avoid reviewing privileged communications. When this is done, if a judge orders the record disclosed, the judge may be willing to limit disclosure to non-privileged portions of the record. Although this approach entails the burden of separating records into privileged and non-privileged sections, and may not persuade all judges, the technique is worth considering.

If it is necessary to take the record to court, consider taking only the portions of the record that will be useful during testimony and leaving the remainder at the office.

If the record is taken to court, the record can remain in a briefcase rather than be taken to the witness stand. Make no mention of the record unless it becomes necessary to refer to it while testifying. Once the record is used during testimony, the attorney for the alleged perpetrator probably has a right to inspect it.

If the record is taken to court and to the witness stand, it may be possible to testify without referring to the record.

Legal advice should be obtained before implementing any of the foregoing suggestions. Some of the recommendations may not be permitted in some states. Additionally, there may be strategic reasons why these practices are not advisable in a particular case. For example, a physician who is familiar with the entire medical record may be permitted to testify to test results or medical findings of other professionals, thus avoiding the need for multiple witnesses to be called. Moreover, it may be important to be familiar with the entire record so you cannot be impeached due to lack of such familiarity.

Child Abuse Reporting Laws Override Confidentiality and Privilege

Child abuse reporting laws require professionals to report suspected child abuse and neglect to designated authorities. The reporting laws override the ethical duty to protect confidential client information. Additionally, the reporting requirement overrides privileges for confidential communications between professionals and patients.

Although reporting laws abrogate confidentiality and privilege, abrogation usually is not complete. In many states, professionals may limit the information they report to the specific information required by law. Information that is not required to be reported remains private.

Psychotherapist's Duty to Warn Potential Victims About Dangerous Clients

In 1974 the California Supreme Court ruled in *Tarasoff v Regents of the University of California*[14] that a psychotherapist has a legal duty to warn the potential victim of a psychiatric patient who threatens the victim. The duty to warn overcomes both the ethical duty to protect confidential information and the psychotherapist-patient privilege. If the therapist fails to take reasonable steps to warn the victim, and the patient carries out the threat, the therapist can be sued.

Since *Tarasoff* was decided, judges have grappled with the difficult question of when professionals have a legal duty to warn potential victims. In most states, the law remains unsettled. Judges generally agree that there is a legal duty to warn some potential victims, but judges have not achieved consensus on when the duty applies. In 1985 California enacted a statute on the subject, which limits the duty to warn to situations in which "the patient has communicated to the psychotherapist a serious threat of physical violence against a reasonably identifiable victim or victims."[15]

Emergencies

In emergencies, a professional may have little choice but to release confidential information without prior authorization from the patient. The law allows release of confidential information in genuine emergencies.

Court-Ordered Examinations

A judge may order an individual to submit to a medical examination or a psychological evaluation to help the judge decide the case. Because everyone knows from the outset that the professional's report will be shared with the judge and the attorneys, the obligation to protect confidential information is limited, and privileges generally do not attach.

Obligation to Report Suspected Abuse and Neglect

Professionals who work with children are required to report suspected abuse and neglect to designated authorities. The list of mandated reporters includes physicians, nurses, mental health professionals, social workers, and child care providers.

Mandated reporters have no discretion whether to report. Reporting is mandatory, not optional. Both civil and criminal penalties may result if a professional fails to report suspected abuse. States protect the identity of reporters. Additionally, states provide immunity from civil liability for individuals who report suspected maltreatment.

The reporting requirement is triggered when a professional possesses a prescribed level of suspicion that a child is abused or neglected. The terms used to describe the triggering level of suspicion vary slightly from state to state and include *cause to believe, reasonable cause to believe, known or suspected abuse,* and *observation or examination which discloses evidence of abuse.* Despite shades of difference, the basic meaning of the reporting laws is the same across the country. Reporting is required when a professional has information that would lead a reasonable professional to believe abuse or neglect is likely.

The duty to report does not require the professional to "know" that abuse or neglect occurred. All that is required is information that raises a reasonable suspicion of maltreatment. A mandated reporter who postpones reporting until all doubt is eliminated probably violates the reporting law and potentially places the child at risk. A substantial number of reporting laws authorize designated professionals to obtain photographs or radiographs of children without parental consent or to conduct other diagnostic tests (eg, STI testing) or collect forensic evidence.

Expert Testimony in Child Abuse Litigation

Expert testimony is provided by physicians, nurses, psychologists, social workers, and other professionals.

Who Qualifies as an Expert Witness

Before a professional may testify as an expert witness, a judge must be convinced that the professional possesses sufficient knowledge, skill, experience, training, and education to qualify as an expert. The professional takes the witness stand and answers questions about education, specialized training, and relevant experience. Typically, the attorney who offers a professional's testimony asks all the questions related to qualifications. Occasionally the judge asks questions. The opposing attorney has the right to question the professional in an effort to persuade the judge that the professional should not be allowed to testify as an expert. Such questioning is called *voir dire.* When the professional's qualifications are obvious, there usually is no voir dire.

The level of expertise required to qualify as an expert witness is relatively low, necessitating only that the expert possess enough specialized knowledge to assist the jury on technical, scientific, or clinical matters that the jury is not equipped to understand on its own. With this minimal threshold in mind, physicians qualify to testify on many matters within their specialty. Thus a pediatrician or an obstetrician-gynecologist would qualify to testify on some aspects of child sexual abuse. A neurosurgeon qualifies to testify on certain aspects of inflicted head injury.

Although a physician who does not specialize in child abuse will pass the relatively low threshold required to provide some forms of expert testimony, physicians who lack advanced training and experience on child maltreatment should be careful to avoid exceeding their level of expertise. The recent move toward establishing board certification for child abuse pediatricians may raise the level of expertise courts will require. Chadwick and Krous[16] suggest the following qualifications for professionals involved in child abuse cases: (a) training and experience in the cause of injuries to children; (b) training, education, or experience as to the particular type of case before the court; (c) membership in relevant medical and professional societies; (d) child abuse and neglect conference presentations or, at a minimum, attendance; and (e) knowledge of relevant publications.

A medical degree is not required to qualify as an expert on some aspects of child abuse. For example, trained and experienced nurse practitioners and nurse examiners routinely qualify to testify as expert witnesses regarding child sexual abuse.

Preparation for Expert Testimony

When a professional prepares to testify, it is important to meet with the attorney for whom the expert will testify. Nothing about pretrial conferences is ethically or legally improper. Chadwick[17] observes, "Face-to-face conferences between…attorneys and [expert witnesses] are always desirable, and rarely impossible."

Preparation includes review of relevant records. The law allows experts to base their testimony on all sources of data that are relied on by experts in the field. The materials do not have to be independently admissible in court. Thus hearsay that would be inadmissible in court may be relied on by an expert in formulating testimony. The expert should review relevant literature and anticipate that the opposing attorney will be at least partially familiar with the literature and may use it to try and impeach testimony during cross-examination.

In preparing to testify, the professional should ask the attorney whether he or she will testify primarily as a fact witness to describe observations and knowledge of the circumstances of the case. The professional also should ask whether the facts as he or she understands them are likely to be chal-

lenged by the opposing attorney. It should also be determined if he or she will be asked to provide an opinion and, if so, whether the opinion is likely to focus on a hotly contested issue in the case. Also important is whether there will be an opposing expert witness. What are the likely defenses in the case? Will testimony be offered during the case in chief or during the case in rebuttal? Are you the only expert for "your side"? What are the style, demeanor, and level of sophistication of opposing counsel? What are areas of permissible and impermissible testimony? Is the case being tried to a judge or to a jury? (When there is no jury, it is called a *bench trial* or *trial to the court.)* Is the case in juvenile, family, or criminal court? What questions will be asked during direct examination and what information needs to be imparted to the judge or jury? What are the anticipated lines of cross-examination? Has the opposing attorney requested to interview you prior to trial? What materials should be brought to court and to the witness stand?

The expert should be familiar with the reports of other expert witnesses. The expert should be prepared to discuss similarities and differences between the expert's opinion and the opinions of other experts, and whether differences between opinions can be reconciled. If an opposing expert has testified on prior occasions, there may be a transcript of the expert's earlier testimony that can be reviewed with an eye toward anticipating what the expert may say in the present case, as well as potential areas where the opposing expert can be cross-examined. In some instances the opposing expert has written articles that can be reviewed.

Preparation includes creating and discussing any exhibits, charts, or demonstrative aids that will be used during testimony. Exhibits may have to be shared with opposing counsel prior to trial.

Forms of Expert Testimony

Expert testimony usually takes several forms: (a) a factual recitation of what the expert observed, tested for, or documented; (b) an opinion; (c) an answer to a hypothetical question; (d) a lecture providing technical or clinical information for the judge or jury; or (e) testimony rebutting another witness or expert who testified previously. Often more than one of these forms is used during testimony.

Opinion Testimony

Expert witnesses are permitted to offer opinions that embrace the "ultimate factual issue" in the case. In a physical abuse case, for example, one ultimate factual issue is whether a child's injuries were accidental or inflicted. When a defendant is on trial for rape, penetration is an issue of ultimate fact.

In physical abuse cases, physicians testify about the nature of a child's injuries, the likely mechanism or cause of injury, the degree of force required to produce injury, whether injuries are consistent with a caretaker's explanation, whether injuries are consistent with child abuse, and whether a child's injuries were inflicted or accidental. An expert may

offer an opinion that a child has a diagnosis of battered child syndrome or shaken baby syndrome. In appropriate circumstances an expert may render an opinion that injuries were probably caused by someone of adult strength, someone who had continuing access to the child, or someone who was with the child immediately before the child became symptomatic. In neglect cases, experts commonly offer an opinion that a child's failure to thrive was caused by parental behavior and not by some medical condition or physical abnormality. In sexual abuse cases, medical experts offer opinions about whether findings of physical examination are consistent with the history of sexual activity. An expert may offer an opinion that a child was penetrated.

The expert must be reasonably confident of the opinion that is offered in court. Lawyers use the term *reasonable certainty* to describe the necessary degree of confidence. Unfortunately, reasonable certainty is not well defined in law. It is clear that expert witnesses may not speculate or guess. It is equally clear that experts do not have to be 100% certain their opinion is correct. (Complete certainty is seldom achieved in medicine or psychology.) Thus reasonable certainty lies somewhere between speculation and certainty—closer to the latter than the former. Skilled child abuse professionals employ a high threshold before they diagnose abuse. The confidence level required to diagnose so serious a matter as child abuse equates, if it does not surpass, the certainty required for reasonable certainty. The expert may be asked to explain to the jury what the expert means by reasonable certainty.

A helpful way to think about the degree of certainty underlying expert opinion is to ask questions that shed light on the strength of the opinion. In formulating the opinion, did the expert consider all relevant facts? Did the expert have adequate understanding of pertinent clinical and scientific principles? Did the expert use methods of assessment that are appropriate, reliable, and valid? Are the expert's assumptions and conclusions reasonable? The California Supreme Court observed, "Like a house built on sand, the expert's opinion is no better than the facts on which it is based."[18]

A Lecture to Educate the Jury

Experts may testify in the form of a lecture that provides the jury with information on technical, clinical, or scientific issues. This form of expert testimony plays an important role in maltreatment litigation. For example, in sexual abuse cases, the defense often asserts that a child's delayed reporting, inconsistent disclosures, or recantation means the child cannot be believed. When the defense attacks the child's credibility this way, judges often allow an expert witness to inform the jury that it is not uncommon for sexually abused children to delay reporting, provide partial or piecemeal disclosures, and recant. Equipped with this information, the jury is in a better position to evaluate the child's credibility.

In physical abuse cases, experts inform the jury about pertinent aspects of anat-

omy and physiology, how the body responds to injury, symptoms associated with injuries, the timing and dating of injuries, the role that the history plays in diagnosis, and other matters. The expert may be asked to summarize relevant literature. With this background information in place, the expert may go on to describe the child in the case on trial, culminating in an opinion on the nature and origin of the child's injuries.

The Hypothetical Question

In some instances, expert testimony is elicited in response to a hypothetical question. The hypothetical question generally asks the witness to assume that certain facts have been established. The judge informs the jurors that they are only to consider the answer to the hypothetical question if all of the facts assumed to be true by the expert are established by other evidence. Consider a physical abuse case in which the testifying expert was the child's treating physician in the hospital. The attorney offering the doctor's testimony says, "Now doctor, let me ask you to assume that all of the following facts are true." The attorney then describes testimony by earlier witnesses regarding the child's condition and symptoms prior to hospitalization, including the child's eating, feeding, and sleeping patterns; the time when the 911 call was placed; the child's condition when the paramedics arrived; and the observations made by the emergency department doctors on admission. The attorney then asks the expert to consider the child's injuries and condition when the expert examined the child at the hospital. The attorney ends by asking, "Doctor, based on these facts, do you have an opinion, based on a reasonable degree of medical certainty, as to when the child was injured in relation to the 911 call?" Alternatively, the hypothetical question might be, "Doctor, assuming that the child had been injured by a mechanism involving violent shaking, how soon after the shaking episode would you expect the child to exhibit symptoms and what would those symptoms look like?"

Attorneys cross-examining expert witnesses often ask hypothetical questions. The cross-examiner may try to undermine the expert's opinion by presenting a hypothetical set of facts that differs from the facts described by the expert. The cross-examiner then asks, "Now doctor, if the hypothetical facts I have suggested to you turn out to be true, would that change your opinion?" Chadwick[17] observes that it is "common to encounter hypothetical questions based on hypotheses that are extremely unlikely, and the witness may need to point out the unlikelihood." When asked about a hypothetical set of facts, be reasonable, but stick to your opinion and do not commit to an answer when the facts suggested by the attorney are not accurate.

Novel Scientific Evidence and the Judge's Responsibility as Gatekeeper to the Use of Scientific Evidence

The judge presiding over a trial is responsible for ensuring that expert testimony is sufficiently reliable to warrant consideration by the jury. Judges realize that while most expert testimony is based on respectable science, occasions

arise when "junk" science is passed off as legitimate. Judges worry that lay jurors may be "too impressed" with highly polished expert testimony that actually stands on shaky ground. To paraphrase the California Supreme Court, quoted earlier, expert testimony is no better than the science on which it is based.[18] Judges understand that with rare exceptions jurors are not scientists, and jurors are not in a good position to critically evaluate the scientific foundation for expert testimony. Moreover, attorneys are often not much better than jurors at separating scientific wheat from chaff, with the result that attorneys too often fail to expose unreliable expert testimony.

With these concerns in mind, in 1923 the Court of Appeals for the District of Columbia fashioned a legal test to evaluate the reliability of novel scientific principles underlying expert testimony.[19] The test was articulated in the famous case of *Frye v United States*,[19] which involved a precursor of the modern polygraph or lie detector. The court ruled that expert testimony based on novel scientific principles cannot be admitted in court until the principles are generally accepted as reliable by the scientific community. This test for scientific evidence became knows as the general acceptance test or simply the *Frye* test for novel scientific evidence.

When an attorney believes expert testimony offered by the opponent is based on unproven (ie, novel) scientific principles, the attorney objects to the testimony and requests a hearing—called a *Frye* hearing—to determine whether the principle is generally accepted as valid in the scientific community. If the judge is persuaded that the expert testimony is indeed based on novel scientific principles, the judge conducts a *Frye* hearing at which expert testimony is received to determine whether the principle is generally accepted. Following the hearing, if the judge finds general acceptance, then the trial resumes and the objected-to expert testimony is allowed. However, if the judge finds that the principles underlying the expert testimony are not generally accepted as reliable, the judge excludes the expert testimony.

For most of the 20th century, *Frye* was the dominant test in the United States for evaluating the admissibility of novel scientific evidence. Over the years, however, particularly in the 1980s, *Frye* was subjected to a steady drumbeat of criticism from judges and scholars. The basic criticism was that *Frye's* requirement of general acceptance had the undesirable effect of excluding scientific evidence that had yet to achieve general acceptance but that was nevertheless sufficiently reliable for use in court. Criticism of *Frye* culminated in the US Supreme Court's 1993 decision in *Daubert v Merrell Dow Pharmaceuticals, Inc.*[20] In *Daubert,* the Supreme Court rejected *Frye* and replaced it with a new test for scientific evidence.

Under *Daubert,* the trial judge is the gatekeeper for *all* scientific evidence, not just novel scientific evidence. As was the case with *Frye,* under *Daubert* an attorney may object that expert testimony is based on unreliable scientific principles and request a hearing, now called a *Daubert* hearing. Unlike *Frye,*

however, where the only issue at the hearing was general acceptance by the scientific community, the judge conducting a *Daubert* hearing considers all evidence that sheds light on reliability.

In *Daubert* the Supreme Court wrote that judges conducting *Daubert* hearings should consider the following factors: (a) Has the scientific principle underlying the proposed expert testimony been subjected to testing under the scientific method? (b) Has the principle been subjected to peer review and publication? (c) Is there an established error rate when using the principle? (d) Are there standards that govern proper use of the principle? (e) Borrowing from *Frye,* is the principle generally accepted as reliable in the scientific community? A scientific principle that has yet to achieve general acceptance may nevertheless be sufficiently reliable for use in court under *Daubert.*

The *Daubert* decision dealt with expert testimony based squarely on science. Following *Daubert* there was uncertainty as to whether *Daubert* applied to expert testimony that combines science and professional judgment and interpretation. Thus does *Daubert* apply to expert testimony from engineers, physicians, and mental health professionals who combine scientific knowledge with professional or clinical judgment? In 1999 the Supreme Court answered in the affirmative with its decision in *Kumho Tire Company, Ltd. v Carmichael.*[21] In *Kumho,* the Supreme Court ruled, *"Daubert's* general holding—setting forth the trial judge's 'gatekeeping' obligation—applies not only to testimony based on 'scientific' knowledge, but also to testimony based on 'technical' and 'other specialized' knowledge."[21] In *Kumho* the court reiterated that the trial judge should consider all evidence shedding light on the reliability of expert testimony. The Supreme Court's rulings in *Daubert* and *Kumho* are only binding on federal courts and do not compel individual states to abandon *Frye*. As of 2006, a slight majority of states had jettisoned *Frye* in favor of *Daubert*.

In most child maltreatment cases involving expert testimony there is no request for a hearing under *Frye* or *Daubert*. The expert gets on the witness stand, is qualified, testifies, is cross-examined, and that is the end of it. *Frye* and *Daubert* do not come up. Indeed, a few states (eg, California and Florida) have a rule that *Frye* and *Daubert* generally do not apply to opinion testimony. *Frye* or *Daubert* only arises when an attorney believes expert testimony offered by the opponent is based on demonstrably unreliable scientific principles. In such cases the attorney requests a *Frye* or *Daubert* hearing in an effort to exclude the expert testimony.

Physical Abuse Cases

When physical abuse is alleged, the most common defense is that the child's injuries were accidental. Expert testimony plays a key role in proving non-accidental injury (the ultimate factual issue). Judges allow physicians to describe the means used to inflict injury. For example, a physician may testify that a skull fracture was probably caused by a blow from a blunt instrument, such as a fist, foot, or board; by striking the child's head against an object; or by propelling the child into a wall, floor, or furniture item. Experts are permitted to estimate the amount of force required to inflict injury and to contrast those types of violent abusive forces against normal caretaking behavior or typical household accidents that do not generate such injurious forces. Experts may describe a child's developmental capabilities and indicate whether a child was capable of producing sufficient forces through their own mobility to self-injure or to place themselves in situations capable of producing serious injury.

Sexual Abuse Cases

Expert testimony in child sexual abuse cases falls into the following categories: (a) expert medical testimony describing presence or absence of physical evidence of sexual abuse, (b) expert psychological testimony offered to prove sexual abuse, (c) expert psychological testimony offered to rehabilitate a child's credibility following an attack on the child's credibility, and (d) expert testimony referring to a psychological syndrome.

Medical and Laboratory Evidence

The medical history obtained from the child and/or caretaker is critical to assessing and diagnosing possible sexual abuse. The medical history is often admissible as evidence in court under the medical diagnosis or treatment exception to the hearsay rule.

Although medical evidence (injury, DNA, STI) is present in only a small percentage of cases, when such evidence exists, judges permit qualified medical experts to describe the evidence. The medical expert describes the physical examination and any pertinent findings. In the absence of medical findings, an expert may testify that absence of physical evidence is not inconsistent with sexual abuse. Testimony explaining that lack of physical evidence does not rule out sexual abuse is important because some jurors believe that a child who was molested would be injured. Moreover, the defense attorney may focus the jury's attention on lack of physical evidence, necessitating expert testimony to help the jury understand that physical evidence is rare in confirmed cases of sexual abuse.

Judges allow experts to describe the results of examinations aided by colposcopy and permit experts to use photographs and other visual aids, such as genital drawings or anatomical dolls, to illustrate their testimony.

Expert Psychological Testimony Offered to Prove Sexual Abuse

Expert psychological testimony offered to prove abuse takes several forms. The expert might testify that a child has a "diagnosis" of child sexual abuse. The expert might eschew diagnostic terminology and testify, "In my opinion, to a reasonable degree of certainty, the child was sexually abused." Alternatively, the expert might state that a child's symptoms are "consistent" with sexual abuse. Whatever form the testimony takes, the purpose is the same: to prove abuse.

Psychological expert testimony offered to prove sexual abuse is controversial.

One critic of such testimony is psychologist Gary Melton, who argues that mental health professionals have no special skill at differentiating sexually abused children from non-abused children. Melton wrote, "There is no reason to believe that clinicians' skill in determining whether a child has been abused is the product of specialized knowledge."[22] Melton asserts that psychological testimony that a child was sexually abused is little more than an opinion the child was telling the truth, and courts reject expert testimony on truthfulness. Melton and Limber argue, "Under no circumstances should a court admit the opinion of a [mental health professional] about whether a particular child has been abused."[23] In a similar vein, Herman wrote, "The current finding of low overall accuracy in [psychological] clinical judgments about unconfirmed allegations of child sexual abuse is consistent with the almost universal consensus among top scientific experts that these evaluations currently have no firm scientific basis."[24] Melton, Herman, and like-minded scholars do not speak for all experts on child sexual abuse. Faller[25] captures the thinking of many clinicians when she writes, "There appears to be a fair amount of consensus among mental health professionals about both the strategy and the criteria for deciding whether a child has been sexually victimized."

Turning from the psychological literature to the courts, appellate courts around the country are divided on the admissibility of psychological testimony as proof of sexual abuse. A few state courts reject such testimony altogether (eg, *Commonwealth v Dunkle*[26]). Most state courts permit one or more forms of psychological expert testimony and reject others (eg, *Fox v State*[27], *State v Kallin*[28]). Most courts permit qualified experts to state that a child's behavior and symptoms are "consistent" with child sexual abuse. Often judges in family and juvenile court are more receptive to psychological expert testimony than judges presiding over criminal trials.

Expert Testimony Offered to Rehabilitate a Child's Credibility

Expert psychological testimony offered to prove that a child was sexually abused is complex and controversial. By contrast, expert testimony intended to rehabilitate a child's credibility is simple and well accepted by most courts. When a child testifies and describes sexual abuse, the defense attorney may cross-examine the child in an effort to undermine (impeach) the child's credibility in the eyes of the jury. A common impeachment strategy is to focus the jury's attention on the fact that the child delayed reporting maltreatment, was inconsistent, or recanted.

Once the child's credibility is attacked this way, the prosecutor is permitted to rehabilitate the child. Judges in most states permit expert rehabilitation testimony to help the jury understand delayed reporting, inconsistency, and recantation.[29] In addition, courts allow expert testimony to explain why some abused children are angry, why some children want to live with the person who abused them, why a victim might demonstrate flat affect following sexual assault, why an abused child might run away from home, and for other purposes.[1]

Expert Testimony Regarding Syndromes

The legal system is comfortable with medical syndromes that are offered in court to prove physical abuse. Thus judges routinely allow expert testimony on battered child syndrome, shaken baby syndrome, and Munchausen syndrome by proxy. When it comes to sexual abuse, however, no syndrome—medical or psychological—detects or diagnoses sexual abuse. Although no psychological syndrome is pathognomonic of sexual abuse, several psychological syndromes play roles in child sexual abuse litigation. Four psychological syndromes are briefly discussed.

Child Sexual Abuse Accommodation Syndrome (CSAAS)

Summit[30] described CSAAS as involving 5 characteristics frequently observed in sexually abused children: (1) secrecy; (2) helplessness; (3) entrapment and accommodation; (4) delayed, conflicted, and unconvincing disclosure; and (5) retraction. Summit's purpose in describing CSAAS was to provide a common language for professionals working to protect sexually abused children. Summit did not intend CSAAS as a diagnostic device. Summit observed, "The accommodation syndrome is neither an illness nor a diagnosis, and it can't be used to measure whether or not a child has been sexually abused."[31] The accommodation syndrome does not detect sexual abuse. Rather, CSAAS assumes that abuse occurred and explains the child's reaction to it. In 2002

Lyon[29] summarized the research supporting the reliability of the CSAAS.

Child sexual abuse accommodation syndrome has a place in the courtroom—not as proof that a child was abused, but as an aid to help explain why some sexually abused children delay reporting their abuse and why some children recant allegations of abuse. When the syndrome is confined to this rehabilitative purpose, the syndrome serves a useful forensic function.

Rape Trauma Syndrome (RTS)

Rape trauma syndrome was described by Burgess and Holmstrom[32] in 1974 as "the acute phase and long-term reorganization process that occurs as a result of forcible rape or attempted forcible rape. This syndrome of behavioral, somatic, and psychological reactions is an acute stress reaction to a life-threatening situation."

Although expert testimony on RTS is used most frequently in litigation involving adult rape victims, RTS is sometimes useful in child sexual abuse litigation. Expert testimony on RTS has been offered by prosecutors for 2 purposes: (1) to prove lack of consent to sexual relations and (2) to explain certain behaviors, such as delay in reporting rape, which jurors might misconstrue as evidence that rape did not occur.

RTS Proving Lack of Consent

In rape prosecutions involving adult victims, the spotlight often focuses on whether the victim consented. Courts are divided on the admissibility of RTS to prove lack of consent. Most courts reject RTS to prove lack of consent. In *People v Taylor*[33] for example, the New York Court of Appeals wrote, "Evidence of rape trauma syndrome does not by itself prove that the complainant was raped." The court concluded, "Evidence of rape trauma syndrome is inadmissible when it inescapably bears solely on proving that a rape occurred." The California Supreme Court reached a similar result in *People v Bledsoe*[34] in which the court ruled, "Expert testimony that a complaining witness suffers from rape trauma syndrome is not admissible to prove that the witness was raped."

In contrast to the New York and California courts, courts in several states conclude that RTS is admissible when the defendant asserts that the woman consented. In *State v Marks*,[35] for example, the Kansas Supreme Court wrote, "When consent is the defense in a prosecution for rape, qualified expert psychiatric testimony regarding the existence of 'rape trauma syndrome' is relevant and admissible."

It should be remembered that when the victim is a child, consent is not generally an issue because children are legally incapable of consenting to sexual relations. However, in some prosecutions involving child victims (eg, forcible rape), consent is an issue.

RTS Explaining a Victim's Behavior After the Attack

Most courts allow expert testimony on RTS to rehabilitate a child or adult victim's credibility after the defense attorney attacks the victim's credibility by emphasizing delayed reporting and other behaviors that jurors might construe as evidence the rape did not occur. In *People v Bledsoe,*[34] for example, the California Supreme Court wrote, "Expert testimony on rape trauma syndrome may play a particularly useful role by disabusing the jury of some widely held misconceptions about rape and rape victims, so that it may evaluate the evidence free of the constraints of popular myths."[34] In *People v Taylor,*[33] the New York Court of Appeals approved expert testimony explaining why a rape victim might not appear upset after the assault.

Courts that allow RTS to explain behaviors observed in rape victims place limits on such evidence. Thus several court decisions state that the expert should describe behaviors observed in rape victims as a group and should not refer to the victim in the case at hand.

Post-traumatic Stress Disorder (PTSD)

Judges generally permit qualified experts to testify that a patient has a diagnosis of PTSD. The form of the expert's testimony varies from case to case. In a given case an expert might be permitted to describe PTSD, discuss the types of trauma that cause the disorder, inform the jury that the victim has PTSD, and explain the victim's specific symptoms.

Parental Alienation Syndrome (PAS)

The most controversial psychological syndrome to find its way to court is Gardner's[36] PAS. Gardner described PAS as a psychiatric disorder observed in some parents fighting over custody of children in divorce court. One parent— the alienating parent—brainwashes the child to revile the other parent. When one divorcing parent accuses the other of abusing their child, PAS is sometimes used by the accused parent to support an argument that the accusation of abuse is a lie.

Parental alienation syndrome has been the subject of harsh criticism in the literature (American Psychological Association,[37] Bruch,[38] Faller,[39] Hoult,[40] Myers[41]). It is clear that PAS does not help distinguish true from false accusations. Given the lack of empirical support for PAS, and the consensus of professional opinion that PAS lacks validity, professionals are advised to avoid reliance on PAS.

Cross-examination and Impeachment of Expert Witnesses

Testifying begins with direct examination. During direct examination, the expert witness answers questions from the attorney who asked the expert to testify. After direct examination, the opposing attorney has the right to cross-examine the expert witness. Cross-examination is sometimes followed by redirect examination. Redirect examination affords the attorney who asked the expert to testify an opportunity to clarify issues that were raised on cross-examination.[42,43]

Positive and Negative Cross-examination

Cross-examination can be broken down into 2 types: positive and negative. With positive cross-examination, the cross-examining attorney does not attack the expert. Rather, the attorney questions the expert in a positive—even friendly—

way, seeking agreement from the expert on certain facts or inferences that may be helpful to the attorney's client. With negative cross-examination, by contrast, the attorney seeks to undermine (impeach) the expert's testimony. A cross-examining attorney who plans to employ both types of cross-examination typically begins with positive questioning in the hopes of eliciting favorable testimony from the expert. Negative cross-examination is postponed until positive cross-examination pans out.

Master the Facts of the Case

The skilled cross-examiner is a master of the facts of the case and shapes questions to manipulate the facts to favor the cross-examiner's client. To avoid manipulation, the expert witness must know the facts of the case as well as or better than the cross-examiner. An expert who fumbles with the facts loses credibility in the eyes of the jury.

Maintain Professional Demeanor

The experienced expert refuses to be cajoled, dragged, or tricked into verbal sparring with the cross-examiner. The professional is at all times just that— professional. Given the aggression of some cross-examiners—aggression that is sometimes laced with error, misinterpretation, and even personal attack— it is a challenge to maintain a calm, professional demeanor on the witness stand. Yet the professional must remember that the jury is looking to him or her for guidance and wisdom. The jury wants a strong expert, but not someone who takes off the gloves and fights it out with the cross-examiner.

This does not mean, of course, that the expert cannot employ pointed responses during cross-examination. The expert should express confidence when challenged and should not vacillate or equivocate in the face of attack. However, the expert should concede weak points and acknowledge conflicting evidence.

To illustrate how difficult it can be to maintain a professional demeanor during cross-examination, consider the following line of questioning by a cross-examiner who is hoping to convince the jury that the expert is not telling "the truth, the whole truth, and nothing but the truth." The cross-examiner asks: "Doctor you have stated your opinion here today haven't you?" "You have cited several research studies in support of your position, correct?" "You are aware that there are several limitations to those studies are you not?" "You are aware that those studies have been critiqued in the professional literature?" "Nevertheless you chose to offer up those studies in support of your opinion?" "You did not disclose each and every limitation about those studies during your testimony on direct examination did you?" "You took an oath to tell the whole truth, did you not?" "Wouldn't you agree that all of these limitations are part of the 'whole truth' that needs to be disclosed when discussing these studies?" "So, if I hadn't brought out these points on cross-examination, the jury would never have learned of these limitations?" "So are we to understand that your understanding of the obligation to tell the 'whole truth' is whatever information you choose to disclose and whatever conflicting information the other side is smart enough to raise?"

The honest, well-informed, well-prepared, ethical expert is understandably outraged at the insinuation contained in the attorney's attack. Yet to respond with moral outrage or, worse, to "lose your cool" undermines the expert's credibility in the eyes of the jury. Take a deep breath and respond with strength and professionalism. Point out that during direct examination you *did* discuss the principle limitations of the studies—you have nothing to hide. You might add, "If there are particular aspects of any of the studies I relied on, please bring them to my attention and I will be happy to discuss them."

Ask for Clarification

Professionals should not answer a question unless they fully understand it. When in doubt, they should ask the attorney to clarify. Such a request does not show weakness. After all, if a question is not understood, you can bet the jury doesn't either. When a cross-examiner's question is 2 or 3 questions in 1, the other attorney may object that the question is "compound." Absent an objection, it is proper for the expert to respond to the question by asking the cross-examiner which of the several questions the attorney would like answered.

Leading Questions During Cross-examination

The key to successful cross-examination is controlling what the witness says in response to the cross-examiner's ques-

tions. With the goal of witness control in mind, the cross-examining attorney asks leading—often highly leading—questions. Unlike the attorney conducting direct examination, who is not supposed to ask leading questions, the cross-examiner has free reign to ask all the leading questions the examiner desires. Indeed, some experienced cross-examiners almost never ask non-leading questions during cross-examination. The cross-examiner seeks to control the expert with leading questions that require short, specific answers, preferably limited to "yes" or "no." The cross-examiner keeps the witness hemmed in with such leading questions, and seldom asks "why" or "how" something happened. "Why" and "how" questions relinquish control to the expert; the relinquishing of control is precisely what the cross-examiner does not want.

When an expert attempts to explain an answer to a leading question, the cross-examiner may interrupt and say, "Please just answer yes or no." If the expert persists, the cross-examiner may ask the judge to admonish the expert to limit answers to the questions asked. Experts are understandably frustrated when an attorney thwarts efforts at clarification. It is sometimes proper to say, "Counsel, it is not possible for me to answer with a simple yes or no. May I explain myself?" Chadwick advises, "When a question is posed in a strictly 'yes or no' fashion, but the correct answer is 'maybe,' the witness should find a way to express the true answer. A direct appeal to the judge may be helpful in some cases."[17] Judges sometimes permit witnesses to amplify their opinion during cross-examination.

Remember that after cross-examination there is redirect examination, during which the attorney who asked you to testify is allowed to ask further questions. During redirect examination, you have an opportunity to clarify matters that were left unclear during cross-examination.

Undermine the Expert's Facts, Inferences, or Conclusions

One of the most effective cross-examination techniques with expert witnesses is to get the expert to agree to the facts, inferences, and conclusions that support the expert's opinion, and then to dispute one or more of those facts, inferences, or conclusions. Consider a case where a physician testifies a child experienced vaginal penetration. The cross-examiner begins by committing the doctor to the facts and assumptions underlying the opinion. The attorney might say, "So doctor, your opinion is based exclusively on the history, the physical examination, and on what the child told you. Is that correct?" "And there is nothing else you relied on to form your opinion. Is that correct?" The cross-examiner commits the doctor to a specific set of facts and assumptions so that when the attorney disputes those facts or assumptions, the doctor's opinion cannot be justified on some other basis.

Once the cross-examiner pins down the basis of the doctor's opinion, the examiner attacks the opinion by disputing one or more of the facts, inferences, or conclusions that support it. The attorney might ask whether the doctor's opinion would change if certain facts were different (a hypothetical question). The attorney might press the doctor to acknowledge alternative explanations for the doctor's conclusion. The attorney might ask the doctor whether experts could come to different conclusions based on the same facts.

Rather than attack the doctor's facts, inferences, and conclusions during cross-examination, the attorney may limit cross-examination to pinning the doctor down to a limited set of facts, inferences, and conclusions, and then, when the doctor has left the witness stand, offer another expert to contradict the data supporting the doctor's testimony.

Learned Treatises

The cross-examiner may seek to undermine the expert's testimony by confronting the expert with books or articles (called *learned treatises*) that contradict the expert. The rules on impeachment with learned treatises vary from state to state. There is agreement on one thing, however. When an expert is confronted with a sentence or a paragraph selected by an attorney from an article or chapter, the expert has the right to put the selected passage in context by reading surrounding material. The expert might say to the cross-examining attorney, "Counsel, I cannot comment on the sentence you have selected unless I first read the entire article. If you will permit me to read the article, I'll be happy to comment on the sentence that interests you."

Bias

The cross-examiner may raise the possibility that the expert is biased. For example, if the expert is part of a multidisciplinary child abuse team, the cross-examiner might proceed as follows:

Q: Now doctor, you are employed by Children's Hospital, isn't that correct?

A: Right.

Q: At the hospital, are you a member of the multidisciplinary team that investigates allegations of child abuse?

A: The team performs medical examinations and interviews. We do not investigate. The police investigate. But yes, I am a member of the hospital's multidisciplinary child abuse team.

Q: Your team regularly performs investigative examinations and interviews at the request of the prosecuting attorney's office, isn't that correct?

A: Yes.

Q: When you complete your investigation for the prosecutor, you prepare a report for the prosecutor, don't you?

A: A report and recommendation is prepared and placed in the child's medical record. On request, the team provides a copy of the report to the prosecutor and, I might add, to the defense.

Q: After your team prepares its report and provides a copy to the prosecutor, you often come to court to testify as an expert witness for the prosecution in child abuse cases, isn't that right, doctor?

A: Yes.

Q: Do you usually testify for the prosecution rather than the defense?

A: Correct.

Q: In fact, would I be correct in saying that you always testify for the prosecution and never for the defense?

A: I am willing to testify for the defense, but so far I have always testified for the prosecution.

Q: Thank you, doctor. I have no further questions.

The cross-examiner is seeking to portray the doctor as biased in favor of the prosecution, but does not ask, "Well then, doctor, isn't it a fact that because of your close working relationship with the prosecution, you are biased in favor of the prosecution?" The cross-examiner knows the answer is "no," so the cross-examiner simply plants seeds of doubt in the jurors' minds and then, when it is time for closing argument, the cross-examiner reminds the jury of the doctor's close working relationship with the prosecution.

Recall that cross-examination is followed by redirect examination. During redirect, the prosecutor might ask, "Doctor, in light of the defense attorney's questions about your job on the multidisciplinary team, are you biased in favor of the prosecution?" The doctor can then set the record straight.

To further insulate against potential claims of bias, the expert should cooperate with opposing counsel and be willing to discuss the case before trial. An expert who refuses to do this is vulnerable to cross-examination questions that expose the lack of cooperation and that give the cross-examiner ammunition to argue that the expert is in league with one side in the case.

Bias can be established by showing that an expert is unwilling to change an opinion when confronted with data that conflict with the opinion. Indicate that you are willing to look at additional data. An open mind is the hallmark of the unbiased expert.

Impeach the Expert Who Violates Ethical Standards

A potentially damaging area of cross-examination involves the use of ethical standards to impeach an expert witness. There are few things that undermine an expert's credibility more rapidly than a suggestion that the expert violated the ethical standards of the expert's profession. The skilled cross-examiner is familiar with the applicable ethical standards and looks for opportunities to use them against you. As part of pretrial preparation, the professional should discuss applicable ethical guidelines with the attorney who asked him or her to testify. It may be advisable to provide the attorney with a copy of the ethical standards.

The Irresponsible Expert

Experts who are knowledgeable, ethical, and honest occasionally have markedly different opinions. In some cases, however, "expert" witnesses offer testimony that is so far off base that it descends into the realm of irresponsible expert testimony. Chadwick and Krous[16] described the following criteria for irresponsible testimony: (a) lack of qualifications to support opinions, (b) unique theories of causation that are contrary to vast medical literature and consensus, (c) unique interpretation of findings, (d) misquoting the literature (or misunderstanding the nature of the science), and (e) blatantly false statements about the science or their qualifications.

Barnes[44] suggested other criteria to gauge irresponsible expert testimony: (a) the expert omits important facts or knowledge that is pertinent to opinions being offered; (b) the expert's opinion lies outside the expert's field of expertise; (c) the expert offers complicated and highly technical testimony in what appears to be a deliberate attempt to confuse the jury; (d) the expert's testimony appears to be scripted or choreographed; (e) the expert's testimony contradicts the expert's own writing on the topic; and (f) the expert misrepresents facts, science, or literature.

In addition to the factors mentioned by Chadwick and Krous[16] and Barnes,[44] the following can be markers of irresponsible expert testimony: (a) the expert relies on literature or data that are controversial and have been subjected to extensive peer critique, but the expert does not acknowledge the controversy; (b) the expert is not current on relevant literature; (c) the expert is unwilling to discuss or concede limitations of the data supporting the expert's testimony; (d) the expert fails to consider injuries in their entirety; (e) the expert focuses only on isolated injuries, ignoring the broader context; and (f) the expert's opinion is predicated on remote possibilities "dressed up" as reasonable medical certainty.

The Child as an Interviewee and a Witness

As discussed previously, psychological expertise plays a role in child sexual abuse litigation. Additionally, psychological expertise is relevant to the following aspects of child maltreatment litigation: children's memory and suggestibility, proper and improper interview techniques, children's competence to testify, testimony from children with intellectual impairment, children's understanding of time, and children's capacity to testify face-to-face with the person accused of abuse.

Interviewing and Suggestibility

Prior to the 1980s, children's suggestibility and the techniques used to interview children were seldom the subject of controversy in child abuse litigation.[45] In the late 1980s and the 1990s, however, concerns about suggestibility and defective interviewing took center stage.[46,47] Today a common defense strategy in child sexual abuse cases is to criticize the way a child was interviewed.[1] The defense argues that suggestive interview questions distorted the child's memory or instilled ideas of maltreatment that never occurred.[48] To support this strategy, defense counsel sometimes offers expert testimony concerning children's suggestibility, memory, and proper interview techniques.

There are several types of behavioral science testimony involving interviewing techniques and children's memory and suggestibility. First, an expert may provide a general description of children's memory and suggestibility. Second, an expert may critique the interview of a particular child. Finally, an expert might be prepared to offer an opinion on whether interview questions affected a particular child's memory or credibility.[49]

American courts are generally receptive to the first 2 types of expert testimony. Thus the Ohio Supreme Court wrote, "A defendant in a child sexual abuse case may present testimony as to the proper protocol for interviewing child victims regarding their abuse…. Most jurors lack the knowledge of accepted practices in interviewing child victims, and expert testimony on the issue is therefore admissible."[50] The Washington Supreme Court approved expert testimony "regarding the effects of specific interview techniques and protocols."[51] Courts generally do not allow experts to opine that interview questions rendered particular children unreliable, viewing such testimony as inappropriate testimony on credibility.

Some courts exclude expert testimony describing children's suggestibility. The Washington Supreme Court wrote in 2004 that the suggestibility of young children is sufficiently well known to the public and that expert testimony on suggestibility may be unnecessary and therefore inadmissible. The court wrote, "The general principle that younger children are more susceptible to suggestion is 'well within the understanding of the jury.' "[51] In the same vein, Lyon wrote, "Juries likely understand that young children are susceptible to coercive and suggestive questions."[46] It remains to be seen whether other courts will adopt the Washington court's conclusion that expert testimony on the basic principle of suggestibility is unnecessary.

Testimonial Competence

Before a person may testify, the judge must determine that the individual is competent. As a practical matter, testimonial competence is only an issue with children, elders, and persons with intellectual disability. Until the 1970s, the law in many US states said that children younger than a specified age—typically 10 or 12—were presumptively incompetent to testify. Each child younger than the specified age had to be questioned by the judge or the attorneys (called a *competency examination)* to determine whether the child possessed the following attributes of testimonial competence: (a) capacity to observe, (b) ability to communicate so as to be understood, (c) sufficient memory capacity to remember events, (d) sufficient intelligence to testify, (e) understanding of the difference between truth and falsehood, (f) appreciation of the duty to tell the truth in court, and (g) understanding that false testimony may result in punishment. Following questioning on these matters, most children were found competent.

Today the law in nearly all states is that every person, regardless of age, is competent to be a witness, and competency examinations are no longer necessary. Yet when questions arise about the competence of particular children, especially young children, judges conduct competency examinations.[1,52]

With training and experience, judges and attorneys conduct effective compe-tency examinations. Expert behavioral science testimony is seldom necessary to assist in the process. In rare instances, a child's competence is so in doubt that the judge orders the child evaluated by a mental health professional who may then be asked to provide expert testimony including recommendations to the court and the attorneys on how to properly question the child.

Testimony From Children With Intellectual Impairment

When testimony from children with mental retardation is offered, the objection is typically that the disability renders the child incompetent. Although a modicum of intelligence is necessary to testify, the law does not require "average" or "normal" intelligence. Children with below average intelligence are permitted to testify if preliminary questioning reveals that they possess the attributes of testimonial competence discussed previously.[53,54]

Children's Understanding of Time

Time is often of the essence in litigation. For example, criminal charges must be filed within the applicable statute of limitations, making it necessary to establish as precisely as possible the date on which the crime occurred. Additionally, the defendant has the right to know with as much precision as possible the date the alleged crime occurred.

When the victim is a child, establishing dates and times is complicated by children's limited understanding of time.[55] Fortunately, judges understand children's difficulty with time.[56] The Utah Supreme Court spoke for itself and other courts when it wrote, "We have also acknowledged that in child sexual abuse prosecutions, identifying the specific date, time, or place of the offense is often difficult owing to the inability of young victims to provide this information. Responding to the realities of cognitive development, we have been less demanding of exact times and dates when young children are involved."[57] Although judges are typically aware of children's limited understanding of time, many jurors are not. In rare cases, therefore, expert testimony is provided to help jurors understand a child's developing understanding of time.

Children's Capacity to Testify Face-to-Face With the Accused

Testifying in court is difficult for child witnesses, although most are able to testify effectively, particularly when they are prepared for the experience. For some children, however, the prospect of testifying just a few feet from the defendant is overwhelming, rendering testimony impossible. Nearly all states have laws that allow select children to testify outside the physical presence of the defendant, typically via closed-circuit television.

When a prosecutor seeks to use closed-circuit testimony for a child witness, the defense typically objects that allowing the child to testify this way violates the defendant's right under the Sixth Amendment to the US Constitution to confront the prosecution's witnesses. The Sixth Amendment guarantees persons accused of crime the right to face-to-face confrontation with the witnesses against them, including children.

In *Maryland v Craig*,[58] the US Supreme Court ruled that the right to face-to-face confrontation is important but not absolute. In select cases, the right to face-to-face confrontation gives way to the state's interest in protecting children from harm. Before face-to-face confrontation may be curtailed, however, the judge must be convinced that face-to-face confrontation is likely to impair the child's ability to testify and/or traumatize the child. State laws and appellate court decisions take several approaches to the evidence required to dispense with face-to-face confrontation.[1] Most appellate court decisions suggest that such evidence include testimony from a mental health expert to support the judge's conclusion. In some states, confrontation may only be curtailed if a face-to-face encounter with the defendant would render the child completely unable to testify. Other states focus less on the child's availability to testify and more on the psychological harm caused by face-to-face confrontation. There is a small body of psychological research on the impact testifying has on children, and this literature is relevant to the judge's inquiry.[59,60]

When balancing a defendant's right to face-to-face confrontation against the potential harm to the child, judges consider numerous factors, including the following. First, if the child had other face-to-face encounters with the defendant and fared poorly, then the judge has data to predict the impact of face-to-face confrontation at trial. Second, what was the child's reaction when testifying was mentioned? If testifying was mentioned at home, in therapy, or in other situations, the child's reaction is relevant. In *Iowa v Lomholt*,[61] a 4-year-old child's therapist testified that the child became upset when discussing abuse. On one occasion, the child wet her pants. When the therapist tried to discuss the defendant, the child resorted to baby talk and tried to distract the therapist. The court ruled that it was proper to allow the child to testify via closed-circuit television. The third factor considered by judges is evidence suggesting that face-to-face confrontation will impair a child's ability to communicate and perhaps, more importantly, the ability to provide accurate and reliable information. Finally, the judge considers evidence that face-to-face confrontation will likely harm a child's mental health. Courts often allow expert testimony to shed light on the probable impact of face-to-face confrontation. The expert in many cases is the child's therapist.

Conclusion

The professions of medicine and law sometimes seem like ships passing in the night, yet if children are to be protected, physicians and attorneys must put aside their differences and work together. Only genuine interdisciplinary cooperation holds realistic hope of reducing the tragic number of abused and neglected children.

References

1. Myers J. *Myers On Evidence In Child, Domestic, And Elder Abuse Cases.* New York, NY: Aspen Law & Business; 2005

2. Jones DPH. *Interviewing the Sexually Abused Child: Investigation of Suspected Abuse.* Gaskell, United Kingdom: Royal College of Psychiatrists; 1992

3. *Crawford v Washington,* 541 US 36 (2004)

4. *Davis v Washington,* 126 US 2266 (2006)

5. *State v Bobadilla,* 709 NW2d 243 (Minn 2006)

6. *State v Blue,* 717 NW2d 558 (ND 2006)

7. *State v Moses,* 119 P3d 906 (Wash Ct App 2005)

8. *Griner v State,* 899 A2d 189 (Md Ct App 2006)

9. *Commonwealth v DeOliveria,* 849 NE2d 243 (Mass 2006)

10. *Hobgood v State,* 926 So2d 847 (Miss 2006)

11. American Medical Association. *Code of Ethics.* http://www.ama-assn.org/apps/pf_new/pf_online?f_n=browse&doc=policyfiles/HnE/E-0.001.HTM&&s_t=&st_p=&nth=1&prev_pol=policyfiles/CEJA-TOC.HTM&nxt_pol=policyfiles/HnE/E-0.001.HTM&. Accessed June 4, 2007

12. American Nurses Association. *Code of Ethics for Nurses.* http://www.nursingworld.org/ethics/ecode.htm. Accessed June 4, 2007

13. Gutheil TG, Appelbaum PS. *Clinical Handbook of Psychiatry and the Law.* New York, NY: McGraw-Hill; 1982

14. *Tarasoff v Regents of the University of California,* 551 P2d 334 (Cal 1976)

15. Cal. Civ. Code 43.92 (1986)

16. Chadwick DL, Krous HF. Irresponsible testimony by medical experts in cases involving the physical abuse and neglect of children. *Child Maltreat.* 1997;2:313–321

17. Chadwick DL. Preparation for court testimony in child abuse cases. *Pediatr Clin North Am.* 1990;37:955–970

18. *People v Gardeley,* 927 P2d 713 (Cal 1997)

19. *Frye v United States,* 293 F 1013 (DC Cir 1923)

20. *Daubert v Merrell Dow Pharmaceuticals, Inc.,* 509 US 579 (1993)

21. *Kumho Tire Company, Ltd. v Carmichael,* 526 US 137 (1999)

22. Melton GB, Petrila J, Poythress NG, Slobogin C. *Psychological Evaluations for the Courts: A Handbook for Mental Health Professionals and Lawyers.* 2nd ed. New York, NY: Gildford; 1997

23. Melton GB, Limber S. Psychologists' involvement in cases of child maltreatment. *Am Psychol.* 1989;44:1225–1233

24. Herman S. Improving decision making in forensic child sexual abuse evaluations. *Law Hum Behav.* 2005;29:87–120

25. Faller KC. *Understanding Child Sexual Maltreatment.* Newbury Park, CA: Sage; 1990

26. *Commonwealth v Dunkle,* 602 A2d 830 (Pa 1992)

27. *Fox v State,* 175 SW3d 475 (Tex Ct App 2005)

28. *State v Kallin,* 877 P2d 138 (Utah 1994)

29. Lyon TD. Scientific support for expert testimony on child sexual abuse accommodation. In: Conte JR, ed. *Critical Issues in Child Sexual Abuse: Historical, Legal, and Psychological Perspectives.* Thousand Oaks, CA: Sage; 2002:107–138

30. Summit RC. The child sexual abuse accommodation syndrome. *Child Abuse Negl.* 1983;7:177–193

31. Meinig MB. Profile of Roland Summit. *Violence Update.* 1992;1:6

32. Burgess A, Holmstrom L. Rape trauma syndrome. *Am J Psychiatry.* 1974;131:981–986

33. *People v Taylor,* 552 NE2d 131 (NY 1990)

34. *People v Bledsoe,* 681 P2d 291 (Cal 1984)

35. *State v Marks,* 647 P2d 1292 (Kan 1982)

36. Gardner RA. *The Parental Alienation Syndrome and the Differentiation Between Fabricated and Genuine Child Sexual Abuse.* Creskill, NJ: Creative Therapeutics; 1992

37. American Psychological Association. *Violence and the Family.* Washington, DC: American Psychological Association; 1996

38. Bruch CS. Parental alienation syndrome and parental alienation: getting it wrong in child custody cases. *Fam Law Q.* 2001;35:527–552

39. Faller KC. The parental alienation syndrome: what is it and what data support it? *Child Maltreat.* 1998;3:100–115

40. Hoult J. The evidentiary admissibility of parental alienation syndrome: science, law, and policy. *Child Leg Rights J.* 2006;26:1–61

41. Myers JEB. *A Mother's Nightmare—Incest: A Practical Legal Guide for Parents and Professionals.* Thousand Oaks, CA: Sage; 1997

42. Brodsky SL. *Coping With Cross-Examination and Other Pathways to Effective Testimony.* Washington, DC: American Psychological Association, 2004.

43. Stern P. *Preparing and Presenting Expert Testimony in Child Abuse Litigation: A Guide for Expert Witnesses and Attorneys.* Thousand Oaks, CA: Sage; 1997

44. Barnes PD. Ethical issues in imaging nonaccidental injury: child abuse. *Top Mag Reson Imaging.* 2002;13:85–93

45. Myers JEB, Diedrich S, Lee D, Fincher KM, Stern R. Professional writing on child sexual abuse from 1900 to 1975: dominant themes and impact on prosecution. *Child Maltreat.* 1999;4:201–216

46. Lyon TD. Expert testimony on the suggestibility of children: does it fit? In: Bottoms BL, Kovera MB, McAuliff BD, eds. *Children, Social Science, and the Law.* New York, NY: Cambridge University Press; 2002:378–411

47. Lyon TD. The new wave in children's suggestibility research: a critique. *Cornell Law Rev.* 1999;84:1004–1086

48. *State v Michaels,* 642 A2d 1372 (NJ 1994)

49. *State v Wigg,* 899 A2d 233 (Vt 2005)

50. *State v Gersin,* 668 NE2d 486 (Ohio 1996)

51. *State v Willis,* 87 P3d 1164 (Wash 2004)

52. Lyon TD. Child witnesses and the oath: empirical evidence. *South Calif Law Rev.* 2000;73:1017–1074

53. *In re Erica A,* 73 Cal App 4th 1390, (Cal 1999)

54. *United States v Benn,* 476 F2d 1127 (DC Cir 1972)

55. Friedman WJ, Lyon TD. Development of temporal-reconstructive abilities. *Child Dev.* 2005;76:1202–1216

56. *United States v Cano,* 61 MJ 74 (CAAF 2005)

57. *State v Taylor,* 116 P3d 360 (Utah 2005)

58. *Maryland v Craig,* 497 US 836 (1990)

59. Goodman GS, Taub EP, Jones DPH, et al. Testifying in criminal court. *Monogr Soc Res Child Dev.* 1992;57:1–163

60. Henry J. System intervention trauma to child sexual abuse victims following disclosure. *J Interpers Violence.* 1997;12:499–512

61. *Iowa V. Lomholt,* No. 4311 At 3 (Iowa Dist. Ct. For Mitchell County July 8, 1996)

Medical and Psychological Sequelae of Child Abuse and Neglect

David Rubin

University of Pennsylvania School of Medicine
Safe Place: The Center for Child Protection and Health,
Children's Hospital of Philadelphia

James A. Feinstein

Children's Hospital of Philadelphia

Carol D. Berkowitz

Department of Pediatrics, Harbor-UCLA Medical Center David Geffen
School of Medicine at UCLA

Introduction

Much attention has been focused on the immediate medical and psychological effects of child abuse and neglect on the victim; less is known about the long-term consequences of child abuse that may manifest themselves in the months to years after abuse or neglect occurs. These long-term effects may be either a direct result of physical trauma (ie, non-accidental head trauma, skeletal trauma) or secondary to the biopsychosocial consequences of child abuse and neglect (ie, psychological, neuropsychiatric, and behavioral impact on health and well-being). It is imperative that health care providers recognize the potential long-term effects of child abuse in order to institute appropriate interventions that reduce or eliminate the associated morbidity and mortality.

In this chapter, we will first review the current literature and research regarding the long-term sequelae of child abuse and neglect. Specifically, we will provide an assessment of the available literature and research, and then review the findings in detail by individual organ systems. Then, because a significant minority of child abuse victims enters the foster care system, we will discuss the long-term medical and psychological consequences children in foster care face. Continuing to use the example of foster care, we will examine interventions and policy changes that have been implemented to improve the medical and mental health care delivered to foster children. Finally, we will introduce the concept of resiliency and its role in preventing or diminishing the long-term effects of child abuse and neglect.

Overview of Research Addressing the Long-term Medical and Psychological Effects of Child Abuse and Neglect

Over the past 20 years, many studies have attempted to identify and investigate the long-term effects of child abuse and neglect on its victims. Most of these data are compiled from patients' recollections during psychological counseling sessions, medical examinations and assessments, or surveys conducted during clinic visits for patients meeting certain screening criteria. However, a large proportion of the published research prior to the 1990s suffers from significant methodological flaws that limit both the reliability and generalizabilty of the data, including the use of select populations, the absence of control populations, the inconsistent definition of neglect and abuse, the presence of multiple confounding variables, and the presence of significant recall and selection biases.[1]

More recently, efforts have been made to address these shortcomings and improve the quality of research examining the long-term effects of child abuse and neglect. Dr Vincent Felitti and his research team[1] developed the Adverse Childhood Experiences

(ACE) instrument (Box 25.1) in order to standardize the way in which clinicians collect information about a patient's lifetime exposure to adverse childhood experiences, including abuse and neglect. Using the ACE instrument, Felitti et al[1-12] conducted several large-scale surveys within the Kaiser-Permanente health system to examine the relationship between adverse childhood events and a variety of health behaviors and outcomes.

The most widely cited of the studies involved a survey of 13,494 adults using the ACE instrument.[1] Each of the respondents also had completed an independent standardized medical evaluation, which allowed researchers to examine the associations between the survey responses and the respondents' health states. More than 50% of the respondents endorsed at least one category on the ACE instrument; 25% reported 2 or more categories of childhood exposures. The study determined that subjects who had endorsed multiple items on the ACE instrument had increased health risks for adult disease (ie, ischemic heart disease, cancer, chronic lung disease, skeletal fractures, and liver disease) and negative health behaviors (ie, alcoholism, smoking, drug abuse, depression, suicide attempts, obesity, inactivity, and sexual promiscuity).[1-12]

Although studies employing the ACE instrument provide the best available data regarding the long-term consequences of child abuse and neglect, the data are subject to certain limitations.[1] Most importantly, the ACE studies suffer from potential recall bias. For example, adults with poor medical

BOX 25.1
Adverse Childhood Experiences (ACE) Instrument[a]

The ACE questionnaire queried 7 categories of specific childhood events and quantified the frequency with which such events were experienced.

Psychological Abuse
While you were growing up during your first 18 years of life, did a parent or other adult in the household

1. Often or very often swear at, insult, or put you down?
2. Often or very often act in a way that made you afraid that you would be physically hurt?

Physical Abuse
While you were growing up during your first 18 years of life, did a parent or other adult in the household

1. Often or very often push, grab, shove, or slap you?
2. Often or very often hit you so hard that you had marks or were injured?

Sexual Abuse
While you were growing up during your first 18 years of life, did an adult or person at least 5 years older ever

1. Touch or fondle you in a sexual way?
2. Have you touch their body in a sexual way?
3. Attempt oral, anal, or vaginal intercourse with you?
4. Actually have oral, anal, or vaginal intercourse with you?

Substance Abuse
While you were growing up during your first 18 years of life, did you

1. Live with anyone who was a problem drinker or alcoholic?
2. Live with anyone who used street drugs?

Mental Illness
While you were growing up during your first 18 years of life

1. Was a household member depressed or mentally ill?
2. Did a household member attempt suicide?

Mother Treated Violently
While you were growing up during your first 18 years of life, was your mother (or stepmother)

1. Sometimes, often, or very often pushed, grabbed, slapped, or had something thrown at her?
2. Sometimes, often, or very often kicked, bitten, hit with a fist, or hit with something hard?
3. Ever repeatedly hit over at least a few minutes?
4. Ever threatened with, or hurt by, a knife or gun?

Criminal Behavior in Household
While you were growing up in the first 18 years of life

1. Did a household member go to prison?

[a]Adapted from Felitti VJ, Anda RF, Nordenberg D, et al. Relationship of childhood abuse and household dysfunction to many of the leading causes of death in adults. The Adverse Childhood Experiences (ACE) Study. *Am J Prev Med*. 1998;14:245–258.

and/or psychological health may be more inclined to link their problems to and lay blame on adverse childhood events. Similarly, adults with good health, but who were also abused as children, may fail to report having experienced adverse childhood events. In both of these cases, the sample population may not be representative of the actual population. Additionally, the associations made between ACE status and long-term health effects are correlations and do not prove causality, although Felitti et al[1-12] demonstrated dose-dependent relationships between the number of ACE categories endorsed and the risk for adult disease and negative health behaviors.

These limitations notwithstanding, the ACE studies, as well as subsequent similarly conducted studies, have provided recent evidence for what is known about child abuse and neglect and its long-term impact on health, as described in the following sections. Although the causal pathways have yet to be elucidated, the data provide clear and compelling evidence that adverse childhood events have long-term consequences on adult health and well-being.[1]

Medical and Psychological Conditions Associated With Childhood Abuse and Neglect

Neurologic/Developmental Conditions

While most inflicted injuries heal with relatively little long-term disability, they can lead either to death or to permanent and severe neurologic problems, including motor deficits, blindness,

seizure, cerebral palsy, or permanent cognitive impairment.[13] Death from inflicted head trauma is reported to occur in approximately 13% to 36% of cases, and exceeds the 6% to 12% mortality rate for non-inflicted head injuries.[13] Children who survive non-inflicted head trauma may suffer from the aforementioned long-term neuro-developmental consequences of head injury.[14,15] Such individuals often require constant supervision and care, which may necessitate placement within medical institutions, posing significant financial and management challenges to society.[14,15]

The neuropathologic changes occurring after traumatic brain injury have been reported.[16] Directly after brain injury, there is often cortical and subcortical injury, including contusion, hemorrhage, hypoxic-ischemic damage, axonal damage, and cerebral edema. As acute lesions resolve, permanent damage becomes evident, including the development of encephalopathies, such as multicystic encephalomalacia, porencephaly, generalized white matter attenuation, diffuse cortical atrophy, microgyria, ulegyria, or hydrocephalus ex vacuo. Non-injured areas may also undergo reorganization, leading to progressive cortical dysplasia with cytoarchitectural disorganization, laminar obliteration, or morphological and functional synaptic reorganization of neurons.[16-20]

The changes occurring in both the damaged and undamaged portions of the brain may influence an abused child's subsequent neurologic and psychological maturation.[16,20] In one prospective longitudinal study of 25 children who suffered from head trauma, after a mean follow-up time of 59 months, investigators found that nearly 68% of the children were neurodevelopmentally abnormal, with 36% of the children having severe disabilities that required skilled care.[13] The various neurologic disabilities present in the study population included speech and language disorders (64%), motor deficits (60%), behavioral problems (52%), visual deficits (48%), and epilepsy (20%).[13] Cognition was also affected in a number of individuals; the mean psychomotor index (normal 100, SD +/- 15) was found to be 69.9 (SD +/- 25.73) and the mean mental development index (normal 100, SD +/- 15) was 74.53 (SD +/- 28.55).[13]

Musculoskeletal Conditions

Both skeletal fractures and burn injuries may lead to functional impairment and disfigurement, although most children recover from such injuries without significant residual disabilities. Victims of physical child abuse who suffer from skeletal fracture(s) routinely have good outcomes; however, some fractures may have a complicated course of recovery and lead to limb-length discrepancies that require further surgical intervention. Burn injuries to the limbs may impair an individual's ability to write, ambulate, or perform activities of daily living. Facial burns may impact an individual's self-esteem, as well as others' perception of the individual (ie, as manifest through the inability to obtain employment, etc). With appropriate

rehabilitation and therapy, however, burn victims with significant injury (up to 40% of the total body surface area) may enjoy a normal quality of life.[21]

Victims who do not suffer the direct consequences of physical abuse may still experience failure to thrive (FTT) or growth impairment.[22] There are reports of child abuse and neglect victims who suffer from psychosocial dwarfism, which is the residual infant-like appearance, wasting, and stunting of growth of affected individuals.[23] With appropriate recognition and intervention, most notably through establishing a nurturing caregiver relationship and living environment, FTT or growth impairment may be reversed.[24] While data suggest that children with abuse-related FTT may catch up in physical growth, children may not make a similar recovery in terms of neurodevelopment.[13,25]

Gastrointestinal Conditions

Multiple reports link gastrointestinal (GI) disturbances (ie, functional abdominal pain, irritable bowel syndrome [IBS], non-ulcer dyspepsia) and diseases (ie, liver disease) to a history of prior sexual abuse.[1,7,26–29] One study reported that the overall prevalence of sexual abuse in GI clinic patients approached 44%.[27] The explanations for this association are myriad. For example, the alteration in patterns of gastric secretion after the delivery of bad news was first reported in 1929[30]; subsequent research has confirmed the effects of psychological stress on GI secretion and GI motility.[31] The physiological basis for these symptoms is believed to be a result of disturbances to neurotransmitter signaling in the GI nervous system.[31] More recently, research in the field of IBS and inflammatory bowel disease (IBD) has demonstrated the effects of severe, sustained life stressors on the modulation of GI symptoms.[32,33]

While the precise etiology of GI symptoms in those with a history of childhood sexual abuse is unknown, current research indicates a higher than normal incidence of GI disturbances in this population.[34] Felitti[34] noted this association when examining the prevalence of GI complaints among survey respondents who had endorsed multiple categories on the ACE instrument. Sixty-four percent of those respondents with a history of adverse childhood events had GI symptoms or complaints, compared with 39% without a history of adverse childhood events.[34] In a similarly designed study, which used a mailed questionnaire, in patients with GI symptoms or complaints, 41% of women and 11% of men reported some type of prior abuse.[26]

In particular, functional abdominal disturbances such as IBS have been noted to occur more frequently among patients with a history of childhood sexual abuse.[26] Irritable bowel syndrome is typically characterized by a history of 3 or more months of recurrent abdominal pain, usually relieved by a bowel movement; changes in the frequency or consistency of stool; disturbed defecation at least 25% of the time (ie, altered stool frequency, form, or passage); and an association with bloating or the sensation of abdominal

distention.[31] Other symptoms reported by patients include nausea, early satiety, dysphagia, lethargy, back pain, thigh pain, urinary frequency, urinary urgency, dyspareunia, and/or symptoms of fibromyalgia.[31]

Initial studies correlating IBS with a history of sexual abuse were based on questionnaires that queried female GI clinic patients about their history of prior sexual abuse, their GI symptoms, and their use of health services. Fifty-three percent of those with functional GI disturbances (ie, IBS) reported a history of sexual abuse, while only 37% of those with organic GI disease (ie, IBD) reported a history of sexual abuse.[27] In a similar study comparing patients with IBS to patients with IBD, 54% versus 5%, respectively, had a history of severe abuse during childhood or sexual assault as an adult.[35] Finally, in a study evaluating 105 subjects with IBS, IBD, or other GI disorders, investigators reported that those patients suffering from IBS had a much higher frequency of sexual abuse as a child when compared with the patients with IBD or other GI disorders.[29]

Other GI diseases have been linked to a history of adverse childhood events, including liver disease.[1,7] In one survey using the ACE instrument, those who endorsed at least one ACE category demonstrated a 1.2- to 1.6-fold increase in the risk of self-reported liver disease; a 2.6-fold increase was observed for respondents who endorsed 6 or more ACE categories.[7] Investigators postulated that this link between liver disease and adverse childhood events is mediated, in part, by the development of adverse health behaviors (ie, alcoholism, drug abuse, sexual promiscuity, etc) that may increase the risk of viral and/or alcohol-induced liver disease.[7] Lending weight to such theory, after adjusting for such adverse health behaviors, the association between adverse childhood events and the development of liver disease was significantly reduced.[7]

Gynecologic Conditions and Sexual Health

The association between gynecologic conditions/sexual health and a history of adverse childhood events has been widely cited in the literature.[1,36–38] Women who report a history of sexual abuse during childhood are at greater risk for acquiring sexually transmitted infections (STIs), experiencing teen pregnancy, having multiple sexual partners, or becoming repeat victims of abuse when compared with individuals without a history of childhood abuse.[37,39–43] The long-term conditions associated with a history of adverse childhood events range from problems with adult sexual adjustment (ie, dissatisfaction with adult sexual relationships, problems with intimacy) to the practice of risky sexual behaviors (ie, sexual promiscuity, drug and alcohol abuse) to the development of actual physical complaints (ie, chronic pelvic pain, fibromyalgia).[11,44]

Victims of sexual abuse during childhood may be at risk for developing disorders of sexual adjustment later in adult life.[45,46] In a randomized, community-based study that queried participants about the impact of child-

hood sexual abuse on their adult sexual relationships, 50% of the respondents reported that a history of incestuous sexual abuse during childhood had affected their sexual adjustment as adults.[37] In particular, female abuse victims who had a history of abuse including sexual intercourse were more likely to experience dissatisfaction with their adult sexual relationships.[37] Victims of childhood sexual abuse have described having problems with intimacy, specifically by experiencing a sense of insecurity or having disorganized attachments,[47,48] which is manifest by an increased incidence of separation and divorce among abuse victims.[49,50]

Felitti et al[1] have investigated the relationship between the presence of adverse childhood events and risky sexual behaviors such as sexual promiscuity, which may increase the risk of developing subsequent medical diseases (ie, STI, pelvic inflammatory disease, human immunodeficiency virus [HIV] infection, etc) and their complications (ie, pain and discomfort, infertility, etc).[1] For example, in one large survey study, investigators estimated the prevalence of having 50 or more sexual intercourse partners to be 6.8% among respondents endorsing 4 or more ACE categories, compared with 3.0% among those endorsing no ACE categories.[1] They demonstrated that subjects who endorsed one ACE category had an adjusted odds ratio (OR) of 1.7 (95% confidence interval [CI] 1.3, 2.3) for having 50 or more sexual intercourse partners. When compared with those subjects endorsing no ACE categories, the odds ratio increased to 3.2 (95% CI

2.1, 5.1) for subjects endorsing 4 or more ACE categories.[1]

Likewise, individuals who report adverse childhood events seem to be at higher risk for contracting STIs.[1,38] In one study, the prevalence of ever having an STI was 16.7% among those respondents endorsing 4 or more ACE categories, compared with 5.6% among those endorsing no ACE categories.[1] Those subjects endorsing a single ACE category have an adjusted odds ratio of 1.4 (95% CI 1.1, 1.7) for ever having had an STI, when compared with those subjects endorsing no ACE categories.[1] The odds ratio increased to 2.5 (95% CI 1.9, 3.2) for those subjects endorsing 4 or more ACE categories.[1] Additionally, when examined in detail, the ACE categories most associated with ever having had an STI were (from most to least) criminal behavior in household, sexual abuse, emotional abuse, and physical abuse.[1]

Certain gynecologic conditions have also been associated with a history of adverse childhood events. Although the data are conflicting, there are reports that chronic pelvic pain (CPP) occurs at an increased frequency among patients who endorse having had some type of adverse childhood event.[51,52] In one often-cited study, when participants who had either CPP, headache, or no pain complaints were questioned about a history of childhood sexual abuse, those individuals suffering from CPP had a significantly higher lifetime prevalence of major sexual abuse (ie, genital-genital contact, penetration) than individuals in the comparison groups.[51] Another similar study demonstrated a significant relationship between experiencing major sexual abuse before the age of 15 years and developing CPP later in life, although there was no significant difference in the lifetime prevalence of sexual abuse between the CPP and comparison groups.[52]

Psychosomatic Conditions, Including Behavior-Related Medical Conditions

Investigators have described the impact of a history of adverse childhood events on the development of psychosomatic and behavioral conditions, which can result in physical medical conditions whose etiology is thought to be, in large part, due to underlying psychological stressors.[1] Such conditions may include obesity, eating disorders, tobacco use, alcohol abuse, and illicit drug use, as well as medical conditions such as fibromyalgia or chronic pain syndromes.[1,51,53] As an example, individuals with a history of adverse childhood events are at increased risk for developing maladaptive eating behaviors, which may subsequently manifest as obesity and/or eating disorders.[54] The etiology of such behaviors is thought to be multifactorial, including the notion of disordered eating as an adaptive coping mechanism[1] and/or having a distorted body image or misperception of weight.[34] Individuals suffering from obesity and/or eating disorders are at increased risk for developing serious long-term health consequences, such as ischemic heart disease or diabetes.

Obesity, which is a public health problem occurring in epidemic proportions, has been associated with a history of adverse childhood events.[1,8,54,55] Felitti et al[1] reported a prevalence of severe obesity (body mass index ≥35) to be 12.0% in study subjects endorsing 4 or more ACE categories, compared with 5.4% among subjects endorsing no ACE categories.[1] In another related study, 60% of patients with a prior history of adverse childhood events were 50 pounds or more over their ideal body weight, compared with 28% of the control group.[34] The severity of obesity was also greater among those with a history of adverse childhood events, with morbid obesity (≥100 pounds over ideal body weight) occurring in 25% of the abused group, compared with 6% of the non-abused group.[34] Two-thirds of the morbidly obese individuals with a history of adverse childhood events reported a history of incest that was temporally related to the onset of obesity.[34]

Similarly, it has been suggested that eating disorders, such as anorexia nervosa and bulimia, are associated with a history of adverse childhood events. A meta-analysis reviewing 53 different studies reported a small yet significant positive relationship between childhood sexual abuse and the development of an eating disorder.[56] In one study that compared 51 bulimic women with 25 female control subjects across multiple dimensions of health, it was discovered that the bulimic women reported a higher frequency of childhood abuse than the control subjects.[57] Additionally, although the bulimic women suffered from a higher baseline level of psychopathology, the investigators noted a dose-dependent relationship between the severity of abuse occurring among all study subjects and the degree of psychopathology present.[57] In another study comparing sexually abused females (who were abused before 16 years of age) with community controls, investigators found that women with a history of sexual abuse suffered more frequently from eating disorders than the control group.[58]

Alcoholism, smoking, and illicit drug use occur at an increased frequency among adult victims of child abuse, perhaps as a coping mechanism; each has deleterious long-term health consequences, such as heart and liver disease, STI (ie, HIV, hepatitis), psychiatric illness, and multiple psychosocial problems.[1,9,12,59,60] Regarding alcoholism, compared with those individuals endorsing no ACE categories, those endorsing one or more ACE categories had a 2- to 4-fold increase in the lifetime risk of heavy drinking, self-reported alcoholism, and marrying an alcoholic, even after adjusting for a family history of alcoholism.[9,60] Regarding smoking, compared with individuals endorsing no ACE categories, those endorsing 5 or more ACE categories had significantly higher risks of early smoking initiation (OR 5.4; 95% CI 4.1, 7.1), lifetime smoking history (OR 3.1; 95% CI 2.6, 3.8), current smoking (OR 2.1; 95% CI 1.6, 2.7), and heavy smoking (OR 2.8; 95% CI 1.9, 4.2).[12] Regarding illicit drug abuse, compared with those individuals endorsing no ACE categories, those endorsing one or more ACE categories had an earlier age of initiation of drug use, as well as a 7- to 10-fold increase in reporting illicit drug use, drug addiction, and parental drug abuse.[59] Investigators controlled for the presence of temporal and secular trends in drug availability, use, and public attitude; the relationship between the ACE score and the initiation of illicit drug use persisted throughout time, suggesting that the observed trends are not simply a product of their era.[59]

A number of other psychosomatic conditions have been associated with a history of adverse childhood events, although supporting published data are relatively lacking. Chronic pain disorders, specifically fibromyalgia, have been linked to abuse occurring during either childhood or adulthood.[61,62] When compared with patients diagnosed with rheumatoid arthritis, patients suffering from fibromyalgia had a significantly higher lifetime prevalence for all forms of child abuse, including sexual, emotional, and physical abuse.[61] The severity of the abuse was significantly correlated with the self-reported measures of physical disability and pain, psychiatric distress, sleep quality, and ability to cope with stress.[61]

Psychiatric and Psychological Conditions

Victims of childhood abuse and neglect have repeatedly been shown to have an increased risk for developing psychiatric and psychological conditions during adulthood, including post-traumatic stress disorder (PTSD), depression, anxiety, dissociative disorder, and suicidality.[6,50,63,64] Indeed, strong evidence exists that early life experiences influence the development of the brain.[3,25,65] Repeated stressors in early

life have been shown to induce long-term biological changes in the central neurobiological systems, in particular by increasing corticotropin-releasing factor, thereby activating the body's physiological response to stress.[25] Complementary theories have been reported in the psychology literature, citing that adult psychopathology in victims of childhood abuse occurs as a consequence of a chronic form of PTSD rooted in chronic neurophysiological changes.[66–68] In 1987 Finkelhor[69] introduced the "traumatogenic model," which specified that childhood sexual abuse induced a range of psychological effects in the victim at the time of abuse, which later manifest themselves as long-term behavioral changes.

Depression is one of the most frequent psychiatric complaints among adult victims of child abuse.[1,6,9] In one large sample using the ACE instrument, individuals who endorsed at least one ACE category had a lifetime prevalence of having had a depressive disorder of 25.8%, compared with 18.5% of individuals endorsing no ACE categories.[6] The number of endorsed ACE categories also demonstrated a dose-response relationship with the likelihood of having had a depressive disorder; in the group of respondents who endorsed 5 or more ACE categories, the prevalence of a lifetime history of depression approached 61%.[6] Even after controlling for the presence of a mentally ill household member during childhood, the association between experiencing adverse childhood events and developing a subsequent depressive disorder remained significant.[6]

Post-traumatic stress disorder and other anxiety-related disorders are observed at increased frequency among adult victims of child abuse and neglect. One large retrospective survey of inner-city women demonstrated that individuals who had experienced either child abuse or adult rape were 6 times as likely to develop probable PTSD, when compared with those without such a history; women who experienced both child abuse and adult rape were 17 times as likely to develop probable PTSD.[70] Other reports have confirmed the presence of dissociative and anxiety symptoms in adults who suffered abuse during childhood.[71,72]

Individuals with a history of adverse childhood events are also at an increased risk for attempting suicide.[10] In one study using the ACE instrument, the prevalence of at least one self-reported suicide attempt was 1.1% among the general population and 3.8% among individuals endorsing at least one ACE category.[10] Overall, females attempted suicide more frequently than men, as did individuals with a lower educational level.[10] The risk of attempting suicide was increased 2- to 5-fold in individuals who endorsed at least one ACE category, with an increasing, graded response for those individuals endorsing more than one ACE category.[10] Although alcoholism, depression, and illicit drug use were strongly associated with suicidal attempts, even after adjusting for these covariates, the relationship between adverse childhood events and suicide attempts was significant.[10]

Medical and Psychological Care of Children in Foster Care

Medical and Psychological Consequences of Foster Care Placement

Foster care placement is a possible consequence of child abuse and neglect and is intimately related to a child's immediate and long-term medical and psychological health and well-being. Of the 3 million children reported for allegations of abuse or neglect each year (4.5% of the child population), 1 in 6 will enter foster care.[73] As of 2004 approximately 523,000 children lived in foster care, a subgroup of an estimated several million children annually who receive child welfare services.[73,74] Many children receiving child welfare services transition in and out of foster care; they experience stays of varying duration and may move frequently among placement settings.

Evidence drawn from decades of research has demonstrated that children living in foster care experience high rates of adverse chronic medical, mental health, behavioral, and developmental health conditions. Most children in foster care have chronic medical problems unrelated to behavioral concerns,[75-78] and the presence of these chronic medical conditions will greatly increase their likelihood of serious emotional problems.[79] The behavioral and mental health concerns are long-standing: A study released by Casey Family Programs[80] in 2005 revealed that 1 of every 2 adult graduates from their foster care program had a serious mental health problem, and 1 in 4 suffered from PTSD well into adulthood.

Despite the magnitude of the medical and psychological health needs for children in foster care, the research has also been consistent in demonstrating that children in foster care rarely receive health services appropriate to their level of medical need.[75,77,78,81–84] The foster care children most at risk for the worst medical,[85,86] developmental,[87] and mental health problems[77,88–96] are also those most likely to experience lengthy stays in foster care and considerable drift from placement to placement. As a result, the children with the greatest health needs are often most at risk for fragmentation in their care. This fragmentation also helps explain why among the 40% to 80% of foster children who have serious behavioral or mental health problems requiring intervention,[77,97–102] only 25% to 66% receive any services.[75,79,103–106] These gaps in medical care provide a suitable target for intervention that may not only improve the current medical and psychological health of children in foster care, but also their adult medical and psychological well-being.

Current Policy to Address the Shortcomings in Medical and Psychological Services for Children in Foster Care

Over the last decade, the consistent documentation of the unmet health needs of children in foster care has led to legislative and policy changes to address the problem. In 1997 Congress enacted the Adoption and Safe Families Act (ASFA, Pub L No. 105-89). The Act had a number of purposes, including (1) strengthening the federal oversight of state systems to promote greater system safety and permanency for children in the child welfare system and (2) improving the quality of foster care in order to ensure health and well-being. In 2000 the Administration for Children and Families initiated a program of Child and Family Service Reviews (CFSRs) to assess the extent to which states have programs in place that promote optimal health, mental health, and development of the children in their care. These CFSRs include specific assessments of whether the health services provided to foster children have met these children's actual physical and mental health needs.

Faced with mounting pressure to improve outcomes for children in foster care, the child welfare system has responded similarly with an increasing number of "joint ventures" and partnerships among health agencies, child welfare agencies, and state Medicaid programs. The Medicaid program has been a major facilitator for these emerging health programs. Medicaid's involvement in the child welfare system is enormous; before entering foster care, nearly 70% of all children were covered by Medicaid, and on entering foster care, most states use Medicaid funds to provide coverage for foster children. Consequently, because of their needs, children in foster care use Medicaid services at rates significantly greater than children not in foster care. Although children in foster care represent less than 3% of all Medicaid enrollees, they account for more than a quarter of all expenditures for mental health[106,107] and 15% of all case management funding within the program.[108]

At the state and local level, collaborations have resulted in strengthened and more coordinated involvement with local health care providers who care for children in foster care. In some of these arrangements, the child welfare system has ensured the referral of all children entering out-of-home care to a single point-of-entry specialty clinic where a child's physical, developmental, and mental health needs can be properly assessed. These specialty programs have depended heavily on Medicaid financing to support comprehensive screening, diagnosis, and case management services that meet the national professional guidelines of the American Academy of Pediatrics, the Child Welfare League of America, and the American Academy of Child & Adolescent Psychiatry.[109] [111] The use of these comprehensive and specialized clinics has been shown to improve the recognition of underlying problems and increase access to developmental and behavioral services.[112]

Several child welfare systems have increased access to mental health services through the availability of on-site health professionals (ie, psychologists, public health nurses) within their child welfare units. Supported primarily through Medicaid funding, these mental health professionals are responsible for providing mental health care screening at the time of enrollment of clinic patients. These mental health professionals coordinate a child's care and refer qualifying children and adolescents for needed mental health services. County child welfare systems that employ such on-site professionals have demonstrated significant improvements in the quality of care delivered to children in foster care. The evidence suggests that agencies using on-site health care professionals are more likely to identify children in greatest need of services and subsequently obtain services for such children.[104]

Future Challenges in Providing Adequate Medical and Mental Health Care to Children in Foster Care

Despite the recent improvements in health care programs offered by the child welfare system, significant challenges remain. First, the quality of both the medical providers and the services available to children in foster care must be evaluated. Although child welfare programs may provide adequate screening for and authorization for mental health care services, if there remains a shortage of mental health providers and/or a significant variation in the quality of services offered, screening may fail to achieve better outcomes. Even then, because of recent changes to the Medicaid program, child welfare and public health systems may find it more difficult to secure case management funding from the Medicaid program, as well as provide the comprehensive array of health care services to meet the needs of their children.[113] In the future, the extent to which states will be able to fulfill the funding needs of child welfare and public health programs remains uncertain.

As a result of future funding uncertainty, public programs will be increasingly forced to consider novel targets for intervention that will improve outcomes for children. Those interventions inevitably will be linked to improving the well-being of foster children by promoting permanency and adoption. For those who remain in foster care, it will involve designing programs that minimize movement between different homes and provide a higher quality of medical care.

The importance of achieving placement stability or permanency for children in foster care is not trivial. Despite efforts to increase permanency and adoption in recent years, nearly half of all children entering foster care will remain in foster care for more than 18 months, and for some, years. Among those who remain in foster care, 1 in 3 will fail to achieve a long-lasting placement during the first 18 months in foster care. For those children who eventually return home, at least 1 in 4 will return to the foster care system within 2 years.[114]

Those children who fail to achieve placement stability or who return to the system multiple times are at the greatest risk for poor health outcomes.[115–118] Developmental theory provides an explanation for why disruptions specifically in the first year of foster care are highly correlated with poor long-term outcomes.[81,85,88,89,118–120] Simply stated, "The result of poorly initiated mental healthcare is that…multiple placements become common as children disrupt ill-prepared and relatively unsupported foster families who soon request relief from the behavior these children manifest. The cycle of multiple placements contributes to an increase in overall behavior pathology (including school difficulties) and fundamentally undermines attempts to provide a consistent environment wherein attachment to caregivers can be nurtured."[99]

While interventions to improve outcomes for children are almost certain to prioritize placement stability and permanency, skepticism remains about how effective such interventions might be. At least half of all children entering foster care have significant behavioral problems that likely influence their ability to achieve stability in out-of-home settings. However, emerging evidence demonstrates that a child's behavioral problems at entry into foster care cannot entirely explain their outcomes. A recent analysis of the National Survey of Child and Adolescent Well-Being demonstrated that nearly 1 in 5 children who were younger, had no behavioral problems, and had no prior child welfare involvement failed to achieve a long-lasting placement during their first 18 months in foster care. Among these low-risk children, the failure to achieve a long-lasting placement was highly detrimental: 18 months into foster care, nearly a third had significant behavioral problems, double the rate of low-risk children who achieved a more stable placement setting from the outset.[121]

Additionally, there is opportunity to influence placement stability at the local level through initiatives not solely aimed at improvement in health care services. For example, 70% of all placement moves in a large county in California were administrative in nature and seemingly unrelated to the behavior of the child; many required a change in caseworker, agency, or an adjudicated decision made irrespective of the child's attachment within a foster home.[122]

While not all of the placement moves in the study were preventable, the effect of administrative practices on placement stability—a topic which beforehand received little attention in the literature—presents an opportunity to improve stability for children in the system. In particular, the study suggested that placement stability might be improved by ensuring the efficiency of placement decisions and administrative practices.

Interventions to improve placement stability, as well as their subsequent impact on placement outcomes, have been relatively unstudied. Because the child welfare and public health systems share the responsibility for ensuring the provision of preventive, therapeutic, and mental health services, collaborative programs will be needed to address these persistent challenges.[103,113] At the same time, however, child welfare systems, independent of collaboration with public health programs, may have other opportunities to improve (1) the efficiency in which their placement decisions are made and (2) the degree to which placement stability is regarded as a critical performance measure as mandated by the federal CFSR. The child welfare system may debate the relative impact of a system-wide performance intervention on improving placement stability because of the myriad factors that contribute to a child's movement between foster homes (ie, a child's behavioral problems, issues with the foster care family, the availability of kinship providers, etc). However, there is evidence that linking placement stability to financial reimbursement for provider agencies may influence rates of stability dramatically.

In Philadelphia, for example, performance-based contracting with foster care agencies resulted in an 84% increase in the rate at which children achieved permanency through reunification, adoption, or permanent legal custody. In addition, movement of children to more restrictive levels of placement or to other foster care agencies decreased by 50%. The child welfare system assumes the responsibility for the well-being of children in foster care. Public stories of poor outcomes among youth in foster care that have been highlighted in our media, in addition to the consistent data demonstrating poor outcomes in adult medical and psychological health, have engaged a public discourse around the well-being of foster children that began with ASFA in 1997, and is likely to continue for the foreseeable future. It remains unclear which interventions will best improve outcomes for children in foster care, but the seeds for change are being sown in communities throughout the country.[123,124] Future research will need to demonstrate whether the instituted programs are effective, as well as to evaluate ways to generalize the most successful programs to larger groups of children nationwide.

Impact of Resiliency and Coping Styles on the Long-term Effects of Child Abuse

In addition to various macro-level interventions and policy changes that may improve the long-term outcomes of child abuse, as demonstrated by the example of children in foster care, there are also individual-level traits that may reduce the development of long-term medical and psychological consequences of adverse childhood events. In particular, the concept of childhood resiliency is believed, in part, to mitigate the effects of adverse events.[125] Coping styles, which are intimately related to the concept of resiliency, can also modulate the effects of abuse.[126] Resiliency includes the following notions: (1) I have people around me who can help, (2) I am a person people can like and love, and (3) I can find ways to solve problems that I face. One of the major tasks of future research in the field of resiliency will be to standardize a working definition of resiliency.[127] Although many studies have attempted to examine the effects of resiliency on mitigating the effects of adverse childhood events, the use of varying definitions and criteria make it difficult to interpret and compare the results.[128–130]

For instance, in one study of female college students, researchers examined the effects of resilience (termed *protective factors*) on adult functioning in victims of childhood sexual abuse. The study found that women with multiple protective factors (ie, self-esteem, self-efficacy, familial and social supports) had a level of functioning and satisfaction with life equal to those women without a history of childhood sexual abuse; individuals with few protective factors and a history of childhood sexual abuse had a lower level of functioning and satisfaction with life.[131] In another study, Perkins and Jones[132] identified several protective factors that seemed to mitigate the effects

of prior abuse on subsequent adolescent risk-taking behavior. These factors included peer group characteristics, school climate, religiosity, adult support, family support, perceptions of the future, and involvement in extracurricular activities. The specific effects of these factors on risk-taking behaviors varied widely. For example, the variance accounted for by different models of protective factors ranged from 2% (for the development of purging eating behaviors) to 26% (for the development of alcohol use and antisocial behavior). Again, as demonstrated by these 2 studies, the broad array of factors examined in the resiliency and coping skills literature makes it difficult to compare and contrast the results; the criteria used to measure these so-called protective factors must be standardized.

Conclusion

Children who experience child maltreatment are at higher risk for developing long-term adverse medical and psychological consequences.[1] In part, this may be due to the inadequacies of the foster care, child welfare, and public health systems in providing medical and psychological care that is (1) delivered in a timely manner, (2) of high quality, and (3) consistent over time. Interventions and policy occurring at the state and national government levels have the potential to improve the long-term health outcomes of foster children, although further research is warranted. For children not in the foster care system, but who go on to develop the known long-term health consequences of child abuse and neglect, it will be imperative for their health care providers to recognize these consequences and intervene with appropriate measures.

References

1. Felitti VJ, Anda RF, Nordenberg D, et al. Relationship of childhood abuse and household dysfunction to many of the leading causes of death in adults. The Adverse Childhood Experiences (ACE) Study. *Am J Prev Med.* 1998;14:245–258

2. Dube SR, Miller JW, Brown DW, et al. Adverse childhood experiences and the association with ever using alcohol and initiating alcohol use during adolescence. *J Adolesc Health.* 2006;38:444,e1–e10

3. Anda RF, Felitti VJ, Bremner JD, et al. The enduring effects of abuse and related adverse experiences in childhood: a convergence of evidence from neurobiology and epidemiology. *Eur Arch Psychiatry Clin Neurosci.* 2006;256:174–186

4. Dong M, Anda RF, Felitti VJ, et al. Childhood residential mobility and multiple health risks during adolescence and adulthood: the hidden role of adverse childhood experiences. *Arch Pediatr Adolesc Med.* 2005;159:1104–1110

5. Dong M, Giles WH, Felitti VJ, et al. Insights into causal pathways for ischemic heart disease: adverse childhood experiences study. *Circulation.* 2004;110:1761–1766

6. Chapman DP, Whitfield CL, Felitti VJ, Dube SR, Edwards VJ, Anda RF. Adverse childhood experiences and the risk of depressive disorders in adulthood. *J Affect Disord.* 2004;82:217–225

7. Dong M, Dube SR, Felitti VJ, Giles WH, Anda RF. Adverse childhood experiences and self-reported liver disease: new insights into the causal pathway. *Arch Intern Med.* 2003;163:1949–1956

8. Williamson DF, Thompson TJ, Anda RF, Dietz WH, Felitti V. Body weight and obesity in adults and self-reported abuse in childhood. *Int J Obes Relat Metab Disord.* 2002;26:1075–1082

9. Anda RF, Whitfield CL, Felitti VJ, et al. Adverse childhood experiences, alcoholic parents, and later risk of alcoholism and depression. *Psychiatr Serv.* 2002;53:1001–1009

10. Dube SR, Anda RF, Felitti VJ, Chapman DP, Williamson DF, Giles WH. Childhood abuse, household dysfunction, and the risk of attempted suicide throughout the life span: findings from the Adverse Childhood Experiences Study. *JAMA.* 2001;286:3089–3096

11. Hillis SD, Anda RF, Felitti VJ, Nordenberg D, Marchbanks PA. Adverse childhood experiences and sexually transmitted diseases in men and women: a retrospective study. *Pediatrics.* 2000;106:e11

12. Anda RF, Croft JB, Felitti VJ, et al. Adverse childhood experiences and smoking during adolescence and adulthood. *JAMA.* 1999;282:1652–1658

13. Barlow KM, Thomson E, Johnson D, Minns RA. Late neurologic and cognitive sequelae of inflicted traumatic brain injury in infancy. *Pediatrics.* 2005;116:e174–e185

14. Keenan HT, Runyan DK, Nocera M. Child outcomes and family characteristics 1 year after severe inflicted or noninflicted traumatic brain injury. *Pediatrics.* 2006;117:317–324

15. Keenan HT, Runyan DK, Nocera M. Longitudinal follow-up of families and young children with traumatic brain injury. *Pediatrics.* 2006;117:1291–1297

16. Marin-Padilla M, Parisi JE, Armstrong DL, Sargent SK, Kaplan JA. Shaken infant syndrome: developmental neuropathology, progressive cortical dysplasia, and epilepsy. *Acta Neuropathol (Berl).* 2002;103:321–332

17. Marin-Padilla M. Developmental neuropathology and impact of perinatal brain damage. I: hemorrhagic lesions of neocortex. *J Neuropathol Exp Neurol.* 1996;55:758–773

18. Marin-Padilla M. Developmental neuropathology and impact of perinatal brain damage. II: white matter lesions of the neocortex. *J Neuropathol Exp Neurol.* 1997;56:219–235

19. Marin-Padilla M. Developmental neuropathology and impact of perinatal brain damage. III: gray matter lesions of the neocortex. *J Neuropathol Exp Neurol.* 1999;58:407–429

20. Marin-Padilla M. Perinatal brain damage, cortical reorganization (acquired cortical dysplasias), and epilepsy. *Adv Neurol.* 2000;84:153–172

21. Druery M, Brown TL, Muller M. Long term functional outcomes and quality of life following severe burn injury. *Burns.* 2005;31:692–695

22. Block RW, Krebs NF. Failure to thrive as a manifestation of child neglect. *Pediatrics.* 2005;116:1234–1237

23. Oates RK. Similarities and differences between nonorganic failure to thrive and deprivation dwarfism. *Child Abuse Negl.* 1984;8:439–445

24. Black MM, Dubowitz H, Hutcheson J, Berenson-Howard J, Starr RH Jr. A randomized clinical trial of home intervention for children with failure to thrive. *Pediatrics.* 1995;95:807–814

25. Teicher MH, Andersen SL, Polcari A, Anderson CM, Navalta CP. Developmental neurobiology of childhood stress and trauma. *Psychiatr Clin North Am.* 2002;25:397–426, vii–viii

26. Talley NJ, Fett SL, Zinsmeister AR, Melton LJ III. Gastrointestinal tract symptoms and self-reported abuse: a population-based study. *Gastroenterology.* 1994;107:1040–1049

27. Drossman DA, Leserman J, Nachman G, et al. Sexual and physical abuse in women with functional or organic gastrointestinal disorders. *Ann Intern Med.* 1990;113:828–833

28. Drossman DA, Talley NJ, Leserman J, Olden KW, Barreiro MA. Sexual and physical abuse and gastrointestinal illness. Review and recommendations. *Ann Intern Med.* 1995;123:782–794

29. Ross CA. Childhood sexual abuse and psychosomatic symptoms in irritable bowel syndrome. *J Child Sex Abus.* 2005;14:27–38

30. Cannon WB. *Bodily Changes in Pain, Hunger, Fear and Rage: An Account of Recent Researches Into the Function of Emotional Excitement.* 2nd ed. New York, NY: D. Appleton and Company; 1920

31. Sleisenger MH, Feldman M, Friedman LS, Brandt LJ. *Sleisenger & Fordtran's Gastrointestinal and Liver Disease: Pathophysiology, Diagnosis, Management.* 8th ed. Philadelphia, PA: Saunders; 2006

32. Bradesi S, McRoberts JA, Anton PA, Mayer EA. Inflammatory bowel disease and irritable bowel syndrome: separate or unified? *Curr Opin Gastroenterol.* 2003;19:336–342

33. Quigley EM. Disturbances of motility and visceral hypersensitivity in irritable bowel syndrome: biological markers or epiphenomenon. *Gastroenterol Clin North Am.* 2005;34:221–233, vi

34. Felitti VJ. Long-term medical consequences of incest, rape, and molestation. *South Med J.* 1991;84:328–331

35. Walker EA, Katon WJ, Roy-Byrne PP, Jemelka RP, Russo J. Histories of sexual victimization in patients with irritable bowel syndrome or inflammatory bowel disease. *Am J Psychiatry.* 1993;150:1502–1506

36. Fromuth ME. The relationship of childhood sexual abuse with later psychological and sexual adjustment in a sample of college women. *Child Abuse Negl.* 1986;10:5–15

37. Mullen PE, Martin JL, Anderson JC, Romans SE, Herbison GP. The effect of child sexual abuse on social, interpersonal and sexual function in adult life. *Br J Psychiatry.* 1994;165:35–47

38. Senn TE, Carey MP, Vanable PA, Coury-Doniger P, Urban M. Characteristics of sexual abuse in childhood and adolescence influence sexual risk behavior in adulthood. *Arch Sex Behav.* 2007;36:637–645

39. Gorcey M, Santiago JM, McCall-Perez F. Psychological consequences for women sexually abused in childhood. *Soc Psychiatry.* 1986;21:129–133

40. Nagy S, DiClemente R, Adcock AG. Adverse factors associated with forced sex among southern adolescent girls. *Pediatrics.* 1995;96:944–946

41. Russell DEH. *The Secret Trauma: Incest in the Lives of Girls and Women.* New York, NY: Basic Books; 1986

42. Springs FE, Friedrich WN. Health risk behaviors and medical sequelae of childhood sexual abuse. *Mayo Clin Proc.* 1992;67:527–532

43. Fergusson DM, Horwood LJ, Lynskey MT. Childhood sexual abuse, adolescent sexual behaviors and sexual revictimization. *Child Abuse Negl.* 1997;21:789–803

44. Gunter J. Chronic pelvic pain: an integrated approach to diagnosis and treatment. *Obstet Gynecol Surv.* 2003;58:615–623

45. Herman JL, Hirschman L. *Father-Daughter Incest.* Cambridge, MA: Harvard University Press; 2000

46. Finkelhor D. *Child Sexual Abuse: New Theory and Research.* New York, NY: Free Press; 1984

47. Jehu D, Gazan M, Klassen C. *Beyond Sexual Abuse: Therapy With Women Who Were Childhood Victims.* New York, NY: Wiley; 1988

48. Briere J, Runtz M. Multivariate correlates of childhood psychological and physical maltreatment among university women. *Child Abuse Negl.* 1988;12:331–341

49. Beitchman JH, Zucker KJ, Hood JE, daCosta GA, Akman D. A review of the short-term effects of child sexual abuse. *Child Abuse Negl.* 1991;15:537–556

50. Mullen PE, Romans-Clarkson SE, Walton VA, Herbison GP. Impact of sexual and physical abuse on women's mental health. *Lancet.* 1988;1:841–845

51. Walling MK, Reiter RC, O'Hara MW, Milburn AK, Lilly G, Vincent SD. Abuse history and chronic pain in women: I. Prevalences of sexual abuse and physical abuse. *Obstet Gynecol.* 1994;84:193–199

52. Lampe A, Solder E, Ennemoser A, Schubert C, Rumpold G, Sollner W. Chronic pelvic pain and previous sexual abuse. *Obstet Gynecol.* 2000;96:929–933

53. Walling MK, O'Hara MW, Reiter RC, Milburn AK, Lilly G, Vincent SD. Abuse history and chronic pain in women: II. A multivariate analysis of abuse and psychological morbidity. *Obstet Gynecol.* 1994;84:200–206

54. Gustafson TB, Sarwer DB. Childhood sexual abuse and obesity. *Obes Rev.* 2004;5:129–135

55. Felitti VJ. Childhood sexual abuse, depression, and family dysfunction in adult obese patients: a case control study. *South Med J.* 1993;86:732–736

56. Smolak L, Murnen SK. A meta-analytic examination of the relationship between child sexual abuse and eating disorders. *Int J Eat Disord.* 2002;31:136–150

57. Leonard S, Steiger H, Kao A. Childhood and adulthood abuse in bulimic and nonbulimic women: prevalences and psychological correlates. *Int J Eat Disord.* 2003;33:397–405

58. Romans SE, Gendall KA, Martin JL, Mullen PE. Child sexual abuse and later disordered eating: a New Zealand epidemiological study. *Int J Eat Disord.* 2001;29:380–392

59. Dube SR, Felitti VJ, Dong M, Chapman DP, Giles WH, Anda RF. Childhood abuse, neglect, and household dysfunction and the risk of illicit drug use: the adverse childhood experiences study. *Pediatrics.* 2003;111:564–572

60. Dube SR, Anda RF, Felitti VJ, Edwards VJ, Croft JB. Adverse childhood experiences and personal alcohol abuse as an adult. *Addict Behav.* 2002;27:713–725

61. Walker EA, Keegan D, Gardner G, Sullivan M, Bernstein D, Katon WJ. Psychosocial factors in fibromyalgia compared with rheumatoid arthritis: II. Sexual, physical, and emotional abuse and neglect. *Psychosom Med.* 1997;59:572–577

62. Finestone HM, Stenn P, Davies F, Stalker C, Fry R, Koumanis J. Chronic pain and health care utilization in women with a history of childhood sexual abuse. *Child Abuse Negl.* 2000;24:547–556

63. Edwards VJ, Holden GW, Felitti VJ, Anda RF. Relationship between multiple forms of childhood maltreatment and adult mental health in community respondents: results from the adverse childhood experiences study. *Am J Psychiatry.* 2003;160:1453–1460

64. Mullen PE, Martin JL, Anderson JC, Romans SE, Herbison GP. Childhood sexual abuse and mental health in adult life. *Br J Psychiatry.* 1993;163:721–732

65. Nemeroff CB. Neurobiological consequences of childhood trauma. *J Clin Psychiatry.* 2004;65(suppl 1):18–28

66. Bryer JB, Nelson BA, Miller JB, Krol PA. Childhood sexual and physical abuse as factors in adult psychiatric illness. *Am J Psychiatry.* 1987;144:1426–1430

67. Craine LS, Henson CE, Colliver JA, MacLean DG. Prevalence of a history of sexual abuse among female psychiatric patients in a state hospital system. *Hosp Community Psychiatry.* 1988;39:300–304

68. Lindberg FH, Distad LJ. Post-traumatic stress disorders in women who experienced childhood incest. *Child Abuse Negl.* 1985;9:329–334

69. Finkelhor D. The trauma of child sexual abuse: two models. *J Interpers Violence.* 1987;4:348–366

70. Schumm JA, Briggs-Phillips M, Hobfoll SE. Cumulative interpersonal traumas and social support as risk and resiliency factors in predicting PTSD and depression among inner-city women. *J Trauma Stress.* 2006;19:825–836

71. Mulder RT, Beautrais AL, Joyce PR, Fergusson DM. Relationship between dissociation, childhood sexual abuse, childhood physical abuse, and mental illness in a general population sample. *Am J Psychiatry.* 1998;155:806–811

72. Fergusson DM, Horwood LJ, Lynskey MT. Childhood sexual abuse and psychiatric disorder in young adulthood: II. Psychiatric outcomes of childhood sexual abuse. *J Am Acad Child Adolesc Psychiatry.* 1996;35:1365–1374

73. *Child Maltreatment 2004: Reports from the States to the National Child Abuse and Neglect Data Systems—National Statistics on Child Abuse and Neglect.* Washington, DC: US Department of Health and Human Services, Administration for Children and Families, Administration on Children, Youth and Families, Children's Bureau 2006. http://www.acf.hhs.gov/programs/cb/pubs/cm04/cm04.pdf

74. *Adoption and Foster Care Analysis and Reporting System.* Washington, DC: US Department of Health and Human Services, Administration for Children and Families, Administration on Children, Youth and Families, Children's Bureau 2005. http://www.acf.hhs.gov/programs/cb

75. US General Accounting Office. *Foster Care: Health Needs of Many Young Children Are Unknown and Unmet.* Washington, DC: US General Accounting Office; 1995. GAO/HEHS-95-114

76. Takayama JI, Wolfe E, Coulter KP. Relationship between reason for placement and medical findings among children in foster care. *Pediatrics.* 1998;101:201–207

77. Halfon N, Mendonca A, Berkowitz G. Health status of children in foster care. The experience of the Center for the Vulnerable Child. *Arch Pediatr Adolesc Med.* 1995;149:386–392

78. Simms MD. The foster care clinic: a community program to identify treatment needs of children in foster care. *J Dev Behav Pediatr.* 1989;10:121–128

79. Rubin DM, Alessandrini EA, Feudtner C, Mandell D, Localio AR, Hadley T. Placement stability and mental health costs for children in foster care. *Pediatrics.* 2004;113:1336–1341

80. Pecora P, Kessler R, Williams J, et al. *Improving Family Foster Care: Findings From the Northwest Foster Care Alumni Study.* Seattle, WA: Casey Family Programs; 2005. http://www.casey.org

81. Simms MD, Dubowitz H, Szilagyi MA. Health care needs of children in the foster care system. *Pediatrics.* 2000;106(suppl 4):909–918

82. Rosenfeld AA, Pilowsky DJ, Fine P, et al. Foster care: an update. *J Am Acad Child Adolesc Psychiatry.* 1997;36:448–457

83. Wyatt DT, Simms MD, Horwitz SM. Widespread growth retardation and variable growth recovery in foster children in the first year after initial placement. *Arch Pediatr Adolesc Med.* 1997;151:813–816

84. Chernoff R, Combs-Orme T, Risley-Curtiss C, Heisler A. Assessing the health status of children entering foster care. *Pediatrics.* 1994;93:594–601

85. Barth RP, Courtney ME, Berrick JD, Albert V. *From Child Abuse to Permanency Planning: Child Welfare Services Pathways and Placements.* New York, NY: Aldine de Gruyter; 1994

86. Groze V, Haines-Simeon M, Barth RP. Barriers in permanency planning for medically fragile children: drug affected children and HIV infected children. *Child Adolesc Soc Work J.* 1994;11:63–85

87. Horwitz SM, Simms MD, Farrington R. Impact of developmental problems on young children's exits from foster care. *J Dev Behav Pediatr.* 1994;15:105–110

88. Newton RR, Litrownik AJ, Landsverk JA. Children and youth in foster care: disentangling the relationship between problem behaviors and number of placements. *Child Abuse Negl.* 2000;24:1363–1374

89. Webster D, Barth RP, Needell B. Placement stability for children in out-of-home care: a longitudinal analysis. *Child Welfare.* 2000;79:614–632

90. Fanshel D, Shinn E. *Children in Foster Care: A Longitudinal Study.* New York, NY: Columbia University Press; 1978

91. Palmer SE. Placement stability and inclusive practice in foster care: an empirical study. *Child Youth Serv Rev.* 1996;18:589–601

92. Pardeck JT. Multiple placement of children in foster family care: an empirical analysis. *Soc Work.* 1984;29:506–509

93. Pardeck JT. *The Forgotten Children: A Study of the Stability and Continuity of Foster Care.* Washington, DC: University Press of America; 1982

94. Landsverk J, Davis I, Ganger W, Newton R. Impact of child psychosocial functioning on reunification from out-of-home placement. *Child Youth Serv Rev.* 1996;18:447–462

95. Cooper CS, Peterson NL, Meier JH. Variables associated with disrupted placement in a select sample of abused and neglected children. *Child Abuse Negl.* 1987;11:75–86

96. Teare JF, Larzelere RE, Smith GL, Becker CY, Castrianno LM, Peterson RW. Placement stability following short-term residential care. *J Child Fam Studies.* 1999;8:59–69

97. Landsverk JA, Garland AF, Leslie LK. *Mental Health Services for Children Reported to Child Protective Services.* Vol 2. Thousand Oaks, CA: Sage Publications; 2002

98. Glisson C. The effects of services coordination teams on outcomes for children in state custody. *Admin Soc Work.* 1994;18:1–23

99. Trupin EW, Tarico VS, Low BP, Jemelka R, McClellan J. Children on child protective service caseloads: prevalence and nature of serious emotional disturbance. *Child Abuse Negl.* 1993;17:345–355

100. Clausen JM, Landsverk J, Ganger W, Chadwick D, Litrownik A. Mental health problems of children in foster care. *J Child Fam Stud.* 1998;7:283–296

101. Urquiza AJ, Wirtz SJ, Peterson MS, Singer VA. Screening and evaluating abused and neglected children entering protective custody. *Child Welfare.* 1994;73:155–171

102. Garland AF, Hough RL, Landsverk JA, et al. Racial and ethnic variations in mental health care utilization among children in foster care. *Child Serv Soc Policy Res Pract.* 2000;3:133–146

103. Burns BJ, Phillips SD, Wagner RH, et al. Mental health need and access to mental health services by youths involved with child welfare: a national survey. *J Am Acad Child Adolesc Psychiatry.* 2004;43:960–970

104. Hurlburt M, Leslie L, Landsverk J, et al. Contextual predictors of mental health service use among children open to child welfare. *Arch Gen Psychiatry.* 2004;61:1217–1224

105. Harman JS, Childs GE, Kelleher KJ. Mental health care utilization and expenditures by children in foster care. *Arch Pediatr Adolesc Med.* 2000;154:1114–1117

106. Halfon N, Berkowitz G, Klee L. Mental health service utilization by children in foster care in California. *Pediatrics.* 1992;89:1238–1244

107. Takayama JI, Bergman AB, Connell FA. Children in foster care in the state of Washington. Health care utilization and expenditures. *JAMA.* 1994;271:1850–1855

108. Geen R, Sommers A, Cohen M. *Medicaid Spending on Foster Children.* Washington, DC: Urban Institute; 2005

109. American Academy of Pediatrics Committee on Early Childhood, Adoption, and Dependent Care. Health care of children in foster care. *Pediatrics.* 1994;93:335–338

110. American Academy of Pediatrics Committee on Early Childhood, Adoption, and Dependent Care. Health care of young children in foster care. *Pediatrics.* 2002;109:536–541

111. Child Welfare League of America. *Standards for Health Care Services for Children in Out-of-Home Care.* Washington, DC: Child Welfare League of America; 1988

112. Horwitz SM, Owens P, Simms MD. Specialized assessments for children in foster care. *Pediatrics.* 2000;106:59–66

113. Rubin D, Halfon N, Raghavan R, Rosenbaum S. *Protecting Children in Foster Care: Why Proposed Medicaid Cuts Harm Our Nation's Most Vulnerable Youth.* Washington, DC: Casey Family Programs; 2005

114. Rubin DM, Hafner L, Luan X, Localio AR. Placement stability and early behavioral outcomes for children in out-of-home care. Paper presented at: Child Protection: Using Research to Improve Policy and Practice; 2005; Washington, DC

115. Pecora PJ, Kessler RC, Williams J, et al. *Improving Family Foster Care: Findings From the Northwest Foster Care Alumni Study.* Seattle, WA: Casey Family Programs; 2005. http://www.casey.org

116. Taussig HN. Children who return home from foster care: a 6-year prospective study of behavioral health outcomes in adolescence. *Pediatrics.* 2001;108:e10

117. Jonson-Reid M, Barth RP. From maltreatment to juvenile incarceration: uncovering the role of child welfare services. *Child Abuse Negl.* 2000;24:505–520

118. Barth RP, Jonson-Reid M. Outcomes after child welfare services: implications for the design of performance measures. *ChildYouth Serv Rev.* 2000;22:763–787

119. James S, Landsverk JA, Slymen DJ. Placement movement in out-of-home care: patterns and predictors. *Child Youth Serv Rev.* 2004;26:185–206

120. Usher CL, Randolph KA, Gogan HC. Placement patterns in foster care. *Soc Serv Rev.* 1999;73:22–36

121. US Department of Health and Human Services. National survey of child and adolescent well-being (NSCAW), 1997–2010. www.acf.hhs.gov/programs/opre/abuse_neglect/nscaw/index.html. Accessed September 26, 2007

122. James S. Why do foster care placements disrupt? An investigation of reasons for placement change in foster care. *Soc Service Rev.* 2004;78:601–627

123. McCarthy J. *Meeting the Health Care Needs of Children in the Foster Care System*. Washington, DC: Georgetown University; 2002

124. McCarthy J, McCullough C. *A View from the Child Welfare System*. Washington, DC: Georgetown University Center for Child & Human Development; 2003. http://gucchd.georgetown.edu/files/products_publications/cw2.pdf

125. Mrazek PJ, Mrazek DA. Resilience in child maltreatment victims: a conceptual exploration. *Child Abuse Negl*. 1987;11:357–366

126. Steel J, Sanna L, Hammond B, Whipple J, Cross H. Psychological sequelae of childhood sexual abuse: abuse-related characteristics, coping strategies, and attributional style. *Child Abuse Negl*. 2004;28:785–801

127. Kinard EM. Methodological issues in assessing resilience in maltreated children. *Child Abuse Negl*. 1998;22:669–680

128. Wright MO, Fopma-Loy J, Fischer S. Multidimensional assessment of resilience in mothers who are child sexual abuse survivors. *Child Abuse Negl*. 2005;29:1173–1193

129. Edmond T, Auslander W, Elze D, Bowland S. Signs of resilience in sexually abused adolescent girls in the foster care system. *J Child Sex Abus*. 2006;15:1–28

130. McGloin JM, Widom CS. Resilience among abused and neglected children grown up. *Dev Psychopathol*. 2001;13:1021–1038

131. Lam JN, Grossman FK. Resiliency and adult adaptation in women with and without self-reported histories of childhood sexual abuse. *J Trauma Stress*. 1997;10:175–196

132. Perkins DF, Jones KR. Risk behaviors and resiliency within physically abused adolescents. *Child Abuse Negl*. 2004;28:547–563

Index